WJ
190
Car

369 0139864

DATE DUE

22/5/13	
9-7-14	
2 1 NOV 2023	

GAYLORD   PRINTED IN U.S.A.

D1422478

Textbook of Female Urology and Urogynecology

Third Edition

Volume 1

Editors-in-Chief

Linda Cardozo MD, FRCOG
Professor of Urogynaecology,
King's College Hospital,
London, U.K.

and

David R Staskin MD
Director, Female Urology and Male Voiding Dysfunction,
St. Elizabeth's Medical Center, Associate Professor of Urology,
Tufts University School of Medicine, Boston, Massachusetts, U.S.A.

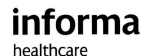

First published in 2001 by Isis Medical Media Ltd, United Kingdom
This edition published in 2010 by Informa Healthcare, Telephone House, 69-77 Paul Street, London EC2A 4LQ, UK.
Simultaneously published in the USA by Informa Healthcare, 52 Vanderbilt Avenue, 7th floor, New York, NY 10017, USA.

A CIP record for this book is available from the British Library.

ISBN-13: 9781841846927

Orders may be sent to: Informa Healthcare, Sheepen Place, Colchester, Essex CO3 3LP, UK
Telephone: +44 (0)20 7017 5540
Email: CSDhealthcarebooks@informa.com
Website: http://informahealthcarebooks.com/

For corporate sales please contact: CorporateBooksIHC@informa.com
For foreign rights please contact: RightsIHC@informa.com
For reprint permissions please contact: PermissionsIHC@informa.com

Typeset by Exeter Premedia Services
Printed and bound in the United Kingdom

Contents

List of Contributors

Paul Abrams
Professor, Bristol Urological Institute, Southmead Hospital, Bristol, U.K.

May Alarab, MBchB MRCOG, MRCPI, MSc
Assistant Professor, Staff, Division of Urogynecology, Department of Obstetrics and Gynecology, and Reconstructive Pelvic Surgery, Mount Sinai Hospital, Toronto, Ontario, Canada

Nadia Ali-Ross
Obstetrics and Gynaecology, Salford Royal Foundation Trust, Greater Manchester, U.K.

Karl-Erik Andersson MD, PhD
Wake Forest Institute for Regenerative Medicine, Wake Forest University School of Medicine, Winston Salem, North Carolina, U.S.A.

Anthony Atala, MD
Department of Urology and Wake Forest Institute for Regenerative Medicine, Wake Forest University School of Medicine, Winston-Salem, North Carolina, U.S.A.

Kaven Baessler
Department of Obstetrics and Gynecology, Charité Hospital, Berlin, Germany

Michael van Balken
Department of Urology, Rijnstate Hospital, Arnhem, The Netherlands

Vanessa Banz
Department of Visceral Surgery and Medicine, University Hospital Berne, Berne, Switzerland

Ahmet Bedestani MD
Fellow, Female Pelvic Medicine and Reconstructive Surgery, Departments of Urology and Gynecology, Louisiana State University Health Sciences Center, New Orleans, Louisiana, U.S.A.

Bary Berghmans PhD, MSC, RPT
Clinical Epidemiologist, Health Scientist, Pelvic Physiotherapist, Pelvic Care Center Maastricht, Maastricht University Medical Center, Maastricht, The Netherlands

Manuel Besendörfer
Section of Coloproctology, Department of Surgery, University of Erlangen, Erlangen, Germany

Jerry G Blaivas MD
Clinical Professor of Urology, Weill Medical College of Cornell University New York, New York, and Adjunct Professor of Urology, SUNY Downstate Medical School, Brooklyn, New York, U.S.A.

Kari Bø
Norwegian University of Sport and Physical Education, Oslo, Norway

JLH Ruud Bosch MD, PhD
Professor and Chairman, Department of Urology, University Medical Center Utrecht, Utrecht, The Netherlands

Sylvia Botros MD, MS
Evanston Continence Center, Division of Urogynecology and Reconstructive Pelvic Surgery, Department of Obstetrics and Gynecology, NorthShore University HealthSystem, Evanston, Illinois, U.S.A.

Catherine S Bradley MD, MSCE
Associate Professor of Obstetrics and Gynecology and of Epidemiology, Division Director, Urogynecology and Reconstructive Pelvic Surgery, University of Iowa Carver College of Medicine, Iowa City, Iowa, U.S.A.

Andrew Browning MBBS, MRCOG
Medical Director, Barhirdar Hamlin Fistula Centre, Barhirdar, Ethiopia

Linda P Brubaker
Section of Urogynecology and Reconstructive Plastic Surgery, Loyola University Medical Center, Maywood, Illinois, U.S.A.

Richard C Bump
Eli Lilly & Co Corporate Center, Indianapolis, Indiana, U.S.A.

Kathryn L Burgio PhD
University of Alabama at Birmingham and Birmingham/Atlanta Geriatric Research, Education, and Clinical Center, Department of Veterans Affairs, Birmingham, Alabama, U.S.A.

Antonio Carbone MD
Department of Urology, First School of Medicine, La Sapienza University–General Hospital, Terracina, Italy

Linda Cardozo MD, FRCOG
Professor of Urogynaecology, King's College Hospital, London, U.K.

Marcus P Carey
Urogynaecology, Royal Women's Hospital, Melbourne, Victoria, Australia

Lesley Carr
Urology, Sunnybrook Health Sciences Centre, Toronto, Ontario, Canada

Rufus Cartwright
Institute of Reproductive and Developmental Biology, Hammersmith Hospital, London, U.K.

Charlotte Chaliha MB BChir, MA MD, MRCOG
Consultant Obsetrician and Gynaecologist, Sub-specialist in Urogynaecology, Royal London and St Bartholomew's Hospitals, London, U.K.

Michael B Chancellor MD
Clinical Professor and Director of Neurology Program, Oakland University William Beaumont School of Medicine, Royal Oak, Michigan, U.S.A.

Christopher R Chapple BSC, MD, FRCS (Urol), FEBU
Consultant Urological Surgeon, Royal Hallamshire Hospital, Honorary Senior Lecturer of Urology, University of Sheffield, Visiting Professor of Urology, Sheffield Hallam University, Adjunct Secretary Responsible for Education, European Association of Urology

Dave Chatoor MBBS, FRCS
Research Fellow in GI Physiology, Gastroenterology, University College Hospital, London, U.K.

Christopher J Chermansky MD
Assistant Professor, Department of Urology, Section of Female Urology and Voiding Dysfunction, Louisiana State University Health Sciences Center, New Orleans, Louisiana, U.S.A.

Nikki Cotterill
Bristol Urological Institute, Southmead Hospital, Bristol, U.K.

Karin Coyne PhD, MPH
United BioSource Corp, Bethesda, Maryland, U.S.A.

Sarah M Creighton MD, FRCOG
Consultant Gynaecologist, Elizabeth Garrett Anderson UCL Institute of Women's Health, University College Hospitals, London, U.K.

Geoffrey W Cundiff MD, FAOCG, FACS, FRCSC
Professor, Department of Obstetrics and Gynaecology, University of British Columbia, Vancouver, British Columbia, Canada

Alfred Cutner
Obstetrics and Gynaecology, University College London Hospitals, London, U.K.

Miriam Dambros
Head of the Geriatric Urology Division, Federal University of São Paulo, São Paulo, Brazil

Melissa C Davies MD, MRCS
Female Urology Fellow, Leicester General Hospital, Leicester, U.K.

Peter Dejong
Gynecology, Groote-Schuur Hospital, Cape Town, South Africa

John OL DeLancey
Pelvic Floor Research Group, Gynecology, University of Michigan Medical School, Ann Arbor, Michigan, U.S.A.

Dirk De Ridder MD, PhD, FEBU
Chairman of the ICS Standardisation Committee, Department of Urology, University Hospitals KU Leuven, Leuven, Belgium

Ananias C Diokno
Department of Urology, William Beaumont Hospital, Royal Oak, Michigan, U.S.A.

Roger R Dmochowski MD
Department of Urologic Surgery, Vanderbilt University Medical Center, Nashville, Tennessee, U.S.A.

Claudine Domoney
Department of Academic Obstetrics and Gynaecology, Chelsea & Westminster Hospital, London, U.K.

Stergios K Doumouchtsis
Department of Pelvic Reconstructive Surgery and Urogynaecology, St George's Hospital, London, U.K.

Richard Dover
Obstetrics and Gynaecology, Royal North Shore Hospital, Sydney, New South Wales, Australia

Marcus Drake
Bristol Urological Institute, Southmead Hospital, Bristol, U.K.

Harold P Drutz MD, FRCS(C)
Professor and Head, Division of Urogynecology, Department of Obstetrics and Gynaecology, University of Toronto, Mount Sinai Hospital, Toronto, Ontario, Canada

Anton Emmanuel BSC, MD, FRCP
Research Fellow in GI Physiology, University College Hospital, London, U.K.

Christopher J Evans PhD, MPH
Director of Economics and Outcomes, Mapi Values, Boston, Massachusetts, U.S.A.

Magnus Fall
Department of Urology, Sahlgrenska University, Göteborg, Sweden

Clare J Fowler
Department of Uro-Neurology, National Hospital for Neurology and Neurosurgery, London, U.K.

Lynette E Franklin MSN, APRN-BC, CWOCN
Department of Urology-Bladder and Pelvic Health Program, Medical University of South Carolina, Charleston, South Carolina, U.S.A.

Robert M Freeman
Professor in Urogynaecology, Peninsula Medical School, Urogynaecology Unit, Directorate of Obstetrics and Gynaecology, Derriford Hospital, Plymouth, U.K.

Michelle M Fynes MD, MRCOG, DU
Lead Consultant Urogynaecologist and Honorary Senior Lecturer, Department of Reconstructive Pelvic Surgery and Urogynaecology, St Georges Hospital, and Medical School University of London, London, U.K.

Bianca A Gago MD
Vanguard Urologic Research Foundation, Houston, Texas, U.S.A.

Roxane Gardner MD, MPH
Assistant Professor of Obstetrics, Gynecology and Reproductive Biology, Harvard Medical School, Department of Obstetrics and Gynecology, Brigham and Women's Hospital, Boston, Massachusetts, U.S.A. and Center for Medical Simulation, Cambridge, Massachusetts, U.S.A.

Mohamed Ghafar MD
Fellow, Female Pelvic Medicine and Reconstructive Surgery, Departments of Urology and Gynecology, Louisiana State University Health Sciences Center, New Orleans, Louisiana, U.S.A.

Robert B Gherman MD
Department of Obstetrics and Gynecology, Division of Maternal/Fetal Medicine, Prince George's Hospital Center, Cheverly, Maryland, U.S.A.

Jason Gilleran MD
Urology, Ohio State University Medical Center, Columbus, Ohio, U.S.A.

Benjamin J Girdler MD
Department of Urology, McKee Medical Center, Loveland, Colorado, U.S.A.

Roger P Goldberg MD, MPH
Clinical Assistant Professor of Obstetrics and Gynecology, University of Chicago Pritzker School of Medicine, Chicago, Illinois, U.S.A. and Division of Urogynecology, NorthShore University HealthSystem, Evanston, Illinois, U.S.A.

David W Goldfarb
Department of Urology, Baylor College of Medicine, Houston, Texas, U.S.A.

Irwin Goldstein MD
Director, Sexual Medicine, Alvarado Hospital, San Diego, California, Director, San Diego Sexual Medicine, Clinical Professor of Surgery, University of California at San Diego, Editor-in-Chief, The Journal of Sexual Medicine, San Diego, California, U.S.A.

Alex Gomelsky MD
Department of Urology, LSU Health Sciences Center, Shreveport, Louisiana, U.S.A.

Ricardo R Gonzalez
Department of Urology, Baylor College of Medicine, Houston Metro Urology, Houston, Texas, U.S.A.

James Gray
Department of Microbiology, Birmingham Women's Hospital, Birmingham, U.K.

Derek Griffiths
Geriatric Continence Unit, Montefiore Hospital, Pittsburgh, Pennsylvania, U.S.A.

Marie-Andrée Harvey MD, MSC, FRCSC, FACOG
Assistant Professor, Department of Obstetrics and Gynaecology and Department of Urology, Queen's University, Kingston General Hospital, Kingston, Ontario, Canada

Hashim Hashim
Bristol Urological Institute, Southmead Hospital, Bristol, U.K.

Jeanette Haslam
Specialist Physiotherapist in Women's Health (Retired), Cumbria, U.K.

Rashel Haverkorn
Urology, University of Texas Southwestern Medical Center, Dallas, Texas, U.S.A.

Bernard T Haylen
Department of Gynaecology, St Vincent's Hospital, Darlinghurst, New South Wales, Australia

John Heesakkers
Radboud University Nijmegen Medical Centre, Department of Urology, Nijmegen, The Netherlands

Sender Herschorn MD, FRCSC
Division of Urology, Sunnybrook and Women's College Health Science Centre, Toronto, Ontario, Canada

Andrew Hextall MD, FRCOG
Consultant Gynaecologist, Department of Urogynaecology, West Hertfordshire Hospitals NHS Trust, St Albans, U.K.

Timothy C Hillard DM, FFSRH, FRCOG
Consultant Obstetrician and Gynaecologist, Poole Hospital, Poole, Dorset, U.K.

Candice Hinote MD
Department of Obstetrics and Gynecology, University of Tennessee at Memphis, Memphis, Tennessee, U.S.A.

Lennox Hoyte
Division of Urogynecology and Pelvic Reconstructive Surgery, University of South Florida College of Medicine, Tampa, Florida, U.S.A.

Kenneth C Hsiao MD
Norcal Urology, Walnut Creek, California, U.S.A.

Christopher Jayne
Urogynecology and Voiding Dysfunction, Rodney A. Appell Center for Continence and Pelvic Health at Vaguard Urologic Institute, Assistant Professor Scott Department of Urology, Baylor College of Medicine, Houston, Texas, U.S.A.

Michael S Ingber
Center for Female Pelvic Medicine and Reconstructive Surgery, Glickman Urological and Kidney Institute, Cleveland Clinic, Cleveland, Ohio, U.S.A.

Swati Jha MRCOG
Department of Urogynaecology, Sheffield Teaching Hospitals NHS Foundation Trust, Sheffield, U.K.

Rob Jones
Bristol Urological Institute, Southmead Hospital, Bristol, U.K.

Saad Juma MD, FACS
Director, Incontinence Research Institute, Encinitas, California, U.S.A.

Scott E Kalinowski
Department of Urology, William Beaumont Hospital, Royal Oak, Michigan, U.S.A.

Mickey M Karram MD
Director, Division of Urogynecology and Pelvic Reconstructive Surgery, Department of Obstetrics and Gynecology, Good Samaritan Hospital, and University of Cincinnati College of Medicine, Cincinnati, Ohio, U.S.A.

Melissa R Kaufman
Department of Urologic Surgery, Vanderbilt University Medical Center, Nashville, Tennessee, U.S.A.

Jonathan D Kaye MD
Georgia Urology, PA, Children's Healthcare of Atlanta, Department of Urology, Emory University School of Medicine, Atlanta, Georgia, U.S.A.

Rohna Kearney
Department of Obstetrics and Gynaecology, Addenbrooke's Hospital, Cambridge, U.K.

Cornelius J Kelleher MD, FRCOG
Department of Obstetrics and Gynaecology, Guy's and St Thomas' Hospital NHS Trust, London, U.K.

Kimberly Kenton MD, MS
Female Pelvic Medicine and Reconstructive Surgery, Obstetrics and Gynecology and Urology, Loyola University Stritch School of Medicine, Maywood, Illinois, U.S.A.

Philip van Kerrebroeck
Department of Urology, University Hospital Maastricht, Maastricht, The Netherlands

Christine Kettle
Department of Obstetrics and Gynaecology, Staffordshire University, Stafford, U.K.

Vik Khullar
Urogynaecology, St Mary's Hospital, London, U.K.

Andrew J Kirsch MD
Georgia Urology, PA, Children's Healthcare of Atlanta, Department of Urology, Emory University School of Medicine, Atlanta, Georgia, U.S.A.

Peter Klarskov MD
Department of Neurology, Copenhagen University Hospital, Herlev, Denmark

Kirsten Kluivers MD
Department of Gynecology, UMC St Radboud, Nijmegen, The Netherlands

Kathleen C Kobashi MD
Co-Director, The Continence Center, Virginia Mason Medical Center, Seattle, Washington, U.S.A.

Zoe Kopp
Outcomes Research, Pfizer, Inc., New York, New York, U.S.A.

Sarah M Lambert MD
Department of Surgery, University of Pennsylvania School of Medicine, Philadelphia, Pennsylvania, U.S.A.

Joseph Lee
Department of Urology, Mercy Hospital for Women, Melbourne, Victoria, Australia

Limim Liao
Department of Urology, China Rehabilitation Research Center, Beijing, China

Fabio Lorenzetti MD, PhD
Geriatric Urology Division, Federal University of São Paulo, São Paulo, Brazil

Kevin R Loughlin
Division of Urology, Brigham and Women's Hospital, Harvard Medical School, Boston, Massachusetts, U.S.A.

Malcolm Lucas MDchM, FRCS
Consultant Urologist, Morriston Hospital, Swansea, U.K. and Honorary Senior Lecturer Swansea University Medical School, Swansea, U.K.

Alvaro Lucioni MD
Fellow, Female Urology, The Continence Center, Virginia Mason Medical Center, Seattle, Washington, U.S.A.

Christopher Maher
Department of Urogynaecology, Royal Women's and Mater Hospital, Brisbane, Queensland, Australia

Tony Mak
Department of Surgery, University Hospital Birmingham, Birmingham, U.K.

Anders Mattiasson
Department of Urology, University Hospital, Lund, Sweden

Klaus E Matzel
Professor, Chirurgische Klinik mit Poliklinik der Universität Erlangen, Section of Coloproctology, Department of Surgery, University of Erlangen, Erlangen, Germany

Jürg Metzger
Department of Visceral Surgery, Cantonal Hospital, Lucerne, Switzerland

John R Miklos
Atlanta Center for Laparoscopic Urogynecology, Vaginal Rejuvenation Center of Atlanta, Atlanta Medical Research, Inc, Atlanta, Georgia, U.S.A.

Richard J Millard
Department of Urology, Prince of Wales Hospital, Sydney, New South Wales, Australia

Ian Milsom MD, PhD
Department of Obstetrics and Gynecology, Sahlgrenska Academy at Gothenburg University, Gothenburg, Sweden

Ash Monga
Department of Urology, Princess Anne Hospital, Southampton, U.K.

Kate H Moore
Associate Professor, Head of Department of Urogynaecology, University of New South Wales, St George Hospital, Sydney, New South Wales, Australia

Robert D Moore
Atlanta Center for Laparoscopic Urogynecology, Vaginal Rejuvenation Center of Atlanta, Atlanta Medical Research, Inc, Atlanta, Georgia, U.S.A.

Jacek Mostwin
James Buchanan Brady Urological Institute, Johns Hopkins Medical Institutions, Baltimore, Maryland, U.S.A.

Diane K Newman RNC, MSN, CRNP, FAAN
Co-Director, Penn Center for Continence and Pelvic Health, Division of Urology, University of Pennsylvania Health System, Philadelphia, Pennsylvania, U.S.A.

Aimee Nguyen MD
Evanston Continence Center, Division of Urogynecology and Reconstructive Pelvic Surgery, Department of Obstetrics and Gynecology, NorthShore University HealthSystem, Evanston, Illinois, U.S.A.

Carl Gustaf Nilsson
Department of Obstetrics and Gynecology, Helsinki University Central Hospital, Helsinki, Finland

Victor W Nitti
Department of Urology, New York University School of Medicine, New York, New York, U.S.A.

Matthias Oelke MD, FEBU
Urologist, Vice-Chairman, Department of Urology, Hannover Medical School, Hannover, Germany

Paulo Palma
Professor and Chairman, Division of Urology, State University of Campinas, São Paolo, Brazil

Demetri C Panayi
Urogynaecology, St Mary's Hospital, London, U.K.

Apurva B Pancholy MD
Fellow, Division of Urogynecology, Department of Obstetrics and Gynecology, Good Samaritan Hospital, Cincinnati, Ohio, U.S.A.

Matthew Parsons MRCOG
Consultant, Department of Urogynaecology, Birmingham Women's Hospital, Edgbaston, Birmingham, U.K.

Francesco Pesce
Urology and Neurology, University of Verona, Verona, Italy

Eckhard Petri
Klinikum Schwerin, Schwerin, Germany

Raymond R Rackley MD
Professor of Surgery, The Cleveland Clinic Lerner College of Medicine of Case Western Reserve University, Center for Female Pelvic Medicine and Reconstructive Surgery, Glickman Urological and Kidney Institute, Cleveland Clinic, Cleveland, Ohio, U.S.A.

Simon Radley
Department of Surgery, University Hospital Birmingham, Birmingham, U.K.

Angie Rantell
Senior Urogynaecology Nurse Specialist, King's College Hospital, London, U.K.

Fiona Reid MD, MRCOG
Consultant Urogynaecologist, The Warrell Unit, St Mary's Hospital, Manchester, U.K.

W Stuart Reynolds
Department of Urologic Surgery, Vanderbilt University Medical Center, Nashville, Tennessee, U.S.A.

Cassio Riccetto
Associate Professor of Urology, Universidade Estadual de Campinas, São Paulo, Brazil

Diaa E Rizk
Department of Urology, Ain Shams University, Cairo, Egypt

Jack R Robertson MD
Urogynecologist and Professor Emeritus, University of Nevada Medical School, Reno, Nevada, U.S.A.

Dudley Robinson MD, MRCOG
Consultant Urogyanecologist Honorary Senior Lecturer, Department of Urogynaecology, King's College Hospital, London, U.K.

Peter Rosier
Department of Urology, University Medical Centre Utrecht, Utrecht, The Netherlands

Eric Rovner
Section of Voiding Dysfunction, Female Urology, and Urodynamics, Department of Urology, Medical University of South Carolina, Charleston, South Carolina, U.S.A.

Matthew P Rutman MD
Assistant Professor of Urology, Columbia University College of Physicians and Surgeons, New York, New York, U.S.A.

Stefano Salvatore
Division of Gyncologic Surgery, Bassini Hospital, University of Milan, Milan, Italy

Peter K Sand MD
Evanston Continence Center, Division of Urogynecology and Reconstructive Pelvic Surgery, Department of Obstetrics and Gynecology, NorthShore University HealthSystems, Evanston, Illinois, U.S.A.

Harriette M Scarpero
Department of Urologic Surgery, Vanderbilt University Medical Center, Nashville, Tennessee, U.S.A.

Werner Schaefer
Continence Research Unit, University of Pittsburgh, Montefiore Hospital, Pitteburgh, Pennsylvania, U.S.A.

Gabriel N Schaer
Kantonsspital, Aarau, Switzerland

Bernhard Schuessler
Department of Obstetrics and Gynecology, Cantonal Hospital, Lucerne, Switzerland

Jane A Schulz MD
Urogynecologist and Associate Professor, Department of Obstetrics and Gynecology, University of Alberta, Edmonton, Alberta, Canada

Chris Sexton PhD
United BioSource Corp, Bethesda, Maryland, U.S.A.

Sagar R Shah
New York University Urology Associates, New York, New York, U.S.A.

Bob L Shull
Scott and White Women's Health Center, Temple, Texas, U.S.A.

Vanja Sikirica PharmD
Associate Director, Health Economics and Reimbursement, Ethicon Medical Devices, Somerville, New Jersey, U.S.A.

William A Silva MD
Division of Urogynecology and Plastic and Reconstructive Surgery, Department of Obstetrics and Gynecology, Good Samaritan Hospital, Cincinnati, Ohio, U.S.A.

Mark Slack FRCOG
Urogynaecology and Pelvic Reconstructive Surgery, Addenbrooke's Hospital, Cambridge, U.K.

Anthony RB Smith
Obstetrics and Gynaecology, St Mary's Hospital for Women and Children, Manchester, U.K.

Ariana L Smith
Division of Urology, Hospital of the University of Pennsylvania, Pennsylvania Hospital, Philadelphia, Pennsylvania, U.S.A.

Howard M Snyder MD
Division of Urology, Children's Hospital of Philadelphia, The University of Pennsylvania School of Medicine, Philadelphia, Pennsylvania, U.S.A.

Anders Spangberg
Department of Urology, University Hospital, Linköping, Sweden

Sushma Srikrishna MRCOG
Subspecialty Trainee in Urogynaecology, Department of Urogynaecology, King's College Hospital, London, U.K.

Edward J Stanford MD, MS
Department of Obstetrics and Gynecology, University of Tennessee at Memphis, Menphis, Tennessee, U.S.A.

David R Staskin MD
Director, Female Urology and Male Voiding Dysfunction, St Elizabeth's Medical Center, Associate Professor of Urology, Tufts University School of Medicine, Boston, Massachusetts, U.S.A.

Arthur M Sterling
Department of Chemical Engineering, Louisiana State University, Baton Rouge, Louisiana, U.S.A.

Michael L Stitely MD
Department of Obstetrics and Gynecology, West Virginia University School of Medicine, Morgantown, West Virginia, U.S.A.

Abdul H Sultan MB.ChB, MD, FRCOG
Obstetrics and Gynaecology, Mayday University Hospital, Croydon, U.K.

Christopher Sutton
Gynaecological Surgery, University of Surry, Royal Surrey County Hospital, Guildford, and Chelsea and Westminster Hospital, London, U.K.

Steven E Swift
Department of Obstetrics and Gynecology, Medical University of South Carolina, Charleston, South Carolina, U.S.A.

Tara Symonds
Outcomes Research, Pfizer, Inc., New York, New York, U.S.A.

Megan Tarr MD
Female Pelvic Medicine and Reconstructive Surgery, Obstetrics and Gynecology and Urology, Loyola University Stritch School of Medicine, Maywood, Illinois, U.S.A.

Alexis E Te
Department of Urology, Weill Medical College, Cornell University, New York, New York, U.S.A.

Ranee Thakar
Obstetrics and Gynaecology, Mayday University Hospital, Croydon, U.K.

Philip Toozs-Hobson
Urogynaecology, Birmingham Women's Hospital, Birmingham, U.K.

Ruben Trochez
Subspecialty Trainee in Urogynaecology, Urogynaecology Unit, Directorate of Obstetrics and Gynaecology, Derriford Hospital, Plymouth, U.K.

Andrea Tubaro MD, FEBU
Department of Urology, Second School of Medicine, La Sapienza University–Sant'Andrea Hospital, Rome, Italy

Renuka Tyagi
Department of Urology, Weill Medical College, Cornell University, New York, New York, U.S.A.

Ulf Ulmsten
Deceased

SS Vasan
Director, Ankur - NeuroUrology and Continence, Director, Manipal Andrology and Reproductive Services, Bangalore, India

Sandip P Vasavada MD
Associate Professor of Surgery, The Cleveland Clinic Lerner College of Medicine of Case Western Reserve University, Center for Female Pelvic Medicine and Reconstructive Surgery, Glickman Urological and Kidney Institute, Cleveland Clinic, Cleveland, Ohio, U.S.A.

Arvind Vashisht
Obstetrics and Gynaecology, University College London Hospitals, London, U.K.

Arne Victor
Medical Product Agency, Uppsala, Sweden

David B Vodušek
Division of Neurology, University Medical Centre, Ljubljana, Slovenia

Manhan Vu DO
Division of Female Pelvic Medicine and Reconstructive Surgery, Department of Obstetrics and Gynecology, NorthShore University HealthSystem, Evanston, Illinois, U.S.A.

Rhonda Walsh MD
Urology Group of New Jersey, West Orange, New Jersey, U.S.A.

Mark D Walters
Professor and Vice Chair of Gynecology, Obstetrics, Gynecology and Women's Health Institute, Cleveland Clinic, Cleveland, Ohio, U.S.A.

Alan J Wein MD
Division of Urology, Hospital of the University of Pennsylvania, Philadelphia, Pennsylvania, U.S.A

Blayne Welk MD, FRCSC
Division of Urology, Sunnybrook and Women's College Health Science Centre, Toronto, Ontario, Canada

Ursula Wesselmann MD, PhD
Edward A. Ernst Endowed Professor of Anesthesiology, Department of Anesthesiology, Division of Pain Treatment, University of Alabama at Birmingham, Birmingham, Alabama, U.S.A.

J Christian Winters MD, FACS
H Eustis Reily Professor of Urology and Gynecology, Chairman, Department of Urology, Louisiana State University Health Sciences Center, New Orleans, Louisiana, U.S.A.

Jean-Jacques Wyndaele MD, PhD
Urologist, Chairman, Department of Urology, University of Antwerp, Antwerp, Belgium

Reena S Yalaburgi
Associate Consultant, Ankur, Bangalore, India

Naoki Yoshimura MD, PhD
Professor of Urology and Pharmacology University of Pittsburgh School of Medicine, Pittsburgh, Pennsylvania, U.S.A.

Stephen A Zderic MD
Department of Surgery, University of Pennsylvania School of Medicine, Philadelphia, Pennsylvania, U.S.A.

Philippe Zimmern MD
Urology, University of Texas Southwestern Medical Center, Dallas, Texas, U.S.A.

Norman R Zinner
Aurologic Medical Corp., Torrance, California, U.S.A.

Foreword

Successful textbooks make it sometimes to a second edition, rarely to a third edition. The criteria have to be that the volume is in demand and that there have been substantial advances. Linda Cardozo and David R Staskin and the contributors are to be congratulated on producing an international, readable, comprehensive, and up to date urogynecological tome—essential reading for the trainee through to the urogynecological consultant and beyond—to the consultant gynecologist, urologist, and continence nurse specialist. The editors acknowledge that urogynecology is a global sub-speciality and have enrolled international contributors who focus on significant research and the clinical advances that have followed from this. There is a logical path from epidemiology, through basic medical science to clinical and investigatory assessment and then management of clinical problems. Important advances such as improvements in continence surgery, the use of prosthetic meshes for prolapse surgery, and the expansion of available drugs for the overactive bladder are included. The editors focus attention on outcome measures, including patient centered goals, and new chapters include cosmetic genital surgery, female sexual dysfunction, and robotic surgery.

Medico-legal problems abound now in all disciplines of medicine and this is recognized by the inclusion of chapters on medical errors and patient safety in the operative room and further chapters on complications of surgery and how to manage them.

The book concludes by summarizing important standardization reports from the international continence society and is a timely reminder that only by speaking the same language can we truly communicate and appreciate the globalization of medicine. This book is a must.

Stuart L Stanton
Professor of Urogynaecology
London University

Preface

We are proud to present a third edition of the *Textbook of Female Urology and Urogynecology* and would like to take this opportunity to thank all those of you who have contributed. We are particularly grateful to our section editors and appreciate how much time and effort they have put in to making this an authoritative comprehensive reference book which will hopefully appeal to both urologists and gynecologists as well as other healthcare professionals involved in the management of pelvic floor problems on both sides of the Atlantic and elsewhere in the world.

We would also like to take this opportunity to thank all those who contributed to the second edition of *Textbook of Female Urology and Urogynecology* which was awarded first prize by the Society of Authors and the Royal Society of Medicine as the best new edition of an edited medical book. We felt that this was a great honor and reflects well on all of you. It is of course this success which has stimulated us to produce this third edition which we hope will be even more successful than the previous two. Once again we have involved the group of authors, some of whom have an international reputation and others are new comers to the field, which we hope has produced a good balance of knowledge, expertise, and writing skills without the polarization of ideas that occurs in many textbooks as a natural product of the contributors' geography, training, and interests. Once again our mission was to produce a comprehensive textbook which would identify past contributions to the field and document and analyze the present state of the art as well as serve as a foundation for future developments in the field.

The text is arranged in sections enabling the reader to access areas of interest and extensive bibliographies are intended to facilitate further study of the subject. The section on surgery has been formatted to serve as both an evidence-based text and atlas and is intended to provide information pertaining to the decision making process as well as the technical aspects of the surgical procedures. We recognize that in this rapidly advancing field it is difficult to remain completely up to date.

As editors we are truly grateful to our publishers who have facilitated the production of this book and once again would like to thank all our authors for the time they have sacrificed outside their working hours to make this project successful. Finally we are most grateful to our patients who place their trust in all of us every day and we hope that this textbook will contribute to their quality of care and to the ability of those who will treat them in the future.

Linda Cardozo
David R Staskin

1   History of Urogynecology and Female Urology

Jane A Schulz, Harold P Drutz, and Jack R Robertson

INTRODUCTION

As we have moved into the new millennium, accompanied by many new advances in the field of urogynecology and reconstructive pelvic surgery, it is appropriate to take time to reflect on the events of the last century, and to make suggestions for future directions. With the significant increase in our postmenopausal female population there is a growing demand for improved quality of life and management of pelvic floor dysfunction. No longer do we contemplate *whether* women will grow older but, rather, *how* they will grow older. The life expectancy for women has almost doubled through the 20th century. In 1923, Professor Sir Arthur Keith, in his Hunterian Lecture on "Man's Posture: It's Evolution and Disorders" (1) stated:

> Every movement of the arms, cough, or strain sets going a multitude of "water hammers" within the abdominal and pelvic cavities. Every impulse sets the bladder knocking at the vaginal exit ... it is the continual repetition of small forces, more frequently than the sudden application of a great effort which wear down the vaginal defense.

Although it has long been recognized that factors such as childbearing and chronic increases in intra-abdominal pressure contributed to pelvic floor prolapse, only recently has there been growing demand to manage all of the resulting problems. Urinary incontinence is now the most common reason for admission to long-term institutionalized centers in Canada and the United States. Billions of dollars are spent every year on nappy (diaper) and pad products, but this does nothing to correct the underlying problem of incontinence.

Since the inception of medical writing, gynecologic and urologic conditions have been reported. The Kahun papyrus, circa 2000 B.C., described diseases of women, including diseases of the urinary bladder. The Ebers papyrus, 1550 B.C., classified diseases by systems and organs. Section 6 includes a prescription for the cure of a woman suffering from disease of her urine, as well as her womb. Urinary fistula is an example of the intimate relationship of the urinary and genital systems in women. Henhenit lived in the court of Menuhotep II, about 2050 B.C. Her mummy, found in 1935, revealed by radiography an extensive urinary fistula (2).

Reviewing the last century of progress in the new subspecialty of urogynecology and reconstructive pelvic surgery proved to be a tremendous, and somewhat daunting, task. Perhaps the quotation that best summarizes the events that have occurred is the opening sentence from Charles Dickens' *A Tale of Two Cities*: "It was the best of times, it was the worst of times." Undoubtedly, we have made tremendous progress in this burgeoning new field; however, a political battlefield was perpetuated with the division of the female pelvic floor between urologists, urogynecologists, gynecologists, and colorectal surgeons. This political feud is cleverly illustrated in the article of Louis Wall and John DeLancey with its well-known drawing of the competing urologist, gynecologist, and colorectal surgeon (3). This is one of the many challenges that must be overcome in providing overall women's healthcare as we move into the 21st century. A multidisciplinary approach to managing female pelvic floor dysfunction must be advocated to provide women with appropriate care in the areas of urinary and fecal incontinence, urogenital aging, conservative management, and reconstructive pelvic surgery (4).

Voltaire, the French philosopher of the "age of enlightenment," said "these truths are not for all men nor for all times." From this we must humbly accept the concept that the truths we believe in today regarding our management of women with pelvic floor disorders must be constantly reassessed and modified with scientific advancements and research. Similarly, the epigram by Alphonse Karr (1849) *"plus ça change plus c'est la même chose"* (the more things change, the more they stay the same) also reflects the changes during the past century especially in the field of surgical intervention, where in many cases we have continued to reinvent the wheel.

HISTORY OF THE INTERNATIONAL UROGYNECOLOGY ASSOCIATION (IUGA)

At the Federation International of Gynecology and Obstetrics (FIGO) meeting in Mexico City in 1976, two medical friends, Professor Axel Ingelman-Sundberg, of Stockholm, Sweden, and Jack Rodney Robertson, of California, U.S.A., met. It was time to form a new society. The objective was to further the urinary health of females and both physicians were deeply involved in this work.

Axel Ingelman-Sundberg, renowned for his research, his pioneering work in gynecologic surgery, and his teaching at the Karolinska Institute in Stockholm, Sweden, was the catalyst. Sweden had been a founding member of FIGO. Axel tried to persuade FIGO to make International Urinary Incontinence a subcommittee, but they declined. In his capacity as Vice President of FIGO, Axel reserved a special room for the formation of the IUGA. He was elected the first president, to serve five years, 1976 to 1980, by the colleagues who registered as members. They were: Abbo Hassan Abbo, M.D., Sudan; Wolfgang Fisher, M.D., East Germany; Bozo Kralj, M.D., Yugoslavia; Oscar Contreras Ortiz, M.D., Argentina; Donald R. Ostergard, M.D., U.S.A.; Eckard Petrie, M.D., West Germany; Jack R. Robertson, M.D., U.S.A.; Mr. Stuart Stanton, M.D., U.K.; Ulf Ulmsten, M.D., Sweden; and David W. Waller, M.D., U.K. Ulf Ulmsten, then professor of Obstetrics and Gynecology in Aarhus, Denmark, was chosen as secretary.

The next meeting followed in Sheffield, U.K., in July 1977, in connection with the local gynecological meeting. At Bergen, Norway, in 1978, IUGA met along with the Scandinavian Congress of Obstetrics and Gynecology. In 1979 in Tokyo, IUGA met again with FIGO; this time IUGA was a special section of the program. In October 1980, IUGA met in New Orleans, organized by Jack Robertson, in connection with the newly formed Gynecological Urology Society (GUS), later to become the American Urogynecological Society (AUGS).

The fifth IUGA meeting was held in Stockholm, September 1981, at the Wenner-Gren Center, famous for Nobel Prize presentations. The banquet was at the Royal Opera House, with a special program by the famous Swedish opera singer, Kerstin Dellert. Jack Robertson was elected president, and served until 1985. Peter Sand, of Chicago, Illinois, became the general secretary. During this time the association was growing in membership.

In the United States, Jack Robertson had found that women were being treated as second class citizens, being examined with male instruments for their incontinence problems. An alarming number of women were incontinent after their hysterectomy surgery. Robertson devised a system of viewing the bladder, using carbon dioxide instead of water. In 1968, he went to Germany and convinced the famous endoscope maker, Karl Storz, who had recently acquired the technique of fiber optics, to produce a female urethroscope to Robertson's specifications. Storz immediately liked the idea of not using water, and made the first Robertson Female Urethroscope. Instead of just resting their instruments upon it, this was the first time doctors could view the female urethra and its pathology. This was the beginning of a pioneering path with Robertson giving seminars to physicians anxious to learn about the female urinary tract, which had not been included in their gynecologic training. An immediate result was a sharp rise in the diagnoses of urethral diverticula.

In 1982 the meeting at Santa Barbara, California, organized by Jack Robertson, was combined with the GUS, organized by Don Ostergard. In 1983 IUGA met in Mainz, Germany, and in 1984, IUGA met at the famous Breakers Hotel in West Palm Beach, Florida.

At the 1985 meeting in Budapest, Hungary, physicians came from behind the Iron Curtain. It was vital for them to present their work at the meeting, as they would rise in professional and, most importantly, pay levels as a result. When one group from Poland presented a problem, the audience asked why ultrasound had not been used, which at that time would have been the obvious method of treatment. The physicians from Poland replied simply, "We do not have ultrasound." Donald Ostergard was elected the third president and presided at the 1986 meeting at Yale University, organized by Ernest Kohorn. Don's memories include "a lot of work organizing individuals to take the financial risks to hold a meeting."

An important event occurred at the 1986 Yale meeting. The *International Urogynecology Journal* was born. Oscar Contreras Ortiz was nominated editor in chief. Donald Ostergard became the first managing editor and later, the editor in chief. He was followed by Linda Brubaker, Mickey Karram, and, now, Peter Dwyer. The first issue, Volume 1, was printed in September 1989 and contained the abstracts of the Riva del Garda meeting. The associate editors, section editors, and editorial board represent countries all around the world.

The 1987 meeting was in Ljubljana, Yugoslavia, organized by Bozo Kralj, of Slovenia, with 200 members worldwide. Bozo became the fourth president at the 1988 memorable meeting at Iguazu Falls, Argentina, hosted by Oscar Contreras Ortiz, who Hans Van Geelen said "made every effort, and succeeded in strengthening social ties." In 1989, Rudolfo Milani hosted the meeting in Riva Del Garda, Italy.

Next elected was Eckhard Petri of Germany, 1990 to 1992, inaugurated at the Stockholm, Sweden, meeting organized by Ulf Ulmsten. Peter Dwyer says of this meeting: "One of the most low key of all the meetings, it was possibly one of the most enjoyable. It was basic but had good science. The chairman's dinner was held in Ulf's department at the Uppsala University cafeteria." The 16th annual IUGA meeting was held in Sydney, Australia, in 1991, and the host and hostess were Jim and Peggy Gibson. They had a fabulous chairman's reception which was held at the farm they owned at the time, called "Stanton Hall."

In 1992, IUGA combined with AUGS, in Boston, Massachusetts, with a lobster bake party at the famous Aquarium. James Gibson, Australia, was elected sixth president. He presided at the 1993 meeting in Nimes, France, which was coordinated with International Continence Society (ICS) in Rome. Gibson organized Organon to give IUGA $10,000 each year for five years for the best presentation at each meeting. He also hosted the Kuala Lumpur meeting in 1995 at which Harold Drutz presided. In 1994, Harold Drutz hosted the meeting in Toronto, Canada, at which he was elected the seventh president. He presided as well at the Kuala Lumpur meeting in 1995, hosted by Jim Gibson, which, he says, was one of the first meetings to make a profit.

In September 1996, the meeting, organized by Paul Riss, was held in Vienna, Austria. This was a glorious site at which Oscar Contreras Ortiz, Buenos Aires, Argentina, was elected eighth president. The 1997 meeting occurred in Amsterdam, arranged with the combined efforts of Hans Van Geelen, Harry Vervest, and Mark Vierhout. The meeting location was planned in Europe as FIGO was in Copenhagen. In 1998, Buenos Aires, Argentina, was the venue for IUGA, hosted by Oscar Contreras Ortiz. Linda Cardozo, London, U.K., was ninth president. In 1999, in Denver, Colorado, Willy Davila organized IUGA with Rick Schmidt of ICS to allow the first combined meeting of the two societies.

The 2000 IUGA meeting in Rome, Italy, organized by Mauro Cervini, chose Hans Van Geelen, from the Netherlands, as president. The largely attended meeting was enlivened by an audience with Pope John Paul II, celebrating the millennium year. The Pope blessed the IUGA in his Papal Address during the meeting. Hans Van Geelen recalls that at an early IUGA meeting the attendance was so small that the members could sit around one round table, discussing the clinical relevance of urodynamics. He too says that "in the beginning, hosting a meeting was a delicate task."

In 2001, the IUGA meeting moved to the southern hemisphere again with Peter Dwyer as host in Melbourne, Australia, combined with the Australian Continence Foundation. Axel Ingelman-Sundberg was awarded a lifetime achievement award, via a live television connection, at the 2001 meeting. The 2002 meeting was held in Prague, with Michael Halaska as organizer. The River Moldau flooded the inner town, and Professor Halaska had to change the venue of the gala dinner, and take out new insurance. In Prague, Peter Dwyer, Melbourne, Australia, was elected president. Peter comments that IUGA became not only a scientific society, but developed a true camaraderie of friendship. He says that the young urogynecologists appreciated the emphasis on the clinic rather than the basic science (rats). Peter writes: "Presenting our own research internationally and getting ideas for our next projects was also very important, and the meetings were great fun."

In 2003, IUGA was back in Buenos Aires, again organized by Oscar Contreras Ortiz. August 2004 saw a spectacular meeting of IUGA in Paris, France, combined for the second time with the ICS. The Chairman's dinner held at Maxim's Restaurant, honored Jack R. Robertson with a lifetime achievement award. The Palais Versailles was the unbelievable site of the gala dinner, all hosted by Bernard Jacquetin for IUGA and Francois Haab for ICS. Paul Riss of Moeding, Austria, was elected to serve as president from 2004 to 2006. Copenhagen, Denmark, was the site of the August 2005 IUGA meeting, organized by Gunnar Lose.

The two old friends, Axel Ingelman-Sundberg and Jack R. Robertson met in Munich, Germany, in August of 2004. The meeting in Copenhagen in 2005 was an exciting meeting at a unique venue with the first discussion of some of newer mesh kits. In 2006, the annual IUGA meeting was in the beautiful historic city of Athens, with many social events being held at some of the ancient historic sites. Professor Oscar Contreras Ortiz received a prestigious lifetime achievement award. The year 2007 found us back across the Atlantic in Cancun Mexico with a stunning gala dinner at sunset on the beach. At the Cancun meeting Professor Donald Ostergard received a lifetime achievement award. Despite difficult weather caused by a number of typhoons, many were still able to attend the 2008 meeting in Taipei, where Professor Harold Drutz was awarded a lifetime achievement award from the IUGA for his ongoing contributions to the society (including the only Canadian to have been president of the society, 1994–1996). The stunning venue of Lake Como, Italy was the site for the 2009 meeting, where Professor Jim Gibson received a lifetime achievement award. The year 2010 will see another joint meeting of the ICS and IUGA hosted by Professors Drutz and Herschorn in Toronto, Canada.

PROGRESS IN THE 20TH CENTURY
Treatment
Marion Sims, in the United States, was one of the first to establish the relationship of urology and gynecology. Determined to cure vesico-vaginal fistulas, he finally used silver wire and announced in 1852 the cure of 252 out of 320 attempts. Howard A. Kelly, the first professor of gynecology at the Johns Hopkins Medical School, believed that gynecology and urology were so closely related that a physician could not be trained in either field and ignore the other. In 1893, he invented a cystoscope, and was the first person to insert urethral catheters under direct vision. Kelly's successor, Guy Hunner described Hunner's Ulcer, which today is called interstitial cystitis. Succeeding Hunner was Houston Everett, whose contribution was the relationship of the urinary tract to cervical cancer. In 1914, Latzko perfected the cure of post-hysterectomy vesical vaginal fistula. Next, Richard TeLinde added water endoscopy to the Hopkins female urology program. Most teaching programs at the time gave little or no exposure to female urology (2).

In 1892, Poussan proposed the concept of urethral advancement for the management of urinary incontinence (5). He suggested "introducing a bougie into the urethra, resecting the external meatus and portion of the urethra, and then after torsion of the canal to one hundred and eighty degrees, it is transplanted to a point just below the clitoris." By the turn of the century, four main treatments for stress urinary incontinence were outlined:

1. injection of paraffin into the region of the urethra;
2. massage and electricity;
3. torsion of the urethra;
4. advancement of the external urethral meatus.

A century later we are still trying to identify the best urethral bulking agent. Although it is no longer paraffin, research with Teflon [poly(tetrafluoroethylene)], silicone, collagen, autologous fat, hyaluronic acid, carbon particles, and various copolymers has failed to identify an ideal medium.

In his landmark paper in 1913 Kelly outlined operations for managing urinary incontinence in women (6). These included the following:

- puncture of the bladder and insertion of a catheter;
- closing the urethra and creating a vesico-abdominal fistula;
- closing the vagina and creating a rectovaginal fistula;
- compression of the urethra with an anterior colporrhaphy;
- periurethral injection of paraffin;
- advancement of the urethral meatus to the clitoris.

Kelly suggested that "the torn or relaxed tissues of the vesical neck should be sutured together using two or three vertical mattress sutures of fine silk linen passed from side to side." In his first publication, he described 16 patients as being well and four patients in whom the procedure was not successful, giving a success rate of 80%. However, further evaluation has revealed that the long term success, using only these sutures to correct stress incontinence falls to roughly 60% (7). This decline is possibly related to gradual postoperative elongation of the smooth muscle in which the sutures were placed (8). With coincident suburethral plication of the pubourethrovaginal ligaments of the urogenital diaphragm, the long-term results of a Kelly plication are significantly better (9).

Sling procedures were pioneered in the early 1900s by three European physicians. Goebell first suggested transplantation of the pyramidalis muscle in 1910 (10). This was followed by Frankenheim who, in 1914, recommended using the pyramidalis or strips of rectus muscle as a suburethral sling by attaching the muscle to overlying fascia (11). In 1917, Stoeckel suggested combining the techniques of Goebell and Frankenheim and adding plication of the vesical neck (12). Throughout the 20th century, there have been many variations of sling procedures described in the literature. In 1907, Giordano suggested the use of the gracilis muscle by wrapping it around the urethra (13). Shortly thereafter, in 1911, Souier described the use of levator ani muscles by placing them between the vagina and urethra (14), and, in 1923, Thompson recommended the use of strips of rectus muscle, surrounded by fascia, to be passed in front of the pubic bones and around the urethra (15). The next key event in the development of surgery to the anterior compartment was the development of the bulbocavernosus muscle fat pad graft by Martius in 1929 (16). This has found wide use in fistula repairs and reconstruction of the anterior vaginal wall. In 1968, John Chasser Moir (17) introduced the concept of the gauze hammock operation as a modification of the original Aldridge (18) sling procedure described in 1942. Chasser Moir recognized that "operations of this type do no more than support the bladder neck and urethrovesical junction and so prevent the undue descent of parts when the woman strains or coughs."

Victor Bonney, in 1923, stated, "Incontinence depends in some way upon a sudden and abnormal displacement of the urethra and urethrovesical junction immediately behind the symphysis" (19). This was followed in 1924 by a description from B.P. Watson of "the muscle sheet that normally supports the base and neck of the bladder" and his statement that "so far as the incontinence of urine is concerned, the important sutures are those which overlap the fascia at the neck of the bladder and so restore it to its normal position." In reviewing Watson's work with anterior colporrhaphy, he was able to obtain "perfect control" in 65.7% of cases, "improvement" in 21.9%, and "no success" in 12.4% (20). These figures are in keeping with others that have been reported for anterior colporrhaphy. Therefore, it was apparent that hypermobility of the bladder neck was an issue, and that the anterior colporrhaphy was not a satisfactory operation for stress incontinence.

The next landmark in genitourinary surgery occurred in 1949 with the publishing of the paper of Marshall, Marchetti, and Krantz on "The correction of stress incontinence by simple vesicourethral suspension." They suggested that this operation was "particularly valuable for patients whose first procedure failed." In their first 44 patients they described 82% of patients with excellent results, 7% with improvement, and an 11% failure rate (21). Shortly thereafter, in 1950, H.H. Fouracre Barns described the "round ligament sling operation for stress incontinence"; this technique was popularized by Paul Hodgkinson (22). In 1961, John Burch first described his modification of the Marshall–Marchetti–Krantz procedure which involved a retropubic colpourethropexy that took the anterolateral aspects of the vault of the vagina and attached them to Cooper's ligament (23). Burch recognized the potential complications of this procedure if done alone including, the creation of an enterocele or rectocele, the development of ventral/incisional hernias, and even the possibility of a vesicovaginal fistula.

Diagnosis and Investigation

As the number of procedures offered for the treatment of stress incontinence increased, there were also significant advances in the urogynecological diagnostic procedures available. In 1882, Mosso and Pellacani described cystometry using a smoked drum and a water manometer (24). An aneroid barometer for cystometric evaluation was developed by Lewis in 1939 (25). Jeffcoate and Roberts, in 1952, introduced the concept of radiographic changes in the posterior urethrovesical angle (26). These changes were further modified in 1956, by Bailey in England, who described seven variations in the urethrovesical angle on radiographic studies (27). Later modifications were performed by Tom Green in the United States in 1962, when he described Green types 1 and 2 incontinence (28). Identification of the posterior urethrovesical angle by lateral bead chain cystography was introduced by Hodgkinson in 1953 (29).

By 1956, Von Garrelts had introduced the concept of uroflowmetry (30). In 1964, Enhorning, Miller, and Hinman combined cystometry with radiographic screening of the bladder (31); this was followed a few years later in 1969 by Brown and Wickham's introduction of urethral pressure profilometry (32). Another landmark occurred in 1971, when Patrick Bates, Sir Richard Turner-Warwick, and Graham Whiteside introduced synchronous cine pressure–flow cystography, with pressure and flow studies (33). This was the beginning of the field of video urodynamics. Equipment was further expanded with the introduction of the microtip transducer, in 1975 by Asmussen and Ulmsten, for measuring urethral closure pressure (34).

Further investigational advances occurred in the latter part of the 20th century. These included the introduction of the Urilos monitor in 1974 by James, Flack, Caldwell, and Smith (35). This device allowed evaluation of the symptom of dampness for whether the fluid lost was urine. In 1981, Sutherst, Brown, and Shawer developed the pad-weighing test as an objective measure of the severity of urinary incontinence (36).

In 1961, Enhorning suggested that "surgical treatment for stress incontinence is probably mainly beneficial because it restores the neck of the bladder and the upper part of the urethra to the influence of intra-abdominal pressure" (37). This introduced the concept of pressure transmission ratios, and the idea that successful operations for stress urinary incontinence worked by restoring the urethrovesical junction to an intra-abdominal position. In 1956, Jeffcoate added further interpretation of our investigative techniques when he attempted to caution gynecologists, stating that "the absence of the posterior urethrovesical angle is merely a sign of incompetence of the internal sphincter. The presence of an angle is a function of the involuntary muscle at the urethrovesical junction, not of the muscle of the pelvic floor" (38), and so the simplistic approach of static cystourethrograms began to be questioned. Green had suggested that if one saw a radiographic diagnosis of type 1 incontinence this could readily be repaired with an anterior colporrhaphy; the type 2 stress incontinence required a retropubic urethropexy. A number of authors, including Drutz in 1978 (39), have confirmed the limited accuracy of static cystourethrograms.

4

By 1953, Paul Hodgkinson had recommended, "If on anteroposterior straining radiograph, the urethrovesical junction is depressed 4 cm below the lower border of the symphysis, I believe the objective of the operation can be accomplished through anterior colporrhaphy" (28). A decade later Hodgkinson commented on the frequency of detrusor dyssynergia, with grade 1 defined as a detrusor contraction in response to coughing and heel bouncing; grade 2 was spontaneous automatic detrusor contractility when recumbent. Hodgkinson recognized the importance of discovering this condition prior to performing any surgery for stress urinary incontinence (40).

Success Rates

As we approached the 1970s, we began to recognize that operative failures in the treatment of stress urinary incontinence involve three areas (41), as follows:

1. incorrect diagnosis and the fact that bladder instability (and not just simple stress incontinence) may have been the cause of the incontinence;
2. the wrong operation may have been chosen and some operations probably give better long-term results;
3. the concept of technical failure.

We recognized that the vaginal approach to primary stress incontinence probably only gave a 50% to 60% success rate, whereas the suprapubic approach gave success rates of at least 80%. J.E. Morgan, in 1973, discussed indications for primary retropubic urethropexy: these included minimal pelvic floor relaxation, chronic chest disease, occupations involving heavy lifting, and patients who were heavily involved in athletics, and obesity (42). In 1970, Hodgkinson stated that "the most durable operation for stress incontinence is a retropubic urethropexy and the least durable is a vaginal repair." Hodgkinson quoted a 92.1% success rate with his own 404 patients that had a retropubic urethropexy (40). The other movement in the 1970s was of the urologists and gynecologists toward endoscopic bladder-neck suspensions such as the Pereyra, Raz, and Stamey suspensions; numerous variations including the Gittes and Cobb-Raagde were described in the literature. In the 1990s, we have now realized that the long-term results of these needle suspension procedures are also not as good as the retropubic procedures.

The 1990s have also seen the advent of minimally invasive sling procedures for stress urinary incontinence. The first of these, the tension free vaginal tape, and the concomitant integral theory of the pathophysiology of incontinence, were described by Ulmsten and Petros in the early 1990s (43,44). There are now multiple variations of this procedure including the transobturator approach. Success rates are reported to be similar to that of the Burch repair (45). More recently, single incision midurethral slings have been advocated although the long-term success of these new procedures is yet to be established.

The great champion of pelvic floor exercises, Arnold Kegel, reported pre- and post-operative benefits of the properly performed exercises (46). Unfortunately, many patients are placed on this regimen only after an unsuccessful surgical procedure.

Robertson, with Bergman and Elia, in 2004, has described an enhancement of Kegel's exercise, when done in a magnetic field, combined with DeLancey's "knack procedure," to give support to the urethra when it is most needed (47).

THE WAY AHEAD

Now as we approach the 21st century, we must consider what lies ahead. The main fields of responsibility as urogynecologists and reconstructive pelvic surgeons include the following:

- education;
- surgery;
- uropharmacology;
- neurophysiology;
- behavior modification;
- collagen;
- ultrasonography/MRI;
- stem cells.

Regarding education, we need to focus on education of our colleagues in obstetrics and gynecology, family practice, geriatrics and community health care, allied health professionals such as nursing and physiotherapy, as well as the public. The awareness must be increased that incontinence is not a normal effect of aging; the many myths, including "everyone gets it" and "it can't be treated," must be dispelled. Urogenital aging must be stressed as part of menopause management, and conservative management in the community should be promoted. The other aspect of education is the training of new subspecialists in the field of urogynecology and reconstructive pelvic surgery. Board certification is now available in Australia and board recognition of training programs has been established in the United States. The IUGA is now establishing international standards for training in conjunction with FIGO and the WHO.

Within the field of surgery for pelvic floor problems, we need to re-evaluate what we do. Over 200 operations have been described for stress incontinence. Randomized controlled trials, with adequate patient numbers and follow-up of at least two years, are required for evaluation of new and existing procedures. The role of bulking agents is still controversial and the ideal medium has yet to be discovered. A variety of fascia and mesh is available for use in pelvic floor reconstructive procedures; however, the long-term durability and consequences of these are still unknown. This includes many new mesh devices and kits for pelvic floor reconstruction. Concerns have been raised about the ethics of some of these newer mesh devices (48). New pharmacologic agents continue to be produced; well designed, placebo controlled trials are mandatory for their evaluation. Neurophysiology is another developing area; work is being done to determine if there are certain factors in labor that lead to irreversible changes to the pelvic floor. Other questions that have been raised include whether abnormalities in the electromyographic patterns predict success or failure of different treatments. We continue to develop new modes of conservative management, including behavior modification and devices; further studies are needed to clarify the specific areas of use for these therapies.

The role of collagen in pelvic floor disorders is a fascinating area. We need both effective qualitative and quantitative assays to determine whether there are certain defects of collagen in patients with pelvic floor dysfunction. Also, we need to establish whether there may be potential genetic markers that may be screened for to determine certain "at-risk" patients. Perhaps there exists a select group of patients that should be counseled to have delivery by caesarean section; this group may also require the use of synthetic materials in reconstruction of their pelvic floor. We need to look at the relationship of collagen to estrogen and the general effects of urogenital aging to see if they are independent factors. Research into genetic components of pelvic floor prolapse is exciting. At Mount Sinai Hospital in Toronto, Dr. May Alarab and her associates have shown that genes that both promote the build-up of extracellular matrix and cause its degradation are different in pre-menopausal women with prolapse compared to controls.

We are in the midst of a revolution in imaging and diagnostic technology. The development of three-dimensional ultrasound (49) and the progress with MRI has allowed a new approach to evaluating defects associated with stress urinary incontinence and pelvic floor disorders. Progress in the field of ultrasound has been hampered by a lack of standardization of terminology; this was recognized by the German Association of Urogynecology, who attempted to make recommendations for standardization of methodology (50). The fact that different methods are used (such as abdominal, perineal, introital, vaginal, and rectal) has further impeded progress in this field. Recent papers have investigated the urethra and surrounding tissues with intra-urethral ultrasonography; the authors have proposed that sphincter measurements can be a prognostic factor in patients who underwent operations for stress urinary incontinence (51). Beco stated that "doppler and color studies will play and increasing role in the evaluation of urethrovesical disorders" (J. Beco, personal communication, November 1996). With new developments in MRI and especially dynamic MRI these techniques will also play a growing role in investigation and research. New ways of investigating urethral function are also appearing with the introduction of the MoniTorr device and measurement of urethral retro-resistance (52).

Stem cell research may introduce a natural type of treatment for stress urinary incontinence that replaces bulking agents.

There is an increasing focus on quality of life tools as a research outcome. National and international societies must continue to promote and support research in the field to advance pelvic floor health for women.

CONCLUSIONS

At the ICS meeting in 1986, Sir Richard Turner-Warwick gave an address in which he defined the urogynecologist as "neither the general urologist nor the general obstetrician and gynecologist, but someone who has special training and expertise in genitourinary problems in women" (53). Today, we should expand this definition to include urogynecology and reconstructive pelvic surgery. Such a physician implies a surgeon with specialized training in the conservative and surgical management of women with urinary and/or fecal incontinence, persistent genitourinary complaints, and disorders of pelvic floor supports.

As Marcel Proust said, "We must never be afraid to go too far, for the truth lies beyond." We must humbly accept that the "truths" that we identify today, certainly will have to be changed in the future. However, if we work collaboratively to produce well-designed scientific research, we should be able to establish truths that stand the test of time in our ongoing quest to improve the quality of life for women with pelvic floor problems.

ACKNOWLEDGMENT

This chapter includes major segments of text adapted from the IUGA Presidential Address given by Professor Harold Drutz at the 21st Annual Meeting of the IUGA held in Vienna in 1996. The text was later published: Drutz HP. The first century of urogynecology and reconstructive pelvic surgery: where do we go from here? Int Urogynecol J 1996; 7: 348–53.

REFERENCES

1. Keith A. Man's posture: it's evolution and disorders. Br Med J 1923; II: 451–54.
2. Robertson JR. Genitourinary Problems in Women. Springfield, IL: Charles C. Thomas, 1978: 6–12.
3. Wall LL, DeLancey JOL. The politics of prolapse: a revisionist approach to disorders of the pelvic floor in women. Perspect Biol Med 1991; 34: 486–96.
4. Nager CW, Kumar D, Kahn M, Stanton SL. Management of pelvic floor dysfunction. Lancet 1997; 350: 1751.
5. Poussan. Arch Clin Bord 1892. No. 1.
6. Kelly HA. Incontinence of urine in women. Urol Cutan Rev 1913; 17: 291.
7. Bergman A, Elia G. Three surgical procedures for genuine stress urinary incontinence: five year follow-up of a prospective randomized study. Am J Obstet Gynecol 1995; 173: 66–71.
8. Wall LL, Norton PA, DeLancey JOL. Practical Urogynecology. Baltimore: Williams and Wilkins, 1993: 153–90.
9. Nichols DH, Randall CL. Vaginal Surgery. Baltimore: Williams and Wilkins, 1996: 218–56.
10. Goebell R. Zur operativen Besierigung der angeborenen Incontinentia vesical. Z Gynäk Urol 1910; 2: 187.
11. Frankenheim P. Zentral Verhandl. d. Deutsch. Geseusch Chir 1914; 43: 149.
12. Stoeckel W. Über die Verwändung der Musculi Pyramidales bei der opeutinen Behandlung der Incontinentia Urinae. 1917; 41: 11.
13. Giordano D. Twentieth Congress Franc de Chir. 1907; 506.
14. Souier JB. Med Rec 1911; 79: 868.
15. Thompson R. Br J Dis Child 1923; 20: 116.
16. Martius H. Sphincter und Harndöurenplastic aus dem Musicailus Bulbocavernosus. Chirurgie 1929; 1: 769.
17. Chasser Moir J. The gauze-hammock operation (a modified Aldridge sling procedure). J Obstet Gynaecol Br Commonw 1968; 75: 1–9.
18. Aldridge AH. Transplantation of fascia for relief of urinary stress incontinence. Am J Obstet Gynecol 1942; 44: 398–411.
19. Bonney V. On diurnal incontinence of urine in women. J Obstet Gynecol Br Emp 1923; 30: 358–65.
20. Watson BP. Imperfect urinary control following childbirth and its surgical treatment. Br Med J 1924; 11: 566.
21. Marshall VF, Marchetti AA, Krantz KE. The correction of stress incontinence by simple vesicourethral suspension. Surg Gynecol Obstet 1949; 88: 509–18.
22. Fouracre Barns HH. Round ligament sling operation for stress incontinence. J Obstet Gynaecol Br Emp 1950; 57: 404–7.

23. Burch JC. Urethrovaginal fixation to Cooper's ligament for correction of stress incontinence, cystocele and prolapse. Am J Obstet Gynecol 1961; 81: 281–90.

24. Mosso A, Pallacani P. Sur les fonctions de la vessie. Arch Ital Biol 1882; 1: 97.

25. Lewis LG. New clinical recording cystometer. J Urol 1939; 41: 638–45.

26. Jeffcoate TNA, Roberts H. Stress incontinence. J Obstet Gynaecol Br Emp 1952; 59: 720–865.

27. Bailey KV. A clinical investigation into uterine prolapse with stress incontinence: treatment by modified Manchester colporrhaphy. Part II. J Obstet Gynaecol Br Emp 1956; 63: 663.

28. Green TH Jr. Development of a plan for the diagnosis and treatment of urinary stress incontinence. Am J Obstet Gynecol 1962; 83: 632–48.

29. Hodgkinson CP. Relationship of female urethra and bladder in urinary stress incontinence. Am J Obstet Gynecol 1953; 65: 560–73.

30. Von Garrelts B. Analysis of micturition: a new method of recording the voiding of the bladder. Acta Chir Scand 1956; 112: 326–40.

31. Enhorning G, Miller E, Hinman F Jr. Urethral closure studied with cine roentgenography and simultaneous bladder-urethral pressure recording. Surg Gynecol Obstet 1964; 118: 507–16.

32. Brown W, Wickham JEA. The urethral pressure profile. Br J Urol 1969; 41: 211–17.

33. Bates CP, Whiteside CG, Turner-Warwick R. Synchronous cine/pressure/flow cystography: a method of routine urodynamic investigation. Br J Radiol 1971; 44: 44–50.

34. Asmussen M, Ulmsten U. Simultaneous urethrocystometry and urethral pressure profile measurements with a new technique. Acta Obstet Gynaecol 1975; 54: 385–6.

35. James ED, Flack F, Caldwell KP, Smith M. Urine loss in incontinence patients: how often, how much? Clin Med 1974; 4: 13–17.

36. Sutherst JL, Brown M, Shawer M. Assessing the severity of urinary incontinence in women by weighing perineal pads. Lancet 1981; 1: 1128–30.

37. Enhorning G. Simultaneous recording of intravesical and intraurethral pressure: a study of urethral closure pressures in normal and incontinent women. Acta Chir Scand 1961; 276(Suppl): 1.

38. Jeffcoate TNA. Bladder control in the female. Proc Roy Soc Med 1956; 49: 652–60.

39. Drutz HP, Shapiro BJ, Mandel F. Do static cystourethrograms have a role in the investigation of female incontinence? Am J Obstet Gynecol 1978; 130: 516–20.

40. Hodgkinson CP, Ayers MA, Drukker BH. Dyssynergic detrusor dysfunction in the apparently normal female. Am J Obstet Gynecol 1963; 87: 717–30.

41. Hodgkinson CP. Stress Urinary incontinence. Am J Obstet Gynecol 1970; 1: 1141–68.

42. Morgan JE. The Suprapubic approach to primary stress incontinence. Am J Obstet Gynecol 1973; 49: 37–42.

43. Petros PE, Ulmsten UI. An integral theory and its method for the diagnosis and management of female urinary incontinence. Scand J Urol Nephrol Suppl 1993; 153: 1–93.

44. Ulmsten U, Petros P. Intravaginal slingplasty (IVS): an ambulatory surgical procedure for treatment of female urinary incontinence. Scand J Urol Nephrol 1995; 29: 75–82.

45. Ward KL, Hilton P. UK and Ireland TVT Trial Group. A prospective multicenter randomized trial of tension-free vaginal tape and colposuspension for primary urodynamic stress incontinence: two-year follow-up. Am J Obstet Gynecol 2004; 190: 324–31.

46. Kegel AH, Powell TH. The physiologic treatment of stress incontinence. J Urol 1950; 63: 808.

47. Bergman J, Robertson JR, Elia G. Effects of a magnetic field on pelvic floor muscle function in women with stress urinary incontinence. Altern Ther Health Med 2004; 10: 70–2.

48. Ross S, Robert M, Harvey MA, et al. Ethical issues associated with the introduction of new surgical devices, or just because we can, doesn't mean we should. J Obstet Gynaecol Can 2008; 30: 508–13.

49. Khullar V, Salvatore S, Cardozo LD, Hill S, Kelleher CJ. Three-dimensional ultrasound of the urethra and urethral sphincter: a new diagnostic technique. Neurourol Urodyn 1994; 13: 352–3.

50. Shaer G, Koelbl H, Voigt R, et al. Recommendations of the German Association of Urogynecology on functional sonography of the lower female urinary tract. Int Urogynecol J 1996; 7: 105–8.

51. Hermans RK, Klein HM, Muller U, Schafer W, Jakse G. Intraurethral ultrasound in women with stress incontinence. Br J Urol 1994; 74: 315–18.

52. Slack M, Culligan P, Tracey M, et al. Relationship of urethral retro-resistance pressure to urodynamic measurements and incontinence severity. Neurourol Urodyn 2004; 23: 109–14.

53. Turner-Warwick R. International Continence Society Proceedings. Boston, MA, USA, 1986.

2 Epidemiology: U.S.A.

Scott E Kalinowski, Benjamin J Girdler, and Ananias C Diokno

INTRODUCTION

Epidemiology is defined as the study of the relationships of various factors determining the frequency and distribution of diseases in a community (1). The epidemiological study of urinary incontinence (UI) has advanced over the past several years. However, most of these studies are cross-sectional. A need exists for more longitudinal studies to evaluate the incidence, remission, risk factors, and prevention of this disease process. The methodologies to evaluate the epidemiology of UI vary greatly. Furthermore, there is no consensus on the definition of UI among investigators dealing with this subject. As a consequence, there is conflicting information, especially in the prevalence rates. Another major issue in studying UI is the fact that incontinence itself is a condition with many varied types, occurring in many different segments of the population. Students of the epidemiology of UI must therefore account for all these variables when evaluating data from these studies.

PREVALENCE OF UI

The prevalence of UI is defined as the probability of being incontinent within the defined population group within a specific period of time. The first comprehensive epidemiologic study of incontinence in the United States was conducted by Diokno et al. (2) in 1983 in Washtenaw County, Michigan. The Medical, Epidemiologic, and Social Aspects of Aging (MESA) study showed the prevalence of incontinence among women 60 years and older living in the community to be 38%. Other more recent studies have agreed with this prevalence rate such as the data reported by Fultz et al. A 14-item questionnaire was returned by 29,903 people of whom 37% reported incontinence in the past 30 days (3).

The prevalence of UI in women increases with age. A postal survey was conducted by Thomas et al. (4) to selected health districts in the London boroughs and neighboring health districts in the late 1970s. In that survey, incontinence was defined as involuntary excretion or leakage of urine in inappropriate places or at inappropriate times twice or more a month, regardless of the quantity of urine lost. Incontinence was further subdivided into regular UI for a loss twice or more per month, and occasional for less than twice per month. The response rate was excellent at 89%. Table 2.1 shows the prevalence rates for regular and occasional incontinence in women aged 15 to more than 85 years. Three age tiers to the prevalence of regular incontinence in women were noted: the first level, 15 to 34 years (prevalence 4–5.5%); the second tier, 35 to 74 years (prevalence 8.8–11.9%); the third, 75 years and older (prevalence 16–16.2%).

Several studies have investigated incontinence in women of different races and found intriguing results. Lower rates of stress and mixed incontinence were reported by African-American women when compared with white women (5). Hispanic and Asian American women have been shown to have equivalent urodynamic stress incontinence rates to white women, whereas the African-American women had higher rates of detrusor overactivity than the other three groups (6). African-American women were found to have statistically significant smaller bladder capacities, smaller maximum cystometric capacities, and higher maximum urethral closure pressures compared to Caucasians (7). A more recent study by Fenner et al. looked at incontinence rates in African-American and Caucasian women in southeastern Michigan. They observed similar racial differences in prevalence, type, and quantity of urine loss, but failed to find support for the belief that risk factors for UI differed between Caucasian and African-American women (8).

INCIDENCE AND REMISSION

Incidence is the probability of becoming incontinent during a defined period of time. Determining the incidence of a condition or disease is helpful in determining the onset of the condition as well as in understanding the risk factors of the condition. The MESA survey established the incidence rate of UI in the United States (9). The incidence rate among women who were continent during the initial baseline interview and became incontinent a year later was 22.4%. For those who remained continent at the one-year follow-up visit, the incidence in the second year of follow-up was 20.2%. Hagglund et al. found a mean 4% annual incidence rate of UI reporting on a Swedish community of 10,500 inhabitants aged between 22 and 50 years (10). An annual incidence rate of 6.3% for people greater than or equal to 40 years old was found in McGrother et al.'s study in the United Kingdom (11). Two thousand twenty-five women older than 65 years in rural Iowa were evaluated by Nygaard and Lemke. The three-year incidence rate for urge incontinence and stress incontinence were 28.5% and 28.6%, respectively (12).

The MESA survey also analyzed the remission rate for UI. The remission rate—that is, women who were incontinent at the baseline (first) interview and became continent during the second interview a year later—was 11.2%. A similar rate (13.3%) of incontinent respondents at the second interview reported being continent a year later at the third interview. Hagglund et al. reported a 4% mean annual remission rate in the same Swedish community as above (10). Nygaard and Lemke's three-year remission rates for urge and stress incontinence were 22.1% and 25.1%, respectively (12). Townsend et al. looked at remission rates in 64,650 women 36 to 55 years of age participating in the Nurses' Health Study II. They reported remission rates of 13.9% at two year follow-up.

Table 2.1 Prevalence of Urinary Incontinence (UI) in Women

Age group (yrs)	Regular UI (%)	Occasional UI (%)	Total UI (%)
15–24	4.0	11.9	15.9
25–34	5.5	20.0	25.5
35–44	10.2	20.7	30.9
45–54	11.8	21.9	32.9
55–64	11.9	18.6	30.5
65–74	8.8	14.6	22.4
75–84	16.0	13.6	29.6
>85	16.2	16.2	32.4

Source: Data adapted from Ref. 4.

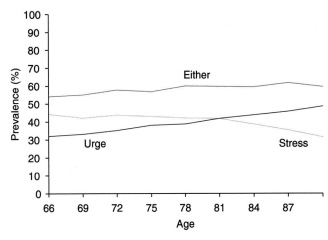

Figure 2.1 Prevalence of incontinence by age groups at baseline. Each age represents the midpoint of a three-year age range. Because of the small number of women above age 90, the graph ends with age range 86–88 years. "Urge" and "stress" refer to women who answered affirmatively to the urge and stress incontinence questions, respectively. "Either" refers to women who reported any incontinence (either urge or stress). Source: Data adapted from Ref. 12.

However, when the group was further delineated by age group they found significantly higher remission rates in women 36 to 45 years of age when compared to those 46 to 55 years of age (17.1% vs. 11.9%) (13).

These findings suggest a proportion of women affected by UI will improve over time without intervention. Because UI can be affected by many factors such as acute illness, seasonal changes, and fluctuating medical illnesses, it can be assumed that when questioned longitudinally many women would report varying degrees and prevalence of incontinence. Implying that for many patients, UI is not necessarily a progressive condition, but rather a dynamic process that may come and go with or without medical or surgical intervention. Further studies are needed to determine which respondents tend to have remission, and which tend to persist or progress. It is also important to consider the possibility of spontaneous remission when reviewing "cure" rates reported in treatment trials and to discuss the possibility of remission/recurrence when counseling patients.

TYPES AND SEVERITY OF UI
Prevalence and Incidence of Types of UI

In epidemiological studies, as in clinical investigations, the type of UI must be defined. In general, incontinence is considered to be of the stress type when the urine loss was experienced at the time of physical exertion (such as coughing, laughing, sneezing, etc.). Urge incontinence is defined as involuntary loss of urine preceded by a sudden urge to void. When the urine loss is associated with both stress and urge, it is considered to be of the mixed type. Because of the difficulty in identifying the overflow type, when the urine loss is associated with neither the stress nor the urge type, the incontinence is labeled "other." However, when the survey respondents were taken one step further into urodynamic testing, the type of incontinence has been classified into the various urodynamic types according to the pathophysiological abnormality.

Interestingly, when urodynamic testing is performed on women with UI, there is often a disconcordance between subjective and objective findings (14–16). Cundiff et al. evaluated 535 women over a ten year period via detailed history and physical exam, urinary diary, and urodynamics. They found that by utilizing symptoms alone, a misdiagnosis would be made in 13% of women reporting only stress incontinence

and 59% of women reporting only urge incontinence (17). Some of this can likely be explained by the artificial nature of office urodynamics and other technical issues, but patient's poor understanding of the different types of UI and incomplete history taking may also be implicated.

The age of onset may be an important factor in the type of UI experienced. Kinchen et al. found the median age of American women reporting stress incontinence was 48 years, mixed incontinence was 55 years, and urge incontinence was 61 years (18). Luber et al. evaluated 642 incontinent women and discovered that stress incontinence was more common in younger women aged 30 to 49 years (78%) versus those aged 50 to 89 years (57%). Urge incontinence predominates in the older population (67%) versus women under the age of 50 years (56%) (19).

According to Nygaard et al., the rate of urge incontinence tends to rise with age, while the rate of stress incontinence decreases somewhat in the oldest age groups, possibly due to lower activity levels (12) (Fig. 2.1).

The MESA survey conducted by Diokno et al. (2) in Washtenaw County, Michigan, reported the prevalence of the types of clinical incontinence encountered among their respondents. The most common type reported by these women aged 60 years and older was the mixed stress and urge type (55.5%), followed by the stress type (26.7%), the urge (9.0%), and other types (8.8%).

A meta-analysis of published studies of UI epidemiology in the world suggested that stress incontinence is the most common form (20). Stress incontinence accounted for almost half of the total worldwide prevalence of UI and mixed incontinence constituted 29% of the total prevalence. The analysis showed that urge incontinence was less common, consistent with the U.S. and European surveys.

Prevalence and Incidence of Severity of UI

In epidemiological studies, severity has been categorized by the frequency of incontinent episodes, by the volume of urine

Table 2.2 Percentage of Severe Incontinence, as Judged by Volume and Frequency of Urine Loss, in 60-Year-Old Women

Volume of urine lost in 24 hrs	No. of days with urine loss				Total percentage[a]
	1–9	10–49	50–299	300–365	
Drops < ½ tsp	16.1	11.6	5.6	3.0	36.3 (135)
½ tsp–<1 tbsp	9.7	9.7	7.5	3.2	30.1 (112)
1 tbsp–<¼ cup	4.6	4.6	5.4	3.2	17.8 (66)
¼ cup or more	2.4	2.4	4.3	6.7	15.8 (59)
Total[a]	32.8 (122)	28.3 (105)	22.8 (85)	16.1 (60)	100.0 (372)

Respondents with mild incontinence were those who reported low frequency (1–9 days/year) and/or small volume (<½ teaspoon/day for <300 days/year); those with severe incontinence were those who reported high frequency (≥300 days/year) and/or large volumes (>¼ cup/day on ≥50 days/year); those respondents with intermediate volume and/or frequency were considered to have moderate incontinence.
[a]Number of patients in parentheses.
Source: Data adapted from Ref. 2.

loss or by the frequency of difficulty in controlling the flow of urine. The Diokno MESA study (2) reported the severity of UI among its 60-year-old respondents in terms of the number of days per year that urine loss was experienced and the volume of urine loss per day. As shown in Table 2.2, if severe or significant UI is considered to be the loss of at least a quarter cup of urine per day on 50 or more days/year, or frequency of incontinence is 300 or more days/year, then 20.4% of women respondents age 60 years and older at the time of the MESA survey had severe incontinence.

The patterns of change in the severity of UI in the MESA survey were also analyzed (9). Based on the severity levels described in Table 2.2, continent respondents who became incontinent were most likely to develop a mild form of incontinence. About half of those who were classified originally as mildly incontinent remained so and very few became severely incontinent. Among those who reported moderate incontinence, most remained moderately incontinent or changed to mildly incontinent, with very few advancing to severe incontinence. Among women who were severely incontinent at baseline, most remained severely incontinent.

Kinchen et al. revealed that over 50% of incontinent respondents have urine loss at least once per week (18). The severity of incontinence symptoms influences a woman's willingness to discuss the symptoms with a physician. Fewer than 20% of women report discussing incontinence with a physician within the past year when symptoms are mild. The proportion increases to 42% of women when symptoms are severe (21).

Prevalence of Voiding Frequency
The prevalence of voiding frequency is receiving greater attention as more and more studies are being conducted for conditions related to bladder dysfunction. For example, pharmacological interventions as well as behavioral techniques aimed at improving bladder function usually affect the frequency of voiding day and night. It is therefore imperative that a comparative standard is available on which to base any observations related to frequency of voiding prior to, during, and after an intervention.

The MESA study has established the distribution of voiding frequency among the elderly (60 years and older) living in a community, who are likely to be the subjects of pharmacological and behavioral interventions aimed at controlling

abnormal voiding (2). It appears that the normal daily frequency of urination in this age group is no more than eight times, as 88% of all our asymptomatic respondents reported that range. To be more specific, 47.3% of asymptomatic women reported that they voided six to eight times, 34.8% voided four or five times, and 5.5% voided one to three times daily. FitzGerald et al. reevaluated the definition of urinary frequency by evaluating 300 asymptomatic women aged 18 to 91 (median 40 years) who volunteered from a large metropolitan community. These women completed a 24-hour log of fluid intake and volumes voided. They found a median of eight voids in 24 hours with 95% of subjects recording less than 13 voids per 24 hours. Their conclusion was that using greater than or equal to eight voids per 24 hours as the definition of "frequency" may be inappropriate, suggesting that "frequency" may be greater than or equal to 13 voids in 24 hours (22). Since the information came from a self-selected group of volunteers that reside in a large metropolitan area, their findings may not represent the true frequency of voiding in the general community.

In an investigation by the Bladder Diary Research Team, 161 asymptomatic women from 19 to 81 years of age were recruited at four independent research sites. Each subject completed a three-day bladder diary to establish normative values based on age and 24-hour urine volumes. They found that there was a statistically significant increase in frequency with increased age and 24-hour volume. They also found a mean of 7.1 voids per 24 hours, with a range of 2 to 13, and that 95% of subjects recorded less than 10.4 voids per 24 hours (23). The same group looked at 92 asymptomatic males from 20 to 84 years of age. They found a mean frequency of 6.6 with a range of 3 to 14 and 95% voiding less than 9.5 times per 24-hours (24). While the numbers are slightly lower than those from the MESA study, they bolster their conclusion that utilizing eight voids as the definition of frequency may be incorrect and may need to be adjusted based on age and 24-hour urine volume.

In terms of nocturia—which was defined as the frequency of being awakened from sleep and getting up to void—93% of asymptomatic women voided no more than twice at night. In contrast, 25% of women with irritative symptoms and 24% of women with difficulty in emptying the bladder voided three or more times each night (2). These data suggest that abnormal bladder function has a significant effect on the frequency of voiding. Incontinent women are voiding much more frequently than continent women. FitzGerald et al. (22) recorded nighttime voids in 44% or their population. Thirty-six percent voided once during the night while 8% voided greater than or equal to two times per night. The number of nighttime voids was dependent only on the patient age.

QUALITY OF LIFE
UI has a significant impact on a woman's quality of life. Fultz et al. examined 174 respondents who were moderately to extremely bothered by stress incontinence symptoms. Of these women 54.4% reported that their symptoms had a moderate to extreme impact on physical activities, 42.7% perceived such impact on confidence, 38.6% on daily activities, and 36.5% on social activities (3). The odds of moderate-to-extreme bother/burden decreased with age and increased with symptom severity.

The relative risk of admission to a nursing home is two times greater for incontinent women according to Thom et al. (25). Over half of all female nursing home residents are reported to have "difficulty controlling urine," and over half need assistance in using the toilet (26).

PREVALENCE OF URODYNAMIC MEASURES AMONG CONTINENT AND INCONTINENT ELDERLY WOMEN
To establish the urodynamic characteristics of both continent and incontinent elderly women living in a community, a series of urodynamic tests were conducted on those MESA respondents who volunteered to undergo such tests (27,28). This study provided information on the prevalence of the various parameters in the urodynamic tests that are of interest in the evaluation of incontinent patients but for which there are no well established data from control subjects. The MESA survey data established the sensitivity and specificity of the various urodynamic tests, from which it was concluded that such tests—including uroflow, cytometrography, static urethral profilometry, and stress cystography—should be used, not to screen and diagnose UI but, rather, to confirm clinical manifestation. Recent studies confirmed the lack of concordance between clinical manifestations and urodynamic findings (14–16).

The MESA survey studied a random sample of non-institutionalized ambulatory elderly women, both continent and incontinent; an initial clinical evaluation was followed by a series of urodynamic evaluations. A total of 258 self-reported continent and 198 self-reported incontinent women underwent the clinical evaluation comprising history taking, physical examination (including pelvic examination) and urinalysis. From these groups, 67 continent and 100 incontinent women underwent urodynamic testing including an initial non-instrumented uroflow test, followed by catheterized post-void volume measurements, followed by filling cystometry, static and dynamic urethral profilometry, provocative stress test, and lateral stress resting and straining cystogram.

Uroflowmetry
The uroflow measures of peak flow rate (PFR) and average flow rate (AFR) were analyzed according to the voided volume at increments of 100 ml. When volume was controlled, the mean PFR and AFR did not differ significantly between respondents who were continent and those who were incontinent. The flow rates did not differ between women with competent sphincters and those with urethral incompetence. The continuity of the urinary stream was not associated with continence status nor with the clinical type of incontinence (i.e., urge, stress, etc.).

Post-Void Residual Volume
A post-void residual volume of 0 to 50 ml was found in 78.1% of continent and 86.5% of incontinent women; 9.7% and 8.4% had residuals of 51 to 100 ml; 2.4% and 1.6% had residuals of 101 to 150 ml, and 9.7% and 3.5% had residuals of 151 ml or more, respectively. There was no statistical difference between continent and incontinent women with regard to prevalence of a residual urine volume greater than 50 ml. This data gives rise to questions regarding the post-void residual volume in relation to the diagnosis of overflow incontinence: the determining factor for overflow incontinence may be the same factor as for urge and/or stress incontinence, and the abnormal post-void residual volume may be coincidental or a contributory factor rather than a primary reason for the incontinence.

Bladder Capacity
Among the women volunteers, 79% of continent volunteers and 64% of incontinent volunteers had a bladder capacity of 300 ml or more; however, this difference in bladder volume between continent and incontinent subjects was not significant. The mean cystometric bladder capacities among 60 to 64-year-old continent and incontinent subjects were 381.8 and 442.7 ml, respectively; for 65 to 69-year-old subjects they were 421.6 and 370.0 ml, for those aged 70 to 74 years they were 410.3 and 414.2 ml; for those aged 75 to 79 years they were 350.3 and 426.8 ml, and for those aged 80 years old or more they were 318.3 and 408.3 ml, respectively. These results refute the notion that the bladder capacity of the elderly is smaller than normal, if we consider a bladder capacity of 300 ml or more to be normal.

Uninhibited Detrusor Contraction
The diagnosis of uninhibited detrusor contraction was based on the definition by the International Continence Society. The overall prevalence of uninhibited detrusor contraction in women was 7.9%; the prevalence of uninhibited detrusor contraction among continent respondents was 4.9%, whereas for incontinent subjects it was 12.2%. The difference between the two prevalence rates was not significant. However, comparison of the bladder capacity between female respondents showed that the capacity in women with uninhibited detrusor contraction was 364 ml, whereas in those without uninhibited contractions it was 404 ml; the difference was statistically significant at p < 0.05. This may explain the increased frequency, urgency, and smaller voided volumes of patients with detrusor overactivity.

Static and Dynamic Urethral Pressure Profilometry (UPP)
The mean functional urethral length (FUL) did not change significantly as the age of the subjects increased, but the values of the maximum urethral pressure (MUP) and the maximum

closure pressure (MCP) showed a significant progressive reduction as age increased (p = 0.002 and p = 0.0003, respectively). This progressive reduction of MUP and MCP reinforces the belief that elderly women are more predisposed to stress urine loss.

The parameters of UPP for supine subjects did not show any significant difference between continence and incontinence. However, for standing subjects, significant differences were observed between continent and incontinent groups with respect to MUP, which was significantly (p = 0.0025) lower in the incontinent compared with the continent group. Likewise, the MCP and the FUL were significantly reduced in standing but not in supine incontinent subjects when compared with the continent group.

The results of dynamic profilometry were reported as either positive (zero or positive reading), corresponding to incontinence, or negative (corresponding to continence). There was no significant difference between incontinent and continent subjects in the supine position, but there was between the groups in the standing position. Despite this significant difference, there was a great deal of overlap between the results for the continent and incontinent groups, invalidating a diagnosis based on this test alone.

Lateral Stress Cystography

Comparison between continent and incontinent subjects and between those with different types of incontinence, with regard to urethral axis, posterior urethrovesical angle (PUV), and distance of urethrovesical junction to the urogenital diaphragm (UGD), showed that incontinent respondents had a significantly (p = 0.001) wider PUV angle than did continent respondents; however, no significant difference was observed between stress and non-stress types of incontinence. There was no difference in the urethral axis and the position of the bladder neck in relation to the UGD between the groups according to continence status or clinical type of incontinence. There was a significantly greater mean PUV angle among incontinent subjects with an incompetent sphincter than among continent subjects with a competent sphincter (p = 0.004); however, neither the measurements of the urethral axis nor the location of the UGD differed between these two groups.

Provocative Stress Test

A provocative cough stress test was found to be significantly correlated to continence and incontinence status and, more specifically, to the stress type of urine loss with or without urge loss (p/ 0.0005). The result of the stress cystogram, when correlated with the stress test, showed a strong association (p = 0.009). A urethral axis of 30 degrees or more is more likely to give rise to a positive stress test than is an axis less than 30 degrees. The stress test can be performed as part of the initial office evaluation and does not require special equipment: there is no morbidity, it is inexpensive and (more importantly) it has extremely high specificity; it should be a part of everyone's initial evaluation. However, a negative test in someone who is experiencing UI does not rule out its existence, as sensitivity of the test often is only 40%.

MEDICAL CORRELATES OF UI

Several medical conditions have been associated with UI in women. Difficulties with physical mobility, lower urinary tract symptoms, bowel problems, and diabetes are more common in women with incontinence. Other factors associated with UI include a family history of incontinence, vaginal childbirth, and estrogen hormone use. Many of these associations were identified through the MESA survey (29).

Patients who used wheelchairs or walking aids, had a diagnosis of arthritis or who had fallen in the past year were defined as having mobility difficulties in the MESA survey. In women with mobility problems, urge incontinence was more common than any other type.

Regarding urinary tract and bowel problems, women with UI had a history of more urinary tract infections, dysuria, hesitancy, urgency, and slow stream than continent women. In addition, those who had more fecal incontinence or constipation had a higher rate of UI. Women with stress incontinence were the least likely of all urinary incontinent patients to lose control of their bowels.

Diabetes effects more than 12% of adults older than 40 and the prevalence increases to 19% of adults older than 60 (30). Diabetic women have a 30% to 70% increased risk of UI (29,31,32). The risk of urge incontinence was increased about 50% among women with diabetes, while they had no increased risk of stress UI (33). The mechanism for the incontinence is unclear. Possibilities include hyperglycemia (34) and microvascular complications causing altered innervation to the bladder (35). Most prior studies on diabetic people with incontinence were conducted on elderly patients with type 1 diabetes who may have had other neurological or urological reasons for their incontinence. A recent cross-sectional analysis of a younger cohort of type 1 diabetics from the Epidemiology of Diabetes Intervention and Complication study demonstrated a twofold greater odds of urge incontinence and 50% greater odds of stress incontinence compared to a matched cohort from the National Health and Nutrition Examination Survey (36). Furthermore, UI was found to be more prevalent than neuropathy, retinopathy, or nephropathy. New data from the prospective, observational Nurses' Health Study cohort of more than 70,000 married registered nurses found type 2 diabetes to be a strong independent risk factor for UI (37,38). In addition, the study found that the risk of incontinence increases with the duration of type 2 diabetes allowing the investigators to conclude that simply delaying the onset of diabetes could have important public health implications. Data from the Diabetes Prevention Program in pre-diabetic women showed that total weekly incontinence at three years was lowest in women randomized to the intensive lifestyle (34%) compared with metformin (48%) or placebo (46%) (39). Weight loss accounted for the largest impact on incontinence in this study, and underscores the difficulty the role of many confounding factors such as parity, stroke, diabetes, age and body weight play in drawing causative conclusions. Further research is needed to define the role diabetes plays in UI and the impact intervention may have on decreasing its incidence.

Females with incontinence more often reported a parent or sibling with UI than continent women. It was also noted that UI patients had a higher rate of personal UI during adolescence versus continent patients.

There is an increased risk of later UI after a vaginal delivery, even after the first delivery (40). An increased risk of surgery for the stress UI is also seen after a vaginal delivery (41). During pregnancy there is an increased prevalence of incontinence, especially in the third trimester, which usually resolves shortly after delivery (42). Possible etiologies are hormonal changes during pregnancy, damage to the pelvic muscles, and nerve injury during labor and delivery (43). It is difficult to identify the specific parturition risk factors as there are many potential, interrelated factors that occur during a single pregnancy and delivery. Most observational studies have demonstrated that cesarean sections are protective against incontinence versus vaginal deliveries (44,45). The EPINCONT study of more than 15,000 Norwegian women demonstrated overall incontinence rates of 10% of nulliparous, 16% of cesarean section, and 21% in vaginal delivery only women (46). However, the protective role of cesarean section diminished when adjusted with increasing age. An interesting study of identical twins at the annual Twins Day Festival in Twinsburg, Ohio, found that vaginal delivery more than doubled the report of stress UI compared to cesarean section (47). In 2007, a systematic review of the literature by Press found that cesarean section reduced the risk of postpartum stress UI from 16% to 9.8% in six cross-sectional studies and from 22% to 10% in 12 cohort studies (48). From this data, they calculated that between 10 and 15 cesarean sections would need to be performed to prevent one woman from developing SUI. Less is known about the cesarean section timing (before labor, in labor but without pushing, or in labor and pushing) and its effect on incontinence. A study of Israeli women one-year after their first delivery found similar stress UI rates in women undergoing vaginal deliveries (10%) and cesarean for obstructed labor (12%) compared to planned cesareans (3%) (49).

Historically estrogen, either vaginal or oral, was thought to improve incontinence episodes in post-menopausal women. The trigone and urethra are covered by nonkeratinized squamous epithelium and these tissues contain estrogen receptors (50) and respond to estrogen (51). There have been many uncontrolled trials demonstrating subjective improvement in incontinence, while a few randomized controlled trials showed no significant difference between control and treatment groups (52,53). Recently, the Heart Estrogen Replacement Study found intriguing UI outcomes when comparing a regimen of conjugated estrogen and medroxyprogesterone acetate with placebo (54). Incontinence improved in 26% of women given placebo compared to 21% assigned to combined estrogen/progestin, whereas 27% worsened in the placebo group compared to 39% receiving hormonal replacement. They concluded the effect of estrogen might be canceled by the progesterone, as progestin has been shown to decrease intraurethral closing pressure.

In the United States, approximately 31% of adults are obese and 33% are overweight, with the most rapid increase among those in the younger (18–29 years) age range (55). Numerous epidemiological studies have demonstrated an association between obesity and stress UI. Women with a median body mass index (BMI) of 28.2 had a higher incidence of UI than those with a BMI of 25.5 (normal range) (56). Odds ratios as high as 1.6 per 5 unit increase in BMI have been demonstrated (55). The additional weight is believed to results in higher pressures on the bladder and causes an increase in urethral hypermobility. In a urodynamic evaluation study of subjects from the Program to Reduce Incontinence by Diet and Exercise trial, BMI had a stronger association with intra-abdominal pressure than with intravesical pressure (57). The authors suggested that increasing weight may push women closer to their threshold for UI episodes, even if their intrinsic continence mechanisms are comparable. Randomized non-surgical weight reduction studies suggest losing 5% or more of body weight can lower UI episodes by as much as 70% (55). In fact, reduction in UI frequency has been suggested to be a powerful motivator for lifestyle modification. UI following gastric bypass surgery has resulted in similar reductions, which correlate significantly with decrease in BMI (55,58).

PATTERNS OF REPORTING OF UI

According to a nationwide, two-staged, cross-sectional postal survey conducted by the NFO Worldgroup (59), 41.6% of incontinent women believed their incontinence was a natural part of growing older and 47.0% accepted it as a part of their life.

Approximately 86% of women reported being bothered by symptoms of UI, with 25.6% reported being moderately bothered, 14.5% very bothered, and 8.5% extremely bothered. Only 44.9% of these incontinent women had ever talked to a physician about it. Those who were more bothered by their symptoms were more likely to have talked to a physician (not bothered, 25.2%; slightly bothered, 37.1%; moderately to extremely bothered, 56.5%). Older women were also more likely to talk to a physician than a younger women (53.5% vs. 39.8%).

Of the incontinent women who spoke with a physician, 42.9% first talked with a family practitioner, 35.1% with an obstetrician-gynecologist, 10.9% with an internist, and 4.4% with an urologist. Of all women who initially spoke with an internist or family practitioner, 19.0% were later referred to a urologist and 17.3% to a gynecologist.

COPING STRATEGIES TO CONTROL UI

Patient self-care practices were also evaluated by the NFO Worldgroup (59). Of all the women surveyed (bothered and non-bothered by UI), 42.1% currently used panty liners, 33.5% used the toilet frequently even when they did not have an urge to urinate, and 29.5% sought out a toilet immediately upon arriving at an unfamiliar location. Of the incontinent women, 23.3% limited their fluid intake and pelvic floor muscle exercises were performed by 19.9% of all UI women and by 20.3% of women with stress symptoms only. Only 6.3% of all the women are currently being treated with prescription medications and 2.1% have had surgery for their UI.

CONTINENT SURGERY AND ITS OUTCOMES

An estimated 126,000 continence surgeries are performed annually in the United States (60). A review of the literature demonstrates that the median proportion of women cured or improved by surgery at one to two years was 78% for anterior repair, 86% for retropubic suspension, and 91% for sling procedures (61). However, the NFO Worldgroup panel evaluated the prevalence and outcomes of continence surgery in community dwelling women via a postal survey (62). Four percent of community dwelling women and 8% of women 60 years or older had a history of continence surgery. The initial satisfaction of surgery was high, but then decreased as time progressed. Of those who had surgery within the past three years, 64% were currently satisfied, where only 41% were satisfied if their surgery was three to five years ago. Seventy-three percent of the women who had surgery reported incontinence in the preceding month, 58% in the preceding week, and 53% who used pads. Of those with recurrent UI, 83% complained of stress incontinence. One-third of the women had their surgery within the last five years.

PREVALENCE OF PELVIC ORGAN PROLAPSE

Pelvic organ prolapse is often a concurrent problem with UI. The prevalence of pelvic prolapse was evaluated by Hendrix et al. in 2002 by analyzing women who enrolled in the Women's Health Initiative Hormone Replacement Therapy Clinical Trial (63). They found in women with a uterus, the rate of uterine prolapse was 14.2%, cystocele was 34.3%, rectocele 18.6%. For the women who had a hysterectomy, the rate of a cystocele was 32.9% and a rectocele was 18.3%. Hispanic women had the highest risk for uterine prolapse and African-Americans had the lowest risk. Finally, parity and obesity were strongly associated with an increased risk of uterine prolapse, cystocele, and rectocele.

ECONOMIC BURDEN OF UI

The direct and indirect financial impact of UI on our health care system is significant. Hu et al. estimated the total cost of UI was $19.5 billion (year 2000 dollars) (64): $14.2 billion was due to community residents and $5.3 billion due to institutional residents. The direct costs for community residents, which included absorbent products, laundry, treatment, and consequences (UTIs, etc.), were $13.66 billion. Indirect costs, which involved lost productivity secondary to missing work, for community residents was estimated to be $553 million, with a $393 million loss for women and $159 million loss for men. For the institutionalized individual, the direct cost is $5.32 billion.

CONCLUSION

UI is a prevalent condition that can affect women of all ages. The incidence is especially high in the elderly population. UI is associated with many medical conditions. Urodynamic testing can help explain the mechanism of UI. Many women with UI think that it is a part of the normal aging process and do not talk to their physicians about this condition. Despite the advancement in medical and surgical treatment of UI, many women's satisfaction rates with the treatment is not as high as some physicians perceive it.

REFERENCES

1. Dorland's Illustrated Medical Dictionary, 26th edn. Philadelphia: WB Saunders, 1985: 451.
2. Diokno AC, Brock BM, Brown MB, et al. Prevalence of urinary incontinence and other urological symptoms in the noninstitutionalized elderly. J Urol 1986; 136: 1022–5.
3. Fultz NH, Burgio K, Diokno AC, et al. Burden of stress urinary incontinence for community-dwelling women. Am J Obstet Gynecol 2003; 189: 1275–82.
4. Thomas TM, Plymat KR, Blannin J, et al. Prevalence of urinary incontinence. Br Med J 1980; 281: 1243–5.
5. Brown JS, Grady D, Ouslander J, et al. Prevalence of urinary incontinence and associated risk factors in postmenopausal women. Heart & Estrogen/Progestin Replacement Study (HERS) Research Group. Obstet Gynecol 1999; 94: 66–70.
6. Duong TH, Korn AP. A comparison of urinary incontinence among African American, Asian, Hispanic and white women. Am J Obstet Gynecol 2001; 184: 1083–6.
7. Graham CA, Mallet VT. Race as a predictor of urinary incontinence and pelvic organ prolapse. Am J Obstet Gynecol 2001; 185: 116–20.
8. Fenner DE, Trowbridge ER, Patel DL, et al. Establishing the prevalence of incontinence study: racial differences in women's patterns of urinary incontinence. J Urol 2008; 179:1455–60.
9. Herzog AR, Diokno AC, Brown MB, et al. Two-year incidences, remissions and change patterns of urinary incontinence in noninstitutionalized older adults. J Gerontol 1990; 45: 67–74.
10. Hagglund D, Walker-Engstrom ML, Larsson G, et al. Changes in urinary incontinence and quality of life after four years. A population-based study of women aged 22–50 years. Scan J Prim Health Care 2004; 22: 112–17.
11. McGrother CW, Donaldson MM, Shaw C, et al. Storage symptoms of the bladder; prevalence, incidence and need for services in the UK. BJU Int 2004; 93: 763–9.
12. Nygaard IE, Lemke JH. Urinary incontinence in rural older women; prevalence, incidence, and remission. J am Geriatr Soc 1996; 44: 1049–54.
13. Townsend MK, Danforth KN, Lifford KL, et al. Incidence and remission of urinary incontinence in middle-aged women. Am J Obstet Gynecol 2007; 197: 167.e1–5.
14. Nager CW, Albo ME, Fitzgerald MP, et al. Reference urodynamic values for stress incontinent women. Neurourol and Urodynam 2007; 26: 333–40.
15. Summitt RL Jr, Stovall TG, Bent AE, Ostergard DR. Urinary incontinence: correlation of history and brief office evaluation with multichannel urodynamic testing. Am J Obstet Gynecol 1992; 166: 1835–40.
16. Walters MD, Shields LE. The diagnostic value of history, physical examination, and the Q-tip cotton swab test in women with urinary incontinence. Am J Obstet Gynecol 1988; 159: 145–9.
17. Cundiff GW, Harris RL, Coates KW, Bump RC. Clinical predictors of urinary incontinence in women. Am J Obstet Gynecol 1997; 177: 262–6.
18. Kinchen K, Gohier J, Obenchain R, et al. Prevalence and frequency of stress urinary incontinence among community-dwelling women. Eur Urol 2002; 40(Suppl 1): 85.
19. Luber KM, Boero S, Choe JY, et al. The demographics of pelvic floor disorders: current observations and future projections. Am J Obstet Gynecol 2001; 184: 1496–501; discussion 1501–3.
20. Hampel C, Wienhold D, Benken N, et al. Definition of overactive bladder and epidemiology of urinary incontinence. Urology 1997; 50(6A Suppl): 4–14.
21. Herzog AR, Fultz NH, Normolle DP, et al. Methods used to manage urinary incontinence by older adults in the community. J Am Geriatr Soc 1989; 37: 339–47.
22. FitzGerald MP, Stablein U, Brubaker L. Urinary habits among asymptomatic women. Am J Obstet Gynecol 2002; 187: 1384–8.
23. Amundsen CL, Parsons M, Tissot B, et al. Bladder diary measurements in asymptomatic females: functional bladder capacity, frequency, and 24-hr volume. Neurourol Urodynam 2009; 26: 341–9.

24. Tissot W, Amundsen CL, Diokno AD, et al. Bladder diary measurements in asymptomatic males: frequency, volume per void, and 24-hr volume. Neurourol Urodynam 2008; 27: 198–204.

25. Thom DH, Haan MN, Van Den Eeden SK. Medically recognized urinary incontinence and risks of hospitalization, nursing home admission and mortality. Age Ageing 1997; 26: 367–74.

26. Nygaard I, Thom DH, Calhoun EA. Urinary incontinence in women. In: Litwin MS, Saigal CS, eds. Urologic Diseases in America. US Government Publishing Office, 2004; (Table 22): 71–103.

27. Diokno AC, Brown MB, Browk BM, et al. Clinical and cystometric characteristics of continent and incontinent noninstitutionalized elderly. J Urol 1988; 140: 567–71.

28. Diokno AC, Normalle DP, Brown MB, et al. Urodynamic tests for female geriatric urinary incontinence. Urology 1990; 36: 431–39.

29. Diokno AC, Brock BM, Herzog AR, et al. Medical correlates of urinary incontinence in the elderly. Urology 1990; 36: 129–38.

30. Harris MI, Flegal KM, Cowie CC, et al. Prevalence of diabetes, impaired fasting glucose, and impaired glucose tolerance in US adults: the Third National Health and Nutrition Examination Survey, 1988–1994. Diabetes Care 1998; 21: 518–24.

31. Brown J, Seeley D, Fong J, et al. Urinary incontinence in older women: who is at risk? Obstet Gynecol 1996; 87: 715–21.

32. Wetle T, Scherr P, Branch LG, et al. Difficulty with holding urine among older persons in a geographically defined community: prevalence and correlates. J Am Geriatric Soc 1995; 43: 349–55.

33. Brown JS, Grady D, Ouslander J, et al. Prevalence of urinary incontinence and associated risk factors in postmenopausal women. Heart and Estrogen/ Progestin Replacement Study (HERS) Research Group. Obstet Gynecol 1999; 94: 66–70.

34. Belis J, Curley R, Lang C. Bladder dysfunction in the spontaneously diabetic male Abyssinian-Hartley guinea pig. Pharmacology 1996; 53: 66–70.

35. Ellenberg M. Development of urinary bladder dysfunction in diabetes mellitus. Ann Intern Med 1980; 92: 321–3.

36. Sarma AV, Kanaya AM, Nyberg LM, et al. Urinary incontinence among women with type 1 diabetes – how common is it? J Urol 2009; 181: 1224–30.

37. Danforth, KN, Townsend MK, Curhan GC, et al. Type 2 diabetes mellitus and risk of stress, urge and mixed urinary incontinence. J Urol 2009; 181: 193–7.

38. Lifford KL, Curhan GC, Hu FB, et al. Type 2 diabetes mellitus and risk of developing urinary incontinence. J Am Geriatr Soc 2005; 53: 1851–7.

39. Brown JS, Wing R, Barrett-Connor E, et al. Lifestyle intervention is associated with lower prevalence of urinary incontinence. Diabetes Care 2006; 29: 385–90.

40. Milsom I, Ekelund P, Molander U, et al. The influence of age, parity, oral contraception, hysterectomy and menopause on the prevalence of urinary incontinence in women. J Urol 1993; 149: 1459–62.

41. Persson J, Wolner-Hanssen P, Rydhstrom H. Obstetric risk factors for stress urinary incontinence: a population based study. Obstet Gynecol 2000; 96: 440–5.

42. Viktrup L, Lose G, Rolgg M, et al. The symptom of stress incontinence caused by pregnancy or delivery in primiparas. Obstet Gynecol 1992; 79: 945–9.

43. Smith AR, Hosker GL, Warrell DW. The role of partial denervation of the pelvic floor in the aetiology of genitourinary prolapse and stress incontinence of urine: a neurophysiological study. Br J Obstet Gynaecol 1989; 96: 24–8.

44. Wohlrab KJ, Radin CR. Impact of route of delivery on continence and sexual function. Clin Perinatol 2008; 35: 583–90.

45. Rogers RG, Leeman LL. Postpartum genitourinary changes. Urol Clin N Am 2007; 34: 12–21.

46. Rortveit G, Daltveit AK, Hannestad YS, et al. Urinary incontinence after vaginal delivery or cesarean section. N Eng J Med 2003; 348: 900–7.

47. Goldberg RP, Abramov Y, Botros S, et al. Delivery mode is a major environmental determinant of stress urinary incontinence: results of the Evanston-Northwestern Twin Sisters Study. Am J Obstet Gynecol 2005; 193: 2149–53.

48. Press JZ, Klein MC, Kaxzorowski J, et al. Does cesarean section reduce postpartum urinary incontinence? A systematic review. Birth 2007; 34: 228–37.

49. Groutz A, Rimon E, Peled S, et al. Cesarean section: does it really prevent the development of postpartum stress urinary incontinence? A prospective study of 363 women one year after their first delivery. Neurourol Urodyn 2004; 23: 2–6.

50. Iosif CS, Batra S, Ek A, et al. Estrogen receptors in the human female lower urinary tract. Am J Obstet Gynecol 1981; 141: 817–20.

51. Van der Kinden MC, Gerretsen G, Brandhorst MS, et al. The effect of estriol on the cytology of urethra and vagina in post-menopausal women with genitourinary symptoms. Eur J Obstet Gynecol Reprod Biol 1993; 51: 29–33.

52. Fantl JA, Bump RC, Robinson D, et al. The Continence Program for Women Research Group. Efficacy of estrogen supplementation in the treatment of urinary incontinence. Obstet Gynecol 1996; 88: 745–9.

53. Jackson S, Shepherd A, Brooks S, et al. The effect of estrogen supplementation in treatment of urinary stress incontinence: a double blind placebo-controlled trial. Br J Obstet Gynaecol 1999; 106: 711–18.

54. Grady D, Brown S Vittinghoff E, et al. HERS Research Group. Postmenopausal hormones and incontinence: The Heart and Estrogen/Progestin Replacement Study. Obstet Gynecol 2001; 97: 116–20.

55. Greer WJ, Richter HE, Bartolucci AA, et al. Obesity and pelvic floor disorders: a systematic review. Obstet and Gynecol 2008; 112: 341–9.

56. Elia G, Dye TD, Scariati PD. Body mass index and urinary symptoms in women. Int Urogynecol J 2001; 12: 366–9.

57. Richter HE, Creasman JM, Myers DL, et al. Urodynamic characterization of obese women with urinary incontinence undergoing weight loss program: the Program to Reduce Incontinence by Diet and Exercise (PRIDE) trial. Int Urogynecol J 2008; 19: 1653–8.

58. Burgio KL, Richter HE, Clements RH, et al. Changes in urinary and fecal incontinence symptoms with weight loss surgery in morbidly obese women. Obstet Gynecol 2007; 110: 1034–40.

59. Diokno AC, Burgio K, Fultz NH, et al. Medical and self-care practices reported by women with urinary incontinence. Am J Manag Care 2004; 10: 69–78.

60. Brown JS, Waetjen LE, Subak LL, et al. Pelvic organ prolapse surgery in the United States, 1997. Am J Obstet Gynecol 2002; 186: 712–16.

61. Leach GE, Dmochowski RR, Appell RA, et al. Female stress urinary incontinence clinical guidelines panel summary report on surgical management of female stress urinary incontinence. J Urol 1997; 158: 875–80.

62. Diokno AC, Burgio K, Fultz NH, et al. Prevalence and outcomes of continence surgery in community dwelling women. J Urol 2003; 170: 507–11.

63. Hendrix SL, Clark A, Nygaard I, et al. Pelvic organ prolapse in the Women's Health Initiative: gravity and gravidity. Am J Obstet Gynecol 2002; 186: 1160–6.

64. Hu TW, Wagner TH, Bentkover JD, et al. Costs of urinary incontinence and over active bladder in the United States: a comparative study. Urology 2004; 63: 461–5.

3 Epidemiology: South America
Paulo Palma, Miriam Dambros, and Fabio Lorenzetti

INTRODUCTION

Worldwide, urinary incontinence (UI) is a common problem which affects 17% to 45% of adult women. The high cost in terms of personal well-being (1) and financial expenditure for both individuals and society (2) makes this syndrome a major public health concern. The most prevalent type is stress incontinence, being responsible for 48% of all cases. After stress incontinence, urge incontinence is the second most prevalent cause of incontinence (17%) (3). Mainly due to shame, taboo, and unawareness of treatment possibilities, only a minority of women suffering from incontinence seek professional help. In daily practice, patients usually seek help only when urine loss leads to significant mental, physical, and social problems, as well as discomfort, often after many years of suffering. The prevalence of UI is the probability of being incontinent within a defined population at a defined point in time, estimated as the proportion of incontinent respondents identified in a cross-sectional survey (4). The WHO defines health not only as the absence of disease, but also a "state of physical, emotional, and social well being" (5). According to the previous International Continence Society definition, UI causes hygienic and social problems (6), and results in quality of life (QoL) impairment, depression, and sexual problems (7). UI has a significant impact on the QoL of 20% of women (8). Epidemiologic studies dealing with UI are sparse and methodologies varied. In South America very little research has been done on this subject, and, as a consequence, there is conflicting information, especially in respect to South American prevalence rates.

ETIOLOGIC FACTORS

It is generally believed that the main etiologic factor leading to UI is one or more vaginal deliveries, with an increase in risk with greater parity (9). Possible etiologies for UI include distension or disruption of the muscles, ligaments, and nerves responsible for bladder control that occurs during vaginal delivery (10). Other authors, however, have found that the occurrence of UI during pregnancy in nulliparous women has a stronger association with persistent incontinence after delivery than with parity (11). This would suggest a more significant effect from pregnancy itself than the process of vaginal delivery. Women who are not exposed to vaginal childbirth by having all their babies by caesarean section (CS) offer the opportunity to check the relative relevance of pregnancy itself, as compared with vaginal delivery, as a risk factor for UI.

Tamanini et al. evaluated women to identify prevalence, associated factors, and risk factors for UI as well as impact on QoL in women seeking for cancer prevention screening. They performed a cross sectional analysis of 646 women who sought cancer prevention screening in an Oncologic Hospital in October 2005 and assessed the prevalence, severity, and impact of UI on QoL by means of International Consultation on Incontinence Questionnaire-Short Form (ICIQ-SF) (12). The mean age was 37.7 years (ranging from 12 to 79) and the general UI prevalence rate reached was 34.8%. The ICIQ-SF final score from the whole population sample was 3.1 (ranging from 0 to 21) increasing to 8.9 in the incontinent group. Age, literacy, diabetes, and hypertension were associated with UI and were identified as risk factors along with frequency of pregnancies (Table 3.1). Family wages per month (<4), neurological diseases, parity, and mode of delivery (vaginal delivery or CS) were not considered risk factors in this study. Elderly women (older than 60 years) had three times the odds of UI compared to those younger than 40 years. Women with hypertension had 1.7 the odds of UI compared to those with no hypertension. UI was highly prevalent among this sample of population in our area. Furthermore, UI caused moderate impairment on QoL (Table 3.2) of women who sought cancer screening. UI should be considered a major public health problem in the studied area. Risk factors identified were age, literacy, diabetes, hypertension, and frequency of pregnancy. Overall, elderly women with hypertension are at a high risk of UI (13).

Latin America has one of the highest rates of CS in the world, with a tendency towards a further increase. Recent estimates indicate that the incidence varies between 16.8% and 40% in most Latin American countries (14), and that this rate is higher in private hospitals than in public hospitals. In addition, the incidence of CS is greater in those Latin American countries with a higher per capita gross domestic product. Although strategies to reduce CS rates have been proposed, very few have been assessed through randomized controlled trials.

URINARY INCONTINENCE, QOL, AND SEXUAL FUNCTION

Recently, many studies have measured the QoL in incontinent patients, using a number of different self administered condition-specific and generic QoL questionnaires. The impact of UI on patients' lives does not appear to be directly related to the volume of urine loss, although it does appear to be related to the overall burden of symptoms (15).

An open prospective study was carried out at our institution, enrolling patients with UI. The aim was to look at the relationship of UI and QoL issues, particularly with respect to altered sexual function. The study population consisted of 30 women aged between 31 and 51 years (mean 43 years). The duration of symptoms ranged from 12 to 53 months. All the patients were multiparous and 60% of women had incomplete elementary education. Two sexual function questionnaires were completed by respondents. The Female Sexual

Table 3.1 Demographic Data on Continent Patients (ICIQ-SF Final Score = 0) as well as Incontinent Patients (3 ≥ ICIQ-SF Final Score ≤ 21) (n = 646)

	Yes		No		
	n	%	n	%	p-Value[a]
Age (years)					
12–40	122	18.9	268	41.6	**0.0002**
41–60	78	12.1	137	21.3	
>60	25	3.9	14	2.2	
Salary per family					
1 a 2 ?	87	13.5	139	21.5	0.3535
3 a 4 ?	90	13.9	186	28.8	
>4 ?	48	7.5	96	14.8	
Diabetes mellitus					
No	213	34	413	66	**0.0164**
Yes	12	60	8	40	
Hypertension					
No	177	32.2	373	67.8	**0.0003**
Yes	48	50.5	47	49.5	
Neurological disease					
No	219	34.9	409	65.1	0.8925
Yes					

Column group header: Urinary incontinence

Abbreviation: ICIQ-SF, International Consultation on Incontinence Questionnaire-Short Form.

Table 3.2 The Impact of QoL on Urinary Incontinence Using the ICIQ-SF Final Score (n = 225)

Impact of QoL	Score	n	%
None	0	45	20
Slight	1–3	75	33.3
Moderate	4–6	45	20
Severe	7–9	20	8.9
Very severe	10	40	17.8

Abbreviations: QoL, quality of life; ICIQ-SF, International Consultation on Incontinence Questionnaire-Short Form.

Table 3.3 Most Frequent Problems Identified in Urinary Incontinence

Problem	Frequency (%)
Bad smell and use of tampon	13 (43)
Involuntary loss and wetness	12 (40)
Surgery indication	2 (07)
Stress incontinence	1 (03)
Urinary frequency	1 (03)
Urine loss in the presence of the husband	1 (03)

Function Index identifies problems related to sexual response and possible dysfunctions, as well as issues related to libido, excitement, lubrication, orgasm, pleasure, and pain. The Impact of UI on the Sexual Response/RJ questionnaire (16,17) identifies the effects of UI on sexual function, social problems, and self-esteem. It also evaluates adaptive changes to cope with urinary symptoms, and sexual behavior before and after the onset of UI.

Of the 30 women participating in the study, 26 (86%) were married and all had only one partner; 19 (63%) were Catholic, and 18 (60%) had incomplete elementary education. Concerning the effects of UI on daily life (Table 3.3), the major problems identified were the bad smell caused by urinary leakage, the need to use pads for 13 patients (43%), and the involuntary loss and wetness for 12 (40%). In addition to the results in Table 3.3, the study also showed that there were significant effects of UI on self-esteem; 11 patients (37%) having the feeling of being less valued, with 17 (57%) women having a worsening of their sexual lives as a result of their urinary symptoms. Twenty-three patients (76%) related that they had urinary loss during sexual intercourse. Among these, 17 (74%) claimed it had a negative influence on their sexual life. Of the 23 patients, 6 (26%) did not complain, 2 (9%) considered it a mild interference, four (17%) evaluated it as moderate, and 11 (48%) indicated it as a severe interference. Regarding the frequency of sexual intercourse before and after the onset of incontinence, 17 patients (57%) expressed altering patterns. Sexual activity changed from weekly to monthly in seven patients (41%), from daily to weekly in five (29%), from daily to monthly in three (18%), from monthly to annual in one (6%), and from weekly to no relationship in one (6%). Differences in sexual function before and after the onset of incontinence were established. Ten variables related to sexuality were studied: desire, excitement, vaginal lubrication, foreplay, masturbation, oral sex in the partner and in the patient, vaginal penetration, anal penetration, and orgasm. Six variables were significantly different following the onset of urinary leakage, with a worsening of sexual desire, masturbation and foreplay, vaginal penetration, anal penetration, and orgasm. Abdo et al. studied the sexual lives of 1502 healthy Brazilian women and concluded that in 34.6% the greatest complaint was a lack of desire and in 29.3% was orgasmic dysfunction (18). These results demonstrated a reasonable degree of sexual dysfunction amongst the general Brazilian population although this appears to be greater in the presence of UI.

Prevalence of Climacteric, Urogenital, and Sexual Symptoms in a Population of Brazilian Women

A cross-sectional, descriptive, population-based study (19) was also carried out at the State University of Campinas on 456 women aged 45 to 60 years, living in Campinas, SP, Brazil, in 1997. Data were collected via home interviews, using structured validated questionnaires. The results showed that climacteric symptoms in the population were highly prevalent and similar to those described in developed Western countries. Figure 3.1 shows the most prevalent symptoms identified. Hot flushes, sweating, and insomnia as expected were significantly more prevalent in peri- and post-menopausal women. The severity of vasomotor and psychological symptoms did not vary according to the menopause phase. Decreased libido was the most frequent sexual complaint. It was also observed that some climacteric complaints were interrelated.

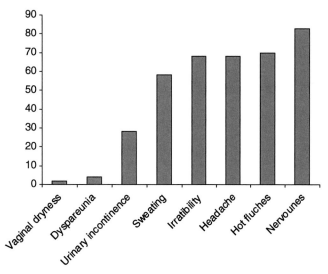

Figure 3.1 The most climacteric and urogenital prevalent symptoms found in the study of Pedro et al. (19).

Table 3.4 Background Data for All Patients Assessed by Guarisi et al. (20)

	Stress urinary incontinence				
	Most times or sometimes (n = 160)		Never (n = 295)		Prevalence ratio
	n	%	n	%	
Age (years)					
45–49	69	40.4	102	59.6	Reference
50–54	50	34.7	94	65.3	0.8
55–60	41	29.3	99	70.7	0.7
Race					
Caucasian	96	37.4	161	62.6	Reference
Black, brown	46	36.8	79	63.2	1.0
Others	18	24.7	55	75.3	0.6
Literacy					
Literate	28	38.9	44	61.1	Reference
Incomplete elementary school	81	33.3	162	66.7	0.9
Complete elementary school	32	39.5	49	60.5	1.0
High school, college	19	32.2	40	67.8	0.8

Source: Data adapted from Ref. 20.

Prevalence of Stress UI (SUI) and its Associated Factors in Perimenopausal Women

A descriptive, exploratory, population-based study with secondary analysis of a population-based household survey on the perimenopause and menopause was conducted among women living in a Brazilian city (20). Through a sampling process, 456 women between 45 and 60 years old were selected. Thirty-five percent of the interviewees complained of SUI although none of the sociodemographic factors studied was associated with the risk of SUI (Table 3.4).

In addition, parity did not significantly alter SUI risk. Other factors, such as previous gynecologic surgery, body mass index, smoking habits, menopausal status, and hormone replacement therapy, were not associated with the prevalence of SUI and there were no racial variations. In the international literature, most prevalence studies are conducted amongst Caucasian women and only few studies have assessed racial differences in the prevalence of UI. In the few studies which have included other racial groups, a significantly larger percentage of Caucasian women appear to report UI compared to African-American or Hispanic women (21). Urodynamic diagnosis showed that SUI was more frequent in Caucasian women compared to African-Americans. However, more research with regard to racial differences in the prevalence of UI is necessary to make significant conclusions regarding inter-racial differences in incontinence.

URINARY INCONTINENCE AMONG ELDERLY PEOPLE IN THE MUNICIPALITY OF SÃO PAULO, BRAZIL

Over the period from 1980 to 2025, the population aged 60 years and over in Latin America and the Caribbean is expected to at least double in size and, in more than half of these countries, to triple in size, before reaching the year 2025 (22). This rapid and accentuated aging of the population will have a significant impact on social, economic, and health demands. Prominent among the health demands will be those relating to chronic diseases and their incapacitating sequelae and other complaints such as UI, which are all included among the so-called "giants of geriatrics," given their negative consequences on QoL among elderly people (23).

The Pan-American Health Organization and WHO (24) coordinated a multicenter study named Health, Well-being, and Aging (SABE study) in elderly people living (over 60 years old) in seven countries of Latin America and the Caribbean. In Brazil, the study population was carried out in São Paulo in the year 2000 and the total Brazilian sample was 2143 people. The data were collected simultaneously, by means of home interviews, using a standardized instrument consisting of 11 thematic sections: personal data, cognitive assessment, heath status, functional status, medications, use of and access to services, family and social support networks, work history and sources of income characteristics of the home, and flexibility and mobility tests (Table 3.5).

The prevalence of self reported UI was 11.8% among men and 26.2% for women. It was verified that among those reporting UI, 37% also reported stroke, 34% depression (Table 3.6). It was found that increasing dependency in the elderly was associated with increasing prevalence of UI. The associated factors found were depression [odds ratio (OR) = 2.49], female (OR = 2.42), advanced age (OR = 2.35), important functional limitation (OR = 2.01). UI is a highly prevalent symptom among the elderly population of the municipality of São Paulo, especially among women. The adoption of preventive measures can reduce the negative effects of the UI.

Table 3.5 Distribution of Elderly People According to the Presence of Urinary Incontinence, Sociodemographic Variables, Health Status, and Functional Status. Municipality of São Paulo, 2000

	60–74 years		≥ 75 years	
	Yes	No	Yes	No
Sociodemographic variables				
Age group	16.5	83.5	33.3	66.7
Sex				
Male	8.9	91.1	23.8	76.2
Female	22.2	77.8	38.6	61.7
Self-reported ethnicity				
White	15.5	84.5	33.3	66.7
Non-white	18.8	81.2	33.6	66.4
Schooling (years)				
Up to 3 years	18.2	81.8	36.2	63.8
4 years or more	15.3	84.7	28.6	71.4
Health status				
Self-reported diseases/conditions				
Diabetes mellitus	23.8	76.2	42.4	57.6
Arterial hypertension	19.9	80.1	36.2	63.8
COPD	20.7	79.3	35.8	64.2
Stroke	31.1	68.9	54.6	45.4
Depression	31.2	68.8	49.8	50.2
Self-reported health status				
Excellent/very good/good	7.1	92.9	22.5	77.5
Regular/poor	25.0	75.0	41.6	58.4
Body mass index				
Low	15.8	84.2	34.2	65.8
Normal	14.7	85.3	26.6	73.4
Overweight	11.9	88.2	36.8	63.2
Obese	24.3	75.7	43.8	56.2
Functional status				
Difficulty in				
Mobility in general	27.2	72.8	60.4	39.6
Going to the bathroom alone	45.1	54.9	73.1	26.9
Doing basic ADLs	32.7	67.3	56.5	43.5
Doing instrumental ADLs	18.4	81.6	35.7	64.3

Abbreviations: ADLs, activities of daily livings; COPD, chronic obstructive pulmonary disease.

Table 3.6 Final Model from Univariate and Multivariate Analysis for the Presence of Urinary Incontinence, According to Sociodemographic, Clinical, and Functional Characteristics of the Elderly People in the Municipality of São Paulo, Brazil, 2000

	Urinary incontinence				
				Confidence interval	
Characteristics	OR[a]	SD	p-Value	Lower limit	Upper limit
Sex					
Female	2.42	0.43	0.0000	1.70	3.43
Age					
75 years and over	2.35	0.33	0.0000	1.78	3.10
Presence of self-reported diseases/conditions					
Depression	2.49	0.43	0.0000	1.77	3.50
Stroke	1.69	0.45	0.049	1.01	2.85
Obesity	1.63	0.27	0.003	1.17	2.26
Diabetes mellitus	1.56	0.29	0.019	1.08	2.25
Functional status					
Difficulty in doing basic activities of daily living	2.01	0.35	0.0000	1.44	2.83

[a]Adjusted OR (95% confidence interval) = OR (95% confidence interval) adjusted using the logistic regression method, one by one for all variables and in the final model only for the significant variables.
Abbreviation: OR, odds ratio.

CONCLUSION

UI is a highly prevalent condition in South America, as it is in many other parts of the world. Very few studies have concentrated on South American populations alone but those that have show a significant impact of UI on the QoL of sufferers.

REFERENCES

1. Thomas TM, Plymat KR, Blannin J, Meade TW. Prevalence of urinary incontinence. Br Med J 1980; 281: 1243–5.
2. Hu TW. Impact of urinary incontinence on health-care costs. J Am Geriatric Soc 1990; 38: 292–5.
3. Norton PA, MacDonald LD, Sedgwick PM, Stanton SL. Distress and delay associated with urinary incontinence, frequency, and urgency in women. Br Med J 1988; 297: 1187–9.
4. Hunskaar S, Burgio K, Dioko AC, et al. Epidemiology and natural history of urinary incontinence. In: Abrams P, Cardozo L, Khoury S, Wein A, eds. Incontinence, 2nd ed. Plymouth: Plymbridge Distributors, 2002: 165.
5. Corcos J, Beaulieu S, Donovan J, et al. Quality of life assessment in men and women with urinary incontinence. J Urol 2002; 168: 896–905.
6. Blaivas JG, Appell RA, Fantl JA, et al. Standards of efficacy for evaluation of treatment outcomes in urinary incontinence: recommendations of the Urodynamic Society. Neurourol Urodyn 1997; 16: 145–7.
7. Hafner RJ, Stanton SL, Guy LA. A psychiatric study of women with urgency and urgency incontinence. Br J Urol 1977; 49: 211–14.
8. Burgio KL, Matthews KA, Engel BT. Prevalence, incidence and correlates of urinary incontinence in healthy middleaged women. J Urol 1991; 146: 1255–9.
9. Foldspang A, Mommsen S, Djurhuus JC. Prevalent urinary incontinence as a correlate of pregnancy, vaginal childbirth, and obstetrics techniques. Am J Public Health 1999; 89: 209–12.
10. Allen RE, Hosker GL, Smith ARB, Warrell DW. Pelvic floor damage and childbirth: a neurophysiological study. Br J Obstet Gynaecol 1990; 97: 770–9.
11. Viktrup L, Lose G, Rolff M, Barfoed K. The symptom of stress incontinence caused by pregnancy or delivery in primiparas. Obstet Gynecol 1992; 79: 945–9.
12. Tamanini JTN, Dambros M, D'Ancona CAL, Palma PCR, Netto NR Jr. Validation of the "International Consultation on Incontinence Questionnaire – Short Form for Portuguese. Rev Saúde Pública 2004; 38: 438–44.
13. Tamanini JT, Tamanini MMM, Mauad LMQ, Auler AMBAP. Urinary incontinence: prevalence and risk factors in women seeking for gynecological cancer revention screenin. BEPA 2006; 3: 34.
14. Osis MJD, Pádua KS, Duarte GA, Souza TR, Faúndes A. The opinion of Brazilian women regarding vaginal labor and cesarean section. Int J Gynecol Obstet 2001; 75: S59–66.
15. Wyman JF, Harkins SW, Choi SC, et al. Psychosocial impact of urinary incontinence in women. Obstet Gynecol 1987; 70: 378–81.
16. Rezende RCA. A Influência da Incontinência Urinária na Resposta Sexual Feminina. Rio de Janeiro: Mestrado em Sexologia da Universidade Gama Filho, M2000. Masters Degree, Brazil: University of Rio de Janeiro.
17. Palma PCR, Thiel RRC, Thiel M, et al. Impacto da incontinência urinária na qualidade de vida e sexualidade feminina. Urodinamica Uroginecologai 2003; 2: 71–6.
18. Abdo CHN, Oliveira WM Jr, Moreira ED, et al. Perfil sexual da população Brasileira: Resultados do Estudo de Com portamento Sexual (ECOS) do Brasileiro. Rev Brasileira de Medicina 2002; 59: 250–7.
19. Pedro AO, Pinto-Neto AM, Costa-Paiva LHS, Osis MJD, Hardy EE. Climacteric syndrome: a population-based study in Brazil. Rev Saúde Publica 2003; 37: 735–42.
20. Guarisi T, Pinto-Neto AM, Osis MJ, et al. Urinary incontinence among climacteric Brazilian women: household survey. Rev Saúde Publica 2001; 35: 428–35.
21. Sze EHM, Jones WP, Ferguson JL, Barker CD, Dolezal JM. Prevalence of urinary incontinence symptoms among Black, White and Hispanic women. Obstet Gynecol 2002; 99: 572–5.
22. Palloni A, Peláez M. Histórico e natureza do estudo. In: Lebrão ML, Duarte YAO, eds. O Projeto SABE no Município de São Paulo: uma abordagem inicial. Brasília: OPAS/Ministério da Saúde, 2003: 15–32.
23. Brasil. Ministério da Saúde. Secretaria de Atenção à Saúde. Departamento de Atenção Básica. Envelhecimento e saúde da pessoa idosa/Ministério da Saúde, Secretaria de Atenção à Saúde, Departamento de Atenção Básica – Brasília: Ministério da Saúde. 2006; 192 (Série A. Normas e Manuais Técnicos) (Cadernos de Atenção Básica, n. 19).
24. Tamanini JTN, Lebrão ML, Duarte YAO, Santos JLF, Laurenti R. Analysis of the prevalence of and factors associated with urinary incontinence among elderly people in the municipality of São Paulo – Study (Health, Well, Being and Aging- Sabe). In press.

4   Epidemiology: Europe
Ian Milsom

INTRODUCTION

Urinary incontinence (UI), overactive bladder (OAB), and other lower urinary tract symptoms (LUTS) are highly prevalent conditions with a profound influence on well-being and quality of life as well as being of immense economic importance for the health service (1–3). Millions of women throughout the world are afflicted (2) and there has been a growing interest in these symptoms in recent years as a consequence of the increased awareness of the human and social implications for the individual sufferer. Population studies have demonstrated that UI is more common in women than men and that approximately 10% of all women suffer from UI (2). Prevalence figures increase with increasing age and in women aged ≥70 years more than 20% of the female population are affected. Inappropriate leakage of urine is perceived by many women but is not always reported to the doctor. However, an increasing awareness of the problem has in recent years attracted more patients to seek advice. In elderly women UI may lead to possible rejection on the part of a relative and may be an important factor in the decision whether or not to institutionalize an elderly person. UI and other LUTS not only causes considerable personal suffering for the individual afflicted but are also of immense economic importance for the health service (3). The annual cost of UI in Sweden, for example, has been reported to account for approximately 2% of the total healthcare budget (1).

URINARY INCONTINENCE

This chapter describes the results of epidemiologic studies performed in Europe. The reported prevalence of UI among women varies widely in different studies due to the use of different definitions, the heterogenicity of different study populations and population sampling procedures. In addition, different definitions of UI have been applied. UI has been defined by the International Continence Society as any involuntary leakage of urine (4). However, some authors have chosen to restrict prevalence figures according to the frequency of involuntary urinary leakage—for example, based only on daily, weekly, monthly, or annual urinary leakage. Thus, for the reasons given above, it is difficult to compare the results of different population studies. However, when reviewing the literature, there is considerable evidence to support the theory that the prevalence of UI in women increases with age, but there are divergent opinions regarding the pattern of this increase (5–34). In a review (2) of population studies from numerous countries the prevalence of UI ranged from approximately 5% to 70%, with most studies reporting a prevalence of any UI in the range of 25% to 45%. For daily incontinence, prevalence estimates typically range between 5% and 15% for middle-aged and older women.

Thomas et al. (5) investigated the prevalence of UI in two London boroughs by a postal survey (Fig. 4.1A). The reported prevalence of UI increased from 5.1% in girls aged 5 to 14 years to 16.2% in 85-year-old women. There was, however, little or no change in prevalence rates up to 35 years of age. The prevalence rates then increased to approximately 10% in the 35 to 44 years age group. There was no significant increase at the time of the menopause but a further increase to approximately 16% occurred in women ≥75 years. On the other hand, Iosif et al. (6) and Jolleys (13) (Fig. 4.1B) reported a maximum prevalence of UI at the time of the menopause. Hannestad et al. (26), in a large Norwegian study, demonstrated an increased prevalence during the perimenopausal years, with prevalence rates being lower both before and after the time of the menopause (Fig. 4.2A).

Conditions in Sweden are extremely favorable for epidemiologic studies, in particular longitudinal studies. The Swedish Population Register, with its personal number system, provides up-to-date information on the total population and can be used to obtain random and, in some cases, representative subgroups of the total population for the purpose of epidemiologic studies. There are several large population-based studies from Sweden describing the prevalence of UI in women. Figure 4.3A illustrates the results from two independent studies of UI in women. In both studies, prevalence was restricted to women who had urinary leakage at least once per week. Although the study performed by Samuelsson and co-workers (24) was undertaken in a rural area and that by Simeonova et al. (26) was carried out in an inner city, there are strong similarities between the results of the two studies, with a linear increase in the prevalence of UI which continues over the perimenopausal years.

In contrast, another Swedish population study (22) (Fig. 4.3B) failed to demonstrate any increase in the prevalence of UI between women aged 46 and 56 years of age (prevalence 12% for both cohorts). The majority of 46-year-old women were premenopausal whereas the majority of 56-year-old women were postmenopausal. There were no differences in prevalence rates between pre- and postmenopausal women within the respective birth cohorts (Fig. 4.4A). Thus there was no evidence to suggest that the prevalence of UI increased at the time of the last menstrual period. However, this is not necessarily synonymous with the fact that the reduction in circulating estrogens is not associated with an increase in the prevalence of UI in women after the menopause.

The prevalence of UI in women has been compared with the prevalence in men of the same age in two large Swedish studies (Fig. 4.3B) (22,34). As can be seen from the results illustrated in Figure 4.3b, there is a higher prevalence of UI in women than in men in all the age groups studied. In general, the

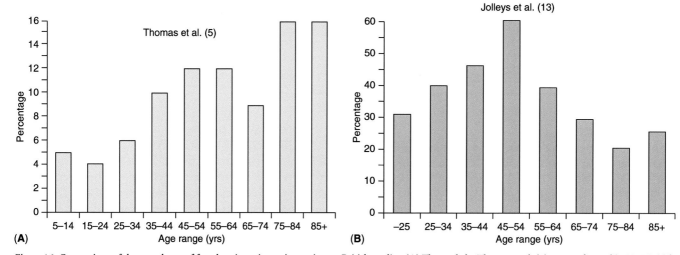

Figure 4.1 Comparison of the prevalence of female urinary incontinence in two British studies. (**A**) The study by Thomas et al. (5) was performed in 9323 British women and (**B**)the study by Jolleys et al. (13) was performed in 833 British women.

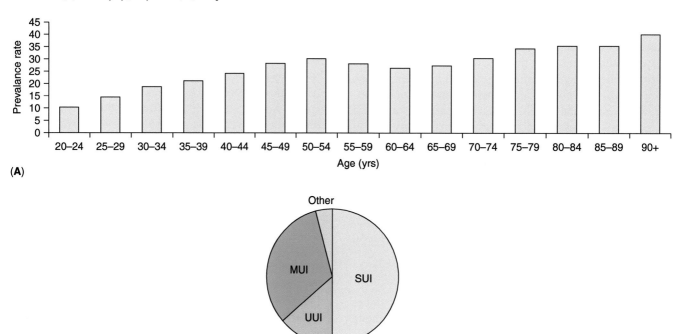

Figure 4.2 Prevalence of urinary incontinence in Norwegian women grouped (**A**) by age, and (**B**) type of incontinence. *Abbreviations*: MUI, mixed urinary incontinence; SUI, stress urinary incontinence; UUI, urge urinary incontinence. *Source*: Based on data from Ref. 26.

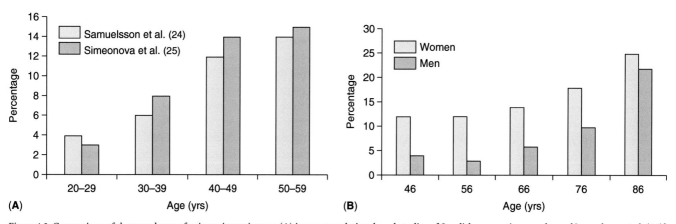

Figure 4.3 Comparison of the prevalence of urinary incontinence: (**A**) in two population-based studies of Swedish women in a rural area [Samuelsson et al. (24)] and in an inner city [Simeonova et al. (25)]; (**B**) in two population-based Swedish studies in women (n = 7459) (22) and men (n = 7763) (48) of the same ages.

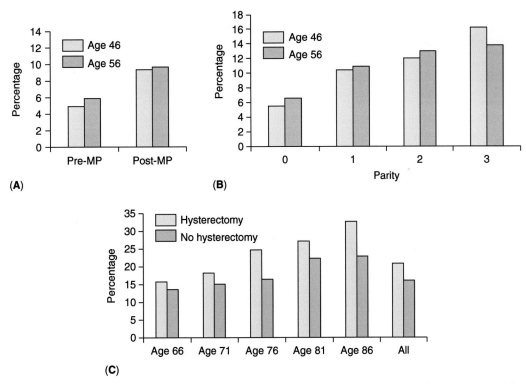

Figure 4.4 Prevalence of urinary incontinence: (**A**) in a random sample of 46- and 56-year-old women grouped according to menopausal (MP) status; (**B**) in a random sample of 46- (n = 1530) and 56-year-old (n = 1638) women grouped according to parity; (**C**) in a random sample of 66-, 71-, 76-, 81-, and 86-year-old women grouped according to history of hysterectomy. *Source*: Data from Ref. 22.

prevalence of UI is approximately three times more common in women than in men.

The majority of the population studies referred to in this chapter have been performed by means of postal questionnaires. In several of the studies, attempts have been made to determine the proportion of women suffering from the different types of urinary leakage, i.e., stress urinary leakage (SUI), urge urinary leakage (UUI), and mixed urinary leakage (MUI). The distribution of the various types of incontinence in the large Norwegian study by Hannestad et al. (26) is shown in Figure 4.2B. In the literature, SUI tends to dominate among younger women while the number of women with urge incontinence and mixed incontinence increases with age.

More recent studies (26,29–34) have added important information on prevalence of incontinence in women younger than 30 and older than 80 years of age, particularly for prevalence of incontinence by type. These studies are consistent with previous studies reporting that older women are more likely to have mixed and urge incontinence while young and middle-aged women generally report stress incontinence. Overall, approximately half of all incontinent women are classified as stress incontinent. A smaller proportion are classified as mixed incontinent and the smallest fraction as urge incontinent. A recent study which included the entire adult age range by Hannested et al. (26) demonstrated a fairly regular increase in prevalence of mixed incontinence across the age range, and a decrease in prevalence of stress incontinence from the 40- to 49-year-old age group through the 60- to 69-year-old group. There is no hard evidence for different prevalences of UI among Western countries. However, comparing prevalence between countries based on separate studies is difficult due to differences in methods and definitions, as well as language, cultural, and social differences. One of the few studies to estimate the prevalence of UI in more than one country found similar prevalences of any UI (41–44%) in three of the four countries examined (France, Germany, and U.K.) but a lower prevalence (23%) in the fourth country (Spain) (27). There was no apparent reason for the lower prevalence in Spain.

UI is, however, not static but dynamic and many factors may contribute to incidence, progression, or remission. There are a few studies describing progression as well as remission, in the short term, of UI in the general population as well as in selected groups of the population. The mean annual incidence of UI seems to range from 1% to 9% while estimates of remission are vary more, 4% to 30% (34–36).

Wennberg et al. (34) studied the prevalence of UI in the same women (aged ≥20 years) over time in order to assess possible progression or regression. A self administered postal questionnaire with questions regarding UI, OAB, and other LUTS was sent to a random sample of the total population of women in 1991. The same women who responded to the questionnaire in 1991 and who were still alive and available in the population register 16 years later were re-assessed using a similar self-administered postal questionnaire. The overall prevalence of UI, increased from 15% to 28% (p < 0.001) from 1991 to 2007 and the incidence rate of UI was 21% while the corresponding remission rate was 34% (Fig. 4.5).

Thus, in summary, when reviewing the literature, there is considerable evidence to support the theory that the prevalence of UI increases in a linear fashion with age as shown

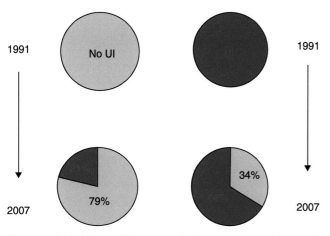

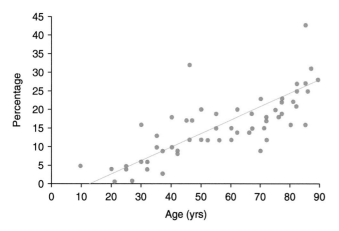

Figure 4.5 The incidence and regression of urinary incontinence (UI) in the same women assessed in 1991 and 2007. *Source*: From Ref. 34.

Figure 4.6 Prevalence of female urinary incontinence (≥1/week) which affected the woman's way of life (summary of 19 population studies, based on Ref. 49).

Table 4.1 Risk Factors for Urinary Incontinence in Women

- Age
- Sex
- Smoking
- Chronic bronchitis, asthma
- Ethnic group
- Obesity
- Pregnancy
- Vaginal delivery
- Collagen defect
- Hysterectomy
- Dementia
- Stroke, Parkinson's disease, etc.
- Physical activity
- Medication
- Constipation
- Diuretics
- Enuresis
- Chronic illness

in Figure 4.6 which includes pooled data from 19 epidemiologic studies where UI was reported to occur at least once per week.

FACTORS INFLUENCING THE PREVALENCE OF UI

Risk factors described in the literature are shown in Table 4.1 (29–31,36,37). For the majority of these risk factors there are at present no controlled trials demonstrating that intervention reduces the incidence, prevalence, or degree of severity of UI.

The influence of various factors on the prevalence of UI was evaluated by means of a postal questionnaire in women aged 46 to 86 years resident in the city of Gothenburg, Sweden (22). Age, parity, and a history of hysterectomy were all correlated to the prevalence of UI which increased in a linear fashion from 12.1% in women 46 years of age to 24.6% in women aged 86 years of age (Fig. 4.3B). The prevalence of UI was greater in parous women compared to nulliparous women, and prevalence increased with increasing parity (Fig. 4.4B). UI was more prevalent in women who had undergone a hysterectomy (Fig. 4.4C). The prevalence of UI was unaffected by the duration of previous oral contraceptive usage and there was no evidence to suggest that the prevalence of UI increased at the time of the last menstrual period.

Several studies suggest that the risk of UI "runs in the family" (28,37,38). Family history studies have found a two to three fold greater prevalence of stress UI among first degree relatives of women with stress UI compared to first degree relatives of continent women. In the Norwegian Nord-Trøndelag health survey (EPINCONT), daughters of mothers with UI had an increased risk of stress incontinence, mixed incontinence, and urgency incontinence (28). In general the risk was somewhat higher for sisters of a woman with UI than for daughters.

A study from the Swedish twin register indicated that heritability contributes to the liability of developing surgically managed pelvic organ prolapse and stress UI. The authors presented evidence that for both disorders genetic and non-shared environmental factors equally contributed 40% of the variation in liability (38). Although study methodology and the magnitude of the risk estimates vary, studies on familial transmission of incontinence are in agreement (28,37): Having a first degree female family member with stress UI increases the risk for an individual becoming afflicted by the same disorder.

OAB and Other LUTS

In recent years, several epidemiological studies have also been conducted in order to better understand the prevalence and the impact of OAB and other LUTS. OAB is defined as the presence of urgency and frequency (either daytime or nighttime), with or without UI (4). OAB is often divided into OAB without UI (OAB$_{dry}$) and those with OAB and UI (OAB$_{wet}$). The reported prevalence of OAB in females varied between 7.7% to 31.3% and, in general, prevalence rates increased with age (39–42). OAB has been shown to be associated with other chronic debilitating illnesses such as depression, constipation and diabetes as well as neurological illnesses. OAB is commonly associated with other LUTS which was well illustrated by the cluster analysis performed by Coyne et al. (43).

The prevalence of OAB symptoms was estimated in a large European study involving more than 16,000 individuals

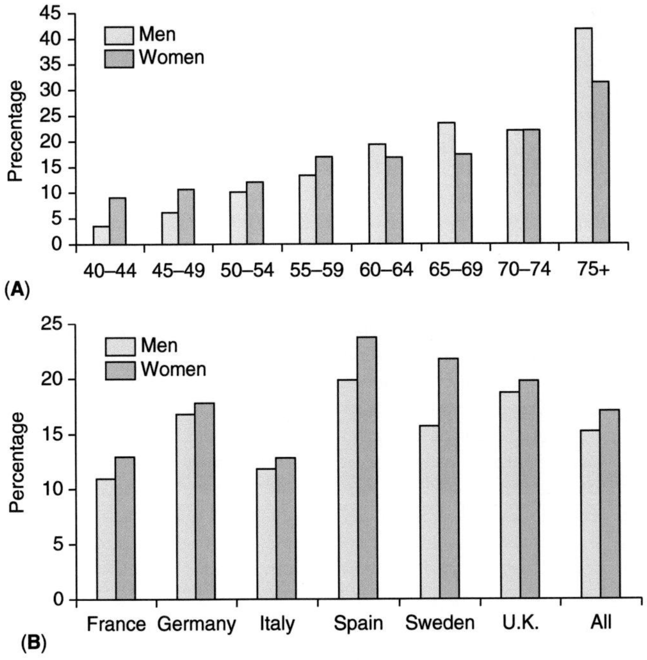

Figure 4.7 Prevalence of overactive bladder symptoms: (**A**) grouped according to age and sex; (**B**) in a random sample of the total population aged ≥40 years from six European countries. *Source*: Adapted from Ref. 39.

		2007			
		No OAB	OAB dry	OAB wet	Total (%)
1991	NO OAB	634	64	93	791 (83%)
	OAB dry	52	24	29	105 (11%)
	OAB wet	14	11	28	53 (6%)
	Total (%)	700 (74%)	99 (10%)	150 (16%)	949 (100%)

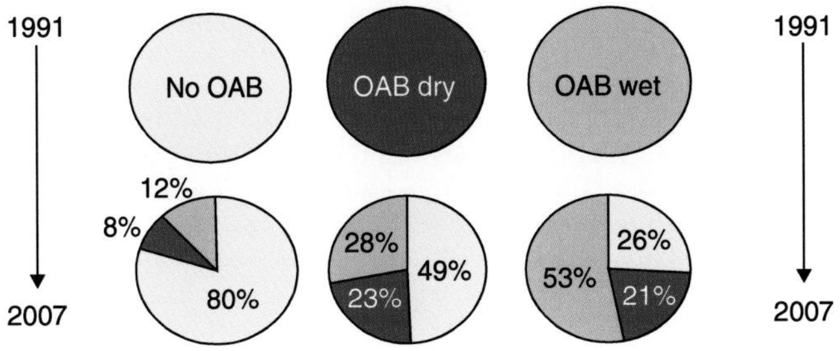

Figure 4.8 The percentage distribution of overactive bladder (OAB) symptoms in the same women assessed in 1991 and 2007. *Source*: From Ref. 34.

(39). Data were collected using a population-based survey (conducted by telephone or face-to-face interview) of men and women aged >40 years, selected from the general population in France, Germany, Italy, Spain, Sweden, and the United Kingdom using a random, stratified approach. The main outcome measures were: prevalence of urinary frequency (>8 micturitions/24 hours), urgency and urge incontinence; proportion of participants who had sought medical advice for OAB symptoms; and current or previous therapy received for these symptoms. The main results of this study are illustrated in Figure 4.7A with the prevalence of OAB symptoms grouped according to age and sex, and in Figure 4.7B grouped according to sex and nationality.

The progression or regression of OAB and other LUTS was studied by Wennberg et al. (34) in the same women (aged ≥20 years) followed over a period of 16 years (from 1991 to 2007). The overall prevalence of OAB, nocturia and daytime micturition frequency of eight or more times per day increased by 9%, 20% ($p < 0.001$), and 3% ($p < 0.05$) respectively from 1991 to 2007. The incidence of OAB was 20 % and the corresponding remission rate 43%. Women with OAB symptoms were classified as OAB dry or wet depending on the presence or absence of concomitant UI. The prevalence of OAB dry did not differ between the two assessment occasions (11% and 10% respectively), but the prevalence of OAB wet increased from 6% to 16% ($p < 0.001$). Among women with No OAB in 1991 the prevalence in 2007 were 8% and 12% for OAB dry and wet, respectively. There was a progression from OAB dry to wet in 28%. Remission from OAB dry or wet to No OAB occurred in 50% and 26% respectively (Fig. 4.8).

SOCIOECONOMIC CONSIDERATIONS

The economic consequences of UI and other LUTS have recently been reviewed (3) and there are now numerous reports to support the statement that UI and LUTS have a huge bearing on health care costs (1,3,44–47). The economic consequences of UI in Sweden in 1990 were assessed by Milsom et al. (1,49). The estimated annual cost for UI in Sweden at that time was 1.8 billion Swedish Crowns. The Swedish Health Care budget for 1990 amounted to 93 billion Crowns. Based on the results of this evaluation, the annual costs of UI in Sweden accounted for approximately 2% of the total healthcare costs.

The mean life expectancy of women in Sweden is at present 83 years, which is higher than in many other Western countries, and 19% of all persons are at present >65 years of age. The proportion of elderly women in many Western countries is currently increasing, and it is estimated that in many European countries there will be a substantial increase in the number of women aged >65 years by the year 2025 (50). Thus, the number of women requiring treatment for UI is expected to increase in the future.

Another important factor to consider, apart from the numerical increase in the number of elderly women, is the fact that many elderly women of today suffer in silence, accepting these symptoms as a normal part of the aging process. Women who are at present 30 and 40 years of age have other demands on their physical condition and will undoubtedly not accept what their older counterparts accepted later in life.

REFERENCES

1. Ekelund P, Grimby A, Milsom I. Urinary incontinence: social and financial costs high. Br Med J 1993; 306: 1344.
2. Milsom I, Altman D, Herbison P, et al. Epidemiology of urinary (UI) and faecal (FI) incontinence and pelvic organ prolapse (POP). In: Abrams P, Cardozo L, Kouhry S, Wein A, eds. Incontinence. Paris: Health Publications Ltd, 2009; 37–111.
3. Moore K, Wei Hu T, Subak L, Wagner T, Deutekom M. Economics of urinary and faecal incontinence, and prolpse. In: Abrams P, Cardozo L, Kouhry S, Wein A, eds. Incontinence. Paris: Health Publications Ltd, 2009; 1685–1712.
4. Abrams P, Cardozo L, Fall M, et al. Standardisation Sub-committee of the International Continence Society. The standardisation of terminology of lower urinary tract function: report from the Standardisation Subcommittee of the International Continence Society. Neurourol Urodyn 2002; 21: 167–78.

5. Thomas TM, Plymat KR, Blannin J, et al. Prevalence of urinary incontinence. Br Med J 1980; 281: 1243–5.

6. Iosif S, Henriksson L, Ulmsten U. The frequency of disorders of the lower urinary tract, urinary incontinence in particular, as evaluated by a questionnaire survey in a gynecological health control population. Acta Obstet Gynecol Scand 1981; 60: 71–6.

7. Vetter NJ, Jones DA, Victor CR. Urinary incontinence in the elderly at home. Lancet 1981; ii; 1275–7.

8. Iosif C, Bekassy Z. Prevalence of genito-urinary symptoms in the late menopause. Acta Obstet Gynecol Scand 1984; 63: 257–60.

9. Campbell AJ, Reinken J, McCosh L. Incontinence in the elderly: prevalence and prognosis. Age Ageing 1985; 14: 65–70.

10. Samsioe G, Jansson I, Mellström D, et al. The occurrence, nature and treatment of urinary incontinence in a 70 year old population. Maturitas 1985; 7: 335–42.

11. Vehkalahti I, Kivelä S-L. Urinary incontinence and its correlates in very old age. Gerontology 1985; 31: 391–6.

12. Berg G, Gottqall T, Hammar M, et al. Climacteric symptoms among women aged 60–62 in Linkö ping, Sweden, in 1986. Maturitas 1988; 10: 193–9.

13. Jolleys J. Reported prevalence of urinary incontinence in women in a general practice. Br Med J 1988; 296: 1300–2.

14. Elving LB, Foldspang A, Lam GW, et al. Descriptive epidemiology of urinary incontinence in 3,100 women aged 30–59. Scand J Urol Nephrol 1989; (Suppl 125): 37–43.

15. Hellström L, Ekelund P, Milsom I, et al. The prevalence of urinary incontinence and incontinence aids in 85-year-old men and women. Age Ageing 1990; 19: 383–9.

16. Molander U, Milsom I, Ekelund P, et al. An epidemiological study of urinary incontinence and related urogenital symptoms in elderly women. Maturitas 1990; 12: 51–60.

17. O'Brien J, Austin M, Parminder S, et al. Urinary incontinence: prevalence, need for treatment, and effectiveness of intervention by nurse. Br Med J 1991; 303: 1308–12.

18. Mäkinen JI, Grönroos M, Kiilholma PJA, et al. The prevalence of urinary incontinence in a randomized population of 5247 adult Finnish women. Int Urogynecol J 1992; 3: 110–13.

19. Rekers H, Drogendijk AC, Valenburg H, et al. Urinary incontinence in women 35 to 79 years of age: prevalence and consequences. Eur J Obstet Gynaecol Reprod Biol 1992; 43: 229–34.

20. Brocklehurst JC. Urinary incontinence in the community: analysis of a MORI poll. Br Med J 1993; 306: 832–4.

21. Lagace EA, Hansen W, Hickner LM. Prevalence and severity of urinary incontinence in ambulatory adults: an UPRNet study. J Fam Pract 1993; 36: 610–14.

22. Milsom I, Ekelund P, Molander U, et al. The influence of age, parity, oral contraception, hysterectomy and the menopause on the prevalence of urinary incontinence in women. J Urol 1993; 149: 1459–62.

23. Seim A, Sandvik H, Hermstad R, et al. Female urinary incontinence – consultation, behaviour and patient experiences: an epidemiological survey in a Norwegian community. Fam Pract 1995; 12: 18–21.

24. Samuelsson E, Victor A, Tibblin G. A population study of urinary incontinence and nocturia among women 20–59 years. Prevalence, well-being and wish for treatment. Acta Obstet Gynecol Scand 1997; 76: 74–80.

25. Simeonova Z, Milsom I, Kullendorff M, et al. The prevalence of urinary incontinence and its influence on the quality of life in women from an urban Swedish population. Acta Obstet Gynecol Scand 1999; 78: 546–51.

26. Hannestad YS, Rortveit G, Sandvik H, et al. A community-based epidemiological survey of female urinary incontinence: the Norwegian EPINCONT study. J Clin Epidemiol 2000; 53: 1150–7.

27. Hunskaar S, Lose G, Sykes D, et al. The prevalence of urinary incontinence in women in four European countries. BJU Int 2004; 93: 324–30.

28. Hannestad YS, Lie RT, Rortveit G, et al. Familial risk of urinary incontinence in women: population based cross sectional study. BMJ 2004; 329: 889–91.

29. Hunskaar S, Burgio K, Diokno A, et al. Epidemiology and natural history of urinary incontinence in women. Urology 2003; 62(4 Suppl 1): 16–23.

30. Papanicolaou S, Hunskaar S, Lose G, Sykes D. Assessment of bothersomeness and impact on quality of life of urinary incontinence in women in France, Germany, Spain and the UK. BJU Int 2005; 96: 831–8.

31. Irwin DE, Milsom I, Kopp Z, Abrams P, Cardozo L. Impact of overactive bladder symptoms on employment, social interactions and emotional well-being in six European countries. BJU Int 2006; 97: 96–100.

32. Heidler S, Deveza C, Temml C, et al. The natural history of lower urinary tract symptoms in females: analysis of a health screening project. Eur Urol 2007; 52: 1744–50.

33. Coyne K, Sexton C, Irwin DE, et al. The impact of overactive bladder, incontinence and other lower urinary tract symptoms on quality of life, work productivity, sexuality and emotional well-being in men and women: results from the EPIC study. BJU Int 2008; 101: 1388–95.

34. Wennberg A, Molander U, Fall M, et al. A longitudinal population-based survey of urinary incontinence, overactive bladder, and other lower urinary tract symptoms in women. Eur Urol 2009; 55: 783–91.

35. Hagglund D, Walker-Engstrom ML, Larsson G, Leppert J. Changes in urinary incontinence and quality of life after four years. A population-based study of women aged 22–50 years. Scand JPrim Health Care 2004; 22: 112–17.

36. Samuelsson EC, Victor FT, Svardsudd KF. Five-year incidence and remission rates of female urinary incontinence in a Swedish population less than 65 years old. Am J Obstet Gynecol 2000; 183: 568–74.

37. Ertunc D, Tok EC, Pata O, et al. Is stress urinary incontinence a familial condition? Acta Obstet Gynecol Scand 2004; 83: 912–16.

38. Altman D, Forsman M, Falconer C, Lichtenstein P. Genetic influence on stress urinary incontinence and pelvic organ prolapse. Eur Urol 2008; 54: 918–22.

39. Milsom I, Abrams P, Cardoza L, et al. How widespread are the symptoms of an overactive bladder and how are they managed? A population-based prevalence study. BJU Int 2001; 87: 760–6.

40. Irwin DE, Milsom I, Hunskaar S, et al. Population-based survey of urinary incontinence, overactive bladder, and other lower urinary tract symptoms in five countries: results of the EPIC study. Eur Urol 2006; 50: 1306–15.

41. McGrother CW, Donaldson MMK, Hatward T, et al. Urinary storage symptoms and comorbidities: a prospective population cohort study in middle-aged and older women. Age Ageing 2006; 35: 16–24.

42. Wagg AS, Cardozo L, Chapple C, et al. Overactive bladder in older people. BJU Int 2007; 99: 502–9.

43. Coyne K, Matza L, Kopp Z, et al. Examining lower urinary tract symptom constellations using cluster analysis. BJU Int 2008; 101: 1267–73.

44. Moller LA, Lose G, Jorgensen T. Incidence and remission rates of lower urinary tract symptoms at one year in women aged 40–60: longitudinal study. BMJ (Clinical research ed.) 2000; 320: 1429–32.

45. Hu T, Wagner T, Bentkover J, et al. Costs of urinary incontinence and overactive bladder in the United States; a comparative study. Urology 2004; 63: 461–5.

46. Reeves P, Irwin D, Kelleher C, et al. The current and future burden and cost of overactive bladder in five European countries. Eur Urol 2006; 50: 1050–7.

47. Irwin DE, Mungapen L, Milsom I, et al. The economic impact of overactive bladder syndrome in six Western countries. BJU Int 2008; 103: 202–9.

48. Malmsten UG, Milsom I, Molander U, et al. Urinary incontinence and lower urinary tract symptoms: an epidemiological study of men aged 45 to 99 years. J Urol 1997; 158: 1733–7.

49. Milsom I. Prevalence and risk factors. In: Treatment of Urinary Incontinence. The Swedish Council on Technology Assessment in Health Care Report on Urinary Incontinence. Stockholm: SBU, 2000.

50. WHO Report. Population Statistics. Geneva: WHO, 1993.

5 Epidemiology: Australia

Richard J Millard and Dudley Robinson

INTRODUCTION

In geographical terms, Australia is the driest continent on earth; regrettably the same cannot be said of its inhabitants. The Australian population is multicultural, having been derived largely from waves of immigrants from Britain and the Mediterranean and Balkan countries for much of its 200 year post-colonization history, and from Asian and Central European countries more recently. Studies show that 5% to 6% of adult Australians have regular or severe urinary incontinence (UI), a prevalence remarkably similar to that reported from other basically Caucasian populations (1,2).

Data regarding prevalence in Australia have been available since a study in Sydney in 1983 (3,4). No systematic study of general prevalence has been conducted since that time. However, the longitudinal Women's Health Australia study, involving over 40,000 women (5), has provided new data on prevalence in women (6) and may yield further data on the incidence of incontinence over the next 10 to 20 years as the cohorts age.

The problem with all surveys aimed at assessing the prevalence of incontinence is how to define UI. Do we wish to know only how many people have regular and severe incontinence, assuming that we could even define what we meant by this term? Alternatively, is it relevant to know about all levels of UI that occur in the community? Is whether the individual chooses to wear an incontinence pad or appliance a good indicator of significant incontinence?

Equally, research into the incidence and prevalence of UI in Australian women has been shown to exhibit significant heterogenicity in the findings due to methodological limitations. Consequently there is a need for future studies to use validated instruments and report age specific data (7). Some of the more recent studies reviewed in this chapter fulfill these criteria.

To circumvent these issues, the 1983 Sydney survey attempted to ascertain the prevalence of all past and present UI and to stratify the type, severity, and frequency of occurrence of the incontinence problems discovered in the study population. The study was designed to ascertain the prevalence of UI in Australia. Prevalence was correlated with age, gender, and socioeconomic stratification. An attempt was made to define at-risk groups, types, and severity of incontinence, and use of protective appliances. A detailed, 38-question, self-report questionnaire was devised and tested for comprehensibility in small focus groups before distribution. A multistage cluster-sampling technique was used to target 3000 adults in 1000 homes, randomly selected from 100 postal districts. All 3000 were telephoned to increase compliance and to check data received, and a total of 1256 completed questionnaires were analyzed.

Three hospitals (1666 beds) and 15 nursing homes (1631 beds) were also surveyed by questionnaires sent to staff, and the data from these establishments were analyzed separately.

A total of 293 individuals admitted to some degree of present UI or leakage by day, and 51 also had some loss of urine at night. In all, 301 persons (24%)—13% of the male and 34% of the female respondents—had some degree of urinary loss. Eight people were incontinent only at night. The male-to-female ratio among those with urinary leakage was 1:2.7, with females accounting for 73% of sufferers. The frequency of urinary loss is shown in Table 5.1.

Leakage was more common in members of blue-collar families (27%) than in members of white-collar families (25%). Students and those in full-time employment tended to have half the prevalence of incontinence (13% and 16%, respectively) reported by the other groups (30–34%). Housewives had the highest prevalence of incontinence overall (40%).

The mean duration of all leakage problems was 8.8 years; 18% reported leakage for less than a year, whereas 23% had had problems for 15 or more years; 17% could not specify the duration of their problem.

The 293 positive respondents were asked to specify circumstances under which they experienced leakage (more than one answer was allowed) (Table 5.2).

All 293 individuals who reported some current degree of leakage were asked to quantify the severity of the urine loss (Table 5.3).

Severe incontinence was twice as common in blue-collar as in white-collar families, but minor degrees of leakage were equally prevalent. The type of incontinence was correlated with severity and frequency of leakage episodes as shown in Table 5.4.

In most cases, incontinence occurred infrequently and was of minor severity. What stands out is the relatively more frequent nature of the leakage of the quiet dribbling incontinence type, which occurs without warning or provocation.

Nocturnal Incontinence

Incontinence at night was reported by 51 (26 female and 25 male) individuals, a prevalence of 4% of the population over the age of 10 years. The frequency of nocturnal incontinence is shown in Table 5.5, correlated with sex and age group.

Treatment Experience

Perhaps reflecting the minor nature of the problem for the majority of the positive respondents, 70% of the 301 with leakage had never sought any treatment. However, 31% of the women and 26% of the men had sought help from

Table 5.1 Frequency of Incontinence Episodes

Frequency	Percentage of respondents		
	Male	Female	Overall
Often wet	2	4	3
Once a day	2	4	3
Once a week	1	3	2
Once or twice a month	0	4	2
Rarely	8	18	13
Never wet	87	66	76

Table 5.2 Circumstances in which Respondents Experienced Leakage

	Percentage of respondents	
	Males (n = 79)	Females (n = 214)
Coughing or sneezing	5	61
Straining or lifting	5	12
Urge	27	35
Giggle	9	30
No warning or provocation	1	7
Postmicturition dribble	59	8
With urinary infections	8	10
Other	8	9
Total[a]	122	172

[a]Respondents may have more than one type of incontinence.

Table 5.3 Quantification of Severity of Urinary Loss in 293 Respondents

	Percentage of respondents		
Urinary loss	Male (n = 79)	Female (n = 214)	Overall
Always wet	0	2	2
Flooding	0	2	1
Moderate loss	8	5	5
Slight loss	25	41	37
Just a spot	66	49	54

general practitioners (24%), from specialists (14%), or from other health professionals (1%). (Respondents may have sought help from more than one healthcare professional.) Those most likely to seek help were over 60 years of age, and either blue-collar or unemployed persons. This may be explained by the fact that it is the elderly and those from blue-collar families who have the highest prevalence of urinary leakage and also the more severe degrees of incontinence.

At the time of the study, 93 people were having treatment for incontinence, representing 31% of the 301 with current leakage. This is similar to the treatment rate reported by Thomas et al. (1). The types of treatment being received were pharmaceutical agents in 33%, appliances in 8%, bladder/muscle training in 13%, and surgery in 24% of patients.

Table 5.4 Percentage Frequency and Severity of Leakage in 293 Respondents Wet by Day[a]

Type of incontinence	Frequency				
	Often	1/day	1/week	2/month	Rarely
Coughing	15	12	9	12	52
Strain	31	7	7	14	41
Urge	20	11	8	10	50
Giggle	15	13	7	8	56
No warning	38	19	6	6	31
Postmicturition	22	15	4	11	48
Other	12	15	4	19	50

	Severity				
	Always	Flood	Moderate	Slight	Drops
Coughing	1	2	2	46	48
Strain	7	3	10	38	41
Urge	1	3	7	35	52
No warning	19	6	6	38	19
Postmicturition	2	2	2	27	69
With UTI	–	–	7	37	56
Other	4	4	8	50	35

[a]A patient may have more than one type of incontinence.
Abbreviation: UTI, urinary tract infection.

Table 5.5 Frequency of Nocturnal Incontinence, Correlated to Sex, and Age Group

Frequency	Overall percentage	No. and sex		Age group (years)				
		M	F	10–29	30–44	45–59	60–74	75+
Most nights	8	2	2	2	0	1	1	0
Once a month	4	2	0	1	0	1	0	0
Occasionally	16	5	3	6	1	1	0	0
Rarely	73	16	21	19	7	8	0	3
Percentage wet in age group				28	8	11	1	3
				5.6	2.3	4.4	1	8

RELATIONSHIP BETWEEN INCONTINENCE AND AGE GROUP

The prevalence of incontinence and its relationship to age group and gender is shown in Figure 5.1 and in Table 5.6. The increased prevalence seen with increasing age is particularly prominent in men over 60 years of age. The normal female preponderance is lost in old age, with a consequent rise in overall prevalence. The high (40%+) prevalence rate in the over-60 age groups is similar to that found in other studies (8) and to the prevalence of incontinence found in nursing homes (9). Those over 60 years of age reported more severe and more frequent episodes of incontinence than did younger people.

Even young women have a higher prevalence of incontinence than young men, and this trend is accentuated after 30 years of age, possibly as a result of pregnancy and childbirth. This was particularly apparent in the rates of stress UI, which increased from 7% in the 10- to 29-year-old group to 26% in 30- to 44-year-old women and to 36% in the 45- to 60-year-old group. These data are similar to those obtained from the Women's Health Australia study (6). The relationship between incontinence type and age group is shown in Table 5.7, which emphasizes the rising prevalence of urge incontinence in the elderly and the high rate of simple stress incontinence in middle age.

The association of age and UI has also been documented in a recent questionnaire based study of 542 community dwelling women aged 24 to 80 years. The overall prevalence of any UI was 41.7% [95% confidence interval (CI): 37.2–45.8] with a response rate of 93.4%. Of the 210 women reporting UI 16% (95% CI: 12.9–19.3) reported stress only, 7.5% (95% CI: 5.2–9.8) reported urge only and 18% (95% CI: 14.7–21.5) reported mixed symptoms. Stress incontinence was found to be most common amongst middle aged women whilst urge incontinence was most common in women over the age of 75 years. Logistic regression revealed a significant association with obesity and parity with stress incontinence. Increasing age, being over weight, and previous hysterectomy was associated with urge incontinence (10).

PRECIPITATING FACTORS

The 301 individuals who were "wet day or night" were requested to identify the "cause" of their leakage problem (Table 5.8). Hysterectomy was blamed for incontinence in 7% of the women, mostly by women from blue-collar families or those off the workforce, compared with only 1% of the women from white-collar families. Incontinence associated with urinary tract infection was also twice as common in women from blue-collar families. The association between incontinence and

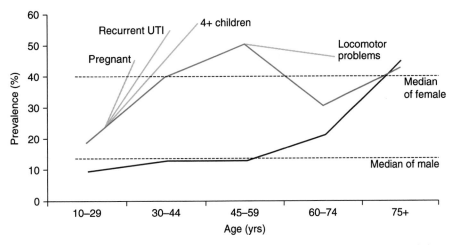

Figure 5.1 Prevalence of incontinence according to age and sex [red line: female (n = 214); blue line: male (n = 79)].

Table 5.6 Prevalence of Incontinence, and Its Relationship to Age Group and Gender

No. of individuals	Age group (years)					
	10–29	30–44	45–59	60–74	75+	Overall
Sample total	498	354	250	117	37	1256
Female	243	194	129	64	21	651
Wet[a]	47	75	64	19	9	214
	(19)	(39)	(50)	(30)	(43)	(33)
Male	255	160	121	53	16	605
Wet[a]	25	20	16	11	7	79
	(10)	(13)	(13)	(21)	(44)	(13)

[a]Percentages in parentheses.

Table 5.7 Relationship Between Incontinence Type and Age Group

Incontinence	Percentage female	Percentage in age group (years)					Overall percentage
		10–29	30–44	45–59	60–74	75+	
Cough/sneeze	97	25	53	63	33	44	46
Strain/lift	86	7	13	12	7	–	10
Urge	78	31	29	28	50	56	33
Giggle	90	29	25	24	13	19	24
No warning	94	6	5	6	3	6	5
Postmicturition	37	26	24	18	23	6	22
With UTI	78	11	12	4	7	13	9
Other	77	14	10	5	7	6	9
No./group size		72/498	97/354	78/250	30/117	16/37	
Prevalence (%)		14	27	31	26	43	30
Percentage of responses/sufferers[a]		150	171	161	143	150	159

[a]A patient may have more than one type of incontinence.
Abbreviation: UTI, urinary tract infection.

Table 5.8 Cause of Leakage Identified by 301 Individuals Who were "Wet Day or Night"

Cause	Percentage of individuals	
	Male	Female
Urinary tract infection	5	13
Hysterectomy	–	7
Childbirth/pregnancy	–	31
Menopause	–	5
Prostatectomy	5	–
Other operation	4	2
Miscellaneous	13	32
No cause identified	69	32

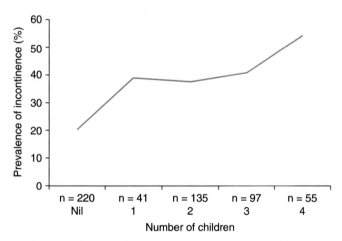

Figure 5.2 Relationship between incontinence and number of children.

hysterectomy and other pelvic surgery has been observed in other studies by Foldspang et al. (11) and Parys et al. (12).

The relationship between incontinence and number of children is shown in Figure 5.2. The first child and pregnancy virtually doubled the prevalence of incontinence in women from 20% to about 40%. There was no change then until the fourth child, when the prevalence rose to 56%. The effect of parity has been noted from other studies (1,2,8,13). Women from blue-collar families were more likely than others to blame childbirth for their incontinence.

A recent study of incontinence during pregnancy was reported by Chiarelli and Campbell (14). In a cross-sectional descriptive study using a five-item structured interview, 336 women were approached and 304 participated (90%): overall, 64% reported stress UI during pregnancy; in the last month of pregnancy 57% reported stress incontinence (with or without urge incontinence); while 42% had urge incontinence (with or without stress incontinence). Among the 195 women experiencing incontinence, 25% lost only a few drops, 57% lost sufficient to dampen the underwear or pad, and 18% reported severe loss. The leakage had started during the first trimester in 8%, in 18% in the second trimester, and in 47% in the last trimester of the most recent pregnancy, whereas, for 20%, leakage had begun in a previous pregnancy, in 6% it began after the birth of a previous child, and only 3% indicated that they had been incontinent before any of their pregnancies. For 49%, leakage was not at all bothersome, 31% found it a little bothersome, 16% quite bothersome, and 4% extremely bothersome.

Chi-square analysis showed four factors to be significantly associated with continence status: previous delivery mode, parity, chronic cough, and bouts of sneezing. Women who had previous vaginal deliveries were 2.5 times more likely to be incontinent than those who had no previous delivery or had only cesarean section. Those who reported previous forceps delivery were 10 times more likely to be incontinent than those with no prior delivery. Only 8% of the women had had their pelvic floor muscles tested during their pregnancy (14).

RISK FACTORS INFLUENCING INCONTINENCE
An analysis of potential risk factors was undertaken. The groups found to be associated with higher rates of incontinence are shown in Table 5.9.

The association between incontinence and cystitis has been noted by Mommsen et al. (15), who found a sixfold increase in experience of incontinence.

A more detailed analysis of risk factors in women has emerged from the Women's Health Australia project (6) (Table 5.10). This longitudinal study involved three cohorts of women: young (age 18–23 years), middle-aged (age 45–50 years), and older (70–75 years) at the time of the baseline survey. The women were selected randomly (5) from the Australian Medicare database covering all women resident in Australia. During 1996, 14.761 young women, 14.070 middle-aged women, and 12.893 older women completed baseline surveys (respectively, 48%, 54%, and 41% of those of each group invited to take part). The baseline questionnaire consisted of 252, 285, and 260 items, respectively, for each of the age cohorts. Participants were asked whether they had leaked urine in the last month "never," "rarely," "sometimes," or "often;" responses other than "never" were taken as indicating incontinence. The advantages of this study were its large sample size and the representative nature of the sample. The limitation was the use of a single non-validated question about leaking urine which fails to differentiate between different types of incontinence.

The prevalence of leaking urine in young women was 12.8% (95% CI: 12.2–13.3); in middle-aged women it was 36.15% (CI 35.2–37.0); and in older women 35.0% (CI 34.1–35.9) (6). These figures are similar to those reported by the earlier Australian prevalence study.

Parity was significantly associated with the prevalence of incontinence in young women but was less strongly correlated in the other age groups. There was a strong association between any degree of constipation and urinary leakage.

In middle-aged women, those with high body mass index (BMI > 25) and constipation were those most likely to experience leakage of urine. Hysterectomy alone had a lower odds ratio (OR) for leakage, whereas women who reported a prolapse repair, either alone or with a hysterectomy, were more likely to leak. Neither current use of hormone replacement therapy nor duration of use was associated with leaking urine.

In the older cohort, the effect of parity was obscured. Pelvic surgery of any kind had a positive association with incontinence. Those with high BMI and those with a history

Table 5.9 Groups Found to be Associated with Higher Rates of Incontinence

Risk factor	Percentage incontinence in group	Percentage incontinence in remainder
Diabetes	36	24
Cerebrovascular accident	25	24
Neurologic disorder	29	24
Locomotor difficulty	45	24
Over 75 years of age	43	24
Recurrent urinary tract infection	55	24
Pregnancy	45	34
Four (or more) children	56	34

Table 5.10 Adjusted Odds Ratios for Variables Associated with Leakage of Urine in Women

	Odds ratio (95% confidence intervals)		
Variable	Young (18–23 years)	Middle-aged (45–50 years)	Older (70–75 years)
Parity			
0	1.00		
1	2.82 (2.37–3.35)	1.58 (1.29–1.93)	0.88 (0.71–1.0)
2	2.59 (1.86–3.61)	1.66 (1.41–1.95)	1.14 (0.96–1.36)
3 or more	4.84 (2.54–9.20)	1.81 (1.54–2.12)	1.16 (0.98–1.36)
Constipation			
Never	1.00		
Rarely	2.13 (1.86–2.42)	2.46 (2.24–2.71)	2.67 (2.38–2.99)
Sometimes	2.86 (2.43–3.36)	2.16 (1.94–2.40)	2.05 (1.82–2.31)
Often	2.66 (2.07–3.40)	2.31 (1.84–3.35)	2.21 (1.87–2.61)
Body mass index			
Underweight <19.9	1.00		
Ideal 20–24.99	1.08 (0.94–1.23)	1.31 1(1.10–1.55)	1.19 (1.00–1.40)
Overweight 25–29.99	1.34 (1.13–1.60)	1.47 (1.23–1.75)	1.39 (1.16–1.65)
Obese 30–40	2.09 (1.67–2.61)	2.05 (1.70–2.46)	1.82 (1.49–2.23)
Very obese >40	1.82 (1.07–3.09)	2.49 (1.84–3.35)	3.29 (2.05–5.29)
Burning and stinging[a]			
Never	1.00		
Rare	2.94 (2.59–3.33)	2.17 (1.96–2.42)	2.45 (2.18–2.76)
Sometimes	4.19 (3.56–4.93)	2.71 (2.35–3.14)	2.99 (2.62–3.41)
Often	4.93 (3.60–6.74)	4.29 (2.85–6.45)	7.97 (5.71–11.12)

Source: Data provided by P. Chiarelli; personal communication and Ref. 6.
[a]Indicative of a history of urinary tract infection.

Table 5.11 Proportion of Incontinent Women in Age Cohorts Who Reported Symptoms of Stress, Urge, or "Other" Incontinence

	Age at time of study		
Type of incontinence	Young (21–26 years) (n = 187)	Middle-aged (48–53 years) (n = 389)	Older (73–79 years) (n = 358)
Stress only (%)	10.7	6.4	2.0
Urge only (%)	2.7	1.3	6.1
Other only (%)	0.0	0.0	0.8
Mixed (%)	86.6	92.3	91.1
Stress, urge, and "other"	63.6	65.3	60.9
Stress and urge	18.2	26.0	26.8
Stress and "other"	3.2	0.8	2.5
Urge and "other"	1.6	0.3	0.8
Any stress symptoms	95.7	98.5	92.2
Any urge symptoms	86.1	92.8	94.7
Any "other" symptoms	68.4	66.3	65.1

Source: Data adapted from Ref. 14.

suggestive of urinary tract infection (burning and stinging) were more likely to report incontinence.

At all ages, women who reported leaking urine had lower scores on the physical and mental component of the Swedish Short Form 36 inventory, suggesting a lower quality of life for these women compared with continent women.

In a follow-up study reported in 2003 (16), the cohorts had aged by five years. The majority of all age groups reported mixed incontinence, most commonly mixtures of stress and urge leakage, almost 80% of wet women over 50 years of age having mixed UI (Table 5.11). The severity of incontinence was as high as or worse than that in older women. Incontinence severity was associated with BMI and this effect involved women with stress UI or urge UI. Other risk factors identified for severity included number of deliveries but there were insufficient numbers of women with large babies for a significant difference to be attributed to the size of the baby. Smoking >20 cigarettes per day was a risk factor (OR 3.34, 95% CI: 1.6, 6.98) in even young women in contrast to other studies that have only shown this association in older cohorts. Urine that burns or stings were often associated with higher adjusted ORs in all age cohorts.

A further longitudinal study based on a cohort of women from the Australian Longitudinal Study of Women's Health, aged 70 to 75 years. In 1996 with nine years follow up has recently been reported. Over this time 14.6% (95% CI: 13.9–15.3) of previously continent women became incontinent. Longitudinal models demonstrated an association between incontinence and dementia, falls, BMI, constipation, lower urinary tract infection, and urogenital prolapse. Stroke and hysterectomy were also found to have weaker associations (17).

Adolescents with chronic lung disease and cystic fibrosis aged 12 to 19 years have been reported to have a high incidence of incontinence (18). Of 55 adolescents, 47% had ever experienced UI and 22% had UI at least twice a month. Median age of onset was 13 (range 7–16 years) and most had leakage associated with coughing (84%) or laughing (64%). Importantly, 42% reported that it sometimes prevented them from doing

Table 5.12 Present Incontinence Among those Recalling Nocturnal Enuresis as a Child

Current	Childhood bedwetter	Childhood non-bedwetter
Percentage wet at night now	11	2
Percentage wet by day now	32	19

effective physiotherapy and 33% said their social life had been affected. Only 58% had told anyone about their problem and only two of 26 girls had talked to their doctor.

PAST EXPERIENCE OF INCONTINENCE IF NO PROBLEM AT PRESENT

The 955 respondents who denied any degree of urinary leakage at the present time were asked to report if they had ever experienced urinary leakage since they were 17 years of age. Replies showed that 16% of men and 30% of women had had previous experience of leakage: In 6% leakage had occurred occasionally and in 17% it had been experienced only rarely. The pattern of previous incontinence was similar to that found among those who admitted to present leakage.

CHILDHOOD INCONTINENCE AND RELATIVE RISK

Of the whole group of 1256 respondents, 21% (269) recalled having problems as a child with bedwetting. The occurrence of this problem was equal in males and females. In addition, 9% (114 respondents, 67% female) recalled having had urinary leakage at school. Bedwetting was apparently more common in white-collar families (25% of whom were affected) than in blue-collar families (where only 20% recalled problems).

Childhood nocturnal enuresis was recalled by 269 individuals. As adults, 11% of these individuals still wet the bed while 32% had diurnal incontinence. Childhood bedwetters accounted for 57% of all those currently wet at night and 30% of all those wet by day (Table 5.12). Childhood bedwetters appeared to carry a fivefold increased risk of nocturnal incontinence in adult life compared with non-bedwetters. They were also at higher risk of developing some degree of UI by day, with 1.7 times the prevalence rate of non-bedwetters. Of 114 respondents (9%) wet at school, 39% were wet by day at the time of the survey, accounting for 15% of all those now wet; 7% of the group now suffer from incontinence at night; and account for 16% of all those now wet at night (Table 5.13). Individuals with incontinence in childhood at school carry a threefold risk of night-time incontinence as an adult and twice the risk of diurnal incontinence than their fellows who had been dry at school.

The epidemiology of childhood enuresis in Australia has been independently studied by Hawkins (19) in 1962 and by Bower et al. (20) in 1996. The former took a sample of 1000 children in one general practice only and found a prevalence of nocturnal enuresis (of one or more nights per week at school age) of 18%; daytime incontinence was not evaluated. The 1996 study by Bower et al. (20) used a self-administered questionnaire distributed to parents with children 5 to 12 years of age at the eight largest polling stations of three electorates. Voting is compulsory in Australia and these electorates were selected to represent voters of high (9000), middle (7600), and lower (9000) socio-economic classification. Of the 3111 parents approached, 2292 (74%) responded. The prevalence rate was 15% for nocturnal enuresis, 2% for isolated day wetting, and 4% for combined day and night wetting; overall, 79% of children were dry, 18.9% had nocturnal enuresis, and 5.5% had daytime incontinence. Whereas daytime wetting did not show a gender bias, 60% of children with enuresis were male, regardless of whether the enuresis was primary or secondary (Table 5.14). The families of only 33.8% of enuretic children had sought professional help for the problem. Family strategies used were reward charts (16%), waking the child to void (30%), fluid restriction (43%), and waiting for maturity (51%). Non-enuretic children woke spontaneously to void at night in 80% of cases; by contrast, enuretic children woke only

49% of the time. There was a significant difference in the incidence of a positive family history between enuretic and dry children: among dry children, 55.5% had no family history, whereas only 30.6% of enuretics had no known family history. These figures corroborate the findings of the earlier general population study (3,4), suggesting that 100,000 children wet the bed each night in Australia.

A more recent population based study of 2856 school age children with incontinence has recently been reported from Sydney. Overall 16.9% reported any daytime incontinence in the previous six months with 64% of cases being very mild, 14.8% mild, 11.6% moderate, and 9.6% severe. Independent risk factors were found to be nocturnal enuresis (OR 7.2; 95% CI: 3.4–15.2), female (OR 5.4; 95% CI: 2.6–11.1), social concerns (OR 3.4; 95% CI: 1.4–8.3), urinary tract infection (OR 5.6; 95% CI: 2.0–15.6), and encopresis (OR 3.3; 95% CI: 1.4–7.7) (21).

PREVALENCE OF SIGNIFICANT INCONTINENCE IN THE POPULATION

The results detailed above indicate that some UI is experienced by many people. The problem has been identification of the rate of troublesome and significant leakage from most of the infrequently wet individuals. Using computer analysis, the entire sample was filtered to exclude all those with rare episodes of leakage and those who had "just a spot" or slight loss of urine only, on infrequent occasions; patients who had leakage only with urinary infections were also excluded. The remainder were considered as having "significant" UI: of these 85 people, 10 were men and 75 were women. The frequency with which they experienced incontinence is shown in Table 5.15.

Infrequent UI was rare in those women over 65 years of age, whereas frequent leakage was unusual in patients under 35 years of age. The degree of wetness experienced is detailed in Table 5.16. Minor leakage volumes were rare over 65 years

Table 5.13 Incontinence Among those Wet at School

Current	Wet at school	Dry at school
Percentage wet at night now	7	2
Percentage wet by day now	39	19

Table 5.14 Prevalence (%) of Enuresis

Type	Male (n = 277)	Female (n = 181)	Overall
Nocturnal enuresis	11.3	7.6	18.9
Daytime wetting	2.7	2.8	5.5
Total	14	10.4	
Frequency	Night	Days	
Every day	2.4	0.6	
2+/week	2.7	0.8	
1/2 weeks	0.9	0.3	
1/month	1.8	0.4	
<1/month	11.1	3.4	

Table 5.15 Frequency of Significant Urinary Incontinence in 10 men and 75 women

Frequency of incontinence	Percentage	
	Male	Female
Often wet	50	25
Once a day	30	27
Once a week	20	25
Once or twice a month	–	23

Table 5.16 Degree of Wetness in Respondents with Significant Urinary Incontinence

Degree of wetness	Percentage	
	Male	Female
Always wet	0	4
Flooding	0	4
Moderate loss	30	11
Slight loss	70	48
Just a spot	0	33

of age. Whereas those "always wet" tended to be younger (<64 years old), the elderly tended to have "moderate loss" or "flooding." Of this group, only 40% of both sexes had ever sought treatment: 30% of each sex had seen their general practitioner, and specialists had seen 30% of the men but only 17% of the women. This low percentage of people seeking treatment reflects the fact that about 40% of each sex needed to wear protective underwear; the remainder managed by hygienic measures alone.

The pattern of incontinence reported by those who were deemed to have significant incontinence is shown in Table 5.17.

Among the men with frequent incontinence, small-volume postmicturition loss was most commonly a complaint of younger men; older men suffered from urge incontinence (especially in the 75+ age group, in which this occurred in 20%). By contrast, females tended to have more than one cause of leakage, with stress incontinence predominant (particularly in middle-aged women). Urge incontinence in women appeared to be equally prevalent at all ages, but its severity grew with advancing years; flooding urinary loss was reported only by those over 50 years of age.

URINARY INCONTINENCE IN PEOPLE IN INSTITUTIONS

A parallel study was conducted to determine the prevalence of incontinence among those in institutional care: 15 nursing homes in the Sydney area were surveyed; one public hospital (824 beds) and two private hospitals (842 beds) were also investigated.

Incontinence in Nursing Homes

The staff of 15 of the larger nursing homes across the city were asked to fill out profiles of their patients' continence status (Table 5.18). Among the 1631 residents of these nursing homes, 596 were incontinent, a prevalence rate of 37%. Most of those who were incontinent were over 70 years of age. The ratio of males to females was close to 1:1, but females outnumbered males in the homes by 2.6:1; as a result there were more wet women than men. Wet men tended to be slightly younger than wet women. The degree of incontinence reported in this group is shown in Table 5.19, correlated with mobility status. There

was no significant difference between the degree of incontinence found in men and women in nursing homes. Residents who were chair-bound tended to have the highest rates of incontinence.

Another Sydney study of 1659 residents of nursing homes found UI affected 77%, and that 25% of nursing staff time was spent dealing with urinary leakage (22). The long-term care of looking after such residents was estimated at AUS $45,000 per annum or AUS $450 million a year.

If the prevalence found in this survey (37%) is applied to the population of all nursing homes in Australia, an estimated 22,000 incontinent individuals might be expected to be found in these establishments.

The importance and association of incontinence and the increasing prevalence of falls in the elderly has also been clearly documented (23) the OR of sustaining a fall is 1.45 (95% CI: 1.36–1.54) in the presence of any type of UI; the OR related to stress incontinence is 1.11 (95% CI: 1.00–1.23) whilst that related to urge incontinence was 1.54 (95% CI: 1.41–1.69). Consequently UI should be considered an important cause of co-morbidity in the elderly and falls prevention programs need to include an assessment of incontinence.

Incontinence in Hospitals

In order to assess the prevalence of incontinence, the staff of one large public hospital and two small private hospitals were asked to make a count of incontinence among their patients. In the public hospital, 3.4% of the 824 patients had incontinence known to the nursing staff and 71% of these were over 71 years of age. This may be an underestimate in that many patients who were able to manage their own incontinence may not have been known to the ward nursing staff.

Table 5.17 Pattern of Incontinence Reported by those Deemed to have Significant Incontinence

	Percentage	
Incontinence type	Male	Female
Coughing or sneezing	–	67
Straining or lifting	–	17
Urge	50	43
Giggle	10	27
No warning or provocation	10	12
Postmicturition dribbling	40	11
Total[a]	110	177

[a]More than one response was allowed.

Table 5.18 Continence Status of Patients in 15 of the Larger Nursing Homes in Sydney

	Percentage		
Degree of wetness	Male	Female	Overall
Always wet	39	40	39
Flooding	15	13	13
Moderate loss	31	35	34
Slight loss	13	10	11
n	194	394	596

Table 5.19 Degree of Incontinence Analyzed by Patient Mobility

	Percentage of patients incontinent				
Mobility	Always wet	Flooding	Moderate	Slight	Overall
Ambulant	10	11	20	44	18
Chair-bound	76	64	54	27	61
Bedridden	8	16	3	–	6
Mobile aided	6	9	23	27	15
n	234	80	200	66	596

In the two small private hospitals, the prevalence of incontinence was 13% and 22%, respectively. There was a high proportion of psychiatric patients, of whom 15% were incontinent; 40% of the geriatric patients in these hospitals were incontinent.

A more recent survey of 447 hospital inpatients confirms these findings. Overall 22% of patients complained of UI, 10% fecal incontinence, 78% nocturia, and 23% urgency. In addition 60% of patients were using a continence product or device. The authors conclude that the management of continence both. In the acute and sub acute care settings were sub optimal and there is a need to raise clinical awareness (24).

PREVALENCE OF INCONTINENCE IN AUSTRALIA

Among adult Australians, 24% of individuals admit to having some urinary loss and 6% of the population have significant or frequent urinary leakage. Of those who currently have no incontinence (76%), 23% have experienced some urinary leakage in their past adult life. Of those who currently suffer some form of leakage, 73% are female, but women account for 88% of those with severe incontinence (M:F ratio = 1:7.5). The female predominance disappears over the age of 60. A summary of the prevalence of incontinence is shown in Table 5.20. If the figures for significant present incontinence are applied to the census figures, it can be estimated that as many as 960,000 adults in Australia may experience regular or severe incontinence; however, fewer than half of these ever seek professional help. Conversely, if prevalence figures of 24% of all women over 18 years are used and applied to current census data, a figure closer to two million incontinent individuals would be more appropriate.

What then is prevalence? Should we only be interested in severe incontinence, or should we screen individuals in the community for lesser degrees of UI which might be amenable to interventions by the family practitioner, thereby perhaps avoiding more major problems later in life? A simple Incontinence Screening Questionnaire was evaluated and correlated with 48-hour pad test data, resulting in only five discriminating questions (25) (Table 5.21).

With an aging population we can anticipate an increase in the probability of UI and in its severity. In addition, with aging comes a change from stress incontinence to urge incontinence and co-morbidity. UI has a considerable financial impact on individuals and the healthcare system. In Australia the total annual cost of UI was estimated at AUS $710 million in 1998 for the 1,835,628 community-dwelling incontinent women over 18 years of age. This represents AUS $387 per incontinent woman, comprising AUS $338.47 million in treatment costs and AUS $371.97 million in personal costs. These costs will escalate to AUS $1.27 billion per annum by 2018 (26). These figures do not include indirect or intangible costs, neither do they include the costs of nursing home care mentioned above.

We cannot afford to ignore the prevalence of incontinence; it is going to cost us or our children dearly. There is a need to emphasize to primary care physicians the importance of identifying at-risk women or those with minor degrees of UI, for which conservative options (pelvic floor exercise programs for stress UI, or bladder training/drug therapy) may be restorative or may prevent deterioration. Clearly, the cost–benefit of early

Table 5.20 Summary of Prevalence of Incontinence in Australia

Incontinence	Percentage of individuals		
	Male	Female	Overall
Childhood enuresis	21	21	21
Past incontinence (in adult life)	16	30	23
All present incontinence	13	34	24
Ever incontinent as an adult	28	53	41
Significant incontinence now	2	11	6

Table 5.21 Predictive Validity of Incontinence Screening Questionnaire

	PPV (%)
Have you leaked urine when	
Coughing/laughing/sneezing	64
On the way to the toilet	68
Waiting to use the toilet	67
Going to the toilet urgently when first feeling the need	67
Going to the toilet "just in case"	68

Abbreviation: PPV, positive predictive value.
Source: Data from Ref. 19.

intervention needs to be evaluated in anticipation of the flood of incontinence with which the profession will be inundated as our population ages.

REFERENCES

1. Thomas TM, Plymat KR, Blannin J, Meade TW. Prevalence of urinary incontinence. Br Med J 1980; 281: 1243–5.
2. Jolleys JV. Reported prevalence of urinary incontinence in women in general practice. Br Med J 1988; 296: 1300–3.
3. Millard RJ. The incidence of urinary incontinence in Australia. Br J Urol 1985; 57: 98–9.
4. Millard RJ. The prevalence of urinary incontinence in Australia: a demographic study in the Sydney area in 1983. Aust Continence J 1988; 4: 92–9.
5. Brown WJ, Bryson L, Byles J, et al. Women's Health Australia: recruitment for a national longitudinal cohort study. Women's Health 1998; 28: 23–40.
6. Chiarelli P, Brown W, McElduff P. Leaking urine—prevalence and associated factors in Australian women. Neurourol Urodyn 1999; 18; 567–77.
7. Botlero R, Urquhart DM, Davis SR, Bell RJ. Prevalence and incidence of urinary incontinence in women; review of the literature and investigation of methodological issues. Int J Urol 2008; 15: 230–34.
8. Milsom I, Ekelund P, Molander U, et al. The influence of age, parity, oral contraception, hysterectomy and menopause on the prevalence of urinary incontinence in women. J Urol 1993; 149: 1459–62.
9. Ouslander JG. Urinary incontinence in nursing homes. J Am Geriatr Soc 1990; 38: 289–91.
10. Botlero R, Davis SR, 10. Botlero R, Davis SR, Urquhart DM, Shortreed S, Bell RJ. Age specific prevalence of, and factors associated with, different types of urinary incontinence in community dwelling Australian women assessed with a validated questionnaire. Maturitas 2009; 62: 134–39.
11. Foldspang A, Mommsen S, Elving L, Lam GW. Parity as a correlate of adult female urinary incontinence prevalence. J Epidemiol Community Health 1992; 46: 595–600.
12. Parys B, Haylen B, Hutton J, Parsons K. The effects of simple hysterectomy on vesicourethral function. Br J Urol 1989; 64: 594–9.
13. Mommsen S, Foldspang A, Elving L, Lam GW. Association between urinary incontinence in women and a previous history of surgery. Br J Urol 1993; 72: 30–7.

14. Chiarelli P, Campbell E. Incontinence during pregnancy: prevalence and opportunities from continence promotion. Aust N Z J Obstet Gynaecol 1997; 37: 66–73.
15. Mommsen S, Foldspang A, Elving L, Lam GW. Cystitis as correlate of female urinary incontinence. Int Urogynaecol J Pelvic Floor Dysfunct 1994; 5: 135–40.
16. Miller YD, Brown WJ, Russell A, Chiarelli P. Urinary incontinence across the lifespan. Neurourol Urodyn 2003; 22: 550–7.
17. Byles J, Millar CJ, Sibbritt DW, Chiarelli P. Living with urinary incontinence: a longitudinal study of older women. Age Ageing 2009; 38; 333–8.
18. Nixon GM, Glazener JA, Martin JM, Sawyer SM. Urinary incontinence in female adolescents with cystic fibrosis. Pediatrics 2002; 110: e22.
19. Hawkins DN. Enuresis: a survey. Med J Aust 1962; 23: 979–80.
20. Bower WF, Moore KH, Shepherd RB, Adams RD. The epidemiology of childhood enuresis in Australia. Br J Urol 1996; 78: 602–6.
21. Sureshkumar P, Jones M, Cumming R, Craig J. A population based study of 2856 school age children with urinary incontinence. J Urol 2009; 181: 808–15.
22. Steel J, Fonda D. Minimising the cost of urinary incontinence in nursing homes. PharmacoEconomics 1995; 7: 191–7.
23. Chiarelli PE, Mackenzie LA, Osmotherly PG. Urinary incontinence is associated with an increase in falls: a systematic review. Aust J Physiother 2009; 55: 89–95.
24. Ostaszkiewicz J, O'Connell B, Millar L. Incontinence: managed or mismanaged in hospital settings? Int J Nurs Pract 2008; 14: 495–502.
25. Gunthorpe W, Brown W, Redman S. The development and evaluation of an Incontinence Screening Questionnaire for Female Primary Care. Neurourol Urodyn 2000; 19: 595–607.
26. Doran CM, Chiarelli P, Cockburn J. Economic costs of urinary incontinence in community dwelling Australian women. Med J Aust 2001; 174: 456–8.

6 Epidemiology: Asia

SS Vasan and Reena S Yalaburgi

INTRODUCTION

Urinary incontinence (UI) is a major clinical problem that has a profound effect on quality of life and activities of daily living (1–3). Women with UI report fear, shame and humiliation, and worry about the odor of urine from pads and wet underclothing (4). UI is physically debilitating and socially incapacitating, and is associated with loss of self-confidence, feelings of helplessness, depression, and anxiety (3).

Many adults suffer from UI, and the financial, physical, emotional, psychological, and social impacts are demoralizing and distressing (5–7). UI has become a costly public health problem (6). In the United States, it is estimated that direct health costs of UI among older people amount to more than US $26 billion per year, an average of US $3565 for each incontinent older person (8). No estimate of this kind is available in Asia.

UI is a general problem among older people (5). Posturination dribble and continuous leakage are both common forms that arise in later life. Many incontinent older people in Asia and elsewhere do not talk about their UI or report it to physicians. This is partly due to their limited understanding of UI, and also because they fear social rejection. Indeed, UI is under-reported and under-diagnosed across all age groups (9–13). Thus no accurate estimate of UI is available for people across the age spectrum. Almost all studies, however, confirm that prevalence increases with adult age (5–11,14–16) and that prevalence is higher among women than among men at all ages (5,7,11,17–19). Prevalence among older people living in institutions also is higher than among their community-dwelling counterparts (5,7,20,21).

The Agency for Health Care Policy and Research in the United States has estimated that 15% to 35% of people aged 60 years and above living in the community have experienced some degree of UI (5,22–25). Burgio and Locher (23) reported that 20% to 30% of older people aged above 65 living in the community suffer from UI. It is also estimated that at least 50% of nursing home residents are incontinent (17,20,23,24,26). Yarnell and St. Leger (27) reported that between 40% and 60% of nursing home residents are incontinent. According to Tobin (28) the higher prevalence of UI among people living in residential care facilities is related to their increased average age and to the increased prevalence of physical and mental morbidity.

Studies of the prevalence of UI suggest that it is widespread among women of all ages (29). The probability of incontinence increases with age (30–32), and the nature of incontinence changes from stress incontinence to urge incontinence (33) with increasing age. This is due to an increased prevalence of multiple disorders and organ dysfunction with increasing age. This change has significant implications for clinical management (34). While stress incontinence is typically managed with strengthening exercises for pelvic floor muscles, with or without neuromuscular electrostimulation and surgery, management of urge incontinence might also include a bladder-training program, transcutaneous electrostimulation aimed at the spinal micturition reflex center, and medications (35,36).

EPIDEMIOLOGY OF UI

Throughout Asia, UI remains a sensitive and taboo subject, and there is a need for more open discussion. For the sufferer, UI brings stigmatization, social embarrassment, loss of self-esteem, and loss of face, all of which prompt widespread under-estimation and under-diagnosis (13). There have been few systematic studies of the prevalence and impact of UI among older people in Asian countries.

This review provides the prevalence and severity of UI within Asia with a discussion of the epidemiology of UI together with a systematic review of prevalence within the community (37–39). Some of the factors assessed include:

- age/gender segments within the population,
- risk factors for incontinence,
- analysis of incontinence prevalence estimates, and
- recommendations for studies to reliably determine the prevalence of incontinence within the Asian population.

In one of the first pioneering studies done in Asia (40), the prevalence and risk factors of UI in a community-residing older population in Japan was assessed by data collected from home visits with a response rate of 95.4%. The prevalence of any degree of UI was 98/1000 in both sexes and 34/1000 of the population was incontinent of urine on a daily basis. Although there was an increasing prevalence with age, the expected greater prevalence in women was not found. Risk factors were, age above 75 years, poor general health as measured by activities of daily living, stroke, dementia, absence of participation in social activities, and lack of life worth living.

In another multi-hospital epidemiological study (41) to elucidate the prevalence and characteristics of UI in elderly inpatients throughout Japan, all patients were evaluated by medical doctors for the following parameters: age, sex, duration of hospitalization, activities of daily living, medical diagnosis, presence or absence of UI, type of UI, and therapy for UI. The prevalence of UI in patients under 70, 70 to 79, 80 to 89, and over 90 years old was 59.3%, 67.7%, 79.8%, and 82.2%, respectively. Overall, 1142 patients (72.0%) suffered from UI. Cerebrovascular disease was the major cause of admission to hospital in patients with UI (37.0%). The most frequent type of UI was functional UI which was seen in patients who were mentally and/or physically unable to go to the bathroom without aid (21.5%). Specifically, 38.1% of patients in geriatric hospitals were diagnosed as having functional UI, in contrast to only 3.9% of patients in non-geriatric units. In patients with dementia, 88.7% were incontinent; whereas in patients without dementia, the prevalence of UI was significantly lower at 51.5% (p < 0.001). Another predisposing factor for UI was urinary tract infection (UTI). The prevalence of UI in patients with and without UTI was 87.8% and 59.5%, respectively (p < 0.001). Almost all patients with poor activities of daily living (who were bedridden) suffered from UI (98.5%). On the other hand, UI was less frequent in patients who could walk (26.9%). Pad (42.8%) and indwelling bladder catheter (18.3%) were the major means of containment of incontinence, whereas behavioral therapy (4.9%) and surgery (0.5%) were not common.

Yoshida et al. (42) examined the prevalence and risk factors of UI and potential factors hindering individuals from seeking treatment for UI among a community-dwelling population aged over 40 years. Data were collected by mailing a 23-item UI questionnaire to a random sample of community-dwelling individuals aged 40 to 75 years (n = 3500) in seven towns of Shiga Prefecture, Japan. The overall response rate was 52.5%. Prevalence of UI for male and female respondents was 10.5% and 53.7%, respectively. The incidence of urge incontinence increased with age in the male group. In women, stress incontinence was prevalent at all ages and the incidence of urge incontinence increased over 70 years of age. UI was more likely as activities of daily living limitations and cystitis increased. Women with a history of hysterectomy or diabetes mellitus and men who had had a stroke were at increased risk for UI. Of those who reported UI, only 3% had ever consulted doctors or other health care professionals concerning it, 25% recognized their condition as a disease and 38% considered it curable by appropriate treatments. In addition, 63% regarded UI as an unavoidable consequence of aging, 63% considered their condition was embarrassing, and 54% were reluctant to seek treatment from a health professional.

Jik-Joen Lee (43) assessed the impact of UI in older Chinese in Hong Kong by a cross-sectional study using face-to-face interviews with a questionnaire mainly composed of closed-ended questions. The study was conducted at two selected elderly homes and one elderly center. The sample was composed of 92 elderly-home residents and 122 elderly-center users. Fultz and Herzog's (18) modified operational definition of severity of UI was used to measure respondents' levels of UI. Specht and Maas's (21) concept of social impact was used to assess respondents' social-life suffering. The reported prevalence of UI increased with adult age, and that the incontinence affected women more than men. About 86.1% of the incontinent respondents experienced negative social impact. There are no statistically significant differences between levels of incontinence and social impact on older respondents' employment, social, family, financial, and physical conditions. Also, no significant difference is found between levels of UI and the reported levels of social impact.

OPERATIONAL DEFINITION OF IMPACT ON SOCIAL LIFE

Specht and Maas's (2001) concept of impact on social life, or social impact, was adopted with modifications. To measure the adverse impact on sufferers with UI, nine complaints were developed and grouped into the following five subscales: employment, social, family, economic, and physical wellbeing.

To measure the level of suffering (a functional issue), an operational definition of social impact was developed using the following dichotomous (yes/no) criteria:

1. Limitation of job opportunities (employment):
   (a) reductions in employment opportunities
2. Negative impact on social life (social):
   (a) restrictions on opportunities for participation in social activities
   (b) restrictions on participation in outings
   (c) need for cumbersome precautions while going out
3. Negative impact on family life (family):
   (a) need for family help
4. Negative impact on finances (economic):
   (a) increase in daily expenditure
5. Negative impact on physical condition (physical well-being):
   (a) fear of odor
   (b) fear of leakage
   (c) affect on personal appearance

It is assumed that moderate to severely incontinent older people experience more impact on their social lives than mildly incontinent people. Contrary to this assumption, this study finds no statistically significant differences in social impact at different levels of UI. Also, there is no significant difference in terms of the impact of moderate to severe incontinence relative to mild incontinence in older sufferers. This is noteworthy as it appears that the level of UI is not a crucial factor in determining impact on older peoples' social lives. The implication is significant; negative impact on incontinent respondents' social lives are basically unique, universal, undeniable, and unavoidable. The social impact is on the whole the same and should be treated as "actual and real."

Theoretically, the result has four possible explanations: adjustment, habituation, social comparisons, and impression management. Moderate to severely incontinent older people may adjust to the adverse impacts of UI as time goes by or through whatever means available to handle the symptoms. The practice of adjustment and the feeling of habituation will actually reduce the significance of social impact. Additionally, moderate to severely incontinent older people frequently rely on social comparisons in making their social-impact appraisals. They assume that the social impact will become increasingly serious for their peers, while theirs will remain stable. The function of adjustment, habituation, and social comparisons is to uphold the self-esteem and self-worth of those with UI. This behavior helps them build up a better self-image and a positive impression among peers.

People with moderate to severe incontinence, suffer from adjustment, habituation, and social comparisons, and impression management may effectively reduce the social impact. Methodologically, measurement and sample problems are two possible reasons for the statistically insignificant differences between the levels of incontinence. First, the measures may not be sensitive enough to detect the difference. Second, the sample is too small to allow for significant and powerful testing of the impact of incontinence. More studies are needed to further explore the social impact between levels of UI.

In a Korean telephone survey of the community by Won Hee Park and colleagues (44) to estimate the prevalence of UI in females between 30 and 75 years, 1300 were interviewed (response rate 86.9%). Overall, UI was reported by 40.8%, and 22.9%, 3.1%, and 14.9% reported pure stress, urge, and mixed UI, respectively. The prevalence of stress, urge, and mixed UI generally did not increase with age. Urge and mixed UI had a greater impact than stress UI on daily tasks (P < 0.001), social life

(P < 0.001), depression or anxiety due to UI (P < 0.001), worry about UI (P < 0.001), sex life (P < 0.001), wear protection due to UI (P = 0.011), and quality of life (P < 0.001). In subjects with pure stress UI, 28.3% reported impaired quality of life compared with 43.9% and 43.8% of subjects with urge and mixed UI. Among these, willingness to seek medical consultation for their problem was seen in 19.1% (stress), 20.0% (urge) and 25.8% (mixed) of urinary incontinent individuals (Tables 6.1 and 6.2).

A study has also been performed to estimate the prevalence rate of UI in a representative sample of women aged 50 to 65 years, using multistage sampling in South Jordan (Karak, Taffileh, Aqaba) in the Middle East (45). The study was to assess the relationship between UI (stress and urge) and the following variables: age and parity, diabetes mellitus, UTI, body mass index (BMI), medications (diuretics), menopause, past history of hys-

Table 6.1 Subject Demographics

Demographics	Total	No incontinence	Stress incontinence	Urge incontinence	Mixed incontinence
Age (yrs)					
30–39	431 (33.1%)	312 (40.5%)	75 (25.2%)	7 (17.5%)	37 (19.1%)
40–49	357 (27.4%)	201 (26.1%)	101 (33.9%)	9 (22.5%)	46 (23.7%)
50–59	234 (18.0%)	123 (16.0%)	56 (18.8%)	6 (15.0%)	49 (25.3%)
60–69	188 (14.4%)	93 (12.1%)	50 (16.8%)	7 (17.5%)	38 (19.6%)
70–79	93 (7.1%)	42 (5.4%)	16 (5.4%)	11 (27.5%)	24 (12.4%)
Occupation					
Agriculture, forestry, or fishery	32 (2.5%)	18 (2.3%)	7 (2.3%)	2 (5.0%)	5 (2.6%)
Self-employed	74 (5.7%)	42 (5.4%)	21 (7.0%)	4 (10.0%)	7 (3.6%)
Blue collar	31 (2.4%)	20 (2.6%)	8 (2.6%)	–	3 (1.5%)
White collar	43 (3.3%)	30 (3.9%)	11 (3.7%)	1 (2.5%)	1 (0.5%)
Housewife	1,072 (82.3%)	633 (82.1%)	243 (81.5%)	30 (75.0%)	166 (85.6%)
Unemployed or others	51 (3.9%)	28 (3.6%)	8 (2.7%)	3 (7.5%)	12 (6.2%)
Education[a]					
Less than middle school	499 (38.5%)	243 (31.8%)	122 (41.2%)	24 (60.0%)	110 (56.7%)
High school	512 (39.6%)	323 (42.3%)	117 (39.5%)	12 (30.0%)	60 (30.9%)
College or above	282 (21.8%)	197 (25.8%)	57 (19.3%)	4 (10.0%)	24 (12.4%)
Income (won/yr)[b]					
>10,000,000	302 (24.5%)	170 (23.3%)	63 (22.0%)	14 (41.2%)	55 (30.6%)
10,000,000–20,000,000	382 (31.0%)	221 (30.3%)	87 (30.3%)	9 (26.5%)	65 (36.1%)
20,000,000–30,000,000	347 (28.2%)	217 (29.7%)	82 (28.6%)	10 (29.4%)	38 (21.1%)
30,000,000 or more	200 (16.3%)	122 (16.7%)	56 (19.1%)	1 (2.9%)	22 (12.2%)
Previous surgery possibly causing incontinence					
Brain or spinal cord	14 (1.1%)	5 (0.6%)	7 (2.3%)	–	2 (1.0%)
Bladder	2 (0.2%)	–	1 (0.3%)	–	1 (0.5%)
Urethra	3 (0.2%)	3 (0.4%)	–	–	–
Uterus	89 (6.8%)	43 (5.6%)	24 (8.1%)	2 (5.0%)	20 (10.3%)
Rectum	5 (0.4%)	5 (0.6%)	7 (2.3%)	–	2 (1.0%)
Co-morbid diseases possibly causing incontinence					
Cerebral infarction	7 (0.5%)	2 (0.3%)	1 (0.3%)	–	4 (2.1%)
Brain or spinal cord injury	4 (0.3%)	1 (0.1%)	1 (0.3%)	–	2 (1.0%)
Other brain or spinal cord diseases	6 (0.5%)	3 (0.4%)	2 (0.7%)	–	1 (0.5%)
Diabetes mellitus	51 (3.9%)	21 (2.7%)	13 (4.4%)	7 (17.5%)	10 (5.2%)
Parkinson's disease	1 (0.1%)	1 (0.1%)	–	–	–
Fecal incontinence	54 (4.1%)	17 (2.2%)	16 (5.4%)	3 (7.5%)	18 (9.3%)

Data presented are numbers (%).
[a]Missing case, 10.
[b]Missing case, 72.

Table 6.2 Prevalence and Frequency of Urinary Incontinence

	Stress incontinence	Urge incontinence	Mixed incontinence
Prevalence according to age cohort (yrs)			
30–39 (n = 431)	75 (25.2%)	7 (17.5%)	37 (19.1%)
40–49 (n = 357)	101 (33.9%)	9 (22.5%)	46 (23.7%)
50–59 (n = 234)	56 (18.8%)	6 (15.0%)	49 (25.3%)
60–69 (n = 188)	50 (16.8%)	7 (17.5%)	38 (19.6%)
70–79 (n = 93)	16 (5.4%)	11 (27.5%)	38 (19.6%)
Total (n = 1303)	298 (100.0%)	40 (100.0%)	194 (100.0%)
Frequency			
Many times a day	6 (2.0%)	2 (5.0%)	9 (4.6%)[a]/8 (4.1%)[b]
A few times a day	1 (0.3%)	2 (5.0%)	17 (8.8%)[a]/13 (6.7%)[b]
About once a day	8 (2.7%)	2 (5.0%)	11 (5.7%)[a]/16 (8.2%)[b]
2–3 times in a wk	13 (4.4%)	4 (10.0%)	24 (12.4%)[a]/22 (11.3%)[b]
>1 in a wk	270 (90.6%)	30 (75.0%)	133 (68.6%)[a]/135 (69.6%)[b]

Data presented are numbers (%).
[a]Stress incontinence.
[b]Urge incontinence.

terectomy, and poor mobility. A questionnaire which was preliminarily tested in a pilot study, and face-to-face interviews were used as the instrument for data collection. Approximately one-third of respondents had UI; 23.1% had stress UI, 26.4% had urge UI, and 18.1% had the mixed type. Prevalence rate of UI was 56.3% for women suffering from UTI and 50% for those who use diuretics. Approximately 54% of women who needed help to move around inside their house complained of UI. High prevalence rates were also observed with parity of five to six (43.5%), menopause (39.7%), obesity (39.3%), and in diabetic women (35%). High prevalence rates of stress incontinence were found in women suffering from UTI (37.5%), in women using diuretics (39.5%), if parity was 5 to 6 (34.8%), and in women with a past history of hysterectomy (28.6%). Stress UI was found to increase with an increase in the BMI. The associations between urge incontinence, BMI, UTI, use of diuretics, and the ability to go around inside the house were all statistically significant.

A survey of 11 cities in 11 different countries by the Asia-Pacific Continence Advisory Board (APCAB) established an overall prevalence of 12.2% (range 4.6–23.1%) among both sexes and all age groups in these communities (46). A Singaporean physician reported prevalence rates of 5% to 15% for UI among older people living in his community (10). In addition, more than one in five older hospital patients suffered from UI, with prevalence among nursing home residents of about 50% (10).

The APCAB study was conducted in Philippines, Singapore, Malaysia, Thailand, and Indonesia, which was later expanded to 11 countries to determine the magnitude of UI in the region. In Thailand, the prevalence was 17%, Taiwan 12%, and the Philippines had a prevalence of 13%. China and Singapore reported the lowest prevalence rate of only 4%.

The study aimed to establish the prevalence of UI, identify the demographic factors related to its occurrence and ascertain the determinants for seeking help for this condition among the female population of Southeast Asia.

A 34-item multiple-choice type questionnaire based assessment was designed to determine presence of UI, defined as the inappropriate leakage of urine, its associated symptoms and the resulting degree of bother, and the action taken to address the condition. This questionnaire was translated into the local dialects and was validated in each country and was administered by medically trained personnel to randomly selected women consulting at outpatient clinics for non-urologic or non-gynecologic problems. The survey was conducted in a total of ten centers: two in the Philippines, one in Singapore, two in Malaysia, one in Indonesia, and four in Thailand.

The first part of the questionnaire included questions on population demographics such as age, civil status, parity, educational attainment, occupation, monthly family income, and place of residence. The general voiding pattern was established by noting the normal daytime and nocturnal voiding frequencies. The main body of the questionnaire focused on establishing the presence of voiding dysfunction, particularly UI and overactive bladder through extensive inquiry on the different symptoms associated with these conditions.

Incontinence as a problem was assessed according to the degree of bother it caused the subject using a scoring system of 0 to 5 (0 as none, 5 as severe). In addition, the need for leakage protection and whether the subject sought help for her condition. The relationship between the occurrence of UI and age, parity, number of vaginal deliveries, occupation, family income, type of toilet used, family history, and place of residence were also analyzed.

Study Population Demographics

Table 6.3 shows the distribution of the study population per country (total respondents 2422). While each age group was well represented (Table 6.4), the population studied was relatively young, with the majority aged below 60 years old and more than 50% younger than 40 years. Forty-four percent of the study population were nulliparous. Among the parous respondents, the majority had had at least two deliveries (Table 6.5). Most of the women were doing office work (Table 6.6). There was a high literacy rate, with more than 85% of the population having had at least a secondary level of education (Table 6.7). The study population was evenly distributed among the income groups (Table 6.8), and at least 60% resided in the urban area (Table 6.9).

Table 6.3 Frequency Distribution of Study Population According to Country

	N	%
Philippines	682	28.2
Singapore	228	9.4
Malaysia	351	14.5
Indonesia	257	10.6
Thailand	904	37.3
Total	2422	100.0

Table 6.4 Frequency Distribution of Study Population According to Age

	N	%
18–28	726	30.0
29–39	676	27.9
40–49	474	19.6
50–59	324	13.4
60–69	153	6.3
≥70	64	2.6
NI	5	0.2
Total	2422	100.0

Abbreviation: NI, not indicated.

Table 6.5 Frequency Distribution of Survey Population According to Parity

	N	%
0	1059	43.7
1	273	11.3
2–4	786	32.5
5–8	260	10.7
>8	40	1.7
NI	4	0.2
Total	2422	100.0

Abbreviation: NI, not indicated.

Table 6.6 Frequency Distribution of Survey Population According to Occupation

	N	%
Manual labor	296	12.2
Office work	1105	45.6
Others	904	37.3
Unemployed	117	4.8
Total	2422	99.9

Table 6.7 Frequency Distribution of Survey Population According to Educational Attainment

	N	%
Never went to school	84	3.5
Primary school	293	12.1
Secondary school	582	24.0
Pre-university	380	15.7
University	652	26.9
Professional education	414	17.1
NI	17	0.7
Total	2422	100.0

Abbreviation: NI, not indicated.

Table 6.8 Frequency Distribution of Survey Population According to Monthly Income

	N	%
A	316	13.0
B	310	12.8
C	493	20.4
D	322	13.3
E	424	17.5
F	375	15.5
NI	182	7.5
Total	2422	100.0

Abbreviation: NI, not indicated.

Table 6.9 Frequency Distribution of Survey Population According to Place of Residence

	N	%
Urban	1473	60.8
Semi-urban	676	27.9
Rural	230	9.5
NI	43	1.8
Total	2422	100.0

Abbreviation: NI, not indicated.

General Voiding Pattern

The voiding pattern of the study population was analyzed according to the frequency of urination (Table 6.10). The majority voided fewer than eight times during the day, with half of this population voiding between four and eight times. Almost all voided fewer than three times during the night, with nearly one-third not voiding at all at night time. Around 72% of the study population voided fewer than eight times per 24 hours.

Prevalence of UI

The prevalence of UI in the study population was 14.8% (359/2422). Nearly half of the incontinent individuals (47.9%) presented with the mixed type. Eighty-one women (22.6%) had stress incontinence while less than 10% presented with urge incontinence (Table 6.11).

INCONTINENCE AS A PROBLEM

The majority of the population who experienced incontinence in this survey was not bothered or, if so, were only mildly bothered by their condition (Table 6.12). However, a major portion (157/359 or 43.7%) felt that protection from leakage was necessary. Of the 359 affected individuals, 150 (41.8%) sought help for their condition.

Table 6.10 Frequency Distribution of Survey Population According to Voiding Frequency: (A) daytime, (B) nighttime, and (C) twenty-four Hour Frequency.

	N	%
(A) Daytime		
1	74	3.1
2–4	917	37.9
4–8	1217	50.2
>8	167	6.9
NI	47	1.9
Total	2422	100.0
(B) Nigthtime		
0	628	2509
1	1027	4204
2–3	667	27.5
>3	73	3.0
NI	27	1.1
Total	2422	99.9
(C) 24-hour		
<8	1737	71.7
≥8	638	26.3
NI	47	1.9
Total	2422	99.9

Abbreviation: NI, not indicated.

Table 6.11 Frequency Distribution of Incontinent Population According to Type of Incontinence.

Type	N	%
Stress	81	22.6
Urge	31	8.6
Mixed	172	47.9
Undetermined	75	20.9
Total	359	100.0

Table 6.12 Frequency Distribution of Incontinent Population According to Degree of Bother.

Bother score	N	%
0—none	130	36.2
1—very mild	94	26.2
2—mild	54	15.0
3—moderate	23	6.4
4—severe	14	3.9
5—very severe	18	5.0
NI	26	7.2
Total	359	99.9

Abbreviation: NI, not indicated.

Factors Related to the Occurrence of UI

Age, parity, mode of delivery or childbirth, number of vaginal deliveries, occupation, family history, and family income were found to be significantly related to the occurrence of UI. The type of toilet used and the place of residence were not found to be related to the occurrence of the condition (Table 6.13).

Age

Increasing age was found to be significantly related to the occurrence of incontinence. By the age of 40 years, the risk for incontinence was found to be increased by 2.5 times (95% CI 2.0–3.1). The odds progressively increased to 2.8 times and 3.4 times at ages 50 and 60 years, respectively.

Parity

The majority of the incontinent population was parous. There was a significant correlation between increasing prevalence of incontinence with higher parity. A woman who has delivered at least once was found to be 2.1 times (95% CI 1.6–2.7) at risk for incontinence compared to the nulliparous. With a parity of more than four, the odds increased to 2.5 times.

Mode of Delivery

There was a higher prevalence of incontinence among those who delivered vaginally, by forceps delivery, or a combination of both; a woman who has given birth vaginally has twice the risk of UI than one who has delivered abdominally.

Number of Vaginal Deliveries

Taking into account vaginal deliveries (including forceps delivery), there was a significant relationship of increasing prevalence of incontinence with a higher number of deliveries. More than one vaginal delivery increased a woman's risk for incontinence to 2.0 times (95% CI 1.6–2.6). The odds increased to 2.6 times when the number of deliveries reached five.

Occupation

The prevalence of incontinence was highest among those doing manual labor (see Table 6.6). This was found to be statistically significant, with a woman who has done manual labor at 1.6 times (95% CI 1.3–2.1) the risk of having incontinence.

Family History

The family history of incontinence was significantly related to the occurrence of the condition. A woman with a positive family history was 2.4 times (95% CI 1.9–3.0) at risk of having the condition as compared to one without.

Family Income

A higher prevalence of incontinence was found among those from the lower income group, which was found to be statistically significant. A woman earning less than "E" had 1.7 times risk (95% CI 1.3–2.2) of having incontinence.

Factors Associated with Seeking Help for UI

Forty-two percent of the incontinent population sought help for their condition, consulting either a specialist or a general practitioner (Table 6.14). Among the factors studied in relation to the likelihood of seeking help for UI, only age and degree of bother were noted to be significant (Table 6.15). Increasing age positively influenced the likelihood of seeking a consultation. A woman of at least 50 years of age is 2.4 times more likely to seek help for her condition compared to a younger woman. This likelihood increases to 2.5 times by age 60 years.

Table 6.13 Demographic Factors and Their Relation with the Occurrence of Urinary Incontinence

Factor	Incontinence[a] Yes	P-value No	Odd's ratio	95% Confidence interval	
Age					
18–28	58	661	<0.001	2.466 (<40 vs. ≥40)	1.959–3.105
29–39	82	587		2.766 (<50 vs. ≥50)	2.178–3.512
40–49	76	397		3.391 (<60 vs. ≥60)	2.491–4.615
50–59	69	248			
60–69	49	103			
>70	24	40			
Parity					
0	104	943	<0.001	3.391 (0 vs. ≥1)	1.648–2.685
1	38	232		(<5 vs. ≥5)	
2–4	133	646			
5–8	69	191			
>8	14	26			
Mode of delivery					
Vaginal only	197	813	<0.001	2.067 (vaginal/forceps vs. caesarian/none)	
Caesarian only	26	160			
Forceps only	3	18			
Combination	25	94			
None	104	945			
Number of vaginal deliveries					
0	131	1111	<0.001	2.025 (≤1 vs. >1)	1.613–2.541
1	34	183			
2–4	108	531			
5–8	69	181			
>8	13	24			
Occupation					
Manual labor	62	231	<0.001	1.645 (manual labor vs. office work/ others)	1.284–2.108
Office work	139	958			
Others	152	752			
Monthly income					
A	30	286	<0.001	1.367 (<F vs. F)	1.021–1.831
				1.682 (<E vs. ≥E)	1.303–2.171
B	56	253			
C	82	406			
D	54	264			
E	43	377			
F	69	302			
Family history					
Yes	174	631	<0.001	2.411	1.924–3.021
No	104	1056			
Type of toilet used					
Sitting	239	1345	NS	NA	NA
Squatting	109	595			
Both	9	86			
Place of residence					
Urban	210	1249	NS	NA	NA
Semi urban	107	566			
Rural	35	194			

[a]Counts may not total to 2422 because category "not available" was not included in the analysis.
Abbreviations: NA, not applicable; NS, not significant.

The incontinent female who is moderately bothered (score of at least 3) is 3.7 times (95% CI 2.0–6.9) more likely to seek consultation for her condition compared to one who is less affected. A severe condition increases this likelihood to 5.1 times (95% CI 2.5–10.4).

Discussion

Prevalence—Comparison with World Figures

The prevalence of UI in this Asian survey is comparable to the Western figures (47–50) and demonstrates the fact that while the condition may not present as a significant problem, UI is

Table 6.14 Frequency Distribution of Incontinent Females Who Sought Help According to Person Consulted

Person consulted	n	%
Herbalist/traditional medical practitioner	19	12.7
General practitioner	34	22.7
Primary health care center	17	11.3
Specialist	37	24.7
Nurse	16	10.7
Others	9	6.0
TMP + GP	5	3.3
TMP + GP + SP	3	2.0
GP + SP	3	2.0
TMP + PHCC	6	4.0
NI	1	0.7
Total	150	100.1

Abbreviations: GP, general practitioner; NI, not indicated; SP, specialist; TMP, traditional medical practitioner; PHCC, primary health care center.

prevalent in the Southeast Asian population. Additionally, this puts into question the presumed fact that UI is more common in those with European versus Pacific ancestry. Thus, it is worthwhile investing time and effort to study the problem, its causes and its management (Figs. 6.1 and 6.2).

Types of Incontinence—Comparison with World Figures
The proportion of females with stress incontinence in relation to the other types appears to be relatively low compared to previous studies citing numbers as high as 50%. This may be due to the fact that the population surveyed is relatively young while stress incontinence is more associated with advancing age. Thus, closer attention to the problem of mixed incontinence may be necessary, it being the more prevalent type among Asian females (51–53).

It must be recognized, however, that the classification of incontinence used in many of these surveys is based mainly on

Table 6.15 Demographic Factors and Their Relation with Seeking Help

Factor	Sought help[a] Yes	No	P-value	Odd's ratio	95% Confidence interval
Age					
18–28	15	43	0.001	2.438 (<50 vs. ≥50)	1.578–3.766
29–39	34	48		2.562 (<60 vs. ≥60)	1.513–4.339
40–49	23	53			
50–59	34	35			
60–69	29	20			
>70	15	9			
Education					
Never went school	13	10	NS	NA	NA
Primary	31	35			
Secondary	37	45			
Pre-university	27	42			
University	30	39			
Professional	12	38			
Monthly income					
A	13	17	NS	NA	NA
B	24	33			
C	37	46			
D	25	31			
E	17	32			
F	21	38			
Place of residence					
Urban	79	131	NS	NA	NA
Semi urban	49	59			
Rural	21	14			
Degree of bother					
0—none	38	93	<0.001	3.740 (<3 vs. ≥3)	2.009–6.961
1—very mild	41	53		5.139 (<4 vs. ≥4)	2.528–10.448
2—mild	25	28			
3—moderate	17	6			
4—severe	10	4			
5—very severe	11	7			

[a]Counts may not total 359 because category "not available" was not included in the analysis.
Abbreviations: NA, not applicable; NS, not significant.

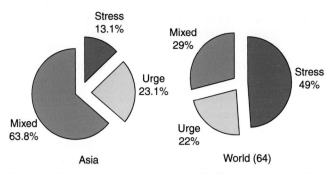

Figure 6.1 Types of urinary incontinence in World and Asia. *Source:* From Ref. 64.

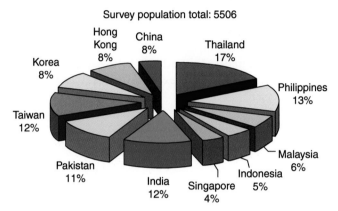

Figure 6.2 Prevalence of urinary incontinence in Asia.

symptoms alone and not on any objective parameter. This is a limitation inherent in the study design, as previous studies have noted that symptoms alone do not accurately classify incontinence. Therefore, further studies must be done to verify the discrepancy in the distribution of the different types of incontinence among Asian females compared to their Western counterparts.

The factors found to be related to the occurrence of incontinence were not unexpected. Older age, higher parity, higher number of vaginal deliveries, the increased physical strain associated with manual labor, and the use of a sitting toilet have all been cited and accepted as contributing to the weakness of the pelvic floor leading to incontinence (54). Aging has been associated with the loss of striated muscle in the area of the urethra leading to impaired continence. The change in the hormonal milieu brought about by aging also affects the ability of the urethral submucosal layer to provide the watertight closure of the female urethra. Childbearing, childbirth (55), and physical straining have been found to cause hypermobility, innervation injuries (56), and connective tissue changes (57) to the pelvic floor leading to loss of support.

Family History, Family Income, and the Occurrence of Incontinence
The significant relation between a positive family history of UI and its occurrence may be indicative of a possible hereditary

component to the disease. A congenital predisposition to UI has been proposed, citing a common collagen makeup of the pelvic floor found among the affected group. However, a more likely explanation is the tendency of the members of one family to be exposed to the same type of work and physical stresses that predispose an individual to UI.

It is difficult to explain the reason behind the relationship between family income and the occurrence of incontinence. This factor may be related to parity, with those belonging in the lower income bracket having a higher parity. In addition, the lower income group tends to do more manual labor. Thus, it may be necessary to test the interdependence of these factors to see the true relationship between income and UI.

Factors Related to Seeking Help—Possible Explanations
The proportion of the incontinent population seeking help in the APCAB study is higher than most study investigators expected since this condition has been regarded as a rare clinical entity among Asians, though the same is not true for studies in other countries (58). While this observation is an interesting finding, this high figure may be due to the fact that this survey is institution-based and the population surveyed may be those who are motivated to seek a medical consult for any disease condition. Therefore, a community-based survey must be undertaken in order to verify this finding.

It is interesting to note that almost one-fifth of those seeking help do so by seeing a traditional medical practitioner. This underscores the high regard the Asian patient still gives to traditional medical science despite decades of Western medicine with its advances. Further studies must be conducted to determine why this is so. This is important in the creation of efficient and effective programs that aim to encourage the affected population to find the solution to their problem.

It is apparent that demographic data are inadequate to fully explain the occurrence of UI and why an affected individual seeks help for the condition. A more objective assessment and a clinical study of the disease must be undertaken to completely understand its pathophysiology. In addition, a deeper and more exhaustive analysis of the attitude of the population toward the disease and the reasons for seeking consult is warranted. Knowledge gained from this will be valuable in future programs and campaigns to increase awareness of UI and to encourage the affected population and the caregivers to address the problem and pursue its solution.

Conclusion
The prevalence of UI among Southeast Asian females appears comparable to worldwide figures. As such, it is a significant and common problem requiring attention. The incontinent female in Southeast Asia is most likely to be older, of higher parity, have delivered vaginally, does manual labor, earns less, has a positive family history for the disorder, uses a squatting toilet, and resides in a rural area. A significant portion of the incontinent population has been noted to seek help. This is most likely composed of the older age group and those who suffer from the condition to a greater degree.

CONCLUSION

The occurrence of UI can be described in terms of prevalence (the number of individuals who have incontinence at a point in time), incidence (the number of individuals who newly develop incontinence in a period of time), and the natural history (whether incontinence improves, stays the same, or worsens over time) (59). Each of these measures varies with factors such as whether the individual is living in the community or in a nursing home and the individual's sex, age, and racial or ethnic group. Severity of incontinence also varies in its frequency and amount. In addition, incontinence has many different causes.

Prevalence of UI in women living in the community increases with age, from 19% at age younger than 45 years to 29% in age 80 years and older; the rate levels off from age 50 to age 70 years, after which prevalence again increases.

Information comparing prevalence in racial or ethnic groups suggests that UI is prevalent in all ethnic groups, with some suggestion of higher rates among white women.

With the exception of prevalence of UI, most estimates of the incidence and prevalence of incontinence in adults are based on relatively small numbers of studies. Because these studies used varying definitions of incontinence and different methods of population sampling, the preceding statistics should be considered to be fairly crude estimates.

Although it is impossible to compare surveys between different time periods, countries, or even authors from the same continent or country, the numbers reported seem higher than actually seen in clinical practice, which could be due many different factors that cause differences in various prevalence rates, which may be due to technical, or cultural differences or due to management strategies offered. Hampel (60), in a meta-analysis, reviewed a series of publications for prevalence rates of incontinence throughout the world, reported stress incontinence as the most prevalent type of all incontinence.

We must have a uniform standardized survey questionnaire (61) that is as applicable in all over the world in developed and developing countries. Without standardizing the questionnaires, we will continue to have reports that may not be meaningful for all interested parties, and it will be impossible to compare the outcomes of different studies. In determining the severity of incontinence, the frequency of UI is important, but equally important is the volume loss. A vast majority of women suffering from stress incontinence with small volume loss will usually cope with their problem and not necessarily seek medical care, whereas an individual who experiences an episode of one big volume loss will be urgently seek help (Tables 6.14 and 6.15). It is therefore imperative that, when obtaining history and performing a survey, volume loss in addition to frequency be part of the information. Recording this information would make it possible to measure the severity on the basis of a combination of these parameters.

The type of urine loss is also of utmost importance (62). We all know that there are different types and that each has its own unique signs and symptoms and unique methods of management. Urge type and mixed stress and urge incontinence appear to be the most common forms of UI in elderly men and women. If we are to understand UI better, we have to know which type we are dealing with. The correlates of UI are well known.

Finally, conventional epidemiologic (63) studies must incorporate issues relevant to all individuals suffering from incontinence, including quality of life (social and emotional well being), financial burden, effects on work and home.

Although UI is common among community-dwelling individuals over 40 years of age, the majority of affected individuals remained untreated due to lack of knowledge and/or a negative perception of UI (64). Thus, community education on UI may be needed to increase the number of UI patients who receive treatment.

ACKNOWLEDGMENTS

"A certain amount of the material in this chapter has been taken from work mentioned in the First Edition by Prof Peter HC Lim and Associate Prof Mela C Lapitan in their chapter on the subject and updated accordingly by this author" and we also acknowledge the assistance of Mr Won-Hee Park in updating this chapter.

REFERENCES

1. Wyman J. The psychiatric and emotional impact of female pelvic floor dysfunction. Curr Opin Obstet Gynecol 1994; 6: 336–9.
2. Hollywood B, O'Dowd T. Female urinary incontinence: another chronic illness. Br J Gen Pract 1998; 48: 1727–8.
3. Grimby A, Milson I, Molander U, et al. The influence of urinary incontinence on the quality of life of elderly women. Age Ageing 1993; 22: 82–9.
4. Lam G, Foldspang A, Elving LB, Mommsem S. Social context, social abstention, and problem recognition correlated with adult female urinary incontinence. Dan Med Bull 1992; 39: 565–70.
5. Bogner HR, Gallo JJ, Sammel MD, et al. Urinary incontinence and psychological distress in community-dwelling older adults. J Am Geriatr Soc 2002; 50: 489–95.
6. White H, Getliffe K. Incontinence in perspective. In: Getliffe K, Dolman M, eds. Promoting Continence: A Clinical and Research Resource, 2nd edn. London, UK: Baillière Tindall, 2003: 1–19.
7. Wyman JF. Treatment of urinary incontinence in men & older women. Am J Nurs 2003; 103 (Suppl): 26–35.
8. Lekan-Rutledge D, Colling J. Urinary incontinence in the frail elderly. Am J Nurs 2003; 103 (Suppl): 36–46.
9. DuBeau C E. Urinary incontinence: taking action against this 'silent epidemic'. Lancet 1995; 346: 94–9.
10. Ee CH. Urinary incontinence in the elderly. In: Chin CM, Lim HCP, eds. Clinical Handbook on the Management of Incontinence, 2nd edn. Singapore: Society for Continence, 2001: 109–26.
11. Gray ML. Gender, race, and culture in research on UI. Am J Nurs 2003; 103 (Suppl): 20–5.
12. Koch T, Hralik D, Kelly S. We just don't talk about it: Men living with urinary incontinence and multiple sclerosis. Int J Nurs Pract 2000; 6: 253–60.
13. Ueda T, Tamaki M, Kageyama S, Yoshimura N, Yoshida O. Urinary incontinence among community-dwelling people aged 40 years or older in Japan: prevalence, risk factors, knowledge and self-perception. Int J Urol 2000; 7: 95–103.
14. Dorey G. Conservative Treatment of Male Urinary Incontinence and Erectile Dysfunction: A Textbook for Physiotherapists, Nurses and Doctors. London, UK: Whurr, 2001.
15. Holroyd-Leduc JM, Mebta KM, Covinsky KE. Urinary incontinence and its association with death, nursing home admission, and functional decline. J Am Geriatr Soc 2004; 52: 712–18.
16. Thakar R, Stanton S. Management of urinary incontinence in women. BMJ 2000; 321: 1326–31.

17. DuBeau CE. Urinary incontinence. In: Evans JG, Williams TF, Beattie BL, Michel J-P, Willcock GK, eds. Oxford Textbook of Geriatric Medicine, 2nd edn. Oxford, UK: Oxford University Press, 2000: 677–89.

18. Fultz NH, Herzog AR. Self-reported social and emotional impact of urinary incontinence. J Am Geriatr Soc 2001; 49: 892–9.

19. Roe B, Doll H. Prevalence of urinary incontinence and its relationship with health status. J Clin Nurs 2000; 9: 178–88.

20. Cooper JW, ed. Urinary Incontinence in the Elderly: Pharmacotherapy Treatment. New York: Pharmaceutical Products Press, 1997.

21. Specht JP, Maas ML. Urinary incontinence: functional, iatrogenic, overflow, teflex, stress, total, and urge. In: Maas ML, Buckwalter KC, Hardy MD, et al., eds. Nursing Care of Older Adults: Diagnoses, Outcomes and Interventions. St. Louis, MO: Mosby, 2001: 252–78.

22. AHCPR (Agency for Health Care Policy and Research) Urinary Incontinence in Adults Guideline Update Panel. Managing acute and chronic urinary incontinence: clinical practice guidelines, quick reference guide for clinicians. Am Fam Physician 1996; 54: 1661–72.

23. Burgio KL, Locher JL. Urinary incontinence. In: Carstensen LL, Edelstein BA, Dornbrand L, eds. The Practical Handbook of Clinical Gerontology. Thousand Oaks, CA: Sage, 1996: 349–73.

24. Burgio KL, Goode PS, Varner RE, et al. Treatment of urinary incontinence: current status and future directions. In: Clair JM, Allman RM, eds. The Gerontological Prism: Developing Interdisciplinary Bridges. Amityville, NY: Baywood, 2000: 281–303.

25. Johnson TM II, Bernard SL, Kincade JE, Defriese GH. Urinary incontinence and risk of death among community-living elderly people: results from the national survey on self-care and aging. J Aging Health 2000; 12: 25–46.

26. Chapple CR, MacDiarmid SA. Urodynamics Made Easy. London, UK: WB Saunders Company, 2000.

27. Yarnell J, St. Leger A. The prevalence, severity, and factors associated with urinary incontinence in a random sample of the elderly. Age Ageing 1979; 8: 81–5.

28. Tobin GW. Incontinence in the Elderly. London, UK: Edward Arnold, 1992.

29. Hunskar S, Arnold EP, Burgio K, et al. Epidemiology and natural history of urinary incontinence. Int Urogynecol J Pelvic Floor Dysfunct 2000; 11: 301–19.

30. Thomas T. Prevalence of urinary incontinence. BMJ 1980; 281: 1243–5.

31. Outlander J. Urinary incontinence in nursing homes. J Am Geriatr Soc 1990; 3: 289–91.

32. Milos I, Eke Lund P, Molander U, et al. The influence of age, parity, oral contraception, hysterectomy and menopause on the prevalence of urinary incontinence in women. J Urol 1993; 149: 1459–62.

33. Herzog A, Fultz N. Prevalence and incidence of urinary incontinence in community dwelling populations. J Am Geriatr Soc 1990; 38: 273–81.

34. Whishaw M. Urinary incontinence in the elderly: establishing a cause may allow a cure. Aust Fam Physician 1998; 27: 1087–90.

35. Wall L, Norton P, Delaney J. Practical Urodynamics. Baltimore: Williams and Wilkins, 1993.

36. Christopher M Doran, Pauline Chiarelli, Jill Cockburn. Economic costs of urinary incontinence in community-dwelling Australian women. MJA 2001; 174: 456–8; Aging (Milano) 1996; 8: 47–54.

37. Millard R, Chiarelli P, Bower W, Szonyi G, Talley N. The Epidemiology of Urinary and Anal Incontinence. A report prepared in three parts (Executive Summary, Part A and Part B) for the Australian Government Department of Health and Ageing, 2001.

38. Chiarelli P, Bower W, Attia J, Sibbrit D, Wilson A. The Prevalence of Faecal Incontinence: A Systematic Review. Report prepared for the Australian Government Department of Health and Ageing, 2002.

39. Chiarelli P, Bower W, Wilson A, Sibbrit D, Attia J. The Prevalence of Urinary Incontinence Within the Community: A Systematic Review. Report prepared for the Australian Government Department of Health and Ageing, 2002.

40. Nakanishi N, Tatara K, Naramura H, et al. Urinary and fecal incontinence in a community-residing older population in Japan. Department of Public Health, Osaka Medical School, Japan. J Am Geriatr Soc 1997; 45: 215–19.

41. Toba K, Ouchi Y, Orimo H, et al. Urinary incontinence in elderly inpatients in Japan: a comparison between general and geriatric hospitals. Aging (Milano) 1996; 8: 47–54.

42. Ueda T, Tamaki M, Kageyama S, Yoshimura N, Yoshida O. Urinary incontinence among community-dwelling people aged 40 years or older in Japan: prevalence, risk factors, knowledge and self-perception. Int J Urol 2000; 7: 95–103.

43. Lee J-J. The impact of urinary incontinence levels on the social lives of older Chinese in Hong Kong. Hallym Int J Aging 2005; 7: 63–80.

44. Myung-Soo Choo, Ja Hyeon Ku, Seung-June Oh. Prevalence of urinary incontinence in Korean women: an epidemiologic survey. Int Urogynecol J 2007; 18: 1309–15.

45. Shakhatreh FMN. Epidemiology of urinary incontinence in Jordanian women. Saudi Med J 2005; 26: 830–5.

46. Lapitan C-MM. Epidemiology of urinary incontinence in Asia. In: Chin CM, Lim H-CP, eds. Clinical Handbook on the Management of Incontinence, 2nd edn. Singapore: Society for Continence, 2001: 1–4.

47. Thomas TM, Plymat KR, Blannin J, Meade TW. Prevalence of urinary incontinence. Br Med J 1980; 281: 1243–5.

48. Jolleys JV. Reported prevalence of urinary incontinence in women in a general practice. Br Med J 1988; 296: 1300–2.

49. Vetter NJ, Jones DA, Victor CR. Urinary incontinence in the elderly at home. Lancet 1981; I: 1275–7.

50. Molander U, Milsom I, Ekelund P, Mellstrom D. An epidemiological study of urinary incontinence and related urogenital symptoms in elderly women. Maturitas 1990; 12: 51–60.

51. Sommer P, Bauer T, Nielson KK, et al. Voiding patterns and prevalence of women. A questionnaire survey. Br J Urol 1990; 66: 12–15.

52. Burgio KL, Matthews KA, Engel BT. Prevalence, incidence and correlates of urinary incontinence in healthy, middle-aged women. J Urol 1991; 146: 1255–9.

53. Payne CK. Epidemiology, pathophysiology and evaluation of urinary incontinence and overactive bladder. Urology 1998; 51(Suppl 2A): 3–10.

54. Shershan S, Ansari RL. The frequency of urinary incontinence in Pakistani women. J Pak Med Assoc 1989; 39: 16–7.

55. Allen RE, Hosker GL, Smith ARB, Warrell DW. Pelvic floor damage and childbirth: a neurophysiological study. Br J Obstet Gynaecol 1990; 97: 770–9.

56. Snooks SJ, Swash M, Setchell M, Henry MM. Injury to innervation of pelvic floor sphincter musculature in childbirth. Lancet 1984; ii: 546–50.

57. Eldabawi A, Yalla SV, Resnick NM. Structural basis of geriatric voiding dysfunction. III. Detrusor overactivity. J Urol 1993; 150: 1650–6.

58. Lapitan MC, Chye PLH. The epidemiology of overactive bladder among females in Asia: A questionnaire survey. Int Urogynecol J 2001; 12: 226–31.

59. Kobelt G, Kirchberger I, Malone-Lee J. Quality of life aspects of the overactive bladder and the effect of treatment with tolterodine. Br J Urol 1999; 83: 583–90.

60. Hampel C, Artibani W, Espuña Pons M, et al. Understanding the burden of stress urinary incontinence in Europe: a qualitative review of the literature. Eur Urol 2004; 46: 15–27.

61. Diokno AC. Epidemiology of urinary incontinence. J Gerontol A Biol Sci Med Sci 2001; 56: M3–4.

62. Bump RC. Racial comparison and contracts in urinary incontinence and pelvic organ prolapse. Obstet Gynecol 1993; 81: 421–5.

63. Maggi S, Minicuci N, Langlois J, et al. Prevalance rate of urinary incontinence in community-dwelling elderly individuals: the Veneto study. J Gerontol A Biol Sci Med Sci 2001; 56: M14–18.

64. Choo MS, Ku JH, Oh SJ, et al. Prevalence of urinary incontinence in Korean women: an epidemiologic survey. Int Urogynecol J Pelvic Floor Dysfunct 2007; 18: 1309–15.

7 Epidemiology of Incontinence in Africa

Peter de Jong and Stephen Jeffery

INTRODUCTION

The impact of urinary incontinence on the lives of African women is very different from the experience on any other continent. Stress and urge urinary incontinence no doubt affect the quality of life of African women, but by far the heaviest burden Africa carries in terms of female urinary incontinence is in the prevailing problem of vesico-vaginal fistulae.

Crippling poverty is the main cause of obstetric fistulae, resulting in a huge burden of disease on individuals who ultimately suffer alone with its devastating sequelae. The obstetric fistula is the one continence problem that is unique to, and especially prevalent in developing countries (1). The occurrence of obstetric fistulae has declined in industrialized countries but they remain both common and problematic in rural Africa. In sub-Saharan Africa the incidence of obstetric fistulae is estimated to be about 124 cases per 100,000 deliveries in rural areas, with virtually no cases in major cities (2). The problem is further highlighted by the fact that the greatest imbalances between the healthcare systems of poor and rich nations are in the areas of HIV and maternal health (3). The fistula problem in third world countries will not be solved until those nations develop effective systems of maternal health care and workable infrastructure. The high prevalence of this condition in many parts of rural Africa highlights this glaring issue as one of the most neglected of modern injustices (4).

Africa has unique problems and challenges. Life expectancy is below 50 years in most countries on the continent compared to the world average of 66 (5). Based on socioeconomic and human development ratings, the United Nations has classified 49 countries as Least Developed Countries (LDCs or Fourth World countries) and currently 34 African countries are currently rated as LDCs. The total population of Africa is estimated at 522 million (6). There are, however, very little data available on the epidemiology of urinary incontinence on the continent. A Medline search using keywords "incontinence," "Africa" followed by a sequential Medline search using "incontinence" and each of the 56 African countries revealed scanty data on incontinence with only a handful of poor quality studies reporting basic epidemiological data such as prevalence. There were 33 papers reporting on fistulae and looking specifically at studies from sub-Saharan Africa, but there were none looking at overactive bladder and only two reporting on stress incontinence.

It is easier to understand why the issue of urinary incontinence, particularly stress and urge urinary incontinence, has received such poor attention over the years when one considers the problem in the context of other major African diseases. Africa has 11% of the world population but 60% of those with AIDS. There are more than one million deaths from malaria and a half a million deaths from tuberculosis each year in Africa (7). Africa also has a large rural-dwelling population and currently only about 37% of Africans live in cities. About 72% of those in Sub-Saharan Africa live in slum conditions. Only 58% of sub-Saharan Africans have safe water supplies and 36% have sanitation. This makes access to even the most basic medical care a challenge (6).

Over the past two decades, Africa has suffered civil wars and unrest, thus preventing the development of infrastructure and basic healthcare. In 1997 there were 8.1 million refugees in Africa and most of these were women and children (8). The consequences of this include poor living conditions and increased violence. Women also carry a very heavy economic burden in Africa. The UN Food and Agriculture Organization (FAO) surveyed the women of nine countries in Africa. They reported that women were involved in 70% of food production and close to 100% of food processing in Africa. Quality of life issues like stress or urge incontinence will often not feature on many women's priority list. African women are also often not empowered to seek help, with little political influence, and this further reduces their access to healthcare.

A major factor affecting the treatment of women with incontinence in Africa is the poor quality of healthcare. Many women do not have access to even the most basic healthcare, not to mention expensive anticholinergic drugs, incontinence pads and mid-urethral tapes. The central region of Kenya has a total of 190 doctors and a doctor-patient ratio of 1:20,715, whilst the north eastern region has only nine doctors with a doctor patient ratio of 1:120,823 (9). Access to specialist services is even more confined, usually limited to the large cities. This equates to reduced access to the necessary skills and resources to investigate and treat women with incontinence. Surgical training is also limited which results in a small number of urologists and gynecologists capable of managing incontinence. Surgical training, or lack thereof, may also increase the risk of developing post-hysterectomy fistula.

There is as yet no subspecialty training program in female urology or urogynecology in Africa (10). South Africa, which leads the way in many fields in African medicine, has only recently formally recognized urogynecology as subspecialty.

FISTULA-RELATED INCONTINENCE

There are two chapters covering urogenital fistula in this volume and for the purposes of this review, the authors will only discuss epidemiological data relating to Africa. There are as yet no comprehensive epidemiological data describing the distribution of fistulae in Africa and almost no population-based studies reporting on the problem. Many of the unfortunate women suffering from this condition are social outcasts, and this further obscures the extent of the disease as well as skewing any data reporting on prevalence and incidence. We are thus left to interpret data collected at large teaching hospitals and fistula centers.

In Ethiopia, 9000 women annually develop a fistula, of which 1200 are repaired. In Ethiopia, Nigeria, and other parts of West Africa, the incidence of fistulae is up to 10 per 1000 births (2). Data from a Nigerian university teaching hospital report 350 cases of vesico-vaginal fistulae per 100,000 deliveries (11). A prospective population study of 19,342 women in West Africa (12) described a prevalence for fistulae of 10.3 per 100,000 urban and 123.9 for rural dwelling women. Extrapolating from these data, the authors estimate a prevalence of 33,451 new obstetric fistulae per year for sub-Saharan Africa.

Large parts of Africa are grossly under-resourced when it comes to obstetric services. Care in labor, which includes prevention of a prolonged first and second stage and intervention for obstructed labor, with recourse to timely caesarean section, is essential in preventing injury to the pelvic floor. Obstetric fistulae usually occur due to delays in women receiving appropriate interventions in labor. Maternal mortality will occur if there is delay in seeking care, delay in arrival at the health care facility, and delay in intervention once arriving at the facility (13). Maternal mortality ratios (MMR) are often considered to be a reflection of obstetric services in a specified country. The reported MMR for the United States of America in 2004 was 13 per 100,000 live births compared with a mean of 900 for Africa as a whole. Rates as high as 1600 for Angola and 1800 for Mali have been reported (14).

Coupled to high maternal mortality rates are high morbidity rates (15). In some regions, where obstructed labor is a major cause of maternal death, the rate of obstetric fistulae may approach the maternal mortality rate (16–18). The "road to obstetric fistula" for many women starts when they have a nutritionally marginal childhood and then marry at puberty, becoming pregnant while still going through adolescence. These girls then labor at home with no access to skilled care (19). Sexual maturity is also achieved before the pelvic girdle is fully grown and an adolescent girl is therefore at greater risk for developing obstructed labor (20).

Sobering data emerged from a sample of women treated for fistula at the renowned Addis Ababa Fistula hospital between 1983 and 1988 (19). The mean age was 22 years, 42% were younger than 20 years of age, 52% had been deserted by their husbands, and 21% lived by begging. Furthermore, 30% had delivered without assistance, and the average labor had lasted 3.9 days. Meyer et al. also report (21) disturbing data from Niger where they investigated the epidemiology of vesico-vaginal fistula in 58 women. The average labor lasted 2.61 days and an average of 1.61 days passed before intrapartum assistance was sought and 91% of babies were stillborn. Kelly and Kwast (22) reported on a sample of 309 women attending the well-known Hamlin Bahirdar Fistula Center in Ethiopia. Of these patients, 82% had traveled at least 700 km for treatment, walking an average of 12 hours and spending an average of 34 hours on a bus, before arriving at the treatment center.

Danso and Martey (16), in a study from Ghana, reporting on 150 fistulae, found that 91% were as a result of a complicated labor and 9% due to gynecological surgery. Twenty-five percent of the women in this study were at least para five which may represent increased birth weight with advanced parity or possible changes in tissue elasticity with age.

Wall and colleagues (1) analyzed 899 obstetric fistula patients from Jos, Nigeria, and found that women with fistulae tended to have been married early (often before menarche), to be short (nearly 80% were less than 150 cm tall), small (mean weight less than 44 kg), to be impoverished, poorly educated, and to live in rural areas. Kelly et al. (19) report that more than 50% of women with fistula in Africa had been rejected by their husbands.

Other causes of fistulae include injuries sustained during complicated gynecologic surgery performed under difficult circumstances, or fistulae resulting from complications of caesarean delivery. These often involve women who arrive at hospital in need of immediate emergency surgery, performed by physicians without adequate operative experience, under circumstances in which they have suboptimal equipment and support. Vesico—uterine fistulas, for example, are frequently the result of complications encountered during caesarean section, rather than direct consequences of prolonged obstructed labor (23). In the study of 164 fistulas reported by Danso and colleagues (16) from Ghana, 150 cases (91.5%) were due to obstetric complications. Of these 150 fistulas, 121 were due to prolonged obstructed labor and 24 were due to complications of caesarean section. A further 12 cases were due to complications of abdominal hysterectomy.

Fistulae may also be caused by accidents or trauma such as penetrating injuries to the vagina and bladder, infection (particurlarly lymphogranuloma venereum, diphtheria, measles, schistosomiasis, tuberculosis), infected bites, foreign bodies, bladder calculi, and cervical cancer (24). In a dated South African study (24) published in 1966, 52 (17%) of 309 fistula were as a result of advanced carcinoma of the cervix. Cervical cancer is the still the most common female malignancy on the continent, and no doubt remains responsible for many cases of vesico-vaginal fistulae.

Much concern has focused recently on genital cutting practices commonly referred to as "female circumcision" or "female genital mutilation" (FGM) (25). About two million African girls per year undergo female genital cutting. It is most prevalent in Somalia, Ethiopia, Sierra Leone, Sudan, and Djibouti. Urinary incontinence may occur if there is direct injury to the bladder or urethra. It may also obstruct the vaginal outlet and hence make fistulae more common following delivery. The literature reporting on the role of FGM in the development of fistula and incontinence remains unclear. Peterman and Johnson (26) could not find a significant relationship in their Demographic and Health Surveys study in Malawi, Rwanda, Uganda, and Ethiopia. Dirie and Lindmark (27) interviewed 290 Somali women between the ages of 18 and 34 who had undergone circumcision. The mean age of the cohort was 22 years. Eighty-eight percent had undergone excision and infundibulation, 6.5% clitoridectomy, and 5.5% excision of the clitoral prepuce. Thirteen percent of the women experienced late complications including pain at micturition, dribble incontinence and poor urine flow.

Various traditional African remedies are also associated with the development of fistulae. The Northern Nigerian practice of "gishri-cutting," involves making a series of vaginal incisions with glass, a blade, or a knife. Between 2% and 13% of women undergoing this gishri-procedure will get a fistula (1). Herbal remedies for various gynecological conditions, which involve

49

the insertion of caustic chemicals vaginally, are also often used by traditional Africa healers (28). The ensuing vaginal fibrosis and stenosis will occasionally lead to fistula formation (29).

The Malawian Demographic and Health Survey, in an attempt to determine the prevalence of fistulae, interviewed 11,698 women and asked if they ever experienced leakage of urine or stool. Seven percent of those women who had had a recent birth and 4 % of those not having had a recent birth reported either fecal or urinary incontinence. This extrapolates into 16 cases per 1000 live births. These symptoms were more likely to occur amongst rural, poor, uneducated women who had endured stillbirths or were victims of sexual violence (30).

Fistulae caused by sexual abuse and rape are a particularly troubling phenomenon (31). Peterman and Johnson (26) used the recent Demographic and Health Surveys in Malawi, Rwanda, Uganda, and Ethiopia to determine the relationship between sexual violence, female genital cutting, and incontinence. Sexual violence was a significant determinant of incontinence in Rwanda and Malawi but not in Uganda. They suggest that elimination of sexual violence will result in up to a 40% reduction of the burden of incontinence. In situations of conflict, refugees and displaced women and girls often have been sexually assaulted. In wartime conditions, sexual violence is a commonly used tactic to intimidate and control. Aid workers have estimated that in war-torn areas, one woman in three is a rape victim and the majority of new non obstetric fistula cases are caused by rape.

NON-FISTULOUS INCONTINENCE

Non-fistula incontinence is overwhelmingly under-investigated, particularly in sub-Saharan Africa. Epidemiological data regarding urge and stress urinary incontinence in Africa is therefore very limited. Studies performed in Egypt (32,33), Morocco (34), and Tunisia (35). Ghana (36), Nigeria (37), and South Africa (38,39) are the only sub-Saharan countries that have any published data on the prevalence or incidence of non-fistulous incontinence.

Investigating incontinence in Africa poses huge problems. There are over 2000 spoken languages and wide cultural differences exist. There are also large variations within some countries. South Africa, for example, has 11 official languages. Standardized validated questionnaires are not available in most countries. El-Azab et al. (32) have made a valuable contribution by validating the UDI-6 and IIQ-7 in Arabic, which is spoken by 178 million Africans living in the north and the horn of the continent. The Arabic IIQ-7 was modified to suit the Egyptian culture. They reported a prevalence of 54% for urinary incontinence using the UDI-6. The prevalence of urge, stress, and mixed incontinence were 15%, 15%, and 25% respectively (33). An important aspect of quality of life was emphasized by this study in that 90% of the subjects stated that the main issue was the inability to pray due to the presence of urinary soiling.

Of the 1000 Moroccan women older than 18 years, sampled by Mikou et al. (34) 271 (27%) reported incontinence in the previous month, with 49% complaining of stress urinary incontinence. A prevalence of 50% for any urinary incontinence has been reported in a study of 500 women in Tunisia (35).

Nel (38) estimated that at least five million South African women suffer from non-fistulous urinary incontinence, yet obstetric fistula are well described in the rural areas of South Africa (39,40). A dated study by Knobel (41) reported a lower prevalence of stress urinary incontinence (SUI) in black women than in Caucasian and Indian women. Assessment techniques, including the availability of questionnaires and urodynamic equipment have changed, and this data therefore needs to be interpreted in that context.

Rienhardt and co-workers interviewed 1207 women in a primary care setting using a questionnaire based on the Leicester MRC Incontinence study survey (Table 7.1). This study showed little difference in the incidence of stress urinary incontinence across different age and color groups (42).

The clinical observation that black women have less stress incontinence than their white counterparts has long been suspected, perhaps on the basis of differences in the quality of connective tissue (43). This impression has been strengthened recently by work by Laborda et al. and Thiem et al. who demonstrated the presence of an elevated elastin content in the tissue of black women (44,45). This issue needs to be clarified by further studies.

Okonkwo et al. (37) have reported on 3963 women presenting to a gynecology clinic with symptoms other than pelvic floor dysfunction in southeastern Nigeria. The pelvic organ prolapse questionnaire (POPQ) was administered to the respondents. The results revealed that 773 (19.5%) respondents had stress incontinence, while 864 (21.8%) had urge incontinence. Exerting uterine fundal pressure in the second stage of labor is common practice by African midwives and in this study women who gave a history of this had a greater risk of reporting a perineal laceration, urinary frequency, urge incontinence, hesitancy, incomplete emptying of bladder, awareness of the protrusion into the vagina, and pain with coitus.

A further study was performed in Ghana (36) on 200 randomly selected women attending for ultrasound. Sixty-two percent of these women had at least one symptom of incontinence. A "paper towel" test was used to objectively detect stress urinary incontinence. Forty-two percent of the women had a positive paper towel test and 80% of these had at least one symptom of incontinence.

A large amount of work remains to be done on non-fistulous urinary incontinence in Africa. Many of the treatment modalities

Table 7.1. Results of an Incontinence Survey in South Africa

	Black	Colored	White
Numbers	411	390	406
Age	41	42	47
Parity	2.9	2.5	1.9
Stress urinary incontinence	9.0	8.2	10.3
Urge incontinence	15.3	12.8	9.9
Urinary urgency	23.4	25.0	15.3
Bothered by symptoms	13.9	12.6	10.6
Has had treatment	9.8	10	11.6

Source: Adapted from Ref. 42.

are costly and thus not accessible to a large proportion of the population. As new treatments emerge, it is hoped that affordability is addressed by the industry to make them accessible to the people of Africa.

CONCLUSION

The huge burden of disease caused by obstetric fistula and its consequences overshadow all other causes of urinary incontinence in Africa. For this reason, the major focus of incontinence is on the epidemiological factors in the genesis of this condition. The road to obstetric fistula includes sociological deprivation, especially the low status of women in the community, poor general infrastructure such as the problems of transport, inadequate health facilities, and retarded rural development. Obstructed labor is by far the most common causative factor of fistulae, and the large numbers of fistulas continue to increase. Other causes include fistula caused by harmful traditional practices, infections, cervical carcinoma, and violence against women. Whilst suffering with incontinence arising from stress urinary incontinence and OAB are severe, the consequence of obstetric fistula are extreme on the continent.

REFERENCES

1. Wall LL, Karshima JA, Kirschner C, Arrowsmith SD. The obstetric vesico-vaginal fistula: characteristics of 899 patients from Jos, Nigeria. Am J Obstet Gynecol 2004; 190: 1011–19.
2. Rectovaginal Fistula and Fecal Incontinence. WHEC Practice Bulletin and Clinical Management Guidelines for healthcare providers. [Available from: www.womenshealthsection.com/content/urogvvf/urogvvf008.php3; accessed February 23, 2009]
3. AbouZahr C, Royston E. Maternal Mortality: A Global Factbook. Geneve: World Helath Organisation, 1991.
4. Graham W. The scandal of the century. Br J Obstet Gynaecol 1998; 105: 375–6.
5. Available from: www.worldbank.org/depweb/english/modules/social/life/index.html; accessed February 23, 2009.
6. Available from: www.wikipedia.org/wiki/Africa; accessed February 23, 2009.
7. Available from: www.who.int/gender/hiv_aids/en; accessed February 23, 2009.
8. Hoyert DL. Maternal Mortality and Related Concepts. National Center for Health Statistics. Vital Health Stat Series, Series 3, No. 33, 2007: 20.
9. Economic Survey 2004. District development plans (2002–2008). 2003 Kenya Demographic and Health Survey.
10. Urogynaecology fellowship training programmes 2008. Int Urogynecol J 2008; 19: 313–31.
11. Harrison KA. Childbearing, health and social priorities: a survey of 22,774 consecutive deliveries in Zaria, northern Nigeria. Br J Obstet Gynaecol 1985; 92(Suppl 5):1–119.
12. Vangeenderhuysen C, Prual A, Ould el Joud D. Obstetric fistulae: incidence estimates for sub-Saharan Africa. Int J Gynecol Obstet 2001; 73: 65–6.
13. Thaddeus S, Maine D. Too far to walk: maternal mortality in context. Soc Sci Med. 1994; 38: 1091–110.
14. Available from: www.unstats.un.org/unsd/Demographic/sconcerns/mortality; accessed February 23, 2009
15. Prual A, Huguet D, Garbin O, Rabé G. Severe obstetric morbidity of the third trimester, delivery and early puerperium in Niamey (Niger). AF J Reprod Health 1998; 2: 10–19.
16. Danso KA, Martey JO, Wall LL, Elkins TE. The epidemiology of genitourinary fistulae in Kumasi, Ghana, 1977–1992. Int Urogynecol J 1996; 7: 117–20.
17. Hilton P. Vesico-vaginal fistulas in developing countries. Int J Gynecol Obstet 2003; 82: 285–95.
18. Hilton P, Ward A. Epidemiological and surgical aspects of urogenital fistulae: a review of 25 year's experience in Southeast Nigeria. Int Urogynecol J 1998; 9: 189–94.
19. Kelly J. Ethiopia: an epidemiological study of vesico-vaginal fistula in Addis Ababa. World Health Stat Q. 1995; 48: 15–7.
20. Moerman ML. Growth of the birth canal in adolescent girls. Am J Obstet Gynecol 1982; 143: 528–53.
21. Meyer L, Ascher-Walsh CJ, Norman R, et al. Commonalities among women who experienced vesicovaginal fistulae as a result of obstetric trauma in Niger: results from a survey given at the National Hospital Fistula Center, Niamey, Niger. Am J Obstet Gynecol 2007; 197: 90. e1–4.
22. Kelly J, Kwast BE. Epidemiological study of vesico-vaginal fistulas in Ethiopia. Int Urogynecol J 1993; 4: 278–81.
23. Porcaro AB, Zicari M, Zecchini Antoniolli S, et al. Vesico uterine fistulas following caesarean section: report on a case, review and update of the literature. Int Urol Nephrol 2002; 34: 335–44.
24. Coetzee T. Lithgow DM, Obstetric fistulae of the urinary tract. J Obstet Gynaecol Br Commonw 1966; 73: 837–44.
25. Gruenbaum E. The Female Circumcision Controversy: An Anthropological Perspective. Philadelphia: University of Pensylvania Press, 2001.
26. Peterman A, Johnson K. Incontinence and trauma: sexual violence, female genital cutting and proxy measures of gynecological fistula. Soc Sci Med 2009; 68: 971–9.
27. Dirie MA, Lindmark G. The risk of medical complications after female circumcision. East Afr Med J. 1992; 69: 479–8.
28. Lawson JB. Birth canal injuries. Proc Royal Soc Med 1968; 61: 22–4.
29. Fahny K. Cervical and vaginal atresia due to packing the vagina with salt after labour. Am J Obstet Gynecol 1962; 84: 1466–9.
30. Johnson K. Incontinence in Malawi: analysis of a proxy measure of vaginal fistula in a national survey. Int J Gynaecol Obstet. 2007; 99(Suppl 1): S122–9.
31. Roy KK, Vaijyanath AM, Sinha A, Deka D, Takkar D. Sexual trauma—an unusual cause of a vesicovaginal fistula. Eur J Obstet Gynecol Reprod Biol 2002; 101: 89–90.
32. El-Azab AS, Mascha EJ. Arabic validation of the Urogenital Distress Inventory and Adapted Incontinence Impact Questionnaires—short forms. Neurourol Urodyn 2009; 28: 33–9.
33. El-Azab AS, Mohamed EM, Sabra HI. The prevalence and risk factors of urinary incontinence and its influence on the quality of life among Egyptian women. Neurourol Urodyn. 2007; 26: 783–8.
34. Mikou F, Abbassi O, Benjelloun A, Matar N, el Mansouri A. Prevalence of urinary incontinence in Moroccan women. Report of 1000 cases Ann Urol (Paris). 2001; 35: 280–9.
35. Ghosh TS, Kwawukume EY Urinary incontinence with effort: surgical management in the maternity ward of a Tunisian military hospital (91 case reports) West Afr J Med. 1993; 12: 141–3.
36. Adanu RM, De Lancey JO, Miller JM, Asante A. The physical finding of stress urinary incontinence among African women in Ghana. Int Urogynecol J Pelvic Floor Dysfunct. 2006; 17: 581–5.
37. Okonkwo JE, Obionu CO, Obiechina NJ. Factors contributing to urinary incontinence and pelvic prolapse in Nigeria. Int J Gynaecol Obstet 2001; 74: 301–3.
38. JT Nel. Urogynaecology in South Africa. Int Urogynecol J. 1999; 10: 275–6.
39. Ramphal S, Kalane G, Fourie F, Moodley J. Obstetric urinary fistulas in KwaZulu-Natal—what is the extent of this tragedy? SAJOG 2007; 13: 92–6.
40. Ramphal SR, Kalane G, Fourie T, Moodley J. An audit of obstetric fistulae in a teaching hospital in South Africa. Trop Doct 2008; 38: 162–3.
41. Knobel J. Stress incontinence in the Black female. S Afr Med J. 1975; 49: 430–2.
42. Reinhardt G, Assassa RP, Van De Walt I. Urinary symptoms and need in women from differing ethnic groups in South Africa. Int Urogynecol J 2003; 14(Suppl 1): S23.
43. Graham CA, Mallett VT. Race as a predictor of urinary incontinence and pelvic organ prolapse. Am J Obstet Gynecol 2001; 185: 116–20.
44. Laborda W, Rienhardt G, Anthony F, Monga A. Why do black African women have a reduced incidence of Stress Incontinence compared to white women? IUJ 2005; 16: S127.
45. Thiem A, Anthony F, Rienhardt G, Monga A. Elevaated elastin content in vaginal tissue of black women compared with white, an explanation for reduced incidence of stress incontinence in black women. IUJ 2006; 17: S60.

8   Tackling the Stigma of Incontinence: Promoting Continence Worldwide
Diane K Newman

INTRODUCTION

It is estimated that a quarter of a billion people worldwide suffer from urinary incontinence (UI) of varying degrees. Despite the considerable impact of incontinence on quality of life (QoL), many people never seek help for their incontinence and are thus uncounted (1,2). There has been extensive research documenting the success of various forms of conservative, pharmacologic, and surgical treatment but reality is that less than 50% of persons with UI seek help (1,3). Many more, especially in less developed countries, do not have help available (4). The psychological consequences of incontinence are well documented and barriers to seeking help have been frequently identified in the literature and include embarrassment, social stigma, and the mistaken belief that incontinence is inevitable, untreatable, and a normal part of aging (5). Public awareness is one method to destigmatize UI and to promote understanding about this widespread condition (6). This chapter will discuss the stigmatization of UI and some examples of what is currently being done worldwide to increase awareness and understanding.

THE BASIS OF STIGMA

The word stigma has been defined in different ways including: "as a mark of disgrace or reproach" and as "a moral or physical blemish that serves to identify a disease or condition." Gartley's (7) definition of stigma is the "recognition of difference based on some distinguishing characteristic or 'mark' and a consequence of devaluation for the person". This definition may more closely describe a person with incontinence. Garcia and colleagues (8) note that persons who are stigmatized are discredited thus reducing the person to a tainted human being. Gartley (9) noted this when she wrote: "It is still difficult to self-identify as a person with the stigma of incontinence." The key feature associated with stigma is that often, the stigmatized person and society represent extreme positions of the condition. Gartley (7,9) also notes that stigma in health care is a subset of stigmatization in society and is costly for all.

Persons with incontinence experience insensitive language, loss of freedom, and endure questions of a sensitive nature. Ignorance and lack of tolerance by, and of, others is common, leading frequently to anger and withdrawal. Whether the condition is visible or apparent to others (e.g., disfigurement) or concealed (e.g., colostomy or incontinence) does not change the way the person with the condition feels or reacts. The stigma associated with incontinence is similar to the stigma in other conditions and is associated with public ignorance and lack of awareness. The "stigma" surrounding bladder and bowel control problems, and the fact that people have many misconceptions about these conditions, prevents patients from seeking care (8). The traditional medical model of care is very much focused at "treatment" but does not empower the sufferer to actually develop strategies to cope with what is often a lifelong condition.

It is possible to understand the longstanding stigma surrounding UI by considering the potential health consequence of incontinence on society (10). Epidemiological and clinical studies of individuals with incontinence indicate that the condition has a considerable impact on overall QoL and well-being. The inability to control urine is one of the most unpleasant and distressing symptoms a person can experience, causing stigmatization and denial of the condition (8). Emotional well-being is impaired, probably as a result of social isolation and feelings of stigmatization produced by the incontinence.

The Social "Taboo" of Incontinence

Given that the process of storing and expelling urine is shaped by social rules for acceptable times and places for elimination, stigma is attached to incontinence. Bladder and bowel continence is an adjustment to the social norm, especially in Western cultures, which have developed acceptable rules and behavior for bladder and bowel emptying (11,12). Our society places a significant emphasis on sanitation and personal hygiene. Discussions of personal hygiene and/or elimination are not part of social conversations, especially in Western cultures. During toilet training, children are inculcated with all the cultural norms and expectations concerning elimination of urine and stool (13). If incontinence occurs in adulthood, persons revive those childhood beliefs and begin to internalize their condition causing a decrease in self-esteem and feelings of shame and of not being "normal" (5). These barriers are shared by the public as well as, by many health care providers. To avoid embarrassment, persons with UI turn to "self-management" rather than "seeking-help" from a doctor or nurse. Unfortunately, factors that promote health seeking behavior for continence issues remain less researched and are complex and multifactorial (4). With chronic problems like urinary and fecal incontinence, it is important to understand what triggers the patient to consult a health care provider (14). Older adults may be keen to seek help if they are concerned that a health issue such as incontinence impacts on their ability to remain independent and living in the community (12). In certain parts of the world, the gender of the person with UI may be a factor in help-seeking behavior and the gender of the health care provider may be a barrier.

The way people react to a person with incontinence is influenced by many factors. The further the person is connected from the sufferer, the more negative attitudes become, as shown in Figure 8.1. As the condition becomes more severe,

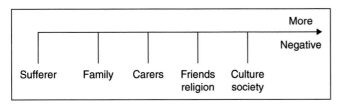

Figure 8.1 Attitudes through society.

Table 8.1 Modifiers of Attitude and Response

Condition	Socio-economic
Severity	Culture
Religion	Sex
Age	Ignorance
Prejudice	Education

the more obvious it becomes to others, and often, therefore, the more the person is likely to be stigmatized (12,8). In addition, attitudes and reactions of both the person with incontinence and those in society who interact with that person may vary according to the age of the person. At the extreme is the newborn child, where incontinence is regarded as a norm, through to childhood bedwetting, all the way to a frail old person in a nursing home. Depending on the age, sex, and social situation of the person, the reaction may well be different. Table 8.1 shows some of the factors that will modify response and attitude to incontinence.

A common phenomenon seen in conditions which have greater stigma (and often are less life threatening) is that they tend to take a much longer time to be reported to a health care provider (e.g., physician) and even longer to family, friends, and others. Breast cancer is a good example where now it is common for a woman to go immediately to a doctor when she identifies a breast lump and to share this finding with family and friends even before the diagnosis is confirmed. Cancer in the past was very much a taboo subject but in the past 10 years we have more public figures coming forward with their health-related issues to give greater insight into cancers such as prostate, colon, etc. While infertility in the past was regarded with shame by the infertile couple, people now know when friends or acquaintances are on an in vitro fertilization (IVF) program. Mental health conditions (particularly depression), HIV, and the AIDS epidemic are gaining more and more acknowledgement in society. Public figures are stepping forward and putting their face and name to such conditions.

It is important to understand how attitudes and stigma changed for these conditions. An important component is breaking the cycle of public and personal ignorance through education and public awareness programs (15). For this to be successful, there needs to be a partnership between healthcare professionals, governments, and industry groups with a vested interest to work together to break the cycle of ignorance and negative attitude (6). Central to this is the availability of funds, either in allocated dollars or "in kind" (e.g., access to advertise-

ments), that represents an ongoing funding source. In the sections below we see examples of how this process is being tackled locally and internationally in order to raise awareness of incontinence, bring a greater opportunity to help, and improve the plight of hundreds of millions of people around the world.

Consumer education in terms of having access to information about incontinence in this age of digital technology is a non-issue, especially for those internet users who tend to have a higher literacy level. In light of the reluctance of those affected by stigmatized illnesses such as incontinence to seek treatment or to ask health care professionals for information, the internet may prove to be a useful tool for patient education and public health outreach. In a national survey of internet users in the United States, Berger and colleagues (16) found a trend among people with a stigmatized illness such as UI to more likely report that using the internet increased their health care utilization and communication with a health care provider.

THE ROLE OF NATIONAL ORGANIZATIONS

As previously mentioned, the stigma associated with incontinence is similar to other conditions and is associated with public ignorance and lack of awareness. Despite all this, it is important to understand how attitudes and stigma have changed for these conditions. An important component is breaking the cycle of public and personal ignorance through education and public awareness programs. As the stigma associated with incontinence is similar to other conditions, and is associated with public ignorance and lack of awareness, educating the public will increase their awareness of the condition. Therefore, it is important to understand how attitudes and stigma have changed for these conditions. There have been some advances in breaking the cycle of public and personal ignorance through education and public awareness programs. Patient advocacy organizations for UI have been formed worldwide to promote awareness.

Continence promotion involves informing and educating the public that incontinence is not inevitable or shameful, but is treatable or at least manageable (4). In the past 15 years, national organizations have been formed under various auspices to tackle issues to do with incontinence awareness, education, and promotion. Table 8.2 provides a list of countries that have national organizations, the organization's name and websites or contact details. While each organization is unique in its mandate, what they have in common is their commitment to improve the situation for persons with incontinence.

Continence promotion is a most challenging endeavor. Although the ratio between affected patient populations and continence national organization funding has not been formally studied, anecdotal information suggests that continence promotion is among the most difficult of medical problems for which to obtain funding. In view of all these challenges, the proliferation of new national continence organizations, especially in Asia, is a validation of both the need for continence promotion and the dedication of those who have recognized and are addressing this need.

Table 8.2 Directory of Continence Organizations

Australia
- Continence Foundation of Australia Ltd
  Website: www.continence.org.au

Austria
- Medizinische Geseelschaft fur Inkontinenhlife Osterreich
  Website: www.inkontinenz.at

Belgium
- U-Control vzw (Belgian Association for Incontinence)

Brazil
- Brazilian Foundation for Continence Promotion
  Email: seabrarios@uol.com.br

Canada
- The Canadian Continence Foundation
  Website: www.canadiancontinance.ca

Czech Republic
- Inco Forum
  Website: www.incoforum.cz/

Denmark
- Kontinensoreningen-Danish Continence Association
  Website: www.kontinens.dk/

Egypt
- Pan Arab Continence Society
  Website: www.pacsoffice.org

France
- Feemes pour Toujourns
  Website: www.femsante.com

Germany
- Deutsche Kontinenz Gesellschaft e.V.
  Website: www.gih.de

Hong Kong
- Hong Kong Continence Society
  Email: emfleung@ha.org.hk

Hungary
- Inko Forum
  Website: www.inkoforum.hu

India
- Indian Continence Foundation
  Website: www.indiancontinencefoundation.org

Indonesia
- Indonesian Continence Society
  Email: urogyn@centrin.net.id

Israel
- National Center for Continence
  Email: ig054@hotmail.com

Italy
- Fondazione Italiana Continenza (The Italian Continence Foundation)
  Website: www.continenza-italia.org
- Associazione Italiana Donne Medico
  Website: www.donnemedico.org
- The Federazione Italiana INCOntinenti
  Website: www.finco.org

Korea
- Korea Continence Foundation
  Website: www.kocon.or.kr

Japan
- Japan Continence Action Society
  Website: www.jcas.or.jp

Malaysia
- Continence Foundation (Malaysia)
  Email: lohcs@medicine.med.um.edu.my

Table 8.2 Directory of Continence Organizations (*Continued*)

Mexico
- Asociacion de Enfremadades Uroginecologicas
  Website: www.asenug.org

Netherlands
- Pelvic Floor Patients Foundation (SBP)
  Website: www.bekkenbodem.net
- Vereniging Nederlandse Incontinentie, Verpleegkundigen
  Website: www.cvnc.nl/

New Zealand
- New Zealand Continence Assn Inc
  Website: www.continence.org.nz

Norway
- Norwegian Society for Patients with Urologic Diseases
  Website: www.nofus.no

Philippines
- Continence Foundation of the Philippines
  Email: dtbolong@skynet.net

Poland
- NTM (INCO) Forum (The Polish Continence Organisation)
  Website: www.ntm.pl

Singapore
- Society for Continence (Singapore)
  Website: www.sfcs.org.sg

Slovakia
- Slovakia Inco Forum
  Website: www.incoforum.sk

South Africa
- Continence Association of South Africa
  Email: casa123@absmail.co.za

Spain
- Association National de Ostomizados e Incontinentes
  Website: www.coalicion.org

Sweden
- SINOBA
  Website: www.sinoba.se

Switzerland
- Schweizerische Gesellschaft fur Blasenschwache
  Website: www.inkontinex.ch

Taiwan
- Taiwan Continence Society
  Website: http://www.tcs.org.tw
  Email: msuuf@ms15.hinet.net

Thailand
- Department of Surgery
  Email: ravkc@mahidol.ac.th

United Kingdom
- The Bladder and Bowel Foundation
  Website: www.bladderandbowelfoundation.org
- Enuresis Resource and Information Centre
  Website: www.eric.org.uk

United States
- American Urological Association Foundation
  Website: http://www.auafoundation.org/
- National Association For Continence
  Website: www.nafc.org
- Simon Foundation for Continence
  Website: www.simonfoundation.org
- International Foundation for Functional Gastrointestinal Disorders
  Website: www.iffgd.org www.aboutincontinence.org

(*Continued*)

National organizations which promote continence are as diverse as the cultures they serve. They represent a wide diversity of models, including consumer-led, company sponsored, professionals only, and organizations which have deliberately set about trying to bring together all relevant stakeholders in a relatively democratic model (4). In every part of the world these organizations play a dynamic role in building both public and professional awareness of this underserved and underreported condition. Most continence organizations are poorly capitalized, being either under- or unfunded (i.e., run by volunteers), and are held together initially by either a dedicated patient advocate or an energized healthcare professional. In most cases this professional is an urologist or nurse whose patient population includes persons with UI. However, despite this limitation, these organizations often provide their country with the first wake-up call that incontinence is common.

A MODEL FOR PARTNERSHIPS
TO PROMOTE CONTINENCE

One of the most supportive government sponsored initiatives for promoting continence is from Australia. The National Continence Management Strategy (NCMS) was established in 1998 by the Australian Government Department of Health and Ageing. Funding of over AUS $33 million has been allocated for the period from 1998 to 2010. More than 120 projects have received funding for research, public awareness activities, continence education, resource development, and continence service development. The Strategy is now in its third phase of activity. A final evaluation report on Phase one and two of the NCMS was released in September 2006 (17,18). In the area of continence awareness, the report noted that recognition of the barriers to help-seeking behavior and identification of the most appropriate terminology and key messages would strengthen awareness raising strategies. The provision of an incontinence specific helpline (the National Continence Helpline) has been an important awareness raising initiative.

THE ROLE OF THE INTERNATIONAL
CONTINENCE SOCIETY

It is understood that for any advocacy group to be successful, there needs to be a partnership between health care professionals, governments, and industry groups with a vested interest to work together to break the cycle of ignorance and negative attitude. Professionals (e.g., urologists, urogynecologists, nurses, physiotherapists, continence advisers) and professional organizations continue to be instrumental in promoting awareness of continence. The International Continence Society (ICS) has addressed the need for partnership through its support of its Continence Promotion Committee (CPC). The CPC is at the forefront of promoting continence awareness on a global front and continues to support national continence organizations and implement new programs to raise continence awareness.

The CPC's multinational and multidisciplinary representation aims to identify broad issues through an international forum that can facilitate translation at the local and national level. As of 2008, there are 47 Continence Organizations in 34 countries world wide with an additional two international patient-based organizations. Table 2 is a directory of ICS-CPC supported national continence organizations. Most of them function as multi-disciplinary bodies. Each year at the ICS's annual meeting, the CPC has held workshops around various themes that have a broad national focus such as prevention; general practitioner education; and promotional strategies. Its relevance, as is the case with each of the national organizations, is to recognize the interface between continence management and continence awareness and promotion. The CPC is increasing continence awareness through new initiatives; specifically a Public Forum on Incontinence and sponsorship of a *World Continence Week* both supported by the ICS.

SUMMARY

Around the world, there has been a goal to "destigmatize" incontinence by promoting awareness through partnerships of healthcare professionals, governments, and industry. This process must continue in order for incontinence to be removed from the list of conditions associated with stigma so that people can and will seek help.

REFERENCES

1. Kinchen KS, Burgio K, Diokno A, et al. Factors associated with women's decisions to seek treatment for urinary incontinence. J Women's Health 2003; 12: 687–98.
2. Shaw C, Das Gupta R, Williams KS, Assassa RP, McGrother C. A survey of help-seeking and treatment provision in women with stress urinary incontinence. BJU International 2006; 97: 752–7.
3. Koch LH. Help-seeking behaviors of women with urinary incontinence: an integrative literature review. J Midwifery Wom Heal 2006; 51: e39–44.
4. Newman DK, Ee CH, Gordon D, Vasan SS, Williams K. Continence promotion, education & primary prevention, In: Abrams P, Cardozo L, Khoury S, Wein A. eds. Incontinence, Proceedings from the 4th International Consultation on Incontinence. Plymouth UK: Health Publication, 2009: 1643–84.
5. Newman DK, Wein AJ. Managing and Treating Urinary Incontinence, 2nd edn. Maryland: Health Professions Press, Baltimore, 2009: 565–84.
6. Newman DK. Community awareness and education. In: Badlani GH, Davila GW, Michel MC, de la Rosette JJMCH. eds. Continence: Current Concepts and Treatment Strategies. London: Springer-Verlag, 2009: 521–32.
7. Gartley CB. Bringing Mohammed to the mountain: educating the community for continence. Urol Nurs 2006a; 26: 387–93.
8. Garcia JA, Crocker J, Wyman JF. Breaking the cycle of stigmatization. J Wound Ostomy Continence Nurs 2005; 32: 38–52.
9. Gartley C. Life with incontinence. Lancet 2006b; 367: 68.
10. Fonda D. Promoting continence as a health issue. Eur Urol 1997; 32: 28–32.
11. Herschorn S, Gajewski J, Schutz J Corcos J. A population-based study of urinary symptoms and incontinence: the canadian urinary bladder survey. BJU International 2007; 101: 52–8.
12. Norton C. Nurses, bowel continence, stigma, and taboos. J Wound Ostomy Continence Nurs 2004; 31: 85–94.

13. Paterson J. Stigma associated with postprostatectomy urinary incontinence. J Wound Ostomy Continence Nurs 2000; 27: 168–73.

14. Norton NJ. The perspective of the patient. Gastroenterology 2004; 126(Suppl 1): S175–9.

15. Fonda D, Newman DK. Tackling the stigma of incontinence—promoting continence worldwide. In: Cardozo L, Staskin D. eds. Textbook of Female Urology and Urogynecology. 2nd edn. United Kingdom: Isis Medical Media, LTD, 2006: 75–80.

16. Berger M, Wagner TH, Baker LC. Internet use and stigmatized illness. Soc Sci Med 2005; 61: 1821–7.

17. McCallum J, Millar L, Burston L, Dong T. Framework for evaluation of the national continence management strategy. Australasian J Ageing 2007; 26(s1): A1–44.

18. Australian Government Initiative, National Continence Management Strategy (NCMS), Evaluation Framework, Victoria University. March, 2008. [Available from: http://www.bladderbowel.gov.au/ncms/indepeval. htm Accessed September 23, 2009].

9 Natural History and Prevention of Urinary Incontinence and Urogenital Prolapse

Ruben Trochez and Robert M Freeman

INTRODUCTION

There are few studies that have prospectively evaluated the natural history of urinary incontinence (UI) and pelvic organ prolapse (POP) in women who have not undergone treatment. Epidemiological studies are described in chapters 2 to 7. A hypothesis for the natural history is presented.

NATURAL HISTORY OF STRESS URINARY INCONTINENCE (SUI)

The association between SUI and parity is well known and, based on the available evidence, the following hypothesis regarding the genesis and natural history can be made [Fig. 9.1, (1)]. This might also be relevant for POP.

Hypothesis for the Genesis of SUI

During pregnancy the endopelvic fascial attachments of the bladder neck and distal sphincter are weakened possibly due to hormonal influences (2). This might be a progesterone effect resulting in reduced urethral closure pressure (3) and connective tissue changes (4). Along with the increasing intra-abdominal pressure from the pregnant uterus, this might increase the risk of SUI antenatally. In fact, incidences of up to 40% have been reported (1) with approximately 20% having severe symptoms (5).

In most cases incontinence *improves* after delivery with an incidence of postpartum SUI of approximately 15% (1). In these cases the onset is rarely "new onset;" it has usually been present during the pregnancy. Why SUI should persist postpartum is unclear, but vaginal delivery is implicated.

If the endopelvic fascial attachments and sphincter function are not damaged at delivery, then the changes seen antenatally are likely to revert to the "non-pregnant" state with the return of urethral function and continence. However, if these structures are damaged or are inherently weak in the *non-pregnant* state, then recovery might not arise.

Support for this hypothesis comes from studies suggesting the presence of a constitutional factor (e.g., weak connective tissue/fascia in women) with SUI (6,7).

For example, there is a known association between connective tissue disorders and UI and POP (e.g., in Marfans and Ehlers–Danlos syndrome) (8).

Also, in women with POP an association with joint hypermobility has been demonstrated suggesting an underlying connective tissue weakness (9).

Should such individuals suffer pelvic floor trauma at delivery then recovery might not be complete resulting in postpartum SUI. This along with further deliveries, ageing, menopause, and muscle weakness seems to increase the risk of long-term incontinence (Fig. 9.1) (10).

Further support for the hypothesis comes from the growing volume of evidence suggesting that *antenatal SUI*, and in particular incontinence *before* a first pregnancy, are high risk factors for the development of incontinence in later years (11–13).

Natural History

As mentioned, there are few studies describing the natural history. A recently published large prospective longitudinal study with 16 years follow up of over a thousand women found considerable rates of both incidence and remission of UI, overactive bladder (OAB), and other lower urinary tract symptoms (LUTS) (14). They reported cumulative incidences of UI and urgency/OAB of 21% and 20%, respectively, with corresponding regressions of 34% and 43%, respectively. However, regression was more frequent in women with mild symptoms, suggesting that clinically relevant UI infrequently improves spontaneously. In a study of women reassessed six years after childbirth (13) there was a rate of new onset incontinence of approximately 30% in women who had been continent at three months postpartum. However, in 27% who were *incontinent* at three months, there was spontaneous remission at six years.

Of particular interest were those women who were incontinent *prior* to pregnancy; there was a markedly increased risk for leakage at six years (odds ratio = 12).

These interesting findings suggest that there are women at-risk of incontinence; while in others there is spontaneous remission. Identification of such individuals might help in prevention of SUI (and POP) if they can be identified at an early stage (see "Childbirth," below).

NATURAL HISTORY OF PROLAPSE

As with SUI, alterations in pelvic organ support leading to prolapse might occur before delivery. Increasing stages of POP with advancing gestation have been reported (15); although this might represent physiologic changes of pregnancy.

The natural history of untreated POP has been assessed in menopausal women as part of the estrogen, progestin trial of the Women's Health Initiative (University of California) (16). Annual pelvic examinations for POP were performed on 412 women (mean 5.7 years) using a (non-validated) classification system. At baseline 31.8% had POP. The annual incidences of new-onset POP were 9, 5, and 7 per 100 woman years for cystocele, rectocele, and uterine POP, respectively. Of interest were the rates of progression and regression.

For *progression*, the rates were 9.5, 13.5, and 1.9 per 100 woman years, respectively. Corresponding figures for *spontaneous regression*, especially grade 1 POP, were: 23.5, 22, and 48,

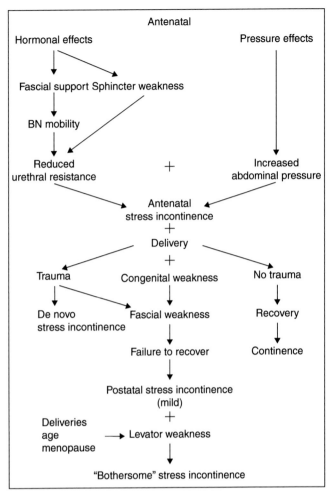

Figure 9.1 Hypothesis for the genesis and natural history of SUI. *Source*: Reproduced from Ref. 1.

suggesting that spontaneous regression is common. Only three women (0.7%) required surgery.

These data suggest that the clinical sign of POP is common and that spontaneous regression occurs in many cases. Treatment might be unnecessary unless the symptoms are bothersome.

Previously, prevalence studies which might have been helpful in identifying the natural history of POP have been hampered by selection bias (e.g., hospital-based populations in developed countries). For example, in such groups 30% to 50% of women seen for other gynecological problems have signs of POP (17,18) but most will be asymptomatic. In older age groups (>70 years) many are symptomatic and approximately 11% will undergo surgery, but there are few data on the numbers treated conservatively (e.g., with pessaries) (19).

In developing countries untreated POP might be more prevalent. For example, in rural Gambia an epidemiological study showed a prevalence of 46%. Only 8 of 152 with "severe POP" (i.e., subjective and objective) accepted the offer of treatment (20). There are no data on the outcome for these untreated women.

If severe and left untreated, POP can sometimes result in obstructed voiding and recurrent urinary infection. This could progress to obstruction of the upper tracts and renal failure.

In a small case series of women with untreated severe POP (i.e., beyond the introitus), all had evidence of bilateral upper tract dilatation, and three had obstructive renal failure. Treatment of POP resolved the renal failure in all but one patient (21). These findings highlight the need for prevention of upper tract changes by early treatment of advanced POP.

Trauma to the cervix and vaginal skin might increase the risk of neoplasia in women with severe POP. However, there are few prospective studies to assess the risk.

PREVENTION

Ideally, the aim of healthcare is prevention rather than cure. Prevention can be classified as *primary* (interventions in asymptomatic individuals to reduce known risk factors for the development of a disease) or *secondary* (to detect symptoms at an early stage and to intervene to stop further development or to improve the prognosis of the condition). To stop recurrence of an illness or preventing it becoming chronic is *tertiary* prevention. In urogynecology there is a paucity of large prospective trials to assess the impact of prevention on incontinence and POP.

There are known predisposing factors such as age, obesity, family history, parity/vaginal childbirth, and surgery. Identification of individuals at-risk might help with implementing preventative measures.

AGE

Although the prevalence of incontinence is increased in the elderly (22), the two do not necessarily have a cause-and-effect relationship; other pathological processes associated with ageing might be responsible. Resnick (23) has created the mnemonic "DIAPPERS" to describe these: Delirium, Infection, Atrophic change, Pharmacological, Psychological, Excess urine output, Restricted mobility, and Stool impaction.

There is a known association between constipation and POP (24), and attention to regular bowel habit, avoiding straining, a high-fiber diet and, if necessary, laxatives might have a positive effect on prevention.

Likewise, management of other risk factors such as chronic cough, smoking, and adjusting medication that has an adverse effect on the bladder, could help incontinence [e.g., diuretics, calcium channel antagonists (that can produce polyuria), non-steroidal anti-inflammatory drugs (that can lead to fluid retention), angiotensin-converting enzyme inhibitors (leading to chronic cough), and sedatives].

Regular toileting, easy access to toilets, restricting fluids (especially caffeine), and prevention of urinary tract infection (e.g., with cranberry juice or vitamin C), might also be effective in prevention of incontinence in the elderly.

Hormone Replacement Therapy (HRT)

There is a definite ageing process in the lower urinary tract (25), resulting in atrophic change and poor urethral function. HRT should in theory prevent LUTS. While this has not been proven objectively in patients with urodynamic stress incontinence (USI) or detrusor overactivity (DO) (26), in postmenopausal women low dose vaginal estradiol appears to improve the symptom of urgency (27); this could be important in prevention although it is not clear if the mechanism of action is on the bladder or the atrophic change.

A Cochrane review suggests that estrogens might help 50% of women with all types of UI compared with 25% on placebo, the effect being most marked in those with urgency incontinence (28).

The effect of HRT on prevention of POP is unknown.

Urgency

Urgency is a distressing symptom for the older patient with restricted mobility, causing panic, and anxiety on the sensation of bladder fullness. Often patients void more frequently to prevent urgency incontinence, which can have the opposite effect, by reducing bladder capacity and worsening the symptoms (29).

Strategies such as explanation, bladder retraining, pelvic floor exercises, easy access to toilets, and the use of bedside commodes might prevent urgency developing into urgency incontinence, and could also prevent falls. There is evidence that patients with urgency incontinence (more than once a week) are at increased risk of falls and bone fracture than in those without (30). These might be preventable.

OBESITY

Obesity is common in women with UI and POP. When defined as "more than 20% above average weight for height and age," obesity has been shown to be more common in patients with USI and DO than in the asymptomatic population (31). Increasing body mass index (BMI) is associated with progression of POP for all three compartments (32).

In pregnancy, an increased BMI has been shown to be an important risk factor for persistent UI *post partum* (33,34).

In theory, weight loss should be preventative. However, studies are often hampered by the failure of subjects to lose weight. One, in morbidly obese women undergoing surgically-induced weight loss, showed subjective and urodynamic improvement in incontinence one year after surgery (35).

In another (a pilot study using diet and behavioral modification), patients losing >5% body weight had a greater reduction in incontinence episodes compared with those who failed to lose weight (36).

In a larger case series of women (BMI > 30) with UI undergoing weight loss by diet, exercise, and drug therapy, reduced incontinence loss (pad test) and improved quality of life have been demonstrated in 42/64 women losing more than 5% body weight (37).

A recent randomized trial in 338 overweight and obese women comparing a program of diet, exercise, and behavior modification with a structured education program found that a mean weight loss of 8% in the intervention group (vs. 1.6% in controls) led to a significant decrease in weekly episodes of incontinence (47% vs. 28%) (38).

It has been recommended by the International Consultation on Incontinence (39) that studies on obesity be given research priority to answer the question whether or not weight loss helps and prevents UI.

The studies that have used incontinence as the primary outcome (36–38) suggest that weight loss can result in improvement

both subjectively and objectively. Weight loss should be recommended as part of the treatment "package" and might also be useful in secondary prevention.

FAMILIAL/GENETIC RISK FACTORS

Identification of risk groups is important and *family history* might be relevant. It has been shown that daughters of women with UI are more likely to develop incontinence themselves (7,40). A small study in four pairs of postmenopausal identical twins with different parity status, i.e., nulliparous/parous for each set of twins, found identical continence status in all four pairs, and a difference greater than one stage on POP quantification assessment in only one set of twins (41), which seems to support a genetic predisposition for both UI and POP rather than parity.

Racial differences have also been demonstrated, with white Caucasian women having an increased risk of SUI (42) and POP (43) compared to African-American women.

Also *childhood symptoms* (e.g., nocturnal enuresis and OAB) might predispose to incontinence in adulthood (44). Identifying and treating these children [e.g., by pelvic floor muscle training (PFMT)], might help to prevent symptoms.

CHILDBIRTH

There is good evidence that vaginal delivery is associated with pudendal nerve injury (45,46). Such nerve damage is also seen in patients with USI (47) and it has therefore been assumed that vaginal delivery alone is responsible for subsequent USI and POP. However, this assumption might not be correct; pregnancy itself might also be responsible (48).

For example, nulliparous women with USI appear to have weak pelvic floor collagen (6) and vaginal delivery in these women might increase the risk of SUI and POP if/when they become pregnant.

Identifying them before, or early in a first pregnancy, might enable preventative measures to be introduced.

Primigravidae with excessive bladder-neck mobility antenatally (a possible marker for weak pelvic floor collagen) appear to be at higher risk of post-partum stress incontinence (49), itself a risk factor for long-term incontinence (10). Antenatal and pre-pregnancy incontinence (11,13) family history of incontinence in pregnancy (40), obesity (34), and persistent postnatal incontinence (50) also appear to be important risk factors.

Intervention of such groups might help with prevention but what this intervention should be is a matter of debate (51). While elective caesarean section might prevent neuromuscular damage (45) and postpartum SUI (52), this latter finding is not consistent with incidences of SUI of up to 16% in patients undergoing caesarean section being reported (5,53).

PFMT might be a less invasive form of prevention. For example, in primigravidae with antenatal bladder neck mobility (49), antenatal PFMT has shown a reduced incidence of postpartum SUI compared with untreated controls (33). Similar results have been seen in "unselected" primigravidae (54).

Post-partum PFMT also seems to be preventative both in the short (55,56) and medium term (57). A Cochrane review with 15 studies involving over 6000 patients found evidence that PFMT can prevent UI in pregnancy [risk ratio (RR) 0.44, 95% CI 0.30–0.65] and postpartum (RR 0.71, 95% CI 0.52–0.97); and is an appropriate treatment for women with postpartum UI (RR 0.79, 95% CI 0.70–0.90) (58). However, the level of intervention, i.e., the PFMT regime, varied greatly in the studies and it remains unclear whether PFMT should be targeted to women at risk (i.e., primiparous women, women with large babies, forceps deliveries, etc.) or should be a population-based intervention.

Longer term studies with six and eight years follow up (59,60) and one review (61) have shown that the initial beneficial effect does not persist, probably due to poor compliance. However the incontinence in those women was not severe enough to require surgery.

As PFMT antenatally and postnatally can be preventative in the short and medium term, Caesarean section might not be necessary except possibly for those women with *severe* incontinence before and/or during the first pregnancy (11,13) or in those with early stage symptomatic prolapse. However prospective studies are required to confirm if this type of delivery will prevent SUI and POP in the long-term.

Can Changing the Management of Labor Help in Prevention of SUI?

This is unlikely as the role of obstetric factors in the genesis of postpartum SUI is unclear. For example, there is conflicting evidence regarding prolonged second stage of labor, birth weight, epidural, episiotomy, and mode of delivery.

Forceps delivery has been implicated (45), but this is not a consistent finding (62). The vacuum/ventouse is arguably less traumatic to the pelvic floor but while one study has suggested that the incidence and severity of SUI one year after forceps delivery was greater than that after spontaneous delivery and vacuum/ventouse (63), this has not been a consistent finding (46).

The role of episiotomy is also unclear. A Cochrane review has failed to show evidence that this prevents UI or prolapse (64).

It would appear that prevention by changing obstetric practice is not possible with the current state of knowledge. However, it might be worthwhile considering earlier delivery (by cesarean section) in short stature primigravidae who have obstructed labor before full dilatation to prevent pelvic floor injury. This might be preferable to prolonged augmentation of labor and instrumental delivery [see the subsection on "Prevention of Obstetric Anal Sphincter Injury (OASI) and Fecal Incontinence" below].

Irritative Symptoms in Pregnancy

Frequency and nocturia are common in pregnancy and probably "physiological," due to the effects of hormonal changes and pressure effects of the pregnant uterus.

For OAB and urgency incontinence in pregnancy, incidences of 8% to 18% have been quoted (5,65). However, the diagnostic accuracy of urodynamics in pregnancy (for DO) is poor (5). A large prospective study of 515 women in their first pregnancy found a high prevalence of frequency and urgency at 12 weeks gestation, 74% and 63%, respectively, which

remained stable during pregnancy (66). However, the majority of women were not bothered by them. Moreover, a year after delivery there was a significant decline in the prevalence of bothersome frequency (67).

A detailed history should identify women with OAB antenatally and bladder retraining might help in secondary prevention. However, few studies have follow-up beyond three months and long-term assessment is necessary to ascertain if symptoms persist. Prevention might not be necessary if they are shown to subside with time.

Prevention of Obstetric Anal Sphincter Injury (OASI) and Fecal Incontinence

Incidence

Fecal incontinence, of either liquid or solid stool, has been reported in 4% of women for the first time postnatally (68). If incontinence of flatus and urgency are added (i.e., "anal incontinence"), this figure is increased (69). Although pudendal nerve injury in labor might be responsible (45,46) occult anal sphincter defects have been identified in 35% of primiparous and 44% of multiparous women on endoanal ultrasonography (70). In 13% and 23%, respectively, there were defecatory symptoms (urgency and/or fecal incontinence). The main obstetric factor associated with symptoms was forceps delivery; caesarean section was protective (70).

Detection of OASI

In women with *recognized* OASI/third-degree tears, 85% have been shown to have residual sphincter damage despite repair at delivery, with 50% being symptomatic (70).

Many remain *unrecognized* with one-third of women having an undetected OASI after their first delivery (69).

It is important that obstetricians and midwives are adequately trained in the identification and treatment of OASI as this might help in prevention of fecal incontinence.

Appropriate methods of defect repair are also important. For example, the "overlap repair" for complete tears seems to be associated with a lower incidence of fecal urgency and deterioration of anal incontinence symptoms compared with "end-to-end" repair (71). Training is therefore recommended.

Identification and repair of OASI might be important in prevention of long-term fecal incontinence. However, prospective follow-up studies are required.

Obstetric Management

Episiotomy might prevent OASI. For example, fewer third- and fourth-degree tears have been seen following *mediolateral* episiotomy (72,73) whereas the risk is increased by *midline* episiotomy (74). The latter should probably be abandoned due to the high risk of OASI. Standard obstetrics textbooks state that a mediolateral episiotomy should be performed at an angle of at least 40°, with most suggesting an angle of between 45° and 60°. However two studies found that most doctors and midwives perform mediolateral episiotomies at a much lesser angulation (75,76). These findings were confirmed by another study (77), which in addition demonstrated that the risk of OASI decreased significantly from 9.7% in women who had episiotomies at <25° to 0.05% in women whose episiotomies

exceeded 45°. The authors estimated a 50% relative risk reduction of OASI for every 6° away from the midline that an episiotomy was performed.

Forceps and Ventouse

Use of the ventouse rather than forceps might help in prevention. While it has been claimed that both are risk factors for OASI (68), other data suggest that ventouse is associated with fewer OASI's compared with forceps (78). In a randomized controlled trial (RCT) of ventouse versus forceps delivery, there was a significant reduction in the incidence of third and fourth degree tears in the ventouse group (79).

However, it might not be the particular instrument which is important but the *indication* for the assisted delivery, e.g., prolonged labor, large baby (45), and occipito posterior position (80) (known risk factors for pelvic floor trauma and OASI).

These factors are outwith the obstetrician's control. Nonetheless, awareness might help in prevention, e.g., by performing an elective 45° episiotomy or, if there are other obstetric indications, e.g., obstructed labor in a woman at risk, delivery by caesarean section.

Subsequent Deliveries

Two prospective studies have shown that in primiparous women with persistent fecal incontinence, the risk of deterioration appears to increase after the second vaginal delivery (81,82). For these women secondary prevention might be achieved by elective caesarean section.

Large retrospective studies using an anatomical rather than a physiological outcome, i.e., recurrence of OASI instead of anal incontinence, have shown that there is a three- to seven-fold increased risk of recurrent OASI with subsequent deliveries (83–85). However, these findings have not been replicated by other equally large retrospective studies (86,87). Further prospective long term studies are required before elective caesarean section can be recommended for secondary prevention in asymptomatic women.

Pelvic Floor Muscle Training

For women without fecal incontinence, PFMT might be preventative. For example, in one study treating women with persistent SUI three months after delivery, lower rates of fecal incontinence were seen compared with controls (50). It is recommended that women with OASI receive supervised PFMT as a form of secondary prevention. However, as with SUI, a randomized trial showed that the significant improvement in fecal incontinence compared to controls at one year (4% vs. 11%) did not persist at six years (12% vs. 13%) irrespective of subsequent deliveries (59).

These research findings have focused the attention of obstetricians and midwives to the potential risk of anal sphincter injury and the possible association with long-term fecal incontinence. This should result in improved awareness, training, and prevention.

Other non-obstetric modifiable risk factors for fecal incontinence including obesity, SUI, and associated medical conditions

such as irritable bowel syndrome have been identified (88,89). Addressing these might also help in prevention.

PREVENTION OF INCONTINENCE AND PROLAPSE FOLLOWING GYNECOLOGICAL SURGERY
Hysterectomy and Incontinence

Urinary tract fistulae are (fortunately) rare, but are not always preventable. A rate of 0.5% to 3% of lower urinary tract injury has been reported at hysterectomy. Many of these are due to congenital abnormalities and distortion of structures caused by disease (90). Preoperative intravenous urography and the use of ureteric catheters in potentially difficult cases might help prevent trauma to the urinary tract.

An increased risk of UI after hysterectomy has also been reported. In a systematic review women over the age of 60 years who had undergone hysterectomy had a higher odds ratio compared with women <60 years (91).

Overall the estimates suggest a 60% increased risk of developing incontinence after hysterectomy. How this can be prevented is unclear but with a reduction in the number of hysterectomies for menorrhagia, by the use of progesterone-containing intra-uterine devices and endometrial ablation, post-hysterectomy incontinence might become less prevalent.

For those patients with *pre-existing* USI who require hysterectomy, consideration might be given to concomitant continence surgery, as *secondary* prevention. This has been shown to improve the chances of continence at one year postoperatively (92). However there is no evidence that this is indicated for primary prevention.

It has been suggested that subtotal hysterectomy might reduce the incidence of UI (93), as the cervix might act as a posterior support for the sphincteric mechanism. It is also thought that division of the cardinal ligaments can result in denervation (94). However RCT's have failed to show any benefit of subtotal over total hysterectomy with regards the onset of UI (95–97).

On the basis of current evidence UI does not seem to be adversely affected *in the short-term* following hysterectomy. However there is an association with incontinence *long-term* (91); therefore, preventative measures need to be investigated.

Hysterectomy and POP

The risk of vaginal vault prolapse and enterocele following hysterectomy has been reported as 3.6 per 1000 person-years. The risk increases from 1% (at 3 years) to 5% (at 15 years) (19). After colposuspension, the incidence of new onset enterocele has a reported incidence of 18% to 30% (98,99).

Possible causes of post-surgical POP include reduced and weakened collagen (9,100) failure to support the vault at hysterectomy or "anteversion" of the anterior vaginal wall following colposuspension. Similarly "retroversion" of the vaginal vault at sacrospinous ligament fixation can result in a high incidence of cystocele (see chap. 91 on "Laparoscopic Sacrocolpopexy"). Prevention will depend on the surgical procedure, the technique, and the strength of the supporting structures.

Attempts to prevent *enterocele*, by performing a Moschowitz procedure, or *vault prolapse* by attaching the round ligaments to the vaginal vault, or *cystocele* by prophylactic anterior repair at sacrospinous fixation, have been tried. Long-term follow-up studies are required to see if these measures are effective in preventing POP after gynecological surgery. However, it is generally accepted that apical support is the key to preventing recurrence of vault prolapse following hysterectomy (101).

Prevention of Urgency Incontinence After Surgery for USI
Mid-Urethral Tapes
There are few data on whether tension free vaginal tape (TVT) has a better effect in prevention of de novo urge symptoms/DO than colposuspension. In a large RCT comparing the two procedures the incidence of *new-onset* urgency and urgency incontinence was <2% for TVT and <5% for colposuspension at five years (102), although this might be an underestimate given the high incidence (over 90%) of preoperative OAB symptoms in both groups in this study.

In a follow-up of patients seven years after TVT, 22.5% had "urge symptoms." In a further 6.3% this was "de novo" (103), similar to the 9.1% incidence reported by other authors (104). In those with *pre-operative* OAB symptoms, 57% resolved after surgery (104).

From these case series it would appear that the incidence of urgency incontinence and OAB after TVT is similar to that reported after colposuspension.

Likewise, the rate of de novo urgency and urgency incontinence after transobturator tape (TOT) seems to be comparable to that of TVT (105,106) and Burch colposuspension (107).

Prevention of "Occult" Incontinence
New onset incontinence is a particularly worrying complication following surgery for POP. It has been shown that 7% to 22% of patients can develop incontinence following POP surgery (108,109).

It is generally acknowledged that the incidence of occult stress incontinence seen pre-operatively, for example following a pessary test, exceeds that actually seen after the procedure (110). Figures range from 23% (111) to 83% (112). However more data are required.

Five prospective studies have investigated several prophylactic anti-incontinence procedures at the time of POP surgery, including Pereyra needle suspension (113), Kelly plication (114), Stamey procedure (115), pubovaginal sling (116), and needle suspension versus endopelvic fascial plication (109). The latter was a small randomized trial which failed to confirm that a concomitant anti-incontinence procedure is preventative. None of these studies have a non-intervention arm ("no anti-incontinence procedure"), which makes difficult to determine and compare the risk of post-operative incontinence with those not having an anti-incontinence procedure.

More recently, the potential role of prophylactic mid-urethral sling (TVT) has been evaluated in two controlled case series which report conflicting results. One small retrospective trial involving 19 patients (117) reported no difference between the groups; while another prospective trial (118) reported significant reduction in the incidence of post-operative incontinence in the women undergoing prophylactic TVT.

The most rigorous study into the prevention of potential/occult incontinence, the CARE study (119), randomized 322 women undergoing sacrocolpopexy into concomitant Burch colposuspension and no intervention. They demonstrated a significant reduction in post-operative stress incontinence at three months, which seems to be maintained at two years (120). The pessary test and pre-operative urodynamics were not very helpful in predicting outcome.

Since these results cannot be extrapolated to other anti-incontinence procedures/POP operations, further research is required.

In the meantime it is advisable to warn patients of the potential risk of incontinence and the possible need for treatment in the future.

The limited evidence suggests that patients with occult/potential SUI are at increased risk of post-operative SUI (121). However there is not enough evidence to counsel patients on prophylactic surgery at present, except possibly for colposuspension at the time of Sacrocolpopexy in light of the CARE study results. However mid-urethral slings might allow for "minimally-invasive" secondary surgery as an "interval" procedure in those who develop "occult" SUI.

Recurrence of SUI After Vault Suspension: Prevention
A rare but potentially distressing scenario is recurrence of SUI following vault prolapse surgery in patients who have had a previously successful colposuspension. While there are fewer of these procedures being performed since the introduction of mid-urethral tapes, nonetheless about 30% of patients will develop symptomatic prolapse requiring surgery with the potential risk of recurrence of SUI. The exact prevalence however is unknown.

A case study has highlighted this risk and suggests methods of prevention (122). For example, measuring that vault elevation (in centimeters from the hymen) pre-operatively which will not result in demonstrable SUI and reproducing it at sacrocolpopexy might prevent this complication.

Also, performing sacrospinous fixation under spinal anesthesia allows the patient to perform a cough stress test, thus enabling alterations in the placement of the sutures to prevent incontinence (122).

How often this complication arises is unclear. However, these reports highlight the need for "vigilance" and to be aware of the possible risk of rendering a patient incontinent again despite previously successful incontinence surgery.

PREVENTION OF FAILED SURGERY FOR INCONTINENCE AND PROLAPSE
Stress Incontinence Surgery
The usually quoted success rates for USI surgery are 80% to 90% (99,123). The difference might be due to the definition of "success" or diagnostic, patient, or technical factors.

Previous incontinence surgery (124) and intrinsic sphincter deficiency (ISD) might be important. For example, a 54%

failure rate has been reported in patients with ISD (125) although this is not a consistent finding (126).

Other predictors of treatment failure two years after surgery for USI including urgency incontinence, more advanced prolapse, and postmenopausal status (not on HRT) have been reported (127). These are difficult to modify but might need to be considered when counseling women on the operative prognosis.

Studies are required to compare the various surgical procedures for ISD, such as slings, colposuspension, injectables, and mid-urethral tapes so that failure can be prevented. A recent randomized trial comparing the efficacy of TVT versus Trans-Obturator Tape (TOT) in women with ISD found that a significantly higher proportion or women in the TOT group had USI at six months follow up (45% vs. 21%) and that more women in the TOT group required repeat sling surgery (128). It therefore seems that TVT might be a more appropriate operation for this group of patients.

The surgical "gold standard" for USI due to bladder-neck "hypermobility" has been the Burch colposuspension (129,130); although the mid-urethral tapes (e.g., TVT) have become popular with comparable short and medium term outcomes (102,103).

Prevention of failed surgery might be achieved by avoiding procedures with a poor success rate (e.g., anterior repair) or those which have not been fully evaluated or failed to show benefit over colposuspension or TVT.

Attention to the above should lead to reduced failure rates with surgery. The old adages are still apt: "the first operation must be the best one" and "we should choose the right operation for the right patient and the right patient for the right operation." The latter will depend on factors such as obesity, age, previous surgery, concomitant prolapse, and DO.

Pelvic Organ Prolapse Surgery

Cystocele/anterior repair has long been known to have a high failure rate (131,132) with incidences as high as 40% being quoted (133). The reasons for failure are unclear and might be related to surgical technique, patient selection, poor tissue collagen, etc.

It is also possible that the anatomical defects associated with cystocele have not been corrected. For example, it is known that in many cases the anatomical defect is a detachment of the paravaginal fascia from the arcus tendineus fascia pelvis/"white line."

It is unlikely that an anterior repair, which is a midline fascial plication, will correct this defect; paravaginal repair might be more appropriate. While success rates of 76% to 97% have been quoted (134), a RCT is required to determine if paravaginal repair produces a better outcome than anterior repair in cases of paravaginal defect.

At present there are no validated tests which will identify these defects either pre- or intra-operatively and whether prevention is possible.

Several surgical techniques have been tried to prevent recurrent POP, mainly aimed at reinforcing apical support (see "Hysterectomy and POP").

The use of grafts/meshes to prevent recurrence of prolapse is becoming increasingly popular despite a lack of supporting evidence on long term efficacy and safety. A recent systematic review on transvaginal mesh kits for vaginal apical prolapse found a high short term success rate (87–95%) anatomically, but an overall high complication rate of up to 18%, including mesh erosion, fistula formation, and necrotizing fasciitis (135). The review did not involve study quality assessment, i.e., the studies included in the review were likely to be of poor methodological quality; and two-thirds of included studies were conference abstracts.

A similar review that compared vaginal mesh kits with traditional vaginal surgery and sacrocolpopexy for apical support (136) also found that complications requiring re-operation and total re-operation rate (i.e., due to complications and recurrent prolapse) were highest in the mesh group, although re-operation rates for recurrent prolapse were lower.

A meta-analysis of mesh repair of the anterior and posterior vaginal wall compartments showed similar results (137) and the authors concluded that the evidence for most outcomes was "too sparse for meaningful conclusions".

Larger RCTs with long term follow up comparing meshes with traditional surgery using both subjective and objective outcomes are therefore required.

PREVENTION OF DO

As the etiology and natural history of DO are unclear, prevention is difficult. There are few studies assessing long term outcomes. Those which exist suggest that OAB is a chronic condition that persists urodynamically and symptomatically (138).

For prevention of post-operative urgency incontinence, accurate diagnosis by urodynamic studies might help avoid unnecessary surgery in patients who have DO and not USI.

It is possible that DO might have its origins in childhood (see section on "Familial/Genetic Risk Factors" above). For example, patients with persistent primary nocturnal enuresis have a high incidence of DO (139). In an attempt to prevent symptoms in their children, some mothers with OAB often "toilet" the children more frequently (140,141). This might be counter-productive as frequent voiding might develop into urgency and urgency incontinence (29).

Although none of the studies cited here are large or the findings conclusive, nonetheless they highlight the need for further investigation in this area.

Should symptoms in childhood be relevant to the etiology of DO then education of parents regarding toileting and bladder drill might be preventative.

Psychological factors have been implicated in the etiology of DO (142,143). Identification together with appropriate psychotherapy, have shown encouraging results (143). This might also prove valuable in prevention.

Anecdotal evidence suggests that a high fluid intake is associated with symptoms of frequency and urgency. Restricting bladder stimulants (e.g., caffeine and alcohol) should be considered.

Finally, the "Integral Theory" suggests that bladder-neck opening (due to a weak anterior vaginal wall) might lead to the development of DO (144). PFMT might therefore have a role in prevention. However, long-term studies are needed to test this hypothesis.

Further research is needed into the etiology of DO, which might be multifactorial. In the meantime, prevention can only be speculative.

CONCLUSIONS

The *natural history of incontinence and POP* requires more study but there is evidence that spontaneous remission occurs.

Effective *prevention* will only be achieved by long-term prospective studies of appropriate interventions in "at-risk" groups. For example:

- Treatment of coexisting factors such as obesity, chronic cough, or constipation, might help in primary and secondary prevention.
- Studies of interventions in children with symptoms, and asymptomatic individuals with a strong family history of incontinence and/or POP.
- Further research is required to assess the preventative effects of hormone replacement in menopausal women.
- Long-term follow-up of patients with incontinence as a result of pregnancy and vaginal delivery is required before elective caesarean section can be recommended for prevention. PFMT seems to have a beneficial effect in "at-risk" groups in the short-term. However, methods to improve compliance are required.
- Attention to the potential risk of incontinence following hysterectomy or POP surgery is suggested. For a patient to be rendered incontinent following unrelated surgery is distressing; measures to identify the risk and prevent this outcome should be considered.
- Further research is required to identify the reasons for poor treatment outcomes (e.g., POP surgery) and measures taken to improve success.

With attention to the above and the natural history, appropriate preventative measures should be found to "protect" women from incontinence and POP.

REFERENCES

1. Freeman RM. The effect of pregnancy on the lower urinary tract and pelvic floor. In: Maclean AB, Cardozo LD, eds. Incontinence in Women. London: RCOG Press, 2002: 334.
2. Swift SE, Ostergard DR. Effects of progesterone on the urinary tract. Int Urogynecol J 1993; 4: 232–6.
3. Van Geelen JM, Lemmens WA, Eskes TK, et al. The urethral pressure profile in pregnancy and after delivery in healthy nulliparous women. Am J Obstet Gynecol 1982; 144: 636–49.
4. Landon CR, Crofts CE, Smith AR, et al. Mechanical properties of fascia during pregnancy: a possible factor in the development of stress incontinence of urine. Contemp Rev Obstet Gynaecol 1990; 2: 40–6.
5. Chaliha C, Kalia V, Stanton SL, et al. Antenatal prediction of postpartum urinary and faecal incontinence. Obstet Gynecol 1999; 94: 689–94.
6. Keane DP, Sims J, Abrams P, Bailey J. Analysis of collagen status in premenopausal nulliparous women with genuine stress incontinence. Br J Obstet Gynaecol 1997; 104: 994–8.
7. Hannested YS, Terje Lie R, Rortvivt T, Hunskaar S. Familiar risk of urinary incontinence: population bases cross-sectional study. BMJ 2004; 329: 889–91.
8. Carley ME, Schaffer J. Urinary incontinence and pelvic organ prolapse in women with Marfan or Ehlers-Danlos syndrome. Am J Obstet Gynecol 2000; 182: 1021–3.
9. Norton PA, Baker JE, Sharp HC, Warenski JC. Genital urinary prolapse and joint hypermobility in women. Obstet Gynecol 1995; 85: 225–8.
10. Thom DH, Van den Eeden SK, Brown JS. Evaluation of parturition and other reproductive variables as risk factors for urinary incontinence in later life. Obstet Gynaecol 1997; 90: 983–9.
11. Dolan LM, Hosker GL, Mallett VT, et al. Stress incontinence and pelvic floor neurophysiology 15 years after the first delivery. BJOG 2003; 110: 1107–14.
12. Viktrup L, Lose G. Lower urinary tract symptoms 5 years after the first delivery. Int Urogynecol J Pelvic Floor Dysfunct 2000; 11: 336–40.
13. Glazener C, Herbison G, Macarthur C, et al. New postnatal urinary incontinence: obstetric and other risk factors in primiparae. BJOG 2006; 113: 208–17.
14. Wennberg A, Molander U, Fall M, et al. A longitudinal population-based survey of urinary incontinence, overactive bladder and other lower urinary tract symptoms in women. Eur Urol 2009; 55: 783–91.
15. O'Boyle AL, O'Boyle JD, Ricks RE, et al. The natural history of pelvic organ support in pregnancy. Int Urogynecol J 2003; 14: 46–9.
16. Handa VL, Garrett E, Hendrix S, et al. Progression and remission of pelvic organ prolapse: a longitudinal study of menopausal women. Am J Obstet Gynecol 2004; 190: 27–32.
17. Samuelsson EC, Victoral FTA, Tibblin G, Svardsudd KF. Signs of genital prolapse in a Swedish population of women 20 to 59 years of age and possible related factors. Am J Obstet Gynecol 1999; 180: 299–305.
18. Swift S. The distribution of pelvic organ support in a population of female subjects seen for routine gynecologic health care. Am J Obstet Gynecol 2000; 183: 277–85.
19. Mant J, Painter R, Vessey M. Epidemiology of genital prolapse: observations from the Oxford Family Planning Association Study. BJOG 1997; 104: 579–85.
20. Scherf C, Morison L, Fiander A, et al. Epidemiology of pelvic organ prolapse in rural Gambia, West Africa. BJOG 2002; 109: 431–6.
21. Aubert J, Goua V, Calaora D, et al. Le retentissement des prolapsus génitaux sur le haut appareil urinaire (impact of genital prolapse on the upper urinary tract). Prog Urol 2000; 10: 107–12.
22. Thomas TM, Plymat KR, Blannin J, Meade TW. Prevalence of urinary incontinence. BMJ 1980; 280: 1243–5.
23. Resnick NM. Geriatric incontinence. Urol Clin North Am 1996; 23: 55–74.
24. Spence-Jones C, Kamm MA, Henry MM, Hudson CN. Bowel dysfunction: pathogenic factor in utero-vaginal prolapse and urinary stress incontinence. Br J Obstet Gynaecol 1994; 101: 147–52.
25. Smith P. Age changes in the female urethra. Br J Urol 1972; 44: 667–76.
26. Fantl JA, Cardozo LD, McClish D, et al. Oestrogen therapy in the management of urinary incontinence in postmenopausal women—a meta-analysis. Obstet Gynecol 1994; 83: 12–18.
27. Benness C, Wise BG, Cutner A, Cardozo LD. Does low dose vaginal oestradiol improve frequency and urgency in postmenopausal women? Int Urogynecol J 1992; 3: 281 (abstract).
28. Moeher B, Hextall A, Jackson S. Oestrogens for urinary incontinence in women [Cochrane Review]. In: The Cochrane Library, Issue 3. Oxford: Update Software, 2003.
29. Frewen WK. The management of urgency and frequency of micturition. Br J Urol 1980; 52: 367–69.
30. Brown JS, Vittinghoff E, Wyman JF, et al. Urinary incontinence. Does it increase risk for falls and fracture? J AM Geriatr Soc 2000; 48: 721–5.
31. Dwyer PL, Lee ETC, Hay DM. Obesity and urinary incontinence in women. Br J Obstet Gynaecol 1988; 95: 91–6.
32. Kudish BI, Iglesia CB, Sokol RJ, et al. Effect of weight change on natural history of pelvic organ prolapse. Obstet Gynecol 2009; 113: 81–8.
33. Reilly ETC, Freeman RM, Waterfield MR, et al. Prevention of postpartum stress incontinence in primigravidae with increased bladder neck mobility: a randomized controlled trial of antenatal pelvic floor exercises. BJOG 2002; 109: 68–76.
34. Rasmussen KL, Krue ES, Johansson LE, et al. Pre-pregnancy obesity—a potent risk factor for urinary symptoms post-partum persisting up to 6–8 months after delivery. Acta Obstet Gynecol Scand 1997; 76: 359–62.

35. Bump RC, Sugerman HJ, Fantl JA, McClish DK. Obesity and lower urinary tract function: effect of surgically-induced weight loss. Am J Obstet Gynecol 1992; 167: 392–9.

36. Subak LL, Johnson C, Whitcomb E, et al. Does weight loss improve urinary incontinence in moderately obese women? Int Urogynecol J 2003; 13: 40–3.

37. Auwad W, Steggles P, Bombieri L, et al. Moderate weight loss in obese women with urinary incontinence: a prospective longitudinal study. Int Urogynecol J Pelvic Floor Dysfunct 2008; 19: 1251–9.

38. Subak LL, Wing R, West DS, et al. Weight loss to treat urinary incontinence in overweight and obese women. N Engl J Med 2009; 360: 481–90.

39. Wilson PD, Bo K, Nygaard IE, et al. Conservative treatment in women. In: Abrams P, Wein A, eds. Second International Consultation on Incontinence. Health Publication Ltd, 2005.

40. Iosif S. Stress incontinence during pregnancy and the puerperium. Int J Gynecol Obstet 1981; 19: 13–20.

41. Buchsbaum GM, Duecy EE. Incontinence and pelvic organ prolapse in parous/nulliparous pairs of identical twins. Neurourol Urodyn 2008; 27: 496–8.

42. Graham CA, Mallett VT. Race as a predictor of urinary incontinence and pelvic organ prolapse. Am J Obstet Gynecol 2001; 185: 116–20.

43. Hendrix SL, Clark A, Nygaard I, et al. Pelvic organ prolapse in the Women's Health Initiative: gravity and gravidity. Am J Obstet Gynecol 2002; 186: 1160–6.

44. Fitzgerald MP, Thom DH, Wassel-Fyr C, et al. Childhood urinary symptoms predict adult overactive bladder symptoms. J Urol 2006; 175: 989–93.

45. Snooks SJ, Swash M, Setchell M, Henry MM. Injury to the innervation of pelvic floor sphincter musculature in childbirth. Lancet 1984; 2: 546–50.

46. Sultan AH, Kamm A, Hudson CN. Pudendal nerve damage during labour: a prospective study before and after childbirth. Br J Obstet Gynaecol 1994; 101: 22–8.

47. Smith ARB, Hosker GL, Warrell DW. The role of pudendal nerve damage in the aetiology of genuine stress incontinence in women. Br J Obstet Gynaecol 1989; 96: 29–32.

48. Stanton SL, Kerr-Wilson R, Harris GV. The incidence of urological symptoms in normal pregnancy. Br J Obstet Gynaecol 1980; 87: 897–900.

49. King JK, Freeman RM. Is antenatal bladder neck mobility a risk factor for postpartum stress incontinence? Br J Obstet Gynaecol 1998; 105: 1300–7.

50. Glazener CMA, Herbison JP, Wilson PD, et al. Conservative management of persistent postnatal urinary and faecal incontinence: randomized controlled trial. BMJ 2001; 323: 593–6.

51. Sultan AH, Stanton SL. Preserving the pelvic floor and perineum during childbirth. Elective caesarean section? Br J Obstet Gynaecol 1996; 103: 731–4.

52. Groutz A, Rimon E, Peled S, et al. Cesarean section: does it really prevent the development of postpartum stress urinary incontinence? A prospective study of 363 women one year after their first delivery. Neurourol Urodyn 2004; 23: 2–6.

53. Rortveit G, Daltveit AK, Hannestad YS, et al. Urinary incontinence after vaginal delivery or cesarean section. N Engl J Med 2003; 348: 900–7.

54. Morkved S, Bo K, Schei B, Salvessen KA. Pelvic floor muscle training during pregnancy to prevent urinary incontinence; a single-blind randomized controlled trial. Obstet Gynecol 2004; 101: 313–19.

55. Chiarelli P, Cockburn J. Promoting urinary continence in women after delivery: randomized controlled trial. BMJ 2002; 324: 1241–4.

56. Wilson P, Herbison GP. A randomized controlled trial of pelvic floor muscle exercises to treat postnatal urinary incontinence. Int Urogynecol J Pelvic Floor Dysfunct 1998; 9: 257–64.

57. Morkved S, Bo K. Effective postpartum pelvic floor muscle training in prevention and treatment of urinary incontinence: a one year follow-up. BJOG 2000; 107: 1022–28.

58. Hay-Smith J, Morkved S, Fairbrother KA, Herbison GP. Pelvic floor muscle training for prevention and treatment of urinary and faecal incontinence in antenatal and postnatal women. Cochrane Database Syst Rev 2008; (4): CD007471. DOI: 10.1002/14651858.CD007471.

59. Glazener CM, Herbison GP, MacArthur C, et al. Randomized controlled trial of conservative management of postnatal urinary and faecal incontinence: six year follow up. BMJ 2005; 330: 337–9.

60. Agur WI, Steggles P, Waterfield M, Freeman RM. The long term effectiveness of antenatal pelvic floor muscle training: eight-year follow up of a randomized controlled trial. BJOG 2008; 115: 985–90.

61. Brostrom S, Lose G. Pelvic floor muscle training in the prevention and treatment of urinary incontinence in women—what is the evidence? Acta Obstet Gynecol Scand 2008; 87: 384–402.

62. Allen RE, Hosker GL, Smith ARB, Warrell DW. Pelvic floor damage and childbirth: a neurophysiological study. Br J Obstet Gynaecol 1990; 97: 770–9.

63. Arya LA, Jackson ND, Myers DL, Verma AV. Risk of new-onset urinary incontinence 1 year after forceps and vacuum delivery in primiparous women. Am J Obstet Gynecol 2001; 185: 1318–24.

64. Carroli G, Belizan J. Episiotomy for vaginal birth (Cochrane Review). In: The Cochrane Library, Issue 4. Chichester, UK: John Wiley and Sons, Ltd., 2004.

65. Cutner A, Cardozo LD, Benness CJ. Assessment of urinary symptoms in early pregnancy. Br J Obstet Gynaecol 1991; 98: 1283–86.

66. van Brummen HJ, Bruinse HW, van der Bom JG, et al. How do the prevalences of urogenital symptoms change during pregnancy? Neurourol Urodyn 2006; 25: 135–9.

67. van Brummen HJ, Bruinse HW, van de Pol G, et al. Bothersome lower urinary tract symptoms 1 year after first delivery: prevalence and the effect of childbirth. BJU Int 2006; 98: 89–95.

68. MacArthur C, Bick DE, Keighley MR. Faecal incontinence after childbirth. Br J Obstet Gynaecol 1997; 104: 46–50.

69. Sultan AH, Kamm MA, Hudson CN. Anal sphincter disruption during vaginal delivery. N Engl J Med 1993; 329: 1905–11.

70. Sultan AH, Kamm MA, Bartram I, Hudson CN. Third degree obstetric anal sphincter tears: risk factors and outcome of primary repair. BMJ 1994; 308: 887–91.

71. Fernando R, Sultan A, Kettle C, Thakar R, Radley S. Methods of repair for obstetric anal sphincter injury. Cochrane Database Syst Rev 2006; (3): CD002866. DOI: 10.1002/14651858.CD002866.pub2.

72. Poen AC, Felt-Bersma RJF, Dekker GA, et al. Third degree obstetric perineal tears: risk factors and the preventative role of mediolateral episiotomy. Br J Obstet Gynaecol 1997; 104: 563–6.

73. De Leeuw JW, Struijk PC, Vierhout ME, Wallenburg HCS. Risk factors for third degree perineal ruptures during pregnancy. Br J Obstet Gynaecol 2001; 108: 383–7.

74. Helwig JT, Thorp JM, Bowes WA. Does midline episiotomy increase the risk of third and fourth-degree lacerations in operative vaginal deliveries? Obstet Gynecol 1993; 82: 276–9.

75. Tincello DG, Williams A, Fowler GE, et al. Differences in episiotomy technique between midwives and doctors. BJOG 2003; 110: 1041–4.

76. Andrews V, Thakar R, Sultan AH, et al. Are mediolateral episiotomies actually mediolateral? BJOG 2005; 112: 1156–8.

77. Eogan M, Daly L, O'Connell PR, et al. Does the angle of episiotomy affect the incidence of anal sphincter injury? BJOG 2006; 113: 190–4.

78. Sultan AH, Johanson RB, Carter JE. Occult anal sphincter trauma following forceps and vacuum delivery. Int J Gynecol Obstet 1998; 61: 113–19.

79. Bofill JA, Rust OA, Schorr SJ, et al. A randomized prospective trial of the obstetric forceps versus the M-cup vacuum extractor. Am J Obstet Gynecol 1996; 175: 1325–30.

80. Combs CA, Robertson PA, Laros RK. Risk factors for third degree and fourth degree perineal lacerations in forceps and vacuum deliveries. Am J Obstet Gynecol 1990; 163: 100–4.

81. Pollack J, Nordenstam J, Brismar S, et al. Anal incontinence after vaginal delivery: a five year prospective cohort study. Obstet Gynecol 2004; 104: 1397–402.

82. Fynes M, Donnelly V, Behan M, et al. Effect of second vaginal delivery on anorectal physiology and faecal continence: a prospective study. Lancet 1999; 354: 983–6.

83. Elfaghi I, Johansson-Ernste B, Rydhstroem H. Rupture of the sphincter ani: the recurrence rate in second delivery. BJOG 2004; 111: 1361–4.

84. Lowder JL, Burrows LJ, Krohn MA, et al. Risk factors for primary and subsequent anal sphincter lacerations: a comparison of cohorts by parity and prior mode of delivery. Am J Obstet Gynecol 2007; 196: 344. e1–5.

85. Spydslaug A, Trogstad LI, Skrondal A, et al. Recurrent risk of anal sphincter laceration among women with vaginal deliveries. Obstet Gynecol 2005; 105: 307–13.

86. Dandolu V, Gaughan JP, Chatwani AJ, et al. Risk of recurrence of anal sphincter lacerations. Obstet Gynecol 2005; 105: 831–5.

87. Edwards H, Grotegut C, Harmanli OH, et al. Is severe perineal damage increased in women with prior anal sphincter injury? J Matern Fetal Neonatal Med 2006; 19: 723–7.

88. Abramov Y, Sand PK, Botros SM, et al. Risk factors for female anal incontinence: new insight through the Evanston-Northwestern twin sister's study. Obstet Gynecol 2005; 106: 726–32.

89. Varma MG, Brown JS, Creasman JM, et al. Fecal incontinence in females older than aged 40 years: who is at risk? Dis Colon Rectum 2006; 49: 841–51.

90. Hendry WF. Urinary tract injuries during gynaecological surgery. In: Studd J, ed. Progress in Obstetrics and Gynaecology, Vol. 5. Edinburgh: Churchill Livingstone, 1985: 362–77.

91. Brown JS, Sawyer G, Tom DH, Grady D. Hysterectomy and urinary incontinence. A systematic review. Lancet 2000; 356: 535–9.

92. Kjeiulff KH, Langenberg PW, Greenaway L, et al. Urinary incontinence and hysterectomy in a large prospective cohort study in American women. J Urol 2002; 167: 2088–92.

93. Kikku P. Supravaginal uterine amputation v hysterectomy with reference to subjective bladder symptoms and incontinence. Acta Obstet Gynecol Scand 1985; 64: 375–9.

94. Parys BT, Haylen BT, Hutton JL, Parsons KF. The effects of simple hysterectomy on vesicourethral function. BJU 1989; 64: 594–9.

95. Thakar R, Ayes S, Clarkson P, et al. Outcomes after total and subtotal hysterectomy. N Engl J Med 2002; 347: 1318–29.

96. Lerman La, Summitt RL, Varner RE, et al. A randomized comparison of total or supracervical hysterectomy: surgical complications and clinical outcomes. Obstet Gynaecol 2003; 102: 453–62.

97. Gimbel H, Zobbe V, Anderson BM, et al. A randomized controlled trial of total compared with subtotal hysterectomy with one year follow-up results. BJOG 2003; 110: 1088–98.

98. Wiskind AK, Crighton SM, Stanton SL. The incidence of genital prolapse after the Burch colposuspension. Am J Obstet Gynecol 1992; 167: 399–405.

99. Jarvis GJ. Surgery for genuine stress incontinence. Br J Obstet Gynaecol 1994; 101: 371–4.

100. Jackson SR, Avery NC, Tarlton JF, et al. Changes in the metabolism of collagen in genitourinary prolapse. Lancet 1996; 347: 1658–61.

101. Ross JW. Apical vault repair, the cornerstone of pelvic vault reconstruction. Int Urogynecol J 1997; 8: 146–52.

102. Ward K, Hilton P, on behalf of the UK and Ireland TVT Trial Group. Tension-free vaginal tape versus colposuspension for primary urodynamic stress incontinence; 5-year follow-up. BJOG 2008; 115: 226–33.

103. Nilsson CG, Falconer C, Rezapour M. Seven-year follow-up of the tension-free vaginal tape procedure for treatment of urinary incontinence. Obstet Gynecol 2004; 104: 1259–62.

104. Segal JL, Vassallo B, Kleeman S, et al. Prevalence of persistent and de novo overactive bladder symptoms after tension-free vaginal tape. Obstet Gynecol 2004; 104: 1263–9.

105. Latthe PM, Foon R, Toozs-Hobson P. Transobturator and retropubic tape procedures in stress urinary incontinence: a systematic review and meta-analysis of effectiveness and complications. BJOG 2007; 114: 522–31.

106. Chene G, Cotte B, Tardieu AS, et al. Clinical and ultrasonographic correlations following three surgical anti-incontinence procedures (TOT, TVT and TVT-O). Int Urogynecol J 2008; 19: 1125–31.

107. Sivaslioglu AA, Caliskan E, Dolen I, Haberal A. A randomized comparison of transobturator tape and Burch colposuspension in the treatment of female stress urinary incontinence. Int Urogynecol J Pelvic Floor Dysfunct 2007; 18: 1015–19.

108. Borstad E, Rud T. The risk of developing urinary stress incontinence after vaginal repair in continent women: a clinical and urodynamic follow-up study. Acta Obstet Gynecol Scand 1989; 68: 545–54.

109. Bump RC, Hurt WG, Theofrastous JP, et al. Randomized prospective comparison of needle colposuspension v endopelvic fascia plication for potential stress incontinence, prophylaxis in women undergoing vaginal reconstruction for Stage III or IV pelvic organ prolapse. Am J Obstet Gynecol 1996; 175: 326–35.

110. Karram MM. What is the optimal anti-incontinence procedure in women with advance prolapse in "potential" stress incontinence? Int Urogynecol J 1999; 10: 1–2 (Editorial).

111. Versi E, Lyell DJ, Griffiths DJ. Videourodynamic diagnosis of occult genuine stress incontinence in patients with anterior vaginal wall relaxation. J Soc Gynecol Investig 1998; 5: 327–30.

112. Veronikis DK, Nichols DH, Wakamatsu MM. The incidence of low-pressure urethra as a function of prolapse-reducing technique in patients with massive pelvic organ prolapse (maximum descent at all vaginal sites). Am J Obstet Gynecol 1997; 177: 1305–13.

113. Bergman A, Koonings PP, Ballard CA. Predicting postoperative urinary incontinence development in women undergoing operation for genitourinary prolapse. Am J Obstet Gynecol 1988; 158: 1171–5.

114. Gordon D, Groutz A, Wolman I, et al. Development of postoperative urinary stress incontinence in clinically continent patients undergoing prophylactic Kelly plication during genitourinary prolapse repair. Neurourol Urodyn 1999; 18: 193–7.

115. Groutz A, Gordon D, Wolman I, et al. The use of prophylactic Stamey bladder neck suspension to prevent postoperative stress urinary incontinence in clinically continent women undergoing genitourinary prolapse repair. Neurourol Urodyn 2000; 19: 671–6.

116. Chaikin DC, Groutz A, Blaivas JG. Predicting the need for anti-incontinence surgery in continent women undergoing repair of severe urogenital prolapse. J Urol 2000; 163: 531–4.

117. de Tayrac R, Gervaise A, Chauveaud-Lambling A, Fernandez H. Combined genital prolapse repair reinforced with a polypropylene mesh and tension-free vaginal tape in women with genital prolapse and stress urinary incontinence: a retrospective case-control study with short term follow up. Acta Obstet Gynecol Scand 2004; 83: 950–4.

118. Liang CC, Chang YL, Chang SD, et al. Pessary test to predict postoperative urinary incontinence in women undergoing hysterectomy for prolapse. Obstet Gynecol 2004; 104: 795–800.

119. Brubaker L, Cundiff GW, Fine P, et al. Abdominal sacrocolpopexy with Burch colposuspension to reduce urinary stress incontinence. N Engl J Med 2006; 354: 1557–66.

120. Brubaker L, Nygaard I, Richter HH, et al. Two year outcomes after sacrocolpopexy with and without Burch to prevent stress urinary incontinence. Obstet Gynecol 2008; 112: 49–55.

121. Haessler AL, Lin LL, Ho MH, et al. Re-evaluating occult incontinence. Curr Opin Obstet Gynecol 2005; 17: 535–40.

122. Bombieri LB, Freeman RM. Recurrence of stress incontinence after vault suspension: can it be prevented? Int Urogynecol J 1998; 9: 58–60.

123. Smith ARB, Daneshgani F, Dmochowski R, et al. Surgery for Urinary Incontinence in Women. In: Abrams P, Cardozo L, Khoury S, Wein A, eds. Incontinence, 3rd Edn. Paris, France. Health Publications Ltd, 2005: 1297–370.

124. Francis LN, Sand PK, Hamrang K, Ostergard DR. Urodynamic appraisal of success and failure after retropubic urethropexy. J Reprod Med 1987; 32: 693–6.

125. Sand PK, Bowen LW, Panganiban R, Ostergard DR. The low pressure urethra as a factor in failed retropubic urethropexy. Obstet Gynecol 1987; 69: 399–402.

126. Richardson DA, Ramahi A, Chalas E. Surgical management of stress incontinence in patients with low urethral pressures. Gynecol Obstet Invest 1991; 31: 106–9.

127. Richter HE, Diokno A, Kenton K, et al. Predictors of treatment failure 24 months after surgery for stress urinary incontinence. J Urol 2008; 179: 1024–30.

128. Schierlitz L, Dwyer PL, Rosamilia A, et al. Effectiveness of tension-free vaginal tape compared with transobturator tape in women with stress

urinary incontinence and intrinsic sphincter deficiency: a randomized controlled trial. Obstet Gynecol 2008; 112: 1253–61.

129. Burch JC. Urethrovaginal fixation to Cooper's ligament for correction of stress incontinence, cystocele and prolapse. Am J Obstet Gynecol 1961; 81: 281–90.

130. Stanton SL, Cardozo LD. Results of the colposuspension operation for incontinence and prolapse. Br J Obstet Gynaecol 1979; 86: 693–9.

131. White GR. Cystocele, a radical cure by suturing lateral sulcus of vagina to white line of pelvic fascia. JAMA 1909; 21: 1707–10.

132. Olsen Al, Smith VJ, Bergstrom JO, et al. Epidemiology of surgically managed pelvic organ prolapse and urinary incontinence. Am J Obstet Gynecol 1997; 89: 501–5.

133. Weber AM, Walters M, Piedmonte M, et al. Anterior colporrhaphy. A randomized trial of three surgical techniques. Am J Obstet Gynecol 2001; 185: 1299–306.

134. Monga A. Fascia; defects and repair. Curr Opinion Obstet Gynaecol 1996; 8: 366–71.

135. Feiner B, Jelovsek J, Maher C. Efficacy and safety of transvaginal mesh kits in the treatment of prolapse of the vaginal apex: a systematic review. BJOG 2009; 116: 15–24.

136. Diwadkar GB, Barber MD, Feiner B, et al. Complication and reoperation rates after apical vaginal prolapse surgical repair: a systematic review. Obstet Gynecol 2009; 113: 367–73.

137. Jia X, Glazener C, Mowatt G, et al. Efficacy and safety of using mesh or grafts in surgery for anterior and/or posterior vaginal wall prolapse: systematic review and meta-analysis. BJOG 2008; 115: 1350–61.

138. Garnett S, Abrams P. The natural history of the overactive bladder and detrusor overactivity. A review of the evidence regarding the long-term outcome of the overactive bladder. J Urol 2003; 169: 843–8.

139. Whiteside CG, Arnold EP. Persistent primary enuresis: an urodynamic assessment. BMJ 1975; 1: 364–7.

140. De Jonge JA. The urge syndrome. In: Kolvin I, MacKeith RC, Meadow R, eds. Bladder Control and Enuresis. Clinics in Developmental Medicine, Nos. 48/49, 1973: 66–9.

141. Foote AJ, Moore KH. Bladder training: should you listen to what your mother says? Neurourol Urodyn 1996; 15: 137–8 (abstract).

142. Freeman RM, McPherson FM, Baxby K. Psychological features of women with idiopathic detrusor instability. Urol Int 1985; 40: 257–9.

143. Macauley AJ, Stanton SL, Stern RS, Holmes DM. Micturition and the mind: psychological factors in the aetiology and treatment of urinary disorders in women. BMJ 1987; 294: 540–3.

144. Petros PEP, Ulmsten U. Role of the pelvic floor in bladder neck opening and closure II: vagina. Int Urogynecol J 1997; 8: 69–73.

10 Medical Error and Patient Safety in Surgery
Roxane Gardner

INTRODUCTION

The impact of surgery-related errors and adverse events has long been felt by surgical patients and their families, surgeons, and their colleagues around the world. The exact number of surgical procedures performed worldwide each year is not known. However, an estimated 234.2 million major surgical procedures were performed globally in 2004 (1). This estimate included surgical procedures performed in a hospital operating room or out-patient surgery facility that required regional or general anesthesia or sedation for pain control. While the number taking place in the hospital versus the out-patient setting was not specified, an estimated seven million perioperative adverse events (based on a 3% peri-operative adverse event rate) and one million surgery-related deaths (based on a 0.5% peri-operative mortality rate) have occurred as a result of these procedures; with about half of adverse events deemed preventable.

Although the number of surgical procedures performed annually in the United States is not precisely known, over 32 million were performed during 2006, with about one fourth taking place in the hospital in-patient setting and the rest in ambulatory surgery clinics, physicians' offices, and hospital-based, out-patient surgical centers (2). Healthy patients deemed at low risk for adverse events are usually selected for out patient procedures. However, the number of surgical mishaps and misadventures is subject to increase with continued growth in the volume of out-patient procedures and less intense oversight of safety measures in these settings. The precise number of in-patient female urology and urogynecology procedures performed in the United States, the European Union, or worldwide in also not known. Oliphant et al. (3) found that age-adjusted rates for in-patient stress urinary incontinence (SUI) procedures performed in the United States between 1979 and 2004 more than doubled from 0.64 to 1.60 per 1000 woman. Their analysis underestimates the true overall and age-adjusted rates of such procedures because the National Hospital Discharge Survey (NHDS) database used for this study excludes federal, military, and Veteran hospital discharge information. Yet, both the overall and age-adjusted rates will likely increase as the population ages since about 20% of the population is expected to be 65 or more years by 2030, the majority being women (4). Although precise numbers of female urology and urogynecology out-patient procedures are not known, Boyles et al. (5) found that female urinary incontinence procedures performed in the out-patient setting doubled between 1994 and 1996 in the United States. Data reflecting more recent experience will soon be available (6) but such procedures are projected to increase in the United States and globally as the population ages, especially in industrialized countries (1). The number of surgical adverse events likely will increase given the projected growth in the aging population with potential co-morbidities, the projected increase in outpatient surgical procedures, and the increasing variety of surgical options, such as minimally-invasive endoscopic procedures, mid-urethral procedures, and injectable implants or bulking agents.

Based on the estimated 3% rate of perioperative adverse events worldwide, growth in preventable adverse events, and harm to patients is inevitable (1). Errors of commission and omission leading to adverse surgical events and patient harm occur across the continuum of patient care, involving knowledge, medical judgment, clinical diagnosis, and decision-making; task performance, interprofessional communication, and teamwork; documentation and medical order entry. As a result, patient safety is now recognized as a serious international public healthcare issue (7). Multidimensional efforts are underway to make healthcare safer for patients and clinicians (7–9). This chapter will provide an overview of medical errors and adverse events, and address some system-wide efforts aimed at preventing their occurrence or mitigating their effects in the surgical setting. Stitely and Gherman in a separate chapter will address specific clinical approaches for improving quality and safety of patient care, such as site verification, prophylaxis for infection, and deep venous thrombosis; the prevention of retained objects, fatigue-related errors; and safe introduction of new technology.

PATIENT SAFETY AND MEDICAL ERRORS

Patient safety, the prevention of harm to patients, is regarded by the Institute of Medicine (IOM) as inseparable from quality of care (10) (pp. 1–18). Safety is the first domain of quality. All patients expect and deserve safe care, freedom from hazards that increase the likelihood of adverse events, or harm. The call to action by the IOM to improve patient safety and decrease medical error came at the heels of two signature studies in the United States. These studies reviewed adverse events in hospitalized patients where prolonged hospital stay or disability occurred in 3.7% in New York (11) and 2.9% in Colorado and Utah (12); and at least 50% of these adverse events were deemed preventable. The landmark study involving Colorado and Utah showed that adverse events were no more likely to occur in surgical versus non-surgical care. However, nearly half of the surgical adverse events involved complications related to surgical technique, wound infections, and post-operative bleeding. Extrapolating the rates of adverse events identified in these studies to the population of all patients hospitalized in the United States during 1997 placed medical errors among the eighth leading cause of death (10) (p. 1), exceeding causes due to car accidents, breast cancer, or AIDS.

The National Health Service (NHS) of the United Kingdom in 2000 addressed the occurrence of healthcare-related adverse events and their impact on patients and their families, clinicians, and NHS organizations (13). In their signature report, *An Organisation with a Memory*, they stated that preventable errors are the result of human error whether intentional or not. Similar appreciation for the relationship between human factors and medical errors, and the subsequent launch of patient safety initiatives occurred in Australia around this same time. Lessons learned from their Australian incident monitoring study of the 1980s (14,15) did much to inform their efforts. Similar awareness and patient safety activities began in New Zealand around 2001 (16); and in Canada during 2002 with their release of a multifaceted action plan to improve patient safety, *Building a Safer System* (17). The WHO discussed patient safety in early 2002, culminating in a resolution by Member States to pay the closest possible attention to patient safety and establish evidence-based systems to improve safety and quality healthcare worldwide (18). Successful efforts in such endeavors led to the formation of the World Health Alliance for Patient Safety in 2004, and the Global Patient Safety Challenge to *Safe Surgery Saves Lives*—improving the safety of surgery around the globe (19).

James Reason asserted in the 1990s that all humans make errors, that errors are inevitable and usually deemed an acceptable price to pay in coping with difficult, complex tasks (20). He described a working framework for human error, highlighting the relationship between various aspects of human cognition and error. His framework differentiates three error types—"skills-based slips and lapses, rule-based mistakes and knowledge-based mistakes," and understanding the differences between these error types helps to identify suitable means by which to intervene and address them (20) (pp. 50–56). Reason described two main approaches by which to deal with the problem of human error, the person approach, and the system approach (21). The person approach embodies the longstanding tradition of targeting and blaming individuals for errors. The systems approach accepts the fallibility of human nature and expects errors. The systems approach scrutinizes how and why defenses fail; and designs ways to trap or minimize the effect of errors via measures that address the person, the team, the workplace, and the institution as a whole. This concept embodies a just culture; one that resonated with the IOM as evidenced by their strong advocacy for such approach to human error, not assigning blame, and building safer health care systems that reliably trap error and mitigate their effects (10) (pp. 155–201). The healthcare industry is highly complex and some 24 hour a day services are more vulnerable to error than others such as intensive care settings, the operating theater, emergency departments, and labor and delivery units. High reliability organizations (HROs) are known to exemplify the systems approach to human error (22).

HIGH RELIABILITY ORGANIZATIONS

A HRO operates in hazardous conditions 24 hours a day under the pressure of time but with fewer than expected accidents, "less than their fair share of adverse events" (22) (pp. 41–50).

Examples of such organizations include naval aircraft carriers, nuclear power plants, off shore oil platforms, and air traffic control systems. More and more hospital emergency units, operating theaters, and perinatal units around the world are striving to transform themselves into HROs. All HROs strive to manage the unexpected with determined mindfulness. Weick and Sutcliffe assert that "good management is mindful management of the unexpected" (22). HROs are characterized by a shared commitment to safety throughout the organization and distinguish themselves by their "collective preoccupation with the possibility of failure." Preoccupation with failure involves anticipating and recognizing where failure can occur, and taking measures to prevent it. Standardizing procedures where possible and taking stock of where and when adverse events and near misses may occur facilitates error prevention or minimizing their effect when they occur. Establishing effective reporting systems further optimizes the ability to identify error and near misses and provides opportunities to learn from them. HROs are not error free, but resilient when error occurs. One way HROs manifest preoccupation with failure is by training their personnel and teams intensively thru drills and simulations (22) (pp. 117–147).

CULTURE OF SAFETY

Importantly, HROs manifest a positive culture of safety. An organization's culture of safety is the product of individual and group values, skills, and behaviors that shape an organization's commitment to and proficiency of their own safety programs (23). A simple way to think about culture is "the way we do things around here and why we do them" (24). Edgar Schein (25) advocates analyzing organizational culture at three levels to better understand that which exits and use the knowledge gained to facilitate change if needed. The first level is comprised of the observable behaviors evident in the workplace; the second consists of the beliefs and values espoused by members within the organization; and perhaps most importantly, within the third level reside the basic underlying assumptions that may be taken for granted, largely subconscious, and not verbalized. According to Schein, these unconscious assumptions may best inform why things unfold within an organization the way they do. As a result, moving from a culture of shame and blame to one that is non-punitive yet preserves accountability can provoke anxiety, present challenging obstacles, and consume resources, especially time. The IOM acknowledged that one of healthcare's biggest challenges in providing reliably safe, high quality care was changing from a culture of shame, and blame to one that is fair and just (10).

Establishing a safe and just culture is not an easy task and cannot be mandated (24). Culture change takes time, and incremental steps will likely be needed to facilitate and solidify the change if it is to be long-lasting. Moreover, professional responsibility and accountability are key elements of the systems approach to error management (26). Individual healthcare providers, surgeons-urologists, urogynecologists, their colleagues, and team mates are not absolved from, but must remain responsible for ethical practice and maintaining competency.

Table 10.1 Practice-Related Issues Contributing to Patient Harm

Issue	Example
Regional variation in (surgical) practice	Deficient or inadequate guidelines, policies, or procedures; lack of adherence to guidelines, policies, or procedures
Uncertainty in clinical care	Presentation Diagnosis Risk assessment Management Response to treatment
Resource limitations	Staff Space Equipment Time
Wishful thinking	"Fallacy of the low risk patient"—continuing to perceive and manage a patient as low risk when their clinical circumstances have become high risk

Source: Modified from Ref. 29.

Table 10.2 Inherent Demands Weakening Defenses to Error

Inherent demands of clinical practice
  Presence demanded in more than one place at the same time
  High clinical volume, largely normal patients
  Increasing growth in elderly population with co-morbidities
  Off-site monitoring of high risk clinical situations
  Poor sign-out
  Protocols inadequate for referrals, consultations, or patient transfers
  Impaired vigilance-distractions, fatigue, etc.
  Hierarchical operations, poor teamwork
  Yielding to patient pressures regarding clinical practice
  Overconfidence (hubris)

Source: Modified from Ref. 29.

Can we "Safety Our Way Out" of Human Error?

In 2005, Young (27) posed the question, can we "safety our way out" of human error? Young referenced Herbert Simon's description of human behavior and decision-making, namely, human minds have a "bounded rationality" (28) for formulating and solving complex problems relative to the size of many problems arising in professional and personal lives. We have human limitations in our behavior and decision-making. Therefore, perfectly rational decisions are often not feasible in real-life due to our limitations, capabilities, and time constraints. It is essential to understand the issues healthcare professionals confront everyday that can contribute to harm while caring for patients if we are to design systems that facilitate provision of safe and high quality healthcare services. We need to appreciate where we are vulnerable to error in our practice and the clinical demands that weaken our defenses.

Veltman (29) identified several practice-related issues that contribute to perinatal harm that are generally applicable to surgical patient harm that may arise in female urology and urogynecology-related care (Table 10.1). He also described some of the inherent demands clinicians manage in the provision of perinatal care that weaken defenses to error. These demands, with some modification to adjust for growth of the aging population and those with co-morbidities, are generally applicable to surgeons of all specialties, affecting the safety and quality of patient care provided in ambulatory settings (office-based procedures), out patient surgery centers, inpatient operating room theaters, and inpatient and outpatient post-operative care settings (Table 10.2).

SOURCES OF ERROR IN SURGERY

Rogers et al. (30) retrospectively analyzed malpractice claims closed between 1986 and 2004, with injury occurring between 1980 and 2002, involving allegations of surgical error. Of 444 claims reviewed from four liability insurers, 258 (58%) were confirmed as being due to surgical error. The majority (76%) were elective procedures, representing a variety of surgical procedures: 74 (~29%) gastrointestinal, 62 (~24%) spinal and non-spinal orthopedic procedures, 18 (7%) hysterectomies, and 12 (5%) genitourinary tract procedures. Most (75%) occurred during the intraoperative period. Just over half of these cases (54%) were due to errors in operative technique, with most (83%) involving more than one clinician. Contributing factors included cognitive errors-judgment or lack of memory or vigilance; lack of technical competence or knowledge; communication breakdowns involving hand-offs, establishing responsibility, clinical supervision, physician–nurse exchange of information, and inability to reach the attending physician. Communication breakdowns were seen in 61 of these 258 cases (24%). Overall, system factors contributed to error in 82%, with inexperience/technical competence and communication being the dominant issues. Patient factors such as excess weight, difficult or unusual anatomy, and behavioral issues also contributed to surgical error.

Surgical Error in Female Urology and Urogynecology

Comprehensive analysis of the sources of error and adverse events and their preventability in female urology and urogynecology procedures are not available. However, Waetjen et al. in 2003 (31) reviewed the 1998 NHDS and 1998 National Census databases to estimate prevalence, morbidity, and mortality rates for SUI inpatient surgery in the United States. Adjusting for population growth, they found a 45% increase in the frequency of such surgery between 1988 and 1998. Overall, retropubic suspension was the most common procedure performed (46%), followed by anterior repair (27%), and other SUI procedures (14%). Mortality from stress incontinence surgery was low at one per 10,000 surgeries. However, 18.3% had one or more complications of which nearly half were due to infection (44%), surgical injury (24%), and bleeding (16%). This analysis was limited to incontinence surgery requiring hospital admission, not accounting for those performed in the outpatient or office-based setting and their associated injuries or adverse events.

Brown et al. (32) in 2002 estimated the prevalence, morbidity, and mortality of pelvic organ prolapse surgery based on the 1997 NHDS and 1997 National Census databases. They confirmed that surgery for pelvic organ prolapse was common, 22.7 per 10,000 women in the United States; and 21% of these included an incontinence procedure. Mortality was uncommon, three per 10,000 surgeries; and 15.5 % of all pelvic organ prolapse surgeries involved complications involving infection (5.4%), bleeding (5.4%), and surgical injury (4.2%).

Gilmore et al. (33) noted in 2006 that the most common major surgery in gynecology worldwide is the hysterectomy. They found a low rate of urinary tract injury (bladder or ureter), ranging from <1 per 1000 (subtotal hysterectomy with or without bilateral salpingo-oophorectomy) to 13 per 1000 surgeries (laparoscopic hysterectomy with or without bilateral salpingo-oophorectomy). Gilmour and Baskett (34) in 2005 had found a low rate of urinary tract injury (three per 1000 surgeries) at benign gynecologic surgery in Canada. However, such injury was associated with a high risk (91-fold) of litigation. A Cochrane review of surgical approach to hysterectomy by Nieboer et al. (35) noted a higher rate of urinary tract injuries with laparoscopic compared to an abdominal approach. David-Montefiore et al. (36) conducted a prospective, observational, multicenter study in France between June and December 2004 of women undergoing hysterectomy for benign disease. Of 634 procedures performed, they found intra- and post-operative complications occurred in 5.8% of the laparoscopic approaches, 8.2% of vaginal approaches, and 18% of abdominal approaches. However, no differences in rates of intraoperative complications were identified regardless of approach. Intraoperative complications included injury to the intestinal tract (~0.8%), urinary tract (~2%), and bleeding (~1%); whereas postoperative complications where more likely due to infection (~1–2%) and bleeding (~2%).

Methods for Mitigating Error and Managing their Effects

Successfully managing routine clinical and crisis situations requires expert knowledge, technical skills, sound decision-making, and optimal teamwork behaviors (37). The following section will address ways to tighten up our defenses against these practice-related issues and clinical demands in order to make surgery safer.

TEAMWORK AND COMMUNICATION

Teamwork is an essential component of HROs (38). The culture of health care, including medical education and residency training programs, has traditionally emphasized individual attainment of a high level of medical knowledge, procedural skills, and abilities, with little emphasis on effective teamwork behaviors and systems approach to problem-solving. Formal instruction and practice of optimal team work behavior for multidisciplinary teams confronting routine and crisis situations was nil to absent in most health profession training programs until about 1990s. The aviation industry was among the first to confront the reality of human error's contribution to accidents and the need for various skilled professionals to learn to work together better and communicate more effectively (39). In light of more than 50 years of research on team work,

Eduardo Salas asked a pivotal question: "How do we turn a team of experts into an expert team?" (40). Team training and cockpit resource management were central components of the aviation industry's initial attempt to answer this question in the early 1980s. Cockpit resource management, now known as "crew" resource management (CRM), focused on acquisition of timely information and optimizing skills in leadership, teamwork behavior, problem-solving, and situation awareness (41). Aviation CRM, better known as "error management" CRM, now focuses on safety and error recognition, management, and recovery. Gaba et al. (37), Helmreich (42), and Shortell et al. (43) adapted the aviation industry's approach to error management to evoke change and improve teamwork and communication among healthcare professionals in several key fields in the 1990s—anesthesia, surgery, and intensive care units. Howard et al. adapted aviation CRM to anesthesia in 1989 and dubbed it as Anesthesia Crisis Resource Management (44), paving the way for dissemination to Anesthesia leadership across the United States and around the world (45–48). Helmreich and associates further facilitated this transformation by integrating principles of organizational behavior and culture (42,49).

The Department of Defense (DoD) of the United States evaluated the impact of their aviation CRM program and found a 20% improvement in mission performance and a 40% reduction in safety-related task errors (50). The DoD adapted their Army Aviation CRM to healthcare in the late 1990s based on potential numbers of lives and dollars saved per year. Risser et al. (51) reviewed closed malpractice claims from a total of eight military and civilian hospital emergency departments, showing that 43% involved poor teamwork and communication. Similar issues were seen in about 60% of the DoD's Obstetrical closed claims-unpublished data. An internal review of Obstetrical closed claims involving Harvard-affiliated hospitals also found 43% had elements of poor teamwork and communication (52). The Joint Commission (53) reported communication failures were the leading root cause in 66% of sentinel events reported between 1995 and 2004, the leading root cause for medication errors, delays in treatment, and wrong-site surgery; and second leading root cause for operative and post-operative events.

Teamwork failures have been identified in surgical malpractice claims. As previously noted, Rogers et al. (30) identified communication breakdowns in 24% of surgical cases. Lingard et al. (54) in 2002 explored the nature of communication in the operating room. Of 35 surgeries and 128 hours of operating room interactions, patterns of conversations were observed as subtle, complex, and socially motivated. Conversations revolved around the following themes of time, safety, sterility, resources, roles, and situation. Tension surfaced regularly and one to four higher tension events arose per procedure. These events had an observable effect on members of the team, including surgical trainees who responded either by withdrawing from conversation or by mimicking their senior surgeon. Both of these responses by trainees had negative implications for effective teamwork.

Lingard et al. (55) subsequently used trained observers to study communication failures in the operating room during

2003. Of 48 surgical procedures and 90 hours of observations, they identified communication failures in about 30% of team exchanges. Such failures included poor timing, incomplete, or inaccurate information exchanged, issues were not resolved or key individuals were excluded. About one-third of these failures were seen to visibly affect system processes and jeapordize patient safety, such as tension amidst the team, inefficiency and delays, workarounds and wasted resources, patient inconvenience, and procedural errors. Such research by Lingard et al. highlights critical aspects of team communication and opportunities for interprofessional training to improve it. They deemed a curriculum to address interprofessional communication across systems and processes to be worthwhile. Interprofessional communication and professionalism in the operating room are areas ripe for research. Tension and the occurrence of higher tension events are inevitable in the operating room. How these moments are managed by members of surgical team, across the hierarchies within and between the disciplines, can directly and indirectly affect the safety of patient care, and surgical outcomes.

Greenberg et al. (56) analyzed 60 closed malpractice claims with communication breakdowns resulting in patient harm (a subset of the 444 closed malpractice claims previously described by Rogers et al. (30). Communication breakdowns were about evenly divided between the pre (38%), intra (30%), and post (32%) operative periods. Verbal communication breakdowns occurred between one transmitter and one receiver, more commonly involving the attending surgeon. Factors associated with these breakdowns included hierarchy and power differentials, and ambiguity about roles and responsibilities. Handoffs and transfer of care were problematic. Failures in resident to attending communication concerned notification of critical information, while attending to attending communication failures were related to inadequate handoffs. About 14% of cases involved intraoperative surgical sponge or instrument miscounts. These investigators proposed a series of triggers for notifying the responsible attending about clinical changes or staff concerns about a patient during the pre and post-operative periods. They estimated 26% to 44% of communication breakdowns would have been prevented if these triggers had been used. They postulated that the use of standardized handoffs and protocols for transferring patients would have prevented 11% to 35% of problematic occurrences. The combination of triggers and standardized transfers or handoffs could potentially prevent half or more of communication breakdowns. Implementation of read-back protocols, closed-loop communication techniques could further augment communication of critical patient information. Interventions aimed at enhancing intraoperative communication were not specifically explored in this analysis. However, they suggested instituting such techniques as standardized team briefings, time-outs, or surgical pauses to improve surgical safety; and exploring technological solutions to mitigate or prevent instrument or sponge miscounts.

Surgical Team Training Interventions
Two recent studies illustrate the impact of interventions aimed at improving communication and teamwork within surgical teams. Haynes et al. (57) evaluated implementation of the WHO surgical safety checklist, a structured communication tool designed to improve communication and consistency of surgical care before administering anesthesia, immediately prior to skin incision and before the patient leaves the operating room. The checklist was used in eight economically and clinically diverse hospitals located across the globe. Significant reductions were seen in death rates (1.5–0.8%, p = 0.003), and intraoperative complications (11–7%, p < 0.001). All sites had reductions in major postoperative complications. Although the reductions were greater in some sites than in others, the checklist program was deemed useful for improving surgical safety in a wide variety of clinical and economic settings worldwide.

McCulloch et al. (58) conducted a single institution (teaching hospital) before and after study of team skills training. They observed a series of laparoscopic cholecystectomy and carotid endarterectomy procedures before and after implementing a nine hour aviation CRM-based teamwork training curriculum. On-site teamwork coaching was provided about twice a week for three months. They also evaluated safety attitude questionnaires (SAQs) pre and post team training intervention. Formal team training led to significantly improved SAQ teamwork climate scores (p = 0.007), improved teamwork performance (p = 0.021) and reductions in technical errors (1.73–0.98 per operation, p = 0.009); and a 40% reduction in non-operative procedural errors. Although the authors acknowledged the limitations in generalizing their results beyond their academic setting, their findings were consistent with those obtained by Morey et al. (59) in their structured team training intervention for emergency department staff. Morey et al. in 2002 had published findings of their prospective, quasi-experimental, multi-center trial of a systematic team training program intervention in the emergency room setting. They reported a significant improvement in team behaviors (p = 0.012); and significant reduction in observed errors (30.9–4.4%, p = 0.039) in those departments participating in team training compared to controls. Significant improvement were also seen in staff attitudes towards teamwork (p = 0.047) and assessment of institutional support (p = 0.04).

Simulation-Based Training of Surgical Teams
Simulation-based training and practice offers a viable means by which to promote safe practice and sharpen procedural and teamwork skills across the spectrum of in-patient and out-patient settings. Formal training and practice of teamwork and procedural skills in simulated operating room settings can obviate relying on the traditional "see one, do one, teach one" approach. Human patient simulation is the medical simulation version of the simulator cockpit, employing an experiential learning model well-suited to adult learners (60). Kolb and Fry positioned four elements of experiential learning in a cycle: concrete experience, observation and reflection, formation of abstract concepts, and testing in new situations. Learners can enter at any point but most enter by means of a specific concrete experience in the context of a particular situation. Gaba incorporated this approach into his Anesthesia CRM curriculum, allowing systematic presentation of a wide variety of

routine and uncommon but critical events in a simulated medical setting (37). Although there is no gold standard team training curriculum in healthcare, the IOM encourages team training programs such as CRM and simulation for personnel who work in critical care areas (10) (p. 173). Medical simulation provides a vehicle by which clinicians can experience an event and reflect and learn in an atmosphere of safety, free of harm to patients.

As stated by Gaba et al. (37), medical simulation, practice, and drills never pose risks to live patients.

Aggarwal et al. (61) asserted in 2004 that practicing team skills enables surgical teams to function in a safer, more efficient manner when crises occur in real life. Moorthy et al. (62) exposed two groups of surgical trainees to a bleeding crisis evolving during a simulated vascular procedure in a simulated operating room. The event was videotaped and used to provide feedback in the immediate post-scenario debriefing. Technical ability in controlling the bleeding was assessed with a global rating scale. Teamwork or "non-technical" skills were assessed using a NOTECHS skills rating scale that was originally developed for aviation and adapted for use in healthcare. Additional metrics included evaluation of communication within the team, amount of time to complete specific tasks, and a surrogate outcome measure of total (simulated) blood lost-amount captured in the canister and weight of blood-soaked sponges. Participants also completed a questionnaire about their perception of the simulation experience. Moorthy et al. found that the simulated scenario was well received and deemed as realistic by the participants. A difference was seen between junior and senior trainees in managing the bleeding crisis, with seniors demonstrating quicker times for recognizing the crisis, and instituting appropriate interventions. Junior trainees were more likely to blindly use and apply clamps to stop the bleeding and experience greater blood loss; and they were less likely to realize their limitations and call for help. There was utility in the variations found between and within groups, potentially for identifying and setting performance standards, and guiding which trainees may need further assistance in skill acquisition and crisis management. NOTECH scores for teamwork did not differ significantly between the groups. The investigators postulated that the wide variability of scores within the groups may be related to the lack of focus on developing effective team skills in surgical training. They acknowledged that further research is needed to assess the construct and content validity of the NOTECHS rating scale.

With Eduardo Salas, Weaver et al. recently evaluated whether or not teamwork improves performance in the operating room-unpublished manuscript (63). They conducted a multi-level evaluation of a medical team training curriculum, "Medical Team Management and Team Strategies, and Tools to Enhance Performance and Patient Safety" (TeamSTEPPS), developed by the DoD in collaboration with the Agency for Healthcare Research Quality. A control group was compared with an intervention group exposed to this structured four hour curriculum with case-based interactive sessions and low-fidelity simulation for practice. They assessed trainee reactions and learning; observed team performance in the operating

room and the degree to which the team training skills were enacted. They reported positive results in the intervention group compared to the control across their multi-level schema. However, they stated generalizing results may be affected by the intervention groups being teams from a single location and from other external factors.

Vincent et al. (64) have long advocated team training as part of a broad-based systems approach to surgical quality and safety. They acknowledge that improving procedural skills may facilitate reductions in mortality from 10% to 1%. However, they also strongly support research aimed at optimizing the surgical environment, equipment design, and understanding subtleties of decision making in the complex operating room environment. Broad-based efforts to improve communication and team performance may be the most important intervention to assist surgical teams in achieving better outcomes for patients. Such efforts would include direct observation, including visual-audio recording, and assessment of surgical team performance and the routine use of full operating theatre simulation targeting all members of the surgical team.

Surgical Simulators for Technical Skills Training

A variety of devices, ranging from simple to complex objects, cadavers, or animal models to elaborate virtual reality (VR) devices, have been developed for training and practice of surgical maneuvers and procedures involving the abdomen and pelvis (65). These include knot-tying or suture placement trainers; pelvic exam training devices such as The Pelvic ExamSim™ (METI®, Saratoga, FL) that has internal sensors and software that feeds information back to the learner about their performance (66); and life-size human patient mannequins for simulating surgical scenarios in a simulated or real operating room environment. It is not yet clear how much physical realism is needed for skills training and assessment of open laparotomy procedures involving major abdominal and pelvic organs, such as hysterectomy, vesico-vaginal fistula repair, or vaginal vault suspensions. Video-simulation, VR, computer screen-based or haptic systems may offer greater opportunities to enhance the realism and may be used in combination with human patient mannequin simulators (67,68). The surgical robot system is revolutionizing surgical practice across a variety of specialties, including urology (69) and gynecology (70). VR-assisted robotic surgery simulators are undergoing validation (71) and full simulations are being developed (72). The total immersion VR-haptic surgical environment, the "surgical holodeck" is an area rich for research and development (73).

Shifting the Paradigm

There is discernable movement in surgical education, shifting from the traditional "see one, do one, teach one" approach to that of "learn and practice on a simulator first." Simulators are steadily being integrated into surgical curriculum for training (74–76), assessment (77–79), and credentialing (80–82) of surgeons. The first hysteroscopy training device was developed in the 1970s (83) and consisted of a surgically removed uterus mounted on a flat base. Semm (84) created the first laparoscopic training device in 1985 for which to practice surgical gestures. The original version had a plexiglass cover allowing trainees to directly view their handiwork; and modern versions employ screen monitors with video-recording capability. The integration of VR technology with endoscopic training devices was proposed by Satava in 1993 (85) and VR has since become integral to a broad range of surgical simulators. Box trainers and VR laparoscopic simulators have been shown to facilitate skill acquisition and training across the spectrum of novice to expert. Such training has translated into improved proficiency in the operating room. The following studies highlight some of the measured steps taken towards this end.

Scott et al. (86) in 2000 evaluated global performance during laparoscopic cholecystectomy and found significantly higher scores among surgical residents who trained with box trainers than those who had not. Fichera et al. (87) in 2005 also noted statistically significant improvements in suture technique and coordination in trainees using the LTS 2000 laparoscopic box trainer. Seymour et al. (88) conducted a randomized, double-blind controlled trial evaluating VR simulator-based training, and found improved performance of skills in the operating room in those with such training. Similar findings were obtained Gallagher et al. (89) and Grantcharov et al. (90). Laparoscopic skills have reportedly improved for novices who trained with either box or VR simulators (91). Grancharov et al. (92) conducted a randomized clinical trial of surgical residents using VR simulators. Surgical skills of residents who trained with the laparoscopic simulator directly translated into better performance in the operating room. Even third year medical students rotating through gynecology and general surgery achieved proficiency whether they trained with laparoscopic box or VR simulators (93). However, students training with laparoscopic VR simulators reached proficiency sooner than those who had not used them.

Aggarawal et al. (94) demonstrated that non-VR simulators can differentiate novice from expert. They evaluated the performance of novice and experienced gynecologists in a series of laparoscopic tasks needed for managing ectopic pregnancy. Novices significantly improvement their surgical performance and experienced gynecologists demonstrated little change over time. Aggarwal and Darzi (95) showed that skills acquired using a VR simulator had high transferability to the porcine model, every hour of training reduced by 2.3 hours the time needed to gain proficiency. Demonstrating transferability to surgical procedures involving real patients, and evaluating cost-effectiveness of such training will be an area of future research. Both Geoffrian (96) and Goff (97) showed simulation-based surgical skills training improved the technical performance of gynecology residents, and such skills translated well to the operating room. They each underscored the need for standardizing simulator-based curriculum to consistently train and assess surgical care in clinical practice.

Kahol et al. (98) evaluated the potential role of surgical warm-ups, pre-procedure short term practice sessions with a simulator, to exercise a surgeon's psychomotor, and cognitive skills. Kahol et al. conducted a series of experiments involving 46 surgeons comprised of novice to senior gynecology and general surgery residents and attending trauma surgeons. The first experiment evaluated impact of the warm-up on surgical proficiency, its relationship with experience, fatigue, and cognitive and psychomotor skills. The second evaluated whether basic skills warm-up improved performance of complex tasks. They found that regardless of level of expertise, all surgeons benefited from the surgical warm ups as a 25% to 45% range in reduction of error was noted. Time required to complete a task was substantially diminished. Warm ups diminished cognitive errors ($p < 0.0004$) and improved performance in all parameters being studied in the fatigued individual. Even though performance improved in the fatigued individual, it did not return to baseline performance levels characteristic of the rested state. These findings suggest that the preoperative warm-ups may become a new surgical standard, assuring optimal care of the patient during surgery.

Decision-Making and Diagnostic Errors

Identifying evidence-based methods that facilitate effective decision-making and reduce diagnostic errors is the next frontier for patient safety (99). Diagnostic error is a diagnosis that is delayed, missed, or wrong, detected by subsequent definitive test or finding. Such errors occur in every specialty, ranging from 2% in perceptual specialties (such as radiology and pathology) to as much as 15% in the clinical specialties (100). Berner and Graber's review of the literature led them to conclude that overconfidence, a trait of human nature, does exist among physicians (100). Physicians believe that diagnostic error exists but underestimate the likelihood of their occurrence, especially in their own decision-making processes. This is evident in physician disregard for decision aids or tools, diagnostic or treatment guidelines, or algorithms. Such overconfidence contributes to diagnostic error. If a clinician is uncertain about a clinical situation then formal or informal consultative assistance is more likely to be requested. However, Berner and Graber believe most cognitive errors arise when cases seem to be routine and physicians are certain about the decisions they have made.

Newman-Toker and Pronovost (99) define misdiagnosis-related harm as preventable harm resulting from delay or failure to treat a condition that is actually present or treating a condition that does not actually exist. Diagnostic errors are frequently not recognized, underreported, and methods for detecting them are lacking. Such errors are often classified as cognitive errors rather than systems errors, a perspective that facilitates attribution of individual blame. Newman-Toker and Pronovost suggest a different approach, taking a five-point action plan that includes developing systems such as computer-based decision support systems to facilitate cognition; grouping errors based on clinical context rather than cognitive defect; emphasizing misdiagnosis-related harm instead of diagnostic error; taking a systems approach to improving workflow; and building cost-effective diagnostic tools or decision aids that may not be perfectly accurate but out perform the human mind. Simulation of diagnostic error-related cases offers safe and practical means by which to better understand the factors contributing to cognitive error in contextually relevant settings; and identify solutions for preventing or mitigating their effect. Likewise, simulation is a practical and safe means by which to assess the efficacy of diagnostic

Table 10.3 Three Generations of Simulation in the Surgical Arena

Generation (time period)	I (1939–1987)	II (1988–2002)	III (2003–2006)	The future
Focus	Adoption and adaptation of aviation simulation to surgery	Simulation curriculum development with validation	Criterion-based training valued over time-based training	Further development of haptics, robotic simulators, intelligent tutoring, and judgment assessment

Source: Based on Ref. 101.

and decision support interventions before they are implemented on a system-wide basis in the clinical setting.

Despite the wealth of information gained thus far, Satava regards surgical simulation as still in its infancy relative to the breadth and scope of its use within the fields of aviation and the military (101,102). He described the evolution of simulation in surgery as the "generations of simulation" (Table 10.3). Generation I encompassed the long period required for adoption and adaptation of simulation into the surgical discipline. Generation II encompassed the recognition that the curriculum and learning objectives should take precedence and guide the use of surgical simulators. Generation III refers to the transition from relying on time or repetition-based metrics in simulation to a criteria-based evaluation of performance. Generation IV involves current and future development and use of haptics, robotic simulator environments; and embedding training and assessment of psychomotor skills and judgment. The future looks bright for shifting the paradigm of surgical training towards one of "continuous, automatic evaluation of performance for every procedure," thus full integration with maintenance of certification.

DISCLOSURE AND APOLOGY

Surgery-related errors are part of the healthcare process and errors are inevitable wherever humans are involved. Much can be done in the aftermath of errors to ensure that information disclosed to patients and their families will be transparent, preserving trust in the patient–doctor relationship, and aid in preventing future errors. Traditional medical education and post-graduate residency and subspecialty training has long overlooked the importance of effective communication and formally helping trainees manage difficult conversation and apologize to a patient who has experienced harm due errors and adverse events.

The Joint Commission stepped forward in 2001 and, as part of the process of hospital accreditation, set standards for disclosing unanticipated outcomes of patient-related events by the provider or institutions (103). The Patient Safety and Quality Improvement Act of 2005 (104) established a confidential, voluntary system in the United States for clinicians to report adverse medical events. Healthcare institutions in the United States and worldwide have since established or are instituting policies for such disclosure and incident reporting systems to capture information about adverse events and near misses (105,106). Disclosure is telling patients important information about their medical care or condition that affects or has the potential their current or future well-being. The

physician is expected to conduct the conversation but may be accompanied by other members of the team; or there may be occasion for some other team member to lead the discussion. Patients prefer to know about unanticipated outcomes and adverse events that may have occurred (107) but a recent survey by Kaldjian et al. (108) identified a gap between physicians' attitudes towards disclosure and what they practice. Surveys were sent to physicians, residents and medical students in the Northeast Mid-Atlantic and Midwest of the United States, and 97% of responders stated they would disclose a hypothetical error resulting in minor harm and 93% would disclose a hypothetical error resulting in major harm to patients. However, only 41% of faculty and residents disclosed an actual error involving minor harm and 5% had disclosed an actual medical error involving major harm-death or disability to a patient. Despite the willingness to disclose medical errors, the actual disclosure of errors by physicians was lagging. Waterman et al. (109) evaluated the impact of medical error on physicians in the United States and Canada and found that physicians experienced anxiety about future errors, loss of confidence, difficulty sleeping, and some feared damage to their reputation. Barriers to disclosure include psychological issues such as the fear of retribution from the patient and colleagues; fear that conversations will not go well; fear of the emotional impact to the patient and self; and beliefs that disclosure is unnecessary, that the unanticipated outcome would have happened anyway, and the outcome is not directly related to the clinician's actions. Legal barriers to disclosure include lack of legal protection about the information conveyed; lack of clarity about what needs to be disclosed and when; and belief that disclosing will not be beneficial if case becomes a malpractice claim. However, from the ethical perspective, patients have a right to know about what happened. Disclosure of unanticipated outcomes, adverse events, or near misses is the ethical imperative. Leape also highlights the therapeutic aspects of disclosure, stating that full disclosure is essential for healing (110), healing for the patient and the patient–doctor relationship and for the clinician involved.

Apology is the expression of regret or remorse for the unanticipated outcome, adverse event, or near miss. Apology shows the humanity and fallibility of clinicians, a therapeutic necessity for healing, and making amends (110). Lazare (111) in 2006 stated that an effective apology should acknowledge the offense, explain the commitment of the offense, express remorse, and offer reparation for the offense. Properly conveyed, the apology should touch on these four elements and be relayed with sincerity, preserving the patient's dignity, and

Table 10.4 Guide for Effective Disclosure and Apology

The "Five Rs" of apology	
Recognition	Understand the patient's feelings and your feelings, the basis for them; and recognize when apology is in order
Regret	Respond with empathy, acknowledge the patient's feelings. Tell them you regret what they are experiencing. Apology does not imply guilt
Responsibility	Take responsibility for what happened and disclose all the details that led to the outcome
Remedy	Make clear to the patient what is being done to remedy the situation, including financial costs or compensation if appropriate
Remain engaged	Continue to provide care for your patient after the outcome, reassuring them you will remain engaged, and available

The "Five As" of making amends	
Accurate	Truthfully and accurately tell the patient that an error has occurred
Answers	Anticipate the patient's needs for answers about the error and what impact it may have on their clinical situation
Accountable	Explain what is known about how the error occurred and accountable about future actions taken to prevent similar errors from occurring
Apology	Apologize to the patient for the error
Acknowledge	Acknowledge the patient's responses about the error and its occurrence, addressing their concerns as they arise

Source: Adapted from Ref. 112.

providing reassurance that the clinician cares about the patient's well-being. Performed this way, such apologies facilitate the healing process. Cravens and Earp (112) highlighted the "Five Rs" and "Five As" for guiding effective disclosure and apology (Table 10.4).

Legislative initiatives that provide legal protection for disclosure and an expression of sympathy or full apology have been drafted or passed, varying in scope, and breadth from region to region worldwide. An expression of sympathy with disclosure is legally protected in some locales, while in others a full apology with disclosure is not admissible in court proceedings. For example, as of December 2008, Pelt and Faldmo (113) reported that 35 states within the United States had enacted apology statutes and three had legislation pending. They regard such statutes as still in their infancy and as yet unclear how well they will stand up in court. It is important to be aware of the statutes that apply to your specific practice location, seeking guidance from your institutional risk managers if you are uncertain of when and how best to proceed.

SUMMARY

Ensuring safety and quality is the responsibility of every member of the surgical team. Achieving a balance of expert knowledge, technical skills, sound decision-making, and optimal teamwork behaviors offers the best approach towards assuring reliably safe, high quality care of our surgical patients. As surgeons, we aspire to provide the safest, highest quality healthcare services. We can no longer rely on the apprenticeship style of learning in urology and gynecology. The literature reviewed here supports surgical teamwork training and simulation for practicing routine and critical procedures and events, improving technical proficiency, and team interactions; and error reduction, recognition, and management. Further research is needed to advance our understanding of what environments best facilitates training and ensures proficiency in technical and teamwork skills, skills that are translatable to the surgical arena. Sound educational objectives will best guide the evolution of simulator technology and the extent to which realism and fidelity is required for training. This chapter has reviewed several ways in which we can safety our way out of error or mitigate their effects despite the constraints of our bounded rationality and the reality that humans make errors. Effective disclosure and apology is integral to this process. A thorough understanding of where surgical practice is vulnerable to error will best inform design of systems-based approaches in education, training and practice, mitigate the clinical demands that weaken our defenses, and facilitate provision of the safest, highest quality surgical care for our patients.

REFERENCES

1. Weiser TG, Regenbogen SE, Thompson KD, et al. An estimation of the global volume of surgery: a modeling strategy based on available data. Lancet 2008; 372: 139–44.
2. U.S. surgical procedure volumes. Medtech Insight. Report No. A606; February 2007.
3. Oliphant SS, Wang L, Bunker CH, Lowder JL. Trends in stress urinary incontinence inpatient procedures in the United States, 1979–2004. AJOG 2009; 200: 521.e1–6.
4. An older and more diverse nation by mid-century. Washington: Census Bureau (US). [Available from: http://www.census.gov/Press-Release/www/releases/archives/population/012496.html].
5. Boyles SH, Weber AM, Meyn L. Ambulatory procedures for urinary incontinence in the United States, 1994–1996. AJOG 2004; 190: 33–6.
6. National Hospital Discharge and Ambulatory Surgery Data. Public use data files. To NSAS 2006 Data Users. [Available from: http://www.cdc.gov/nchs/about/major/hdasd/nhds.htm].
7. National Audit Office. A Safer Place for Patients: Learning to Improve Patient Safety. London: Stationary Office, 2005: 1–86.
8. Institute of Medicine. Patient Safety, Achieving a New Standard of Care. Washington, DC: National Academy Press, 2004.
9. World Health Organization. World Alliance for Patient Safety: Forward Program 2005. Geneva: World Health Organization, 2004. [Available from: http://www.who.int/patientsafety/en/brochure_final.pdf].
10. Institute of Medicine. To Err is Human, Building a Safer Health System. Washington, DC: National Academy Press, 2000.
11. Thomas EJ, Studdert DM, Burstin HR, et al. Incidence and types of adverse events and negligent care in Utah and Colorado in 1992. Med Care 2000; 38: 261–71.
12. Brennan T, Leape L, Nan M, et al. Incidence of adverse events and negligence in hospitalized patients: results of the Harvard Medical Practice Study I. N Engl J Med 1991; 324: 370–76.
13. National Audit Office. Organisation with a Memory: Report of an Expert Group on Learning from Adverse Events in the NHS. London: Stationary Office, 2000.
14. Webb RK, Currie M, Morgan CA, et al. The Australian Incident Monitoring Study: an analysis of 2000 incident reports. Anaesth Intensive Care 1993; 21: 520–8.

15. Runciman WB, Moller J. Iatrogenic injury in Australia. Adelaide: Australian Patient Safety Foundation, 2001. [Available from: http://www.apsf.net.au/dbfiles/Iatrogenic_Injury.pdf].

16. Davis P, Lay-Yee R, Briant R, et al. Adverse Events in New Zealand Public Hospitals: Principle Findings from a National Survey. Wellington, NZ: Ministry of Health, 2001. [Available from: http://www.moh.govt.nz/moh.nsf/pagesmh/1240?Open].

17. National Steering Committee on Patient Safety. Building a Safer System: A National Integrated Strategy for Improving Patient Safety in Canadian Health Care. Ottawa, ON, 2002.

18. World Health Organization. World Alliance for Patient Safety. Forward Programme 2005. Geneva, Switzerland: WHO Press, 2004.

19. World Health Organization. Safe Surgery Saves Lives—Background Paper Draft. Geneva, Switzerland: WHO Press, 2006.

20. Reason J. Human Error. USA: Cambridge University Press, 1990: 148.

21. Reason J. Human error: models and management. BMJ 2000; 320: 768–70.

22. Weick KE, Sutcliffe KM. Managing the Unexpected: Assuring High Performance in an Age of Complexity. San Francisco: John Wiley & Sons, Inc., 2001: 1–23.

23. Weick KE, Sutcliffe KM. Managing the Unexpected: Assuring High Performance in an Age of Complexity. San Francisco: John Wiley & Sons, Inc., 2001: 128.

24. Carroll JS, Quijada MA. Redirecting traditional professional values to support safety: changing organizational culture in health care. Qual Saf Health Care 2004; 13 Suppl 2: ii 16–21.

25. Schein EH. Organizational Culture and Leadership, 2nd ed. San Francisco: Jossey-Bass, 1992: 25–37.

26. Walton M. Creating a "no blame" culture: have we got the balance right? Qual Saf Health Care 2004; 13: 163–4.

27. Young T. Presidential address: human error, patient safety and tort liability crise: the perfect storm. AJOG 2005; 193: 506–11.

28. Simon HA. Reason in Human Affairs. Stanford: Stanford University Press, 1983.

29. Veltman L. Getting to Havarti. ObGyn 2007; 110: 1146–50.

30. Rogers SO, Gawande AA, Kwaan M, et al. Analysis of surgical errors in malpractice closed claims at 4 liability insurers. Surgery 2006; 140: 25–33.

31. Waetjen LE, Subak LL, Shen H, et al. Stress urinary incontinence surgery in the United States. Obstet Gynecol 2003; 101: 671–6.

32. Brown JS, Waetjen LE, Subak LL, et al. Pelvic organ prolapse surgery in the United States, 1997. AJOG 2002; 186: 712–6.

33. Gilmore DT, Das S, Flowerdew G. Rates of urinary tract injury from gynecologic surgery and the role of intraoperative cystoscopy. Obstet Gynecol 2006; 107: 1366–72.

34. Gilmour DT, Baskett TF. Disability and litigation from urinary tract injuries at benign gynecologic surgery in Canada. Obstet Gynecol 2005; 105: 109–14.

35. Nieboer TE, Johnson N, Barlow D, et al. Surgical approach to hysterectomy for benign gynaecological disease. Cochrane Database of Systematic Reviews 2006, Issue 2. Art. No.: CD003677. DOI: 10.1002/14651858.CD003677.pub3.

36. David-Montefiore E, Rouzier R, Chapron C, Darai E, and the Collegiale d'Obstetrique et Gynecologie de Paris-Ile de France. Surgical routes and complications of hysterectomy for benign disorders: a prospective observational study in French university hospitals. Hum Reprod 2007; 22: 260–65.

37. Gaba DM, Fish KJ, Howard SK. Crisis Management in Anesthesiology. New York: Churchill Livingstone Inc., 1994: 5–45.

38. Baker DP, Day R, Salas E. Teamwork as an essential component of high-reliability organizations. HSR 2006; 41: 1576–98.

39. Helmreich RL, Merritt AC. Safety and error management: the role of Crew Resource Management. In: Hayward BJ, Lowe AR, eds. Aviation Resource Management. Aldershot, UK: Ashgate, 2000: 107–19.

40. Salas E, Cannon-Bowers JA, Johnston JH. How can you turn a team of experts into an expert team: emerging training strategies. In: Zsambok CE, Klein G eds. Naturalistic Decision Making. Mahwah, NJ: Lawrence Erlbaum Associates, 1997: 359–70.

41. Helmreich RL, Merritt AC, Wilhelm JA. The evolution of crew resource management training in commercial aviation. Int J Aviat Psychol 1999; 9: 19–32.

42. Helmreich RL. On error management: lessons learned from aviation. BMJ 2000; 320: 781–5.

43. Shortell SM, Zimmerman JE, Rousseau DM, et al. The performance of intensive care units: does good management make a difference? Med Care 1994; 32: 508–25.

44. Howard SK, Gaba DM, Fish KJ, et al. Anesthesia crisis resource management training: teaching anesthesiologists to handle critical incidents. Aviat Space Environ Med 1992; 63: 763–70.

45. Holzman RS, Cooper, JB, Gaba DM, et al. Anesthesia crisis resource management: real-life simulation training in operating room crises. J Clin Anesth 1995; 7: 675–87.

46. Blum RH, Raemer DB, Carroll JS, et al. Crisis resource management training for an anaesthesia faculty: a new approach to continuing education. Med Educ 2004; 38: 45–55.

47. Cooper JB. The APSF: 20-year anniversary of the first patient safety organization—past, present and future. Anesthesia Patient Safety Foundation Newsletter 2007; 22: 1. [Available from: http://www.apsf.org/resource_center/newsletter/2007/spring/01_20year.htm].

48. Cooper JB, Davies JM, Desmonts JM, et al. 1986 Meeting of the International Committee for Prevention of Anesthesia Mortality and Morbidity. Can J Anaesth 1988; 35: 287–93.

49. Sexton JB, Thomas EJ, Helmreich RL. Error, stress, and teamwork in medicine and aviation: cross sectional surveys. BMJ 2000; 320: 745–49.

50. Grubb G, Morey JC, Simon R. Sustaining and advancing performance improvements achieved by crew resource management training. Paper presented at the Eleventh International Symposium on Aviation Psychology, Dayton OH. April 2001.

51. Risser DT, Rice MM, Salisbury ML, et al. The potential for improved teamwork to reduce medical errors in the emergency department. The MedTeams Research Consortium. Ann Emerg Med 1999; 34: 373–83.

52. Risser D, Marcus R, Groff H. Proactive risk management for obstetrical teams. FORUM (Risk Management Foundation, Harvard Medical Institutes) 2001; 21: 9–11.

53. Smith JI, ed. The Joint Commission Guide to Improving Staff Communication. Joint Commission Resources Inc., 1st edn. August 2005.

54. Lingard L, Reznick R, Espin S, Regehr G, DeVito I. Team communication in the operating room: talk patterns, sites of tension, and implications for novices. Acad Med 2002; 77: 232–37.

55. Lingard L, Espin S, Whyte S, et al. Communication failures in the operating room: an observational classification of recurrent types and effects. Qual Saf Health Care 2004; 13: 330–4.

56. Greenberg CC, Regenbogen SE, Studdert DM, et al. Patterns of communication breakdowns resulting in injury to surgical patients. J Am Coll Surg 2007; 204: 533–40.

57. Haynes AB, Weiser TG, Berry WR, et al. A Surgical safety checklist to reduce morbidity and mortality in a global population. N Engl J Med 2009; 360: 491–9.

58. McCulloch P, Mishra A, Handa A, et al. The effects of aviation-style non-technical skills training on technical performance and outcome in the operating theatre. Qual Saf Health Care 2009; 18: 109–15.

59. Morey JC, Simon R, Jay GD, et al. Error reduction and performance improvement in the emergency department through formal teamwork training: evaluation results of the MedTeams project. Health Serv Res 2002; 37: 1553–81.

60. Kolb DA, Fry R. Toward an applied theory of experiential learning. In: Cooper C, ed. Theories of Group Process. London: John Wiley, 1975.

61. Aggarwal R, Undre S, Moorthy K, Vincent C, Darzi A. The simulated operating theatre: comprehensive training for surgical teams. Qual Saf Health Care 2004; 13; i27–32.

62. Moorthy K, Munz Y, Forrest D, et al. Surgical crisis management skills training and assessment: a stimulation-based approach to enhancing operating room performance. Ann Surg 2006; 244: 139–47.

63. Weaver SJ, Rosen MA, DiazGranados D, et al. (unpublished manuscript-under review). Does teamwork improve performance in the operating room?: a multi-level evaluation. Direct correspondence to: esalas@ist.ucf.edu

64. Vincent C, Moorthy K, Sarker SK, Chang A, Darzi AW. Systems approaches to surgical quality and safety: from concept to measurement. Ann Surg 2004; 239: 475–82.

65. Gardner R, Raemer D. Simulation in obstetrics and gynecology. Obstet Gynecol Clin N Am 2008; 35: 97–127.

66. Pugh CM, Youngblood P. Development and validation of assessment measures for a newly developed physical examination simulator. JAMIA 2002; 9: 448–60.

67. Hammoud M, Gruppen L, Erickson SS, et al. To the point: reviews in medical education online computer assisted instruction materials. Amer J ObGyn. 2006; 194, 1065-9.

68. Gaba DM. The future vision of simulation in health care. Qual Saf Health Care 2004; 13: 2–10.

69. Wexner SD, Bergamaschi R, Lacy A, et al. The current status of robotic pelvic surgery: results of a multinational interdisciplinary consensus conference. Surg Endosc 2009; 23: 438–43. [Epub 2008 Nov 27].

70. Visco AG, Advincula AP. Robotic gynecologic surgery. Obstet Gynecol 2008; 112: 1369–84.

71. Sethi AS, Peine WJ, Mohammadi Y, Sundaram CP. Validation of a novel virtual reality robotic simulator. J Endourol 2009; 23: 503–8.

72. Albani JM, Lee DI. Virtual reality-assisted robotic surgery simulation. J Endourol 2007; 21: 285–7.

73. Lee CH, Sofia del Castillo AL, Bowyer M, et al. Towards an immersive virtual environment for medical team training. Stud Health Tech Informat 2007; 125: 274–9.

74. Vassiliou MC, Ghitulescu GA, Feldman LS, et al. The MISTELS program to measure technical skill in laparoscopic surgery: evidence for reliability. Surg Endosc 2006; 20: 1432–2218.

75. Chou B, Handa VL. Simulators and virtual reality in surgical education. Obstet Gynecol Clin Am 2006; 33: 283–96.

76. Julian TM, Rogers RM. Changing the way we train gynecologic surgeons. Obstet Gynecol Clin N A 2006; 33: 237–46.

77. The AAMC Project on the Clincal Education of Medical Students. Association of the American Medical Colleges, Washington, DC, 2005. [Available from: http://www.aamc.org/meded/clinicalskills/]. Accessed March 26, 2009.

78. Accreditation Council for Graduate Medical Education: Outcome Project: General Competency and Assessment. Common program requirements. [Available from: http://www.acgme.org/outcome/comp/compCPRL.asp]. Accessed March 26, 2009.

79. ACGME Program Requirements of Graduate Medical Education in Surgery, Residency Review Committee, Accreditation Council for Graduate Medical Education, Chicago, IL, 2008.

80. "ABS to require ACLS ATLS, and FLS for General Surgery Certification." American Board of Surgery. August 15, 2008. [Available from: http://home.absurgery.org/default.jsp?news_newreqs&ref=index_pd]. Accessed March 26, 2009.

81. "METI and ABPS team up to develop world's first American Board of Disaster Medicine Certification Examination." American Board of Physician Specialties. March 27, 2006. [Available from: http://www.abpsga.org/events/past_news.html?story=42]. Accessed March 26, 2009.

82. Ziv A, Rubin O, Sidi A, Berkenstadt H. Credentialing and certifying with simulation. Anesthesiology Clin 2007; 25: 261–9.

83. US 4001952 (1977) (Inventor: Kleppinger, T. (Reading, PA)).

84. Semm K. [Pelvi-trainer, a training device in operative pelviscopy for teaching endoscopic ligation and suture technics]. Geburtshilfe Fraueheilkd 1986; 46: 60–2 (German).

85. Satava RM. Virtual reality surgical simulator: the first steps. Surg Endosc 1993; 7: 203–5.

86. Scott D, Bergen P, Rege R, et al. Laparoscopic training on bench models: better and more cost effective than operating room experience? J Am Coll Surg 2000; 191: 272–83.

87. Fichera A, Prachand V, Kives S, Levine R, Hasson H. Physical reality simulation for training laparoscopists in the 21st century. A multispecialty, multi-institutional study. JSLS 2005; 9: 125–9.

88. Seymour NE, Gallagher AG, Roman SA, et al. Virtual reality training improves operating room performance: results of a randomized, double-blinded study. Ann Surg 2002; 236: 458–64.

89. Gallagher A, Lederman A, McGlade K, et al. Discrimitive validity of the minimally invasive surgical trainer in virtual reality (MIST-VR) using criteria levels based on expert performance. Surg Endosc 2004; 18: 660–5.

90. Grantcharov T, Bardram L, Funch-Jensen P, et al. Learning curves and the impact of previous operative experience on performance on a virtual reality simulator to test laparoscopic surgical skills. Am J Surg 2003; 285: 146–9.

91. Munz Y, Kumar B, Moorthy K, et al. Laparoscopic virtual reality and box trainers: is one superior to the other? Surg Endosc 2004; 18: 485–94.

92. Grantcharov T, Kristiansen V, Bendix J, et al. Randomized clinical trial of virtual reality simulation for laparoscopic skills training. Br J Surg 2004; 91: 146–50.

93. Kanumuri P, Ganai S, Wohaibi EM, et al. Virtual reality and computer-enhanced training devices equally improve laparoscopic surgical skill in novices. J Soc Laparoendosc Surg 2008; 12: 219–26.

94. Aggarwal R, Tully A, Grantcharov T, et al. Virtual reality simulation training can improve technical skills during laparoscopic salpingectomy for ectopic pregnancy. Br J Obstet Gynaecol 2006; 113: 1382–7.

95. Aggarwal R, Darzi A. From scalpel to simulator: a surgical journey. Surgery 2009; 145: 1–4.

96. Geoffrian R. Standing on the shoulders of giants: contemplating a national curriculum for surgical training in gynaecology. J Obstet Gynaecol Can 2008; 30: 684–95.

97. Goff BA. Changing the paradigm in surgical education. Obstet Gynecol 2008; 112: 328–32.

98. Kahol K, Satava RM, Ferrara J, Smith ML. Effect of short term pretrial practice on surgical proficiency in simulated environments: a randomized trial of the "preoperative warm-up" effect. J Am Coll Surg 2009; 208: 255–68.

99. Newman-Toker DE, Pronovost PJ. Diagnostic errors-the next frontier for patient safety. JAMA 2009; 301: 1060–2.

100. Berner ES, Graber ML. Overconfidence as a cause of diagnostic error in medicine. Am J Med 2008; 121(Suppl 5A): S2–23.

101. Satava RM. The future of surgical simulation and surgical robots. Bull Am Coll Surg 2007; 92: 13–19.

102. Satava RM. Historical review of surgical simulation-a personal reflection. World J Surg 2008; 32: 141–8.

103. The Joint Commission. Standard R1.01.02.01, Comprehensive Accreditation Manual for Hospitals. 2009.

104. Patient Safety and Quality Improvement Act of 2005, Public Law 109-041. S 544, 109th US Congress. 2005.

105. Kalra J, Massey KL, Mulla A. Disclosure of medical errors: policies and practice. J R Soc Med 2005; 98: 307–9.

106. Kalra J, Neufeld H, Mulla A. Disclosure of medical errors: a view through a global lens. Clin Invest Med 2007; 30(Suppl): S33–4.

107. Gallagher TH, Waterman AD, Ebers AG, Fraser VJ, Levinson W. Patients' and physicians' attitudes regarding the disclosure of medical errors. JAMA 2003; 289: 1001–7.

108. Kaldjian LC, Jones EW, Wu BJ, et al. Disclosing medical errors to patients: attitudes and practices of physicians and trainees. J Gen Intern Med 2007; 22: 988–96.

109. Waterman AD, Garbutt J, Hazel E, et al. The emotional impact of medical errors on practicing physicians in the United States and Canada. Jt Comm J Qual Patient Saf 2007; 33: 467–76.

110. Leape L. Full disclosure and apologydan idea whose time has come. Physician Exec 2006; 16–18.

111. Lazare A. Apology in medical practice. JAMA 2006; 296: 1401–4.

112. Cravens C, Earp JL. Disclosure and apology: patient-centered approaches to the public health problem of medical error. NC Med J 2009; 70: 140–6.

113. Pelt JL, Faldmo LP. Physician error and disclosure. Clin Obstet Gynecol 2008; 51: 700–8.

11 Patient Safety in the Operating Room

Michael L Stitely and Robert B Gherman

OVERVIEW

The landmark paper "To err is human" by Kohn et al. brought national attention to the issue of patient safety in medical care. It is estimated that medical error contributes to 44,000 to 98,000 deaths per year in hospitalized patients (1). Patient safety initiatives are being widely implemented to improve patient safety. Many of these initiatives have not been shown to statistically reduce the prevalence of poor medical outcomes. Due to the relative rarity of poor outcomes and death, many of the implemented safety initiatives measure surrogate markers for safety and quality such as antibiotic dosing and timing for prophylaxis and time from diagnosis to treatment for acute myocardial infarction (2).

Medical errors in the operating room (OR) environment can cause significant morbidity and mortality. The OR can be a high-pressure environment with time constraints affecting performance even further. It is a complex multifaceted system with built-in capacity for system failures in addition to individual provider surgical error. This article is intended to review a system-based approach to the reduction of errors encountered in the OR environment.

PATIENT SAFETY WHILE PREPARING THE PATIENT FOR SURGICAL PROCEDURES

The provision of safe surgical care starts well before the patient reaches the OR. The planned surgical procedure and operative site should be clearly documented in any preoperative charts or records. There should be consistency between chart documents, OR schedules, and surgical consent forms. Of course, if the initial office chart contains an error, all subsequent documents generated from this information will likely contain the same error. Therefore, timely and accurate documentation of the diagnosis and surgical plan at the time of the initial patient encounter is imperative.

In January 2009 the Joint Commission revised the universal protocol for preventing wrong site, wrong procedure, wrong patient surgery (3). This universal protocol includes several steps to verify the location of the procedure and the identity of the patient.

The first step in the process is the pre-procedure verification. This process includes a verification of the correct patient, procedure site, and procedure. This process is completed at the time of procedure scheduling and is to be repeated at the preadmission encounter and at the time of admission. This verification is also repeated at any time responsibility for the patient's care is transferred to another provider. Is important to note that this is a multidisciplinary process and the participation and involvement of the patient in addition to members of the surgical care team is invaluable.

The second step of the preprocedure verification occurs in the preoperative area. Here, a checklist is completed to verify the completeness and accuracy of patient care documentation, consent forms, relevant diagnostic tests, and images, and to ensure that all implants, devices, and special equipment are available. This is also an appropriate time to ensure the availability of deep venous thrombosis (DVT) prophylaxis and antibiotic prophylaxis, if indicated.

The third step involves marking the operative site. A designated member of the operative team marks the procedure site with their initials in the preoperative staging area. The mark is placed at or near the procedure or incision site. The mark should be able to withstand removal during skin preparation and draping.

Due to the nature of pelvic reconstructive surgery including minimally invasive technology and intra-orifice location of operative sites, surgical site marking is often impractical for such cases. An alternative method of site verification is recommended for such cases, such as a special temporary wristband identifying the procedure and laterality of the procedure.

Once in the operating theater, patient identity, surgical procedure and site marking, consent forms, patient position, availability of relevant images, and need for antibiotic prophylaxis are verified by a surgical "timeout" process. The actual process is standardized by the individual institution and is designed to include the surgeon, anesthetist, circulating nurse, and OR technician. Communication is verbal and policies should include a mechanism for addressing inconsistent responses regarding the patient's identity or planned procedure. If multiple surgical procedures or surgical teams are involved, the timeout process should be repeated. The operative record should include documentation of the timeout process.

A multisite, multi-national study published in January 2009 by Haynes and colleagues illustrates the beneficial effects of utilizing a surgical safety checklist (4). This study evaluated over 7000 surgical patients before and after the implementation of a surgical safety checklist based upon the checklist developed by the World Health Organization (Table 11.1) (5). The elements of the checklist are verified before the induction of anesthesia, before skin incision, and prior to the patient leaving the OR. Overall complications were significantly reduced from 11% to 7% and the in-hospital death rate fell from 1.5% to 0.8% after the routine implementation of the checklist. There was also a significant reduction in the rate of surgical site infection (6.2–3.4% P value <0.001) and unplanned return to the OR (2.4–1.8% P value 0.047) after implementation of the checklist process (4).

Table 11.1 World Health Organization Surgical Safety Checklist

Before induction of anesthesia Sign in	Before skin incision Time out	Before patient leaves operating room Sign out

• Patient has confirmed
  o Identity
  o Site
  o Procedure
  o Consent
• Site marked/not applicable
• Anesthesia safety check completed
 	
• Pulse oximeter on patient and functioning
 	
Does patient have a:
 	
Known allergy?
• No
• Yes
 	
Difficult airway/aspiration risk?
• No
• Yes and equipment/assistance available
 	
Risk of >500 ml blood loss (7 ml/kg in children)?
• No
• Yes, and adequate intravenous access and fluids planned
	• Confirm all team members have introduced themselves by name and role
	
	• Surgeon, anesthesia professional, and nurse verbally confirm
	  o Patient
	  o Site
	  o Procedure
	Anticipated critical events
	  • Surgeon reviews: What are the critical or unexpected steps, operative duration, anticipated blood loss?
	  • Anesthesia team reviews: Are there any patient-specific concerns?
	  • Nursing team reviews: has sterility (including indicator results) been confirmed? Are there equipment issues or any concerns?
	Has antibiotic prophylaxis been given within the last 60 minutes?
	• Yes
	• Not applicable
	
	Is essential imaging displayed?
	• Yes
	• Not applicable
		Nurse verbally confirms with the team:
		• The name of the procedure recorded
		• That instrument, sponge, and needle counts are correct (or not applicable)
		• How the specimen is labeled (including patient name)
		• Whether there are any equipment problems to be addressed
		
		• Surgeon, anesthesia professional, and nurse review the key concerns for recovery and management of this patient

This checklist is not intended to be comprehensive. Additions and modifications to fit local practise are encouraged.
Source: Reproduced by permission of the World Health Organization from http://www.who.int/patientsafety/safesurgery/tools_resources/SSSL_Checklist_finalJun08.pdf

PREVENTION OF SURGICAL SITE INFECTION

Surgical site infections are a significant source of postoperative morbidity, mortality, and increased length of hospital stay. Many surgical site infections are potentially preventable outcomes. It has been estimated that 500,000 surgical site infections occur per year in the United States alone (6).

Patient factors such as poor nutrition, diabetes, and obesity are known to contribute to postoperative infections, however surgical technique and patient preparation can reduce the occurrence of such infections.

In 1999, the Centers for Disease Control (CDC) released guidelines outlining methods of reducing surgical site infections. A number of these measures are presently tracked by the Joint Commission's surgical care improvement project. The following is a summary of the CDC recommendations (7):

Hair removal: Preoperative hair removal should not be performed unless the presence of hair will interfere with the performance of the procedure. If hair removal is necessary, it should be removed immediately prior to the operation. Hair removal should be performed with electric clippers and not a razor.

Preoperative shower: Preoperative showering with antiseptic solutions decrease bacterial colony counts (8). Multiple

exposures to chlorhexidine may be required to achieve desired antiseptic concentrations. However, no convincing evidence to date shows that bathing with preoperative antiseptic solutions reduces surgical site infections (8).

Skin preparation: Numerous agents are available for preoperative skin preparation. The most common agents are povidone iodine or chlorhexidine containing agents. These products can also be combined with alcohol. Chlorhexidine has an increased residual effect as compared to povidone iodine (9). Povidone iodine is inactivated when exposed to blood or serum proteins (10). Alcohol prep solutions are flammable in the presence of ignition sources if they are not allowed to dry completely prior to the initiation of the procedure. Allergic reactions can occur with both povidone iodine and chlorhexidine. Severe desquamating reactions have been reported after the vaginal application of chlorhexidine (11).

The combination of alcohol and chlorhexidine may be superior to the use of povidone iodine alone. A randomized trial by Bibbo et al. showed a reduction in bacterial colonization after application of chlorhexidine and alcohol as compared to povidone iodine alone when preparing surgical sites on the foot and ankle (12). The effects on surgical site infection are still unknown.

Antimicrobial Prophylaxis

Surgical site infections occur in up to 5% of clean extra abdominal cases and up to 20% of intra-abdominal cases (13). Morbidity, mortality, and hospital costs are significantly increased in patients who develop postoperative infection (14). The effectiveness of antibiotic prophylaxis in gynecologic surgery has been clearly demonstrated in multiple randomized clinical trials and meta-analyses (15–18).

The theory of the mechanism of action of antibiotic prophylaxis relies upon an improved ability of the body's host defenses to remove inoculated bacteria from the surgical site. To best accomplish this, the antibiotic must be administered within 60 minutes of the start of the procedure (19). Ideally, the choice of agent should be inexpensive, have a broad spectrum of activity, not be routinely used for the treatment of surgical site infection, and have a low incidence of side effects. The agent should be chosen to cover the flora most often exposed to the planned surgical site. For example, the skin flora frequently contaminates a skin incision with *Staphylococcus epidermidis* or *Staphylococcus aureus*, while entry into the vagina can contaminate the surgical site with a mixed flora of aerobic, anaerobic, and bowel flora.

In most cases, a single dose of prophylactic antibiotic is sufficient. Additional doses are indicated for lengthy procedures (more than twice the half-life of the prophylactic agent) and for cases when blood loss exceeds 1500 ml. Antibiotic prophylaxis should not extend beyond 24 hours postoperatively.

The appropriate antibiotic regimens for vaginal cases includes a first or second generation cephalosporin (cefazolin or cefoxitin 1 to 2 g intravenous) or clindamycin 600 mg intravenous with or without an aminoglycoside for those with IgE mediated beta-lactam allergies (2). For laparoscopic or open cases, without entering the urinary tract, prophylaxis is unnecessary (20). For open or laparoscopic cases with entry into either the vagina or urinary tract, prophylaxis with a first or second generation cephalosporin or an aminoglycoside and clindamycin is indicated (20).

Prevention of DVT

DVT is a common complication of pelvic surgery. Pulmonary thromboembolism is a major cause of nonsurgical death in patients following pelvic surgery. A strategy of prophylaxis for DVT can significantly reduce the incidence of this devastating complication.

Risk Factors for DVT

Major risk factors for the development of DVT include trauma or surgery, immobilization, malignancy, pregnancy, increasing age, pharmacologically administered estrogen, nephrotic syndrome, obesity, inherited thrombophilia, and central venous catheterization (21).

When assessing risk preoperatively, both patient factors and the planned procedure should be taken into account. DVT prophylaxis strategy can be planned based upon risk stratification.

A variety of procedures are available within the spectrum of surgical therapy for female urinary incontinence and pelvic organ prolapse. Some procedures, such as cystoscopy or sling procedures, confer a low risk of DVT in otherwise low-risk patients. Other procedures may incur higher risks such as sacrocolpopexy or anterior or posterior colporrhaphy.

DVT prophylaxis strategies include early ambulation, intermittent pneumatic compression, subcutaneous heparin, or low molecular weight heparin injections.

Randomized controlled trials have shown that both intermittent pneumatic compression (22) and subcutaneous heparin or low molecular weight heparin are effective for reducing the incidence of DVT in surgical patients (23,24).

With any surgical patient there are concerns with bleeding risks when pharmacologic DVT prophylaxis is utilized. A study by Clarke-Pearson et al. showed no statistically significant difference in bleeding complications between patients receiving low-dose heparin compared to controls receiving no DVT prophylaxis (25). Likewise, Maxwell and colleagues showed no difference in bleeding complications when utilizing low molecular weight heparin or pneumatic compression devices for DVT prophylaxis (26).

It has been shown that heparin induced thrombocytopenia can result in up to 6% of patients if prophylaxis extends for longer than four days (25).

A strategy for DVT prophylaxis is presented in evidence-Based clinical practice guidelines published by the American College of Chest Physicians (21). Low-risk patients are patients under 40 years of age with no additional risk factors undergoing minor surgery with a short operating time when the patient is expected to ambulate soon after surgery. For these patients early ambulation alone is sufficient for DVT prophylaxis (27).

Moderate risk patients are those undergoing minor surgery with additional risk factors or patients between 40 and 60 years of age undergoing any surgical therapy. For patients with moderate risk, DVT prophylaxis can be instituted with either pneumatic compression, or low dose heparin or prophylactic dose low molecular weight heparin.

High-risk patients include those patients who are older than age 60, or between 40 and 60 years old with additional risk factors.

The highest risk category includes patients with multiple risk factors such as age, malignancy, or prior venous thromboembolism.

Expert opinion recommends combination therapy with pneumatic compression plus low-dose heparin or low molecular weight heparin for patients at high risk or at highest risk (27). There is presently no randomized controlled trials assessing the efficacy of combination therapy in gynecologic or urologic surgery, but cost analysis data (28) and trials in neurosurgery (29) suggest benefit from combination DVT prophylaxis.

Subacute Bacterial Endocarditis Prophylaxis

Recommendations for the prevention of infective endocarditis have recently undergone significant changes. The administration of antibiotics solely to prevent endocarditis is no longer recommended for patients who undergo a genitourinary tract or gastrointestinal tract procedure (30).

Perioperative Beta Blockers

Previously published guidelines encourage the use of perioperative beta blockers to reduce the risk of myocardial infarction and perioperative death in high risk patients undergoing noncardiac surgery (31).

However, a recent large randomized controlled trial that assigned patients to perioperative extended release metoprolol or placebo found a significant increased risk of death and stroke in patients receiving perioperative metoprolol (32).

The practice of routinely administering perioperative beta blockers in patients with risk factors for cardiac ischemia should be reevaluated, with the notable exception of those patients already taking such medication prior to surgery (33).

PATIENT SAFETY DURING THE SURGICAL PROCEDURE

The surgical patient is at risk of injury during the performance of the operation due to events such as retained instrumentation, surgeon fatigue or distraction, electrosurgical burns, medication errors, or fire. Systems based approaches may be able to reduce such risk.

Retained Foreign Bodies

Retained foreign bodies for surgical procedures occur in up to 1 per 8801 to 1 per 18,760 surgical procedures (34). The risk is highest for operations involving an open body cavity. Extrapolating these numbers to overall case numbers means that a foreign body will be retained in more than 1500 surgical procedures annually in the United States (34).

Risk factors that significantly increased the risk for retained foreign bodies include increased body mass index of the patient, emergency operation, involvement of more than one surgical team, unexpected change in the operation, and the omission of a sponge and instrument count (34). In Gawande's report of retained sponges and instruments, it was noted that the sponge and instrument counts were documented as correct in 88% of cases of retained foreign bodies after surgery. Despite the imperfection of this method, the counting of sponges and instruments is still a useful process the prevention of retained foreign bodies during surgery.

The identification of patients at risk allows the surgical team to selectively screen these patients by x-ray. Gawande et al. estimated that 300 radiographs would need to be performed to detect one retained foreign body in such at risk patients (34). Given the catastrophic complications that can arise from an undetected retained item, this approach seems reasonable. Of course, all items used in surgery must be radio opaque or contain radio opaque markers for such an approach to be effective.

Several organizations have adopted best practices to prevent retained surgical instrumentation. The Association of periOperative Registered Nurses describes the following recommended practices (35):

1. Sponges should be counted on procedures in which the possibility exists that a sponge could be retained. Sponges should be counted before the procedure, before cavity closure, before wound closure, and at skin closure or procedure end. Counts should also be performed at the time the scrub or circulator is permanently relieved from the case.
2. Sharps and other miscellaneous items should be counted on all procedures. The timing of the counts should be the same as in item number one.
3. Instruments should be counted for all procedures which the likelihood exists that an instrument could be retained. Counts should be performed before the procedure, before wound closure and at the time of permanent relief of the scrub or circulator when feasible.
4. Additional measures for investigation, reconciliation, and prevention of retained surgical items should be taken.

In the event of a count discrepancy the surgical team should be notified to assist in locating the missing item. This should include (patient condition permitting): inspection of the surrounding area including the floor, drapes, linen, kick buckets, and trash receptacles. If the item is not located, an intraoperative x-ray should be obtained prior to the patient leaving the operating theater. All measures undertaken to locate the missing item should be documented in the patient record.

It should be noted that plain film x-ray is not capable of detecting all cases of retained foreign material, especially sponges or needles. In a study using pig cadavers, Ponrartana and colleagues noted that only 29% of retained needles less than 10 mm in length were detected on abdominal x-ray (36). Needles less than 13 mm in length are unlikely to cause injury if they are retained in the patient and cannot be retrieved (37).

It is also important to note that both plain film intraoperative x-rays and even computed tomography can fail to detect retained sponges (38), also referred to as gossypiboma.

Dossett and colleagues formulated a cost-effectiveness model of routine radiographs for all emergent open cavity operations (39). They concluded that it was cost-effective to perform routine abdominal radiographs for such emergent cases. However, the model included assumptions that radiographic methods would have 100% sensitivity and that is known to be an inaccurate assumption.

It is well known that surgical counts (40) and radiographs (38) are imperfect tools in the detection and prevention of retained surgical items. Several emerging new technologies may represent significant improvement to current prevention strategies. A randomized controlled trial utilizing barcoded sponges was performed by Greenberg and colleagues (41). The barcode system detected more counting discrepancies than did traditional counting. The discrepancies included misplaced and miscounted sponges. The only sponges detected that remained in the patient (3) were in the barcoded group.

Preliminary studies have evaluated the utility of using radiofrequency identification technology (RFID) to account for surgical sponges. Rogers et al. studied the use of RFID labeled sponges in an animal model. The RFID tags were detectable when within the body cavity of a pig and were detectable while submerged in water, although the detection

range decreased in both instances. Of note, the RFID tags were clearly visible on x-ray due to the metallic content of the antenna materials (42).

Macario et al. tested RFID technology in eight patients undergoing abdominal or pelvic surgery in blinded fashion (43). An RFID labeled sponge was placed into a randomly assigned quadrant of the abdomen and the wound edges were pulled together but not sutured. The blinded member of the surgical team then scanned the abdomen externally with the detection wand. In all eight cases, the wand was able to detect and locate the sponge within one minute.

Additional research is necessary to determine if either of these promising new technologies can reduce the occurrence rate of retained objects during surgery.

PREVENTION OF SURGICAL FIRES

The three elements necessary to promote and maintain a fire: fuel, oxidizer, and an ignition source, are commonly present in the operating theater. The ignition source is almost always the electrosurgery unit or a laser. The fuel can include surgical drapes or prep solutions and the source of the oxidizer is the supplemental oxygen delivered to the patient.

It is estimated that approximately 100 OR fires occur every year (44).

The highest risk surgical procedures with respect to fire in the OR involve procedures on the head, neck, or within the airway (45).

Being distant from supplemental oxygen sources makes pelvic reconstructive procedures less likely to result in OR fires. However, numerous case reports of fires associated with alcohol containing skin preps have been reported from various specialties (45,46).

What is noted from these prior occurrences is that the prep solution must be allowed to dry prior to draping the patient. The vapors from the alcohol containing prep solutions can accumulate beneath the drapes or even saturate paper draping material, providing a volatile fuel source that can be easily ignited by a laser or electrosurgical device in explosive fashion.

Careful attention to the separation of ignition sources, fuel, and oxidizer is imperative to reducing the risk of fire in the operating theater.

INTRAOPERATIVE MEDICATION ERRORS

Medication ordering and delivery systems in the surgical care setting typically differ from systems designed for other areas within a hospital. In the surgical care setting, medications are often administered directly to the patient by the physician and the medication is often dispensed from a sterile field.

Verbal intraoperative medication orders and verbal orders issued during urgent or emergent situations increase the risk of transcription errors and decrease the utilization of decision support features available in many electronic medical record systems.

Because aqueous solutions of medications cannot be definitively visually identified once removed from their original vial or ampoule, all basins or syringes containing medications or solutions must be properly labeled at the time of transfer of the solution.

Strategies that can be used to ensure safe intraoperative medication administration include: active communication and read back of all verbal medication orders, established protocols and orders for commonly used medications and solutions, clear communication of the patient's weight in both pounds and kilograms to avoid dose calculation errors, and having the pharmacy dispense medications in sterile unit dose amounts that contain a preprinted secondary label. The secondary label should be affixed to any basin or syringe that the medication is transferred to (47).

Clear and effective communication between the surgeon, scrub technician, circulating nurse, and anesthesia provider is also essential to providing safe intraoperative medication delivery.

Fatigue

Fatigue is known to have a detrimental effect on cognitive and physical performance. Driving while sleepy correlates with the risk of having a serious road traffic accident (48).

Despite clear evidence that sleep deprivation and fatigue affect human performance, the medical profession still routinely allows physicians to provide patient care services after working extended shifts. A recent survey of obstetric/gynecology (OB/GYN) physicians in Wisconsin noted that only 18% of physicians had restrictions from performing major surgery after a night on call (49).

Two studies assessed the effect of sleep deprivation upon fine motor skills and performance on surgical simulators. Ayalon and Friedman studied OB/GYN residents' performance after a 24-hour call by testing residents utilizing a Purdue pegboard (50). They demonstrated a statistically significant decrement in performance post call as compared to pre call.

Rotas et al. performed a study comparing the effects of sleep deprivation after being on call, after a night of rest, or after ingesting alcohol on simulated laparoscopic performance (51). In their study of OB/GYN residents, the sleep deprived group showed a similar number of surgical errors as a group that ingested alcohol. Both of these groups had a significant increase in the number of surgical errors as compared to the well rested group.

Given the clear evidence of the effects of fatigue on surgical performance, it is best to avoid performing scheduled major surgery during times when fatigue or sleep deprivation are anticipated or expected.

Distraction

The ready availability of communication with a surgeon regarding emergent or urgent concerns for other patients is a necessity. However, excessive paging or telephone calls into the OR can inhibit communication within the room and cause unnecessary distractions of the surgical team. Beepers, radios, phone calls, and nonessential conversation should be postponed until the critical portions of the procedure are completed (52).

IMPLEMENTING NEW TECHNOLOGY

The addition of new surgical techniques, materials, and instrumentation can enhance and improve patient outcomes. The successful adoption of new techniques and materials requires quality research to ensure patient safety and efficacy.

Prior to performing new surgical procedures or utilizing the technology, it is imperative that a surgeon obtain adequate training in the techniques and obtain assistance or supervision by a more experienced colleague until the physician demonstrates competency in the technique or with the new device (53).

One example of evolving new procedures includes the advent of surgical mesh kits to treat pelvic organ prolapse. In three years, there have been over 1000 reports of adverse events associated with the transvaginal placement of surgical mesh (54). The most frequent complications included vaginal erosion, infection, and pain. Specific guidance from the U.S. Food and Drug Administration suggests that physicians obtain specialized training for each specific mesh placement technique and be aware of its risks. Vigilance is also required in the surveillance for potential adverse events.

A review of risk factors for rejection of synthetic mesh material used for suburethral slings showed a significant decrease in mesh erosions after practice changes included the administration of prophylactic antibiotics and a second vaginal wash with antiseptic solution (55).

Another recent technologic advance is the use of robot assisted laparoscopy. This technique is still in the early stages of its implementation curve. This technology has been utilized extensively for hysterectomy, prostatectomy, and sacrocolpopexy. Although long-term outcome data are limited, this evolving technology has the potential to reduce blood loss and decrease length of hospital stay (56).

Safe expansion and implementation of this technology will require adequate training and supervision during the learning curve, and ongoing maintenance of competence for practicing physicians.

SUMMARY

Providing safe patient care in the surgical setting is an evolving process from both a research and an implementation standpoint. Emerging technology may help to improve safety in the urologic and gynecologic OR. The laparoscopic robot and radiofrequency identification counting technologies appear to be promising. Each institution should develop processes and systems that address potentially preventable surgical errors such as wrong site surgery, surgical site infection, DVT, retained instrumentation, medication administration errors, and errors related to surgeon distraction and fatigue. Tracking and reporting the outcomes of such measures is important on both a local and global level so that effective interventions can be shared with peer institutions.

REFERENCES

1. Kohn LT, Corrigan JM, Donaldson MS. To Err Is Human: Building a Safer Health System. Washington, DC: National Academy Press, 2000: 26.
2. The Joint Commission. Specifications Manual for National Hospital Inpatient Quality Measures. Version 2.5, 2008.
3. The Joint Commission National Patient Safety Goals, 2008: 25–9.
4. Haynes AB, Weiser TG, Berry WR, et al. Safe Surgery Saves Lives Study Group. A surgical safety checklist to reduce morbidity and mortality in a global population. N Engl J Med 2009; 360: 491–9.
5. World Alliance for Patient Safety. WHO Guidelines for Safe Surgery, 1st edn. Geneva: World Health Organization, 2008.
6. Nichols RL. Preventing surgical site infections: a surgeon's perspective. Emerg Infect Dis 2001; 7: 220–4.
7. Mangram AJ, Horan TC, Pearson ML, Silver LC, Jarvis WR. Guideline for prevention of surgical site infection, 1999. Centers for Disease Control and Prevention (CDC) Hospital Infection Control Practices Advisory Committee. Am J Infect Control 1999; 27: 97–132.
8. Edmiston CE Jr, Krepel CJ, Seabrook GR, et al. Preoperative shower revisited: can high topical antiseptic levels be achieved on the skin surface before surgical admission? J Am Coll Surg 2008; 207: 233–9.
9. Peterson AF, Rosenberg A, Alatary SD. Comparative evaluation of surgical scrub preparations. Surg Gynecol Obstet 1978; 146: 63–5.
10. Ritter MA, French ML, Eitzen HE, Gioe TJ. The antimicrobial effectiveness of operative-site preparative agents: a microbiological and clinical study. J Bone Joint Surg Am 1980; 62: 826–8.
11. Shippey SH, Malan TK. Desquamating vaginal mucosa from chlorhexidine gluconate. Obstet Gynecol 2004; 103(5 Pt 2): 1048–50.
12. Bibbo C, Patel DV, Gehrmann RM, Lin SS. Chlorhexidine provides superior skin decontamination in foot and ankle surgery: a prospective randomized study. Clin Orthop Relat Res 2005; 438: 204–8.
13. Bratzler DW, Houck PM. Surgical Infection Prevention Guideline Writers Workgroup. Antimicrobial prophylaxis for surgery: an advisory statement from the National Surgical Infection Prevention Project. Am J Surg 2005; 189: 395–404.
14. Kirkland KB, Briggs JP, Trivette SL, Wilkinson WE, Sexton DJ. The impact of surgical-site infections in the 1990s: attributable mortality, excess length of hospitalization, and extra costs. Infect Control Hosp Epidemiol 1999; 20: 725–30.
15. Duff P, Park RC. Antibiotic prophylaxis in vaginal hysterectomy: a review. Obstet Gynecol 1980; 55(5 Suppl): 193S–202S.
16. Mittendorf R, Aronson MP, Berry RE, et al. Avoiding serious infections associated with abdominal hysterectomy: a meta-analysis of antibiotic prophylaxis. Am J Obstet Gynecol 1993; 169: 1119–24.
17. Tanos V, Rojansky N. Prophylactic antibiotics in abdominal hysterectomy. J Am Coll Surg 1994; 179: 593–600.
18. DiLuigi AJ, Peipert JF, Weitzen S, Jamshidi RM. Prophylactic antibiotic administration prior to hysterectomy: a quality improvement initiative. J Reprod Med 2004; 49: 949–54.
19. Burke JF. The effective period of preventive antibiotic action in experimental incisions and dermal lesions. Surgery 1961; 50: 161–8.
20. Wolf JS, Bennett CJ, Dmochowski RR, et al. Best practice statement on urologic surgery antimicrobial prophylaxis. American Urological Association, 2007.
21. Geerts WH, Bergqvist D, Pineo GF, et al.; American College of Chest Physicians. Prevention of venous thromboembolism: American College of Chest Physicians Evidence-Based Clinical Practice Guidelines, 8th edn. Chest 2008; 133(6 Suppl): 381S–453S.
22. Clarke-Pearson DL, Synan IS, Hinshaw WM, Coleman RE, Creasman WT. Prevention of postoperative venous thromboembolism by external pneumatic calf compression in patients with gynecologic malignancy. Obstet Gynecol 1984; 63: 92–8.
23. Pezzuoli G, Neri Serneri GG, Settembrini P, et al. Prophylaxis of fatal pulmonary embolism in general surgery using low-molecular weight heparin Cy 216: a multicentre, double-blind, randomized, controlled, clinical trial versus placebo (STEP). STEP-Study Group. Int Surg 1989; 74: 205–10.
24. Collins R, Scrimgeour A, Yusuf S, Peto R. Reduction in fatal pulmonary embolism and venous thrombosis by perioperative administration of subcutaneous heparin. Overview of results of randomized trials in general, orthopedic, and urologic surgery. N Engl J Med 1988; 318: 1162–73.
25. Clarke-Pearson DL, DeLong ER, Synan IS, Creasman WT. Complications of low-dose heparin prophylaxis in gynecologic oncology surgery. Obstet Gynecol 1984; 64: 689–94.
26. Maxwell GL, Synan I, Dodge R, Carroll B, Clarke-Pearson DL. Pneumatic compression versus low molecular weight heparin in gynecologic oncology surgery: a randomized trial. Obstet Gynecol 2001; 98: 989–95.

27. Forrest JB, Clemens JQ, Finamore P, et al. Best practice statement for the prevention of deep vein thrombosis in patients undergoing urologic surgery. American Urological Association, 2008.

28. Dainty L, Maxwell GL, Clarke-Pearson DL, Myers ER. Cost-effectiveness of combination thromboembolism prophylaxis in gynecologic oncology surgery. Gynecol Oncol 2004; 93: 366–73.

29. Agnelli G, Piovella F, Buoncristiani P, et al. Enoxaparin plus compression stockings compared with compression stockings alone in the prevention of venous thromboembolism after elective neurosurgery. N Engl J Med 1998; 339: 80–5.

30. Nishimura RA, Carabello BA, Faxon DP, et al. ACC/AHA 2008 guideline update on valvular heart disease: focused update on infective endocarditis: a report of the American College of Cardiology/American Heart Association Task Force on Practice Guidelines. J Am Coll Cardiol 2008; 52: 676–85.

31. Eagle KA, Berger PB, Calkins H, et al. ; American College of Cardiology; American Heart Association. ACC/AHA guideline update for perioperative cardiovascular evaluation for noncardiac surgery—executive summary: a report of the American College of Cardiology/American Heart Association Task Force on Practice Guidelines (Committee to Update the 1996 Guidelines on Perioperative Cardiovascular Evaluation for Noncardiac Surgery). J Am Coll Cardiol 2002; 39: 542–53.

32. POISE Study Group, Devereaux PJ, Yang H, Yusuf S, et al. Effects of extended-release metoprolol succinate in patients undergoing noncardiac surgery (POISE trial): a randomised controlled trial. Lancet 2008; 371: 1839–47.

33. Sear JW, Giles JW, Howard-Alpe G, Foëx P. Perioperative beta-blockade, 2008: what does POISE tell us, and was our earlier caution justified? Br J Anaesth 2008; 101: 135–8.

34. Gawande AA, Studdert DM, Orav EJ, Brennan TA, Zinner MJ. Risk factors for retained instruments and sponges after surgery. N Engl J Med 2003; 348: 229–35.

35. AORN Recommended Practices Committee. Recommended practices for sponge, sharps, and instrument counts. AORN J 2006; 83: 418, 421–6, 429–33.

36. Ponrartana S, Coakley FV, Yeh BM, et al. Accuracy of plain abdominal radiographs in the detection of retained surgical needles in the peritoneal cavity. Ann Surg 2008; 247: 8–12.

37. Gibbs VC, Coakley FD, Reines HD. Preventable errors in the operating room: retained foreign bodies after surgery—Part I. Curr Probl Surg 2007; 44: 281–337.

38. Cima RR, Kollengode A, Garnatz J, et al. Incidence and characteristics of potential and actual retained foreign object events in surgical patients. J Am Coll Surg 2008; 207: 80–7.

39. Dossett LA, Dittus RS, Speroff T, May AK, Cotton BA. Cost-effectiveness of routine radiographs after emergent open cavity operations. Surgery 2008; 144: 317–21.

40. Greenberg CC, Regenbogen SE, Lipsitz SR, Diaz-Flores R, Gawande AA. The frequency and significance of discrepancies in the surgical count. Ann Surg 2008; 248: 337–41.

41. Greenberg CC, Diaz-Flores R, Lipsitz SR, et al. Bar-coding surgical sponges to improve safety: a randomized controlled trial. Ann Surg 2008; 247: 612–16.

42. Rogers A, Jones E, Oleynikov D. Radio frequency identification (RFID) applied to surgical sponges. Surg Endosc 2007; 21: 1235–7.

43. Macario A, Morris D, Morris S. Initial clinical evaluation of a handheld device for detecting retained surgical gauze sponges using radiofrequency identification technology. Arch Surg 2006; 141: 659–62.

44. Batra S, Gupta R. Alcohol based surgical prep solution and the risk of fire in the operating room: a case report. Patient Saf Surg 2008; 2: 10.

45. American Society of Anesthesiologists Task Force on Operating Room Fires, Caplan RA, Barker SJ, Connis RT, et al. Practice advisory for the prevention and management of operating room fires. Anesthesiology 2008; 108: 786–801.

46. Meltzer HS, Granville R, Aryan HE, et al. Gel-based surgical preparation resulting in an operating room fire during a neurosurgical procedure: case report. J Neurosurg 2005; 102(Suppl 3): 347–9.

47. Association of Perioperative Registered Nurses. Best practices for safe medication administration. AORN J 2006; 84(Suppl 1): S45–56.

48. Nabi H, Guéguen A, Chiron M, et al. Awareness of driving while sleepy and road traffic accidents: prospective study in GAZEL cohort. BMJ 2006; 333: 75.

49. Schauberger CW, Gribble RK, Rooney BL. On call: a survey of Wisconsin obstetric groups. Am J Obstet Gynecol 2007; 196: 39.e1–39.e4.

50. Ayalon RD, Friedman F Jr. The effect of sleep deprivation on fine motor coordination in obstetrics and gynecology residents. Am J Obstet Gynecol 2008; 199: 576.

51. Rotas M, Minkoff H, Min D, Feldman J. The effect of acute sleep deprivation and alcohol consumption on simulated laparoscopic surgery. (Published abstract) Obstet Gynecol 2007; 109(Suppl 4): 9S.

52. American College of Obstetricians and Gynecologists. ACOG Committee Opinion #328: patient safety in the surgical environment. Obstet Gynecol 2006; 107(2 Pt 1): 429–33.

53. Stumpf PG. Practical solutions to improve safety in the obstetrics/gynecology office setting and in the operating room. Obstet Gynecol Clin North Am 2008; 35: 19–35.

54. U.S. Food and Drug Administration. FDA Public Health Notification: Serious Complications Associated with Transvaginal Placement of Surgical Mesh in Repair of Pelvic Organ Prolapse and Stress Urinary Incontinence. Issued October 20, 2008.

55. Persson J, Iosif C, Wølner-Hanssen P. Risk factors for rejection of synthetic suburethral slings for stress urinary incontinence: a case-control study. Obstet Gynecol 2002; 99: 629–34.

56. Visco AG, Advincula AP. Robotic gynecologic surgery. Obstet Gynecol 2008; 112: 1369–84.

Section Introduction: The Role of Patient Reported Outcome Measures and Health Economics

Cornelius J Kelleher

INTRODUCTION

Patient reported outcomes (PROs) are important for the assessment of all patients with disorders of the urinary tract, bowel, and pelvic floor. The principles of assessment described in the following chapters and the questionnaires themselves are likely to form a part of all clinical studies in these fields. Understanding the development of questionnaires, what to use and when will greatly enhance the ability of a reader to evaluate their own clinical practice, develop a meaningful clinical study, and critically evaluate the research of others.

The flow of chapters is designed to guide the reader through the basics of design and development through to a detailed analysis of the instruments available for the assessment of a wide range of different disorders. Only by understanding what is available and the purpose for which it was originally designed can a user thoroughly utilize the potential of these measures. The final chapter in this section discusses the issue of health economics, making sense of the definitions used in this field, and explaining how both to interpret and to design a health economic study.

The first chapter from Coyne is perhaps the most important in this section. The concept of PRO measures is introduced and the psychometric process of questionnaire design is described in detail. The chapter guides the reader from item selection to validation in a logical and thoughtful manner.

Coyne describes the difference between generic and condition specific measures and why both are needed. Methods of questionnaire administration, scoring, the meaning of minimal important difference, quality adjusted life years (QALYs), and linguistic validation are described. Perhaps of greatest value to those less familiar with PRO measures is the advice on how to select and use a questionnaire in a clinical study or trial.

The next chapter in the section describes the questionnaires available for the health related quality of life assessment, assessment of patients with urinary incontinence, and other forms of lower urinary tract dysfunction. The chapter discusses the psychometric properties, advantages, and disadvantages of each questionnaire. In addition this section also covers questionnaires assessing symptom bother and specific questionnaires to assess individual symptoms such as urinary urgency.

In the following chapter, Kopp and Brubaker use a similar format to discuss in detail questionnaires used for screening as well as those to measure treatment satisfaction, expectations and goal achievement. This is a new and important role for PRO tools.

The authors discuss the value of screening in clinical practice and clinical trials. The ethics of screening for non life threatening conditions are discussed and the potential benefits for patients of doing so are described. Increasingly we are aware that setting appropriate expectations for patients improves satisfaction with treatment. The concepts of goal assessment, goal setting, and goal achievement are described, and how this can be performed with patient interactive tools. Satisfaction tools for the assessment of medical and surgical treatments are discussed and currently available tools described.

Domoney and Symonds chapter on "Questionnaires to Assess Sexual Function" addresses the importance of standardized questionnaires completed by the patient for the assessment of embarrassing personal problems. Sexual problems are very commonly associated with pelvic organ prolapse (POP) and bowel and bladder dysfunction. Fifty to sixty percent of urogynecology research participants are sexually active and up to 64% of these have a label of female sexual dysfunction.

The topics of sexual activity, sexual difficulties, problems of arousal, desire, and sexuality are discussed. The varied models of sexual behavior and the huge variation of normal sexual behavior are explored.

The next chapter in this section from Emmauel covers assessment of disorders of the lower bowel. In many ways bowel and bladder problems are closely related. Research into questionnaires to assess bowel dysfunction lags some way behind that of the lower urinary tract. Anal incontinence and evacuatory disorders are often considered together, and the complexity of causes of bowel dysfunction and overlap with other disorders has hampered the development of specific focused measures.

The difficulty of developing such measures is related to the huge range of normal and the overlap of disorders affecting the bowel and other aspects of pelvic floor dysfunction. Questionnaire most frequently used are discussed in detail.

In the following chapter Slack evaluates the assessment tools for patients with POP. For many reasons, not least of which being the multitude of new surgical procedures for POP repair, this is an area desperately needing PRO questionnaires. Several questionnaires are in development and those in use are described in this chapter. Inevitably there is overlap with preceding chapters as many patients with POP have associated bowel, bladder, or sexual problems.

Avery and Abrams in their chapter summarize the development to date of the International Consultation on Incontinence modular questionnaire (ICIQ). The ICIQ was conceived after the first International Consultation on incontinence in France in 2000. At that time questionnaire development was expanding rapidly and the ICIQ was seen as a means of establishing an international standard tool. Over the years the project has evolved from a single questionnaire to assess patients with urinary incontinence, to a modular questionnaire format covering all aspects of lower urinary tract, bowel, POP, and sexual dysfunction. This does not mean that the questionnaires described in the preceding chapters have been superceded, as many have been adopted and included in the ICIQ modular format. The process of choosing the right questionnaire for a study, how to ask for help from the ICIQ team, and future module design is outlined in this chapter.

Lastly but by no means least Moore's chapter on health economics written from a clinicians' perspective will come as a welcome relief for all those who feel the need to understand heath economics but are overwhelmed by the complexity. She describes how to understand the terminology and what to expect from a health economic analysis. The ethics and funding of research to evaluate treatments which will ultimately generate company profits is also explored.

If you ever wanted to understand the difference between a cost of illness, cost minimization analysis, cost consequence analysis, cost effectiveness analysis, cost utility analysis, and cost benefit analysis this is essential reading. The process of decision analysis and economic modeling, and how to practically conduct a cost utility analysis in your own practice is described.

This is an important section in a large textbook written by world renowned specialists in their designated areas. This is essential reading for anyone involved in clinical research but also for those who read the research of others or merely want to improve the clinical assessment of the patients they see every day.

12 Patient Reported Outcomes: From Development to Utilization

Karin Coyne and Chris Sexton

INTRODUCTION

A patient reported outcome (PRO) is any report coming directly from patients, without interpretation by physicians or others, about how they function or feel in relation to a disease or treatment (1,2). The field of PRO research has evolved considerably over the last 30 years from an initial focus on quality of life (QOL) to a more multi-faceted study of different aspects of disease and therapeutic impact with a comprehensive theoretic framework, accepted methods, and diverse applications (3). As medical treatments have progressed from life-saving benefits to QOL improving benefits, PROs have become increasingly important to patients and healthcare providers.

Traditionally, the clinical history has been used to gain a summary view of the symptoms patients' experience; however, clinical histories often do not assess patient impact or patient perception of their condition. As such, patient-administered PRO measures have increasingly been used to support the clinical history and provide information about outcomes patients consider important. The science of developing and validating such PRO measures is the focus of this chapter.

In providing a method for the standardized collection of data, or an objective assessment of a subjective phenomenon, PROs represent the most important clinical review of the patient experience of a condition, disease, or set of symptoms. In the clinical setting, PROs can be used to inform clinicians' and patients' decisions about treatments (4,5). In the context of research and clinical trials, PROs can serve as a primary efficacy or key secondary endpoint in order to evaluate treatment effects from the patient perspective (2,6).

Importantly, patients' perceptions of outcomes associated with urogynecologic health are greatly influenced by their personal beliefs about their condition and their understanding of the availability of various treatments (7). Assessment of patient goals may be useful to patients and their clinicians in determining treatment options. For example, women with pelvic floor dysfunction who undergo treatment have been shown to have a variety of desired subjective goals that relate to their short and long-term treatment satisfaction (8).

PROs are especially valuable in assessing symptoms that may be bothersome but cannot be fully assessed without direct report from the patient, such as pelvic floor disorder, urinary symptoms, fatigue associated with gynecologic cancer, and aspects of bowel and sexual function. The use of PROs in the measurement of urogynecological health can help provide a context for what is driving treatment-seeking behavior and inform decisions about treatment options. Although urogynecological symptoms perceived by the patient or caregiver or partner do not necessarily translate into a definitive diagnosis (9), the quantification of symptoms and their impact coupled with observations in the clinical setting can be used to better consider treatment options and to assess treatment outcomes. This chapter will provide an overview of the types of PRO measures and review the PRO development and validation process from a scientific and regulatory perspective.

TYPES OF PROS
Generic and Condition-Specific PRO Measures

PRO measures generally fall into two broad categories: generic and condition-specific. Generic measures are designed to assess outcomes in a broad range of populations (e.g., both healthy as well as ill individuals). These instruments are generally multidimensional and tend to assess the physical, social, and emotional dimensions of life. An example of this type of instrument is the Medical Outcomes Study SF-36 Health Status Profile (SF-36) (10).

Condition-specific measures are designed to assess the impact of specific diseases or conditions and include items more specific to the particular condition or population being studied. Condition-specific measures can be similar to generic instruments in that they assess multiple outcome dimensions. Examples of frequently used condition-specific instruments in urogynecology include the Functional Assessment of Cancer Therapy-Ovarian (11), the Pelvic Floor Impact Questionnaire (12), the Incontinence Impact Questionnaire, the King's Health Questionnaire (KHQ) (13), and the Overactive Bladder Questionnaire (OAB-q) (14). In general, there has been a growing trend to include condition-specific outcome measures in the clinical trial and research setting due to their enhanced sensitivity to change and the need to minimize participant burden.

Importantly, the type of measures selected for inclusion in a research study will depend on the goals of the intervention and the specific research questions to be addressed. Important considerations about the instrument include what is being measured (concept and form), who is being assessed (target population), when the assessment is occurring (study design and frequency of assessment), and how it is being administered (mode) (6). In practice, clinical trials that include PROs usually incorporate a combination of PRO measures most relevant to the study population and intervention and prioritize the selection of these instruments according to the resource constraints and staff and participant burden. In the clinical setting, PROs can be used to provide information about symptoms of disease to aid physicians in selecting therapies.

CLASSIFICATIONS OF PROS

The term "PRO" is often used to refer to a number of different aspects of patient-based assessment. It is important to distinguish between the concept being measured, the instrument used to assess the concept, and the outcome as analyzed in a clinical trial, or "endpoint" (2). For example, when assessing

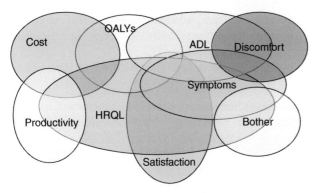

Figure 12.1 Patient reported outcomes assessment areas. *Abbreviations*: ADL, activities of daily living; HRQL, health related quality of life assessment; QALYs, quality adjusted life years. *Source*: From Ref. 56.

urogenital pain in relation to sex, urogenital pain intensity is the concept, decrease in pain intensity is the outcome, and change over a certain time interval in pain intensity (as represented by a 10 cm visual analog scale) is the data point that is used in the statistical analysis.

As shown in Figure 12.1, outcomes that can be assessed directly from the patient frequently overlap. The most broad category is health related quality of life assessment (HRQL), which, at a minimum, measures physical, psychological (including emotional and cognitive), and social functioning. Examples of urogynecologic-specific HRQL measures were provided above. Outcomes that frequently overlap with HRQL include the experience and frequency of symptoms (e.g., pain, urinary incontinence); the bother and discomfort associated with these symptoms; the impact of symptoms on activities of daily living (ADLs); treatment satisfaction; and cost considerations, such as work productivity, cost, and quality adjusted life years (QALYs). A brief description of each of these outcomes, with examples of instruments used in urogynecology, is provided below.

Symptom Frequency and Bother

As stated previously, many symptoms in urogynecology are best understood based on direct report from the patient. For example, symptoms are defined by the International Continence Society as "the subjective indicator of a disease or change in condition as perceived by the patient, caregiver, or partner and may lead him/her to seek help from health care professionals" (9). Instruments designed to elicit patient report of symptoms can assess a number of different dimensions, including presence/absence, frequency [e.g., how often patients experience a specific symptom; e.g., Pelvic Floor Distress Inventory (PFDI-20) (15,16)], and severity or bother [e.g., the Symptom Bother scale of the OAB-q (14) and the Urogenital Distress Inventory (17)].

Discomfort and ADL

Discomfort and/or pain are common outcome measures for many therapeutic areas. As such, measures of pain or discomfort are typically adapted from other generic measures [e.g., Brief Pain Inventory (18,19)] for specific urogynecology conditions. ADL (e.g., ability to dress and feed oneself) are

infrequently assessed within urogynecology as such concepts, if pertinent, are incorporated into condition-specific HRQL measures.

Treatment Satisfaction

Patient satisfaction with treatment is the subjective, individual evaluation of treatment effectiveness and/or the service provided by the healthcare system. At its most basic level, satisfaction is a comprehensive evaluation of several dimensions of health care based on patient expectations and provider and treatment performance. Measures of satisfaction can include evaluation of accessibility/convenience, availability of resources, continuity of care, efficacy, finances, humaneness, information gathering and giving processes, pleasantness of surroundings, and perceived quality/competence of health care personnel (20). As an outcomes measure, patient satisfaction allows health care providers to assess the appropriateness of treatment according to patient expectations. In chronic diseases, where patients must continually adhere to treatments, patient satisfaction may be the distinguishing outcome among treatments with comparable efficacy (21). Two examples of patient satisfaction outcome measures are the Benefit, Satisfaction, and Willingness to Continue (BSW) measure (22) and the Overactive Bladder Satisfaction (OAB-S) measure (23,24). The BSW is a single item overall satisfaction measure whereas the OAB-S is a multi-item, multi-domain satisfaction measure. Generally, responsiveness cannot be assessed in this domain as there is no baseline assessment of patient satisfaction with treatment as no treatment has been given.

Productivity

The assessment of work productivity is particularly relevant for conditions that impact women in their working years (<65). Currently, there are no condition-specific PROs for work productivity for urogynecologic conditions, however generic measures, such as the Work Productivity and Activity Impairment (WPAI) (25) are typically adapted to the specific patient population [e.g., the WPAI: Irritable Bowel Syndrome (26)]. Productivity impact is an important construct to measure; however there are many cultural and gender considerations in assessing this construct. Particularly notable is the complexity surrounding the assessment of productivity for those who work in the home but are not currently employed—a heterogeneous group predominantly composed of women and older people.

Cost and Economic Assessments

Cost and economic assessments are not necessarily PROs, as many cost evaluations are conducted using currently existing economic data and claims databases. However, cost data are occasionally collected from patients to obtain cost information that is relevant to the patient (e.g., costs paid by the patient for urinary incontinence pads). The key to obtaining cost data from patients is to ensure that the questions asked are clear, easy to read, and understandable. Additionally, other relevant cost information must be collected as needed from other sources (e.g., claims databases) to fully evaluate economic impact.

QALY

Increasingly, HRQL outcome measures are being used in the development of QALY measures. A QALY is a universal health outcome measure applicable to all individuals and all diseases, which combines gains or losses in both life quantity (mortality) and life quality (morbidity) and enables comparisons across diseases and programs. QALYs are widely used for cost-utility analysis (27). In the past decades, economic evaluation has been increasingly important for the decision maker to decide which treatment or intervention is more cost-effective, in order to allocate limited healthcare resources soundly. The aim of economic evaluation is to compare interventions in terms of their costs and benefits, including their patient outcome impact. Health benefits can be quantified as QALYs, which has become a standard measure and is now recommended in most of health economics guidelines as the method of choice (28). For example, algorithms have been derived to convert the OAB-q and KHQ to QALYs (29,30).

Conceptual Congruency

As described above, there are a variety of PRO instruments that differ in underlying construct measured. Thus, an essential component of selecting a PRO is to ensure consistency with the clinical purpose and objectives of the study. For example, if the goal is to assess treatment satisfaction, then a treatment satisfaction measure must be incorporated into the study design as a PRO. The matching of appropriate PRO selection with one's desired outcome is critical to success when assessing PROs.

PRO QUESTIONNAIRE DEVELOPMENT AND VALIDATION

To ensure that the results obtained with PROs are clinically useful, data must be gathered using valid and reliable instruments. The development of a PRO is a rigorous, scientific process designed to provide confidence that the PRO is measuring what it is intended to measure, that it does this reliably, and is appropriate for use in the patient or population group under investigation. The process begins by determining the intent and

purpose of the PRO and culminates in studies that demonstrate the measure's validity, reliability, and responsiveness in the intended patient population. The specific steps required for developing a PRO questionnaire are outlined in Figure 12.2.

Determining Questionnaire Intent and Purpose

The first task in developing a PRO measure is to determine why a new outcome measure is needed. Given the current number of disease-specific questionnaires available in the field of incontinence and related pelvic disorders, a new PRO measure must fill a need that has not already been met by an existing instrument. Once the need for the measure is recognized, its purpose and clinical usefulness need to be considered in order to inform the validation design. For example, a symptom measure would be developed and validated differently from a treatment-satisfaction measure because of the different concepts evaluated by these outcomes.

The development stage would focus on the outcome of interest (e.g., symptoms patients experience and the significance of each symptom, or what issues patients consider when determining how satisfied they are with treatment), with the items derived directly from patient statements and relating to the outcome of interest.

Developing Items and Assessing Content Validity

Designing a clinically useful PRO measure involves more than just developing a series of questions. In addition to obtaining clinician input and reviewing the literature to better understand the disease, questionnaire items should be developed based on carefully planned qualitative research with patients (2,31). Qualitative research is critical to documenting the content validity of an instrument. Content validity refers to the qualitative assessment of whether the questionnaire captures the range of the concept it is intended to measure among the patient population for which it is intended (32). For example, does a measure of symptom severity capture all the symptoms that patients with a

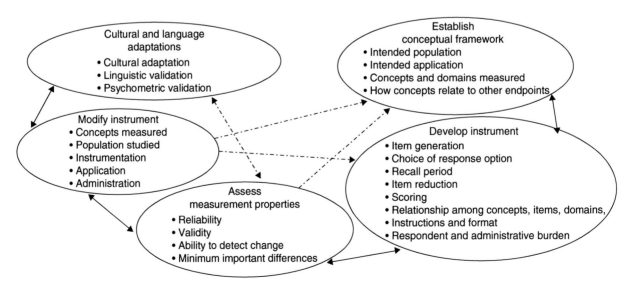

Figure 12.2 Developing guidance issues: the patient-reported outcome development process. *Source:* From Ref. 1.

particular condition have, and if so, is the measure capturing the items in a manner meaningful to patients? To obtain content validity, patients (and clinical experts to some extent) review the measure and judge whether the questions are clear, unambiguous, and comprehensive (6).

Qualitative research methods can involve focus groups, semi-structured one-on-one interviews, and/or cognitive debriefing interviews (1,31,33). Focus groups, which typically involve six to ten people with a common attribute, such as a disease, can have advantages over individual interviews in that descriptions of the patient experience are enriched by participants' responses to the comments of others (6). Conversely, personal or sensitive topics may be better suited for one-on-one interviews or gender-specific groups. Focus groups and one-to-one interviews should be conducted by moderators with experience in qualitative methods, following a semi-structured interview or discussion guide.

There are three types of focus groups and/or semi-structured interviews commonly used to inform PRO instrument selection or development: exploratory, developmental, and confirmatory (6). *Exploratory* focus groups or semi-structured interviews are conducted before instrument selection or development to provide insight into the patient experience of a disease in order to better understand a PRO concept(s). Data collected at this stage can be used to determine the relevance of concepts to patients. Building on this, *developmental* focus groups are designed to explicitly capture patient descriptions of the proposed concept of measurement, including the themes, topics, and language that patients use in describing their experience. Careful consideration at this point should be given to the questionnaire intent and purpose. For example, if a measure is intended to assess symptom bother, interview questions should be designed to elicit the words and phrases patients use to describe the impact of their condition. Rather than using clinical terminology which patients may not understand, the words used during the focus groups or interviews should be common to patients. Moderator prompting should be designed to elicit emergent information rather than leading participants to prespecified responses. Finally, evaluative or *confirmatory* focus groups or interviews can be conducted to provide documentation that an existing instrument is appropriate for a given purpose and patient population. Qualitative data obtained in confirmatory focus groups can be used to map content, words, phrases, and themes to items from existing and/or newly developed instruments.

Saturation is defined as the point at which no substantially new themes, descriptions of concepts, or terms are introduced as additional focus groups or interviews are conducted (34). The exact number of focus groups or interviews needed to reach saturation is determined by the number of concepts elicited, the complexity of these concepts, and the attributes of the patient population (e.g., age, severity). Although larger sample sizes (i.e., additional focus groups/interviews) may provide additional confirmation of the findings, it is important to recognize that there is a point at which additional qualitative research fails to provide new information—this is the point of saturation (6). Saturation of concepts can be documented through a saturation grid (see Table 12.1).

Table 12.1 Example Saturation Grid

Stress urinary incontinence symptoms	Group 1	Group 2	Group 3
Leak urine while coughing	X		X
Leak urine while laughing	X		
Leak urine when sneezing	X	X	X
Leak urine when lifting something		X	X

Notes: No new concept emerged after Group 2; conceptual saturation for this set of concepts is demonstrated.

After questionnaire items have been generated, the newly drafted questionnaire should be reviewed by other patients and experts to ensure its *readability* and provide additional evidence of *content validity*. Cognitive debriefing interviews are one-on-one interviews designed to uncover problems in the social-cognitive processes involved in completing a questionnaire (35).

During cognitive debriefing interviews, patients are typically asked to review and respond to the questionnaire items and are then interviewed about what each item meant to them as they completed the questionnaire. The results are used to make modifications in the words or phrases in the items, response options, recall period, and instructions or format of the instrument in order to improve ease of administration and enhance the validity (6). This process is also important when reviewing or adapting an existing measure to meet the needs of a new patient population. The adapted questionnaire must be validated on its own in the target population; the validity of the original questionnaire does not apply to an adapted measure. Saturation should be demonstrated in the cognitive debriefing process in a similar way to that used in the initial focus group or one-on-one interview process used to generate items. Also valuable for content validity review is a listing of all changes made to each item in the instrument development process, the rationale for decisions to drop or change items, and a record of items added or dropped (2).

Determining the Mode of Administration of a Questionnaire

Once items have been generated, the mode of administration must be considered. Will the measure be completed by the patient (i.e., self-administered) or administered by an interviewer (i.e., interviewer-administered)? How the questionnaire will be completed needs to be determined before the validation stage because mode of administration can affect patient responses. For highly personal or intimate questions or questions regarding satisfaction, a self-administered questionnaire is recommended to avoid response bias. Questionnaires that are self-administered are preferable to interviewer-administered questionnaires because the data collection burden is reduced and patients are more likely to provide unbiased information on self-administered questionnaires. Importantly, if a questionnaire has been validated for a particular mode of administration, this does not make the questionnaire valid for all modes of administration. Each mode of administration should be validated separately. This applies to varying modes of self-administration such as going from pen and paper to electronic; the new mode of administration needs to be demonstrated as equivalent to the initial mode of administration.

PRO PSYCHOMETRIC PROPERTIES

All PRO measures must demonstrate *reliability*, *validity*, and *responsiveness*, which are described in detail below. This can be accomplished in several ways:

1. Perform a stand-alone cross-sectional study to validate the questionnaire in the patient population for which it was designed;
2. Administer the untested questionnaire in a clinical trial and use the baseline data to perform psychometric validation (the end-of-study data can also be used to evaluate responsiveness); or
3. Perform a stand-alone longitudinal study with an intervention to determine the instrument's psychometric performance and responsiveness in a non-clinical trial setting.

The following psychometric properties must be tested for and demonstrated in a validated questionnaire.

Reliability refers to the ability of a measure to produce similar results when assessments are repeated (i.e., Is the measure reproducible?) (36–38). Reliability is critical to ensure that change detected by the measure is due to the treatment or intervention and not due to measurement error (38).

Test-retest reliability, or reproducibility, indicates how well results can be reproduced with repeated testing. To assess test-retest reliability, the same patient completes the questionnaire more than once, at baseline and again after a period of time during which the impact of symptoms is unlikely to change (e.g., a few days or weeks) (38). The Spearman's correlation coefficient and intraclass correlation coefficient are used to demonstrate reproducibility. For group data, a Spearman's correlation coefficient or an intraclass correlation coefficient of at least 0.70 demonstrate good test-retest reliability (38).

Internal consistency reliability is another measure of reliability that indicates how well individual items within the same domain (or subscale) correlate (36,39). Cronbach's alpha coefficient is used to assess internal consistency reliability, with higher alphas indicating greater correlation (40,41). Typically, Cronbach's alpha should be greater than 0.70 to indicate good internal consistency reliability (3,38).

Interrater reliability indicates how well scores correlate when a measure is administered by different interviewers or when multiple observers rate the same phenomenon (36). Demonstration of interrater reliability is not necessary for self-administered questionnaires but is necessary for instruments based on observer ratings or using multiple interviewers. A correlation of 0.80 or higher between raters indicates good interrater reliability (42).

Validity refers to the ability of an instrument to measure what it was intended to measure (3,36,38). A measure should be validated for each specific condition or outcome for which it will be used. For example a measure designed to assess stress incontinence would not be valid for OAB unless it were specifically validated in patients with OAB symptoms.

Evidence of content validity, convergent validity, discriminant validity, and criterion validity typically are required to validate a questionnaire (36). As described previously in relation to qualitative research, content validity is a qualitative assessment of whether the questionnaire captures the range of the concept it is intended to measure. Construct-related validity refers to evidence that an instrument behaves in a way that is consistent with the theoretical implications associated with the constructs being measured (3).

Convergent validity is demonstrated by the extent to which the measure correlates with other measures designed to assess similar constructs (43). *Discriminant validity* refers to the degree to which the scale does not correlate with other measures designed to assess dissimilar constructs, or is able to discriminate between constructs that should be related (43). Stronger relationships should be seen with the most closely related constructs and weaker relationships seen with less-related constructs (38). Another common method for examining construct-related validity is to evaluate whether a questionnaire can differentiate between known patient groups (e.g., those with mild, moderate, or severe disease) (3); generally, measures that are highly discriminative among known groups are also highly responsive (44).

Criterion validity reflects the correlation between the new questionnaire and an accepted reference, or gold standard (3,45). One difficulty in establishing criterion validity is that a gold-standard measure might not be available (3). When criterion validity can be established with an existing measure, the correlation should be 0.40 to 0.70; correlations approaching 1.0 indicate that the new questionnaire may be too similar to the gold-standard measure and therefore redundant (3).

Responsiveness indicates whether the measure can detect change in a patient's condition (3,38). An important aspect of responsiveness is determining not only whether the measure detects change but whether the change is meaningful to the patient. This can be done by determining the minimal important difference (MID) of the measure. The MID is the smallest change in a PRO questionnaire score that would be considered meaningful or important to a patient (46,47). A treatment that is statistically significantly better than another may not necessarily have made a meaningful difference to the patient; the MID indicates whether the treatment made such a difference from a patient perspective (46,47).

Unfortunately, there is no scientific test for MID as it is an iterative process that typically involves two methodologies: an anchor-based approach and a distribution-based approach (48,49). With the anchor-based approach, the MID is determined by comparing the measure to other measures (or "anchors") that have clinical relevance, such as a global measure of well-being or perception of treatment benefit (47). With the distribution-based approach, the MID is determined

by the statistical distributions of the data, using analyses such as effect size, one-half standard deviation, and standard error of measurement (48,49).

LINGUISTIC AND CULTURAL VALIDATION

Increasingly, PRO questionnaires are required to be used in a number of different populations and settings; however, questionnaires and their psychometric properties are not necessarily transferable (50,51). A measure that is valid and reliable for a particular language and culture may not prove so when used in a different population. Linguistic and cultural adaptation of a questionnaire occur during the development phase before validation, or it can be done after the questionnaire is validated in the language in which it was initially developed, with the latter being the more common approach. Ensuring the linguistic and cultural validity of a questionnaire is especially important for measures used in multinational clinical trials.

The principal steps in adapting a measure for different languages and cultures are as follows:

1. two forward translations of the original instrument into the new language;
2. quality-control procedures that may include a backward translation (translating the instrument back into the original language) (52);
3. adjudication of all translated versions;
4. discussion by an expert panel to ensure clarity of the translated questionnaire; and
5. testing the translated instrument in monolingual or bilingual patients to ensure that it measures the same concepts as the original instrument (39,51,52).

However, if a backward translation of the measure does not produce a semantically equivalent instrument, then the instrument may need to be developed in the target language, rather than just translated (52).

After cultural and linguistic validation, PROs should also be psychometrically validated within the target language. Thus, reliability, validity, and responsiveness need to be assessed with each language translation to confirm the same measurement properties are present in the translated language(s) to ensure psychometric equivalence. If psychometric equivalence is not present (e.g., not achieving similar or better results in new language translation), the cultural and linguistic translations need to be re-evaluated and perhaps revisions made to the existing instrument or a new instrument may need to be developed.

Regulatory Oversight

As clinicians and scientists have begun to appreciate and accept PROs as appropriate outcome measures, regulatory authorities have issued guidance documents on current best practices in the development and implementation of PRO in clinical trial settings (1,53). Both the Food and Drug Administration (FDA) and the European Agency for the Evaluation of Medicinal Products (EMEA) have released documents acknowledging the importance of PROs in clinical trials and providing recommendations about their use (1,31). For PROs to be acceptable outcome measures for regulatory authorities, documentation of measurement properties must be present as well as qualitative evidence of inclusion of the patient perspective and understanding of the PRO. Importantly, a cohesive endpoint model that stipulates how the PRO is related to the specific intervention must also be developed and presented to the regulatory authorities. It is strongly suggested that regulatory authorities be contacted early in the process of selecting a PRO for clinical trials to ensure regulatory acceptance of the PRO measure.

Questionnaire Modification

Most PROs have been developed for use with members of the general population or urology/gynecology patients with the specific condition (e.g., incontinence, OAB, pelvic organ prolapse). However, specific patient groups may experience particular problems or have unique needs that need to be addressed within the PRO (for example, children, frail elderly, spinal cord injuries, or those who are severely disabled). As such, a new questionnaire or modifications to an existing questionnaire may be needed which would require additional investigation and to establish relevance and content validity among the specific patient group. This situation also occurs when using a PRO to assess an outcome within a new patient population for which the PRO was not developed. Coyne et al. evaluated several sexual health outcome measures to establish content validity of the PROs among women with OAB (54). Since none of the PRO had been developed among women with OAB, this qualitative step was essential to evaluate relevance of the sexual health measures among this patient group.

Importantly, any modifications of established questionnaires may result in changes (sometimes substantial) in the psychometric performance of the instrument. Consequently, all modified instruments should be qualitatively reviewed first by the target patient population to ensure patient understanding and relevance as well as be subjected to the same psychometric testing as that employed in developing a completely new instrument. Specifically, modified instruments should report information regarding the instrument's content validity, construct validity, reliability, and test-retest reliability, at a minimum, and sensitivity to change, in intervention studies.

SELECTING PRO MEASURES FOR CLINICAL TRIALS AND CLINICAL PRACTICE

The previous sections have provided an overview of PRO measure development and validation. But how does a researcher choose which instruments are most appropriate for a particular research study and/or clinical assessment? As there are many available PROs, it is of utmost importance to select the PRO measure that is relevant and applicable to one's desired outcome. The goal is to develop a conceptually adequate, yet practical PRO battery given the study population, the specific intervention, and the study design. If an intervention is designed to reduce symptom bother, then a relevant PRO would be a symptom bother measure. Multiple PROs can be included in a research study; however, the designation of the PRO as a primary or secondary endpoint must be a priori. In addition, issues of staff and participant burden, time constraints, and resources should be considered in the selection of a PRO measure.

Study Design Considerations

There are several protocol concerns that must be taken into account when implementing PRO measures in research studies, including the length of the study, the frequency of contact with the study participants, the timing of clinical assessments, the complexity of the trial design, the number of participants enrolled, and participant and staff burden. The goal of the PRO investigation is to "fit" the PRO measures to the protocol without compromising either the study objective or design. For example, if the study design is complex with frequent participant contacts and multiple clinical measures, it may be necessary to keep the PRO measures at a minimum or to reduce the number of times the PRO is assessed (e.g., baseline and end of study rather than during all participant contacts) to minimize participant and staff burden. At the same time, however, PROs must be viewed as an important variable in the overall trial design and cannot be devalued in the data collection process. Consequently, PRO measures cannot be altered or reduced to accommodate study design as such alterations may yield potentially less reliable measures or may seriously diminish the integrity of the overall study design and yield useless information. The frequency with which PRO will need to be assessed in a research study will depend upon the nature of the condition or intervention being investigated and the expected effects (both positive and negative) of treatment. At a minimum, as with all measurements collected in a research study, a baseline and end of study assessment should be completed. In addition, other PRO assessments should be timed to match expected changes in functioning due to the intervention, the condition, or the disease itself.

It is critical to specify key population demographics that could influence the choice of instruments, the relevant dimensions of PRO to be assessed, and the mode of administration. Thus, age, gender, educational level, the language(s) spoken, and cultural diversity should be carefully considered prior to selecting PRO measures. For example, a cohort of patients over the age of 70 may have more vision problems than middle-aged persons, making self-administered questionnaires potentially difficult. Ethnically diverse groups also require measures that have been validated across different cultures and/or languages.

CONCLUSION

PROs provide vital information regarding disease impact and treatment outcomes from the patient's perspective that is critical for urogynecologists. The development of a PRO questionnaire is an iterative, time-consuming process that involves many steps. As such, developing a new questionnaire is not a task that should be undertaken lightly. Prior to questionnaire development, ensure that there is a need for a new questionnaire and that existing PRO measures do not meet current needs or cannot be modified to meet current needs. If a new scale needs to be developed, ensure that the guidelines proposed by the FDA and EMEA on developing PROs are followed and that the appropriate expertise in questionnaire development and psychometrics is available to your research team in order to guide the questionnaire development process.

REFERENCES

1. Food and Drug Administration. Guidance for industry on patient-reported outcome measures: use in medical product development to support labeling claims. Federal Register 2009; 74: 65132–3.
2. Patrick DL, Burke LB, Powers JH, et al. Patient-reported outcomes to support medical product labeling claims: FDA perspective. Value Health 2007; 10(Suppl 2): S125–37.
3. Lohr KN. "Assessing health status and quality-of-life instruments: attributes and review criteria. Qual Life Res 2002; 11: 193–205.
4. Penson RT, Wenzel LB, Vergote I, Cella D. Quality of life considerations in gynecologic cancer. FIGO 6th Annual Report on the Results of Treatment in Gynecological Cancer. Int J Gynaecol Obstet 2006; 95(Suppl 1): S247–57.
5. Valderas JM, Kotzeva A, Espallargues M, et al. The impact of measuring patient-reported outcomes in clinical practice: a systematic review of the literature. Qual Life Res 2008; 17: 179–93.
6. Leidy NK, Vernon M. Perspectives on patient-reported outcomes: content validity and qualitative research in a changing clinical trial environment. Pharmacoeconomics 2008; 26: 363–70.
7. Marschall-Kehrel D, Roberts RG, Brubaker L. Patient-reported outcomes in overactive bladder: the influence of perception of condition and expectation for treatment benefit. Urology 2006; 68(Suppl 2): 29–37.
8. Hullfish KL, Bovbjerg VE, Gibson J, Steers WD. Patient-centered goals for pelvic floor dysfunction surgery: what is success, and is it achieved? Am J Obstet Gynecol 2002; 187: 88–92.
9. Abrams P, Cardozo L, Fall M, et al. The standardisation of terminology in lower urinary tract function: report from the standardisation subcommittee of the International Continence Society. Urology 2003; 61: 37–49.
10. Ware Jr. JE, Kosinski M, Bayliss MS, et al. Comparison of methods for the scoring and statistical analysis of SF-36 health profile and summary measures: summary of results from the Medical Outcomes Study. Med Care 1995; 33(Suppl 4): AS264–79.
11. Basen-Engquist K, Bodurka-Bevers D, Fitzgerald MA, et al. Reliability and validity of the functional assessment of cancer therapy-ovarian. J Clin Oncol 2001; 19: 1809–17.
12. El-Azab AS, Abd-Elsayed AA, Imam HM. Patient reported and anatomical outcomes after surgery for pelvic organ prolapse. Neurourol Urodyn 2009; 28: 219–24.
13. Kelleher CJ, Pleil AM, Reese PR, Burgess SM, Brodish PH. How much is enough and who says so? The case of the King's Health Questionnaire and overactive bladder. Br J Gynaecol 2004; 111: 605–12.
14. Coyne K, Revicki D, Hunt T, et al. Psychometric validation of an overactive bladder symptom and health-related quality of life questionnaire: the OAB-q. Qual Life Res 2002; 11: 563–74.
15. Barber MD, Kuchibhatla MN, Pieper CF, Bump RC. Psychometric evaluation of 2 comprehensive condition-specific quality of life instruments for women with pelvic floor disorders. Am J Obstet Gynecol 2001; 185: 1388–95.
16. Barber MD, Walters MD, Bump RC. Short forms of two condition-specific quality-of-life questionnaires for women with pelvic floor disorders (PFDI-20 and PFIQ-7). Am J Obstet Gynecol 2005; 193: 103–13.
17. Shumaker SA, Wyman JF, Uebersax JS, McClish D, Fantl JA. Health-related quality of life measures for women with urinary incontinence: the Incontinence Impact Questionnaire and the Urogenital Distress Inventory. Continence Program in Women (CPW) Research Group. Qual Life Res 1994; 3: 291–306.
18. Cleeland CS, Ryan KM. Pain assessment: global use of the brief pain inventory. Academy of Medicine 1994; 23: 129–38.
19. Keller S, Bann CM, Dodd SL, et al. Validity of the brief pain inventory for use in documenting the outcomes of patients with noncancer pain. Clin J Pain 2004; 20: 309–18.
20. Krowinski W, Steiber S. Measuring Patient Satisfacion. American Hospital Publishing, 1996.
21. Weaver M, Patrick DL, Markson LE, et al. Issues in the measurement of satisfaction with treatment. Am J Manag Care 1997; 3: 579–94.

22. Pleil AM, Coyne KS, Reese PR, et al. The validation of patient-rated global assessments of treatment benefit, satisfaction, and willingness to continue—the BSW. Value Health 2005; 8(Suppl 1): S25–34.

23. Piault E, Evans C, Marcucci G, et al. Patient satisfaction: international development, translatability assessment and linguistic validation of the OAB-S, an overactive bladder treatment satisfaction questionnaire. ISPOR 8th Annual European Congress, Florence, Italy. Value Health, 2005; 8: A88.

24. Piault E, Evans CJ, Espindle D, et al. Development and validation of the Overactive Bladder Satisfaction (OAB-S) Questionnaire. Neurourol Urodyn 2008; 27: 179–90.

25. Reilly MC, Zbrozek AS, Dukes EM. The Validity and reproducibility of a work productivity and activity impairment instrument. Pharmacoeconomics 1993; 4: 353–65.

26. Reilly MC, Bracco A, Ricci J-F, Santoro J, Stevens T. The validity and accuracy of the work productivity and activity impairment questionnaire–irritable bowel syndrome version (WPAI:IBS). Aliment Pharmacol Ther 2004; 20: 459–67.

27. Berger M. Health Care Cost, Quality and Outcomes. ISPOR Book of Terms, 2003: 195–97.

28. Ingolf G, Joanna C, Jackie B. Quality-adjusted life-year lack quality in pediatric care: a critical reiew of published cost-utility studies in child health. Pediatrics 2005; 115: e600.

29. Brazier J, Czoski-Murray C, Roberts J, et al. Estimation of a preference-based index from a condition-specific measure: the King's Health Questionnaire. Med Decis Making 2008; 28: 113–26.

30. Yang Y, Brazier J, Tsuchiya A, Coyne K. Estimating a preference-based single index from the overactive bladder questionnaire. Value Health, 2008.

31. Revicki DA. FDA draft guidance and health-outcomes research. Lancet 2007; 369: 540–2.

32. Wynd CA, Schmidt B, Schaefer MA. Two quantitative approaches for estimating content validity. West J Nurs Res 2003; 25: 508–18.

33. Hays RD, Anderson R, Revicki D. Psychometric considerations in evaluating health-related quality of life measures. Qual Life Res 1993; 2: 441–9.

34. Creswell JW. Qualitative Inquiry and Research Design: Choosing Among Fie Methods. Thousand Oaks, CA: Sage Publications, Inc., 1998.

35. Willis G. Cognitve Interviewing. Thousand Oaks, CA: Sage Publications, Inc., 2005.

36. Carmines EG, Zeller RA. Reliability and Validity Assessment. Beverly Hills, Calif: Sage Publications, 1979.

37. Murawski MM, Miederhoff PA. On the generalizability of statistical expressions of health related quality of life instrument responsiveness: a data synthesis. Qual Life Res 1998; 7: 11–22.

38. Frost MH, Reeve BB, Liepa AM, Stuffer JW, Hays RD. What is sufficient evidence for the reliability and validity of patient-reported outcome measures? Value Health 2007; 10: 94–105.

39. Guyatt GH, Juniper EF, Walter SD, Griffith LE, Goldstein RS. Interpreting treatment effects in randomised trials. BMJ 1998; 316: 690–3.

40. Cronbach L. Coefficient alpha and the internal structure of tests. Psychometrika 1951; 16: 297–334.

41. Kazis LE, Anderson JJ, Meenan RF. Effect sizes for interpreting changes in health status. Med Care 1989; 27(Suppl 3): S178–89.

42. Landis JR, Koch GG. The measurement of observer agreement for categorical data. Biometrics 1977; 33: 159–74.

43. Campbell DT, Fiske DW. Convergent and discriminant validation by the multitrait-multimethod matrix. Psychol Bull 1959; 56: 81–105.

44. Revicki DA, Osoba D, Fairclough D, et al. Recommendations on health-related quality of life research to support labeling and promotional claims in the United States. Qual Life Res 2000; 9: 887–900.

45. Allen MJ, Yen WM. Introduction to Measurement Theory. Long Grove, IL: Waveland Press, Inc., 1979, 2002.

46. Wyrwich KW, Bullinger M, Aaronson N, et al. Estimating clinically significant differences in quality of life outcomes. Qual Life Res 2005; 14: 285–95.

47. Revicki D, Hays RD, Cella D, Sloan J. Recommended methods for determining responsiveness and minimally important differences for patient-reported outcomes. J Clin Epidemiol 2008; 61: 102–9.

48. Wyrwich KW, Tierney WM, Wolinsky FD. Further evidence supporting an SEM-based criterion for identifying meaningful intra-individual changes in health-related quality of life. J Clin Epidemiol 1999; 52: 861–73.

49. Norman GR, Sridhar FG, Guyatt GH, Walter SD. Relation of distribution- and anchor-based approaches in interpretation of changes in health-related quality of life. Med Care 2001; 39: 1039–47.

50. Witjes WP, de la Rosette JJ, Donovan JL, et al. The International Continence Society "Benign Prostatic Hyperplasia" study: international differences in lower urinary tract symptoms and related bother. J Urol 1997; 157: 1295–300.

51. Eremenco SL, Cella D, Arnold BJ. A comprehensive method for the translation and cross-cultural validation of health status questionnaires. Eval Health Prof 2005; 28: 212–32.

52. Herdman M, Fox-Rushby J, Badia X. A model of equivalence in the cultural adaptation of HRQoL instruments: the universalist approach. Qual Life Res 1998; 7: 323–35.

53. EMEA CfPMP. Note for Guidance on the Clinical Investigation of Medicinal Products for the Treatment of Urinary Incontinence. London, 2002.

54. Coyne KS, Margolis MK, Brewster-Jordan J, et al. Evaluating the impact of overactive bladder on sexual health in women: what is relevant? J Sex Med 2007; 4: 124–36.

13 Patient Reported Outcome Questionnaires to Assess Health Related Quality of Life and Symptom Impact

Cornelius J Kelleher

There are a variety of patient reported outcome (PRO) measures available for use in clinical practice and research that assess a broad range of concepts. It would be unusual for any clinical study of patients with lower urinary tract symptoms (LUTS) to not include at least one PRO questionnaire. This chapter will cover three types of PRO namely health related quality of life symptom bother, and urgency specific measures. Screener satisfaction goal assessment tools are described in chapter 14. PROs to evaluate sexual and bowel dysfunction are described in chapters 15 and 16. There is inevitable overlap between this chapter that regarding the International Consultation on Incontinence (ICI) modular questionnaire wherever possible repetition has been avoided. If the reader is using this chapter to select a questionnaire for use in a clinical study it is important that this chapter is read with reference also to the other chapters regarding PROs. The design validation usage of PROs has been described in detail by Coyne and Sexton in chapter 12 and will not be repeated here. All of the questionnaires included in this chapter are largely Grade A or B as outlined in the recently published Fourth International Consultation on Incontinence (1). For the sake of clarity, the grading of questionnaires adopted from the ICI fourth consultation is outlined below. To the extent that it is possible, it is advisable to use questionnaires of the highest possible grade providing they meet the requirements of the study or evaluation undertaken (Table 13.1).

Although for the purpose of this chapter I have divided the questionnaires into three groups—health related quality of life measures, symptom bother scales, and urgency specific questionnaires—there are areas of overlap. Some questionnaires [e.g., King's Health Questionnaire (KHQ) (2), overactive bladder questionnaire (OAB-q) (3)] have questions covering each of these areas. As stressed previously, it is important when selecting questionnaires that the content of the questionnaire is understood and the purpose of questioning is suited by the chosen measure. For studies that focus on specific symptoms (e.g., urgency) and wish to assess many facets of this symptom, urgency specific or OAB specific questionnaires will be invaluable, and overall symptom bother questionnaires advisable. As a general rule most studies will use a health related quality of life measure, an overall symptom bother measure, and additional symptom specific scales. Care must be exercised to avoid questionnaire overload, and only questionnaires that are deemed useful should be chosen.

Clearly there are many questionnaires to choose from and determining the most fitting option requires some guidance.

1. Try to select a Grade A questionnaire if available
2. Understand questionnaire content

There is no replacement for reading and understanding the content of the questionnaire, layout of the questionnaire, the scoring system, the présentation, and how the questionnaire is completed.

3. What is the target population?
   What is the intended age range, and are the respondents men, women or both? Are the target population patients with specific lower urinary tract problems or patients with mixed diagnoses?

4. Where is the study to be carried out?
   Is there a need for linguistically validated versions of the questionnaire, of particular importance for multinational studies, or inner city studies with mixed cultural populations.

5. How often will the questionnaire be completed?
   Is there any benefit of using a complex and longer questionnaire when a short form questionnaire would offer adequate information. This is particularly important in busy clinical settings or when patients are expected to complete many other questionnaires at the same time.

6. Has the questionnaire previously been used successfully?
   Use if possible questionnaires that have a proven track record in the area that you intend to study. If many studies of stress incontinent patients or patients with overactive bladder have utilized a questionnaire, did it respond as expected and was the choice of questionnaire good?

7. Are there specific issues that you need to investigate?
   If you need to investigate certain issues make sure the questionnaire you choose has appropriate questions and covers the problem in sufficient depth. If, for example, a study of nocturia is performed does the questionnaire suitably cover aspects of sleep deprivation, tiredness, work impact, etc?

8. Is the questionnaire recognized by the audience, governmental, or regulatory body that will review or credit the results produced?
   This may seem obvious but is extremely important. Check before starting clinical trials and studies that the outcomes used will be accepted if necessary by the appropriate regulatory agencies. Stringent criteria for design and validation of questionnaires are usually required and it is normally desirable that validation data is available in a country specific fashion. Is the questionnaire recognized and widely used in the country where the study is conducted? Will the audience recognize and understand the questionnaire and results when you present your study?

Table 13.1 Criteria for Recommendation of Questionnaires for Urinary Incontinence (UI) and UI/Lower Urinary Tract Symptoms (LUTS) at the Fourth Consultation 2009

Grade of recommendation	Evidence required (published)
Recommended (Grade A)	Validity, reliability, and responsiveness established with rigor in several data sets
Recommended (Grade A^new)	Validity, reliability, and responsiveness indicated with rigor in one data set
(Grade B)	Validity, reliability, and responsiveness indicated but not with rigor. Validity and reliability established with rigor in several data sets. To be used if suitable questionnaires not available in ICIQ modular format or Grade A or Grade A new

Abbreviations: ICIQ, International Consultation on Incontinence Questionnaire.

It is not possible to be too prescriptive; however, careful planning is the key to any successful study. Questionnaires should be regarded as tools and you should choose "the sharpest and best tools in the box" for an appropriate task. It would be recommended that potential users obtain a copy of the questionnaire, and review the established literature concerning prior usage of the questionnaire in clinical studies.

HEALTH-RELATED QUALITY OF LIFE MEASURES

The term quality of life is used widely in research, often without any clear definition. It is linked to the WHO definition of health which refers to a state of physical, emotional, and social well-being, and not just the absence of disease or infirmity (4). "Health-related quality of life" (HRQL) has been defined as including "those attributes valued by patients including their resultant comfort or sense of well-being; the extent to which they were able to maintain reasonable physical, emotional, and intellectual function; the degree to which they retain their ability to participate in valued activities within the family, in the workplace and in the community" [Wenger and Furberg, quoted in (5)]. This lengthy definition helps to emphasize the multidimensional nature of quality of life and the importance of considering each individual's perception of their own situation in the context of non-health related aspects such as jobs, family, and other life circumstances.

HRQL PROs are multi item questionnaires that usually collect information on various aspects or "domains" relating to a patient's life. These domains may relate to sleep, energy, emotions, social life, work life, sexual problems, etc., but vary to some extent between the different questionnaires. The results are usually presented as impairment in individual domains and for intervention studies improvement in the respective domains after treatment. It is possible for some of the questionnaires to provide a summary score "overall HRQL" but this

means that the value of measuring the individual domains is lost in the overall presentation of results.

There are two major types of HRQL PRO: generic and condition specific. These are discussed by Coyne in chapter 12. Generic questionnaires are designed to assess all patients with all conditions and are also used as population survey tools. They allow comparison of different patients with different medical problems but are often insufficiently sensitive to measure clinically relevant change when applied to patients with lower urinary tract dysfunction. For the purpose of this chapter only condition specific HRQL questionnaires are discussed (i.e., in this context questionnaires designed for the assessment of HRQL amongst patients with LUTS).

As HRQL questionnaires cover many different domains they tend to be longer and consequently require greater time for completion than single item or summary measures. When time constraints exist and or questionnaires are to be completed on many different occasions, or multiple questionnaires are to be used, this may be an important consideration. Overall the value of such questionnaires far outweighs these considerations. Some of the questionnaires do have a short form version which allows them to overcome this potential problem. It is important to look at the short form version in detail to ensure that you are able to collect the information you require and do not sacrifice clarity for the sake of brevity.

Coyne and Sexton discuss the issue of questionnaire responsiveness in their chapter with reference to minimal important difference (MID). This refers to the smallest change in PRO score that would be deemed clinically meaningful to a patient. MID values have been calculated for both the KHQ and the OAB-q and are commonly used in data analysis and presentation of PRO results (6).

One drawback of multi domain questionnaires is their inability to probe with great detail into any specific problem. This issue is discussed by Domoney and Symonds in their chapter on sexual dysfunction. Greater detail requires greater number of questions which would make HRQL questionnaires excessively lengthy and cumbersome. It is for this reason that studies will often employ a HRQL questionnaire in addition to specific questionnaires to measure in greater depth problems such as sexual dysfunction, sleep disorder, dépression, etc. when these issues are selective important outcomes to measure.

A final consideration for your study may be the requirement for economic data within your analysis. This topic is addressed in detail by Kate Moore in her chapter on health economics. In her chapter she discusses the use of quality adjusted life years (QALYs). HRQL questionnaires (mainly generic HRQL questionnaires) can be used to generate QALYs. Similar analyses have been performed for condition specific questionnaires and modeling to generate a QALY from the KHQ has been published (7).

In Table 13.2 the major condition specific health related quality of life questionnaires for the assessment of patients with lower urinary tract dysfunction are listed in alphabetical order. Their purpose, psychometric properties, translation availability, and recommended ICI grade are also listed. Some of the more commonly used Grade A questionnaires are listed below.

Table 13.2 Summary of Urinary Incontinence (UI), Overactive Bladder (OAB), and Lower Urinary Tract Symptoms (LUTS) Patient Reported Outcome (PRO) Measures—Health Related Quality of Life (HRQL)

PRO name/ grade	Purpose of tool	Population sample	Reliability		Validity				Responsiveness (Treatment duration)	Psychometric validation in other languages	Available languages
			Internal consistency	Test-retest	Content	Criterion	Concurrent	Discriminant			
BFLUTS (Bristol Female Lower Urinary Tract Symptoms questionnaire). Currently the ICIQ-FLUTS (International Consultation on Incontinence Questionnaire-Female Lower Urinary Tract Symptoms) (8) Grade A	To assess female LUTS, particularly UI, measure impact on quality of life and evaluate treatment outcome	Women, incontinence	√	√	√		√				BFLUTS translated in 10 languages. http://www.iciq.net/ICIQ.FLUTS.html
Contilife® (Quality of Life assessment Questionnaire Concerning Urinary Incontinence) (55) Grade B	To assess the impact of UI on quality of life. Originally developed in French and designed for women with UI (urge, stress, and mixed UI)	Women, SUI	√				√		√	√	Contilife translated in 11 languages. http://proqolid.org/instruments/quality_of_life_assessment_questionnaire_concerning_urinary_incontinence_contilife_r
DAN-PSS-1 (Danish Prostatic Symptom Score) (14) Grade A	To evaluate males with LUTS suggestive of uncomplicated BPH	Men, BPH	√	√	√		√				DAN-PSS-1 translated in 9 languages http://proqolid.org/instruments/danish_prostatic_symptom_score_dan_pss_1

Instrument	Purpose	Population							Translation
EPIQ (Epidemiology of Prolapse and Incontinence questionnaire) (56) Grade B	Developed and validated in English and Spanish to assess the presence or absence of AI, OAB, SUI, and pelvic organ prolapse in female population	Women, PFD	√	√	√	√			√ Translated in English and Spanish
IBS (Incontinence Bothersome Scale) (57) Grade C	One item questionnaire to assess the quality of life in women with UI.	Women, UI	√	√		√			None found
ICIQ-UI Short Form (58) Grade A	To assess the symptoms and impact of UI in clinical practice and research	Men and women, urinary symptoms	√	√	√	√	√ (8 weeks)	√	ICIQ-UI SF translated in 38 languages http://proqolid.org/instruments/international_consultation_on_incontinence_questionnaire_urinary_incontinence_short_form_iciq_ui_short_form
ICSmale (International Continence Society-male) (ICIQ-MLUTS) (International Consultation on Incontinence Questionnaire-Male Lower Urinary tract Symptoms) (58) Grade A	To provide a thorough evaluation of the occurrence and bothersomeness of LUTS and their impact on the lives of men with BPH	Men with LUTS and possible BPH	√	√		√	√		ICSmale translated in 11 languages. http://proqolid.org/instruments/icsmale_icsmale

(Continued)

Table 13.2 Summary of Urinary Incontinence (UI), Overactive Bladder (OAB), and Lower Urinary Tract Symptoms (LUTS) Patient Reported Outcome (PRO) Measures—Health Related Quality of Life (HRQL) *(Continued)*

PRO name/grade	Purpose of tool	Population sample	Reliability		Validity				Responsiveness (Treatment duration)	Psychometric validation in other languages	Available languages
			Internal consistency	Test-retest	Content	Criterion	Concurrent	Discriminant			
ICSQoL (International Continence Society-Benign Prostatic Hyperplasia study quality-of-life) (59) Grade A	To assess impact of lower urinary tract symptoms on the lives of men with LUTS	Men with LUTS and possible BPH	√	√	√		√			√	ICSQoL translated in 11 languages http://proqolid.org/instruments/international_continence_society_benign_prostatic_hyperplasia_study_quality_of_life_icsqol__1
IIQ (Incontinence Impact Questionnaire) (60) Grade A	Developed to describe the severity of incontinence in a population. Used to assess the impact of UI on HRQL. Primarily been evaluated in patients with stress incontinence	Women, UI, SUI	√	√	√		√		√ (12 Weeks)	√	Available in English and Turkish
IIQ-7 (IIQ-short form) (52) Grade A	Used to assess the impact of UI on HRQL	Validation study on men after radical prostatectomy who had UI			√	√	√			√	Available in English and Turkish
IOQ (Incontinence Outcome Questionnaire) (61) Grade C	Developed for assessing HRQL after surgery for SUI	Women SUI			√	√			√		None found

Questionnaire	Purpose	Population									Languages/Source
I-QOL (ICIQ-Uiqol) (Urinary Incontinence-Specific Quality of Life Instrument) (62) Grade A	To assess quality of life of women with UI	Men, UI	√	√		√				√	I-QOL translated in 35 languages http://proqolid.org/instruments/urinary_incontinence_specific_quality_of_life_instrument_i_qol
KHQ (ICIQ-LUTSqol) (King's Health Questionnaire) (2,63) Grade A	To assess the impact of lower urinary tract symptoms including UI on HRQL. Developed in a clinical perspective to evaluate incontinence in women	Men and women, OAB	√	√	√	√	√	√	√ (12 Weeks)	√	KHQ translated in 45 languages. http://proqolid.org/instruments/king_s_health_questionnaire_khq
LIS (Leicester Impact Scale) (64)	A condition specific quality of life measure for males and females with urinary storage symptoms of urgency, frequency, nocturia, and incontinence. Was originally developed for women with incontinence only	Men and women, LUTS	√	√	√	√	√		√		None found
N-QoL (ICIQ-Nqol (Nocturia Quality of Life questionnaire) (65) Grade A	To assess the impact of nocturia on the quality of life of patients	Men and women	√	√		√	√	√	√	√	N-QoL translated in 17 languages www.prolutssh.com

(Continued)

Table 13.2 Summary of Urinary Incontinence (UI), Overactive Bladder (OAB), and Lower Urinary Tract Symptoms (LUTS) Patient Reported Outcome (PRO) Measures—Health Related Quality of Life (HRQL) (*Continued*)

PRO name/ grade	Purpose of tool	Population sample	Reliability		Validity				Responsiveness (Treatment duration)	Psychometric validation in other languages	Available languages
			Internal consistency	Test-retest	Content	Criterion	Concurrent	Discriminant			
OAB-q SF (3) Grade A	A shortened version of the OAB-q to evaluate both continent and incontinent symptoms of OAB and their impact on HRQL	Men and women OAB	√	√			√	√	√ (12 Weeks)	√	OAB-q SF translated in 40 languages www.prolutssh.com
OAB-q (ICIQ-OABqol) (Overactive Bladder Questionnaire) (3) Grade A	To evaluate both continent and incontinent symptoms of OAB and their impact on HRQL. Developed from focus groups of men and women, clinician opinion, and a thorough literature review	Continent and incontinent OAB	√		√	√	√	√	√ (12 Weeks)	√	OAB-q translated in 41 languages www.prolutssh.com
PRAFAB (Protection, Amount, Frequency, Adjustment, Body Image) (66,67) Grade A	Five item questionnaire widely used in the Netherlands by physiotherapists and researchers used to evaluate treatment effects for UI in women	Women, UI	√	√	√		√		√	√	English, Arabic, and Dutch

IHI (Urinary Incontinence Handicap Inventory) (68) Grade C	Elderly women, UI due to detrusor instability	To identify difficulties patients may be experiencing because of their incontinence	√			√		None found
UISS (Urinary Incontinence Severity Score) (69) Grade A	Women, UI	Designed by the Finnish Gynecological Society's urogynecologic working group to assess symptom severity and impact UI on everyday life	√ √	√	√	√		None found
UQ (Urgency Questionnaire) (70,71) Grade B	Women, OAB	To assess the severity and impact of urinary urgency symptoms on HRQL. VAS scale is used to measure the impact of urinary urgency on overall quality of life, the severity of urgency the intensity of urgency and the discomfort experienced in conjunction with urgency	√	√	√	√	√ (10 Days)	None found

(Continued)

Table 13.2 Summary of Urinary Incontinence (UI), Overactive Bladder (OAB), and Lower Urinary Tract Symptoms (LUTS) Patient Reported Outcome (PRO) Measures—Health Related Quality of Life (HRQL) (*Continued*)

PRO name/ grade	Purpose of tool	Population sample	Reliability		Validity				Responsiveness (Treatment duration)	Psychometric validation in other languages	Available languages
			Internal consistency	Test-retest	Content	Criterion	Concurrent	Discriminant			
Urolife (BPHQoL9) (Benign Prostatic Hypertrophy Health-related Quality of Life Questionnaire) (72) Grade A	To assess the impact of BPH and its treatment on the quality of life of patients	Men, BPH	√	√	√		√		√	√	UROLIFETM/ BPHQoL9 translated in 11 languages http://proqolid.org/ instruments/ benign_prostatic_ hypertrophy_ health_related_ quality_of_life_ questionnaire_ urolife_sup_tm_ sup_bphqol9
YIPS (York Incontinence Perceptions Scale) (73) Grade C	To measure the psychosocial aspects of UI	Women UI	√	√	√		√				None found

Bristol Female Lower Urinary Tract Symptoms (BFLUTS) and BFLUTS-Short Form (SF)

The long form of BFLUTS (8,9) was developed for use with women, following the pattern established for the questionnaire developed for the international continence society-benign prostatic hyperplasia (ICS-"BPH") study. The questionnaire covers the occurrence and bothersomeness of symptoms relating to incontinence and other lower urinary tract symptoms. It has shown good levels of validity and reliability and has been increasingly used in epidemiological and outcome studies (10–12). Validity, reliability, and responsiveness have been demonstrated, and a scored short form has been produced, which is now the recommended version (13).

Danish Prostatic Symptom Score (DAN-PSS)

This questionnaire was designed in Denmark to measure the degree to which men are bothered by urinary symptoms (14,15). A composite score is achieved by the multiplication of the "symptom" by the "bother" score, with a total range of 0 to 108. A computer version of this questionnaire has been validated and patients seemed to appreciated more this new version than the paper version (16). It is primarily a questionnaire for the assessment of the occurrence and bothersomeness of a wide range of LUTS in men.

International Continence Society (ICS)*male* and ICS*male* SF

The ICS*male* questionnaire contains 22 questions on 20 urinary symptoms and, for most questions, the degree of problem that the symptom causes (9). It has exhibited acceptable levels of validity, reliability, and sensitivity to change following a range of treatments including surgery, minimally invasive therapies, and drug treatments (9,17,18). This long version has been largely replaced now by a scored short-form—ICS*male* SF (19). It is primarily a questionnaire for the assessment of the occurrence and bothersomeness of a wide range of LUTS in men.

Incontinence Impact Questionnaire (IIQ) and IIQ-7

This questionnaire was developed to assess the psychosocial impact of urinary incontinence in women and consists of 30 items (24 on the degree to which incontinence affects activities and six on the feelings engendered) (20–22). Scores are obtained overall or for four subscales determined by factor and cluster analyses: physical activity, travel, social relationships, and emotional health. The IIQ has been found to have acceptable levels of reliability and validity across a range of studies (23,24). The IIQ has also been produced in a short form comprising seven items, also with evidence of validity and reliability (25). Responsiveness of the IIQ has been assessed in several intervention studies (26).

International-Quality of LIfe (I-QOL)

This questionnaire was designed to be used in clinical trials to measure the impact of incontinence on men and women (27). Psychometric information on translated versions of the I-QOL have been reported for French, Spanish, Swedish, German, Korean, and Thai language versions (28–30). Other cultural and linguistic adaptations are available but have not been validated. In all countries, the use of three subscales, and an overall summary score was confirmed to be useful.

Kings Health Questionnaire (KHQ)

The KHQ consists of three parts (2). The first section contains two questions measuring general health and overall health related to urinary symptoms. The second section includes 19 questions divided into seven domains of quality of life: incontinence impact, role limitations, physical limitations, social limitations, personal relationships, emotions, sleep and energy, and severity coping measures. The third section of the questionnaire comprises 11 questions measuring the bother or impact of urinary symptoms. The KHQ has demonstrated reliability and validity in men and women and is available in 39 languages (31–36). Sensitivity to change has been shown successfully in clinical trials where it has been used to assess the HRQL improvement following treatment for patients with OAB, urodynamic stress incontinence (USI), and mixed incontinence symptoms (37–40). A minimally important difference has been derived to establish clinically meaningful interpretations of the KHQ scores and a QALY measure has been derived from KHQ scoring (6,7).

Leicester Impact Scale (LIS)

The LIS is a condition-specific HRQL measure for men and women assessing the symptoms of urgency, frequency, nocturia, and incontinence. It is an interviewer-administered tool so it is not a true PRO as interviewer administration can introduce potential bias into the patient responses. The LIS does have utility in the clinical and research settings (41).

Overactive Bladder Symptom and Health-related Quality of life (OAB-q) and OAB-q SF

The OAB-q is a 33-item questionnaire developed to assess the Symptom Bother (8 items) and HRQL impact of OAB (25 items and 4 domains: Coping, Concern/Worry, Sleep, and Social Interaction.) (3). It has demonstrated reliability, validity, responsiveness in multiple clinical studies of men and women (42). A minimally important difference has been derived (43) to establish clinically meaningful interpretations of the OAB-q scores and a QALY measure has been derived from OAB-q scoring (44). The 19-item short-form (OAB-q SF) is a six-item symptom bother scale and 13-item HRQL scale that is a single score which has also demonstrated reliability, validity, and responsiveness to change (45). The OAB-q was the basis for the OAB-V8 Awareness Tool to screen for symptoms of OAB (46) and has been used in a Parkinson disease patient population (47).

Urogenital Distress Inventory (UDI) and UDI-6

This questionnaire was developed in the U.S.A. with women to assess the degree to which symptoms associated with incontinence are troubling (21). It contains 19 lower urinary tract symptoms and has been shown to have high levels of validity, reliability, and responsiveness in community-dwelling women with incontinence, and women over 60 years of age (48). Responsiveness to changes in clinical status as or a result of treatment have been reported in a number of areas: comparing abdominal and vaginal prolapse surgery (49), and the use of a simple urethral occlusive device (50).

A short-form version of the UDI (UDI-6 short form) has been shown to be valid and reliable in older adult males and females (51,52), with demonstrated responsiveness to reconstructive pelvic surgery, tension-free vaginal tape (53), and imipramine (54).

ASSESSING SYMPTOM BOTHER
AND OVERALL BOTHER

Bother questionnaires assess the impact or bother of symptoms rather than their presence or absence. Although superficially simplistic patients make many valued judgements to score these questionnaires and to patients they are a hugely important assessment of condition severity. These measures, particularly the patient perception of bladder condition (PPBC) are frequently used in clinical studies and clinical trials. They are short and relatively easy to complete and usually appear to be clinically meaningful.

Measures that can be used to assess how bothered patients are by urinary symptoms are included in Table 13.3. The PPBC (74) and the UDI are the only Grade A recommended instruments. There are several Grade B and C measures which assess bother for incontinence and LUTS.

PPBC

The PPBC is a single item questionnaire designed to rapidly assess patients' perception of their bladder condition (74).

The questionnaire asks patients to choose one of six statements that best describes their present bladder condition. The scale was validated during two large 12-week clinical studies evaluating the efficacy and tolerability of Tolterodine in patients with OAB. Patients taking part in the studies completed the PPBC, OAB-q, KHQ, and bladder diaries. Baseline and week 12 data was used for statistical analysis. PPBC scores were well correlated with OAB-q questionnaire scores and bladder diary variables. Correlations of the KHQ and PPBC were significant for all KHQ domains with the exception of the general health perception domain. The scale was found to be responsive to change in OAB symptoms and to have discriminant validity as reflected in the OAB-q, KHQ score, and bladder diary changes. The PPBC has also shown to have good test retest reliability (74). This scale has been widely used in studies evaluating the use of drug therapy in patients with OAB (75–77).

UDI-6

The UDI-6 is a six item questionnaire that assesses the presence and bother of six lower urinary tract symptoms (82). The UDI-6 assesses types of incontinence, frequency, difficulty emptying bladder, and pain/discomfort in the lower abdomen/genitalia. The response options are zero to three. The instrument has demonstrated validity, reliability, and responsiveness (78).

ASSESSING THE IMPACT OF URGENCY

Several instruments have been developed specifically to assess urinary urgency, which is defined by the International Continence Society as "the complaint of a sudden compelling desire to pass urine which is difficult to defer" (82). Urgency is the principle symptom of OAB (78), and, as such, assessing the effect of treatment on this symptom and its impact on HRQL is important. With any measure designed to evaluate urgency, patients must be able to distinguish between the normal desire to urinate (urge) and the difficult-to-postpone need to urinate (urgency) (83,84). Wording thus becomes critical in the development of urgency assessment measures. Chapple and Wein (85) make a case for describing urgency as a "compelling desire to void in which patients fear leakage of urine" as a means of distinguishing this abnormal sensation from the normal need to void. However, some patients may have a sensation of urgency without fear of leakage, further complicating attempts to define urgency. Importantly, with some of these scales, patients have the option of indicating that they experienced urge urinary incontinence (UUI) (an event) rather than the strongest feeling of urgency (a sensation) itself. In such cases, patients who have severe urgency, but not UUI, do not have an option for endorsing the highest (worst) value, because they are not incontinent. Urgency severity scales that include a UUI response option thus may be less useful than those that do not because such scales are trying to measure two things at once, both urgency and UUI.

Several instruments have been developed to assess urinary urgency and these are summarized in Table 13.4. Given no urgency measures have a Grade A rating, a brief summary of each urgency measure is presented below.

Urgency Perception Scale was designed for use in clinical trials to evaluate patient-perceived urgency (86). This instrument consists of a single question asking patients to describe their typical experience when they feel the need to urinate. The three possible responses are: "I am usually not able to hold urine," "I am usually able to hold urine until I reach the toilet if I go immediately," and "I am usually able to finish what I am doing before going to the toilet" (86). This scale was validated in a clinical trial evaluating the efficacy of tolterodine in treating OAB symptoms; however, its limited responsiveness may preclude its usefulness in clinical practice (87).

Indevus Urgency Severity Scale asks patients to rate their level of urgency on a four-point scale, from zero (no urgency) to four (extreme urgency discomfort that abruptly stops all activity/tasks) (88). The scale has been validated in a clinical trial of trospium in patients with OAB (88), but Chapple et al. (87) question whether this scale actually measures urgency or just the normal urge to void.

Urinary Sensation Scale is a five-point scale ranging from one (no urgency; can continue activities until it is convenient to use the bathroom) to five (urge incontinence; extreme urgency discomfort, cannot hold urine and have a wetting accident before arriving at the bathroom) (89). The content validity of this scale was established through a physician survey and patient interviews (89).

Table 13.3 Summary of Urinary Incontinence (UI), Overactive Bladder (OAB), and Lower Urinary Tract Symptoms (LUTS) Patient Reported Outcome (PRO) Measures—Symptom Bother

PRO name/ grade	Purpose of tool	Population sample	Reliability		Validity				Responsiveness (Treatment duration)	Psychometric validation in other languages	Available languages
			Internal consistency	Test-retest	Content	Criterion	Concurrent	Discriminant			
PGI-I and PGI-S (Patient Global Impression of Severity and of Improvement) (79) Grade C	Two single-question global indexes to measure symptom bother related to urinary incontinence	Women, SUI					√		√ (12 Weeks)		None found
POSQ (Primary OAB Symptom Questionnaire) (71) Grade C	To assess which symptom of OAB is the most bothersome to patients	Men and women, OAB		√	√						None found
PPBC (Patient Perception of Bladder Condition) (74) Grade A	To assess patients' subjective impression of their current urinary problems. Developed for patients with urinary problems as a global assessment of bladder condition and is recommended as a global outcome measure for urinary incontinence by the European Medicine Evaluation Association	Men and women		√			√		√	√	PPBC is translated in 22 languages www.prolutssh.com
SSI and SII (Symptom Severity Index and Symptom Impact Index for stress incontinence in women) (80) Grade C	To measure stress incontinence severity and impact or bother-some of symptoms. This questionnaire was developed and administered to women undergoing stress incontinence surgery	Women, SUI		√	√		√			√	SSI and SII translated in five languages http://proqolid.org/instruments/symptom_severity_index_and_symptom_impact_index_for_stress_incontinence_in_women_ssi_and_sii

(*Continued*)

Table 13.3 Summary of Urinary Incontinence (UI), Overactive Bladder (OAB), and Lower Urinary Tract Symptoms (LUTS) Patient Reported Outcome (PRO) Measures—Symptom Bother (*Continued*)

PRO name/grade	Purpose of tool	Population sample	Reliability		Validity				Responsiveness (Treatment duration)	Psychometric validation in other languages	Available languages
			Internal consistency	Test-retest	Content	Criterion	Concurrent	Discriminant			
UI-4 (Urinary Incontinence-4 Questionnaire) (81) Grade C	To assess how patients are bothered by urinary incontinence	Women, UI					√				Available only in Spanish http://www.ncbi.nlm.nih.gov/pubmed/10488609?ordinalpos=3&itool=EntrezSystem2.PEntrez.Pubmed.Pubmed_ResultsPanel.Pubmed_RVDocSum
UDI (Urogenital Distress Inventory) (60) Grade B	To assess symptom bother related to UI. UDI is meant to complement the IIQ, was developed at the same time as the IIQ	Women, UI, SUI	√	√	√		√	√		√	Available in 3 languages (English, Italian, and Arabic)
UDI-6 (Urogenital Distress Inventory-6) (78) Grade A	To assess LUTS bother, including incontinence, in women	Women	√	√	√	√			√	√	Available in 3 languages (English, Turkish, and Arabic)

Abbreviations: AI, All incontinence; BPH, benign prostatic hyperplasia; I-QOL, international-quality of life; PFD, pelvic floor disorders; SUI, stress urinary incontinence; VAS, visual analog score.

Table 13.4 Summary of Urinary Incontinence (UI), Overactive Bladder (OAB), and Lower Urinary Tract Symptoms (LUTS) Patient Reported Outcome (PRO) Measures—Urgency

PRO name/ grade	Purpose of tool	Population sample	Reliability Internal consistency	Reliability Test-retest	Validity Content	Validity Criterion	Validity Concurrent	Validity Discriminant	Responsiveness (Treatment duration)	Psychometric validation in other languages	Available languages
IUSS (Indevus Urgency Severity) (88) Grade A	Used to quantify the level of urgency associated with each toilet void as measured during standard voiding diaries	OAB with urgency incontinence, men and women		√	√	√	√		√ (12 Weeks)		None found
SUIQ (Stress/Urge Incontinence Questionnaire) (92) Grade C	Two item questionnaire used to differentiate between symptoms of stress and urge urinary incontinence	Women, UI		√			√				None found
UDI (Urogenital Distress Inventory) (60) Grade B	To assess symptom bother related to UI. UDI is meant to complement the IIQ, was developed at the same time as the IIQ	Women, UI, SUI	√	√	√		√	√		√	Available in three languages (English, Italian, and Arabic)
UPS (Urgency Perception Score) (93) Grade C	Self-report five item OAB questionnaire used for grading the urge to void and assessing the reason why individuals usually void	Men and women		√	√		√	√		None found	None found
UPS (Urgency Perception Scale) (85) Grade B	To assess the severity of urgency—whether or not urgency; the sudden and compelling desire to urinate should have a severity measure is debated. The UPS was designed for use in clinical trials to evaluate patient perceived urgency	OAB (double-blind), men and women			√		√		√		None found

(Continued)

Table 13.4 Summary of Urinary Incontinence (UI), Overactive Bladder (OAB), and Lower Urinary Tract Symptoms (LUTS) Patient Reported Outcome (PRO) Measures—Urgency (*Continued*)

PRO name/ grade	Purpose of tool	Population sample	Reliability		Validity				Responsiveness (Treatment duration)	Psychometric validation in other languages	Available languages
			Internal consistency	Test-retest	Content	Criterion	Concurrent	Discriminant			
URIS-24 (Urge Impact Scale) (94) Grade C	To assess of the impact of the most common form of UI in older persons	Older persons, UI	√	√	√		√				None found
URS (Urgency Rating Scale) (95) Grade C	5-point scale to be used concurrently with voiding diaries to measure the level of urgency associated with each micturiation. Advocated by the EMEA CPMP	Psychometric evaluation not reported									None found
USS (Urinary Sensation Scale) (96) Grade C	To assess the impact of urgency with patients with OAB	Urologists or urogyne-cologists, Survey respon-dents with OAB symptoms	N/A	N/A	√	N/A	N/A	N/A	N/A		None found
UU Scale (10-item scale to measure urinary urgency) (97) Grade B	10 item questionnaire use to measure UU	Men and women		√			√		√	None found	None found

Abbreviations: EMEA CPMP; European medicines evaluation agency committee for proprietary medicinal products; SUI, stress urinary incontinence.

Urgency Rating Scale recommended by the European Medicines Evaluation Agency, consists of a five-point rating scale to be rated with every void, ranging from one (no urgency; I felt no need to empty my bladder but did so for other reasons) to five (urge incontinence; I leaked before arriving at the toilet). This scale was used in a tolterodine clinical trial, in which responses on this scale were used to calculate sum urgency, a measure that accounts for changes in both urgency and frequency (90,91).

CONCLUSION

Questionnaire design is a complex and lengthy process and reinventing the wheel unnecessary for the vast majority of cases. A careful read of the chapter by Cotterill and Abrams will reveal that many of the questionnaires discussed in this and the chapter by Kopp and Brubaker have been adopted by the International Consultation as modules for the ICIQ.

There are clearly many different questionnaires and types of questionnaires from which to choose. Plan a study carefully with respect to what you expect to measure, which populations you intend to survey, and read the content of a questionnaire carefully. The value of spending time to make an informed and careful decision will however always be worth the effort.

REFERENCES

1. Patient Reported Outcome Assessment in Report of the 4th International Consultation on Incontinence. Health publications Ltd, 2009: 363–412.
2. Kelleher CJ, Cardozo LD, Khullar V, Salvatore S. A new questionnaire to assess the quality of life of urinary incontinent women. Br J Obstet Gynaecol 1997; 104: 1374–9.
3. Coyne K, Revicki D, Hunt T, et al. Psychometric validation of an overactive bladder symptom and health-related quality of life questionnaire: the OAB-q. Qual Life Res 2002; 11: 563–74.
4. World HO. Definition of Health. Geneva: WHO, 1978.
5. Naughton MJ, Shumaker SA. Assessment of health-related quality of life. In: Furberg CD, ed. Fundamentals of Clinical Trials. St. Louis: Mosby Press, 1996: 185.
6. Kelleher CJ, Pleil AM, Reese PR, Burgess SM, Brodish PH. How much is enough and who says so? The case of he King's Health Questionnaire and overactive bladder. British Journal of Gynaecology 2004; 111: 605–12.
7. Brazier J, Czoski-Murray C, Roberts J, et al. Estimation of a preference-based index from a condition-specific measure: the King's Health Questionnaire. Med Decis Making 2008; 28: 113–26. Epub 2007 Jul 19.
8. Jackson S, Donovan J, Brookes S, et al. The Bristol Female Lower Urinary Tract Symptoms questionnaire: development and psychometric testing. Br J Urol 1996; 77: 805–12.
9. Donovan JL, Abrams P, Peters TJ, et al. The ICS-"BPH" Study: the psychometric validity and reliability of the ICSmale questionnaire. Br J Urol 1996; 77: 554–62.
10. Swithinbank LV, Donovan JL, du Heaume JC, et al. Urinary symptoms and incontinence in women: relationships between occurrence, age, and perceived impact. Br J Gen Pract 1999; 49: 897–900.
11. Swithinbank LV, Donovan JL, Rogers CA, Abrams P. Nocturnal incontinence in women: a hidden problem. J Urol 2000; 164: 764–6.
12. Temml C, Haidinger G, Schmidbauer J, Schatzl G, Madersbacher S. Urinary incontinence in both sexes: prevalence rates and impact on quality of life and sexual life. Neurourol Urodyn 2000; 19: 259–71.
13. Brookes ST, Donovan JL, Wright M, Jackson S, Abrams P. A scored form of the Bristol Female Lower Urinary Tract Symptoms questionnaire: data from a randomized controlled trial of surgery for women with stress incontinence. Am J Obstet Gynecol 2004; 191: 73–82.
14. Hansen BJ, Flyger H, Brasso K, et al. Validation of the self-administered Danish Prostatic Symptom Score (DAN-PSS-1) system for use in benign prostatic hyperplasia. Br J Urol 1995; 76: 451–8.
15. Meyhoff HH, Hald T, Nordling J, et al. A new patient weighted symptom score system (DAN-PSS-1). Clinical assessment of indications and outcomes of transurethral prostatectomy for uncomplicated benign prostatic hyperplasia. Scand J Urol Nephrol 1993; 27: 493–9.
16. Flyger HL, Kallestrup EB, Mortensen SO. Validation of a computer version of the patient-administered Danish prostatic symptom score questionnaire. Scand J Urol Nephrol 2001; 35: 196–9.
17. Abrams P, Donovan JL, de la Rosette JJ, Schafer W. International Continence Society "Benign Prostatic Hyperplasia" study: background, aims, and methodology. Neurourol Urodyn 1997; 16: 79–91.
18. Donovan JL, Brookes ST, de la Rosette JJ, et al. The responsiveness of the ICSmale questionnaire to outcome: evidence from the ICS-"BPH" study. BJU Int 1999; 83: 243–8.
19. Donovan JL, Peters TJ, Abrams P, et al. Scoring the short form ICSmale SF questionnaire. International Continence Society. J Urol 2000; 164: 1948–55.
20. Lee PS, Reid DW, Saltmarche A, Linton L. Measuring the psychosocial impact of urinary incontinence: the York Incontinence Perceptions Scale (YIPS). J Am Geriatr Soc 1995; 43: 1275–8.
21. Shumaker SA, Wyman JF, Uebersax JS, McClish D, Fantl JA. Health-related quality of life measures for women with urinary incontinence: the Incontinence Impact Questionnaire and the urogenital distress inventory. Continence Program in Women (CPW) Research Group. Qual Life Res 1994; 3: 291–306.
22. Wyman JF, Harkins SW, Choi SC, Taylor JR, Fantl JA. Psychosocial impact of urinary incontinence in women. Obstet Gynecol 1987; 70: 378–81.
23. Corcos J, Behlouli H, Beaulieu S. Identifying cut-off scores with neural networks for interpretation of the incontinence impact questionnaire. Neurourol Urodyn 2002; 21: 198–203.
24. Dmochowski RR, Sand PK, Zinner NR, et al. Comparative efficacy and safety of transdermal oxybutynin and oral tolterodine versus placebo in previously treated patients with urge and mixed urinary incontinence. Urology 2003; 62: 237–42.
25. Blanc E, Hermieu JF, Ravery V, et al. Value of the use of a questionnaire in the evaluation of incontinence surgery. Prog Urol 1999; 9: 88–94.
26. FitzGerald MP, Kenton K, Shott S, Brubaker L. Responsiveness of quality of life measurements to change after reconstructive pelvic surgery. Am J Obstet Gynecol 2001; 185: 20–4.
27. Wagner TH, Patrick DL, Bavendam TG, Martin ML, Buesching DP. Quality of life of persons with urinary incontinence: development of a new measure. Urology 1996; 47: 67–71.
28. Chaisaeng S, Santingamkun A, Opanuraks J, Ratchanon S, Bunyaratavej C. IQOL: translation & reliability for use with urinary incontinence patients in Thailand. J Med Assoc Thai 2006; 89(Suppl 3): S33–9.
29. Oh SJPH, Lim SH, Hong SK. Translation and linguistic validation of Korean version of the incontinence quality of life(I-QoL) instrument. J Korean Continence Soc 2002; 6: 10–23.
30. Patrick DL, Martin ML, Bushnell DM, et al. Quality of life of women with urinary incontinence: further development of the incontinence quality of life instrument (I-QOL). Urology 1999; 53: 71–6.
31. Badia LCD, Conejero S. Validity of the King's Health questionnaire in the assessment of quality of life of patients with urinary incontinence. The King's Group. Med Clin (Barc) 2000; 114: 647–52.
32. Okamura K, Usami T, Nagahama K, Maruyama S, Mizuta E. "Quality of life" assessment of urination in elderly Japanese men and women with some medical problems using International Prostate Symptom Score and King's Health questionnaire. Eur Urol 2002; 41: 411–9.
33. Yip SK, Chan A, Pang S, et al. The impact of urodynamic stress incontinence and detrusor overactivity on marital relationship and sexual function. Am J Obstet Gynecol 2003; 188: 1244–8.
34. Homma YAT, Yoshida M, et al. Validation of Japanese version of QOL questionnaire for urinary incontinence. Journal of NBS 2002; 13: 247–2.
35. Homma YGM, Ando T, Fukuhara S. Development of the Japanese version of QOL questionnaires for urinary incontinence. Jpn J NBS 1999; 10: 225–36.
36. Tamanini JT, D'Ancona CA, Botega NJ, Rodrigues Netto N, Jr. Validation of the Portuguese version of the King's Health Questionnaire for urinary incontinent women. Rev Saude Publica 2003; 37: 203–11.
37. Liu JF, Wang QZ, Hou J. Surgical treatment for cancer of the oesophagus and gastric cardia in Hebei, China. Br J Surg 2004; 91: 90–8.

38. Plachta Z, Adamiak A, Jankiewicz K, Skorupski P, Rechberger T. Quality of life after mid-urethra polypropylene tape sling surgery (IVS, TVT) in female stress urinary incontinence. Ginekol Pol 2003; 74: 986–91.

39. Rufford J, Hextall A, Cardozo L, Khullar V. A double-blind placebo-controlled trial on the effects of 25 mg estradiol implants on the urge syndrome in postmenopausal women. Int Urogynecol J Pelvic Floor Dysfunct 2003; 14: 78–83.

40. Wang AC, Wang YY, Chen MC. Single-blind, randomized trial of pelvic floor muscle training, biofeedback-assisted pelvic floor muscle training, and electrical stimulation in the management of overactive bladder. Urology 2004; 63: 61–6.

41. Shaw C, Matthews RJ, Perry SI, et al. Validity and reliability of a questionnaire to measure the impact of lower urinary tract symptoms on quality of life: the Leicester Impact Scale. Neurourol Urodyn 2004; 23: 229–36.

42. Coyne KS, Matza LS, Thompson C, Jumadilova Z, Bavendam T. The responsiveness of the OAB-q among OAB patient subgroups. Neurourol Urodyn 2007; 26: 196–203.

43. Coyne KS, Matza LS, Thompson CL, Kopp ZS, Khullar V. Determining the importance of change in the overactive bladder questionnaire. J Urol 2006; 176: 627–32.

44. Yang Y, Brazier J, Tsuchiya A, Coyne K. Estimating a Preference-Based Single Index from the Overactive Bladder Questionnaire. Value Health, 2008.

45. Coyne K, Lai JS, Zyczynski T, et al. An Overactive Bladder Symptom and Quality-of-Life Short Form: Development of the Overactive Bladder Questionnaire (OAB-q) Short Form (SF). France: ICS Paris, 2004.

46. Coyne KS, Zyczynski T, Margolis MK, Elinoff V, Roberts RG. Validation of an overactive bladder awareness tool for use in primary care settings. Adv Ther 2005; 22: 381–94.

47. Palleschi G, Pastore AL, Stocchi F, et al. Correlation between the overactive bladder questionnaire (OAB-q) and urodynamic data of Parkinson disease patients affected by neurogenic detrusor overactivity during antimuscarinic treatment. Clin Neuropharmacol 2006; 29: 220–9.

48. Robinson D, Pearce KF, Preisser JS, et al. Relationship between patient reports of urinary incontinence symptoms and quality of life measures. Obstet Gynecol 1998; 91: 224–8.

49. Roovers JP, van der Vaart CH, van der Bom JG, et al. A randomised controlled trial comparing abdominal and vaginal prolapse surgery: effects on urogenital function. Bjog 2004; 111: 50–6.

50. Simons AM, Dowell CJ, Bryant CM, Prashar S, Moore KH. Use of the Dowell Bryant Incontinence Cost Index as a post-treatment outcome measure after non-surgical therapy. Neurourol Urodyn 2001; 20: 85–93.

51. Dugan E, Cohen SJ, Robinson D, et al. The quality of life of older adults with urinary incontinence: determining generic and condition-specific predictors. Qual Life Res 1998; 7: 337–44.

52. Uebersax JS, Wyman JF, Shumaker SA, McClish DK, Fantl JA. Short forms to assess life quality and symptom distress for urinary incontinence in women: the incontinence impact questionnaire and the urogenital distress inventory. Continence Program For Women Research Group. Neurourol Urodyn 1995; 14: 131–9.

53. Vassallo BJ, Kleeman SD, Segal JL, Walsh P, Karram MM. Tension-free vaginal tape: a quality-of-life assessment. Obstet Gynecol 2002; 100: 518–24.

54. Woodman PJ, Misko CA, Fischer JR. The use of short-form quality of life questionnaires to measure the impact of imipramine on women with urge incontinence. Int Urogynecol J Pelvic Floor Dysfunct 2001; 12: 312–5.

55. Amarenco G, Arnould B, Carita P, et al. European psychometric validation of the CONTILIFE: a Quality of Life questionnaire for urinary incontinence. Eur Urol 2003; 43: 391–404.

56. Lukacz ES, Lawrence JM, Buckwalter JG, et al. Epidemiology of prolapse and incontinence questionnaire: validation of a new epidemiologic survey. Int Urogynecol J Pelvic Floor Dysfunct 2005; 16: 272–84.

57. Abdel-Fattah M, Ramsay I, Barrington JW. A simple visual analogue scale to assess the quality of life in women with urinary incontinence. Eur J Obstet Gynecol Reprod Biol 2007; 133: 86–9.

58. Avery K, Donovan J, Peters TJ, et al. ICIQ: a brief and robust measure for evaluating the symptoms and impact of urinary incontinence. Neurourol Urodyn 2004; 23: 322–30.

59. Donovan JL, Kay HE, Peters TJ, et al. Using the ICSQoL to measure the impact of lower urinary tract symptoms on quality of life: evidence from the ICS-"BPH" study. International Continence Society-Benign Prostatic Hyperplasia. Br J Urol 1997; 80: 712–21.

60. Hagen S, Hanley J, Capewell A. Test-retest reliability, validity, and sensitivity to change of the urogenital distress inventory and the incontinence impact questionnaire. Neurourol Urodyn 2002; 21: 534–9.

61. Bjelic-Radisic V, Dorfer M, Tamussino K, et al. The incontinence outcome questionnaire: an instrument for assessing patient-reported outcomes after surgery for stress urinary incontinence. Int Urogynecol J Pelvic Floor Dysfunct 2007; 18: 1139–49.

62. Bushnell DM, Martin ML, Summers KH, et al. Quality of life of women with urinary incontinence: cross-cultural performance of 15 language versions of the I-QOL. Qual Life Res 2005; 14: 1901–13.

63. Reese PR, Pleil AM, Okano GJ, Kelleher CJ. Multinational study of reliability and validity of the King's Health Questionnaire in patients with overactive bladder. Qual Life Res 2003; 12: 427–42.

64. Shaw C, Matthews RJ, Perry SI, et al. Validity and reliability of a questionnaire to measure the impact of lower urinary tract symptoms on quality of life: the Leicester Impact Scale. Neurourol Urodyn 2004; 23: 229–36.

65. Abraham L, Hareendran A, Mills IW, et al. Development and validation of a quality-of-life measure for men with nocturia. Urology 2004; 63: 481–6.

66. Hendriks EJ, Bernards AT, Berghmans BC, de Bie RA. The psychometric properties of the PRAFAB-questionnaire: a brief assessment questionnaire to evaluate severity of urinary incontinence in women. Neurourol Urodyn 2007; 26: 998–1007.

67. Hendriks EJ, Bernards AT, de Bie RA, de Vet HC. The minimal important change of the PRAFAB questionnaire in women with stress urinary incontinence: results from a prospective cohort study. Neurourol Urodyn 2008; 27: 379–87.

68. Rai GS, Kiniors M, Wientjes H. Urinary incontinence handicap inventory. Arch Gerontol Geriatr 1994; 19: 7–10.

69. Stach-Lempinen B, Kujansuu E, Laippala P, Metsanoja R. Visual analogue scale, urinary incontinence severity score and 15 D–psychometric testing of three different health-related quality-of-life instruments for urinary incontinent women. Scand J Urol Nephrol 2001; 35: 476–83.

70. Coyne KSML, Versi E. Urinary Urgency: Can "Gotta Go" Be Measured? 10th Annual Conference of the International Society for Quality of Life Research. Prague, Czech Republic: Quality of Life Research, 2003: 828.

71. Matza LS, Thompson CL, Krasnow J, et al. Test-retest reliability of four questionnaires for patients with overactive bladder: the overactive bladder questionnaire (OAB-q), patient perception of bladder condition (PPBC), urgency questionnaire (UQ), and the primary OAB symptom questionnaire (POSQ). Neurourol Urodyn 2005; 24: 215–25.

72. Lukacs B, Comet D, Grange JC, Thibault P. Construction and validation of a short-form benign prostatic hypertrophy health-related quality-of-life questionnaire. BPH group in general practice. Br J Urol 1997; 80: 722–30.

73. Lee PS, Reid DW, Saltmarche A, Linton L. Measuring the psychosocial impact of urinary incontinence: the York Incontinence Perceptions Scale (YIPS). J Am Geriatr Soc 1995; 43: 1275–8.

74. Coyne KS, Matza LS, Kopp Z, Abrams P. The validation of the patient perception of bladder condition (PPBC): a single-item global measure for patients with overactive bladder. Eur Urol 2006; 49: 1079–86.

75. Capo JP Jr., Laramee C, Lucente V, Fakhoury A, Forero-Schwanhaeuser S. Solifenacin treatment for overactive bladder in Hispanic patients: patient-reported symptom bother and quality of life outcomes from the VESIcare open-label trial. Int J Clin Pract 2008; 62: 39–46.

76. Chapple C, DuBeau C, Ebinger U, Rekeda L, Viegas A. Darifenacin treatment of patients >or = 65 years with overactive bladder: results of a randomized, controlled, 12-week trial. Curr Med Res Opin 2007; 23: 2347–58.

77. Staskin DR, Rosenberg MT, Dahl NV, Polishuk PV, Zinner NR. Effects of oxybutynin transdermal system on health-related quality of life and safety in men with overactive bladder and prostate conditions. Int J Clin Pract 2008; 62: 27–38.

78. Lemack GE, Zimmern PE. Predictability of urodynamic findings based on the urogenital distress inventory-6 questionnaire. Urology 1999; 54: 461–6.

79. Yalcin I, Bump RC. Validation of two global impression questionnaires for incontinence. Am J Obstet Gynecol 2003; 189: 98–101.

80. Black N, Griffiths J, Pope C. Development of a symptom severity index and a symptom impact index for stress incontinence in women. Neurourol Urodyn 1996; 15: 630–40.

81. Badia Llach XCDD, Perales Cabañas L, Pena Outeriño JM, et al. The development and preliminary validation of the IU-4 questionnaire for the clinical classification of urinary incontinence. Actas Urol Esp 1999; 23: 565–72.

82. Abrams P, Cardozo L, Fall M, et al. The standardisation of terminology in lower urinary tract function: report from the standardisation sub-committee of the International Continence Society. Urology 2003; 61: 37–49.

83. Staskin DR. The urge to define urgency: a review of three approaches. Current urology reports. 2004; 5: 413–5.

84. Brubaker L. Urinary urgency and frequency: what should a clinician do? Obstet Gynecol 2005; 105: 661–7.

85. Chapple CR, Wein AJ. The urgency of the problem and the problem of urgency in the overactive bladder. BJU Int 2005; 95: 274–5.

86. Cardozo L, Coyne KS, Versi E. Validation of the urgency perception scale. BJU Int 2005; 95: 591–6.

87. Chapple CR, Artibani W, Cardozo LD, et al. The role of urinary urgency and its measurement in the overactive bladder symptom syndrome: current concepts and future prospects. BJU Int 2005; 95: 335–40.

88. Bowden ACS, Sabounjian L, Sandage B, Schwiderski U, Zayed H. Psychometric validation of an Urgency Severity Scale (IUSS) for Patients with Overactive Bladder. 33rd Annual Meeting of the International Continence Society. Florence, Italy: Neurourology and Urodynamics, 2003: 531–2.

89. Brewster JLGZ, Green H, Jumadilova Z, Coyne K. Establishing the Content Validity Of The Urinary Sensation Scale (USS). International Society For Pharmacoeconomics and Outcomes Research. Washington, DC: Value in Health, 2005: 418–9.

90. European Agency for the Evaluation of Medicinal Products CfPMP. Note for Guidance on the Clinical Investigation of Medicinal Products for the Treatment of Urinary Incontinence. Report No.: CPMP/EWP/18/01. London, December 2002.

91. Coyne KSML, Thompson C, et al. A Comparison of Three Approaches to Analyze Urinary Urgency as a Treatment Outcome. 35th Annual Meeting of the International Continence Society. Montreal, Canada, 2005.

92. Bent AE, Gousse AE, Hendrix SL, et al. Validation of a two-item quantitative questionnaire for the triage of women with urinary incontinence. Obstet Gynecol 2005; 106: 767–73.

93. Blaivas JG, Panagopoulos G, Weiss JP, Somaroo C, Chaikin DC. The urgency perception score: validation and test-retest. J Urol 2007; 177: 199–202.

94. DuBeau CE, Kiely DK, Resnick NM. Quality of life impact of urge incontinence in older persons: a new measure and conceptual structure. J Am Geriatr Soc 1999; 47: 989–94.

95. European Agency for the Evaluation of Medicinal Products CfPMP. Note for Guidance on the Clinical Investigation of Medicinal Products for the Treatment of Urinary Incontinence in Women. November 2001.

96. Coyne KS, Tubaro A, Brubaker L, Bavendam T. Development and validation of patient-reported outcomes measures for overactive bladder: a review of concepts. Urology 2006; 68(2 Suppl): 9–16.

97. Al-Buheissi S, Khasriya R, Maraj BH, Malone-Lee J. A simple validated scale to measure urgency. J Urol 2008; 179: 1000–5.

14 PRO Questionnaires to Screen and Measure Satisfaction, Expectations, and Goal Achievement

Zoe S Kopp, Christopher J Evans, and Linda P Brubaker

INTRODUCTION

This chapter reviews patient-reported outcome (PRO) questionnaires that assist urogynecologists in patient screening, setting realistic patient expectations that lead to goal achievement and assessing satisfaction with treatment. Symptom condition screeners identify health conditions in patients who may benefit from treatment. Satisfaction questionnaires and goal achievement measures help clinicians understand the patients' point of view regarding their treatment goals so that clinicians can increase the probability of a successful outcome. Other chapters in this section focus on PROs that assess function, health-related quality of life (HRQL), the development of PROs and their effective implementation in clinical trials.

As with other PROs, the development of screeners, expectation, goal assessment, and satisfaction questionnaires must be done scientifically following recommended development guidelines and must have been psychometrically validated to ensure that results are accurate (1–3). The development process steps—from conceptual design through cognitive debriefings, psychometric, and linguistic validation—are described in detail in chapter 12 (Coyne and Sexton). Prior to using a PRO in clinical trials or clinical practice, it is important to verify the validity of multiple aspects of the tool, including the way in which it was developed, administration (paper or electronically), the population in which it is to be used (elderly, surgical, etc.), and the usage setting (clinical practice vs. research). Prior to using PROs in multilingual environments, the tool should be linguistically validated instead of merely translated.

SCREENING TOOLS (SCREENERS)

Patient-completed screeners can facilitate appropriate diagnosis and treatment in urogynecological clinical practice. Most clinicians recognize that many patients find it difficult to articulate their health issues for a variety of reasons such as embarrassment about their problem or lack of medical knowledge or language barrier. Providing questionnaires that screen for common urogynecological conditions to patients before their medical consultation can help focus the medical visit. In this section validated screeners, their individual strengths and weaknesses, and how to obtain them are presented.

Compared to other PROs, screeners have additional criteria they must satisfy in order to be considered sound measurement tools. When choosing and interpreting results of screeners the sensitivity and specificity of the measures should be considered. Sensitivity is the probability of a positive screener score in a patient with the condition. That is, how likely is someone with the condition to score positive? At the same time the screener should have a high likelihood of correctly identifying individuals without the condition—specificity.

Lower Urinary Tracts Symptoms (LUTS) Screeners

To improve the detection of incontinence, overactive bladder (OAB), and other LUTS, several screening questionnaires have been developed (Table 14.1). These tools help patients self-describe symptoms and facilitate diagnosis of LUTS by the clinician. Only the bladder self-assessment questionnaire (B-SAQ) has been designed to screen for general LUTS rather than solely symptoms of one condition. The majority of patients with LUTS have mixed urinary symptoms, and therefore a questionnaire which can detect more than one symptom complex may be more functional as a screening tool in clinical practice than a highly specific questionnaire. The Leiscester Impact Scale, OAB-V8, OAB-symptom score, and questionnaire for urinary incontinence diagnosis are all validated, short, simple to understand and complete, and easy to interpret; however, the Leiscester Impact Scale is interviewer, not patient administered. Importantly, with screeners, responsiveness is not assessed, however, the sensitivity and specificity of each tool is critical. The International Consultation on Incontinence has evaluated many LUTS questionnaires and you can obtain their questionnaires at www.iciq.net (4).

In this section, we describe details of some of the most commonly used screeners along with some of their practical applications.

B-SAQ or Bladder Control Self-Assessment Questionnaire

The B-SAQ instrument was developed by a European panel of experts in lower urinary tract dysfunction as a screening tool to evaluate the presence of bothersome LUTS in women (5). The final instrument was validated and showed good reliability, validity, and sensitivity/specificity. The questionnaire was further translated and validated in 14 languages.

Interstitial Cystitis Symptom Index (ICSI)

The O'Leary–Saint ICSI assesses global IC symptom severity, with scores ranging from 0 to 20. This is based on four questions that measure the severity of day and night-time urinary frequency, urgency, and bladder pain over the past month (6). The content of the questionnaire was developed from literature review, patient focus groups, and input from clinicians with expertise in the diagnosis and treatment of IC. Internal consistency and test–retest reliability were found to be high for the scale. The ICSI has been further validated as an IC/painful bladder syndrome (PBS) symptom measure in a randomized, double-blind clinical trial of pentosan poly-

Table 14.1 LUTS Screeners Overview

PRO name/grade	Purpose of tool	Population sample	Reliability		Validity					Sensitivity/ specificity	Validation in other languages	Available languages
			Internal consistency	Test–retest	Content	Criterion	Concurrent	Discriminant				
B-SAQ (bladder self-assessment questionnaire) or bladder control self-assessment questionnaire (BCSQ) (5)	A screening tool for the presence of bothersome LUTS in women	Women	√	√		√	√	√		√	√	B-SAQ translated in 14 languages. Available from: http://www. mapi-research. fr/i_03_list_urol.htm
Interstitial cystitis symptom index (6)			√	√	√							
I-PSS (international prostate symptom score) (16)	Eight-item questionnaire used to capture the severity of urinary symptoms related to benign prostatic hyperplasia. Originally developed from the American Urological Association symptom index	Men	√	√			√			√	√	I-PSS translated into 40 languages. Available from: http://proqolid. org/instruments/ international_prostate_symptom_score_i_pss
Incontinence screening questionnaire (17)	Five item questionnaire developed to screen for incontinence in women	Women, UI		√				√		√		None found
The Leicester urinary symptom questionnaire (18)	A condition-specific screener of storage LUTS (urgency, frequency, nocturia, and incontinence) was originally developed for women with incontinence only	Men and women, LUTS	√	√	√		√					None found

(*Continued*)

Table 14.1 LUTS Screeners Overview (*Continued*)

PRO name/grade	Purpose of tool	Population sample	Reliability		Validity					Sensitivity/ specificity	Validation in other languages	Available languages
			Internal consistency	Test–retest	Content	Criterion	Concurrent	Discriminant				
Medical, epidemiological, and social aspects of aging questionnaire (10)	A 15 item screening tool for UI in female pelvic medicine and reconstructive surgery patients	Women, UI		√							√	Translated in English and Spanish. Available from: http://www.ncbi.nlm.nih.gov/pubmed/17576498?ordinalpos=2&itool=EntrezSystem2.PEntrez.Pubmed.Pubmed_ResultsPanel.Pubmed_RVDocSum
OAB-SS (overactive bladder symptom score) (19)	A seven item questionnaire validated to measure overall symptom severity due to the four index symptoms of OAB	Men and women, LUTS with or without OAB	√	√	√			√		√		None found
OAB-V8 (OAB awareness tool) (20)	An eight-item screening tool for use in a primary care setting to identify patients who may have OAB	Men and women, OAB			√	√				√	√	OAB-V8 is translated in 32 languages. Available from: http://www.prolutssh.com
PUF patient symptom scale (pelvic pain, urgency, and frequency) (14)	To evaluate patients with suspected IC/PBS	Women and women, IC/PBS								√	√	PUF available in English and Spanish. Available from: http://www.ncbi.nlm.nih.gov/pubmed/15833505?ordinalpos=3&itool=EntrezSystem2.PEntrez.Pubmed.Pubmed_ResultsPanel.Pubmed_RVDocSum

								Available in German
Questionnaire for urinary incontinence diagnosis (21)	Six item questionnaire used to diagnose stress and/or urge types of UI	Women, UI and SUI	√	√	√	√		
Three incontinence questions questionnaire (22)	A three item questionnaire used to classify urge and stress incontinence	Women, UI	Psychometric evaluation not reported			√		
UI (urinary incontinence score) (23)	Developed in German used to asses UI	Women, UI			√			√
Urinary symptom profile (24)	To assess urinary symptoms in male and female with stress, urge, frequency, or urinary obstructive symptoms for use in clinical practice to complement clinical measures and diagnosis	Men and women stress UI (SUI), urge UI, frequency, low stream, combined symptoms	√	√				

Abbreviations: PRO, patient-reported outcome; LUTS, lower urinary tracts symptoms; IC/PBS, interstitial cystitis/painful bladder syndrome.

117

sulfate sodium in patients with IC (7). In addition to good test–retest reliability, internal consistency, and construct validity, the ICSI was found to be responsive to change: patients who reported a 75% improvement in symptoms had a 48% mean reduction in total ICSI score, and patients who reported a 100% improvement had a 77% reduction in total ICSI score from baseline to end of treatment. A score of 0 to 6 has been suggested as indicative of mild symptoms, 7 to 14 of moderate symptoms, and 15 to 20 of severe symptoms (8). However, the ICSI lacks sufficient specificity for use as a diagnostic tool (9). In addition, the reliability of a one-month time-frame for the accurate recall of IC symptom severity has not been tested.

Medical, Epidemiological, and Social Aspects of Aging Questionnaire (MESA)

The MESA is a 15 item tool developed to screen for urinary incontinence and other urinary symptoms in non-institutionalized women (10). Frequency of symptoms is measured on a four-point scale from "never" to "often" with higher scores indicating more frequent symptoms. There are two subscales: six items that assess stress incontinence and nine items for urge incontinence and other urinary symptoms; each subscale was rescored to have a range from 0 to 100 (11).

OAB-V8/OAB Awareness Tool

The OAB-V8/OAB awareness tool has been adapted from the OAB-questionnaire (OAB-q); which is a 33 item questionnaire which assesses symptom bother and HRQL impact of OAB (12). The OAB-V8 is an eight-item questionnaire, which evaluates the symptoms of OAB; namely, urinary frequency, nocturia, urgency, and urge incontinence. Responses are graded on a six point Likert scale. Patients with an overall score of eight or more are directed to seek medical advice. This questionnaire is validated for use by men and women (13).

Pelvic Pain and Urgency/Frequency (PUF)

The PUF questionnaire is an eight-question scale that measures both the severity of IC/PBS symptoms, including PUF and dyspareunia, and the degree to which patients are bothered by them (14).

Kushner and Moldwin evaluated the ability of the PUF, along with the ICSI to screen for IC/PBS among patients attending a urology clinic prior to diagnosis (9). They found that while both tools could adequately distinguish IC from other urinary tract pathologies and therefore aid in the diagnosis of IC/PBS, neither demonstrated sufficient specificity to serve as a sole diagnostic indicator. A score of 13 or greater was found to provide the best sensitivity–specificity ratio for the PUF. As a result of Kushner and Moldwin's findings and concerns with diagnostic short-comings of the potassium sensitivity test, Brewer et al. sought to test the validity of the PUF as a diagnostic tool by correlating scores with cystoscopy with hydrodistension (C-HD) (15). C-HD is conducted under anesthesia, allowing examination of the bladder for abnormalities such as glomerulations or Hunner's ulcers indicative of IC, although this method too has limitations as a diagnostic

for IC. In this study, the PUF was not found to be predictive of positive findings at HD, and also failed to correlate with the severity of IC/PBS findings among those with evidence of the disease.

Although the PUF was developed to be patient-reported, its content was developed by clinicians without patient input. While the scale provides good coverage of the key symptoms of IC/PBS, it includes clinical language such as "urethra" and "perineum" which may not be well understood by patients. Additionally, the layout of the questions may be confusing to patients. Thus, the validity of the PUF as a patient-reported, symptom-based diagnostic tool remains in question.

SEXUAL DYSFUNCTION

There are several screeners that can be used to detect sexual dysfunction. PRO questionnaires have been developed to detect hypoactive sexual desire disorder (HSDD), female sexual arousal disorder (FSAD), female orgasmic disorder (FOD), and pain on intercourse (dyspareunia) (Table 14.2)

Sexual Function Questionnaire (SFQ)

The SFQ developed by Quirk et al. was designed to detect HSDD, FSAD, FOD, and dyspareunia in clinical studies (25). Further validation of the SFQ was undertaken to determine its usefulness as a screener. This research has shown that the SFQ can distinguish between the presence and absence of specific female sexual dysfunction (FSD) symptoms in a large sample of different clinical populations (26). The SFQ consist of 34 questions in two scales, one on sexual activity and the other sexual life with a four week recall period.

Hypoactive Sexual Desire Disorder Screener

The four-item HSDD screener was developed to screen specifically for presence or absence of HSDD in women 18 years and older (27).

Three of the items address desire and one-item addresses level of distress. The HSDD screener was developed and validated in women with HSDD, as confirmed by clinician diagnosis. The HSDD is self-administered in approximately two minutes, has five-point Likert scale and three month recall period.

Sexual Function Questionnaire 28

The 28-item SFQ28 was developed as a screening tool for FSD and also as an efficacy measure in women 18 years and older (25,26). The SFQ has six domains, four of which are specific to the four main types of FSD: FSAD, FOD, HSDD, and pain disorder. The other two domains address "enjoyment" and "partner" issues. The instrument was developed and validated in a broad spectrum of women with FSD. The SFQ is self-administered in approximately 10 minutes, has five-point Likert scale and a four week recall period. An abbreviated 15-item version is also available, which captures information on the four main types of FSD: FSAD, FOD, HSDD, and pain. The other two domains of "enjoyment" and "partner" have been removed.

Table 14.2 Sexual Dysfunction Screeners Overview

PRO name/grade	Purpose of tool	Population sample	Reliability		Validity				Sensitivity/ specificity	Validation in other languages	Available languages
			Internal consistency	Test-retest	Content	Criterion	Concurrent	Discriminant			
HSDD (hypoactive sexual desire disorder screener) (27)	Four-item developed to screen specifically for presence or absence of HSDD in women 18 years and older	Women with HSDD, as confirmed by clinician diagnosis	√	√			√		√	√	Translated in three languages available. Available from: http://www.prolutssh.com/ftranslate.html
Sexual function questionnaire (25)	34 items to detect HSDD, female sexual arousal disorder, female orgasmic disorder, and dyspareunia in clinical studies	Women, female sexual dysfunction (FSD)	√	√				√	√	√	Persian. Available from: http://www.ijrm.ir/library/upload/article/23-28.pdf
Sexual function questionnaire 28 (13,25)	28-item developed as a screening tool for FSD and also as an efficacy measure in women 18 years and older	Women, FSD						√	√	√	Translated in 21 languages available. Available from: http://www.prolutssh.com/ftranslate.html

Abbreviation: PRO, patient-reported outcome.

MEASURING PATIENT SATISFACTION AND EXPECTATIONS
Background

Patient satisfaction is the subjective, personal evaluation of treatments, health service, and health care providers. Although frequently reduced to a single, one dimensional item in clinical practice—"Are you satisfied with your treatment?"—satisfaction with medical treatment represents a complicated construct, which includes efficacy, side effects, accessibility/convenience, availability of resources, continuity of care, cost, availability of information on the disease, information giving, and pleasantness of surroundings and quality/competence of health care providers (28). At its most basic level, satisfaction is a comprehensive evaluation of several dimensions of health care based on patient expectations and provider and treatment performance.

As an outcomes measure, patient satisfaction allows health care providers to assess the appropriateness of treatment according to patient expectations. Although the importance of patient satisfaction assessment is often ignored, it plays a key role in assessing outcomes. In chronic diseases, where patients must live with treatment, patient satisfaction may the distinguishing outcome (29). Evidence suggests that patient satisfaction may be more sensitive to change than quality of life in clinical trials in chronic diseases (30).

Satisfaction with treatment provides information on treatment effectiveness (31) and is believed to affect clinical outcome (32). It has been shown that high levels of patient satisfaction with medication correlates with treatment compliance; maintenance of a relationship with a specific provider; and disclosure of important medical information (33). High levels of satisfaction have also been positively associated with good health status, fewer medical encounters, and shorter hospital stays (34). In contrast, dissatisfaction with medication may impact a patient's likelihood to register formal complaints about services; engage in legal action against a clinic or provider; or provide unfavorable publicity about a clinic (35). Preliminary work suggests satisfaction with pain treatment can influence patient behavior, particularly regarding their intention to continue to take medications (36).

Satisfaction, if measured correctly, differs from other patient reported, clinician reported, and objective outcome measures, in that it addresses the influence that expectations can have on satisfaction. For instance, health status instruments measure the outcomes of treatment (whether they be physiological, symptoms, or impact); satisfaction assessments measure the level of satisfaction with these outcomes given a level of expectations about treatment outcome. The role that expectations play in satisfaction assessments cannot be minimized: a patient with high expectations for treatment outcome may remain dissatisfied even after "successful" treatment because the patient's expectations for treatment benefit were not in alignment with what could be reasonably expected in terms of efficacy. Similarly, a patient with low expectations for treatment benefit can end up extremely satisfied with the treatment regardless of whether or not it worked simply because any treatment benefit, even small, is seen as meeting low expectations. Although the role of expectations in satisfaction assessments cannot be ignored, they can be accounted, or controlled for by ensuring that patient expectations are measured at the time a patient initiates treatment.

As in other areas, the use of satisfaction assessments in urogynecological clinical practice can provide complementary information to other PRO measures and provide information that may be useful in understanding why a patient may or may not remain adherent to treatment.

There are both generic and condition specific questionnaires to assess patient satisfaction with urogynecological treatment. There are three generic questionnaires: the Treatment Satisfaction Questionnaire for Medication (TSQM), Benefit, Satisfaction, and Willingness (BSW), and the Satisfaction with Medication Questionnaire (SAT-MED-Q) and the OAB-satisfaction (OAB-S), which is a condition specific satisfaction measure for OAB. Of the four measures, only the OAB-S adequately addresses the role of expectations in satisfaction assessments. Generally responsiveness cannot be assessed as there is no baseline assessment of patient satisfaction with treatment as no treatment has been given. Table 14.3 below presents a summary of generic and disease specific satisfaction instruments identified in urogynecology and their reliability, validity, and availability.

Benefit, Satisfaction, and Willingness Questionnaire (BSW)

This three-item questionnaire is designed to assess treatment benefit, patient satisfaction with treatment, and patient willingness to continue treatment. The BSW questionnaire was validated using data from three 12-week placebo-controlled trials of tolterodine in patients with OAB (37). In this validation study correlations were seen between patient-reported treatment satisfaction and improvements in the OAB-q, the King's health questionnaire, and micturition variables.

The Treatment Satisfaction Questionnaire for Medication (TSQM)

The TSQM is a general measure of treatment satisfaction with medication suitable for use in a wide variety of medication types and illness conditions. Version one of the questionnaire contains four scales: side effects (four items), effectiveness (three items), convenience (three items), and global satisfaction (three items). It has been demonstrated to be psychometrically sound and valid measure of patients' satisfaction with medication (38). Version 2 of the questionnaire is slightly shorter (39). Psychometric tests of the two measures have shown they perform equivalently when predicting measures of concurrent validity.

The Satisfaction with Medication Questionnaire (SAT MED-Q)

The SAT-MED-Q is a 17-item questionnaire with six dimensions: treatment effectiveness, convenience of use, impact on daily activities, medical care, global satisfaction, and undesirable side effects. The SAT-MED-Q has been demonstrated to be a reliable and valid measure of treatment satisfaction; however, the sensitivity to change has yet to be established (40).

Table 14.3 Summary of Urogynecological PRO Measures of Patient Satisfaction

PRO name	Purpose of tool	Population sample	Reliability		Validity				Responsive-ness (treatment duration)	Psychometric validation in other languages	Available languages
			Internal consistency	Test–retest	Content	Criterion	Concurrent	Discriminant			
BSW Benefit and Satisfaction with Treatment, and Willingness to continue (37)	To capture patients' perceived benefit, satisfaction with treatment, and the willingness to continue treatment	Men and women, OAB					√	√	√		Available from: www.prolutssh.com
OAB-S (Overactive Bladder Satisfaction Questionnaire) (41,42)	To assess patients' satisfaction with OAB treatment including/or not medication. The pre-medication module is designed to assess the patient's expectations with treatment and impact of OAB on patient's day to day life	Men and women, OAB	√	√	√		√	√		√	US English, US Spanish
Satisfaction with Medication Questionnaire (40)	To assess patients' satisfaction with medications		√		√		√	√			English, Spanish for Spain
Treatment Satisfaction with Medication Questionnaire (38,39)	To assess patients' satisfaction with medications	Arthritis, asthma, depression, type 1 diabetes, high cholesterol, hypertension, migraine, psoriasis, and pharmacy patients	√		√		√	√		√	Available from: http://www.quintiles.com/elements/media/files/tsqm-language-availability.pdf

Abbreviation: PRO, patient-reported outcome.

The OAB Treatment Satisfaction Questionnaire

The OAB-S is a five domain questionnaire which evaluates urine control expectations, impact on daily living with OAB, OAB control, fulfilment of OAB medication tolerability, and satisfaction with control. Internal reliability coefficients were good (Cronbach's alpha 0.76–0.96), and test–retest reliability has been established (reliability coefficients 0.72–0.87) (41,42). Cultural and linguistic differences were considered early in the development process, and the OAB-S is available in over 16 languages (43).

GOAL ATTAINMENT SCALING (GAS)

Background

GAS was first introduced in the 1960s by Kiresuk and Sherman (1968) (44). It was created to assess health outcomes in mental health settings, but has in recent years been expanded to other therapeutic areas. This technique is used to measure clinically important change in numerous settings, especially those which require an individualized and multidimensional approach to treatment planning and outcome. Most notably, GAS has been used to assess drug trials for the treatment of Alzheimer's disease (45,46) and has been recently expanded to include evaluations in urogynecology (47,48). The advantage that GAS offers is its responsiveness to change: GAS has been found to be more responsive to change than the measures commonly used in evaluating effectiveness of a specialized intervention (49). The validity and reliability of GAS has been demonstrated in the areas of elderly care (50), chronic pain (51), and cognitive rehabilitation (52).

Goal attainment scaling differs from traditional quality of life measures and satisfaction assessments in several ways. First, it represents an individualized approach to measurement that augments information gained from standardized outcome measures. The chief weakness to standardized PRO measures is that it requires that patients to answer a fixed set of questions—essentially a "one size fits all" approach to assess quality of life. If the measure is well developed and validated (such as the OAB-q and the OAB-S) it can be assumed that the content is generally relevant to patients; however, even with these measures there is no adjustment for the individual or a particular situation. Under goal attainment scaling, the outcome scales are tailored specifically to the individual. Individuals select their own goals for treatment and only rate the symptoms or impacts that they experience: there is no need to rate symptoms or impacts that patients do not care about or never experience. In this sense, GAS represents the purest form of a PRO: only those areas each patient finds important are measured and evaluated.

Second, the role of patient expectations is central to GAS. Under traditional quality of life evaluations, expectations for treatment outcomes are largely ignored. Under satisfaction assessments, the role is made more explicit; however, expectations data in satisfaction assessments are usually only analyzed to determine how much of the change in satisfaction was due to pre-treatment expectations vis-à-vis actual treatment efficacy. Under the GAS methodology, the goals or the expectations patients have about treatment benefit are something that

is seen to be actively managed. If patients set unrealistic treatment goals and their expectations for treatment benefit can never be achieved, it is up to the health care provider to separate unrealistic goals from realistic goals and explain to patients what their treatment can actually achieve (53). In this way, patients are expected to remain adherent to treatment because they understand that some of their goals will never be achieved, while others may obtained with treatment. For instance, if a patient understands from the outset that their goal of cure is unrealistic, then they may remain happy with a treatment that only alleviates symptoms with few side effects.

The third advantage of GAS is that although it is a very individualized approach to measuring PROs it may still be employed in clinical trial settings. Although this appears counterintuitive because one patient's goals may differ from another patient's goals both in terms of number of goals and the types of goals, GAS scores may be combined by treatment group into a summary score utilizing standardized z-based scoring. Although GAS should not be used to derive an absolute level of an outcome (a health status score), it can be used to track achievement: either at an individual level or group level.

Goal attainment scaling involves a multi-step approach which begins with the identification of goals by the patients. Patients are involved in the goal setting and weighting of the importance of goals and communicating the goals to their health care provider (54). At the initial assessment, patients list their goals and the importance of each goal to them (e.g., 1 = fairly important, 2 = very important, and 3 = extremely important; the score of 0 is not allowed because that would mean that the goal was not important to the patient and therefore not necessary to be included in the list of goal). For the next step, anticipated or expected outcome levels are discussed by patients with their health care provider: goals that are unrealistic may be eliminated and the health care provider resets patient expectations for treatment benefit. Finally, a time for the assessment of treatment goal attainment is determined. During this assessment period, goal attainment is rated according to the following: if the goal was achieved as predicted, this is scored 0; achievement above the level predicted is scored at +1 ("somewhat better than expected or predicted") or +2 ("much better than expected or predicted"); no change or achievement below the expected level is scored as −1, and a worsening of the target function is scored as a −2.

Goal achievement has been used in five studies in the area of urogynecological conditions. The studies are best described as preliminary investigations into how goal setting and attainment play a role in this area. The use of GAS in urogynecological conditions is developing rapidly and the usefulness, validity, and reliability in these conditions is still being evaluated.

The earliest investigation was by Hullfish et al. (55). In this study, patients were asked to describe five personal goals for pelvic floor surgery which were rated on a five-point scale. After surgery (three months, one and three years), patients assessed their goals and either agreed or disagreed that the goals were met. Agreement was rated as +1 and strong agreement was rated as +2; disagreement was rated as −1 and strong disagreement was rated as –2. The validity of the assessment in pelvic floor surgery was partially established by relating Incontinent Impact Questionnaire-7 and the urogenital distress inventory-6 scores to goal achievement.

Elkadry et al. (56) found that women's goals for reconstructive pelvic surgery are personal and highly subjective, and that the decision to undergo surgery is based on specific patient-selected goals. In a follow up to this work, Mahajan et al. (57) examined goals and satisfaction in an urge incontinence population. Patients were asked to list their goals and at follow-up patients were asked to identify the degree to which each goal was achieved one year post surgery (completely to not at all). The study found that failure to meet goals was associated with long-term dissatisfaction with surgery.

In the area of IC/PBS GAS has been employed to determine if patients' treatment goals are unique (58). This study found over 140 separate goals with a mean number of four goals per patient with pain, frequency, and nocturia being the most frequently described goals. Based on these findings a new GAS instrument is in development in this area.

In the area of OAB and LUTS, a new measure of goal attainment scaling has been developed: the self-assessment goal achievement (SAGA) questionnaire (47). Due to the fact that early research found that some patients have difficulty formulating goals, interviews with LUTS patients were conducted to identify the most bothersome symptoms. These symptoms were incorporated in the first part of the SAGA tool as a fixed assessment of nine symptom goals. In the second part of SAGA, in line with traditional goal attainment scaling measures, patients can record any other goals that they have related to their LUTS. At follow-up patients rate the level of goal achievement on each of the goals they selected. Further validity and reliability testing of SAGA is needed before it can be recommended for use in clinical studies.

CONCLUSION

The accurate screening for, and the importance of understanding patient expectations, goals, and satisfaction, is increasingly recognized as a critical element in judging overall outcomes in urogynecological conditions. The increasing availability of validated PRO screeners that can assist clinicians and researchers with assessing symptoms and conditions has the potential to greatly enhance communication amongst clinicians and patients, as well as amongst researchers. Validated tools that assist with assessing expectations, goal setting, and achievement, and measurement of satisfaction can be incorporated into clinical and research practice. This is a high-impact area for continued research as clinicians and patients alike seek to improve their understanding of each other's expertise and seek mutually reasonable treatment plans that results in satisfied patients with an improved quality of life. This chapter should facilitate inclusion of appropriate PRO screening and outcomes tools as part of routine assessment in clinical practice. In future urogynecological research measuring expectations, satisfaction, and goal attainment as primary or co-primary outcomes should be considered as part of a complete assessment of urogynecological treatment.

REFERENCES

1. Food & Drug Administration (FDA). Guidance for Industry—Patient-Reported Outcome Measures: Use in Medical Product Development to Support Labeling Claims. Silver Spring, MD: FDA, 2006.
2. Turner R, Quittner A, Parasauraman B, Kallich J, Cleeland C. The Mayo/FDA Patient-Reported Outcomes Consensus Meeting. Patient-Reported Outcomes: Instrument Development and Selection Issues. Value Health 2007; 10(Suppl 2): S86–93.
3. Frost M, Reeve B, Leipa A, Stauffer J, Hays R. The Mayo/FDA Patient-Reported Outcomes Consensus Meeting Group. What is sufficient evidence for the reliability and validity of patient-reported outcome measures? Value Health 2007; 10(Suppl 2): S94–105.
4. Abrams P, Cardozo L, Khoury S, Wein A. Incontinence, 4th edn. Paris: Health Publication Ltd., 2009.
5. Basra R, Artibani W, Cardozo L, et al. Design and validation of a new screening instrument for lower urinary tract dysfunction: the bladder control self-assessment questionnaire (B-SAQ). Eur Urol 2007; 52: 230–7.
6. O'Leary MP, Sant GR, Fowler FJ Jr, Whitmore KE, Spolarich-Kroll J. The interstitial cystitis symptom index and problem index. Urology 1997; 49(Suppl 5A): 58–63.
7. Lubeck DP, Whitmore K, Sant GR, Alvarez-Horine S, Lai C. Psychometric validation of the O'Leary–Sant interstitial cystitis symptom index in a clinical trial of pentosan polysulfate sodium. Urology 2001; 57(Suppl 1): 62–6.
8. Nickel JC, Barkin J, Forrest J, et al. Randomized, double-blind, dose-ranging study of pentosan polysulfate sodium for interstitial cystitis. Urology 2005; 65: 654–58.
9. Kushner L, Moldwin RM. Efficiency of questionnaires used to screen for interstitial cystitis. J Urol 2006; 176: 587–92.
10. Diokno AC, Brock BM, Brown MB, Herzog AR. Prevalence of urinary incontinence and other urological symptoms in the noninstitutionalized elderly. J Urol 1986; 136: 1022–5.
11. Young A, Fine P, McCrery R, et al. Spanish language translation of pelvic floor disorders instruments. Int Urogynecol J 2007; 18: 1171–8.
12. Coyne K, Revicki D, Hunt T, et al. Psychometric validation of an overactive bladder symptom and health-related quality of life questionnaire: the OAB-q. Qual Life Res 2002; 11: 563–74.
13. Roovers JP, van der Vaart CH, van der Bom JG, et al. A randomised controlled trial comparing abdominal and vaginal prolapse surgery: effects on urogenital function. BJOG 2004; 111: 50–6.
14. Parsons CL, Dell J, Stanford EJ, et al. Increased prevalence of interstitial cystitis: previously unrecognized urologic and gynecologic cases identified using a new symptom questionnaire and intravesical potassium sensitivity. Urology 2002; 60: 573–8.
15. Brewer ME, White WM, Klein FA, Klein LM, Waters WB. Validity of pelvic pain, urgency, and frequency questionnaire in patients with interstitial cystitis/painful bladder syndrome. Urology 2007; 70: 646–9.
16. Barry MJ, Fowler FJ Jr, O'Leary MP, et al. The American Urological Association symptom index for benign prostatic hyperplasia. The Measurement Committee of the American Urological Association. J Urol 1992; 148: 1549–57; discussion 64.
17. Gunthorpe W, Brown W, Redman S. The development and evaluation of an incontinence screening questionnaire for female primary care. Neurourol Urodyn 2000; 19: 595–607.
18. Shaw C, Matthews RJ, Perry SI, et al. Validity and reliability of an interviewer-administered questionnaire to measure the severity of lower urinary tract symptoms of storage abnormality: the Leicester Urinary Symptom Questionnaire. BJU Int 2002; 90: 205–15.
19. Blaivas JG, Panagopoulos G, Weiss JP, Somaroo C. Validation of the overactive bladder symptom score. J Urol 2007; 178: 543–7; discussion 7.
20. Coyne KS, Zyczynski T, Margolis MK, Elinoff V, Roberts RG. Validation of an overactive bladder awareness tool for use in primary care settings. Adv Ther 2005; 22: 381–94.
21. Bradley CS, Rovner ES, Morgan MA, et al. A new questionnaire for urinary incontinence diagnosis in women: development and testing. Am J Obstet Gynecol 2005; 192: 66–73.
22. Brown JS, Bradley CS, Subak LL, et al. The sensitivity and specificity of a simple test to distinguish between urge and stress urinary incontinence. Ann Intern Med 2006; 144: 715–23.

23. Gaudenz R. [A questionnaire with a new urge-score and stress-score for the evaluation of female urinary incontinence (author's transl)]. Geburtshilfe Frauenheilkd 1979; 39: 784–92.

24. Haab F, Richard F, Amarenco G, et al. Comprehensive evaluation of bladder and urethral dysfunction symptoms: development and psychometric validation of the urinary symptom profile (USP) questionnaire. Urology 2008; 71: 646–56.

25. Quirk FH, Heiman JR, Rosen RC, et al. Development of a sexual function questionnaire for clinical trials of female sexual dysfunction. J Wom Health Gend Base Med 2002; 11: 277–89.

26. Quirk F, Haughie S, Symonds T. The use of the sexual function questionnaire as a screening tool for women with sexual dysfunction. J Sex Med 2005; 2: 469–77

27. Leiblum S, Symonds T, Moore J, et al. A methodology study to develop and validate a screener for hypoactive sexual desire disorder in postmenopausal women. J Sex Med 2006; 3: 455–64.

28. Krowinski W, Steiber S. Measuring Patient Satisfaction, 2nd edn. Chicago: American Hospital Publishing, 1996: 15.

29. Weaver M, Patrick DL, Markson LE, et al. Issues in the measurement of satisfaction with treatment. Am J Manag Care 1997; 3: 579–94.

30. Weinberger M, Oddone EZ, Henderson WG. Does increased access to primary care reduce hospital readmissions? Veterans Affairs Cooperative Study Group on Primary Care and Hospital Readmission. N Engl J Med 1996; 334: 1441–7.

31. Cousins M, Wall PD, Melzack R, eds. Textbook of Pain: Acute and Postoperative Pain, 3rd edn. Philadelphia: Churchill Livingstone, 1994.

32. Kehlet H. The importance of post operative pain relief. Acta Anaesthesiol Scand 2002; 37(Suppl 100): 122–3.

33. American Pain Society Quality of Care Committee. Quality improvement guidelines for the treatment of acute pain. J Am Med Ass 1995; 274: 1874–80.

34. McCracken L, Klock A, Mingay D. Assessment of satisfaction with treatment for chronic pain. J Pain Symptom Manage 1997; 14: 292–9.

35. Carroll K, Atkins P, Herold G. Pain assessment and management in critically ill postoperative and trauma patients: a multisite study. Am J of Crit Care 1999; 8: 105–17.

36. Horowicz-Mehler N, Evans C, Crawford B, et al. Structural equation modeling in a trial of rheumatoid arthritis patients: indicators of satisfaction with pain medication and intention to comply with treatment. Poster presented at the Annual European Congress of Rheumatology; June 12–15, 2002; Stockholm, Sweden.

37. Pleil AM, Coyne KS, Reese PR, et al. The validation of patient-rated global assessments of treatment benefit, satisfaction, and willingness to continue—the BSW. Value Health 2005; 8(Suppl 1): S25–34.

38. Atkinson M, Sinha A, Hass S, et al. Validation of a general measure of treatment satisfaction, the treatment satisfaction questionnaire for medication (TSQM), using a national panel study of chronic disease. Health Qual Life Outcomes 2004; 2: 1–13.

39. Atkinson M, Kumar R, Cappelleri J, Hass S. Hierarchical construct validity of the treatment satisfaction questionnaire for medication (TSQM version II) among outpatient pharmacy consumers. Value Health 2005; 8(Suppl): S9–24.

40. Ruiz M, Pardo A, Rejas J, et al. Development and validation of the treatment satisfaction with medicinces questionnaire (SATMED-Q). Value Health 2008; 11: 913–26.

41. Piault E, Evans CJ, Espindle D, et al. Development and validation of the overactive bladder satisfaction (OAB-S) questionnaire. Neurourol Urodyn 2008; 27: 179–90.

42. Piault E EC, Marcucci G, Kopp Z, Brubaker L, Abrams P. Patient satisfaction: international development, translatability assessment and linguistic validation of the OAB-S, an overactive bladder treatment satisfaction questionnaire. ISPOR 8th Annual European Congress. Florence, Italy: Value in Health, 2005. p. A88.

43. Acquadro C, Kopp Z, Coyne KS, et al. Translating overactive bladder questionnaires in 14 languages. Urology 2006; 67: 536–40.

44. Kiresuk T, Sherman R. Goal attainment scaling: a general method of evaluating comprehensive community mental health programs. Community Ment Health J 1968; 4: 443–53.

45. Rockwood K, Stolee P, Howard K, Mallery L. Use of goal attainment scaling to measure treatment effects in an anti-dementia drug trial. Neuroepidemiology 1996; 15: 330–8.

46. Rockwood K, Song F, Gorman M. Attainment of treatment goals by people with Alzheimer's disease receiving galantamine: a randomized controlled trial. CMAJ 2006; 174: 1099–105.

47. Brubaker L, Kopp Z, Piault E, et al. Development of a Self-Assessment Goal Achievement (SAGA) Questionnaire in urinary disorders. Presented at International Continence Society; August 20–24, 2007; Rotterdam, The Netherlands.

48. Fianu-Jonasson A, Brubaker L, Kelleher V, et al. Understanding Swedish patients' expectations for treatment of their urinary symptoms. Presented at: Nordic Urogynecological Association; May 14–16, 2009; Reykjavik, Iceland.

49. Rockwood K, Stolee P, Fox R. The use of goal attainment scaling in measuring clinically important change in the frail elderly. J Clin Epidemiol 1993; 46: 113–18.

50. Stolee P, Stadnyk K, Myers A, Rockwood K. An individualized approach to outcome measurement in geriatric rehabilitation. J Gerontol A Biol Sci Med Sci 1999; 54: M641–7.

51. Zaza C, Stolee P, Prkachin K. The application of goal attainment scaling in chronic pain settings. J Pain Symptom Manag 1999; 17: 55–64.

52. Rockwood K, Joyce B, Stolee P. Use of goal attainment scaling in measuring clinically important change in cognitive rehabilitation patients. J Clin Epidemiol 1997; 50: 581–8.

53. Marschall-Kehrel D, Roberts R, Brubaker L. Patient-reported outcomes in overactive bladder: the influence of perception of condition and expectation for treatment benefit. Urology 2006; 68(Suppl 2A): 29–37.

54. Ashford S, Turner-Stokes L. Goal attainment for spasticity management using botulinum toxin. Physiother Res Int 2006; 11: 24–34.

55. Hullfish K, Bovbjerg V, Steers W. Patient-centered goals for pelvic floor dysfunction surgery: long-term follow-up. Am J Obstet Gynecol 2004; 191: 201–5.

56. Elkadry E, Kenton K, FitzGerald M, Shott S, Brubaker L. Patient-selected goals: a new perspective on surgical outcome. Am J Obstet Gynecol 2003; 189: 1551–8.

57. Mahajan S, Elkadry E, Kenton K, Shott S, Brubaker L. Patient-centered surgical outcomes: the impact of goal achievement and urge incontinence on patient satisfaction one year after surgery. Am J Obstet Gynecol 2006; 194: 722–8.

58. Payne C, Alle T. Goal achievement provides new insight into interstitial cystitis/painful bladder syndrome symptoms and outcomes. Neurourol Urodyn 2009; 28: 13–17.

15 Questionnaires to Assess Sexual Function
Claudine Domoney and Tara Symonds

Patient reported outcome (PRO) measures to assess sexual function are perhaps those of most significant value, as this sphere of activity is one of the most difficult in which to capture information that is meaningful. These instruments, if designed well, may incorporate the functional aspects of sexuality, the symptom severity, and the impact on quality of life. The WHO has defined sexual health as a state of physical, emotional, mental, and social well-being in relation to sexuality, (and) not merely the absence of disease, dysfunction, or infirmity (1), and therefore an important reflector of global wellbeing. However there are great differences in the perception of clinicians and patients when discussing sexual outcomes. What is important for the patient may not be easily communicated to the doctor. Monitoring the effect of treatment or interventions on sexual parameters has generally been relatively crude to date. Questions which appear comfortable for doctor and patient to discuss may have little bearing on the true change in sexual activity. On the background of a varied population whose sexual backgrounds may be diverse, determining the right method of assessment is crucial for measuring the desired data. As 11% of women have surgical treatment for pelvic floor dysfunction (PFD) (2), it is now the time to determine the impact of the disease process and its treatment on sexual function.

WHY USE QUESTIONNAIRES?
Traditionally gynecologists and urologists have asked questions of their patients pertaining to sex that are comfortable for both to ask and answer. The enquiry may be directed to areas perceived by clinicians as influenced by the disease or condition and that may reasonably be expected to improve with intervention. These include sexual activity, often phrased as frequency of penetrative vaginal intercourse, and pain or dyspareunia. More qualitative components of sexual function may be more difficult to assess unless posed in questionnaire format. Asking about orgasm frequency or quality, satisfaction, arousal, and sexual desire may be difficult for some clinicians and patients, particularly if they perceive they have had inadequate training (3,4). As these factors frequently vary between couples depending on length and quality of relationship, age of both partners, and menopausal or peripartum status, a questionnaire that is sensitive enough to determine these factors may be important if trying to determine the impact of an intervention such as surgery.

It is likely that issues of lesser concern to individuals were previously focused on and this underestimates the true incidence of sexual difficulties. At present it appears vaginal measurements in urogynecological patients do not predict function (5). Investigations such as urodynamic measures, pelvic blood flow, 4D ultrasound, vaginal plethysmography, and nerve conduction studies may give quantitative values to compare population or study groups but evaluation of their relationship to sexual function is in its infancy. Whether they will ever graduate to useful clinical measurements with respect to sexuality is arguable. "The vagina may say yes but the mind says no"—physical measures to assess state of arousal such as blood flow, lubrication do not reproducibly correlate with subjective sense of arousal.

PFD is common with up to one-third of premenopausal and half of postmenopausal women having some form of PFD, which may then lead to a reduction in quality of life, the most important outcome. However sexual problems are also highly prevalent, with a North American study reporting that up to 43% of women and 31% of men aged between 18 and 59 admitted a problem in the previous year (6). British studies have indicated the prevalence of sexual problems in primary care is high with 22% of men and 40% of women being diagnosed with a sexual dysfunction, although this was poorly recognized or documented (7). Yet when the degree of distress or bother is considered the proportion with a sexual problem approximately halves in many studies (8). Clearly it is important for the pelvic surgeon to be able to evaluate the changes in PFD that prevent sexual activity or reduce satisfaction from those that are common in the general population. Questionnaires that are sensitive enough to detect these differences and the modification that can be expected from urogynecological interventions must be developed when considering these factors.

FEMALE SEXUAL FUNCTION
Designing instruments to measure sexuality requires a model to promote understanding of female (and male) sexuality and its deviations. Over the 20th century, models of human sexual behavior have been proposed and classification of normal and abnormal became a clinical and arguably measurable entity. However, the norms for function and activity are varied and at present there is debate over how medicalization of human sexual behavior has been propagated by the prospect of pharmaceutical intervention. Yet there is also a drive from women as expectation of a full and satisfying sexual life has been raised, with over half of one study of 1805 European menopausal women stating it was important (9). Many other international studies of older populations reinforce these findings (10,11).

The Masters and Johnson human sexual response cycle model from the 1960's details the changes occurring during sexual activity based on observations from laboratory based sexual encounters (12). This has been developed into other models over the last 30 years but more recently an International Consensus Group on female sexual dysfunction (FSD) has expanded these female sexuality models to include the importance of intimacy and sexual stimuli on innate sexual drive (13,14). This contrasts to the linear human sexual response model of Masters and Johnson more in keeping with male sexuality, with an inbuilt sexual drive, i.e., libido and desire to be involved in sexual behavior that precedes excitement and arousal. Women in contrast to men may only achieve orgasm in 50% of penetrative intercourse and a further 20% with external stimulation.

The International Consensus Group model of female sexuality indicates that a spontaneous sexual drive to be involved in sexual activity does not need to be present for satisfactory relationships to be maintained. The content of sexual activity of women *may* be less goal driven than that of men. Therefore it is important to understand the other features influencing an individual woman's ability to be sexual in order to explain why she may be experiencing difficulties. How much urogynecological complaints contribute to this may not be clear to the clinician or patient themselves. Sexuality is modulated by many factors and normal features of life, including life events, reproductive events, health, relationships, and cultural factors. Female sexuality is a complex interplay of physiological, psychological, and cultural factors. A well developed questionnaire may be able to detect the effect of PVD on sexual function and activity, its effect on quality of life and the changes in sexual function after interventions.

FEMALE SEXUAL DYSFUNCTION

At present the most accepted international definitions of FSD have been determined by the International Consensus Conference panel modification of the framework of the International Classification of Diseases-10 and Diagnostic and Statistical Manual of Mental Disorders of the American Psychiatric Association (DSM-IV). These areas are defined as four separate categories but with significant comorbidity: sexual desire disorders (hypoactive desire disorder [HSDD] or aversion disorder), female sexual arousal disorder (FSAD), female sexual orgasmic disorder or female orgasmic disorder (FSOD/FOD), and pain disorders (dyspareunia, vaginismus, noncoital pain disorders). The quantification of these disorders including the identification and qualification of pain can be adapted for clinical and research settings. Specific dysfunctions can be diagnosed if the domains within an instrument correspond with a current model and are sufficiently sensitive. Before choosing an instrument for use, the outcomes sought should be clarified and therefore ensure its fitness for purpose. Diagnosing FSD or a specific disorder may not be important and global sexual function the only important issue. Questionnaires may be designed to give a composite score that can be broken down into domains to diagnose or screen for a specific dysfunction (e.g., FSFI) or a global score for comparison, with non diagnostic domains (e.g., PISQ). Those that are diagnostic are likely to be longer unless screening for a particular disorder (e.g., Brief PFSF for HSDD).

FSD in Urogynecology

It is clear that the minority of physicians caring for women with PFDs screen for sexual dysfunction at present. Surveys have reported this is due to lack of time, lack of treatment options, the older age of many of the patient groups, and the perceived lesser importance of this aspect of functioning (3,4). However there is objective evidence that pelvic floor problems adversely affect sexual relationships and sexuality, making it important clinicians are aware. Most studies report that 50% to 60% of urogynecology research participants are sexually active. Up to 64% may be labeled with FSD (15) but this may not take into account the degree of distress which is pivotal in the diagnosis of dysfunction. There is a reluctance on the part of patients to seek help which may be mitigated by the doctors comfort and ability to communicate about such personal matters. It may be easier for both doctor and patient to use a questionnaire to detect these difficulties. However, this can also be perceived as an avoidance tactic for having to engage in offering therapeutic interventions when problems are identified by means of a more remote screening tool, particularly if the outcome of interest is measurement of the effect of an intervention such as surgery. Questionnaires also help to reduce the time constraint of the doctor-patient interaction by having patients complete questionnaires whilst waiting for the consultation. Furthermore, in the area of sex, some degree of removal from embarrassment may result in more valuable answers. Yet as all clinicians would agree, these instruments are no replacement for the consultation, but should be interpreted and integrated with the patients complaints.

Up to 50% of women with urinary incontinence complain of coital incontinence with approximately one-third admitting it compromises their sexual health (16). This has been reported widely as impacting on quality of life (17) yet surgical cure of this complaint is not always reported to improve sexual function (18). Similar findings have been reported with pelvic organ prolapse procedures although the huge variation in technique and individual patient findings may be potential confounding factors (19). This may in part depend on the tools used to measure this outcome as demonstrated by the lack of change of the behavioral/emotive domains of the disease specific questionnaire, pelvic organ prolapse and incontinence sexual questionnaire (PISQ) (20).

OUTCOME MEASURES

Since the launch of sildenafil in 1998 for the treatment of erectile dysfunction (ED) there has been significant growth in male and female sexual health research, which has resulted in the development of numerous new assessment measures, both objective and subjective.

Objective Measures

There have been numerous objective measures developed to diagnose and assess erectile function [e.g., Doppler Ultrasonography, Penile Brachial Index (21)], but penile tumescence using RigiScan has been the most widely used (22). Diagnosis and assessment of men with premature ejaculation has relied on the use of time (stop-watch assessment) to ejaculation (intra-vaginal latency time). For women, objective measures have been developed such as vaginal photoplethysmography and doppler ultrasonography (23). Objective assessment of sexual function in men with ED show good agreement with subjective assessments, considered to be because of the obvious biofeedback loop of the ridigity of the penis. However, in women agreement between the objective and subjective assessment of sexual function has not been as easy to demonstrate and may be due to it being multi-dimensional compared to the uni-dimensionality of ED.

Subjective Measures

Subjective measures of sexual health have flourished over the past 10 years. For assessing ED the gold standard measure is the international index of erectile function (24,25), for men with premature ejaculation there is no gold standard equivalent but there are a number of measures to choose from and were reviewed recently by Althof and Symonds (2007) (26). Assessment of women's sexual health has tended to use sexual inventories, which capture all elements of the female sexual function cycle (FSAD, FOD, HSDD, and Pain) [e.g., sexual function questionnaires (SFQ) (27); female sexual function index (FSFI) (28), see Table 15.1 for detailed listing of measures].

Clinician Measures

Evaluation of change in sexual function status can be assessed using clinician interview, which benefits from an in-depth discussion of all aspects of the individuals sexual history or problem. However, standardization of an interview is difficult if trying to use this approach in the evaluation of a new treatment and probably has most utility in diagnosis, although even in diagnosis there will be issues with concordance and reliability between clinicians due to the complex diagnostic criteria for FSD. Utian et al. (2005) (29) successfully developed a structured diagnostic method for diagnosing FSD and Derogatis et al. (2008) (30) have recently developed a standardized clinician assessment for diagnosing hypoactive sexual desire disorder— women's sexual interest diagnostic interview.

In evaluating the outcome of treatments for both male and FSD, small lab-based studies have generally relied on an initial clinician diagnosis of sexual dysfunction, followed by an objective assessment. Larger, randomized controlled trials, have used similar clinician diagnosis of dysfunction but subjective measures of outcome due to ease of use.

DIFFICULTIES SPECIFIC TO SFQS IN PFD

Neither pelvic floor nor sexual dysfunction are seen as life threatening disorders and therefore may have been neglected in the past. There is now a priority for assessing patient outcomes rather than that of the clinician in an attempt to improve health care provision for these patient groups. Until relatively recently the only tools available for urogynecologists and urologists to use were generic questionnaires validated in the general population. Prior to the use of these questionnaires which may have previously been considered outside of the remit of surgeons, self designed items focusing on the clinicians area of interest such as dyspareunia, frequency of penetrative intercourse, and coital incontinence were quantified in trials. As a result it is not clear what effect surgical interventions have on sexual functioning as the results are highly variable depending on how the questions are asked and to whom, and over what time frame. The rate of sexual activity and the causes of change needs to include assessment of partner factors, which more often determine sexual activity in a relationship (31). Pain as an endpoint may be particularly misleading given that it is widely reported by younger women as a significant factor in their sexual problems compared to older women who are more likely to report other physical features of intercourse as problematic. Sixty percent of women in their 30's had intermittent dyspareunia and one-third persistent (32) whereas another study suggested lubrication was the most important issue for older women (33).

Table 15.1 Female Sexual Dysfunction Patient Reported Outcome measures

Patient reported outcome	No. of items	Domains	Psychometric evaluation	Diagnostic use
Brief index of sexual functioning for women	22	Desire, arousal, frequency of sexual activity, receptivity, pleasure, satisfaction, sexual problems	Partial	No
Changes in sexual functioning questionnaire	35 (14)	Desire-frequency, desire-interest, pleasure, arousal, orgasm	Full	Yes
Female sexual function index	19	Desire, arousal, lubrication, orgasm, pain, satisfaction	Full	Yes
Short form of the personal experience questionnaire	9	Desire, arousal, dyspareunia, partner's sexual problems	Full	Yes
Sexual function questionnaire	28	Desire, arousal-lubrication, arousal-cognitive, arousal-sensation, orgasm, pain, enjoyment, partner	Full	Yes
Profile of female sexual function	37	Desire, arousal, orgasm, self-image, concerns, responsiveness, pleasure	Partial	No
Monash female sexual satisfaction questionnaire	12	Receptivity, arousal, lubrication, orgasm, sexual pleasure, sexual satisfaction	Partial	Yes (total score only)
Prolapse and incontinence sexual questionnaire (PISQ31 or 12)	31 (12)	Behavioral-emotive, physical, partner related	Full	No

Full: Factor analysis for domain structure, internal consistency, test–retest reliability, convergent validity, known-groups validity, responsiveness. Partial: One or more of the above was not completed.

Asking patients about sex is likely to yield information as sexual difficulties are less often spontaneously reported. However questionnaires may produce more reproducible answers and less embarrassment. Subjective information can be gathered in an objective manner. If screening is the aim, three simple questions have been shown to be as effective as detailed interview (34).

Are you sexually active?

Are there any problems?

Do you have any pain with intercourse?

This pain may be interpreted as physical or psychosomatic and for many patients may not be distinguishable.

What a more sophisticated instrument should aim to clarify would be the presence of symptoms, their severity, and/or frequency. In addition, it should aim to assess how the patient feels and its impact on activities of daily living and social, psychological, and emotional wellbeing. With respect to sexual function for instance, the difference between the ability to become aroused compared to the feelings about arousal. Condition specific questionnaires will further assess the impact of the condition on function. Therefore general and condition specific questionnaires seek different endpoints. Generic questionnaires may elucidate the differences in various conditions and allow comparison with control populations without the condition whereas condition specific questionnaires will ideally be designed to elucidate the small differences in patients with a condition such as PFD (35). This may be further distinguished in PFD sufferers, such as a comparison between those with urinary incontinence and fecal incontinence, depending on validation of the instrument. Sexual function measurement with non-validated tools results in inaccurate and inconsistent results.

Questions within other condition specific quality of life measures may be validated but yield limited information about sexual function and activity such as the Kings health questionnaire (KHQ) and the incontinence impact questionnaire (IIQ). If more global functioning is the endpoint of interest or more likely to be acceptable to the patient group this may be more appropriate but the information and conclusions regarding sexual functioning more limited.

When developing these tools it is also important to determine how often these questions are going to be answered, how easily they can be misinterpreted and, especially with sexual function, how acceptable and suitable they are. During the validation process or in a paid clinical trial, patients may be more inclined to answer intrusive questions than in general clinical practice. If questions are routinely not answered or if questionnaires are left substantially incomplete (e.g., because the first question asks about penetrative intercourse without stipulating that further questions do not rely on the presence of a partner), the tool will be effectively useless. Additionally most questionnaires available are only validated in heterosexual relationships.

If the group that are sexually inactive secondary to their pelvic floor problems are excluded, the proportion that improve will not be readily determinable. For this reason, recognition of the length of recall regarding previous sexual intercourse and/or activity when choosing a tool is imperative. One month,

three months, or six months are the usual time frames and some are clearly inappropriate in some settings such as perioperatively. Yet for those women having sexual intercourse once a month [the mean frequency for British heterosexual couples aged 45–55 years (36)], although quality may be more important than quantity, the weighting of frequency in the score could potentially wrongly determine FSD.

With respect to urogynecological problems it is useful to evaluate other confounding factors including age, menopausal status and possibly length of relationship and partner functionality. The perception of the partner as reported by the index patient can have a bearing on function as women tend to protect their sexually dysfunctional partners by developing a corresponding dysfunction such as loss of desire to mask their partners inability, for instance, to maintain an erection or ejaculate.

DEVELOPMENT OF SFQS

Developing useful questionnaires is an involved and expensive process. The initial process of conceptualization requires the input of clinician and patient. The fundamentals of survey questions requires item development and evaluation. It can be argued that the only valid perspective is that of the patient but if the instrument is to be used by surgeons, it needs to incorporate factors of relevance to their practice. A clinician judging the impact of an operation may want to know that a woman has a noncoital pain disorder such as vulvodynia only to be able to counsel that patient she is unlikely to be cured from this complaint by her prolapse surgery.

The words used in items need to be appropriate to ask or identify the same aspect of behavior that the clinician is interested in. The shared understanding may need to be tested in focus groups, particularly with respect to sex where both clinicians and patients use surrogate phrases. An example may be the use of the word libido which for many lay people means all aspects of sexual function—desire, arousal, erection. The words, sentences, and response choices used need to be clear. Simpler, shorter questions with depersonalized answers to sensitive issues are more likely to produce answers that patients are willing to divulge.

Any instrument requires validation and also reliability testing (content/face, construct and criterion—see chapter 12 on PRO development). Further validation is recommended in distinct cultural groups since sex/sexual relationship is especially culturally determined.

QUESTIONNAIRES TO ASSESS FEMALE SEXUALITY

Over the years both generic and condition-specific measures have been developed for assessing sexual (dys)function in men and women; below is an overview of some of the generic measures, condition-specific measures for assessing FSD, and disease-specific measures for use in PFD.

Generic

The Derogatis inventory of sexual functioning (37) and the Golombok Rust inventory of sexual satisfaction (38) are earlier measures designed to capture the essence of sexual behavior and sexual dysfunction in both men and women. However, with the surge in research looking to develop suitable pharmacological treatment(s) for FSD, a number of simple PROs have been developed over the past 10 to 15 years and are summarized in Table 15.1.

The Brief Index of Sexual Functioning for Women (BISF-W) (39,40), a 22-item measure, was developed for use in large clinical trials and assesses a number of concepts: Thoughts/desire, arousal, frequency of sexual activity, receptivity/initiation, pleasure/orgasm, relationship satisfaction, and problems affecting sexual function. It covers a wide range of concepts and assesses the two main sexual dysfunctions—desire and arousal—but validation of the measure is questionable. A follow-up study by Mazer has produced a new scoring algorithm but needs further validation.

The changes in sexual functioning questionnaire (CSFQ) was designed to measure illness and medication effects on sexual functioning (41,42). There are male and female versions. The female version comprises 35 items, forming five domains: sexual desire/frequency, sexual desire/interest, sexual pleasure, sexual arousal, and sexual orgasm. The CSFQ can assess sexual functioning in both clinical and non-clinical samples, particularly depressed patients, and has shown sensitivity to change (43). Recently, a short form (14 items) was developed and validated to allow easier use in clinical practice (44).

Condition-Specific FSD Measures
The female sexual function index was developed by an international panel of experts to apply to all types of FSD and was initially validated in an FSAD population (28). Meston (2003) (45) has since shown its validity in women with FOD and HSDD. The FSFI can also be used to classify women with either FSAD, FOD, or HSDD (46). This was the first measure to show validity across the differing FSD sub-types rather than just in a general dysfunctional group and as such has been used in a number of studies to assess outcome [e.g., Blumel et al., 2008 (47); Bradford and Meston, 2007 (48); Ito et al., 2006 (49)]. It has frequently been used in PFD studies.

The Short Personal Experiences Questionnaire was adapted from the Personal Experiences Questionnaire and was developed to capture the components of female sexual function for menopausal women in nine items: desire, arousal, dyspareunia; and also an assessment of partner's sexual problems (50). The measure was subsequently validated in a group of sexually active women, women with a sexual dysfunction, and women attending a psychiatric clinic (51). However, the number of subjects was small: n = 115, n = 17, and n = 16, respectively, and particularly draws into question the robustness of the cut-off score to indicate sexual dysfunction.

The SFQ was developed using extensive input from women with a sexual dysfunction (n = 22) and from those who were sexually functional (n = 60). Additionally, the interviews were conducted across seven countries (U.K., U.S.A., Australia, the Netherlands, Denmark, France, and Italy) to determine if cultural background affected the way women described their sexual health/function; consistency of reporting was found. Comprehensive validation resulted in 28-items assessing the following concepts: desire, arousal-lubrication, arousal-sensation, orgasm, pain, enjoyment, and partner. The SFQ has also been developed to screen for likelihood of sexual dysfunction, across each of the functional domains (desire, arousal-lubrication, arousal-sensation, orgasm, pain) (52). Confirmation of the pain cutoff scores is required because there were few women with sexual pain used in the assessment. An abbreviated 15-item version is also available.

The Profile of Female Sexual Dysfunction (PFSF) was developed through patient interviews and focus groups with women from Europe and North America and who were either naturally or surgically post-menopausal and had low desire (53). The measure was then further evaluated multinationally in surgically menopausal women with HSDD. Item analysis resulted in seven domains (sexual desire, arousal, orgasm, sexual pleasure, sexual concerns, sexual responsiveness, and sexual self-image) across 37-items. The validity and reliability of the PFSF in naturally menopausal women with HSDD has also been demonstrated (54), although scale structure still needs to be confirmed for this population. A brief seven-item version has also been validated for screening use with HSDD in surgically menopausal women.

The most recently published measure for assessing women's sexual function is the Monash female sexual satisfaction questionnaire (MFSSQ) and was developed specifically to assess acute therapeutic effects (55). The 12-item measure was developed from 10 interviews with women, which led to domains of receptivity, arousal, lubrication, sexual pleasure, sexual satisfaction, and orgasm. Validation was conducted in pre and post-menopausal women who were dissatisfied with their sexual function. The MFSSQ can be used to screen women dissatisfied with their sexual dysfunction but cut-scores for the separate domains has yet to be determined. Reliability of the orgasm and receptivity domains were not ideal and should be explored further. Responsiveness of the scale was not reported.

Disease-Specific Questionnaires for Use in Women with PFD
SFQs should seek to evaluate the impact of PFD on sexual function, and ultimately the subsequent impact of intervention. The few questions relating to sex in other quality of life questionnaires give a score of overall impact on quality of life (KHQ, IIQ, ePAQ [electronic personal assessment questionnaire]) and are therefore less suitable to examine sexual impact in detail. General questionnaires will analyze function in general populations but may not be sensitive enough to detect subtle changes. Confounders such as age and menopausal status need to be accounted for and could alter the suitability of a particular instrument. For these reasons, disease-specific measures are the gold standard (Table 15.2).

There are two validated condition specific SFQs for PFD available to date: PISQ and the International Consultation On Incontinence Questionnaire Vaginal Symptoms (ICIQ-VS) (56). Unfortunately neither is validated in women with rectal symptoms. The PISQ is currently the most widely used. Both have undergone construct validity and reliability testing to establish internal validity but the ICIQ-VS has not undergone external validation. The PISQ has been validated in more

129

Table 15.2 Factors to be Considered When Choosing Sexual Function Assessment Questionnaires for Patients with Pelvic Floor Disorders

Patient factors	Clinician factors
Length/number of other questionnaires	Length/number of other questionnaires
Acceptability	Consistency
Validity/reliability	Validity/reliability
Simplicity	Reproducibility
Relevance	Captures outcomes of interest
Cultural validity	Generic/condition specific/ disease-specific
Language	Self/interviewer administered

languages than the ICIQ-VS and therefore to date may be more suitable for international use.

The PISQ (31 items) has three domains: behavioral-emotive (frequency, orgasm, satisfaction), physical, and partner related (patient perception of). This has detected an improvement in sexual function in 70% of patients post surgical repair of PFD, with an increase in physical and partner related domains but no significant change in orgasm, desire, or arousal. Many studies using non-disease-specific tools have shown no change which may be in part due to their lack of sensitivity or could really suggest limited change with surgery. The PISQ results correlate well with established general questionnaires including the FSFI and sexual history form function (SHF)12 (57). It also differentiates depression associated with poor sexual function. Higher scores in the PISQ indicate better function. Normative scores established with general population testing established a mean score of 94, maximum being 124. There is a short form PISQ 12 (58), which correlates well with PISQ 31 scores. The normative scores in PISQ 12 in the general population without prolapse or incontinence is 40, maximum score 48. The PISQ 12 scores can be multiplied by 2.58 to equal a PISQ 31 score. Increasing severity of PFD is generally associated with reduced PISQ scores. The PISQ however has its limitations. It cannot diagnose FSD at present although as stated above, global normative values have been determined. It is not suitable for women in same sex relationships. As it excludes all women not engaging in penetrative intercourse and does not screen for other sexual activity, it may underestimate the impact of PFD. The International Urogynecology Association is currently in the process of developing a revision of the PISQ 31 to address issues considered important by an expert panel—the PISQ-R—to establish an internationally acceptable SFQ for use in women with PFD for clinical and research purposes.

The FSFI, a measure to assess FSD (see above for further details), has also been extensively used in urogynecological studies. One study investigating the effects of vaginal surgery on women with PFD concluded that domain scores changed but overall the scores did not improve (59). The authors suggest one problem replaces another—altered vaginal anatomy before surgery to dyspareunia post surgery. This demonstrates the possible unsuitability of these general SFQs for the PFD

patient groups where emphasis of a disease-specific measure should perhaps be in assessing dyspareunia, which measures such as the FSFI do inadequately due to the importance given to assessing the two main sub-types of FSD: FSAD and HSDD. The FSFI has also detected up to half of women with interstitial cystitis/painful bladder syndrome or recurrent urinary tract infection have a diagnosis of FSD with a deterioration in desire, lubrication, and satisfaction but no difference in arousal or orgasm (60). Yet a North American epidemiological validated questionnaire did not find a significant association between PFD and sexual activity or satisfaction (61). Overall the use of non-validated and generic questionnaires makes urogynecological studies of sexual function difficult to compare and the results if contradictory, inconclusive. Therefore when determining the right tool to be used, the outcomes of value should be carefully considered to ensure that these are adequately captured.

CLINICAL PRACTICE VS. CLINICAL TRIALS

Ascertaining which measure to use will be based on the setting and the research question under consideration. For instance, if the measure is to be used in clinical practice to monitor patient outcome then a short instrument would be more realistic to mitigate the time burden for both clinician and patient (e.g., short-form CSFQ). If, however, the aim is to test a new therapeutic agent in a clinical trial the most relevant measure regardless of length would be the best to ensure all aspects of FSD are captured in the most robust manner possible (e.g., FSFI, SFQ). Alternatively a clinician may wish to use a measure to help screen for potential sexual function problems and would then need to look for a short measure that can also provide guidance on likelihood of FSD or even in relation to a particular FSD sub-type (e.g., SFQ). Regardless of setting, when choosing a measure, ensuring appropriate information of interest is obtained is essential. Then an assessment of the measures validity and reliability in the population of interest to the clinician should be evident.

CONCLUSION

The tendency of women to become less interested in sex and men less able to perform with age may be distinguishable with well designed instruments. It is important to evaluate engagement in sexual activity and the reasons why it may have ceased or become less satisfying in women with PFD. The distress caused by these difficulties and its alleviation by urogynecological interventions is the information sought by clinicians and that should guide management of patients. In the area of sexual function, the only reproducible and consistent method of reporting these outcomes is with well designed, validated questionnaires.

REFERENCES

1. Declaration of Alma-Ata. International Conference of Primary Health Care. USSR: Alma-Ata, 1978. [Available from: http://www.who.int/hpr/archive/docs/almaata.html].
2. Olsen AL, Smith VJ, Bergstrom JO, Colling JC, Clark AL. Epidemiology of surgically managed pelvic organ prolapse and urinary incontinence. Obstet Gynecol 1997; 89: 501–6.

3. Pauls RN, Kleeman SD, Segal JL, et al. Practice patterns of physician members of the American urogynecologic society regarding female sexual dysfunction: results of a national survey. Int Urogynecol J Pelvic Floor Dysfunct 2005; 16: 460–7.

4. Roos AM, Thakar R, Sultan AH, Scheer I. Female sexual dysfunction: are urogynecologists ready for it? Int Urogynecol J Pelvic Floor Dysfunct 2009; 20: 89–101.

5. Weber AM, Walters MD, Schover LR, Mitchinson A. Vaginal anatomy and sexual function. Obstet Gynecol 1995; 86: 946–9.

6. Laumann E, Paik A, Rosen R. Sexual dysfunction in the United States: prevalence and predictors. JAMA 1999; 281: 537–44.

7. Nazareth I, Boynton P, King M. Problems with sexual function in people attending London general practitioners: cross sectional study. BMJ 2003; 327: 423–6.

8. Shifren JL, Monz BU, Russo PA, Segreti A, Johannes CB. Sexual problems and distress in United States women. Obstet Gynecol 2008; 112: 970–8.

9. Nappi NE, Nijland EA. Women's perception of sexuality around the menopause: outcomes of a European telephone survey. Eur J Obstet Gynecol Reprod Biol 2008; 137: 10–16.

10. AARP: www.research.aarp.org/health/mmsexsurvey

11. Beckman N, Waern M, Gustafson D, Skoog I. Secular trends in seld reported sexual activity and satisfaction in Swedish 70 year olds: cross sectional survey of four populations, 1971–2001. BMJ 2008; 337: 151–4.

12. Masters WH, Johnson VE. Human sexual response. Boston: Little Brown, 1966.

13. Basson R, Berman J, Burnett A, et al. Report of the international consensus development conference on female sexual dysfunction: definitions and classifications. Urology 2000; 163: 888–93.

14. Basson R, Althof S, Davis S, et al. Summary of te recommendations on sexual dysfunction in women. J Sex Med 2004; 1: 24–34.

15. Pauls RN, Segal JL, Silva WA, et al. Sexual function in women presenting to a urogynecology practice. Int Urogynecol J Pelvic Floor Dysfunct 2006; 17: 576–80.

16. Temml C, Haidinger G, Schmidbauer J, et al. Urinary incontinence in both sexes: prevalence rates and impact on quality of life and sexual life. Neurourol Urodyn 2000; 19: 259–71.

17. Pons ME, Clota MP. Coital incointence: impact on quality of life as measured by Kings health questionnaire. Int Urogynecol J 2008; 19: 621–5.

18. Glavind K, Tetsche MS. Sexual function in women before and after suburethral sling operation for stress urinary incontinence: a retrospective questionnaire study. Acta Obstet Gynecol Scand 2004; 83: 965–8.

19. Gheilmettii T, Kuhn P, Dreher EF, Kuhn A. Gynaecological operatons: do they improve sexual life? Eur J Obstet Gynecol Reprod Biol 2006; 129: 104–10.

20. Rogers RG, Kammerer-Doak D, Villarreal A, Coates K, Qualls C. A new instrument to measure sexual function in women with urinary incontinence and pelvic organ prolapse. Am J Obstet Gynecol 2001; 184: 552–8.

21. Broderick GA. Evidence based assessment of erectile dysfunction. Int J Impot Res 1998; 10(Suppl 2): S64–73; discussion S77–9.

22. Bradley WE, Timm GW, Gallagher JM, Johnson BK. New method for continuous measurement of nocturnal penile tumescence and rigidity. Urology 1985; 26: 4–9.

23. Gerritsen J, van der Made F, Bloemers J, et al. The clitoral photoplethysmograph: a new way of assessing genital arousal in women. J Sex Med 2009; 6: 1678–87.

24. Rosen RC, Riley A, Wagner G, et al.The international index of erectile function (IIEF): a multidimensional scale for assessment of erectile dysfunction. Urology 1997; 49: 822–30.

25. Rosen RC, Cappelleri JC, Gendrano N. The international index of erectile function (IIEF): a state-of-the-science review. Int J Impot Res 2002; 14: 226–44.

26. Althof SE, Symonds T. Patient reported outcomes used in the assessment of premature ejaculation. Urol Clin North Am 2007; 34: 581–9, vii.

27. Quirk FH, Heiman JR, Rosen RC, et al. Development of a sexual function questionnaire for clinical trials of female sexual dysfunction. J Womens Health Gend Based Med 2002; 11: 277–89.

28. Rosen R, Brown C, Heiman J, et al. The female sexual function index (FSFI): a multidimensional self-report instrument for the assessment of female sexual function. J Sex Marital Ther 2000; 26: 191–208.

29. Utian WH, MacLean DB, Symonds T, et al. A methodology study to validate a structured diagnostic method used to diagnose female sexual dysfunction and its subtypes in postmenopausal women. J Sex Marital Ther 2005; 31: 271–83.

30. DeRogatis LR, Allgood A, Rosen RC, et al. Development and Evaluation of the Women's Sexual Interest Diagnostic Interview (WSID): a structured interview to diagnose hypoactive sexual desire disorder (HSDD) in standardized patients. J Sex Med 2008; 5: 2827–41.

31. Cain VS, Johannes CB, Avis NE, et al. Sexual functioning and practices in a multi-ethnic study of midlife women: baseline results from SWAN. J Sex Res 2003; 40: 266–76.

32. Glatt AE, Zinner SH, McCormack WM. The prevalence of dyspareunia. Obstet Gynecol 1990; 75(3 Pt 1): 433–6.

33. Bachmann GA, Leiblum SR. Sexuality in sexagenarian women. Maturitas 1991; 13: 43–50.

34. Plouffe L. Screening for sexual problems through a simple questionnaire. Am J Obstet Gynecol 1985; 151: 166–9.

35. Kelleher CJ, Cardozo LD, Khullar V, Salvatore S. A new questionnaire to assess the quality of life of urinary incontinent women. BJOG 1997; 104: 1374–9.

36. Johnson AM, Mercer CH, Erens b, et al. Sexual behaviour in Britain: partnership practices, and HIV risk behaviours. Lancet 2001; 358: 1835–42.

37. Derogatis LR, Melisaratos N. The DSFI: a multidimensional measure of sexual functioning. J Sex Marital Ther 1979; 5: 244–81.

38. Rust J, Golombok S. The GRISS: a psychometric instrument for the assessment of sexual dysfunction. Arch Sex Behav 1986; 15: 157–65.

39. Taylor JF, Rosen RC, Leiblum SR. Self-report assessment of female sexual function: psychometric evaluation of the brief index of sexual functioning for women. Arch Sex Behav 1994; 23: 627–43.

40. Mazer NA, Leiblum SR, Rosen RC. The brief index of sexual functioning for women (BISF-W): a new scoring algorithm and comparison of normative and surgically menopausal populations. Menopause 2000; 7: 350–63.

41. Clayton AH, McGarvey EL, Clavet GJ. The changes in sexual functioning questionnaire (CSFQ): development, reliability, and validity. Psychopharmacol Bull 1997; 33: 731–45.

42. Clayton AH, McGarvey EL, Clavet GJ, Piazza L. Comparison of sexual functioning in clinical and nonclinical populations using the changes in sexual functioning questionnaire (CSFQ). Psychopharmacol Bull 1997; 33: 747–53.

43. Bobes J, Gonzalez MP, Bascarán MT, et al. Evaluating changes in sexual functioning in depressed patients: sensitivity to change of the CSFQ. J Sex Marital Ther 2002; 28: 93–103.

44. Keller A, McGarvey EL, Clayton AH. Reliability and construct validity of the changes in sexual functioning questionnaire short-form (CSFQ-14). J Sex Marital Ther 2006; 32: 43–52.

45. Meston CM. Validation of the female sexual function index (FSFI) in women with female orgasmic disorder and in women with hypoactive sexual desire disorder. J Sex Marital Ther 2003; 29: 39–46.

46. Wiegel M, Meston C, Rosen R. The female sexual function index (FSFI): crossvalidation and development of clinical cutoff scores. J Sex Marital Ther 2005; 31: 1–20.

47. Blumel JE, Del Pino M, Aprikian D, et al. Effect of androgens combined with hormone therapy on quality of life in post-menopausal women with sexual dysfunction. Gynecol Endocrinol 2008; 24: 691–5.

48. Bradford A, Meston C. Correlates of placebo response in the treatment of sexual dysfunction in women: a preliminary report. J Sex Med 2007; 4: 1345–51.

49. Ito TY, Polan ML, Whipple B, Trant AS. The enhancement of female sexual function with ArginMax, a nutritional supplement, among women differing in menopausal status. J Sex Marital Ther 2006; 32: 369–78.

50. Dennerstein L, Lehert P, Dudley E. Short scale to measure female sexuality: adapted from McCoy female sexuality questionnaire. J Sex Marital Ther 2001; 27: 339–51.

51. Dennerstein L, Anderson-Hunt M, Dudley E. Evaluation of a short scale to assess female sexual functioning. J Sex Marital Ther 2002; 28: 389–97.

52. Quirk F, Haughie S, Symonds T. The use of the sexual function questionnaire as a screening tool for women with sexual dysfunction. J Sex Med 2005; 2: 469–77.

53. McHorney CA, Rust J, Golombok S, et al. Profile of female sexual function: a patientbased, international, psychometric instrument for the assessment of hypoactive sexual desire in oophorectomized women. Menopause 2004; 11: 474–83.

54. Derogatis L, Rust J, Golombok S, et al. Validation of the profile of female sexual function (PFSF) in surgically and naturally menopausal women. J Sex Marital Ther 2004; 30: 25–36.

55. Davison SL, Bell RJ, La China M, Holden SL, Davis SR. Assessing sexual function in well women: validity and reliability of the Monash women's health program female sexual satisfaction questionnaire. J Sex Med 2008; 5: 2575–86.

56. Price N, Jackson SR, Avery K, Brookes ST, Abrams P. Developement and psychometric evaluation of the ICIQ vaginal symptoms questionnaire: the ICIQ-VS. BJOG 2006; 113: 700–12.

57. Schover L, Jensen S. Sexuality and chronic illness: a comprehensive approach. J Am Geriatr Soc 1988; 36: 520–4.

58. Rogers RG, Coates KW, Kammerer-Doak D, et al. A short form of the Pelvic Organ Prolapse/Urinary Incontinence Sexual Questionnaire (PISQ-12). Int Urogynecol J 2003; 14: 164-8. [Erratum Int Urogynecol J 2004; 15: 219.]

59. Pauls RN, Silva WA, Rooney CM, et al. Sexual function after vaginal surgery for pelvic organ prolapse and urinary incontinence. Am J Obstet Gynecol 2008; 97: 622e1–7.

60. Salonia A, Zanni G, Nappi RE, et al. Sexual dysfunctionis common in women with lower urinry tract symtoms and urinary incontinence: results of a cross sectional study. Eur Urol 2004; 45: 642–8.

61. Lukacz ES, Whitcomb EL, Lawrence JM, et al. Are sexual activity and satisfaction affected by pelvic floor disorders? Analysis of a community based survey. Am J Obstet Gynecol 2007; 197: 88 e1–6.

16 Questionnaires to Assess Bowel Function

Anton Emmanuel and Dave Chatoor

INTRODUCTION

The gold standard for assessment of gut symptoms will always be a focused comprehensive clinical history. By contrast, research endeavors require symptom score and qualitative assessment tools. This serves both as confirmation of the inclusion or entry criteria, and as a monitor of outcome with intervention. Increasingly, however, the role of these instruments is extending into the clinical setting. This chapter will review the symptom specific tools which have focused on the distinct, but occasionally overlapping symptoms of fecal incontinence and rectal evacuation difficulties. There are particular issues that make questionnaire assessment of bowel function complex: The normal range of bowel function in the population is great both within individuals and between individuals, and there is frequent overlap between bowel disturbance and other pelvic floor disorders (in particular urinary incontinence and gynecological prolapse). Consequently instruments in this field are likely to lack a degree of sensitivity or specificity for the specific bowel disorders such as irritable bowel syndrome (IBS), inflammatory bowel disease (IBD) evacuation disorder, and constipation.

QUESTIONNAIRES TO ASSESS SYMPTOMS AND QUALITY OF LIFE IMPACT OF FECAL INCONTINENCE

Several questionnaires have been developed to identify the severity of fecal incontinence and its impact on quality of life. Some of the questionnaires used for other pelvic disorders also include items to cover fecal incontinence in view of the well established overlap between urogynecological and rectal symptoms (1–3). Similarly, items relating to fecal incontinence have often been included in questionnaires relating to common gastro-intestinal disorders such as IBS and IBD (4,5). Anal incontinence has a huge number of potential etiologies (6) and bowel evacuation is intrinsically related to pelvic floor function (7). Thus, it is appropriate to consider assessment of both bowel evacuation and control synchronously. Evacuatory dysfunction may result from a variety of underlying pathologies including outlet obstruction, slow transit, or other mechanical, pharmacological, metabolic, endocrine, and neurogenic abnormalities (2,8). The pattern of symptoms (whether passive fecal soiling or urge incontinence) and the degree of nuisance (to liquids and gas only, or solids too) are important as they often reflect the underlying causation (6). Thus, urgency (the inability to defer defecation) and urge incontinence are thought to indicate loss of voluntary control due to impaired external anal sphincter function, whereas passive incontinence is thought to indicate impairment of the smooth muscle of the internal sphincter (9).

The complexity of causes and the overlap with other pelvic floor function has meant little energy has been put into optimizing the questionnaire and scoring systems available. Certainly many of the much used colorectal instruments fall short compared to the highest standards of questionnaire development (10). For example, the widely used Wexner score does not have published data related to its psychometric properties. The International Consensus on Incontinence (11) recommended the following schema to assess the quality of questionnaires, and this will be adopted for this chapter:

- *Grade A—highly recommended*: Validity, reliability, and responsiveness established with rigor.
- *Grade B—recommended*: Validity and reliability established with rigor, or validity, reliability, and responsiveness indicated.
- *Grade C—with potential*: Early development—further work required and encouraged.

Quality of Life

Fecal Incontinence Quality of Life Scale (Grade B)
The 29-item Fecal Incontinence Quality of Life (12) Scale developed and tested by Rockwood et al. measures the impact of fecal incontinence over four scales of quality of life: lifestyle (10 items), coping/behavior (9 items), depression/self-perception (7 items), and embarrassment (3 items). It was developed to be treatment responsive. A panel of colorectal surgeons and researchers generated items. The questionnaire showed good discriminant validity, with significant differences between 118 patients with fecal incontinence and 72 controls with other gastrointestinal disorders. Convergent validity was assessed by comparison with responses in the SF-36, which showed significant correlations between domains of the two instruments. Test–retest reliability at a mean interval of eight days was satisfactory, with alpha values for the four scales of 0.8 to 0.96. Internal consistency of the four scales was >0.7. The instrument does not measure physical symptom severity and has not been tested in asymptomatic controls, but appears to offer a valid and reliable measure of the impact of fecal incontinence on quality of life in men and women with this condition. Its use in an unscreened population is not yet reported, and, despite the original rationale for its development, no responsiveness data have yet been produced.

Manchester Health Questionnaire (Grade B)
This questionnaire (13) consists of items modified from questions about urinary incontinence from the King's health questionnaire (KHQ) (14). It uses the same basic structure and format but items have a 5-point response scale (rather than the four-point scale in the KHQ). It includes a symptom severity scale, within 31 items in eight subscales of quality of life: general health, incontinence impact, role, physical function, social

function, personal function, emotional problems, sleep, and energy. Face validity was assessed by interviewing 15 patients with fecal incontinence. Test–retest reliability was good (Pearson correlation > 0.8 in all domains). Test–retest abnormality was assessed at a mean interval of 20 days, with a Cronbach's alpha > 0.7 in all domains tested, indicating adequate internal consistency. There were also significant correlations with subscales of the SF-36. Once again, the utility of the questionnaire in unscreened individuals, and the sensitivity to change is also not yet established. The Manchester Health Questionnaire has also been shown to be valid for telephone interview (15).

Birmingham Bowel and Urinary Symptoms Questionnaire (BBUS-Q) (GRADE B)

This is a 22-item self-report questionnaire developed to evaluate symptoms of both bowel and urinary dysfunction, specifically in women (16,17). Items were generated by a panel of clinicians (urogynecological and colorectal) and scientists and following review of existing instruments in the literature. It was then evaluated in a mixed group of 141 asymptomatic women and 489 patients: Most were awaiting hysterectomy, some were post-hysterectomy, and some had been referred to hospital with functional bowel and/or urinary symptoms. Content validity has been shown for four-factor domains: constipation, evacuatory function, anal incontinence, and urinary symptoms. Comparison of content between these domains shows acceptable internal structure. The gold standard for structural and physiological assessment of anorectal symptoms is controversial; nevertheless comparison with clinical, anorectal physiological, videoproctographic, and whole gut transit time supported the instrument's criterion validity. The standard for fecal incontinence is endoanal ultrasound (6), and it is unfortunate that this has never been cross-validated with the BBUS-Q. Key domain question analysis and Cronbach's alphas have shown internal consistency and equally kappa values and limits of agreement also shown good test–retest reliability. Some responsiveness data have been produced, but this is a relatively new instrument, and further reports of use as both a research and clinical tool are awaited. This questionnaire also forms a core element in an electronic pelvic floor symptoms assessment questionnaire [electronic personal assessment questionnaire (e-PAQ)].

Wexner Scores (GRADE C)

Scoring systems for incontinence and constipation were developed from the Cleveland clinic with the twin purposes of providing quantitative data about colorectal function and assessment of treatment effectiveness (18,19). The incontinence score grades type of incontinence (solid, liquid, and gas) as well as quantifying frequency form "never" to "always" and a grid-type score is arrived at. This can be totaled, with a range from 0 (no incontinence) to 20 (severe incontinence). The constipation score (details below) was derived from a group of patients referred for anorectal testing, a summarized from a starting point of 100 constipation-related symptoms. The score ranges from 0 (normal) to 30 (severe constipation). The scores are validated for completion by the clinician. The psychometric properties of the scores have not been established.

St. Mark's Incontinence Score (GRADE C)

This five question scale provides a score for the assessment of the severity of fecal incontinence (20). It comprises five questions concerned with fecal leakage, bowel urgency, use of pads, medication, and interference with activities. The validation process entailed comparing the performance of this novel tool with Wexner, Pescatori (21) and a commercial, unvalidated scale (the American Medical Systems score) in small groups of patients. There was good inter-instrument correlation and also a good relationship with a diary card and objective "clinical impression." In addition, a smaller cohort of patients completed the score after surgical treatment, and it was found to be a treatment-responsive score. A more recent study of 390 patients with fecal incontinence compared subjective visual analog scale scores to the St. Marks score and showed only moderate correlation regardless of type of incontinence, age, or gender (22). One-third of these patients also underwent biofeedback and only 65% of patients reported subjective changes reflected in the St. Marks score (22).

Pescatori Incontinence Score (GRADE C)

This scoring system (21) has been comparatively little used since its first description in 1992. It uses a number–letter system to describe type of incontinence (letters A, B, and C for flatus/mucus, liquid, and solid, respectively; numbers 1, 2, and 3 for occasional, weekly, and daily incontinence, respectively). The first description was in a heterogenous group of 335 patients, with no comparisons with other scores being made. One-third of these patients underwent surgical treatment for their incontinence and the instrument was shown to be treatment-responsive.

MAYO Fecal Incontinence Survey (GRADE C)

This questionnaire was designed for the assessment of fecal incontinence and associated symptoms (23). It also aimed to assess the risk factors for developing the symptoms. The 13-item questionnaire is based on previously validated instruments from the Mayo Clinic, based on the local Olmsted County population (24–26). Initial validation and reliability testing was carried out in 94 patients. Reliability and validity were assessed by telephone interview in 41 patients and by mailed questionnaire in 34. The kappa values were >0.59, indicating reasonable reliability and validity, but was very low for some domains. Data on responsiveness are not available.

Elderly Bowel Symptom Questionnaire (EBSQ) (GRADE C)

The Mayo group have also reported on the reliability and validity of the EBSQ in both clinic attendees to a medical outpatients and community based elderly subjects (26). There was a 77% response rate to the postal survey, suggesting reasonable patient acceptability. Test–retest reliability was also acceptable, with a median kappa value of 0.65.

Fecal Incontinence and Constipation Assessment (GRADE C)

This 98 item questionnaire (27) was another modification of existing instruments (23,24,26) by the Mayo group. Assessment was made of frequency and type of incontinence, the number of perineal protective devices used daily leakage, and the severity of urgency. Urgency was rated by asking subjects whether they were incontinent because they had great urgency and could not reach the toilet on time; responses included never, sometimes, often, and usually. The questionnaire was validated in 83 hospital attending patients, 20 of whom completed six month re-test validity. The reproducibility values were acceptable, with a kappa value of 0.8 and concurrent validity of 0.59.

Postpartum Flatal and Fecal Incontinence Quality of Life Scale (GRADE C)
Cockell et al. conducted one-hour interviews with 10 women identified as having fecal or flatal incontinence after childbirth (28). Using these interviews, the authors used qualitative analyzes to modify the fecal incontinence quality-of-life scale and added new items. Further evaluation of the scale is awaited, including a treatment response analysis from a planned study of surgical repair of obstetric sphincter injuries.

QUESTIONNAIRES TO ASSESS SYMPTOMS AND QUALITY OF LIFE IMPACT OF BOWEL EVACUATION DIFFICULTY

Patient Assessment of Constipation Quality of Life (GRADE B)
This questionnaire was developed to assess the burden of symptoms and their change over time with treatment (29). It consists of a 28-item questionnaire, and a 5-point Likert scale. Its content was derived form patient focus groups, streamlined by clinicians. It has five subscales addressing worries and concerns (11 items), physical discomfort (4 items), psychosocial discomfort (8 items), and satisfaction (5 items). It assesses quality of life issues well, and is an internally consistent and reproducible measure (with the exception of its satisfaction subscale). It was validated cross culturally in the U.S.A., France, the Netherlands, Belgium, Canada, U.K., and Australia. It however, focuses less on specific symptoms and their severity (30).

To address severity, the authors have developed it to be used with the symptom severity measure: the constipation symptom assessment instrument [patient assessment of constipation symptom (PAC-SYM)], another sister questionnaire which has 12 items under three subscales assessing: stool symptoms, rectal symptoms, and abdominal symptoms. It also has good internal consistency and retest reliability. It was also able to assess responders and nonresponders showing its response to change as discriminant validity. Both are, but the authors expect some synergy between these two measures (30).

Wexner Constipation Score (GRADE C)
This is one of the most commonly used questionnaires for constipation to date (19). It was first published in 1996 and still used in many studies to date, initially meant to give an objective measure of constipation based on weighted subjective symptomatic complaints. It has eight questions and a global scale (0–30), with constipation defined if the sore is >15. The only mention of validation was the comparison of 50 constipated to 50 nonconstipated patients, finding that 96% of patients with constipation were correctly predicted, it was then applied to 232 patients with constipation, with 97% of these

scoring > 15. This questionnaire has gained acceptance because of its wide use, but initially has had no convergent, or divergent validity testing, it also has little quality of life focus.

The Chinese Constipation Questionnaire (GRADE C)
This has been developed as a tool for the Chinese population for assessing symptoms, their severity and outcome of treatment in a simple measure (31). It initially started with 30 questions and after several steps involving patient interviews and retesting, reduced to 24 questions, these were applied to 111 patients with constipation and 110 healthy controls. Through a logistic regression analysis six questions were chosen as these represented the discriminating questions that provided the greatest separation between controls and constipated patients. The final questionnaire consisted of a composite score of these six questions (0–21, with ≥5 defined as constipated). It was shown to be comprehensive by 88% of subjects, highlighting its content validity, reliable on test–retesting with a correlation coefficient 0.7 and internally consistent with a Cronbach's-alpha coefficient of 0.792. It provided a 91% specificity and 91% sensitivity and correlated negatively with the SF-36, showing the inverse relationship with quality of life, highlighting its construct validity. Twenty constipated patients were given polyethylene glycol and again the questionnaire showed discriminant validity with improvement in symptoms (Kendall's tau = 0.69, p = 0.001). This questionnaire is a simple validated measure for the Chinese population which can be used as an outcome measure.

Constipation Severity Instrument (GRADE C)
This is a recently validated tool by Varma et al. (32) which was developed to address the major components of constipation with 16 questions (5-point Likert scale) under three subscales: colonic inertia (assessing slot transit symptoms), pain (addressing IBS-C pain symptoms), and obstructive defecation (evacuation difficulty symptoms). It was validated using 191 patients with constipation symptoms and 103 control patients. Its subscales are reliable; based on its internal consistency it has good discriminant validity compared to control subjects. There was good correlation as a measure of convergent validity compared with the PAC-SYM and poor correlation with non-bowel related questionnaires, suggesting good divergent validity. Subscale scores were inverse to quality of life measures on the SF-36. Physical and mental subscales, suggesting a good association, though it contains no specific subscales for quality of life. This questionnaire has potential use in studies and clinical scenarios where patients present with varied subtypes of constipation syndromes.

Gastro-Intestinal Quality of Life Index (GRADE C)
This instrument was designed to measure quality of life in patients with gastrointestinal disease (33), and has been widely used. It does not have any items specific to fecal incontinence, but does have some related to constipation.

Obstructive Defection Syndrome (ODS) Score
The ODS score was developed as a simple measure for outcome of procedures for evacuation difficulty (34). The score assesses

straining, incomplete emptying, use of enemas/laxatives, vaginal/perineal digitation and constipation on a 5-point Likert scale, with a range from 0 to 20 (normal to complete obstructed defecation). It was described by Renzi for identifying patients suitable for the STARR procedure (stapled transanal rectal resection) initially described by Longo for treating ODS with a circular stapler with resection of both the rectocele and intussusception (35). Patients were chosen if their score was greater than or equal to 12, together with other parameters of evacuation difficulty. It was used postoperatively as an outcome measure—with excellent scoring (0–3), good (406), adequate (7–9), and poor (10–20). It is unclear how these ranges were defined. There have also been modifications to the score, with unbalanced weighting—particularly for items such as laxative and enema use which are allocated disproportionately high scores (34). It has no quality of life items and is unvalidated. Nevertheless, it has been used in the context of assessing surgical procedures. A validated simple "evacuation difficulty" specific tool is still awaited.

Neurogenic Bowel Dysfunction Score (GRADE B)

This score was developed specifically to assess the effectiveness of management strategies in patients with bowel dysfunction secondary to central nervous system disease, specifically spinal cord injury (36). None of the available instruments listed above have been validated for use in those with spinal injury or cauda equina syndrome. The other questionnaires also fail to take into account the unique problem of the combination of constipation and fecal incontinence in spinal cord injury (SCI). The questionnaire was derived by being applied to 424 Danish spinal injury individuals, reproducibility, and validity being checked in 20 and 18 patients, respectively. Based on the odds ratios for associations between items and quality of life, the most reflective items from a possible list of 39 were included in the final instrument. These were: frequency of bowel movements (0–6 points); headache, perspiration, or discomfort before or during defecation (0–2 points); medications for constipation (0–2 points each); time spent on each defecation (0–7 points); frequency of digital stimulation or evacuation (0–6 points); frequency of fecal incontinence (0–13 points); medication used for fecal incontinence (0–4 points); flatus incontinence (0–2 points); and perianal skin problems (0–3 points). With a maximum potential score of 32, the authors described four groups according to severity: very minor dysfunction (0–6 points), minor dysfunction (7–9), moderate dysfunction (10–13), and severe dysfunction (>13).

CONCLUSION

A number of instruments have been described to assess the inter-related colorectal functions of evacuation disturbance and fecal incontinence. However, the number of instruments betrays their generally low quality. Future directions will focus on the burden of specific subgroups (such as the neurogenic bowel dysfunction score), assessment of quality of life, and validation with psychometric performance. A final complicating issue is the need to establish validity for each language, given the subtle differences in cultural and linguistic expectations of bowel function.

REFERENCES

1. Nygaard I, Barber MD, Burgio KL, et al. Pelvic floor disorders network. Prevalence of symptomatic pelvic floor disorders in US women. JAMA 2008; 300: 1311–16.
2. Soligo M, Salvatore S, Emmanuel AV, et al. Patterns of constipation in urogynecology: clinical importance and pathophysiologic insights. Am J Obstet Gynecol 2006; 195: 50–5.
3. Meschia M, Buonaguidi A, Pifarotti P, et al. Prevalence of anal incontinence in women with symptoms of urinary incontinence and genital prolapse. Obstet Gynecol 2002; 100: 719–23.
4. Francis CY, Morris J, Whorwell PJ. The irritable bowel severity scoring system: a simple method of monitoring irritable bowel syndrome and its progress. Aliment Pharmacol Ther 1997; 11: 395–402.
5. Drossman DA, Leserman J, Li ZM, et al. The rating form of IBD patient concerns: a new measure of health status. Psychosom Med 1991; 53: 701–12.
6. Chatoor D, Taylor SJ, Cohen CR, Emmanuel AV. Fecal incontinence. Br J Surg 2007; 94: 134–44.
7. Craggs MD, Balasubramaniam AV, Chung EAL, Emmanuel AV. Aberrant reflexes and function of the pelvic organs following spinal injury in man. Auton Neurosci 2006; 126–127: 355–70.
8. Emmanuel AV. Constipation. In: Bloom S, ed. Handbook of Gastroenterology. Reading: Harwood Academic Publishers, 2000.
9. Engel AF, Kamm MA, Bartram CI, Nicholls RJ. Relationship of symptoms in faecal incontinence to specific sphincter abnormalities. Int J Colorectal Dis 1995; 10: 152–5.
10. Woolf SH. Practice guidelines, a new reality in medicine. II. Methods of developing guidelines. Arch Intern Med 1992; 152: 946–52.
11. Staskin D, Hilton P, Emmanuel A, et al. Initial assessment of incontinence. In: Abrams P, Cardozo L, Khoury S, Wein A, eds. Incontinence, 3rd edn. Plymouth, UK: Health Publications, 2005: 485.
12. Rockwood TH, Church JM, Fleshman JW, et al. Fecal Incontinence Quality of Life Scale: quality of life instrument for patients with fecal incontinence. Dis Colon Rectum 2000; 43: 9–16.
13. Dillman DA, Sangster, RL, Tarnai, J, et al. Understanding differences in people's answers to telephone and mail surveys. In: Braverman MT, Slater JK, eds. Advances in Survey Research, Vol. 70. San Francisco: Jossey-Bass, 1996: 110.
14. Rockwood TH, Sangster RL, Dillman DA. The effect of response categories on questionnaire answers: context and mode effects. Sociol Methods Res 1997; 26: 118–40.
15. Kwon S, Visco AG, Fitzgerald MP, et al.; Pelvic Floor Disorders Network (PFDN). Validity and reliability of the Modified Manchester Health Questionnaire in assessing patients with fecal incontinence. Dis Colon Rectum 2005; 48: 323–34.
16. Hiller L, Radley S, Mann CH, et al. Development and validation of a questionnaire for the assessment of bowel and urinary tract symptoms in women. Br J Obstet Gynaecol 2002; 109: 413–23.
17. Hiller L, Bradshaw HD, Radley SC, Radley S. A scoring system for the assessment of bowel and lower urinary tract symptoms in women. British J Obstet Gynaecol 2003; 109: 424–30.
18. Jorge JMN, Wexner SD. Etiology and management of fecal incontinence. Dis Colon Rectum 1993; 36: 77–97.
19. Agachan F, Chen T, Pfeifer J, Reissman P, Wexner SD. A constipation scoring system to simplify evaluation and management of constipated patients. Dis Colon Rectum 1996; 39: 681–5.
20. Vaizey CJ, Carapeti E, Cahill JA, Kamm MA. Prospective comparison of faecal incontinence grading systems. Gut 1999; 44: 77–80.
21. Pescatori M, Anastasio G, Bottini C, et al. New grading system and scoring for anal incontinence. Evaluation of 335 patients. Dis Colon Rectum 1992; 35: 482–7.
22. Maeda Y, Parés D, Norton C, Vaizey CJ, Kamm MA. Does the St. Mark's incontinence score reflect patients' perceptions? A review of 390 patients. Dis Colon Rectum 2008; 51: 436–42. [Epub 2008 Jan 25].
23. Reilly TW, Talley NJ, Pemberton JH, Zinsmeister AR. Validation of a questionnaire to assess fecal incontinence and associated risk factors fecal incontinence questionnaire. Dis Colon Rectum 2000; 43: 146–54.
24. Talley NJ, Phillips SF, Melton LJ III, Wiltgen C, Zinsmeister AR. A patient questionnaire to identify bowel disease. Ann Intern Med 1989; 111: 671–4.

25. Locke GR, Talley NJ, Weaver AL, Zinsmeister AR. A new questionnaire for gastroesophageal reflux disease. Mayo Clin Proc 1994; 69: 539–47.

26. O'Keefe EA, Talley NJ, Tangalos EG, Zinsmeister AR. A bowel symptom questionnaire for the elderly. J Gerontol 1992; 47: Ml16–21.

27. Bharucha AE, Locke GR III, Seide BM, Zinsmeister AR. A new questionnaire for constipation and faecal incontinence. Aliment Pharmacol Ther 2004; 20: 355–64.

28. Cockell SJ, Oates-Johnson T, Gilmour DT, Vallis TM, Turnbull GK. Postpartum flatal and fecal incontinence quality-of-life scale: a disease- and population-specific measure. Qual Health Res 2003; 13: 1132–44.

29. Marquis P, De La Loge C, Dubois D, McDermott A, Chassany O. Development and validation of the patient assessment of constipation quality of life questionnaire. Scand J Gastroenterol 2005; 40: 540–51.

30. Frank L, Kleinman L, Farup C, Taylor L, Miner P Jr. Psychometric validation of a constipation symptom assessment questionnaire. Scand J Gastroenterol 1999; 34: 870–7.

31. Chan AO, Lam KF, Hui WM, et al. Validated questionnaire on diagnosis and symptom severity for functional constipation in the Chinese population. Aliment Pharmacol Ther 2005; 22: 483–8.

32. Varma MG, Wang JY, Berian JR, et al. The constipation severity instrument: a validated measure.Dis Colon Rectum 2008; 51: 162–72. [Epub 2008 Jan 3].

33. Eypasch E, Williams JL, Wood-Dauphinee S, et al. Gastrointestinal quality of life index: development, validation and application of a new instrument. Br J Surg 1995; 82: 216–22.

34. Longo A. Obstructed defecation because of rectal pathologies. Novel surgical treatment: stapled transanal rectal resection (STARR). Proceedings of the 14th Annual International Colorectal Disease Symposium, 2003.

35. Renzi A, Izzo D, Di Sarno G, Izzo G, Di Martino N. Stapled transanal rectal resection to treat obstructed defecation caused by rectal intussusception and rectocele. Int J Colorectal Dis 2006; 21: 661–7.

36. Krogh K, Christensen P, Sabroe S, Laurberg S. Neurogenic bowel dysfunction score. Spinal Cord 2006; 44: 625–31.

17 International Consultation on Incontinence Modular Questionnaire (ICIQ)

Nikki Cotterill and Paul Abrams

WHAT IS THE INTERNATIONAL CONSULTATION ON INCONTINENCE MODULAR QUESTIONNAIRE (ICIQ)?

The first International Consultation on Incontinence was held in 1998 to provide evidence based recommendations regarding all aspects of incontinence care and research. Committees of experts were convened to encompass all the relevant subject areas. These individuals were from multidisciplinary backgrounds and represented the worldwide scientific community and the range of specialities involved. Each committee was tasked with performing a systematic review of the relevant medical literature in order to make recommendations for clinical practice and research. One such committee responsible for the review of symptom and quality of life assessment identified numerous published questionnaires for the assessment of urinary incontinence (UI). Grades of recommendation regarding their use were applied based on their degree of validation in the published literature (1). The use of questionnaires with the highest levels of validation was encouraged in clinical practice and research to enable robust evaluation of symptoms and their impact on quality of life and to facilitate the comparison of results across studies. It was also suggested that there was a need for a universally applicable, brief and simple UI questionnaire to be developed and used widely across the population in clinical practice and research—the ICIQ-UI Short Form (2). Such an instrument would facilitate comparisons between findings in different settings and studies and was supported by the ICI Scientific Committee (3).

An advisory board was convened to steer development of this questionnaire and whilst not included in the review at the first consultation, the lack of questionnaires available for bowel symptoms and incontinence, and vaginal symptoms such as prolapse, was recognized. The decision was taken to expand the project to enable the recommendation and development of, where required, high quality, fully validated questionnaires for all lower pelvic dysfunction related to incontinence. The ICIQ project was then established to include a wider spectrum of urinary, bowel, and vaginal symptoms and their impact on quality of life.

AIMS AND OBJECTIVES

The ICIQ's objectives are to provide consensus on the use of published questionnaires for the assessment of lower pelvic symptoms and their impact on quality of life. Three aims underpin the ICIQ in order to achieve clarity over questionnaire use:

- To recommend high quality self-completion questionnaires according to evidence of validation;
- To promote wider use of questionnaires to standardize assessment of lower pelvic dysfunction and its impact on quality of life, in order to;

- Facilitate communication in different patient settings and different patient groups.

HOW IS THE ICIQ DEVELOPED?

Development of the ICIQ is achieved in two ways:

- inclusion of existing high quality questionnaires with the author's permission, or
- production of new questionnaires.

Inclusion into the ICIQ is based on a principal factor: evidence of a questionnaire's robust validation. Psychometric testing of questionnaires for use in clinical practice and research is considered essential to afford confidence in the results obtained (4). This is of particular importance where decisions regarding treatment or research outcomes are made. There are three main components to standard psychometric evaluation:

- Validity—indicates that the instrument is a valid measure of the concept in question;
- Reliability—indicates that the instrument can measure the concept in a reproducible and consistent manner;
- Sensitivity to change—indicates that the instrument is able to detect real change in the concept under evaluation (4–9).

To achieve these standards requires considerable time and effort. Production of a new questionnaire therefore is only undertaken when there is a specific requirement for the new instrument, and when available instruments are inadequate.

METHODS OF ICIQ DEVELOPMENT

ICIQ questionnaire production follows a standard protocol incorporating mixed methodology.

Qualitative studies are undertaken to achieve the aims of both patients and clinical relevance dependent on the nature of the questionnaire. Issues required for clinical evaluation may be more readily identified by clinical experts particularly where specific clinical manifestations are required to infer diagnosis, for example, urinary urgency and frequency are symptoms characteristic of overactive bladder (OAB) (10). Potential respondents, symptomatic patients for example, are often better placed to identify issues related to quality of life evaluation as they can reflect on their own lived experience (11). There is inevitably overlap between these groups however. This process ensures that the most pertinent issues for evaluation are identified. The value of conducting qualitative enquiry is also in establishing the most appropriate phraseology and terminology for self-report questionnaires (12). This approach provides a sound evidence base for questionnaires to go on and be evaluated using rigorous quantitative methods.

Parallel studies are conducted to evaluate different aspects of validity, reliability, and sensitivity to change in subgroups of potential respondents (e.g., outcome following conservative and surgical treatments). These sub-studies provide larger datasets on which to conduct numerous statistical analyses in order to make decisions regarding the most robust measurement question items to retain in the final version of the questionnaire. Further consultations with clinicians and potential respondents are conducted to ensure the final version of the questionnaire reflects clinical and patient relevance while displaying the most robust psychometric properties.

The ICIQ's international nature requires that translations are available, which is also conducted according to an established protocol involving structured translation and back translation to ensure the original meaning of the questionnaire is retained. Over 40 language versions are now provided across available ICIQ modules.

HOW TO USE THE ICIQ

Fourteen ICIQ modules/questionnaires are currently available for use, with further modules in development, (discussed in detail below). Clinicians or researchers are able to select modules to compile a tailored questionnaire set that meets their study/clinical practice requirements to achieve complete evaluation.

In order to simplify this, modules have been categorized to aid selection (Table 17.1).

The ICIQ recommends the use of a "core" or "symptom-specific" module and an "add-on" quality of life measure, in all patient evaluations for both clinical practice and research. Symptom alleviation may not indicate a difference in impact on quality of life and so the evaluation of both is recommended to encompass all relevant aspects to the individual (13,14). This approach can also target treatment to the most bothersome component of a symptom complex. The features of each module are summarized below to inform decisions regarding questionnaire selection.

Table 17.1 International Consultation on Incontinence Modular Questionnaire (ICIQ) Modular Structure

Condition	Recommended modules	Optional modules	Recommended add-on modules			
			QoL	Generic QoL	Sexual matters	Post-treatment
A) Core modules						
Urinary symptoms	Males: ICIQ-MLUTS Females: ICIQ-FLUTS	Males: ICIQ-MLUTS LF Females: ICIQ-FLUTS LF	ICIQ-LUTSqol	SF-12	Males: ICIQ-MLUTSsex Females: ICIQ-FLUTSsex	ICIQ-satisfaction*
Vaginal symptoms and sexual matters	ICIQ-VS		ICIQ-VSqol*	SF-12		
Bowel symptoms	ICIQ-B		ICIQ-BSqol*	SF-12		
Urinary incontinence (UI)	ICIQ-UI short form	ICIQ-UI LF^a	ICIQ-LUTSqol	SF-12	Males: ICIQ-MLUTSsex Females: ICIQ-FLUTSsex	
B) Specific patient groups						
Nocturia	ICIQ-N		ICIQ-Nqol	SF-12	Males: ICIQ-MLUTSsex Females: ICIQ-FLUTSsex	
Overactive bladder (OAB)	ICIQ-OAB		ICIQ-OABqol	SF-12	Males: ICIQ-MLUTSsex Females: ICIQ-FLUTSsex	
Neurogenic	ICIQ-spinal cord disease*			SF-12		
Long-term catheter users	ICIQ-LTC*					
Children	ICIQ-CLUTS*		ICIQ-CLUTSqol*			

* In development.

Recommended Modules

Core Modules

This group of questionnaires provides assessment of core symptoms of lower pelvic dysfunction:

- Lower urinary tract symptoms (male and female specific versions): ICIQ-MLUTS/ICIQ-FLUTS.
- Vaginal symptoms (female version only): ICIQ-VS.
- Bowel symptoms focusing on anal incontinence (male and female applicable version): ICIQ-B.
- UI (male and female applicable version): ICIQ-UI short form.

Each module provides a comprehensive yet brief instrument for measurement of the stated symptoms and associated "bother." The bother items attached to individual symptoms enable the individual to indicate areas causing the most impact on quality of life, as perceived by them. This can be a more sensitive indicator of treatment outcome than frequency of symptoms alone (Fig. 17.1).

The characteristics of the core ICIQ modules are summarized below.

Core Modules Available for Use

ICIQ-MLUTS

Purpose	Comprehensive assessment of male lower urinary tract symptoms and associated bother
Availability	Available for use Published evidence of validity, reliability, and sensitivity to change (15,16)
Domains/items	Voiding Incontinence Individual items evaluating frequency and nocturia
Number of items	13
Available translations	26
Scoring system	0–20 voiding symptoms subscale 0–24 incontinence symptoms subscale Bother scales are not incorporated in the overall score but indicate impact of individual symptoms for the patient
Derived from	ICS*male*SF (15)

ICIQ-FLUTS

Purpose	Comprehensive assessment of female lower urinary tract symptoms and associated bother
Availability	Available for use Published evidence of validity, reliability, and sensitivity to change (17)
Domains/items	Filling Voiding Incontinence
Number of items	12
Available translations	19
Scoring system	0–15 filling symptoms subscale 0–12 voiding symptoms subscale 0–20 incontinence symptoms subscale Bother scales are not incorporated in the overall score but indicate impact of individual symptoms for the patient
Derived from	Bristol Female Lower Urinary Tract Symptoms Questionnaire-Short Form (BFLUTS-SF) (17)

ICIQ-VS

Purpose	Comprehensive assessment of vaginal symptoms and associated bother
Availability	Available for use Published evidence of validity, reliability, and sensitivity to change (18)
Domains/items	Vaginal symptoms Sexual matters Quality of life
Number of items	14
Available translations	2
Scoring system	0–53 vaginal symptoms subscale 0–58 sexual matters subscale 0–10 overall impact on quality of life subscale Bother scales are not incorporated in the overall score but indicate impact of individual symptoms for the patient
Derived from	Newly developed module

5a. Do you have to rush to the toilet to urinate?

Never ☐ 0
Occasionally ☐ 1
Sometimes ☐ 2
Most of the time ☐ 3
All of the time ☐ 4

5b. How much does this bother you?
Please ring a number between 0 (not at all) and 10 (a great deal)

0 1 2 3 4 5 6 7 8 9 **10**
Not at all — A great deal

Figure 17.1 Example of an ICIQ question item.

ICIQ-B

Purpose	Comprehensive assessment of male/female bowel symptoms, predominantly anal incontinence, and associated impact on quality of life
Availability	Available for use
	Evidence to suggest validity, reliability, and sensitivity to change awaiting publication
Domains/items	Bowel pattern
	Bowel control
	Quality of life
Number of items	21
Available translations	2 in production
Scoring system	1–21 bowel pattern subscale
	0–28 bowel control subscale
	0–26 impact on quality of life subscale
	Bother scales are not incorporated in the overall score but indicate impact of individual symptoms for the patient
Derived from	Newly developed module

ICIQ-UI Short Form

Purpose	Comprehensive assessment of male/female UI
Availability	Available for use
	Published evidence of validity, reliability, and sensitivity to change (2).
Domains/items	UI including items on frequency and amount of leakage along with overall interference
	A self-diagnostic item invites respondents to indicate the cause of incontinence
Number of items	4
Available translations	32
Scoring system	0–21 UI score
	Self-diagnostic item not scored
Derived from	Newly developed module

Specific Patient Groups

This group of questionnaires provides assessment of some specific conditions or symptom complexes such as nocturia and overactive bladder (OAB). This category also includes specific patient groups (e.g., children). These instruments contain only question items associated with the symptom complex or have been developed specifically for use in a specific group. These questionnaires therefore are only utilizable in the stated populations and would need further evaluation for use in other groups.

- Nocturia (male and female applicable version): ICIQ-N.
- OAB (male and female applicable version): ICIQ-OAB.
- Patients with spinal cord disease: ICIQ-spinal cord disease.
- Patients using long term catheters: ICIQ-LTC.
- Lower urinary tract symptoms in children: ICIQ-CLUTS.

Bother items are included for all except the children's questionnaire.

The characteristics and developmental progress of the ICIQ modules for use in specific patient groups are summarized below.

Specific Patient Group Modules Available for Use
ICIQ-N

Purpose	Comprehensive assessment of symptoms of nocturia and associated bother
Availability	Available for use
	Evidence of validity, reliability, and sensitivity to change (15–17)
Domains/items	Frequency
	Nocturia
Number of items	2
Available translations	30
Scoring system	0–8 total score of both items
	Bother scales are not incorporated in the overall score but indicate impact of individual symptoms for the patient
Derived from	ICS*male*SF/BFLUTS-SF (15,17)

ICIQ-OAB

Purpose	Comprehensive assessment of symptoms of OAB and associated bother
Availability	Available for use
	Evidence of validity, reliability, and sensitivity to change (15–17)
Domains/items	Frequency
	Nocturia
	Urgency
	Urge incontinence
Number of items	4
Available translations	22
Scoring system	0–16 total score of all items
	Bother scales are not incorporated in the overall score but indicate impact of individual symptoms for the patient
Derived from	ICS*male*SF/BFLUTS-SF (15,17)

Specific Patient Group Modules in Development
ICIQ-Spinal Cord Disease

Purpose	Assessment of urinary symptoms and impact on quality of life associated with specific management devices and related bother
Current status	Draft instrument prepared
	Content validity testing and full psychometric validation to be commenced
Development methodology	Items generated by clinical experts and patients managing urinary symptoms with varying devices
Domains/items	Bladder function
	Issues associated with specific management devices
	Sexual matters
	Quality of life
Derived from	Newly developed module

ICIQ-LTC

Purpose	Assessment of urinary symptoms and impact on quality of life associated with long term urethral catheterization and related bother
Current status	Draft instrument prepared
	Content validity completed and full psychometric validation underway
Development methodology	Items generated by clinical experts and patients managing urinary symptoms with long term catheters
Domains/items	Coping strategies
	Social functioning
	Attitudes
	Body image
Derived from	Newly developed module

ICIQ-CLUTS

Purpose	Assessment of urinary symptoms in children
Current status	Draft instrument prepared and has undergone content validity testing
	Further validity testing underway in the U.K., Italy, and Germany
	Reliability and sensitivity to change evaluation to be commenced
Development methodology	Items generated by clinical experts
	Criterion validity evaluated by comparison with gold standard clinical parameters
Domains/items	Urinary symptoms and incontinence
Derived from	Newly developed module

Recommended Add-on Modules

Core Modules

This group of questionnaires incorporates quality of life and sexual matters modules. They are recommended to be completed as stand alone questionnaires or alongside core or specific symptom evaluations. The core symptom modules described above contain bother items indicating impact on quality of life directly related to symptoms. Quality of life questionnaires cover more specific issues that are a consequence of symptoms (e.g., limiting activities and affecting relationships). The combination of symptom assessment with associated bother, and a quality of life assessment provides a more complete evaluation of the patient's experience (14,19). In addition, given the nature of lower pelvic dysfunction, sexual matters can also be affected and questionnaires are available for this further evaluation where appropriate.

- Quality of life associated with lower urinary tract symptoms (male and female applicable version): ICIQ-LUTSqol.
- Quality of life associated with vaginal symptoms (female version only): ICIQ-VSqol.
- Quality of life associated with bowel symptoms (male and female applicable version): ICIQ-BSqol.
- Sexual matters associated with lower urinary tract symptoms (male and female specific versions): ICIQ-MLUTSsex/ICIQ-FLUTSsex.

- Sexual matters associated with vaginal symptoms are included in the symptom questionnaire (ICIQ-VS) as the issues were considered too intrinsically linked to separate for evaluation.
- Sexual matters associated with bowel symptoms are included in the symptom and quality of life questionnaire (ICIQ-B) as the issues were considered too intrinsically linked to separate for evaluation.

Bother associated with impact items are included as this can be very personal and quite unrelated to the frequency of the issue alone.

The characteristics and developmental progress of the ICIQ recommended add-on modules for use alongside the core questionnaires are summarized below.

Add-on Modules Available for Use

ICIQ-LUTSqol

Purpose	Detailed assessment of quality of life issues associated with urinary symptoms and related bother
Availability	Available for use
	Published evidence of validity, reliability, and sensitivity to change (20).
Domains/items	Life restrictions
	Emotional aspects
	Preventive measures
Number of items	22
Available translations	45
Scoring system	0–76 total score of all items
	0–10 overall impact on everyday life subscale
	Bother scales are not incorporated in the overall score but indicate impact of individual quality of life aspects for the patient
Derived from	King's Health Questionnaire (20)

ICIQ-MLUTSsex

Purpose	Assessment of male sexual matters associated with urinary symptoms and related bother
Availability	Available for use
	Published evidence of validity, reliability, and sensitivity to change (16,21)
Domains/items	Erection and ejaculation issues
	Overall interference
Number of items	4
Available translations	24
Scoring system	0–12 total score of all items
	0–10 overall impact on sexual matters subscale
	Bother scales are not incorporated in the overall score but indicate impact of individual symptoms for the patient
Derived from	ICSmaleSF (15,16,21)

ICIQ-FLUTSsex

Purpose	Assessment of female sexual matters associated with urinary symptoms and related bother
Availability	Available for use
	Published evidence of validity, reliability, and sensitivity to change (22)
Domains/items	Pain and leakage with sexual intercourse
	Overall interference
Number of items	4
Available translations	18
Scoring system	0–14 total score of all items
	Bother scales are not incorporated in the overall score but indicate impact of individual symptoms for the patient
Derived from	BFLUTS (22)

Add-on Modules in Development

ICIQ-VSqol

Purpose	Detailed assessment of quality of life issues associated with vaginal symptoms and related bother
Current status	Draft instrument prepared and has undergone content validity testing
	Data collection ongoing
Development methodology	Items generated by clinical experts and patients with vaginal symptoms
	Content validity testing with potential respondents and clinical experts
	Multi-center postal administration to potential respondents for validity, reliability, and sensitivity to change data collection
Domains/items	Life restrictions
	Emotional aspects
Derived from	Newly developed module

ICIQ-BSqol

Purpose	Detailed assessment of quality of life issues associated with bowel symptoms and related bother
Current status	Data collection complete and final analysis underway
	Evidence to suggest validity, reliability, and sensitivity to change
Development methodology	Items generated by clinical experts and patients with anal incontinence (12)
	Extensive content validity testing with potential respondents and clinical experts
	Multi-center postal administration to potential respondents for validity, reliability, and sensitivity to change data collection
Domains/items	Life restrictions
	Emotional aspects
	Preventive measures/coping strategies
Derived from	Newly developed module

Specific Patient Groups

In the same manner as the symptom modules, quality of life modules are available for specific symptom complexes.

- Quality of life associated with nocturia (male and female applicable version): ICIQ-Nqol.
- Quality of life associated with OAB (male and female applicable version): ICIQ-OABqol.

The characteristics of the ICIQ recommended add-on modules for use in specific patient groups are summarized below.

Specific Patient Group Add-on Modules Available for Use

ICIQ-Nqol

Purpose	Detailed assessment of quality of life issues associated with nocturia
Availability	Available for use
	Published evidence of validity, reliability, and sensitivity to change (23)
Domains/items	Issues associated with sleep disturbance
	Life restrictions
	Preventive measures
Number of items	13
Available translations	27
Scoring system	0–48 total score of all items
	or
	0–24 sleep/energy subscale
	0–24 bother/concern subscale
	0–10 overall interference caused by nocturia subscale
Derived from	N-QoL (23)

ICIQ-OABqol

Purpose	Detailed assessment of quality of life issues associated with OAB
Availability	Available for use
	Published evidence of validity, reliability, and sensitivity to change (24)
Domains/items	Life restrictions
	Emotional aspects
	Measure to accommodate OAB
Number of items	26
Available translations	33
Scoring system	0–150 total score of all items
	0–10 overall impact on everyday life subscale
Derived from	OAB-q (24)

Optional Modules

This category includes lengthier questionnaires for more exploratory evaluation of the core symptoms of lower pelvic dysfunction. While these questionnaires are suitable for use in clinical practice they have not been shortened for clinical efficiency and are therefore more widely used in research studies where exploration of a broader range of symptoms may be desired and more feasible.

- ICIQ-MLUTS Long Form/ICIQ-FLUTS Long Form.
- ICIQ-UI Long Form.

The characteristics of the ICIQ optional modules available for use and progress of one module in development are summarized below.

143

Optional Modules Available for Use
ICIQ-MLUTS Long Form

Purpose	Detailed assessment of male lower urinary tract symptoms and associated bother
Availability	Available for use
	Published evidence of validity, reliability, and sensitivity to change (15,21)
Domains/items	Varied lower urinary tract symptoms
Number of items	23 (including the 13 items within the ICIQ-MLUTS)
Available translations	29
Scoring system	1–84 total score of all items
	Bother scales are not incorporated in the overall score but indicate impact of individual symptoms for the patient
Derived from	ICS*male* (16,21)

ICIQ-FLUTS Long Form

Purpose	Detailed assessment of female lower urinary tract symptoms and associated bother
Availability	Available for use
	Published evidence of validity, reliability, and sensitivity to change (17,22)
Domains/items	Varied lower urinary tract symptoms
Number of items	18 (including the 12 items within the ICIQ-FLUTS)
Available translations	7
Scoring system	0–69 total score of all items
	Bother scales are not incorporated in the overall score but indicate impact of individual symptoms for the patient
Derived from	BFLUTS (22)

Optional Module in Development
ICIQ-UI Long Form

Purpose	Detailed assessment of perceived causes of UI
Current status	Draft instrument prepared and has undergone content validity testing
	Data collection ongoing
Development methodology	Items generated by clinical experts and patients with UI
	Extensive content validity testing with potential respondents and clinical experts
	Postal administration to potential respondents for validity, reliability and sensitivity to change data collection
Domains/items	For each perceived cause of incontinence (for example, physical activity) the frequency, amount and degree of bother are evaluated
Derived from	Newly developed module

Post-Treatment Module

The issue of post-treatment satisfaction evaluation is being explored from various perspectives. To date, a fully validated questionnaire for generic use among individuals undergoing varied treatments for all lower pelvic dysfunction has not been fully validated. The feasibility of an ICIQ module for this purpose is undergoing exploration to establish if satisfaction following treatment can be characterized by a set of common question items applicable to all treatments. An alternative suggestion is that satisfaction may be simply assumed by alleviation of symptoms or improvement in quality of life. Ongoing studies will provide further evidence on which to make suggestions regarding post treatment evaluation.

UPTAKE OF THE ICIQ

Use of the ICIQ in clinical practice and research has been encouraging in achieving the aims of standardized, high quality assessment for symptoms of lower pelvic dysfunction and their impact on quality of life. More than 550 requests for use of the various modules have been recorded and over 70 related publications have been identified. The most widely applied module is the ICIQ-UI short form (ICIQ), which is closely followed by the ICIQ-FLUTS reflecting the fact that most applications relate to the evaluation of female urinary symptoms. The ICIQ has most commonly been applied to clinical and general practice settings, alongside its considerable uptake in the research setting.

CONCLUSION

The ICIQ modular questionnaire project provides a series of standardized questionnaires for the assessment of lower pelvic dysfunction and its impact on quality of life. The ICIQ provides clarity over which questionnaires to use by recommending only those with evidence of high quality and robust psychometric validation data, including validity, reliability, and sensitivity to change. This assurance provides the user with confidence in the results obtained. This is particularly important in clinical practice and research where treatment decisions or trial outcomes increasingly rely on this source of evidence. Increasing awareness of the ICIQ aims to promote increased usage of standardized questionnaires thereby facilitating communication and more widespread comparisons between different treatments and in different patient groups worldwide.

REFERENCES

1. Donovan J, Naughton M, Gotoh M, et al. Symptom and quality of life assessment. In: Abrams P, Khoury S, Wein A, eds. Incontinence: Proceedings of the First International Consultation on Incontinence, June 28–July 1, 1998, 1st edn. Plymouth: Health Publication Ltd, 1999: 295–331.
2. Avery K, Donovan J, Peters T, et al. ICIQ: a brief and robust measure for evaluating symptoms and impact of urinary incontinence. Neurourol Urodyn 2004; 23: 322–30.
3. Abrams P, Avery K, Gardener N, Donovan J. The international consultation on incontinence modular questionnaire: www.iciq.net. J Urol 2003; 175: 1063–6.
4. Streiner DL, Norman GR. Health Measurement Scales: A Practical Guide to Their Development and Use, 3rd edn. New York: Oxford University Press, 2004.
5. Oppenheim AN. Questionnaire Design, Interviewing and Attitude Measurement, 2nd edn. London: Continuum, 1992.
6. Bowling A. Research Methods in Health: Investigating Health in Health Services, 2nd edn. Maidenhead: Open University Press, 2002.
7. Boynton PM, Greenhalgh T. Selecting, designing, and developing your questionnaire. BMJ 2004; 328: 1312–15.
8. Saw SM, Ng TP. The design and assessment of questionnaires in clinical research. Singapore Med Journal 2001; 42: 131–5.
9. Donovan J, Bosch JLHR, Gotoh M, et al. Symptom and quality of life assessment. In: Abrams P, Cardozo L, Khoury S, Wein A, eds. Incontinence: Proceedings of the Third International Consultation on Incontinence, June 26–29, 2004, 3rd edn. Plymouth: Health Publication Ltd, 2005: 519–84.

10. Peat J. Health Science Research: A Handbook of Quantitative Methods. London: Sage Publications, 2002.

11. Rapley M. Quality of Life Research: A Critical Introduction, 1st edn. London: SAGE Publications Ltd, 2003.

12. Cotterill N, Norton C, Avery KNL, Abrams P, Donovan JL. A patient centered approach to developing a comprehensive symptom and quality of life assessment of anal incontinence. Dis Colon Rectum 2008; 51: 82–7.

13. Weber AM, Abrams P, Brubaker L, et al. The standardization of terminology for researchers in female pelvic floor disorders. Int Urogynecol J 2001; 12: 178–86.

14. Fairclough DL. Patient reported outcomes as endpoints in medical research. Stat Methods Med Res 2004; 13: 115–38.

15. Donovan J, Peters TJ, Abrams P, et al. Scoring the short form ICSmaleSF questionnaire. J Urol 2000; 164: 1948–55.

16. Donovan J, Brookes ST, De La Rosette JJMCH, et al. The responsiveness of the ICSmale questionnaire to outcome: evidence from the ICS-'BPH' study. BJU International 1999; 83: 243–8.

17. Brookes ST, Donovan J, Wright M, Jackson S, Abrams P. A scored form of the Bristol female lower urinary tract symptoms questionnaire: data from a randomized controlled trial of surgery for women with stress incontinence. Am J Obstet Gynaecol 2004; 191: 73–82.

18. Price N, Jackson SR, Avery K, Brookes ST, Abrams P. Development and psychometric evaluation of the ICIQ vaginal symptoms questionnaire: the ICIQ-VS. BJOG 2006; 113: 700–12.

19. Abrams P, Artibani W, Gajewski JB, Hussain I. Assessment of treatment outcomes in patients with overactive bladder: importance of objective and subjective measures. Urology 2006; 68(Suppl 2a): 17–28.

20. Kelleher CJ, Cardozo L, Khullar V, Salvatore S. A new questionnaire to assess the quality of life of urinary incontinent women. BJOG 1997; 104: 1374–9. 1997.

21. Donovan J, Abrams P, Peters TJ, et al. The ICS-'BPH' study: the psychometric validity and reliability of the ICSmale questionnaire. BJU International 1996; 77: 554–62.

22. Jackson S, Donovan J, Brookes ST, et al. The bristol female lower urinary tract symptoms questionnaire: development and psychometric testing. BJU International 1996; 77: 805–12.

23. Abraham L, Hareendran A, Mills I, et al. Development and validation of a quality-of-life measure for men with nocturia. Urology 2004; 63: 481–6.

24. Coyne KS, Revicki D, Hunt TL, et al. Psychometric validation of an overactive bladder symptom and health-related quality of life questionnaire the OAB-q. Qual Life Res 2002; 11: 563–74.

18 Questionnaires to Assess Pelvic Organ Prolapse

Vanja Sikirica and Mark Slack

INTRODUCTION

Pelvic organ prolapse (POP) is a common disorder affecting 20% to 30% of parous women (1,2) many of whom are asymptomatic (up to 80%) (3). In addition to symptoms directly related to their prolapse patients may present with bowel, bladder, or sexual symptoms as discussed in the previous chapters in this section. These may or may not be directly attributable to POP (4). Many women with POP are managed conservatively but surgical intervention is also commonly employed as a first line measure or when conservative therapy has failed. Surgical treatment is associated with the risk of complications, failure to relieve patients' symptoms or meet their treatment expectations, and longer term POP recurrence (5).

It is essential to obtain an accurate anatomic assessment, symptom assessment, and bother assessment when determining the correct treatment strategy. It is also important to help the patient distinguish which symptoms are due to the prolapse and which ones have their origin in bowel, bladder, and sexual dysfunction unrelated to their POP. A number of questionnaires are available to assess POP and augment information obtained from the clinical assessment. These are discussed in this chapter. In addition, for patients who have symptoms related to the bladder, bowel, or sexual function, questionnaires described in detail in the preceding chapters may also be appropriate. Screening questionnaires and goal assessment tools previously described would also apply to patients with POP.

PLACE OF INSTRUMENTS
Clinical Note Taking

Traditional clinical history taking provides a summary view of the symptoms of POP experienced by the patient and the impact these have on their lives. The intimate nature of some of these complaints may affect the quality of questioning and the accuracy of patient response (6).

This is important as it may well be the more intimate and personal issues that bother the patient the most and are therefore the most important to cure. A thorough clinical assessment must also record in a reproducible and understandable fashion the nature and extent of the POP that needs correction. This is particularly important for clinical studies where the extent of prolapse prior to an intervention needs to be accurately known in order to determine anatomical improvement. Good documentation and assessment should however apply equally to clinical practice, clinical studies, and clinical trials.

Finally, questioning must not omit symptoms related to the bladder, bowel, and sexual function, even if these issues are not initially volunteered by the patient.

A clinical interview should always assess the bother of symptoms to the patient and conclude with a sensible management plan. This is the most critical part of the assessment and must be individualized to achieve the best outcome. Intervention may vary from simple reassurance to complex surgery but engaging the patient and offering realistic and achievable treatment expectations is the key to clinical success. It is insufficient to view the patient with POP as a simple anatomical abnormality which requires surgical correction.

STANDARDIZED POP ASSESSMENT INSTRUMENTS
Methods of Administration

A common means to avoid biases introduced by clinician note taking is to systematically administer standardized, validated, and reliable POP instruments. Instruments may be self-administered in the healthcare setting, mailed to patients to complete prior to the visit, completed online or via phone, or administered by a member of the medical team. The method of administration of the questionnaire will affect both the response rate and the accuracy of the response (7,8). Self administration of the questionnaire is probably the most accurate means of assessing the patient perspective because they are not affected by inter-observer variability (9).

Self-administered patient reported outcome (PRO) questionnaires can be completed in a paper format or can be electronically administered. One of the advantages of the electronic version is that they can skip irrelevant sections when the response to the primary question is negative and improve accuracy of results (7). Additionally computer administered questionnaires will usually provide a concise printed summary. Used as part of the clinical assessment this method can save valuable time for both the patient and clinician and allow more time to be dedicated to discussing other treatment issues.

An electronic Personal Assessment Questionnaire-Pelvic Floor (ePAQ-PF) was developed from earlier paper forms and has been shown to provide a reliable and valid measure of urinary, bowel, vaginal, and sexual symptoms (10,11). It has also been shown to be sensitive to change in vaginal symptoms in women undergoing prolapse surgery (12). The simple format supports unsupervised self-completion; levels of missing data are low and satisfaction ratings from patients high.

Potential disadvantages of the ePAQ-PF include the cost of technology (portable or stationary), infrastructure to collect PRO data, and patient technological know-how, especially since the majority of POP women who present for surgery are elderly (7,10).

Due to time, economic constraints, and patient factors the administration of PRO questionnaires is often not possible in clinical practice. The administration of multiple PROs

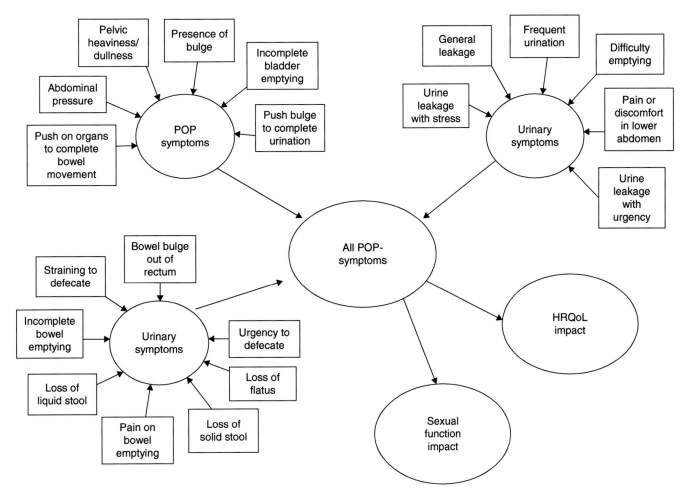

Figure 18.1 An example of a possible conceptual framework for a POP instrument (based on the PFDI-20). *Abbreviations*: POP, pelvic organ prolapse; PFDI, pelvic floor distress inventory; HRQoL, health related quality of life. *Source:* Reproduced from Ref. 25, with persmission from Elsevier.

leads to increased patient burden and decrease response rates and accuracy of responses (13,14). Nevertheless, whenever logistically possible, PROs should be used to ensure a consistent means of evaluating the presence and severity of POP symptoms, impact on quality of life (QoL), and satisfaction following intervention.

INSTRUMENT SELECTION

Instrument selection has been discussed in detail by Coyne in her earlier chapter in this section; suffice to say the clinician should choose the correct instrument based on its intended use and the concept(s) they are trying to measure (9).

There are a number of instruments available for the assessment of POP within multiple conceptual areas. Figure 18.1 presents an example of a conceptual framework one might hypothesize in considering a surgical POP repair. There are clearly significant areas of overlap within each of these individual concepts. The design of all questionnaires needs to follow standard psychometric process as outlined previously (9,15–17).

Table 18.1 lists questionnaires available to assess the various problem areas of patient with POP and these are discussed within this chapter. It is important to consider how many questionnaires to administer to individual patients. Too many can lead to a degree of patient fatigue and possibly erroneous answers. A long POP questionnaire may be suitable for a

research study where patients are encouraged by the research team and given appropriate time to complete their instruments, but may be too cumbersome for day-to-day clinical practice. The ePAQ has been validated for use in the clinical setting (12,18). The electronic version allows direct input to a database while paper based PRO questionnaires often have to be entered onto the computer adding to the administrative burden.

The recall period of the instrument should also be considered when selecting an instrument. It is important to consider factors that may affect patient recall and create a recall bias. For instance, pivotal traumatic events can often be recalled with accuracy while the subtle waning of a symptom over a few months may not be noticed from memory. Validated instruments take this into consideration and test for this. An example in POP is that the Pelvic Floor Distress Inventory (PFDI) and Pelvic Floor Impact Questionnaire (PFIQ) instruments have a three-month recall period which has been validated to have appropriate recollection of symptom acuity, events, and impact on QoL (19,20). Equally it is important that questionnaires are responsive to change after treatment, and are completed after a suitable time interval in order that clinically meaningful improvement in symptoms will have taken place (21). This is particularly important when evaluating conservative treatments which may take some time to show clinical benefit.

Table 18.1 Summary of Reliable and Validated PRO Instruments for Pelvic Organ Prolapse (POP) or POP-Associated Conditions

POP
Pelvic Floor Distress Inventory (PFDI) and (PFDI-20) (19,20)
POP Distress Inventory (19,20)
Pelvic Floor Impact Questionnaire (PFIQ) and (PFIQ-7) (19,20)
Prolapse Quality of Life Questionnaire (P-QoL) (29)
Sheffield Prolapse Symptoms Questionnaire (SPS-Q) (30)
Electronic Pelvic Floor Assessment Questionnaire (e-PAQ-PF) (10)
Urinary incontinence
Incontinence Severity Index (ISI) (31)
International Consultation on Incontinence Questionnaire Short Form (ICIQ-SF) (32)
Urogenital Distress Inventory (UDI) (33) and (UDI-6) (34)
Bristol Female Lower Urinary Tract Symptom Questionnaire (BFLUTS) (35)
Incontinence Impact Questionnaire (IIQ) (33) and (IIQ-7) (34)
Incontinence Quality of Life Questionnaire (I-QOL) (36)
Urge Incontinence Impact Questionnaire (Urge IIQ) (37)
Kings Health Questionnaire (KHQ) (38)
Fecal incontinence (colorectal-anal)
Wexner Scale (39)
Fecal Incontinence Severity Index (FISI) (40)
Cleveland Clinic Fecal Incontinence Score (41)
Fecal Incontinence QoL Scale (FIQL) (42)
Manchester Health Questionnaire (43)
Sexual (dys)function
Prolapse and Incontinence Sexual Function Questionnaire (PISQ) (44) and (PISQ-12) (45)
Sexual Quality of Life-Female (SQOL-F) (46)
Female Sexual Function Index (FSFI) (47)
McCoy's Female Sexual Function Questionnaire (MFSQ) (48)

Note: Text in bold italic font represents the symptoms, text in bold font represents the QoL, and text in italic font represents both.
Abbreviation: PRO, patient reported outcome.

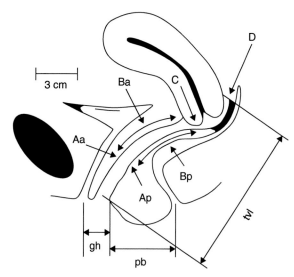

Figure 18.2 Six sites (points *Aa*, *Ba*, *C*, *D*, *Bp*, and *Ap*), genital hiatus (*gh*), perineal body (*pb*), and total vaginal length (*tvl*) used for pelvic organ support quantitation. *Source*: Reproduced from Ref. 25, with permission from Elsevier.

For an overall assessment of POP symptoms or QoL it is essential that any single instrument (or battery of individual instruments) cover all aspects of prolapse, urinary, bowel, and sexual function. Use of existing standardized and validated instruments is preferable to developing a new or modified instrument. Changes to a questionnaire such as the addition or deletion of scales or use in a different population are considered an instrument modification (7,22). This will require re-validation for context and/or content (9,23).

There following sections in this chapter will address instruments in the following areas:

1. Anatomic measures of POP
2. Symptom questionnaires
3. QoL questionnaires
   - Generic
   - Disease specific
4. Sexual function questionnaires
   - Generic
   - Disease specific

ANATOMIC MEASURES OF POP

There are a few tools available to measure the degree of POP. It is important to note that these are purely clinician reported outcome (CRO) measures and the patient is not asked any questions in relation to the measure. The degree of POP should be evaluated by a standardized measurement system clearly defined relative to anatomic points of reference. The Baden–Walker measure is an older measure that relies on total vaginal length (24). Because of the subjective nature of this measure it has in large part been replaced by the Pelvic Organ Prolapse-Quantification (POP-Q) system (25). The POP-Q is based on two types of anatomic points in order to measure the degree of POP; a fixed reference point and defined points to measure with respect to the reference point.

Fixed Point for Reference

It is essential to provide a fixed anatomical landmark that can be consistently and precisely identified in the evaluation of POP. The hymen serves as the fixed point of reference used throughout the POP-Q. Visually, the hymen provides a precisely identifiable landmark for reference. While the location of the hymen can be variable, it remains the best landmark available. The anatomic position of the six defined points for measurement should be centimeters above or proximal to the hymen (negative number) or centimeters below or distal to the hymen (positive number) with respect to the location of the hymen being defined as zero. For example, a cervix that protruded 3 cm distal to the hymen would be +3 cm.

Defined Points for POP Measurement

The POP-Q is a site-specific system that has been adapted from several classifications. Six points (two on the anterior vaginal wall, two in the superior vagina, and two on the posterior vaginal wall) are located with reference to the hymen (Fig. 18.2). The position of points Aa, Ba, Ap, Bp, C, and (if applicable) D with reference to the hymen should be measured and recorded.

Positions are expressed as centimeters above or proximal to the hymen (negative number) or centimeters below or distal to the hymen (positive number) with the plane of the hymen being defined as zero. Reporting of POP-Q scores should clearly specify the patient position and technique of use when taking the measurements. Scores are grouped into an ordinal set of stages. Stages represent adjacent categories that can be ranked in an ascending sequence of magnitude from stage 0 to IV. As is true for an ordinal scale, the categories are assigned arbitrarily and the intervals between them cannot be actually measured. Nevertheless, for accurate description or comparison of populations or to compare various treatment options, such a system is necessary. For a complete reference of the POP-Q development and validation see Ref. 25.

SYMPTOMS INSTRUMENTS FOR POP

In contrast to anatomic measurement via CRO instruments, POP symptom measures fall under the definition of PROs. The U.S. FDA defines a PRO as "a measurement of any aspect of a patient's health status that comes directly from the patient (i.e., without the interpretation of the patient's responses by a physician or anyone else)" (9). PROs can provide additional information to alter clinical knowledge about an intervention in addition to the clinician perspective and/or physiologic measures. This is important because improvements in anatomical measures of a condition may not necessarily correspond to improvements in how the patient functions or feels. For example, improvements in POP-Q stages in terms of anatomic repair, may not correlate well with improvements in urinary or bowel symptoms (26–28). What is most important to women is not necessarily what is wrong with the anatomy; it is the symptoms that causes them to present for care. Often their chief complaint is physically having a "vaginal bulge" or "lump," or "something falling out" or a sensation of such (20,29). However these patients often present with symptoms relating to bowel, bladder, and sexual dysfunction that may or may not be related to the POP. Reliable and validated instruments exist to assess the presence, severity, and/or bother each of these five areas of symptoms and are presented in Table 18.1.

Conceptually, since POP affects a number of different organs [e.g., stress urinary incontinence (SUI), overactive bladder, etc.], it is technically possible for clinicians to choose many different instruments from the four sections listed in Table 18.1. However, choosing an instrument which incorporates many symptom areas into one, such as the PFDI or PFIQ, has inherent efficiencies. Such instruments decrease or eliminate the need to have separate scoring instructions and possible duplication of concepts or items between instruments (e.g., urogenital distress inventory-6 is already part of the PFDI-20). In addition, they offer less patient burden and take less time to administer. However, it is important not to confuse this with only using a part of a validated questionnaire, changing a measurement scale, or changing the order or content of a questionnaire. This should be avoided whenever possible as this can change its psychometric properties of the instrument and invalidate the scoring, or interpretation of results (9,16,17).

QUALITY OF LIFE OR IMPACT MEASURES

PRO instruments can range from simple concepts such as the purely symptomatic instruments mentioned above, to more complex concepts like the ability to carry out activities of daily living, or still further, multi-dimensional concepts such as health related QoL (HRQoL). A HRQoL instrument is generally accepted to be a multi-concept (e.g., multi-domain) instrument that can capture physical, psychological, social (or other) components within a given disease state or condition (49,50). There are two types of PRO's applicable to measure HRQoL within the POP area, generic, and condition-specific.

Generic HRQoL instruments are broad in their scope of questioning to assess impact on various aspect of life impact. Generic HRQoL measures are used to assess HRQoL in numerous diseases and patient populations, most often chronic in nature (51). The advantage of generic instruments is that they allow for comparisons across different groups or illnesses. The two generic HRQoL instruments that have been used most frequently in women with POP are the SF-36 and the Euro QoL (ED-5Q) (19,52). Another advantage of either of these generic HRQoL instruments can be used by national health systems as a common measure of utility for either economic payer evaluations (e.g., cost as the numerator and QoL/utility as the benefit for the denominator) (53,54). However, generic HRQoL instrument may lack sensitivity to the unique aspects of a specific disease and how it impacts the life of an affected POP population (17,52). Specifically, some studies have shown that generic HRQoL instruments do not always show improvement in overall HRQoL after a surgical POP repair (20).

Condition-specific HRQoL instruments are created to be a more targeted measure of the disease-specific impact on HRQoL. By definition, condition-specific instruments provide a deeper assessment of specific concepts critical to the disease that they where designed for (55). Their primary advantage is that they tend to be more responsive to change than generic instruments (19). However, comparison across disease states is clearly not possible.

The scores measured on a HRQoL instrument are an important source of information for the clinician. They can serve to identify the effect of an intervention on a patient's disease-specific QoL or on their overall (e.g., general) QoL. Once the physician is able to examine the QoL scores, they can be applied in clinical practice to determine the meaning and clinical relevance to the patient.

As before, a clinician should choose the instrument that is most relevant for their practice or research question. For instance, the physical condition (prolapse), can affect the patient's body image, which may in turn affect her ability to perform common activities (walking, exercise, intercourse, etc.). Once again, the conceptual framework serves to determine the inter-relationships between the various concepts being evaluated. The community-centered theory illustrates how the conceptual framework forms the basis of and also predicts the associations among various concepts (51). For example, the physical effects of a POP disease are central (e.g., bulge, incontinence, pressure, etc.) to more distal concepts such as psychological and emotional functioning (e.g., activities of daily living, social activities, nervousness, or depression, etc.) (56). Hence, the actual impact of the POP may extend into multiple areas of life, far beyond the physiological condition. A few QoL instruments that illustrate this include the prolapse-QoL which measures both symptoms and their impact to the QoL and the PFIQ which measures impact only Table 18.1.

SEXUAL FUNCTION

Sexual function or dysfunction is an important treatment consideration in POP. It is generally perceived that adequate sexual functioning is important for overall life satisfaction and general QoL (57,58). It represents concepts from sexual activity (yes/no) to more complex concepts such as physical (e.g., orgasm, dyspareunia, etc.), behavioral/emotive (e.g., enjoyment, desire, fear of intercourse, etc.), or partner related (e.g., closeness with partner due to sexual function, conversing, etc.). Although a number of valid and reliable sexual function questionnaires exist, the number of POP-specific sexual function instruments is quite limited. The only condition-specific sexual function questionnaire for women with POP or urinary incontinence is the Pelvic Organ Prolapse and Incontinence Sexual Function Questionnaire (PISQ) (44,45). The PISQ is valid and reliable and the original instrument contains 31 items within three conceptual domains: behavioral/emotive, physical, and partner-related. The PISQ-31 is designed for use in sexually active women with POP and/or SUI. Subsequently a short form has been developed which contains 12 items- and has shown to correlate well with the long-form.

As before, it is important to match what aspects of sexual function the clinician and/or patient are most interested in. For example, the PISQ asks about concepts that may not be related to the women's POP condition (e.g., "Does your partner have a problem with erections that affects your sexual ability?"). If an investigator is more interested in the patient's perspective rather than their partner's perspective, a general sexual function questionnaire may be more suitable in this situation. For example, the Sexual Quality of Life-Female has shown good reliability and validity and asks a different question—Have lost confidence in myself as a sexual partner?—which is answered on a six-point scale from "completely agree" to "completely disagree" (46). Again, the literature review, conceptual model and forethought into what concepts should be measured is the key part of instrument selection process that will help elucidate what the clinician truly wants to capture.

TIPS, TRICKS, AND THE STATE OF SCIENCE OF POP INSTRUMENTS

There are a number of important considerations to be aware of in the selection and use of PROs. Just because an instrument has been published or "used a lot before" does not mean that it is reliable. Appropriate principles of instrument development are not routinely taught in medical school and so it is natural to rely on the referral or recommendations of colleagues in the selection of instruments. As mentioned before, the literature should be reviewed and a psychometrician or statistician consulted before selecting an instrument. It is important to keep an eye out for instrument development that

does not introduce patient involvement from the outset. Failure to do this will create unclear content validity of the instrument. Instruments based solely on literature and clinician opinion but intended for patient use are considered incomplete in the eyes of the FDA and likewise should be considered the same in the eyes of clinical practice.

Clinicians often have doubts about the amount of error associated with the use of a purely subjective measure. It is important to realize that all measures will have some error. Even the most objective measures have a degree of sensitivity and specificity that must be considered when considering their role in routine practice (e.g., annual mammogram for women of a given age) or in combination with other lab measures or tests. Similarly, the amount of error and variability of response should also be assessed. The reliability and validity of the instrument must always be assessed and applicability to the population at hand must always be reconsidered rather than just plugging in previous instruments. Sometimes, analogous diseases may have instruments which can overlap sufficiently within the POP disease state to make them worthy of consideration. Examples of this include SUI instruments, fecal incontinence, or sexual dysfunction. For instance, sexual dysfunction has a multi-factorial and possibly multi-etiological basis, one of which is POP. Assessing sexual dysfunction within POP via sexual dysfunction instruments that inherently have some POP patients from their original validation study can be a viable option to consider, if the instrument has shown good psychometric properties. It is also important to remember that in the treatment of conditions such as POP, the chief complaint is subjective, therefore a subjective measure can be the strongest means of assessing improvement alone or alongside other objective measures. The persistence of a symptom after an intervention may occur for many different reasons. The patient is always the final arbiter of their disease and symptoms.

It is extremely important to realize what represents a meaningful change in score in an instrument. For example, a mean change of 10 points may be large numeric number change on the PISQ-12 and it can even be statistically significant. However what does this mean clinically? A clinically meaningful threshold of change needs to be established. Again, in comparison to other common chronic diseases, POP instruments are only now beginning to establish minimally important difference measures where the scores of an instrument are correlated to a global subjective measure of change instrument to find the threshold where a change in score indicates that a patient is subjectively better after their POP intervention. It is important to establish these both for research and practice purposes and at the present state, the POP literature lacks much of this.

Overall, the practicing clinician or researcher stands to gain from improved insights into the anatomic, symptomatic, or HRQoL impact that are of critical importance to their medical treatment decisions. The practicing clinician only has 15 to 20 minutes to complete a history and examination. The use of standardized instruments can greatly help this process and in so doing add consistency to POP practice. The use of electronic questionnaires facilitates this process and can save staff time in the clinic. The use of such a service online will also help with the triage process (59).

Management of POP is about improving symptoms in a patient with the condition. As such CRO and PRO collection and measurement is highly relevant to the practicing POP clinician as they give a degree of measurement of the condition and allow assessment that the changes to the anatomy have on the patient's perspective of treatment effectiveness, and so provide a measure of the success of the intervention or procedure.

REFERENCES

1. Samuelsson EC, Victor FT, Tibblin G, Svardsudd KF. Signs of genital prolapse in a Swedish population of women 20 to 59 years of age and possible related factors. Am J Obstet Gynecol 1999; 180(2 Pt 1): 299–305.
2. Hendrix SL, Clark A, Nygaard I, et al. Pelvic organ prolapse in the Women's health initiative: gravity and gravidity. Am J Obstet Gynecol 2002; 186: 1160–6.
3. Subak LL, Waetjen LE, van den Eeden S, et al. Cost of pelvic organ prolapse surgery in the United States. Obstet Gynecol 2001; 98: 646–51.
4. Tegerstedt G, Maehle-Schmidt M, Nyren O, Hammarstrom M. Prevalence of symptomatic pelvic organ prolapse in a Swedish population. Int Urogynecol J Pelvic Floor Dysfunct 2005; 16: 497–503.
5. Subramanian D, Szwarcensztein K, Mauskopf JA, Slack MC. Rate, type, and cost of pelvic organ prolapse surgery in Germany, France, and England. Eur J Obstet Gynecol Reprod Biol 2009; 144: 177–81.
6. Avery KN, Bosch JL, Gotoh M, et al. Questionnaires to assess urinary and anal incontinence: review and recommendations. J Urol 2007; 177: 39–49.
7. Coons SJ, Gwaltney CJ, Hays RD, et al. Recommendations on evidence needed to support measurement equivalence between electronic and paper-based patient-reported outcome (PRO) measures: ISPOR ePRO Good Research Practices Task Force report. Value Health 2009; 12: 419–29.
8. Rosenbaum A, Rabenhorst MM, Reddy MK, Fleming MT, Howells NL. A comparison of methods for collecting self-report data on sensitive topics. Violence Vict 2006; 21: 461–71.
9. Guidance for Industry Patient-Reported Outcome Measures: Use in Medical Product Development to Support Labeling Claims, February 2006.
10. Radley SC, Jones GL, Tanguy EA, et al. Computer interviewing in urogynaecology: concept, development and psychometric testing of an electronic pelvic floor assessment questionnaire in primary and secondary care. BJOG 2006; 113: 231–8.
11. Jones GL, Radley SC, Lumb J, Jha S. Electronic pelvic floor symptoms assessment: tests of data quality of ePAQ-PF. Int Urogynecol J Pelvic Floor Dysfunct 2008; 19: 1337–47.
12. Jones GL, Radley SC, Lumb J, Farkas A. Responsiveness of the electronic Personal Assessment Questionnaire-Pelvic Floor (ePAQ-PF). Int Urogynecol J Pelvic Floor Dysfunct 2009; 20: 557–564.
13. Ulrich CM, Wallen GR, Feister A, Grady C. Respondent burden in clinical research: when are we asking too much of subjects? IRB Ethics and Human Research 2005; 27: 17–20.
14. Boynton PM. Administering, analysing, and reporting your questionnaire. BMJ 2004; 328: 1372–5.
15. Cook T, Campbell DT. Quasi-Experimentation: Design and Analysis Issues for Field Settings. Boston, MA: Houghton Mifflin, 1979.
16. Bland JM, Altman DG. Statistics notes: validating scales and indexes. BMJ 2002; 324: 606–7.
17. Guyatt GH, Feeny DH, Patrick DL. Measuring health-related quality of life. Ann Intern Med 1993; 118: 622–9.
18. Jha S, Radley S. Patient experience of an electronic questionnaire in clinical practice. UKCS Poster Presentation, Birmingham, 2007.
19. Barber MD, Kuchibhatla MN, Pieper CF, Bump RC. Psychometric evaluation of 2 comprehensive condition-specific quality of life instruments for women with pelvic floor disorders. Am J Obstet Gynecol 2001; 185: 1388–95.
20. Barber MD, Walters MD, Bump RC. Short forms of two condition-specific quality-of-life questionnaires for women with pelvic floor disorders (PFDI-20 and PFIQ-7). Am J Obstet Gynecol 2005; 193: 103–13.
21. Crosby RD, Kolotkin RL, Williams GR. Defining clinically meaningful change in health-related quality of life. J Clin Epidemiol 2003; 56: 395–407.
22. Wild D, Grove A, Martin M, et al. Principles of good practice for the translation and cultural adaptation process for patient-reported outcomes (PRO) measures: report of the ISPOR task force for translation and cultural adaptation. Value Health 2005; 8: 94–104.
23. Stephenson NL, Herman JA. Pain measurement: a comparison using horizontal and vertical visual analogue scales. Appl Nurs Res 2000; 13: 157–8.
24. Baden W, Walker T. Surgical repair of vaginal defects. Philadelphia: JB Lippincott, 1992.
25. Bump RC, Mattiasson A, Bo K, et al. The standardization of terminology of female pelvic organ prolapse and pelvic floor dysfunction. Am J Obstet Gynecol 1996; 175: 10–17.
26. Swift SE. The distribution of pelvic organ support in a population of female subjects seen for routine gynecologic health care. Am J Obstet Gynecol 2000; 183: 277–85.
27. Swift SE, Pound T, Dias JK. Case-control study of etiologic factors in the development of severe pelvic organ prolapse. Int Urogynecol J Pelvic Floor Dysfunct 2001; 12: 187–92.
28. Swift S. Current opinion on the classification and definition of genital tract prolapse. Curr Opin Obstet Gynecol 2002; 14: 503–7.
29. Digesu GA, Khullar V, Cardozo L, Robinson D, Salvatore S. P-QOL: a validated questionnaire to assess the symptoms and quality of life of women with urogenital prolapse. Int Urogynecol J Pelvic Floor Dysfunct 2005; 16: 176–81; discussion 81.
30. Bradshaw HD, Hiller L, Farkas AG, Radley S, Radley SC. Development and psychometric testing of a symptom index for pelvic organ prolapse. J Obstet Gynaecol 2006; 26: 241–52.
31. Hanley J, Capewell A, Hagen S. Validity study of the severity index, a simple measure of urinary incontinence in women. BMJ 2001; 322: 1096–7.
32. Avery K, Donovan J, Peters TJ, et al. ICIQ: a brief and robust measure for evaluating the symptoms and impact of urinary incontinence. Neurourol Urodyn 2004; 23: 322–30.
33. Shumaker SA, Wyman JF, Uebersax JS, McClish D, Fantl JA. Health-related quality of life measures for women with urinary incontinence: the incontinence impact questionnaire and the urogenital distress inventory. Continence Program in Women (CPW) Research Group. Qual Life Res 1994; 3: 291–306.
34. Uebersax JS, Wyman JF, Shumaker SA, McClish DK, Fantl JA. Short forms to assess life quality and symptom distress for urinary incontinence in women: the incontinence impact questionnaire and the urogenital distress inventory. Continence Program for Women Research Group. Neurourol Urodyn 1995; 14: 131–9.
35. Jackson S, Donovan J, Brookes S, et al. The Bristol female lower urinary tract symptoms questionnaire: development and psychometric testing. Br J Urol 1996; 77: 805–12.
36. Patrick DL, Martin ML, Bushnell DM, et al. Quality of life of women with urinary incontinence: further development of the incontinence quality of life instrument (I-QOL). Urology 1999; 53: 71–6.
37. Lubeck DP, Prebil LA, Peeples P, Brown JS. A health related quality of life measure for use in patients with urge urinary incontinence: a validation study. Qual Life Res 1999; 8: 337–44.
38. Kelleher CJ, Cardozo LD, Khullar V, Salvatore S. A new questionnaire to assess the quality of life of urinary incontinent women. Br J Obstet Gynaecol 1997; 104: 1374–9.
39. Jorge JM, Wexner SD. Etiology and management of fecal incontinence. Dis Colon Rectum 1993; 36: 77–97.
40. Rockwood TH, Church JM, Fleshman JW, et al. Patient and surgeon ranking of the severity of symptoms associated with fecal incontinence: the fecal incontinence severity index. Dis Colon Rectum 1999; 42: 1525–32.
41. Hull TL, Floruta C, Piedmonte M. Preliminary results of an outcome tool used for evaluation of surgical treatment for fecal incontinence. Dis Colon Rectum 2001; 44: 799–805.

42. Rockwood TH, Church JM, Fleshman JW, et al. Fecal incontinence quality of life scale: quality of life instrument for patients with fecal incontinence. Dis Colon Rectum 2000; 43: 9–16; discussion 7.

43. Bug GJ, Kiff ES, Hosker G. A new condition-specific health-related quality of life questionnaire for the assessment of women with anal incontinence. BJOG 2001; 108: 1057–67.

44. Rogers RG, Kammerer-Doak D, Villarreal A, Coates K, Qualls C. A new instrument to measure sexual function in women with urinary incontinence or pelvic organ prolapse. Am J Obstet Gynecol 2001; 184: 552–8.

45. Rogers RG, Coates KW, Kammerer-Doak D, Khalsa S, Qualls C. A short form of the Pelvic Organ Prolapse/Urinary Incontinence Sexual Questionnaire (PISQ-12). Int Urogynecol J Pelvic Floor Dysfunct 2003; 14: 164–8; discussion 8.

46. Symonds T, Boolell M, Quirk F. Development of a questionnaire on sexual quality of life in women. J Sex Marital Ther 2005; 31: 385–97.

47. Rosen R, Brown C, Heiman J, et al. The female sexual function index (FSFI): a multidimensional self-report instrument for the assessment of female sexual function. J Sex Marital Ther 2000; 26: 191–208.

48. McCoy NL. The McCoy Female Sexuality Questionnaire. Quality of Life Research 9: Suppl 1: 739–745.

49. Spitzer WO. State of science 1986: quality of life and functional status as target variables for research. J Chronic Dis 1987; 40: 465–71.

50. Naughton M, Shumaker SA. Assessment of health-related quality of life. In: Furberg CD, ed. Fundamentals of Clinical Trials. St. Louis: Mosby, 1997: 185.

51. Ware JE Jr, Sherbourne CD. The MOS 36-item short-form health survey (SF-36). I. Conceptual framework and item selection. Med Care 1992; 30: 473–83.

52. Naughton MJ, Donovan J, Badia X, et al. Symptom severity and QoL scales for urinary incontinence. Gastroenterology 2004; 126(1 Suppl 1): S114–23.

53. EuroQol—a new facility for the measurement of health-related quality of life. The EuroQol Group. Health Policy 1990; 16: 199–208.

54. Brazier J, Roberts J, Deverill M. The estimation of a preference-based measure of health from the SF-36. J Health Econ 2002; 21: 271–92.

55. Barber MD. Questionnaires for women with pelvic floor disorders. Int Urogynecol J Pelvic Floor Dysfunct 2007; 18: 461–5.

56. Alonso J, Ferrer M, Gandek B, et al. Health-related quality of life associated with chronic conditions in eight countries: results from the International Quality of Life Assessment (IQOLA) Project. Qual Life Res 2004; 13: 283–98.

57. Laumann EO, Paik A, Rosen RC. Sexual dysfunction in the United States: prevalence and predictors. JAMA 1999; 281: 537–44.

58. Laumann E, Gagnon JH, Michael RT, Michaels S. The social organization of sexuality: sexual practices in the United States. Chicago (IL): University of Chicago Press, 1994.

59. Jha S, Radley S, Farkas A. The virtual urogynaecology clinic. IUGA, Tapiei. Oral Poster Presentation, 2008.

19 Economic Aspects of Urinary Incontinence
Kate H Moore

INTRODUCTION

Because health economics is sometimes considered a rather "dry" subject, this chapter is written from the clinician's perspective in an attempt to make the concept "come alive" for continence practitioners. We all need to become more aware of the costs of the treatments that we routinely recommend. We also need to be able to judge whether a new treatment is truly cost effective.

The reason for this is that as our population becomes more aged, the prevalence of urinary incontinence (UI) is likely to relentlessly increase, but our health care budget will probably not keep pace with the demand for continence services. Most countries in the developed world have "controlled" budgets for health. As we all know, the prevalence of lethal conditions such as cardiovascular disease and stroke is also rising with the aging population. Because incontinence is not generally lethal, we must be able to compete with clinicians in other fields of medicine for increasingly precious health care funds.

The recent dilemma of medicated stents for coronary artery disease is a good example. Five years ago, the evidence appeared to show that inserting a medicated stent was a good way to avoid coronary artery bypass graft (CABG) surgery, resulting in large savings to the health economy. The need for long term clopidegrel therapy, with its associated hemorrhagic risks if the patients needed urgent surgery for another condition, was considered a "necessary evil" to allow this cost saving. However in the last year or so, it was found that, in the long term, these medicated stents were still likely to occlude, so the patient was no better off. Now with the passage of time, the pendulum is swinging back to CABG surgery, because it is more cost effective over the long term. Nevertheless, CABG surgery is very expensive and now has been functionally "validated" from an economic perspective (although formal economic studies have not been concluded for all aspects of the above changes).

To some extent, the transition from open Burch colposuspension, moving to laparoscopic colposuspension to allow early discharge with cost savings, then onto the tension-free vaginal tape (TVT) with its re-usable instruments but equivalent if not better efficacy and cost savings, is analogous. In actual fact, long term data is not yet available for the laparascopic procedure. A head to head cost comparison of laparoscopic colposuspension versus TVT has not been conducted. Nevertheless, with the advent of the TVT and trans-obturator procedures, it would seem that we have achieved the same cost savings but with a more robust cure rate, at least in the first 9 to 10 years of the TVT. Attempts to further "mimimalize" bladder neck surgery with the recent "mini" procedures will certainly need long term cost and efficacy data before their true value can be judged.

One of the major issues facing urogynecologists is the fact that the very companies who create and manufacture new surgical devices are the people we look to for funding of clinical trials of these products. Certainly such companies are seriously interested in efficacy data (witness the recent withdrawal of the "minimalistic" TVT Secure device by Gynecare). However, surgical supply companies are not likely to conduct economic analyses for general publication, nor to sponsor this type of work. As business entrepreneurs, they must conduct market analysis and calculate what the market will bear, to thus determine whether they can realistically introduce a new product and still make an appropriate degree of profit. Similar practical constraints limit the ability of pharmaceutical companies to embark upon economic studies when introducing new drugs for incontinence, although government purchasing agents in many countries are now demanding some economic data in order to place new pharmacotherapies onto the government subsidy list.

In order to make sense of what is going on economically, as each new product is introduced to the market (and some are discarded) the continence clinician needs to have a basic understanding of economic analysis in our field. This chapter will deal only with UI in women, in keeping with the subject of this textbook, and also because economic data about fecal incontinence and prolapse is very limited.

Also, because a formal survey of the economics of incontinence has recently been undertaken by a team of health economists and continence clinicians for the International Consultation on Incontinence (1), the present chapter gives a more clinically based summary of economic matters. The chapter is divided into two parts. Part one describes how to interpret an economic study, and part two outlines how to conduct an economic analysis. Throughout each part, important examples will be given from the literature, followed by a summary of important economic analyses in the last decade.

PART ONE: HOW TO INTERPRET AN ECONOMIC STUDY IN THE CONTINENCE FIELD
The Problem of Perspective

The perspective taken by any author in writing any economic analysis is fundamental to interpreting their analysis. For example, pharmaceutical companies often undertake "willingness to pay" (WTP) studies (see below for details of this method) because they are most interested in knowing what patients will pay "out of pocket" for a new medication, if it provides a theoretical degree of symptom relief. But "WTP" studies only consider the patients' perspective and their out of pocket expenses, with no calculation for the government subsidy provided for many drugs in many countries (see below for further discussion).

Surgical authors often look at the costs of a new procedure versus the old standard procedure, but if one looks at these reports critically, they often have a very short term perspective, i.e., 6 to12 months. We only have to remember the "honeymoon" success of the Stamey/Gittes/Raz procedures in the late 1980's, which soon gave way to large failure rates, to be reminded of this important axiom. One cannot stress strongly enough that at least two years, and preferably five years of outcome and economic data should be looked at, before concluding that a new treatment is superior to the old one.

The final note of caution concerns economic models, such as the decision tree and the Markov model. Clinical (non-academic) urogynecologists probably don't realize that an economist can design a Markov model to include whatever input parameters, success rates, procedural costs etc., they wish. Now of course most economists would "fill in" the data in their model with published outcomes from the literature. The problem comes when there is no data to use. Economists may then turn to some theoretical constructs desired from another part of medicine, that really doesn't relate to urogynecology, and try to "plug in the numbers" based on their analogy. This can have unfortunate consequences (see discussion on Markov model on p. 156).

The Different Types of Economic Studies Available: Cost of Illness (COI) Vs. "Economic Analysis" Studies

When reading an economic study, to start with, we need to consider whether one is looking at a COI study, or an analysis of the benefit of one treatment compared with another (hereafter called an economic analysis).

A COI study just simply tabulates all the costs of the incontinence being studied. Usually these studies have three parts. Firstly they consider the *direct costs* of incontinence, which comprise the personal and treatment costs of the condition. The patient's perspective is usually taken first, for personal costs of continence products/laundry/barrier creams etc. Then the "payer" perspective is usually taken, for the costs of investigations and treatments. The payer is often a government body, except in the United States where a combination of Medicare/Medicaid and private insurance payers will be considered. Often investigations and treatments involve some out of pocket "co-payment" from the patient [see Table 19.1, and Dowell et al. (2) for more detail].

As can be seen in Table 19.1, the "payer" for this broad range of direct costs varies considerably, especially in the treatment section. For example, patients in a Public Hospital in most Commonwealth/European countries would seldom have any notion of operating theater fees, as the hospital budget is derived from taxpayer revenue. However, almost all Americans would have a very clear notion of just how costly operating theater fees can be.

Another aspect of the *direct cost* of incontinence, which is not always considered, is the cost of the consequences of being incontinent. Part of the reason that these costs may be missed is that they are controversial. For example, the literature now contains several reports that incontinent people are 26% more likely to fall and 34% more likely to sustain a fracture, than non incontinent people (3). This may occur because they are

Table 19.1 Direct Costs of Incontinence

Personal costs	Incontinence pads, disposable or re-usable laundry costs for re-usable products + urine stained clothes/sheets
	Dry cleaning of urine stained clothes
	Replacement of urine stained clothes
	Cleaning/replacing uriniferous carpets/furniture
	Barrier creams etc., to prevent urine excoriation of skin
	Bed pads, disposable or re-usable
Treatment costs	Specialist visits (urogynecologist, urologist, geriatrician)
	Urodynamic tests, renal/post void ultrasounds
	Mid stream urine cultures, other laboratory tests
	Pharmacotherapy costs
	Physiotherapy/nurse continence advisor treatments
	Catheters for CISC
	Vaginal devices e.g., dish pessaries, contiform
Surgical costs	Anesthetic costs/preop workup
	Surgeons fees
	Theater fees
	Inpatient bed stay fees
	Postop followup, treatment of complications

Abbreviation: CISC, Clean intermittent self-catheterization.

rushing to the toilet with urgency (4), or because they slip over when the urine renders the floor wet. However, this subject was initially quite controversial.

More controversial is the issue of whether incontinence can precipitate admission to a nursing home. The paper by Thom et al. (5) is frequently quoted to show that the risk of admission to a nursing home for an incontinent women age > 65 is twice that of a non-incontinent woman, which of course has huge cost implications. However, the actual study focused upon women who had either Parkinsonism, dementia, stroke, depression, or congestive heart failure, *with or without incontinence.* This would accord with clinical experience(i.e., UI in an otherwise *non-frail* elderly woman does not usually provoke nursing home admission); it is the incontinence on top of the co-morbidities which may provide the "final insult."

The "top down" versus "bottom up" approach to COI: Readers should be aware that many COI studies (and also economic models that are discussed in the next section) can compile their cost data in two ways. The "top down" approach uses large national databases for costs (such as Diagnostic Related Groups in United States/Australia, or the Health Care Resource Group in the United Kingdom) combined with national prevalence data, to give an overall estimate of national expenditure for a particular condition. This is also known as "gross costing." For example see Hu et al. (6). The alternative approach is to conduct individual, face to face enquiries about costs and utilization of resources in a sample of, say, 100 typical patients. This is known as the "bottom up" approach, which is of course more accurate, but much more costly as a researcher has to actually interview all these patients about their incontinence costs in a systematic fashion [for example see (2)]. This method is also known as micro-costing.

Secondly, the *indirect costs* of the condition are considered. These comprise costs arising from the individual losing productivity (e.g., time off work) and the implications for society. In the late 1990's, preliminary data began appearing regarding the impact of incontinence upon working women (7), including teachers (8) and soldiers (9). Between 21% and 33% of such working women suffered from incontinence. The effects upon their productivity included loss of concentration, interference with job performance, needing to take time from work for frequency of micturition, and the tendency to fluid restrict on the job. Nocturia with sleep disturbance leading to impaired daytime performance was also noted.

More recently, Faltz et al. (10) obtained postal questionnaires from 2326 employed American women: 37% had leaked urine in the past month. Severity (on Sandvik index) was slight 52%, moderate 40%, severe 8%. The impact of incontinence upon ability to concentrate, performance of physical activities, self confidence, and ability to complete tasks without interruption increased with the severity of the leak and affected nearly 75% of all those with severe leak status. Similarly, Wu et al. (11) studied the work loss burden of women with overactive bladder (OAB). Absenteeism was 15% higher among 3077 OAB employees compared to 6154 controls. Multivariate analysis showed that OAB subjects had 4.4 more days off work than non-OAB subjects, yielding an excess cost of U.S. $1220 per OAB employee per annum.

A further *indirect cost* of incontinence that is poorly measured to date is the cost of care provided by spouses and informal caregivers. Langa et al. (12) analyzed a large American dataset and estimated the yearly cost of informal continence care at U.S. $6 billion (1998 dollars), or about U.S. $2000 to $4000 per annum for women and men whose incontinence was severe enough to warrant using pads.

Thirdly, a COI study should consider the *intangible costs* of the condition such as pain from urine excoriation or depression from the psychological impact of longstanding unpredictable incontinence. Urge incontinence is known to have a strong association with depressive symptoms (13) which occurs in 60% of those with idiopathic urge incontinence compared to 14% of those with pure stress incontinence, but the economic/cost utility impact of this has not been studied.

Many COI studies have now been published for most European and Commonwealth countries, for example Sweden (14,15), Italy (16), France (17), the United States (18–20), and Australia (2,21,22).

COI studies are now considered somewhat "passe" within the field of health economics. Nevertheless, the urogynecologist should be mindful that few COI studies have been published for fecal incontinence, and very few for prolapse treatments [See (1)].

Formal Economic Analyses
As described, COI studies are not formal economic analyses because they simply summate the costs of the condition for a given population. COI studies provide little information about how to allocate scarce funds for treating particular conditions, because the COI study does not measure the "value" of the treatments under study. The following paragraphs give an overview of the true economic analyses available, ending with focus on the most desirable type, which is a cost utility analysis (CUA).

Cost Minimization Analysis (CMA)
In a CMA study, the costs of alternative health care strategies are compared but we assume at the beginning of the study that the benefits of the two options are very likely to be equivalent. When the two treatments actually prove to be equivalent in their outcomes, complications and patient satisfaction, then a CMA is sufficient; the cheapest intervention is to be desired.

For example, our group undertook a randomized controlled trial of the urogynecologist versus the nurse continence advisor (NCA), in the performance of conservative continence therapy for any mild to moderate incontinence. Nurses were able to give prescriptions for anticholinergic drugs that the urogynecologists had written at the enrollment visit. We hypothesized that the outcomes for each clinician would be similar, which proved true. As might be expected, the nurses were a great deal cheaper, despite the same result (23). CMA studies are actually not that common in the literature.

Cost Consequence Analysis (CCA)
The CCA is a variation on CMA. It tests the hypothesis that a new treatment may result in a greater decrease in health care utilization than a standard treatment. Unfortunately, whether the new treatment gives any benefit in outcome is not assessed, so CCA is not recommended.

Cost Effectiveness Analysis (CEA)
The term CEA covers a broad type of economic analyses wherein the effectiveness is measured by a general health outcome. One can perform a CEA with a narrow outcome such as a pad test but you will miss other important effects. Therefore we generally prefer the use of quality adjusted life years (QALYs) as the most appropriate health outcome in CEA. Once you include QALYs in your analysis, the study becomes known as a CUA.

Cost Utility Analysis
The CUA study is a type of CEA wherein QALYs are used as the outcome measure, to compare two different treatments for the same condition. Gold et al. (24) and Drummond et al. (25) have published texts that discuss standard techniques for conducting a CUA. In the field of medicine, the CUA is now considered to be the gold standard. Utilities capture all potential benefits of an intervention and allow comparisons with other health conditions, which is vitally important. The "bottom line" of both the CEA and the CUA are represented by the incremental cost-effectiveness ratio (ICER). The ICER represents the average cost of the intervention group minus the average cost of the control group. This amount is then divided by the average utility of the intervention group minus the average utility of the control group (see section "Part Two: How to Conduct an Economic Analysis and What Have We Learned from Analyses in the Last Two Decades," for full formula).

155

Cost Benefit Analysis (CBA)

CBA involves measuring the benefits in dollars (or other currency). When everything is measured in dollars, optimal choice can be found by addition and subtraction. However, it is difficult to measure benefits in dollars, and many researchers, policymakers, and clinicians avoid placing a dollar value on life. CBA is rarely used in medicine.

Decision Analysis: Economic Modeling

The above mentioned methods of economic analysis generally involve "real data," e.g., that taken from a randomized clinical trial or even a prospective observational study of one treatment versus the costs of "no intervention." However, there are other forms of economic analysis that involve the construction of a theoretical model, that is then filled in with, or "populated" with samples of data taken from the previous literature.

The two most common of these are the decision analysis, which involves making a decision tree, and a broader based (more all-encompassing) Markov model. In both cases, the first step in the analysis is to identify the structure of the clinical problem, i.e., make a list of all the likely decision alternatives, all the clinical outcomes, and a sequence of events. Then one assigns a mathematical probability to all chance events (e.g., 50% likelihood of cure, 12% likelihood of death, etc.). In step three, one assigns an outcome measure such as a QALY to all outcomes. In the fourth step, one performs the mathematical calculation of the expected utility for each strategy; this may reveal the preferred strategy. Finally one has to test how "robust" the model is (how sensitive the outcomes would be to changes in the input parameters) by performing sensitivity analyses. A range of different inputs such as cure rates are changed, e.g., from 50% to 75%, to see if the model still holds true.

The *decision tree* is easy to understand. A group of patients with a certain type of incontinence enter into theoretical pathway along which they will undergo treatments and have a variety of outcomes. As they pass along the tree, various limbs of the tree branch off—each of these branches is called a "node." A "decision node" is a branching off where the patient or the doctor makes a decision about what kind of treatment to have/administer. A "chance node" is a fork in the tree where a range of chance events occur that the patient or doctor may have little control over, such as "cure," "partial response," "non-response," or complete failure (or they may encounter a complication, such as death, nursing home admission etc.). The final events on the end of the branches of the tree are called the "terminal nodes."

A frequently quoted example of a decision analysis study in the field of incontinence was conducted in 2000 by Weber et al. (26). The authors constructed a model to examine the cost effectiveness of preoperative urodynamic testing in women with prolapse and stress incontinence (with or without complaints of urgency, frequency, nocturia), compared with basic office evaluation (i.e., by history and examination). The costs in the model were "filled in" from U.S. government (Medicare/Medicaid) data.

Figure 19.1 shows the first half of their decision tree, the square box represents the decision node, and the round circles represent the chance nodes (although this was not stated in the original legend).

The relevant efficacy data were obtained from published literature, which yielded a calculation that office testing versus urodynamic testing gave the same cure rate for UI in this group of patients (96%). They calculated that basic office testing was more cost effective than urodynamics, so long as the prevalence of detrusor overactivity (DO) was greater than 8%, or if the cost of urodynamics was more than U.S. $103 (which even in 2000 would be a cheap urodynamic test). The paper is often quoted because it concluded that urodynamic tests are not cost effective for women who have a main complaint of stress incontinence with prolapse. However the model was not necessarily applicable to routine clinical practice because the chosen continence procedure was an abdominovaginal sling and the quoted prevalence of DO in patients with a main complaint of stress leakage has been criticized.

A *Markov model* is slightly superior to a decision tree because it allows the dimension of time to come into the analysis. The decision tree, as shown above, assumes that the chance of particular events such as cure/partial cure/failure is stable over time. However, we know only too well that UI treatments may "look good" immediately after they are given (new drugs, or surgery), but often begin to fail over the longer term. The receptor for the drug may become "resistant," or the surgical sutures may dissolve/become remodeled. Markov models are set up to allow one to incorporate such changes over time. Patients can go through various cycles of moving from one treatment state to another over time. The likelihood of moving from one state to another is given a mathematical probability (using techniques derived from matrix algebra). The final option is to become dead, a state from which they cannot move.

The author of the Markov model needs to define health states and the probability of moving from one to another, as in a decision tree. But also, the author determines the cycle length, or time period overwhich one moves between states (e.g., weeks to months for pharmacotherapy, months to years for surgical studies). The outcome measure regarding treatment effect is the QALY.

A frequently quoted Markov model for elderly home dwelling women with stress incontinence was performed in 1996 by Ramsey et al. (27). Such women were treated by three options; "behavioral therapy" (presumably pelvic floor muscle training), pharmacotherapy with phenylpropanolamine and estrogen, and surgery by needle suspension. Failed surgery was treated by artificial urethral sphincter. All options were based upon the Agency for Health Care Policy and Research guidelines which were widely recognized at the time.

The Markov model is shown in Figure 19.2. In this model, 100 elderly stress incontinent women were treated as above and could move from their initial state (incontinent, living at home) to one of four possible states: (*i*) cured; (*ii*) continued incontinence, at home; (*iii*) continued incontinence but moved to a nursing home; or (*iv*) death. Each Markov cycle ran for one year and the simulation was run for 10 years.

This Markov model has been criticized because phenylpropanolamine with estrogen is no longer used, needle suspensions

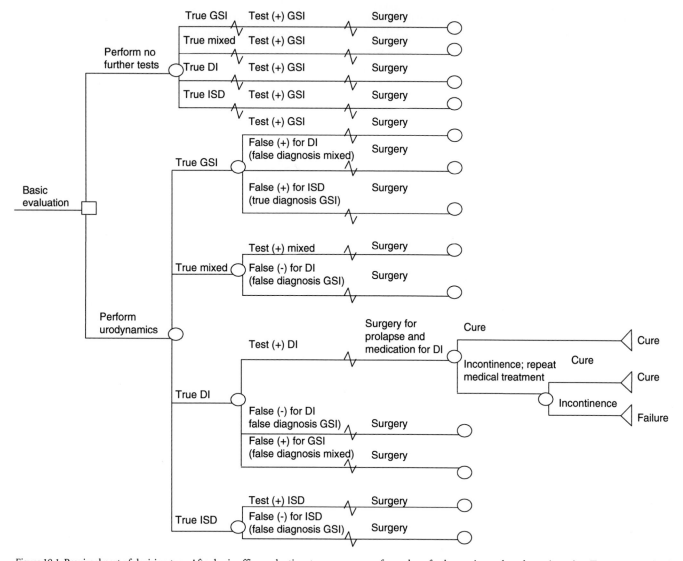

Figure 19.1 Proximal part of decision tree. After basic office evaluation, two groups were formed, no further testing and urodynamic testing. Treatment was instituted according to assigned diagnoses, outcome of treatment was estimated. "Surgery" comprised surgery for prolapse and sling procedure for urinary incontinence. *Abbreviations*: GSI, genuine stress incontinence; DI, detrusor instability; ISD, intrinsic sphincter deficiency. *Source*: From Ref. 26.

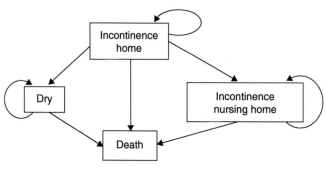

Figure 19.2 Markov model cycle.

the benefits of therapy over the costs of nursing home admission, and was one of the earliest Markov models published in this field.

Before we conclude this section on how to interpret an economic analysis, a few words are needed about the concept of WTP. This method involves giving a group of patients a questionnaire about how much money they would be willing to pay, from their own income, to achieve a given reduction in incontinence. For example (28):

Imagine that a new drug, free of side-effects, against incontinence becomes available, that is not paid for by the state. This new drug reduces the number of times per day you need to go to the bathroom and number of urinary leakages per day by one quarter (25%); this means that if you, for instance, at present need to go to the bathroom 12 times per day and you have four urinary leakages per day, this will be reduced to nine bathroom visits and three urinary leakages per day. Would you choose to take this new drug if you, out of your income, have to pay nine pounds per month (or 100 Swedish krona)?

are no longer considered effective, and the fall back surgery, artificial sphincter, is not widely used for failed needle suspension. This highlights the fact that the author of a Markov model can choose any treatments to "populate" the model that they wish, based upon their reading of the current literature. However the Ramsey model does provide useful insight into

The price can be varied up or down, and the leakage reduction is usually then varied up to 50% benefit.

The authors found that the median amount patients were willing to pay ranged from 240 krona for 25% reduction and 470 krona for 50% reduction. However the authors pointed out that measuring WTP in the Swedish population is difficult, because healthcare costs and the cost of incontinence pads are paid for by the state in Sweden, so patients will not have figured in these costs in their willingness to spend disposable income. Indeed economists dislike WTP, because such questionnaires survey people about their preferences and intents, but do not observe actual behavior. Thus the preferred economic method remains CUA.

PART TWO: HOW TO CONDUCT AN ECONOMIC ANALYSIS AND WHAT HAVE WE LEARNED FROM ANALYSES IN THE LAST TWO DECADES
How to Conduct a CUA
Clearly, the CUA is now the gold standard in economic analyses. The following paragraphs explain ten key points that must be included in a CUA—a how-to guide to achieving the appropriate minimum standard for performing and reporting CUAs. Each point should be explicitly covered in every study (1).

1. The **research question, i.e., the hypothesis that treatment A will be more effective per unit of QALY than treatment B**, must be clearly stated. All CUAs must compare at least two different therapies. One of these should comprise the current standard practice. For example when comparing surgeries for stress incontinence, one of the comparators should be a longstanding method; avoid comparing two *new* methods side by side.

2. The **time frame over which costs and benefits are measured should be long enough to capture the economic impact of an intervention** and all relevant future health outcomes such as treatment failure or complications. Pharmacology studies of 12 weeks duration give very little real economic information, and surgical complications/failures seldom emerge in less than one to two years.

3. **The perspective used by the author must be clearly stated.** Total society perspective (all payers) is the optimum ("gold standard"). Other perspectives, such as the payer or the patient's out of pocket expenses, may be useful but must be stated clearly. When reading an economic analysis of continence treatments, usually comparing an older standard therapy with something new, one must be very careful. The writer may inadvertently have used a narrow perspective, for example, just looking at the treatment costs from the hospital provider perspective as regards savings in bed days or theater consumables.

4. **Probabilities** are needed for each "chance" event, if you are constructing a Markov model or a decision tree (i.e., chance of cure or chance of an adverse event). These should come from meta-analyses of randomized clinical trials (or from individual clinical trials if no meta-analysis).

5. **Costs** should be described in detail, including exactly how the "charges," "bills," or co-payments were derived. The year of the cost data should be given, because studies are often not published until months or years after the data was actually collected.

6. **Outcome measure:** Measures of effectiveness depend on the type and objectives of analysis. QALYs are the gold standard, as described previously in this text in chapter 12.

7. **Analytic model:** If a real clinical study is not being used, but a Markov model or decision tree is being constructed, then each intervention must be described and possible courses of events identified, including the expected course of disease, treatments, complications, and outcomes.

8. **Discounting:** Since the value of both costs and benefits may decrease over time, discounting is used to calculate the present value of money and health states that will occur in the future. Future costs and utilities should be discounted to present value; 3% per year is a recommended starting point.

9. **Incremental analysis:** The purpose of a CUA is to describe the relative value of one health care strategy compared to another. An ICER is the incremental cost divided by the incremental effectiveness of intervention a compared to intervention b, and is calculated as follows.

$$ICER = \frac{\text{Average cost}_{\text{intervention a}} - \text{Average cost}_{\text{intervention b}}}{\text{Average utility}_{\text{intervention a}} - \text{Average utility}_{\text{intervention b}}}$$

Averages should be used (not medians), because we want to see the effect of statistical outliers. The "leverage" of the outliers should then be tested in a sensitivity analysis.

10. **Sensitivity analysis:** A sensitivity analysis should allow the reader to understand whether the conclusion of the analysis would hold true if either the costs or the probabilities (of cure or complications) were to vary substantially. For example if one treatment costs 5000 Euro and has a cure rate of 90%, and the second treatment costs 2000 Euro with a cure rate of 80%, then the ICER will assess whether the resultant benefit in QALY/quality of life makes the first treatment worthwhile. The author should then vary the costs and the cure rates in the model, to see how much variation in real life would be allowed for the conclusion to remain valid.

What Have We Learned from Economic Analyses in the Past Decade?
This overview of our current state of knowledge about incontinence costs is organized according to the type of incontinence (stress, urge, or mixed). Conservative treatments will be considered followed by surgical treatments.

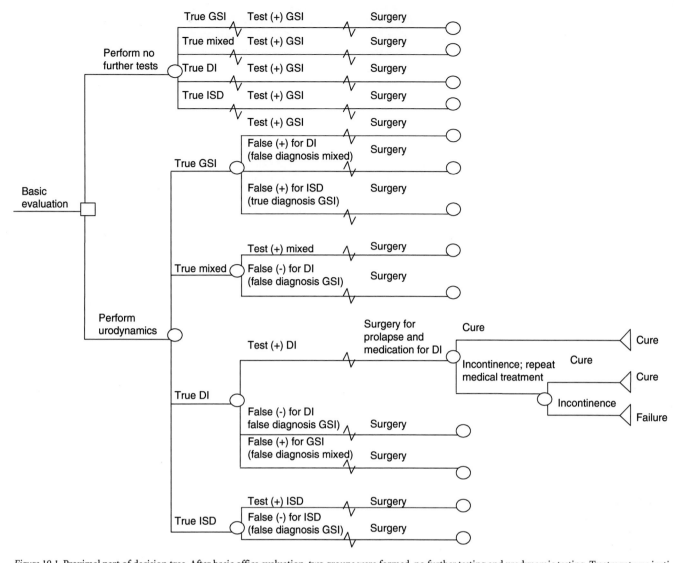

Figure 19.1 Proximal part of decision tree. After basic office evaluation, two groups were formed, no further testing and urodynamic testing. Treatment was instituted according to assigned diagnoses, outcome of treatment was estimated. "Surgery" comprised surgery for prolapse and sling procedure for urinary incontinence. *Abbreviations*: GSI, genuine stress incontinence; DI, detrusor instability; ISD, intrinsic sphincter deficiency. *Source*: From Ref. 26.

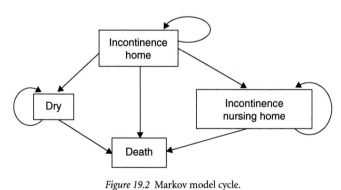

Figure 19.2 Markov model cycle.

are no longer considered effective, and the fall back surgery, artificial sphincter, is not widely used for failed needle suspension. This highlights the fact that the author of a Markov model can choose any treatments to "populate" the model that they wish, based upon their reading of the current literature. However the Ramsey model does provide useful insight into

the benefits of therapy over the costs of nursing home admission, and was one of the earliest Markov models published in this field.

Before we conclude this section on how to interpret an economic analysis, a few words are needed about the concept of WTP. This method involves giving a group of patients a questionnaire about how much money they would be willing to pay, from their own income, to achieve a given reduction in incontinence. For example (28):

Imagine that a new drug, free of side-effects, against incontinence becomes available, that is not paid for by the state. This new drug reduces the number of times per day you need to go to the bathroom and number of urinary leakages per day by one quarter (25%); this means that if you, for instance, at present need to go to the bathroom 12 times per day and you have four urinary leakages per day, this will be reduced to nine bathroom visits and three urinary leakages per day. Would you choose to take this new drug if you, out of your income, have to pay nine pounds per month (or 100 Swedish krona)?

The price can be varied up or down, and the leakage reduction is usually then varied up to 50% benefit.

The authors found that the median amount patients were willing to pay ranged from 240 krona for 25% reduction and 470 krona for 50% reduction. However the authors pointed out that measuring WTP in the Swedish population is difficult, because healthcare costs and the cost of incontinence pads are paid for by the state in Sweden, so patients will not have figured in these costs in their willingness to spend disposable income. Indeed economists dislike WTP, because such questionnaires survey people about their preferences and intents, but do not observe actual behavior. Thus the preferred economic method remains CUA.

PART TWO: HOW TO CONDUCT AN ECONOMIC ANALYSIS AND WHAT HAVE WE LEARNED FROM ANALYSES IN THE LAST TWO DECADES
How to Conduct a CUA

Clearly, the CUA is now the gold standard in economic analyses. The following paragraphs explain ten key points that must be included in a CUA—a how-to guide to achieving the appropriate minimum standard for performing and reporting CUAs. Each point should be explicitly covered in every study (1).

1. The **research question, i.e., the hypothesis that treatment A will be more effective per unit of QALY than treatment B**, must be clearly stated. All CUAs must compare at least two different therapies. One of these should comprise the current standard practice. For example when comparing surgeries for stress incontinence, one of the comparators should be a longstanding method; avoid comparing two *new* methods side by side.

2. The **time frame over which costs and benefits are measured should be long enough to capture the economic impact of an intervention** and all relevant future health outcomes such as treatment failure or complications. Pharmacology studies of 12 weeks duration give very little real economic information, and surgical complications/failures seldom emerge in less than one to two years.

3. **The perspective used by the author must be clearly stated.** Total society perspective (all payers) is the optimum ("gold standard"). Other perspectives, such as the payer or the patient's out of pocket expenses, may be useful but must be stated clearly. When reading an economic analysis of continence treatments, usually comparing an older standard therapy with something new, one must be very careful. The writer may inadvertently have used a narrow perspective, for example, just looking at the treatment costs from the hospital provider perspective as regards savings in bed days or theater consumables.

4. **Probabilities** are needed for each "chance" event, if you are constructing a Markov model or a decision tree (i.e., chance of cure or chance of an adverse event). These should come from meta-analyses of randomized clinical trials (or from individual clinical trials if no meta-analysis).

5. **Costs** should be described in detail, including exactly how the "charges," "bills," or co-payments were derived. The year of the cost data should be given, because studies are often not published until months or years after the data was actually collected.

6. **Outcome measure:** Measures of effectiveness depend on the type and objectives of analysis. QALYs are the gold standard, as described previously in this text in chapter 12.

7. **Analytic model:** If a real clinical study is not being used, but a Markov model or decision tree is being constructed, then each intervention must be described and possible courses of events identified, including the expected course of disease, treatments, complications, and outcomes.

8. **Discounting:** Since the value of both costs and benefits may decrease over time, discounting is used to calculate the present value of money and health states that will occur in the future. Future costs and utilities should be discounted to present value; 3% per year is a recommended starting point.

9. **Incremental analysis:** The purpose of a CUA is to describe the relative value of one health care strategy compared to another. An ICER is the incremental cost divided by the incremental effectiveness of intervention a compared to intervention b, and is calculated as follows.

$$ICER = \frac{\text{Average cost}_{\text{intervention a}} - \text{Average cost}_{\text{intervention b}}}{\text{Average utility}_{\text{intervention a}} - \text{Average utility}_{\text{intervention b}}}$$

Averages should be used (not medians), because we want to see the effect of statistical outliers. The "leverage" of the outliers should then be tested in a sensitivity analysis.

10. **Sensitivity analysis:** A sensitivity analysis should allow the reader to understand whether the conclusion of the analysis would hold true if either the costs or the probabilities (of cure or complications) were to vary substantially. For example if one treatment costs 5000 Euro and has a cure rate of 90%, and the second treatment costs 2000 Euro with a cure rate of 80%, then the ICER will assess whether the resultant benefit in QALY/quality of life makes the first treatment worthwhile. The author should then vary the costs and the cure rates in the model, to see how much variation in real life would be allowed for the conclusion to remain valid.

What Have We Learned from Economic Analyses in the Past Decade?

This overview of our current state of knowledge about incontinence costs is organized according to the type of incontinence (stress, urge, or mixed). Conservative treatments will be considered followed by surgical treatments.

Stress Incontinence

There has been surprisingly little economic data generated about conservative treatment for stress incontinence. Neuman et al. (29) calculated the physiotherapy treatment costs for 274 women with stress incontinence in Australia. A median of 5 [interquartile range (IQR) 4–6] treatments were given, for a median cost of AU $250 (IQR 206–295). Of the patients who completed therapy, 84% were dry on a stress test. Improvement was seen on Kings health questionnaire, but utilities were not collected. This appears to be the first prospective study of physiotherapy costs for stress incontinence. Monz et al. (30) studied total costs of physiotherapy treatment in France, Germany, Spain, Sweden, and the United Kingdom. These ranged from 64 Euro to 467 Euro (for a range of 4–10 prescribed visits).

As regards conservative therapy for urge and mixed incontinence, Williams et al. (31), of the Leicestershire U.K. MRC Incontinence Study Team undertook a large randomized controlled trials (RCT) of conservative therapy. Personal and treatment costs were measured (year 2001). A sample of 3746 men and women were randomized in a 4:1 ratio to either treatment by a specialist NCA (who provided conservative therapy and urodynamic testing) or access to routine continence care by their general practitioner and local continence nurse. Cure at six months occurred in 28% versus 19% (95% CI 5–13, p < 0.001). The intervention costs at six months (252 pounds, IQR 234–268) were greater than the routine costs (73 pounds, IQR 53–93). Cost utilities were not collected.

Subak et al. (20) performed a "bottom up" analysis of the personal "routine care" costs (pads and laundry questionnaire) of incontinence in 293 women age over 40 who had stress or urge leak more than three times per week, wanted help, but had not been treated in the previous three months. Quality of life was tested by Health Utilities Index Mark 3 and WTP for incontinence was determined. Women were willing to pay U.S. $70 per month for 100% reduction in the frequency of incontinence. WTP increased 2.3-fold in the highest income bracket compared to the lowest. WTP for improvement exceeded the routine care costs by three to seven fold.

Ho et al. (22) performed a "bottom up" study of the short and long-term direct costs of conservative and surgical management of childbirth-related stress and mixed UI in 150 women. During active treatment in the unit, patients with stress UI treated conservatively incurred a median cost of AU $658 per capita (IQR 476–1191 AU$) compared to a median cost of AU $6870 per capita for surgical treatment (IQR 6320–7508 AU$). Similar cost difference was seen for the two treatment options for mixed incontinence. Of regular clinic attendees, 39% of conservatively treated and 78% of surgically treated patients were cured. At 6 to 13 years follow up, treatment expenditure was measured by postal questionnaire. Of 82 women with a known address, 43 (52%) responded to the survey, of whom 46% remained cured. The median treatment cost for the total group of postnatal incontinence (irrespective of continence status) was AU $885 per capita per annum (IQR 338–2589).

Before moving on to the cost effectiveness of surgical treatments, a few words about *vaginal devices* are needed. Although a range of such continence devices are available (such as Contigard vaginal sponge, Introl bladder neck support device, Femassist urethral occlusive device, and Contiform vaginal ring), economic analyses of these are uncommon. However, a good lesson about the importance of such economic testing can be learned from the story of the Femassist device.

When it was first launched, the device was estimated to cost AU $12.50 (in 1997, then about 8 Euros) and was to be changed weekly by the patient. Staff from our unit developed an incontinence cost index (2) then measured incontinence costs before and after using the Femassist (32). The median person costs fell from AU $6.52 per week (IQR 1.5, 10.6) down to a median of 1.57 per week (IQR 0.84–4.89). Thus the savings provided by the device in this group of 100 women with moderate leakage on pad test (typical of those who might want to use it) was not equivalent to the cost of the device. Unfortunately production of the device ceased about 10 years later.

As regards *surgery for stress incontinence*, Cody et al. (33) performed a systematic review of the cost effectiveness of TVT versus other standard surgeries for stress incontinence. Using a Markov model, the TVT dominated the open colposuspension (lower costs with similar QALYs) within five years. The authors pointed out that there were no RCT data beyond two years however. Wu et al. (34) also developed a Markov model to compare TVT versus colposuspension at 10 years, with similar findings but with a similar proviso that no such long term data exist. Much of the economic data used in the Markov models arose from the now-famous RCT of Manca et al. (35), which compared TVT to open colposuspension at six months. Procedural and convalescence resource use costs were collected directly from the 344 trial participants, then health care consumption was estimated from the British NHS data, along with QALYs (on the EQ-5D) The TVT saved 243 pounds per patient and gave slightly higher QALY benefits (0.01 units of QALY). Dumville et al. (36), compared laparoscopic versus open colposuspension as part of a RCT. Analysis of costs and QALYs (on EQ-5D) at six months revealed a mean increase of 372 pounds for the laparoscopic procedure, but a QALY benefit of 0.005, yielding an ICER of 744,000 pounds at six months.

Urge Incontinence

As regards *conservative therapy of urge incontinence*, there have been no cost effectiveness studies of first line therapy, bladder retraining. However, many "economic studies" of pharmacotherapy have been undertaken, albeit many are of uncertain economic quality as they are funded by the relevant pharmaceutical company.

The Food and Drug Administration of the United States does not evaluate economic data when looking at a new drug, but insurance companies or government purchasers often require such data. In the United Kingdom, the National Institute for Health and Clinical Excellence (NICE) does require economic review; they have withheld approval for new drugs that have an ICER greater than £30,000 per QALY.

An independently funded study by Ko et al. (37), performed economic evaluation of five antimuscarinic drugs [both immediate release "usual" form and extended release (ER) forms] for the treatment of OAB. They compared oxybutynin, ER-oxybutynin, transdermal oxybutynin, tolterodine, ER tolterodine, trospium, solifenacin, and darifenacin. Solifenacin had the lowest costs and greatest effectiveness for OAB. However, their analysis did not comply with the ten steps recommended for CEA (see page 158). The perspective was that of the payer (rather than a societal perspective), the time frame was too short (3 months) and complete continence was the main effectiveness measure (rather than QALYs).

Most economic studies in this field compare oxybutynin to tolterodine. Guest et al. (38) compared the cost-effectiveness of oxybutynin, oxybutynin ER, and tolterodine. A six-month decision model was devised, using the payer's perspective and short-term clinical endpoints (daily incontinence episodes and daily voids). Oxybutynin ER appeared to be the most cost-effective treatment. Getsios et al. (39), conducted two economic evaluations comparing oxybutynin ER to tolterodine, and found that oxybutynin ER may be cost-effective to tolterodine. Hughes and Dubois (40), undertook a cautiously worded CEA model. O'Brien et al. (41), performed a CEA using a one year Markov model regarding tolterodine for patients who discontinued oxybutynin, using the payer perspective. The incremental cost per QALY was CA $9982 (year of costs not stated) the sensitivity analysis suggested that the conclusion was valid across a range of input data.

Getsios et al. (42) reviewed economic studies for OAB, highlighting the limitations, including a lack of comparison between drugs and behavioral training. The UTIN group (43) is currently conducting a clinical trial comparing behavioral treatments to medications for urge incontinence. This important study will measure costs and utilities, and through a NIH-funded substudy, separate researchers will conduct parallel economic evaluation of this trial.

As regards *surgery for DO*, Wielink et al. (44), examined the costs of sacral anterior root stimulation versus routine care costs for 51 patients with spinal cord lesions. At that time, the Brindley stimulator was being used. The baseline pre-implantation costs were U.S. $1965 per annum. The implantation costs of the procedure and hospital stay were U.S. $13,933. After implantation, direct routine care costs dropped to U.S. $593 per annum. The Nottingham health profile scores did not reveal significant benefit but other scores related to incontinence impact showed benefit. The long term model showed the stimulation implantation to be cheaper than routine care after eight years.

More recently, the economic impact of the InterStim sacral nerve stimulator in 65 patients (45) yielded a 73% reduction in average annual office visit expenses and a 30% reduction in drug expenditures. A Cochrane review of sacral neuromodulation implanted devices (46) www.thecochranelibrary.com reported that no formal economic analysis of this treatment has been undertaken. Similarly Kalsi et al. (47) studied the costs of botox injections for OAB patients, but QALYs were not measured.

SUMMARY AND CONCLUSIONS

Looking at the past two decades of economic studies for UI, we have certainly come a long way. Twenty years ago, we were still trying to establish the basic COI in a range of countries and health care models. In the last ten years, as some continence clinicians have developed collaboration with health economists, we are beginning to see formal economic analyses of some of the more important questions in this field.

Twenty years ago, doctors essentially controlled the health care budget. As long as we could show efficacy and safety, the treatment was eventually implemented even though there might be preliminary delay.

As government bodies such as NICE (and American insurance companies/Health maintanence organizations) gain ever more control of the outflow of monies to patients and health services, we need to generate economic data to show that a new treatment is not just more effective, but is more cost effective, than the old standard. If we clinicians don't generate the raw data, then the health economists will create "top down" economic simulations such as decision trees or Markov models, to be used instead of real economic data from randomized controlled trials. If the conclusions drawn from such theoretical models don't mirror real life data, we have only ourselves to blame for the lack of true economic data, and for the health policies that may be derived from these mathematical models.

ACKNOWLEDGMENTS

I wish to thank my co-authors of the recent ICI chapter entitled "Economics of Urinary and Fecal Incontinence and Prolapse; Report of the 4th International Consultation on Incontinence," TW Hu, L Subak T, Wagner, and M Deutekom, for their shared intellectual input, some of which will have distilled into the present chapter however unintentionally.

REFERENCES

1. Moore KH, Hu TW, Subak L, Wagner TH, Deutekom M. Economics of urinary and faecal incontinence, and Prolapse. Report of 4th International Consultation on Incontinence. In: Abrams P, Cardozo L, Koury S, Wein A, eds. Incontinence. Plymouth: Health Publications Ltd., 2009: 1685–712.
2. Dowell CJ, Bryant CM, Moore KH, Simons AM. Calculation of the direct costs of urinary incontinence: the DBICI, a new test instrument. Brit J Urol 1999; 83: 596–606.
3. Brown J, Vittinghof E, Wyman J, et al. Urinary incontinence: does it increase risk for falls and fractures? Study of Osteoporotic Fractures Research Group. J Am Geriatr Soc 2000; 48: 721–5.
4. Wagner T, Hut, Bentkover J, et al. Estimated economic costs of overactive bladder in the US. Urology 2003; 61: 1123–8.
5. Thom DH, Haan MN, Van den Eeden SK. Medically recognized urinary incontinence and risks of hospitalization, nursing home admission and mortality. Age Ageing 1997; 26: 367–74.
6. Hu TW, Wagner TH, Bentkover JD, et al. Costs of urinary incontinence and overactive bladder in the United States: a comparative study. Urology 2004; 63: 461–5.
7. Palmer MH, Fitzgerald S, Berry SJ, Hart K. Urinary incontinence in working woman: an exploratory study. Women Health1999; 29: 67–80.
8. Nygaard JE, Linder M. Thirst at work—an occupational hazard? Int Urogynecol J Pelvic Floor Dysfunction 1997; 8: 3.40–3.
9. Davis G, Sherman R, Wong MF, et al. Urinary incontinence among female soldiers. Military Med 1999; 164: 182–7.
10. Faltz N, Girts T, Kinchen K, et al. Prevalence, management and impact of urinary incontinence in the workplace. Occup Med (Lond) 2005; 55: 552–7.
11. Wu EQ, Birnbaum H, Marynchenko M, et al. Employees with overactive bladder: work loss burden. J Occup Environ Med 2005; 47: 439–46.

12. Langa KM, Fultz NH, Saint S, Kabeto MU, Herzog AR. Informal care giving time and costs for urinary incontinence in older individuals in the United States. J Am Geriatr Soc 2002; 50: 733–7.

13. Zorn BH, Montgomery H, Pieper K, Gray M, Steers WD. Urinary incontinence and depression. J Urol 1999; 102: 82–4.

14. Milsom I, Fall M, Ekelund P. Urinary incontinence an expensive national disease. Lakartidningen 1992; 89: 1772–4.

15. Samuelsson E, Mansson L, Milsom I. Incontinence aids in Sweden: users and costs. Brit J Urol Int 2001; 88: 893–8.

16. Tediosi F, Parazzini F, Bortolotti A, Garattini L. The cost of urinary incontinence in Italian women: a cross sectional study. Pharmacoeconomics 2000; 17: 71–6.

17. Ballanger P, Rischmannp. Incontinence urinaire de la femme: evaluation et traitment. Prog Urol 1995; 5: 739–63.

18. Wagner T, Hu T. Economic costs of urinary incontinence in 1995. Urology 1998; 51; 355–61.

19. Wilson L, Oark GE, Luc KO, Brown JA, Subak LL. Annual costs of urinary incontinence. Obstet Gynecol 2001; 98: 398–406.

20. Subak LL, Brown JS, Draus SR, et al., Diagnostic Aspects of Incontinence Study Group. The costs of urinary incontinence for women. Obstets & Gynecol 2006; 107: 908–16.

21. Doran CM, Chiarelli P, Cockburn J, et al. Economic costs of urinary incontenince in community-dwelling Australian Women. Med J Aust 2001; 174: 456–8.

22. Ho MT, Kuteesa W, Short A, Eastwood A, Moore KH. Personal and treatment costs of childbirth related incontinence. Neurourol & Urodyn 2006; 25: 513–14.

23. Moore KH, O'sullivan RJ, Simons A, et al. Randomized controlled trial of nurse continence advisor therapy versus standard urogynaecology regime for conservative incontinence treatment: efficacy, costs and two year follow up. Brit J Obstet & Gynae 2003; 110: 649–57.

24. Gold MR, Siegel JE, Russell LB, Weinstein MC, eds. Cost-Effectiveness in Health and Medicine. Oxford: Oxford University Press, 1996.

25. Drummond MF, O'brien B, Stoddart GL, Torrance GW. Methods for the Economic Evaluation of Health Care Programmes, 2nd edn. Oxford: Oxford University Press, 1997.

26. Weber AM, Walters MD. Cost effectiveness of urodynamic testing before surgery for women with pelvic organ prolapse and stress urinary incontinence. Am J Obstet Gynecol 2000; 183: 1338–46.

27. Ramsey SD, Wagner TH, Bavendam TG. Estimated costs of treating stress urinary incontinence in elderly women according to the AHCPR clinical practice guidelines. Am J Man Care 1996; 2: 147–54.

28. Johannesson M, O'Conor RM, Kobelt-Nguyen G, Mattiasson A. Willingness to pay for reduced incontinence symptoms. Brit J Urol 1997; 80: 557–62.

29. Neumann PD, Grimmer KA, Grant RE, Gill VA. The costs and benefits of physiotherapy as first-line treatment for female stress urinary incontinence. Aust N Z J Public Health 2005; 29: 416–21.

30. Monz B, Hampel C, Porkes S, et al. A description of health care provision and access to treatment for women with urinary incontinence in Europe—a five country comparison. Maturitas 2005; 52S: S3–12.

31. Williams KS, Assessa RP, Cooper NJ, et al. and the Leicestershire MRC Incontinence Study Team. Clinical and cost-effectiveness of a new nurse-led continence service: a randomised controlled trial. Br J Gen Pract 2005; 55: 696–703.

32. Simons AM, Dowell CJ, Bryant CM, Prashar S, Moore KH. Use of the Dowell Bryant incontinence cost index as a post-treatment outcome measure. Neurourol & Urodyn 2001; 20: 85–93.

33. Cody J, Wyness L, Wallace S, et al. Systematic review of the clinical effectiveness and cost-effectiveness of tension-free vaginal tape for treatment of urinary stress incontinence. Health Technol Assess 2003; 7: iii, 1–189.

34. Wu JM, Visco AG, Weidner AC, Myers ER. Is Burch colposuspension ever cost-effective compared with tension-free vaginal tape for stress incontinence? Am J Obstet Gynecol 2007; 197: 62.e1–5.

35. Manca A, Sculpher MJ, Ward K, Hilton P. A cost-utility analysis of tension-free vaginal tape versus colposuspension for primary urodynamic stress incontinence. BJOG 2003; 110: 255–62.

36. Dumville JC, Manca A, Kitchener HC, et al. COLPO study group. Cost-effectiveness analysis of open colposuspension versus laparoscopic colposuspension in the treatment of urodynamic stress incontinence. BJOG 2006; 113: 1014–22.

37. Ko Y, Malone DC, Armstrong EP. Pharmacoeconomic evaluation of antimuscarinic agents for the treatment of overactive bladder. Pharmacotherapy 2006; 26: 1694–702.

38. Guest JF, Abegunde D, Ruiz FJ. Cost effectiveness of controlled-release oxybutynin compared with immediate-release oxybutynin and tolterodine in the treatment of overactive bladder in the UK, France and Austria. Clin Drug Investig 2004; 24: 305–21.

39. Getsios D, Caro JJ, Ishak KJ, et al. Oxybutynin extended release and tolterodine immediate release: a health economic comparison. Clin Drug Investig 2004; 24: 81–8.

40. Hughes DA, Dubois D. Cost-effectiveness analysis of extended-release formulations of oxybutynin and tolterodine for the management of urge incontinence. Pharmacoeconomics 2004; 22: 1047–59.

41. O'brien BJ, Goeree R, Bernard L, Rosner A, Williamson T. Cost-effectiveness of tolterodine for patients with urge incontinence who discontinue initial therapy with oxybutynin: a Canadian perspective. Clin Ther 2001; 23: 2038–49.

42. Getsios D, El-Hadi W, Caro I, Caro JJ. Pharmacological management of overactive bladder: a systematic and critical review of published economic evaluations. Pharmacoeconomics 2005; 23: 995–1006.

43. UTIN study group. Design of the behavior enhances drug reduction of incontinence (BE-DRI) study. Contemp Clin Trials 2007; 28: 48–58.

44. Wielink G, Essink-Bot ML, Van Kerrebroeck PH, Rutten FF. Sacral rhizotomies and electrical bladder stimulation in spinal cord injury. Eur Urol 1997; 31: 441–6.

45. Aboseif SR, Kim DH, Rieder JM, et al. Sacral neuromodulation: cost considerations and clinical benefits. Urology 2007; 70: 1069–74.

46. Herbison GP, Arnold EP. Sacral neuromodulation with implanted devices for urinary storage and voiding dysfunction in adults, 2009. [Available from: www.thecochranelibrary.com].

47. Kalsi V, Popat RB, Apostolidis, et al. Cost consequence analysis evaluating the use of butulinum neurotoxin—a in patients with detrusor overactivity based on clinical outcomes observed at a single UK centre. European Urology 2006; 49: 519–27.

20 Anatomy
John OL DeLancey

FUNCTIONAL ANATOMY OF THE LOWER URINARY TRACT

The inseparable relationship between structure and function in living organisms is one of the common themes found in biology. The anatomy and clinical behavior of the lower urinary tract exemplify this immutable link. The following descriptions are intended to offer a brief overview of some clinically relevant aspects of lower urinary tract structure that help us understand the normal and abnormal behavior of this system. Because of the importance of the pelvic floor to lower urinary tract function, comments on the structure of the lower urinary tract organs are followed by a section describing the structure of the pelvic floor as it relates to micturition, continence, and pelvic organ support.

The lower urinary tract can be divided into the bladder and urethra. At the junction of these two continuous, yet discrete, structures lies the vesical neck. This hybrid structure represents that part of the lower urinary tract where the urethral lumen traverses the bladder wall before becoming surrounded by the urethral wall. It contains portions of the bladder muscle, and also elements that continue into the urethra.

The vesical neck is considered separately because of its functional differentiation from the bladder and the urethra. The spatial relationships of this region are illustrated in Figure 20.1 and described in Table 20.1.

Bladder

The bladder consists of the detrusor muscle, covered by an adventitia and serosa over its dome, and lined by a submucosa and transitional cell epithelium. The muscular layers of the detrusor are not discrete; nevertheless, in general, the outer and inner layers of the detrusor musculature tend to be longitudinal, with an intervening circular—oblique layer.

Two prominent bands on the dorsal aspect of the bladder form one of the prominent landmarks of detrusor musculature (1). They are derived from the outer longitudinal layer and pass beside the urethra to form a loop on its anterior aspect, called the detrusor loop. On the anterior aspect of this loop, some detrusor fibers leave the region of the vesical neck and attach to the pubic bones and pelvic walls; these are called the pubovesical muscles and are discussed below.

Trigone

Within the bladder there is a visible triangular area known as the vesical trigone. The two ureteral orifices and the internal urinary meatus form its apices. The base of the triangle, the interureteric ridge, forms a useful landmark in cystoscopic identification of the ureteric orifices. This triangular elevation is caused by the presence of a specialized group of smooth muscle fibers that lie within the detrusor and arise from a separate embryologic primordium. They are continuous above with the ureteral smooth muscle (2); below, they continue down the urethra. In addition to their visible triangular elevation, these muscle fibers form a ring inside the detrusor loop at the level of the internal urinary meatus (3) (Fig. 20.2).

Some fibers continue down the dorsal surface of the urethra and lie between the ends of the U-shaped striated sphincter muscles of the urethra. These smooth muscle fibers of the trigone are clearly separable from those of the detrusor by the smaller size of their fascicles and greater density of surrounding connective tissue. The mucosa over the trigone frequently undergoes squamous metaplasia and therefore differs from that in the rest of the bladder. The circumferential distribution of the trigonal ring fibers at the vesical neck might contribute to closure of the lumen of the vesical neck in this area, but its role has yet to be fully elucidated.

Urethra

The urethra holds urine in the bladder and is therefore an important structure that helps determine urinary continence. Although for many years the urethra was thought to be relatively unimportant in the cause of stress urinary incontinence recent research has indicated that it is actually the primary factor responsible for stress incontinence. Proper matching of cases with stress incontinence and true asymptomatic controls has revealed that more than 50% of stress incontinence is directly attributable to maximum urethra closure pressure (4).

The urethra is a complex tubular viscus extending below the bladder. In its upper third it is clearly separable from the adjacent vagina, but its lower portion is fused with the wall of the latter structure. Embedded within its substance are a number of elements that are important to lower urinary tract function; their locations are summarized in Table 20.1 (5). MRI is being used more frequently to visualize the components of the urethra and suggests functional interpretations of findings in an effort to correlate clinical anatomy with pathophysiology of incontinence (6–8).

Striated Urogenital Sphincter

The outer layer of the urethra is formed by the muscle of the striated urogenital sphincter (Figs. 20.3 and 20.4) which is found from approximately 20% to 80% of the total urethral length (measured as a percentage of the distance from the internal meatus to the external meatus). In its upper two-thirds, the sphincter fibers lie in a primarily circular orientation; distally, they leave the confines of the urethra and either encircle the vaginal wall as the urethrovaginal sphincter or extend along the inferior pubic ramus above the perineal membrane (urogenital diaphragm) as the compressor urethrae. This muscle is composed largely of slow-twitch muscle

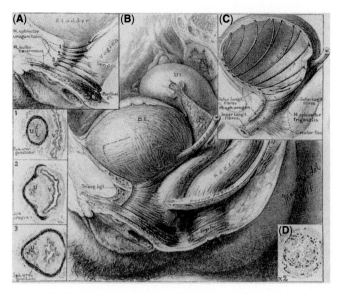

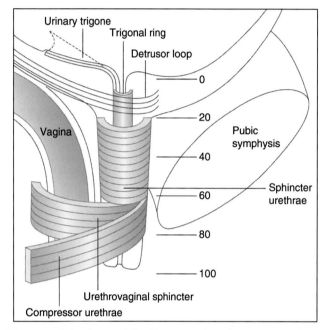

Figure 20.1 The lower urinary tract, including the striated urogenital sphincter muscle. Panel (**A**) shows the components of the striated urogenital sphincter muscle with the numbered elements 1, 2, & 3 shown below in cross section. Panel (**B**) represents the relationship of the urethral muscles to the surrounding pelvic organs. Panel (**C**) displays the fiber direction of muscles within the detrusor. Panel (**D**) indicates the urethra's vascularity in cross section.

Table 20.1 Topography of Urethral and Paraurethral Structures[a]

Approximate location[b]	Region of the urethra	Paraurethral structures
0–20	Intramural urethra	Urethral lumen traverses the bladder wall
20–60	Midurethra	Sphincter urethrae muscle
		Pubovesical muscle
		Vaginolevator attachment
60–80	Perineal membrane	Compressor urethrae muscle
		Urethrovaginal sphincter muscle
80–100	Distal urethra	Bulbocavernosus muscle

[a]Smooth muscle of the urethra was not considered.
[b]Expressed as a percentage of total urethral length.
Source: Reproduced from Ref. 5 with permission.

fibers (9), which are well suited to maintaining the constant tone exhibited by this muscle. In addition, voluntary muscle activation increases urethral constriction during times when increased closure pressure is needed. In the distal urethra, this striated muscle compresses the urethra from above; proximally, it constricts the lumen. Studies of skeletal muscle blockade suggest that this muscle is responsible for approximately one-third of resting urethral closure pressure (10).

Recent research has shown that the amount of striated muscle declines considerably with age (11). This is associated with a decline in innervating nerves (12). First vaginal delivery also results in changes in electromyographic patterns of striated sphincter musculature that is consistent with impaired muscular function persisting for at least six months beyond delivery (13).

Figure 20.2 Striated urogenital sphincter muscle and trigonal musculature within the bladder base and urethra (cut in sagittal section). The ruler indicates the locations of structures along the urethral length.

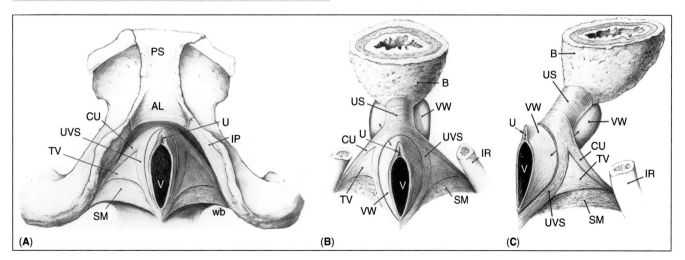

Figure 20.3 Striated urogenital sphincter muscle seen from below after removal of the perineal membrane (**A**) and pubic bones (**B,C**). *Abbreviations*: AL, arcuate pubic ligament; B, bladder; CU, compressor urethrae; IP, ischiopubic ramus; IR, ischiopubic ramus; PS, pubic symphysis; SM, smooth muscle; TV, transverse vaginal muscle; U, urethra; US, urethral sphincter; UVS, urethrovaginal sphincter; V, vagina; VW, vaginal wall. *Source*: Reproduced from Ref. 43 with permission.

163

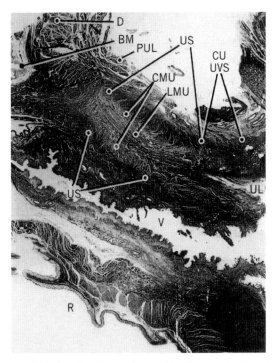

Figure 20.4 Sagittal section from a 29-year-old cadaver, cut just lateral to the midline and not quite parallel to it. The section contains tissue nearer the midline in the distal urethra where the lumen can be seen at the vesical neck. *Abbreviations*: BM, bladder mucosa; CMU, circular smooth muscle of the urethra; CU, compressor urethrae; D, detrusor muscle; LMU, longitudinal smooth muscles of the urethra; PUL, pubourethral ligament; R, rectum; UL, urethral lumen; US, urethral sphincter; UVS, urethrovaginal sphincter; V, vagina. *Source*: Reproduced from Ref. 5 with permission.

Urethral Smooth Muscle

The smooth muscle of the urethra is contiguous with that of the trigone and detrusor, but can be separated from these other muscles on embryologic, topographical, and morphologic grounds (3,14). It has an inner longitudinal layer, and a thin outer circular layer, with the former being by far the more prominent of the two (Fig. 20.5). The layers lie inside the striated urogenital sphincter muscle, and are present throughout the upper four-fifths of the urethra. The configuration of the circular muscle suggests a role in constricting the lumen, and the longitudinal muscle may help to shorten and funnel the urethra during voiding.

Submucosal Vasculature

Lying within the urethra is a surprisingly well-developed vascular plexus that is more prominent than one would expect for the ordinary demands of so small an organ (15). These vessels have been studied in serial reconstruction by Huisman (3), who has demonstrated the presence of several specialized types of arteriovenous anastomosis. They are formed in such a way that the flow of blood into large venules can be controlled to inflate or deflate them. This would assist in forming a watertight closure of the mucosal surfaces, and offer the possibility of rapid increases in their filling from the pressure on the abdominal vessels that supply them. Occlusion of the arterial inflow to these venous reservoirs has been shown to influence urethral closure pressure (10). In addition, these appear to be hormone sensitive (3), which may help to explain some individuals' response to estrogen supplementation.

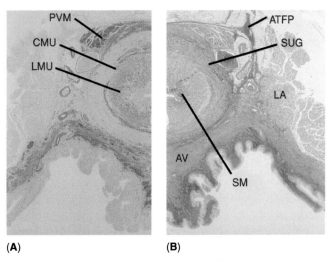

(A)   **(B)**

Figure 20.5 Axial midurethral actin immunoperoxidase histologic section for smooth muscle (**A**) and mirrored Mallory trichrome histologic section (**B**) from the same specimen. A few small spots are identified in the submucosa (SM). The longitudinal (LMU) and circular (CMU) smooth muscle of the urethra, the pubovesical muscle (PVM) and the smooth muscle layer of the anterior vaginal wall (AV) are easily identified on the actin-stained immunoperoxidase preparation whereas the striated urogenital sphincter muscle (SUG) does not stain with actin. *Abbreviations*: ATFP, arcus tendineus fasciae pelvis; LA, levator ani muscles.

Mucosa

The mucosal lining of the urethra is continuous above with the transitional epithelium of the bladder and below with the non-keratinizing squamous epithelium of the vestibule. This mucosa shares a common derivation from the urogenital sinus with the lower vagina and vestibule. Like these other areas, its mucosa is hormonally sensitive and undergoes significant change, depending on its state of stimulation.

Connective Tissue

In addition to the contractile and vascular tissue of the urethra, there is a considerable quantity of connective tissue interspersed within the muscle and the submucosa. This tissue contains both collagenous and elastin fibers. Studies that have sought to abolish the active aspects of urethral closure have suggested that the non-contractile elements contribute to urethral closure (3). However, it is difficult to study the function of these tissues because there is no specific way to block their action pharmacologically or surgically.

Glands

A series of glands are found in the submucosa, primarily along the dorsal (vaginal) surface of the urethra (16). They are most concentrated in the lower and middle thirds, and vary in number. The location of urethral diverticula (which are derived from cystic dilation of these glands) follows this distribution, being most common distally and usually originating along the dorsal surface of the urethra. In addition, their origin within the submucosa indicates that the fascia of the urethra must be stretched and attenuated over their surface, and indicates the need for its approximation after diverticular excision.

Vesical Neck

The term "vesical neck" is both a regional and a functional one, as previously discussed. It does not refer to a single anatomic entity; it denotes that area, at the base of the bladder, where the urethral lumen passes through the thickened musculature of the bladder base. Therefore, it is sometimes considered as part of the bladder musculature, but it also contains the urethral lumen studied during urethral pressure profilometry. It is a region where the detrusor musculature, including the detrusor loop, surrounds the trigonal ring and the internal urinary meatus.

The vesical neck has come to be considered separately from the bladder and urethra because it has unique functional characteristics. Specifically, sympathetic denervation or damage of this area results in its remaining open at rest (17); when this happens in association with stress incontinence, simple urethral suspension is often ineffective in curing this problem (18).

Functional Terms

A number of terms have been used to describe functional units within the vesicourethral unit, based upon radiographic observations of the activities of these viscera. The term "extrinsic continence mechanism" or "external sphincteric mechanism" usually refers to that group of structures that respond when an individual is instructed to stop the urine stream. The two phenomena observed during this effort are a constriction of the urethral lumen by the striated urogenital sphincter and an elevation of the vesical neck, caused by contraction of the levator ani muscles, as described below. The intrinsic continence mechanism then consists of the structures which lie within the vesical neck, and which are not specifically activated by contraction of the voluntary muscles. It is this system that fails in patients whose vesical neck can be seen to be open at rest.

PELVIC FLOOR

The position and mobility of the bladder and urethra are recognized as important to urinary continence (19). Although urethral support plays a secondary role in causing stress incontinence it is still an independent and important factor (4). Because these two organs are limp and formless when removed from the body, they must depend upon attachments to the pelvic floor for their shape and position. Fluoroscopic examination has shown that the upper portions of the urethra and vesical neck are normally mobile structures, whereas the distal urethra remains fixed in position (20,21). The pelvic floor muscles and fasciae determine these aspects of support and fixation. The term "pelvic floor" is used in different ways by different authors. Sometimes, especially in the colorectal field, the term is used to refer to the levator ani muscles. In this chapter, it will be given its broader interpretation because the anatomic term "pelvic diaphragm" serves to identify levator ani muscles and their covering fascia, leaving the term "pelvic floor" to identify the complex structural unit that lies at the bottom of the abdominal cavity.

The pelvic floor consists of several components lying between the pelvic peritoneum and the vulvar skin. These are (from above downwards) the peritoneum, viscera and endopelvic fascia, levator ani muscles, perineal membrane, and external genital muscles. The eventual support for all of these structures comes from their connection to the bony pelvis and its attached muscles. The viscera are often thought of as being supported by the pelvic floor; however, they are actually a part of it. Through such structures as the cardinal and uterosacral ligaments and the pubocervical fascia, the viscera have an important role in forming the pelvic floor.

Endopelvic Fascia

The Viscerofascial Layer

The top layer of the pelvic floor is provided by the endopelvic fascia that attaches the pelvic organs to the pelvic walls, thereby suspending the pelvic organs (22–24). Because this layer is a combination of the pelvic viscera and the endopelvic fascia, it is referred to here as the viscerofascial layer. It is common to speak of the fasciae and ligaments alone, separate from the pelvic organs as if they had a discrete identity; however, unless these fibrous structures have something to attach to (the pelvic organs), they can have no mechanical effect.

On each side of the pelvis the endopelvic fascia attaches the uterus and vagina to the pelvic wall (Figs. 20.6–20.8). This fascia forms a continuous sheet-like mesentery, extending from the uterine artery at its cephalic margin to the point at which the vagina fuses with the levator ani muscles below. The part that attaches to the uterus is called the parametrium and that which attaches to the vagina, the paracolpium.

The parametria are made up of what are clinically referred to as the cardinal and uterosacral ligaments (25,26).

Although the cardinal and uterosacrals are termed "ligaments" and "fasciae," they are not the same type of tissue as that seen in the "fascia" of the rectus abdominis muscle or in the ligaments of the knee, both of which are composed of parallel collagen fibers forming dense, regular, connective tissue. The cardinal ligament consists of blood vessels, nerves, and fibrous connective tissue, and can be thought of as mesenteries that supply the genital tract bilaterally. The uterosacral ligament contains a specific body of smooth muscle not

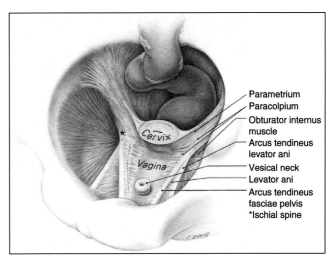

Figure 20.6 Supportive tissues of the cervix and upper vagina. Bladder has been removed above the vesical neck.

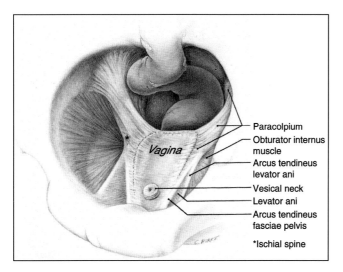

Figure 20.7 Vagina and supportive structures drawn from dissection of a 56-year-old cadaver after hysterectomy. The paracolpium extends along the lateral wall of the vagina. *Source*: Reproduced from Ref. 24 with permission.

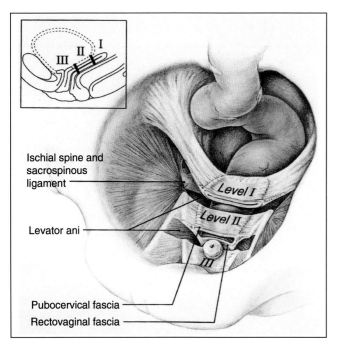

Figure 20.8 Level I (suspension) and level II (attachment). In level I the paracolpium suspends the vagina from the lateral pelvic walls. Fibers of level I extend both vertically and posteriorly towards the sacrum. In Level II, the vagina is attached to the arcus tendineus fasciae pelvis and superior fascia of levator ani. *Source*: Reproduced from Ref. 24 with permission.

contained in the cardinal ligament that attaches to the dorsal surface of the cervix. The ridge formed by these tissues when the uterus is elevated is visible when the cul de sac is viewed from above and is the most familiar view of this structure, but looks entirely different when the uterus is drawn downward, the action that demonstrates its supportive function.

The structural effect of the cardinal and uterosacral ligaments is most evident when the uterine cervix is pulled downwards with a tenaculum, as occurs during dilation and

curettage, or pushed downwards, as during laparotomy. After a certain amount of descent within the elastic range of the fascia, the parametria become tight and arrest the further cervical descent. Similarly, downward descent of the vaginal apex after hysterectomy is resisted by the paracolpia. The fact that these ligaments do not determine the position of the uterus in normal healthy women is attested to by the observation that the cervix may be pulled down to the level of the hymen with little difficulty (27).

Although it is traditional to focus attention on the ligaments that suspend the uterus, the attachments of the vagina to the pelvic walls are equally important and are responsible for normal support of the vagina, bladder, and rectum, even after hysterectomy. The location of damage to these supports determines whether a woman has a cystocele, rectocele, or vaginal vault prolapse; understanding the different characteristics of this support helps in the understanding of the different types of prolapse that can occur.

After hysterectomy the upper two-thirds of the vagina is suspended and attached to the pelvic walls by the paracolpium (24). This paracolpium has two portions (see Fig. 20.8): the upper portion (level I) consists of a relatively long sheet of tissue that suspends the vagina by attaching it to the pelvic wall; in the mid-portion of the vagina, the paracolpium attaches the vagina laterally and more directly to the pelvic walls (level II). This attachment stretches the vagina transversely between the bladder and rectum and has functional significance. The structural layer that supports the bladder ("pubocervical fascia") is composed of the anterior vaginal wall and its attachment through the endopelvic fascia to the pelvic wall. It is not a layer separate from the vagina, as sometimes suggested, but is a combination of the anterior vaginal wall and its attachments to the pelvic wall. Similarly, the posterior vaginal wall and endopelvic fascia (rectovaginal fascia) form the restraining layer that prevents the rectum from protruding forwards, blocking formation of a rectocele. In the distal vagina (level III) the vaginal wall is directly attached to surrounding structures without any intervening paracolpium: anteriorly it fuses with the urethra, posteriorly with the perineal body, and laterally with the levator ani muscles.

Damage to the upper suspensory fibers of the paracolpium causes a type of prolapse that differs from damage to the mid-level supports of the vagina: defects in the support provided by the mid-level vaginal supports (pubocervical and rectovaginal fasciae) result in cystocele and rectocele, whereas loss of the upper suspensory fibers of the paracolpium and parametrium is responsible for development of vaginal and uterine prolapse. These defects occur in varying combinations and this variation is responsible for the diversity of clinical problems encountered within the overall spectrum of pelvic organ prolapse.

Loss of level II support occurs because of detachment of the arcus tendineus from the ischial spine rather than from the pubic bone (28). This allows the trapezoidal-shaped anterior vaginal wall to swing downward, resulting in the characteristic cystocele seen clinically. There is also some failure of the midline vaginal wall in these patients and the relationship between these two defects remains to be clarified.

Pelvic Diaphragm

Subjecting connective tissue to constant force will stretch any such tissue within the body. Skin expanders used in plastic surgery stretch the dense and resistant dermis to extraordinary degrees, and flexibility exercises practiced by dancers and athletes elongate leg ligaments with as little as 10 minutes of stretching a day. Both of these observations underscore the malleable nature of connective tissue when subjected to force over time. If the ligaments and fasciae within the pelvis were subjected to the continuous stress imposed on the pelvic floor by the great weight of abdominal pressure, they would stretch; this stretching does not occur because the pelvic floor muscles close the pelvic floor and carry the weight of the abdominal and pelvic organs, preventing constant strain on the ligaments. Recent research has demonstrated the importance of levator ani muscle defects in the occurrence of pelvic organ prolapse (29). Fifty-five percent of women with prolapse have major injuries to their levator ani muscles. Only 16% of the normal population have this level of injury. Therefore women with prolapse are much more likely to have major levator muscle injury. This injury is associated with loss of levator contraction force and a larger urogenital hiatus. There is also evidence that poorly functioning levator ani muscles are associated with surgical failure (30).

Below the viscerofascial layer is the levator ani group of muscles (31) (Fig. 20.9). They have a connective tissue covering on both superior and inferior surfaces, known as the superior and inferior fasciae of the levator ani, respectively. When these muscles and their fasciae are considered together, the combined structure is termed the pelvic diaphragm. Although there have been disagreements about the terminology for this muscle, recent review of the literature shows good unanimity regarding anatomy, and a consistent nomenclature based on standardized anatomic terminology is possible (32).

The levator ani consists of two portions: the pubovisceral muscle and the iliococcygeal muscle (33,34). Laterally, the iliococcygeus arises from a fibrous band on the pelvic wall [arcus tendineus levator ani (ATLA)] and forms a relatively horizontal sheet that spans the opening within the pelvis and provides a shelf on which the organs may rest. The muscle inserts into the iliococcygeal raphe that is connected to the inner surface of the coccyx and sacrum. The pubovisceral muscle is a thick U-shaped muscle, the ends of which arise from the pubic bones on either side of the midline, and inserts into, or forms a sling around, the urethra, vagina, and rectum. This portion includes both the pubococcygeus and puborectalis portions of the levator ani. The pubococcygeus muscle lies medial to the puborectalis. It has several identifiable portions, each with a specific insertion point: the puboperineal muscle attaching to the perineal body, the pubovaginal muscle where the fibers of the levator attach to the elevator ani muscle as they pass by its lateral margin, and the puboanalis part where fibers insert into the space between the internal and external anal sphincter. The puborectalis muscle originates near the pubic bone, possibly from the superior surface of the perineal membrane, and forms a sling dorsal to the anorectal angle, just cranial to the external anal sphincter.

The opening within the levator ani muscle through which the urethra and vagina pass (and through which prolapse occurs) is called the urogenital hiatus of the levator ani. The rectum also passes through this opening; however, because the levator ani muscles attach directly to the anus, it is not included in the name of the hiatus. The hiatus, therefore, is bounded ventrally (anteriorly) by the pubic bones, laterally by the levator ani muscles and dorsally (posteriorly) by the perineal body

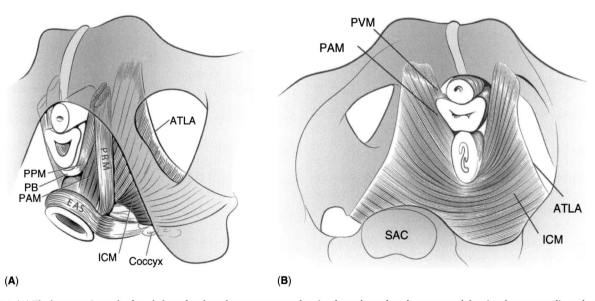

(A)   **(B)**

Figure 20.9 (**A**) The levator ani muscles from below after the vulvar structures and perineal membrane have been removed showing the arcus tendineus levator ani (ATLA), external anal sphincter (EAS), puboanal muscle (PAM), perineal body (PB) uniting the two ends of the puboperineal muscle (PPM), iliococcygeal muscle (ICM), and puborectal muscle (PRM). The urethra and vagina have been transected just above the hymenal ring. (**B**) The levator ani muscle seen from above looking over the sacral promontory (SAC) showing the pubovaginal muscle (PVM; other abbreviations as in Fig. 20.9A). The urethra, vagina, and rectum have been transected just above the pelvic floor. Note: The internal obturator muscles have been removed to clarify levator muscle origins. *Source:* Reproduced from Ref. 32 with permission. ©DeLancey 2003.

and external anal sphincter. The normal baseline activity of the levator ani muscle keeps the urogenital hiatus closed: it squeezes the vagina, urethra and rectum closed by compressing them against the pubic bone and it lifts the floor and organs in a cephalic direction.

The levator ani muscles have constant activity (35), like that of other postural muscles. This continuous contraction is similar to the continuous activity of the external anal sphincter muscle and closes the lumen of the vagina in a way similar to that by which the anal sphincter closes the anus. This constant action eliminates any opening within the pelvic floor through which prolapse could occur and forms a relatively horizontal shelf on which the pelvic organs are supported (36,37).

Interaction Between Muscle and Connective Tissue

The interaction between the pelvic floor muscles and the supportive ligaments is critical to pelvic organ support. Recent biomechanical modeling has demonstrated the interaction between muscle and connective tissue supports indicating that each has its own contribution to supporting the pelvic organs. This coupled with the recent demonstration of the high association between levator ani damage and pelvic organ prolapse confirms the importance of understanding the relationship of musculature support and connective tissue support (38,39). As long as the levator ani muscles function properly, the pelvic floor is closed and the ligaments and fascia are under no tension; the fasciae simply act to stabilize the organs in their position above the levator ani muscles. When the pelvic floor muscles relax or are damaged, the pelvic floor opens and the vagina lies between the high abdominal pressure and low atmospheric pressure; in this situation it must be held in place by the ligaments. Although the ligaments can sustain these loads for short periods of time, if the pelvic floor muscles do not close the pelvic floor then the connective tissue must carry this load for long periods and will eventually fail to hold the vagina in place. Song and colleagues have recently shown that there is a decrease in collagen type III in premenopausal women with stress incontinence, suggesting that less flexibility of connective tissue may be associated with greater likelihood of eventual loss of vaginal support (40).

This support of the uterus has been likened to a ship in its berth, floating on the water attached by ropes on either side to a dock (41). The ship is analogous to the uterus, the ropes to the ligaments, and the water to the supportive layer formed by the pelvic floor muscles. The ropes (ligaments) function to hold the ship (uterus) in the center of its berth as it rests on the water (pelvic floor muscles). If, however, the water level were to fall so far that the ropes would be required to hold the ship without the support of the water, the ropes would break. The analogous situation in the pelvic floor involves the pelvic floor muscles supporting the uterus and vagina that are stabilized in position by the ligaments and fasciae: once the pelvic floor musculature becomes damaged and no longer holds the organs in place, the connective tissue fails because of significant overload.

Perineal Membrane and External Genital Muscles

In the anterior portion of the pelvis, below the pelvic diaphragm, is a dense triangular membrane containing a central opening called the perineal membrane (urogenital diaphragm). This lies at the level of the hymenal ring and attaches the urethra, vagina, and perineal body to the ischiopubic rami. Just above the perineal membrane are the compressor urethrae and urethrovaginal sphincter muscles, previously discussed as part of the striated urogenital sphincter muscle.

Recent dissection show the intimate relationship between the perineal membrane and the levator ani muscle. These are in close proximity and so the action of the muscle certainly could influence the poition of the perineal membrane (42).

The term "perineal membrane" replaces the old term "urogenital diaphragm," reflecting more accurate recent anatomic information (43). Previous concepts of the urogenital diaphragm show two fascial layers, with a transversely orientated muscle between them (the deep transverse perineal muscle). Observations based on serial histology and gross dissection, however, reveal a single connective tissue membrane, with these muscles and the levator ani muscles lying immediately above. The correct anatomy explains the observation that pressures during a cough are greatest in the distal urethra (44,45), where the compressor urethrae and urethrovaginal sphincter can squeeze the lumen in anticipation of a cough (46). The perineal membrane has been visualized in normal women by MRI examination (8).

Position and Mobility of the Urethra

When the importance of urethral position to determining urinary continence was recognized, anatomic observations revealed an attachment of the tissues around the urethra to the pubic bones. These connections were referred to as the pubourethral ligaments (47) and were found to be continuous with the connective tissue of the perineal membrane (48). Further studies (46,49,50) have expanded these observations and revealed several separate structural elements contained within these—tissues that have functional importance to urinary—continence (51).

As mentioned earlier in this chapter, urethral support is dynamic rather than static. Fluoroscopic and topographic observations (20,21) suggest that urethral position is determined both by attachments to bone and by those to the levator ani muscles. The role of the connection between the ureteral supports and those to the levator ani is probably more important than previously thought, for the following reasons:

- The resting position of the proximal urethra is high within the pelvis, some 3 cm above the inferior aspect of the pubic bones (52) (Fig. 20.10) and above the insertion of the "posterior pubourethral ligaments" which attach near the lower margin of the pubic bones (47).
- Maintenance of this position would be best explained by the constant muscular activity of the levator ani. In addition, the upper two-thirds of the urethra is mobile (20,21,53) and under voluntary control.
- At the onset of micturition, relaxation of the levator ani muscles allows the urethra to descend and obliterates the posterior urethrovesical angle (Fig. 20.10).
- Resumption of the normal tonic contraction of the muscle at the end of micturition returns the vesical neck to its normal position.

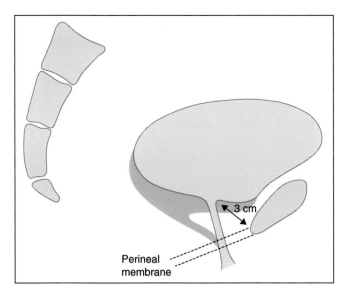

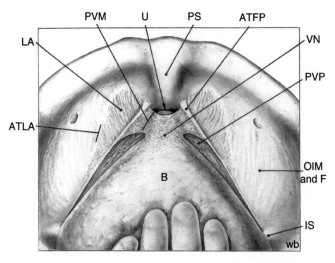

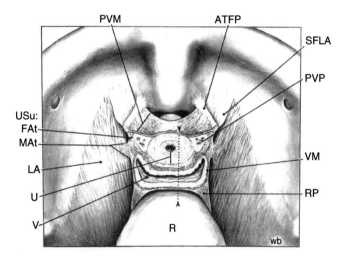

Figure 20.10 Topography and mobility of the normal proximal urethra and vesical neck based upon resting (■) and voiding (■) in nulliparae.

Figure 20.11 Space of Retzius (drawn from cadaver dissection). Pubovesical muscle (PVM) can be seen going from vesical neck (VN) to arcus tendineus fasciae pelvis (ATFP) and running over the paraurethral vascular plexus (PVP). *Abbreviations:* ATLA, arcus tendineus levator ani; B, bladder; IS, ischial spine; LA, levator ani muscles; OIM and F obturator internus muscle and fascia; PS, pubic symphysis; U, urethra. *Source:* Reproduced from Ref. 56 with permission.

Figure 20.12 Relationship of the supportive tissues of the urethra (USu) to the pubovesical muscles (PVM). Cross-section of the urethra (U), vagina (V), arcus tendineus fasciae pelvis (ATFP), and superior fascia of levator ani (SFLA) just below the vesical neck (drawn from cadaver dissection). The PVM lie anterior to the urethra, and anterior and superior to the paraurethral vascular plexus (PVP). The USu ("the pubourethral ligaments") attach the vagina and vaginal surface of the urethra to the levator ani (LA) muscles (MAt, muscular attachment) and to the superior fascia of the LA (FAt, fascial attachment). *Abbreviations:* R, rectum; RP, rectal pillar; VM, vaginal wall muscularis. *Source:* Reproduced from Ref. 56 with permission.

As previously mentioned, urethral support is not as important as previously been thought but does still influence urinary incontinence. It is probably most influential in the youngest women with stress urinary incontinence because they have relatively good urethral function. As urethral function declines with age the role that maximum urethral closure pressure begins to predominate. In women with de novo stress incontinence after first birth, injury to the levator ani muscle is seen twice as often as individuals who deliver and are continent (54). Later on in life this seems, however, to disappear (4).

The anterior vaginal wall and urethra arise from the urogenital sinus and are intimately connected. The support of the urethra does not depend on attachments of the urethra itself to adjacent structures, but on the connection of the vagina and periurethral tissues to the muscles and fasciae of the pelvic wall. Surgeons are most familiar with seeing this anatomy through the space of Retzius, and this view is also helpful in understanding urethral support (Fig. 20.11). On either side of the pelvis, the arcus tendineus fasciae pelvis (ATFP) is found as a band of connective tissue attached at one end to the lower one-sixth of the pubic bone, 1 cm from the midline, and at the other end to the ischial spine. The anterior portion of this band lies on the inner surface of the levator ani muscle that arises some 3 cm above the ATFP. Posteriorly, the levator ani arises from a second arcus, the ATLA, which fuses with the ATFP near the ischial spine.

The layer of tissue that provides urethral support has two lateral attachments: a fascial attachment and a muscular attachment (Fig. 20.12). The fascial attachments of the urethral supports connect the periurethral tissues and anterior vaginal wall to the ATFP and have been termed the paravaginal fascial attachments (49). The muscular attachment connects these same periurethral tissues to the medial border of the levator ani muscle. These attachments allow the normal resting tone of the levator ani to maintain the position of the vesical neck, supported by the fascial attachments (Fig. 20.13). When the muscle relaxes at the onset of micturition, it allows the vesical neck to rotate downwards to the limit of the elasticity of the fascial attachments; at the end of micturition, contraction allows it to resume its normal position.

Also within this region are the pubovesical muscles, which are extensions of the detrusor muscle (1,55,56). They lie within connective tissue; when both muscular and fibrous elements are considered together they are termed the pubovesical ligaments, in much the same way that the smooth muscle of the ligamentum teres is referred to as the round ligament (see Figs. 20.4, 20.5, 20.11, and 20.12). Although the terms

169

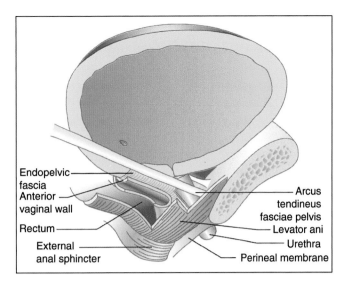

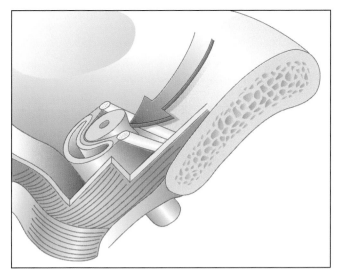

Figure 20.13 Lateral view of the pelvic floor structures related to urethral support, seen from the side in the standing position cut just lateral to the midline. Note that windows have been cut in the levator ani muscles, vagina, and endopelvic fascia, so that the urethra and anterior vaginal walls can be seen.

Figure 20.14 Lateral view of pelvic floor with the urethra, vagina, and fascial tissues transected at the level of the vesical neck, drawn from three-dimensional reconstruction indicating compression of the urethra by downward force (arrow) against the supportive tissues indicating the influence of abdominal pressure on the urethra (arrow).

"pubo-vesical ligament" and "pubourethral ligament" have sometimes been considered to be synonymous, the pubovesical ligaments are different structures from the urethral supportive tissues. Fibers of the detrusor muscle are able to undergo great elongation, and these weak tissues are, therefore, not suited to maintain urethral position under stress. In addition, they run in front of the vesical neck rather than underneath it, where one would expect supportive tissues to be found. It is not surprising, therefore, that these detrusor fibers do not differ, in stress-incontinent patients, from those in patients without this condition (57). The tissues that support the urethra are separated from the pubovesical ligaments by a prominent vascular plexus, and are easily parted from them. Rather than supporting the urethra, the pubovesical muscles may be responsible for assisting in vesical neck opening at the onset of micturition by contracting to pull the anterior vesical neck forwards, as some have suggested (58).

This mechanism influences incontinence by determining how the urethra is supported, not by how high or low the urethra is in the pelvis. In examining anatomic specimens, simulated increases in abdominal pressure reveal that the urethra lies in a position where it can be compressed against the supporting hammock by rises in abdominal pressure (Fig. 20.13). In this model, it is the stability of this supporting layer under the urethra rather than the height of the urethra that determines stress continence. In an individual with a firm supportive layer, the urethra would be compressed between abdominal pressure and pelvic fascia (Fig. 20.14) in much the same way that the flow of water through a garden hose can be stopped by stepping on and compressing it against underlying paving. If, however, the layer under the urethra becomes unstable and does not provide a firm backstop against which the urethra can be compressed by abdominal pressure, the opposing force that causes closure is lost and the occlusive action is diminished. This latter situation is similar to an attempt to stop the flow of water through a garden hose by stepping on it while it lies on soft soil.

The structural and functional aspects of the body must always be in agreement. As new functional observations are made of the lower urinary tract, it will be necessary to re-examine our anatomic concepts; doubtless, some of the structural arrangements described in this chapter will be corrected, expanded upon, and improved. This will continue to enhance our ability to understand the variety of patients with lower urinary tract dysfunction, and will improve our ability to restore normal urinary control.

REFERENCES
1. Gil Vernet S. Morphology and Function of the Vesico-Prostato-Urethral Musculature. Italy: Edizioni Canova Treviso, 1968.
2. Woodburne RT. The ureter ureterovesical junction and vesical trigone. Anat Rec 1965; 151: 243–9.
3. Huisman AB. Aspects on the anatomy of the female urethra with special relation to urinary continence. Contrib Gynecol Obstet 1983; 10: 1–31.
4. DeLancey JO, Trowbridge ER, Miller JM. Stress urinary incontinence relative importance to urethra support and urethra closure pressure. J Urol 2008; 179: 2286–90.
5. DeLancey JOL. Correlative study of paraurethral anatomy. Obstet Gynecol 1986; 68: 91–7.
6. Macura KJ, Genadry RR, Bluemke DA. MR imaging of the female urethra and supporting ligaments in assessment of urinary incontinence: spectrum of abnormalities. Radiographics 2006; 26: 1135–49.
7. Elsayes KM, Mukundan G, Narra VR, et al. Endovaginal magnetic resonance imaging of the female urethra. J Comput Assist Tomogr 2006; 30: 1–6.
8. Brandon CJ, Lewicky-Gaupp C, Larson KA, Delancey JO. Anatomy of the perineal membrane as seen in magnetic resonance images of nulliparous women. Am J Obstet Gynecol 2009; 200: 583 e1–6.
9. Gosling JA, Dixon JS, Critchley HOD, Thompson SA. A comparative study of the human external sphincter and periurethral levator ani muscles. Br J Urol 1981; 53: 35–41.
10. Rud T, Anderson KE, Asmussen M, et al. Factors maintaining the intraurethral pressure in women. Invest Urol 1980; 17: 343–7.
11. Perucchini D, DeLancey JO, Ashton-Miller JA, et al. Age effects on urethral striated muscle. I. changes in number and diameter of striated muscle fibers in the ventral urethra. Am J Obstet Gynecol 2002; 186: 351–5.

12. Pandit M, DeLancey JO, Ashton-Miller JA, et al. Quantification of intramuscular nerves within the female striated urogenital sphincter muscle. Obstet Gynecol 2000; 95(6 Pt 1): 797–800.

13. Weidner AC, South MM, Sanders DB, Stinnett SS. Change in urethral sphincter neuromuscular function during pregnancy persists after delivery. Am J Obstet Gynecol 2009; 201: 529 e1–6.

14. Dröes JTPM. Observations on the musculature of the urinary bladder and urethra in the human foetus. Br J Urol 1974; 46: 179–85.

15. Berkow SG. The corpus spongiosum of the urethra: its possible role in urinary control and stress incontinence in women. Am J Obstet Gynecol 1953; 65: 346–51.

16. Huffman J. Detailed anatomy of the paraurethral ducts in the adult human female. Am J Obstet Gynecol 1948; 55: 86–101.

17. McGuire EJ. The innervation and function of the lower urinary tract. J Neurosurg 1986; 65: 278–85.

18. McGuire EJ. Urodynamic findings in patients after failure of stress incontinence operations. Prog Clin Biol Res 1981; 78: 351–60.

19. Hodgkinson CP. Relationships of the female urethra in urinary incontinence. Am J Obstet Gynecol 1953; 65: 560–73.

20. Muellner SR. Physiology of micturition. J Urol 1951; 65: 805–10.

21. Westby M, Asmussen M, Ulmsten U. Location of maximum intraurethral pressure related to urogenital diaphragm in the female subject as studied by simultaneous urethrocystometry and voiding urethrocystography. Am J Obstet Gynecol 1982; 144: 408–12.

22. Ricci JV, Thom CH. The myth of a surgically useful fascia in vaginal plastic reconstructions. Q Rev Surg Obstet Gynecol 1954; 2: 261–3.

23. Uhlenhuth E, Nolley GW. Vaginal fascia a myth? Obstet Gynecol 1957; 10: 349–58.

24. DeLancey JOL. Anatomic aspects of vaginal eversion after hysterectomy. Am J Obstet Gynecol 1992; 166: 1717–28.

25. Range RL, Woodburne RT. The gross and microscopic anatomy of the transverse cervical ligaments. Am J Obstet Gynecol 1964; 90: 460–7.

26. Campbell RM. The anatomy and histology of the sacrouterine ligaments. Am J Obstet Gynecol 1950; 59: 1–12.

27. Bartscht KD, DeLancey JOL. A technique to study cervical descent. Obstet Gynecol 1988; 72: 940–3.

28. DeLancey JOL. Fascial and muscular abnormalities in women with urethral hypermobility and anterior vaginal wall prolapse. Am J Obstet Gynecol 2002; 187: 93–8.

29. DeLancey JO, Morgan DM, Fenner DE, et al. Comparison of levator ani muscle defects and function in women with and without pelvic organ prolapse. Obstet Gynecol 2007; 109(2 Pt 1): 295–302.

30. Vakili B, Zheng Yt, Loesch H, et al. Levator contraction strength and genital hiatus as risk factors for recurrent pelvic organ prolapse. Am J Obstet Gynecol 2005; 192: 1592–8.

31. Dickinson RL. Studies of the levator ani muscle. Am J Dis Women 1889; 22: 897–917.

32. Kearney R, Sawhney R, DeLancey JO. Levator ani muscle anatomy evaluated by origin-insertion pairs. Obstet Gynecol 2004; 104: 168–73.

33. Lawson JON. Pelvic anatomy. I. Pelvic floor muscles. Ann R Coll Surg Engl 1974; 54: 244–52.

34. Lawson JON. Pelvic anatomy. II. Anal canal and associated sphincters. Ann R Coll Surg Engl 1974; 54: 288–300.

35. Parks AG, Porter NH, Melzak J. Experimental study of the reflex mechanism controlling muscles of the pelvic floor. Dis Colon Rectum 1962; 5: 407–14.

36. Berglas B, Rubin IC. Study of the supportive structures of the uterus by levator myography. Surg Gynecol Obstet 1953; 97: 677–92.

37. Nichols DH, Milley PS, Randall CL. Significance of restoration of normal vaginal depth and axis. Obstet Gynecol 1970; 36: 251–6.

38. Chen L, Ashton-Miller JA, Hsu Y, DeLancey JO. Interaction among apical support, levator ani impairment, and anterior vaginal wall prolapse. Obstet Gynecol 2006; 108: 324–32.

39. Chen L, Ashton-Miller JA, DeLancey JO. A 3D finite element model of anterior vaginal wall support to evaluate mechanisms underlying cystocele formation. J Biomech 2009; 42: 1371–7.

40. Song Y, Hong X, Yu Y, Lin Y. Changes of collagen type III and decorin in paraurethral connective tissue from women with stress urinary incontinence and prolapse. Int Urogynecol J Pelvic Floor Dysfunct 2007; 18: 1459–63.

41. Paramore RH. The uterus as a floating organ. The Statics of the Female Pelvic Viscera. London: HK Lewis, 1918: 12–15.

42. Stein TA, DeLancey JO. Structure of the perineal membrane in females: gross and microscopic anatomy. Obstet Gynecol 2008; 111: 686–93.

43. Oelrich TM. The striated urogenital sphincter muscle in the female. Anat Rec 1983; 205: 223–32.

44. Hilton P, Stanton SL. Urethral pressure measurement by microtransducer: the results in symptom-free women and in those with genuine stress incontinence. Br J Obstet Gynaecol 1983; 90: 919–33.

45. Constantinou CE. Resting and stress urethral pressures as a clinical guide to the mechanism of continence in the female patient. Urol Clin North Am 1985; 12: 247–58.

46. DeLancey JOL. Structural aspects of the extrinsic continence mechanism. Obstet Gynecol 1988; 72: 296–301.

47. Zacharin RF. The anatomic supports of the female urethra. Obstet Gynecol 1968; 21: 754–9.

48. Milley PS, Nichols DH. Relationship between the pubo-urethral ligaments and the urogenital diaphragm in the human female. Anat Rec 1971; 170: 81–3.

49. Richardson AC, Edmonds PB, Williams NL. Treatment of stress urinary incontinence due to paravaginal fascial defect. Obstet Gynecol 1981; 57: 357–62.

50. DeLancey JOL. Structural support of the urethra as it relates to stress urinary incontinence: the hammock hypothesis. Am J Obstet Gynecol 1994; 170: 1713–20.

51. el-Sayed RF, Morsy MM, el-Mashed SM, Abdel-Azim MS. Anatomy of the urethral supporting ligaments defined by dissection, histology, and MRI of female cadavers and MRI of healthy nulliparous women. AJR Am J Roentgenol 2007; 189: 1145–57.

52. Noll LE, Hutch JA. The SCIPP line—an aid in interpreting the voiding lateral cystourethrogram. Obstet Gynecol 1969; 33: 680–9.

53. Jeffcoate TNA, Roberts H. Observations on stress incontinence of urine. Am J Obstet Gynecol 1952; 64: 721–38.

54. DeLancey JO, Miller JM, Kearney R, et al. Vaginal birth and de novo stress incontinence: relative contributions of urethral dysfunction and mobility. Obstet Gynecol 2007; 110(2 Pt 1): 354–62.

55. Woodburne RT. Anatomy of the bladder and bladder outlet. J Urol 1968; 100: 474–87.

56. DeLancey JOL. Pubovesical ligament: a separate structure from the urethral supports (pubo-urethral ligaments). Neurourol Urodyn 1989; 8: 53–62.

57. Wilson PD, Dixon JS, Brown ADG, Gosling JA. Posterior pubo-urethral ligaments in normal and genuine stress incontinent women. J Urol 1983; 130: 802–5.

58. Power RMH. An anatomical contribution to the problem of continence and incontinence in the female. Am J Obstet Gynecol 1954; 67: 302–14.

21 Embryology of the Female Urogenital System and Clinical Applications
Sarah M Lambert and Stephen A Zderic

INTRODUCTION

The first goal of this chapter is to provide an overview of the embryologic events that lead to formation of the upper lower urinary tract in women. Normal female lower urinary tract development cannot be discussed in isolation from that of rectum, anus, and vagina. Therefore a good deal of attention will be focused on the embryology of the perineum. Traditional embryology writings were highly descriptive anatomic treatises based on observations two dimensional line drawings. The modern world of developmental biology is changing this rapidly as embryology may now be imaged in three dimensions over time using a wide range of mice with targeted genetic anomalies. The second goal of this chapter, therefore, is to briefly discuss the genetic molecular signals that enable these complex structures to develop. The third goal of this chapter is to provide clinical examples of malformations that arise when deviations from this path of normal development occur.

EARLY EMBRYOGENESIS

After initial conception, the resultant zygote undergoes a series of cell divisions. If this process occurs properly, the embryo ultimately implants within the endometrial wall of the uterine cavity. Pluripotent stem cells then begin to differentiate into three basic germ cell layers. By 22 days of gestation, the embryo is a disc-shaped structure containing the three germ cell layers: the ectoderm lined amniotic cavity, the mesoderm, and the endoderm arising within the yolk sac. At the cranial and caudal ends the ectoderm and endoderm are in direct contact, and these bilaminar areas are described as the oropharyngeal and cloacal membranes (Fig. 21.1A) (1). With further growth this disc folds progressively both craniocaudally and laterally, resulting in yolk sac invagination. Over the ensuing six weeks the yolk sac tubularizes and differentiates into the stomach, small intestine, and large intestine completing this process by week 10 of embryonic development (1). During the course of this yolk sac tubularization, the intestines are extruded from the abdominal cavity by means of the incompletely developed anterior abdominal wall. Simultaneously with the abdominal wall closure, the developing intestine returns to the abdominal cavity, and undergoes a 245 degree anticlockwise rotation about the superior mesenteric artery. This process is complete by 10 weeks of age, and explains why the cecum is found in the right lower quadrant.

The development of the ureters, bladder, and urethra starts at the caudal end of the embryo at the cloacal membrane and within the adjacent mesenchyme. Via differential growth rates of the adjacent mesenchyme, the distal primitive hindgut begins to form a dilated chamber known as the cloaca. To appreciate the development of the lower urinary tract and female perineum, one must understand the transition from the 4 mm (4-week) to the 36 mm (10-week) embryo as the cloaca is partitioned into anterior (urogenital) and posterior (rectal) components.

DIVISION OF THE CLOACA

Following invagination of the yolk sac at day 28, the primitive hindgut begins to form a dilated chamber, referred to as the cloaca. From this develops a ventral outgrowth orientated towards the umbilicus referred to as the allantois (Fig. 21.2A). At this stage, the cloacal membrane which separates the internal cloaca (lined with endoderm derived from the yolk sac) from the external cloaca (composed of ectoderm) remains intact (2). Part of the allantois will contribute to bladder development; those portions closest to the umbilicus will atrophy forming the urachus. However, in order for these structures to form, the internal cloaca must be partitioned into the ventral (urogenital) and dorsal (rectal) cloaca. This division of the cloaca begins during the fifth week within the upper portions of the chamber and is completed during the seventh week of gestation with resulting rupture of the cloacal membrane (Fig. 21.2B) (2). The exact mechanisms are still debated. Rathke (3) claimed that this partition takes place by median fusion of two lateral ridges of the cloacal wall in a caudal direction, whereas Tourneux (4) described a descending septum fusing with the cloacal membrane. In contrast, more recent studies described this process as a fusion of the surrounding mesoderm of the incorporated parts of the yolksac and allantois (5,6). Irrespective of the exact mechanism, by the beginning of the eighth week of gestation, the cloaca has been divided into anterior (ventral) and posterior (dorsal) components, and there is free communication between the internal and external cloaca due to the rupture of the cloacal membrane.

Many cellular signaling pathways are required for normal cloacal differentiation. Using a murine model of fetal exposure to all trans retinoic acid on the ninth day of conception, Sasaki et al. (7), demonstrated that all fetal survivors had a short tail and imperforate anus. In females this was manifest as a common cloaca in which the urethra, vagina, and rectum merged. The process of normal cloacal differentiation appears to be under the control of the sonic hedgehog (Shh) signaling pathway. Shh immunoreactivity was prominent in the rectal, urethral, and bladder epithelium in normal mice, but was absent in those with ano rectal malformations (ARM). Bone morphogenic protein type 4 (BMP4) immunoreactivity was noted in the mesenchyme below the epithelium staining for Shh expression in normal mice, but was absent in the population with ARM. In a second model using a knockout mouse model for Shh, Sukegawa et al. demonstrated that Shh signaling is critical to the concentric development of the hindgut (8). Recent

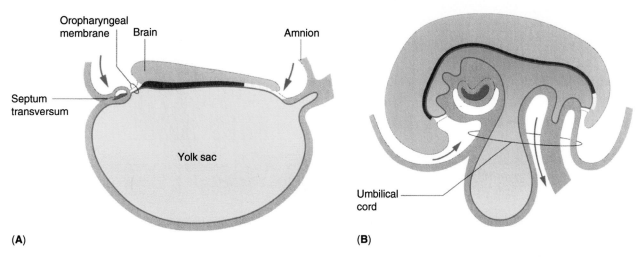

(A)

(B)

Figure 21.1 (**A**) Sagittal section of the discoid 22-day-old embryo, showing the relationship of the yolk sac to the neural and mesenchymal layers prior to the fold-ing. The arrows show the direction of the subsequent folding that takes place by day 28. The oropharyngeal and cloacal membranes are already developing at the cranial and caudal ends of the neural tube. (**B**) Sagittal section of the embryo at day 28, showing the residual yolk sac contained within the developing umbilical cord. The second smaller extension of the yolk sac into the cord (which forms the basis of the allantois) can be seen. The cloacal membrane is just to the right of the umbilical cord. *Source*: From Ref. 2.

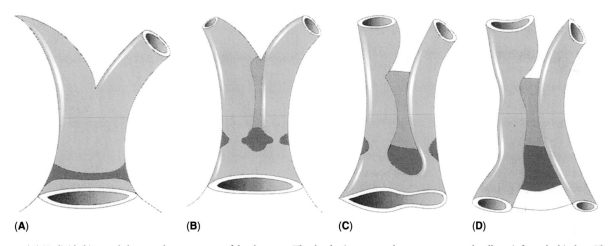

(A)   **(B)**   **(C)**   **(D)**

Figure 21.2 (**A**) Undivided internal cloaca at the 4 mm stage of development. The developing urorectal septum separates the allantois from the hindgut. The allan-toic extension to the left leads to the umbilical cord and the future navel; this extension forms the basis of the urachal remnant. (**B**) Division of the internal cloaca is completed in this sequence, and the cloacal membrane has now ruptured, allowing for communication between the internal and external cloacal chambers. (**C**) With further growth, the external cloaca is partitioned by an extension of the urorectal septum and an ingrowth of the genital folds. (**D**) Fusion of the genital folds in the midline completes the separation of the urethra anteriorly from the rectum posteriorly. *Source*: From Ref. 2.

murine models demonstrate that Wnt5a and Axin2, both downstream of the Shh signaling, are absent in mice with ARM providing evidence of their importance in normal cloa-cal development (9). Cloacal malformations occur to due to disruption of these signaling pathways during gestation. The mechanism of disruption delineates the type of malforma-tion. For example, mice lacking two zinc finger transcritpion factors, Gli2 or Gli3, that participate in Shh signaling display imperforate anus, rectourethral fistula, and anal stenosis (10). It is becoming increasingly clear that complex epithelial mesenchymal interactions are critical to normal cloacal differentiation.

Simultaneously with the septation of the internal cloaca, the external cloaca also undergoes partitioning in order for the normal perineum to develop and the process of external sexual differentiation begins. Partitioning of the external cloaca begins in part as a distal extension of the urorectal septum

(Fig. 21.2C) coupled to an inward migration of the genital folds to create the short female perineal body and median raphe (Fig. 21.2D). In contrast in males, the perineal body is elongated, and there is an anterior deflection of the proximal urethra; a process that is regulated by androgens. This phase also marks the onset of Müllerian differentiation in the female embryo.

Normal perineal and external genital development also arise from a complex epithelial mesenchymal interaction. While androgens are critical to the resulting male phenotype, genital patterning is initiated two weeks prior to testosterone synthe-sis in part through Shh dependent signaling pathways. These concepts are nicely demonstrated in a mouse with a deletion of Shh expression; external genitalia are absent and a primitive cloaca develops instead (Fig. 21.3) (11). It appears that with with Shh deletion, there is also a concomitant downregula-tion of BMP2, BMP4, Fgf8, Fgf10, and Wnt5a, and increased

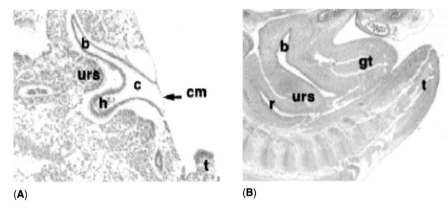

(A)   **(B)**

Figure 21.3 (**A**) Midsagittal section taken through a mouse embryo with a deletion of Shh expression shows a persistent cloaca (c) covered by a thin cloacal membrane (cm). The bladder (b) and hindgut (h) are partially separated by the urorectal septum (urs). The proximal portion of the tail (t) can be seen. (**B**) In comparison a midsagittal section taken through a wild type embryo showing almost complete separation of the bladder and urogenital sinus from the rectum (r). *Abbreviation:* gt, genital tubercle. *Source:* From Ref. 11.

apoptosis occurs within the genitalia (11). Clearly some of the pathways leading to genital development must be androgen dependent of which Ephrin B signaling in the developing urethral seam is one such example (12).

MÜLLERIAN DIFFERENTIATION

Müllerian ducts develop in both sexes during embryogenesis. Murine genetic studies have revealed many homeodomain transcription factors that are involved in Müllerian development including Pax2, Pax8, Lim1, Emx2, Hoxa13, and Dach1. Some of these transcription factors have an important role in regulating Wolffian development as well. In Lim1-null mice, ovarian development still occurs but the female neonates lack uteri and fallopian tubes providing further evidence of the specific effects upon the Müllerian ducts themselves (13). Additionally, many signaling molecules are required for normal Müllerian development. Wnt9b and Wnt4 act as paracrine signals. Wnt9b is expressed in the Wolffian duct epithelium and is required for Müllerian duct elongation (14). Retinoic acid, a derivative of vitamin A is also necessary for Müllerian developement; Retinoic acid receptor alpha beta two knockout mice lack Müllerian ducts (15). Normal development of the female genital tract requires specific interactions between both transcription factors and signaling molecules. Aberrations in these signaling pathways lead to many of the genital abnormalities observed clinically.

By week 6 the Müllerian ducts form from the intermediate mesoderm located laterally to the Wolffian ducts and develop along the anterior-posterior axis of the embryo. These ducts are composed of epithelial cells, mesenchymal cells, and coelomic epithelial cells that form three distinct cellular layers. Recent lineage tracing experiments in chickens and mice reveal that these three layers are all derived from different populations of coelomic epithelium without any direct cellular contribution from the Wolffian ducts (16). Although cells derived from the Wolffian duct do not contribute to the Müllerian duct, cell-cell signaling between the Müllerian duct and the Wolffian duct, such as Wnt9b and Wnt4, induces Müllerian development. Indeed, close contact with the Wolffian duct is necessary for Müllerian duct elongation (17). The Müllerian

ducts begin as solid cords that likely tubularize on the basis of apoptosis during their differentiation. Proximal parts of these ducts form the fallopian tubes; distally, they fuse in the midline producing the uterus, cervix, and proximal two-thirds of the vagina (18). By week 7, the caudal ends of the Müllerian ducts migrate through the urorectal septum to penetrate the posterior aspect of the urethra at the Müllerian tubercle between the two openings of the Wolffian ducts (Fig. 21.4) (18). The urethra and Müllerian structures terminate in the common urogenital (UG) sinus (Fig. 21.4B) prior to the separation of the urethra and vagina that proceeds as a result of differential growth (Fig. 21.4C) and an anterior turn of the distal urethra (Fig. 21.4D). Failures in distal migration of the Müllerian ducts to form the UG sinus may result in distal vaginal atresia.

It is important to appreciate the interaction between the Wolffian and Müllerian systems leading to formation of the UG sinus. The Wolffian ducts serve to guide the Müllerian ducts to the UG sinus, and are carried towards the perineum in the lateral walls of the vagina and undergo involution in the course of normal differentiation. The Wolffian ducts can remain as appendix vesiculosa, epoophoron, paroophoron, or as Gartner's ducts. If they fail to involute properly, they can remain as small cysts within the lateral vaginal wall or the cervix. Occasionally, these remnants become larger and infected, and present clinically as Gartner's duct cysts. This embryology is also clinically relevant because the ureteral buds arise from the Wolffian system as a result the lateral walls of the vagina are a potential site for the rare insertion of an ectopic ureter.

SMOOTH MUSCLE DIFFERENTIATION

The female urothelium is composed of endoderm derived from the ventral cloacal chamber created by the division of the cloaca by the urorectal septum (19). The connective tissue and smooth muscle are subsequently derived from adjacent mesenchyme. The developing urethra and bladder contain no muscle in the early stages of development and the endoderm of the UG sinus remains a single layer of epithelium up to the seventh week and then gradually assumes the appearance of transitional epithelium in the third month. The earliest muscle

174

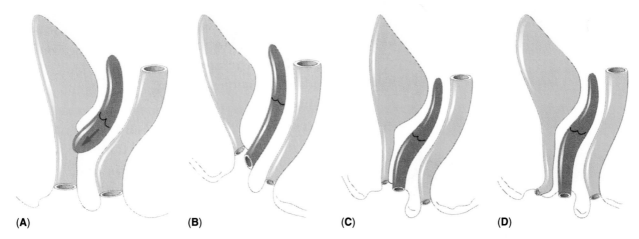

(A)   (B)   (C)   (D)

Figure 21.4 (**A**) The Müllerian ducts migrate to and penetrate the posterior urethra at week 7. The Müllerian ducts are guided to this point in the posterior urethra by the Wolffian ducts. (**B**) The ducts migrate caudally, and the urogenital sinus becomes a shallow channel. At this point there is a good separation between the urethra and vagina. (**C**) With continued growth the urogenital sinus disappears, as both the urethra and vaginal introitus are now at the perineal surface. The distal vagina is formed from sinus epithelium which streams into the vaginal vault. (**D**) With continued growth, the urethra turns anteriorly to reach its final location. *Source*: From Ref. 18.

layers arise within the bladder, and the urethral smooth muscle layers are induced one week later implying that these smooth muscle bodies are distinct entities despite their close approximation at the bladder neck (19). This should not be particularly surprising given the pharmacologic differences and functional demands between these two intravescial regions of smooth muscle.

The mechanism by which epithelial mesenchymal interactions induce smooth muscle development has been described. Using fetal rat primitive mesenchyme transfered below the renal capsule in nude mice, Baskin et al. demonstrated, that a transformation of this mesenchyme into smooth muscle was possible only if urothelium was also implanted simultaneously (20,21). The growth factors secreted by such epithelial regions are powerful driving forces for differentiation. In another murine model, it was observed that urethral urothelium implanted in a primitive limb bud, could induce additional digits to develop (11). Further morphological growth of smooth muscle development is accompanied by complex serial changes in muscle specific protein expression and cell turnover, as shown in a detailed study of mouse detrusor development (22).

DEVELOPMENT OF THE SPHINCTERS

Little data exists regarding the development of the internal or smooth muscle sphincter (i.e., the bladder neck). In contrast more efforts have been expended in trying to better characterize the development of the striated external sphincter. Evidence supports the notion of transdifferentiation from smooth to striated muscle which could then account for the development of the external sphincter (23). As an alternative explanation, anatomic observations in female fetal specimens confirm that by nine weeks of gestation, there is a condensation of undifferentiated mesenchyme immediately adjacent to the urethra. By 10 weeks of gestation this mesenchyme had differentiated into striated muscle which formed the omega shaped external sphincter (24,25). In this study, there was no evidence for

concentric development of this striated muscle group followed by a selective loss of muscle to produce the omega shape characteristic of this sphincter. Similar observations were reported by Yucel et al. (26) who also noted that this striated sphincter is always distinct from the levator muscle group, and commented on the innervation of this sphincter by both myelinated fibers and neurons that strained positively for nNOS (27). A recent study examining 28 female fetuses confirmed the presence of the external urethral sphincter primordium at week 9 of gestation. Additionally, at week 15 the smooth sphincter and rhabdosphincter could be clearly identified. Both muscular complexes were located in the middle third of the urethra but only the muscle fibers of the smooth sphincter intermingled with the detrusor muscle (28).

DEVELOPMENT OF THE TRIGONE AND UPPER URINARY TRACT

The pronephros develops at the fourth week and differentiates into the mesonephric ducts and the mesonephros. The mesonephros consists of glomeruli and tubules, which open into the mesonephric (Wolffian) ducts which are derived from the pronephric ducts. The mesonephric ducts extend caudally and drain into the cloaca (1), and an outgrowth of the ducts near their insertion at the cloaca gives rise to the ureteric buds (Figs. 21.5 and 21.6) (29,30). The ureteric buds grow cranially until they contact the metanephric mesenchyme at which point a series of complex reciprocal interactions between the bud and the mesoderm result in differentiation to the metanephros and ultimately a functioning kidney; fetal urine production is evident by the ninth week of gestation. The initiation location of the ureteric bud is critical for formation of the trigone, development of a normal vesicoureteral junction, and ultimately for the formation of a normal kidney. Over 30 years ago, Mackie and Stephens (31) proposed the ureteral bud hypothesis which stated that a bud arising from an abnormal location along the Wolffian duct would lead to abnormal nephrogenesis (Fig. 21.7) (32). They proposed that if the bud appeared too

175

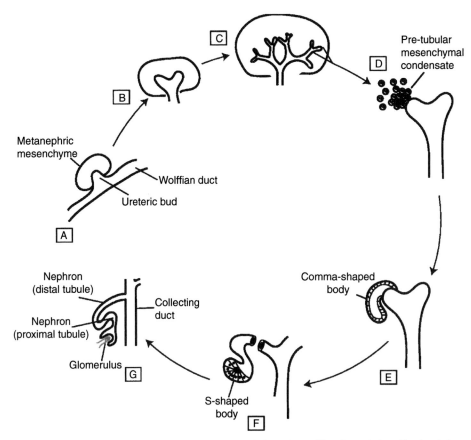

Figure 21.5 Stages of the renal branching morphogenesis: (**A**) Ureteric bud outgrowth from the Wolffian duct is induced by signals from the metanephric mesenchyme. (**B, C**) Invasion of the metanephric mesenchyme by the ureteric bud results in branching. (**D**) At the tips of the branches, the epithelium induces the mesenchyme to form pre-tubular aggregates, which are stimulated to undergo mesenchymal to epithelial transformation through the formation of comma-shaped (**E**) and S-shaped (**F**) bodies to form components of the nephron. (**G**) The renal tubules merge with the epithelial and vascular components of the glomerulus. *Source*: From Ref. 29.

close to the cloaca, it would ultimately be incorporated into the trigone in a very lateral position leaving it more prone to reflux and in extreme cases, abnormal nephrogenesis would occur. Clinically this might manifest in the neonate who presents with antenatally diagnosed hydronephrosis, who in the first days of life undergoes a voiding cystourethrogram (VCUG) demonstrating high grade reflux, and who on sonography has an abnormal renal parenchyma and an elevated creatinine. They also noted that if the bud arose too far away from the cloaca, it would be carried out into an ectopic position either within the bladder neck, urethra, or even the lateral walls of the vagina in females. Again, this ectopic ureter would subserve a tiny amount of renal parenchyma which in many instances would also be dysplastic.

The embryologic development of the trigone continues to be a source of some debate. The trigone was traditionally thought to be of mesodermal origin. In order for the ureteric bud to become incorporated into the developing UG sinus, the common nephric duct must become absorbed into this sinus. Thus it would stand to reason that at least part of the trigone is of mesodermal origin. However recent studies using transgenic mice suggest that in fact the trigone is of endodermal origin (33). Normal trigonal development is essential to the prevention of vesicoureteral reflux, a common clinical entity in young girls. Therefore, the development of the trigone itself

deserves examination. Historically, the trigone was believed to originate from the common nephric duct and the ureter (34). Yet, others postulated that the detrusor muscle contributed to the trigone (35). Examination of murine models recently demonstrated that the majority of the trigone is derived from the detrusor muscle but interdigitating ureteral fibers do contribute to the final trigonal structure. These data were obtained via immunohistochemical analysis of both murine and human fetal tissue (36). Apoptosis plays an integral role in trigone formation; the common nephric duct undergoes apoptosis resulting in separation of the ureter from the Wolffian duct and apoptosis is required to create a patent ureteral orifice (37–39). It is likely that the final position of the ureteral orifice also depends on the growth of the bladder itself (40).

The kidney develops as a result of complex reciprocal signaling between the ureteric bud and the primitive metanephric mesenchyme (29). Once this signaling is initiated, the bud elongates to penetrate the blastema, and the process of branching begins. In order for the final form of a single human kidney to have 500,000 to one million nephrons, the ureteral bud must undergo branching morphogenesis (Fig. 21.5) (29). Iterative branching with of the ureteral bud must occur about 15 times during human development in order to lead to this number of nephrons. As this division of the terminal ureteral bud takes place to produce a tree-like struc-

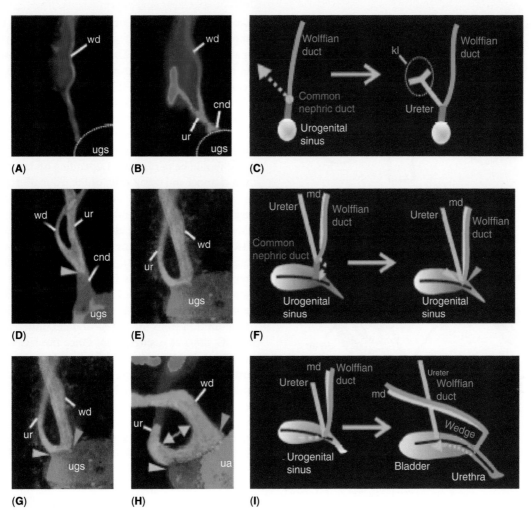

Figure 21.6 Visualization of the three stages of ureter maturation in vivo in a *Hoxb7*-GFP mice, that express green fluorescent protein in epithelia of the fetal excretory system. (**A–C**) Ureteric bud formation and outgrowth: The distal ureter (ur) remains attached to the Wolffian duct (wd). The distal ureter starts to separate from the primitive bladder (ugs) by a terminal Wolffian duct segment, the common nephric duct (cnd). (**D–F**) Vertical displacement: distal ureter descends and contacts the urogenital sinus. The yellow arrow indicates the common nephric duct. Broken yellow arrow shows downward movement of the ureter towards the urogenital sinus. Yellow and green arrowheads indicate final position of distal ureter and Wolffian duct. (**G–I**) Lateral displacement: The distal ureter separates from the Wolffian duct and moves to the final position at bladder base. Yellow and green arrowheads mark the position of distal ureter and Wolffian duct before and after separation. Double-headed yellow arrow indicates epithelial wedge, an epithelial outgrowth, which facilitates the separation. Color code for C, F, I: Wolffian duct and trigonal wedge: green, urogenital sinus: grey, Müllerian duct: pink, common nephric duct: red, kidney and ureter: blue. *Abbreviation*: md, Müllerian duct. *Source*: From Ref. 30.

ture, lateral branches diffferentiate into terminal bifid branches. In these terminal bifid branches, the ureteral bud tip will attach itself to a nephron, and remove itself from further bifurcations. This attachement of bud to a primitive nephron then initiates the formation of the full nephron. Critical to this view is the notion that the final population of nephrons is ultimately determined by the branching and proper functioning of the ureteral bud, a view espoused by Mackie and Stephens over 30 years ago (31). Equally critical to establishing normal renal function is the acquisition of the renal artery(ies) and subsequent vascular development [for a more detailed review of renal development, the reader is referred to Shah et al. (29)].

With current methods of molecular biology, the complex chemistry underlying these reciprocal interactions is being clarified, and several examples are offered here. Transcription factor PAX2 is expressed during normal kidney development and activates Wnt4 gene expression. PAX2 knockout mice are anephric while a heterozygous PAX2 mutation results in a 60% decrease in Wnt4 mRNA (41). In vitro studies have shown that Glial Derived Neurotrophic Factor (GDNF) secreted by the metanehpric mesenchyme serves to induce ureteric budding (32). This is supported by the observation that the ureters and kidney do not develop in GDNF knockout mice. It has also been shown that gene products that antagonize GDNF expression such as FOXc1 (Fig. 21.8) (32) or BMP4 (42) can result in multiple bud formation and duplex collecting systems. There is also a role for retinoic acid mediated signaling in the development of the ureteral buds and trigone as shown in a model using targeted deletion of the retinoic acid receptors (30). Abnormal vesicoureteral development has also been demonstrated in the presence of targeted RET overexpression (43), or the deletion of the type two angiotensin receptor (44).

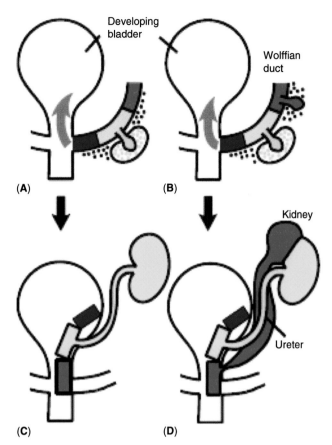

Figure 21.7 The ureteral bud hypothesis described by Mackie and Stephens in 1975 (ref. 31). (**A, B**) Normal kidney development: Single ureteral bud is induced and grows into the nephric mesenchyme (small dots). The caudal end of the Wolffian duct is incorporated into the developing bladder (red arrow). The yellow marked region contributes to the trigone, the green one to the urethra and blue for the lateral bladder. (**C, D**) Ectopic ureter development: a second, ectopic ureteral bud is induced more anteriorly than normal (green region at Wolffian duct), interacts with the adjacent nephrogenic mesenchyme giving rise to a duplex system. This ectopic ureter opens into the urethra with abnormal outflow and development of hydroureter. *Source:* From Ref. 32.

CLINICAL EXAMPLES

UG Sinus

Persistence of the UG sinus can occur as an isolated malformation or in association with other conditions such as congenital adrenal hyperplasia. In these patients the urethra and the vagina converge in a short common channel, and the convergence is close to the perineum. In some cases the voided urine is trapped within the vagina, resulting in hydrocolpos. These patients may present with a palpable pelvic mass requiring decompression, infection of obstructed urine, or overflow incontinence. The rectum is often displaced anteriorly, but it functions normally. A review of Figure 4 should allow the reader to understand the embryological basis for this anomaly. The distal Müllerian ducts fuse with the urethra and then migrate caudally during normal perineal development. Arrest of this distal migration at any point will result in a UG sinus as the fused urethra and vagina drain into a common channel. On physical examination the vaginal introitus is absent with a single opening in the urethral position, although the labia majora and minora might be normal in appearance. UG sinuses are usually separated into those with a low confluence, or short common channel, and

those with a high confluence, or long common channel. Separation into these two categories dictates the type of surgical repair can be performed. The distance from the bladder neck to the confluence is also paramount in determining the surgical technique and outcome (45).

The diagnosis of a UG sinus is confirmed radiographically with a retrograde contrast injection (i.e., a genitogram; Fig. 21.9). If the genitogram is inconclusive and does not reveal the level of confluence, a cystoscopy and retrograde contrast study should be performed. Depending on length of the common channel and complexity of related malformations different surgical procedures are available. The objectives of the surgical repair are separation of urinary and genital tract allowing normal voiding and creation of an adequate vaginal introitus. A UG sinus with a low confluence can be managed with a "cutback" operation, together with an inverted U-flap to prevent introital stenosis (46). When the common channel exceeds 3 cm the modified total UG sinus mobilization is the preferred approach (47,48). This technique avoids separation of the urethra from the vagina and circumferentially dissects the UG sinus as a single unit. Once the UG sinus has been mobilized distally, a perineal flap can be introduced into the posterior wall of the vagina providing a normal caliber vaginal opening. The UG sinus moblization technique has been modified since the original description. Rink and colleagues advocate utilizing the mobilized sinus tissue to create a mucosal vestibule or a posterior vaginal flap (49). Additionally these authors have described a partial urogenital mobilization that limits dissection to remain distal to the pubourethral ligament in hopes of avoiding dissection around the innervation of the urinary sphincter and clitoris (50). Depending on the length of the common channel and related anatomic malformations a more complex surgical repair may be necessary (51,52).

Case—A one-day-old female was noted to have a palpable mass in her lower abdomen, and songraphy revealed distended fluid filled collections in her pelvis. On physical exam, her lower abdomen was filled with a tense mass, the rectum was normally placed, but no vaginal introitus could be appreciated. Via the one opening near her introitus, a genitogram was performed (Fig. 21.9), demonstrating a common UG sinus with a bifurcation leading to the bladder and a dilated vagina. A subsequent endoscopic examination revealed the anatomy shown in Figure 21.9, and allowed for a plan of reconstruction to be developed. Using a posterior sagittal approach, the urethrovaginal trifurcation was divided, and the UG sinus was converted into the urethra. The vaginas were then mobilized, and moved down into the perineum with a perineal skin flap being used to complete the vaginoplasty.

Common Cloaca

Rarely patients may present with a common cloaca in which the urethra, vagina, and rectum converge into one common sinus that exits at the perineum. Many of these patients often present with the associated findings of spinal cord tethering and a neurogenic bladder. The association of these anomalies was initially described in 1961 by Duhamel and termed caudal regression syndrome (53). As the somites develop from cranial to caudal during early gestation, it is possible that a

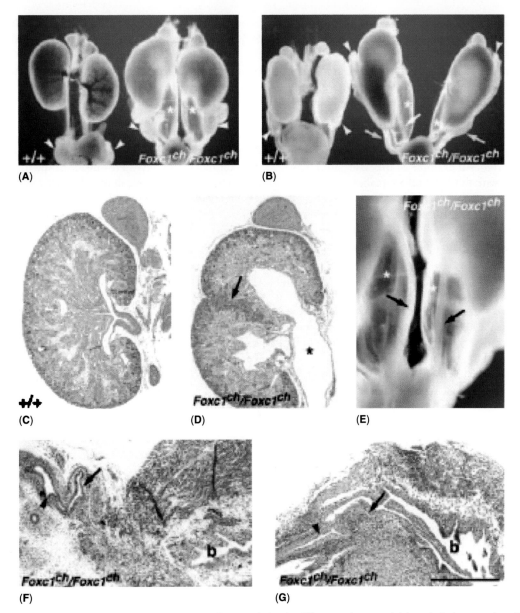

Figure 21.8 Kidney and ureter abnormalities in mice homozygous for Foxc1[ch]. (**A, B**) Wild-type and mutant: (**A**) in male, hydroureter (asterisks) and testis (white arrowheads) located more anteriorly in the mutant compared to wild-type; (**B**) in female, with hydroureter (asterisks) and normal ureter (white arrow) behind, and mutant ovaries located more anteriorly (white arrowheads). Section of wild-type (**C**) and mutant (**D**) kidneys with a duplex kidney in the mutant and clear boundary of the peripheral metanephrogenic mesenchyme (black arrow). The upper part of the kidney connects to the hydroureter (black asterisk). (**E**) Dorsal view of mutant kidney with normal ureters (black arrows) and ectopic hydroureter (white asterisks). (**F, G**) Sections showing abnormal position of hydroureters in mutants: (**F**) in male, hydroureter (arrow) does not connect to bladder (b); (**G**) in female, hydroureter (arrow) ends blindly, while normal ureter (arrowhead) connects to bladder (b). *Source*: From Ref. 32

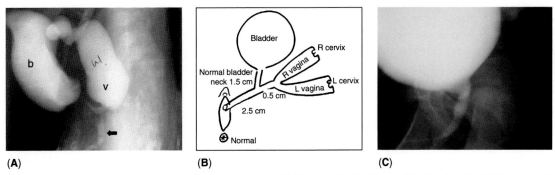

Figure 21.9 (**A**) Genitogram demonstrating a common urogenital sinus (arrow) dividing into bladder (b) and dilated vagina (v). (**B**) Summary of the anatomy as revealed by endoscopic examination. (**C**) Postoperative result after reconstruction and conversion of the urogenital sinus into urethra.

cloaca represents a late defect in somite development and a milder form of caudal regression syndrome. Rodent models have demonstrated that a retinoic acid teratogen can results in spina bifida, imperforate anus, gentourinary anomalies, omphalocele, and limb abnormalities when administered on gestational day 8 (equivalent to gestational week 4 in humans) (54,55). In contrast, administration of the same teratogen on gestational day 9 results in anal atresia, urethral atresia, and tail deformities providing evidence that these anomalies are part of a spectrum (56). An example of this association may be found in patients with the vertebral anomalies, anal atresia, cardiac anomalies, tracheo-esophageal fistula, esophageal atresia, renal anomalies, radial/limb anomalies syndrome. Neonates born with this anomaly require a multidisciplinary including general surgery, urology, and often neurosurgery and orthopedics.

Congenital Vaginal Anomalies

Though rare, a variety of congenital vaginal anomalies have been described in the urologic and gynecologic literature. Such anomalies include transverse vaginal septums, vaginal duplication, distal vaginal atresia, and vaginal agenesis. Increasingly these diagnoses may be made in the neonatal period because of the widespread use of prenatal sonography. Ultrasound can reveal hydrocolpos, duplications, or associated anomalies, such as unilateral renal agenesis, that raise suspicion for a vaginal anomaly. In contrast other vaginal anomalies may become manifest only with the onset of puberty. A thorough medical history and physical examination in conjunction with pelvic ultrasonography and magnetic resonance imaging (MRI) can usually determine the exact diagnosis (57). The constellation of vaginal agenesis, or the absence of the proximal vagina, and unilateral renal agenesis is the classic description of Mayer-Rokitansky-Kuster-Hauser syndrome (18). This association between anomalies of renal and vaginal development can be related to the complex relationship between the Wolffian ducts and Müllerian ducts . Disturbances in the paracrine signaling required for normal development of the genitourinary tract in women can likely result in abnormal renal and vaginal development. Thus it is not surprising that a condition in which ipsilateral and or bilateral vaginal agenesis or stenosis is associated with unilateral renal agenesis.

Case—A previously healthy and normally developed 12-year-old female presented with multiple one week episodes of abdominal pain occurring on a monthly basis; she was amenorrheic. Breast development was present as was pubic hair, and the urethra was normally placed above a blind ending vaginal introitus. Further imaging with ultrasound and MRI revealed a huge hematocolpos with dilated fallopian tubes on both sides (Fig. 21.10) without any other malformations of the upper or lower urinary tract. Evaluation under anesthesia revealed a complete distal atresia of the vagina; the vaginal to perineal surface distance was measured at 10 cm. She was managed with a combined laparoscopic mobilization of the proximal vagina, with a simultaneous perineal exploration and vaginal pull-through in combination with a perineal skin flap.

The normal urethral development seen in this case illustrates the concept that there was most likely a failure of fusion between the distal Müllerian ducts and the urethra (Fig. 21.4). Subsequently urethral migration proceeded distally leaving the distal Müllerian remnants in a position far from the perineal body. Normal urethral migration to the perineum is also seen in patients with androgen resistance syndromes despite the absence of the upper two thirds of the vagina, uterus, and fallopian tubes.

Ectopic Ureter

A ureter that opens anywhere outside of the trigone is considered ectopic and is the result of a displaced ureteric bud. Ureteric buds that develop very low along the mesonephric duct will be sited in a laterocranial ectopic position, often associated with a significant vesicoureteral reflux. In contrast, if a bud develops high along the mesonephric duct, it bypass the trigone and insert within the urethra, vestibule, or vagina. An ectopic ureter can drain a single system (58), but about 70% are associated with complete ureteral duplication with the ectopic ureter draining the upper moiety of a complete pyeloureteral duplication. Complete ureteral duplication occurs when two separate ureteral buds arise independently from the mesonephric duct. A duplex kidney is induced when these two buds meet the metanephric blastema. During the development of the trigone, the most cranial ureter that drains the upper moiety of the duplex kidney rotates inwardly on its long axis and crosses the lower pole ureter. A normal duplex kidney develops, if the two ureters originate close to each other and both ureteral orifices terminate on the trigone. However if the ureteral buds arise from widely separate positions on the mesonephric duct, the upper pole ureter is incorporated into the UG sinus at a later stage of development, and the resulting orifice is situated in an ectopic position, inferior to the trigone. This accounts for the Meyer Weigert law which states that the upper pole ureter shall always be found distal to that ureter which drains the lower renal unit. Mackie and Stephens (31) have postulated that induction of the metanephric blastema either too caudally or too cranially along the metanephric blastema, will result in renal dysplasia. This is the reason for impaired renal function of the renal unit draining into an ectopic ureter, whereas refluxing ureters most often drain normally functioning renal units.

If the ureter opens below the internal sphincter the ectopic ureter can present with incontinence. If the ureteric bud arises very high along the mesonephric duct it fails to become incorporated into the lower urinary tract and remains confluent with the mesonephric duct. These vestiges of the mesonephric system track along the lateral vagina wall and may become clinically manifest as Gartner's duct cysts. This also provides an embryologic basis for the rare vaginal ectopic ureter. Approximately one-half of female patients with ectopic ureters present with continuous dribbling of urine, despite normal bladder emptying due to the normally situated ipsilateral or contralateral ureteral orifices (58,59). If the ectopic ureter is draining a dysplastic or hypoplastic kidney or upper pole, infection or vaginal discharge may be the only complaint. Today, most of these cases are diagnosed by prenatal ultrasound, since most ectopic ureters are associated with sigificant hydronephrosis. On occasion this diagnosis is not established

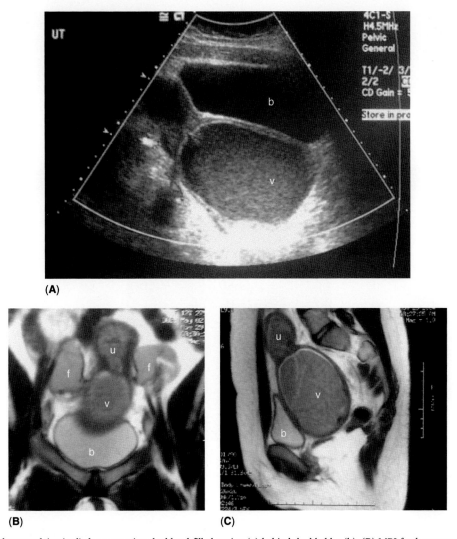

Figure 21.10 (**A**) Pelvic ultrasound (sagittal) demonstrating the blood filled vagina (v) behind the bladder (b). (**B**) MRI furthermore revealed dilated fallopian tubes (f) on both sides. (v) vagina, (u) uterus. (**C**) MRI in coronal view

before toilet training and some patients are mistakenly diagnosed with voiding dysfunction.

The traditional imaging workup included a cyclic VCUG which demonstrates reflux into the ectopic ureter in 70% to 80% of cases, and an iv urogram or CT scan. More recently the application of MR-urography has provided a global view of the malformation, including the renal dysplasia, and dilated ureter, even in the presence of diminished renal function (60). Depending on renal function the treatment varies from ureterureterostomy in duplicated systems, upper pole resection with or without ureterectomy, various ureteroneocystostomy procedures, or nephroureteroectomy.

Case—A seven-year-old female presented to the urology clinic for evaluation of continuous urinary incontinence. A renal bladder ultrasound ordered by her pediatrician was reviewed and found to be normal. She voided at regular intervals and was not constipated. A voiding log confirmed her good voiding habits and a urinary flow rate revealed a normal bell shaped curve with no residual urine as determined by office sonography (Fig. 21.11). An MRI urogram was obtained which confirmed the presence of a small upper pole duplica-

tion associated with an ectopic ureter to the urethra. Following an upper pole partial nephrectomy, she reported immediate continence of urine.

In rare instances bilateral ureteral budding may occur at a cranial location along the mesonephric duct and result in bilateral ectopic ureters. These patients present with total urinary incontinence, a deficient internal sphincter, and a non compliant bladder with small capacity. These cases serve to illustrate the importance of bladder cycling to the aquisition of normal capacity and compliance, a concept that has been confirmed in fetal experimental models (61). For these patients, urinary continence will require complex surgery most often consisting of a bladder neck reconstruction, ureteral reimplantation, and augmentation.

Ureterocele

A ureterocele is a cystic dilation of the lower end of the ureter which protrudes into the bladder. The origin of the defect begins in the eighth week of gestation. This anomaly has been attributed to a failure of Chwalle's epithelial membrane to regress during the incorporation of the ureteral bud into

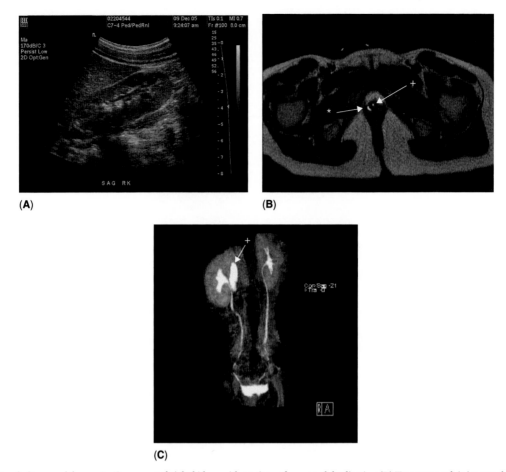

Figure 21.11 (**A**) Renal ultrasound demonstrating a normal right kidney with no signs of a ureteral duplication (**B**) Transverse pelvic images showing the insertion of the ectopic ureter (*) into the urethra adjacent to the foley catheter (+) placed at the time of the MRI urogram. (**C**) Coronal sections of the abdomen on MRI showing a ureteral duplication (+). At surgical exploration this ureter was found to connect with a tiny remnant of renal parenchyma.

developing trigone (62). Ureteroceles are associated with duplex systems in 80% of cases, and girls are affected four times more frequently than boys (63,64). Since most ureteroceles are associated with hydronephrosis, the vast majority of these patients are now being diagnosed with antenatal ultrasound (65). Prenatal diagnosis and management of duplex system ureteroceles are beneficial to decrease morbidity and potential adverse outcomes related to infection (66). Clinically, ureteroceles are the most common cause of retention in female infants (67).

The initial workup of these patients should include n renal and bladder ultrasound, a VCUG to detect whether there is associated reflux, and a renal scan to determine the functional contribution of the system (especially in the case of the rare single system ureterocele). Patients with ureteroceles have a high incidence of associated vesicoureteral reflux into the ipsilateral lower pole and less commonly the contralateral collecting system (68). The presence or absence of reflux may affect the type of surgical intervention performed and therefore must be established. A large number of options exist for management of these patients: complete upper and lower urinary tract reconstruction, upper pole heminephrectomy (simplified approach) and ureterocele decompression and observation, and endoscopic incision (69–72). While endoscopic decompression may be definitive treatment for intravesical

ureteroceles, partial nephrectomy appears to be more definitive for extravesical ureteroceles. Other groups advocate primary endoscopic puncture even for patients with ectopic and duplex ureteroceles, because a third of patients are definitively treated and early decompression is presumed to reduce the risk of pyelonephritis (71).

Incontinence may be seen after the initial treatment of ectopic ureteroceles and is thought to be related to iatrogenic bladder neck or external urinary sphincter injury at surgery. However, Ewalt et al. observed that, in patients treated by partial nephrectomy alone, 10% subsequently developed urinary stress incontinence, despite the abscence of any bladder neck surgery (73). It seems that large ureteroceles are capable of significantly distorting the developing bladder neck and urethra, which will not become apparent until the system is decompressed by whatever means used. In a more recent study (74) the authors concluded that children with ectopic ureteroceles presenting with incontinence are at high risk for a high capacity bladder with incomplete emptying and bladder dysfunction following bladder neck procedures. They concluded that this was not related to the operative intervention, but rather an integral part of the disorder.

Case—An 11-year-old continent girl presented with recurrent febrile urinary tract infections. Sonography revealed duplications of both kidneys and a large ectopic ureterocele draining the upper moiety of the right kidney. The VCUG demonstrated right sided reflux into both moieties on the right side. An endoscopic examination revealed a ureterocele that extended into the bladder neck and upper one-third of the urethra. An endosopic puncture and decompression of the ureterocele was performed. Postoperatively the patient experienced moderate stress incontinence that she had not manifested preoperatively and a VCUG revealed persisting right high grade reflux. A right sided common sheath reimplant, ureterocele excision, and bladder neck reconstruction were performed. Five years later she remains continent, and free of infections off antibiotic prophylaxis.

This clinical evidence would suggest that once a large ectopic ureterocele is deflated, function of the bladder neck and urethra may impaired due to distortion of these structures by the long standing distention.

REFERENCES

1. Moore KL, Persuad TVN. The Developing Human: Clinically Oriented Embryology, 5th edn. Philadelphia: Saunders, 1993: 71–92.
2. Stephens FD, Smith ED, Hutson JM. Normal Embryology of the Cloaca. In: Congenital Anomalies of the Kidney, Urinary, and Genital Tract, 2nd edn. London: Martin Dunitz Ltd, 2002: 3–12.
3. Rathke H. Abhandlungen zur Bildungs-und Entwicklungsgeschichte der Tiere. Leipzig, 1832.
4. Tourneux F. Sur les premiers developpements du cloaques du tubercule genital et de l'anus chez l'embryon de mouton. J Anat 1888; 24: 503–17.
5. Vermeij-Keers C, Hartwig NG, van der Werff JF. Embryonic development of the ventral body wall and its congenital malformations. Semin Pediatr Surg 1996; 5: 82–9.
6. Nievelstein RA, van der Werff JF, Verbeek FJ, et al. Normal and abnormal embryonic development of the anorectum in human embryos. Teratol 1998; 57: 70–8.
7. Sasaki Y, Iwai N, Tsuda T, Kimura O. Sonic hedgehog and bone morphogenetic protein 4 expressions in the hindgut region of murine embryos with anorectal malformations. J Pediatr Surg 2004; 39: 170–3; discussion 170–3.
8. Sukegawa A, Narita T, Kameda T, et al. The concentric structure of the developing gut is regulated by Sonic hedgehog derived from endodermal epithelium. Development 2000; 127: 1971–80.
9. Nakata M, Takada Y, Hishiki T, et al. Induction of Wnt5a-expressing mesenchymal cells adjacent to the cloacal plate is an essential process for its proximodistal elongation and subsequent anorectal development. Pediatr Res 2009; 66: 149–54.
10. Mo R, Kim JH, Zhang J, et al. Anorectal malformations caused by defects in sonic hedgehog signaling. Am J Pathol 2001; 159: 765–74.
11. Perriton CL, Powles N, Chiang C, et al. Sonic hedgehog signaling from the urethral epithelium controls external genital development. Dev Biol 2002; 247: 26–46.
12. Lorenzo AJ, Nguyen MT, Sozubir S, et al. Dihydrotestosterone induction of EphB2 in the female genital tubercle mimics male pattern of expression during embryogenesis. J Urol 2003; 170: 1618–23.
13. Kobayashi A, Shawlot W, Kania A, Behringer RR. Requirement of Lim1 for female reproductive tract development. Dev 2004; 131: 539–49. [Epub 2003 Dec 24].
14. Carroll TJ, Park JS, Hayashi S, et al. Wnt9b plays a central role in the regulation of mesenchymal to epithelial transitions underlying organogenesis of the mammalian urogenital system. Dev Cell 2005; 9: 283–92.
15. Mendelsohn C, Lohnes D, Décimo D, et al. Function of the retinoic acid receptors (RARs) during development (II). Multiple abnormalities at various stages of organogenesis in RAR double mutants. Development 1994; 120: 2749–71.
16. Guioli S, Sekido R, Lovell-Badge R. The origin of the Mullerian duct in chick and mouse. Dev Biol 2007; 302: 389–98. [Epub 2006 Oct 3].
17. Orvis GD, Behringer RR. Cellular mechanisms of Mullerian duct formation in the mouse. Dev Biol 2007; 306: 493–504. [Epub 2007 Mar 27].
18. Stephens FD, Smith ED, Hutson JM. Müllerian and Wolffian Anomalies. Congenital Anomalies of the Urinary and Genital Tracts, 2nd edn. London: Martin Dunitz Ltd, 2002: 50–62.
19. Parrot TS, Gray SW, Skandalakis JE. The Bladder and Urethra. Embryology for Surgeons: The Embryological Basis for the Treatment of Congenital Anomalies, 2nd edn. Baltimore: Williams & Wilkins, 1994: 671–8.
20. Baskin LS, Hayward SW, Young P, Cunha GR. Role of mesenchymal-epithelial interactions in normal bladder development. J Urol 1996; 156: 1820–7.
21. Baskin L, Disandro M, Li Y, et al. Mesenchymal-epithelial interactions in bladder smooth muscle development: effects of the local tissue environment. J Urol 2001; 165: 1283–8.
22. Smeulders N, Woolf AS, Wilcox DT. Smooth muscle differentiation and cell turnover in mouse detrusor development. J Urol 2002; 167: 385–90.
23. Borirakchanyavat S, Baskin LS, Kogan BA, Cunha GR. Smooth and striated muscle development in the intrinsic urethral sphincter. J Urol 1997; 158: 1119–22.
24. Sebe P, Schwentner C, Oswald J, et al. Fetal development of striated and smooth muscle sphincters of the male urethra from a common primordium and modifications due to the development of the prostate: an anatomic and histologic study. Prostate 2005; 62: 388–93.
25. Ludwikowski B, Oesch Hayward I, Brenner E, Fritsch H. The development of the external urethral sphincter in humans. BJU Int 2001; 87: 565–8.
26. Yucel S, Baskin LS. An anatomical description of the male and female urethral sphincter complex. J Urol 2004; 171: 1890–7.
27. Yucel S, De Souza A, Jr., Baskin LS. Neuroanatomy of the human female lower urogenital tract. J Urol 2004; 172: 191–5.
28. Sebe P, Fritsch H, Oswald J, et al. Fetal development of the female external urinary sphincter complex: an anatomical and histological study. J Urol 2005; 173: 1738–42; discussion 1742.
29. Shah MM, Sampogna RV, Sakurai H, et al. Branching morphogenesis and kidney disease. Development 2004; 131: 1449–62.
30. Batourina E, Choi C, Paragas N, et al. Distal ureter morphogenesis depends on epithelial cell remodeling mediated by vitamin A and Ret.[erratum appears in Nat Genet 2002; 32: 331]. Nat Genet 2002; 32: 109–15.
31. Mackie GG, Stephens FD. Duplex kidneys: a correlation of renal dysplasia with position of the ureteral orifice. J Urol 1975; 114: 274–80.
32. Kume T, Deng K, Hogan BL. Murine forkhead/winged helix genes Foxc1 (Mf1) and Foxc2 (Mfh1) are required for the early organogenesis of the kidney and urinary tract. Development 2000; 127: 1387–95.
33. Thomas JC, Demarco RT, Pope JC. Molecular biology of ureteral bud and trigonal development. Curr Urol Rep 2005; 6: 146–51.
34. Wesson M. Anatomical, embryological and physiological studies of the trigone and bladder neck. J Urol 1925; 4: 280.
35. Meyer R. Normal and abnormal development of the ureter in the human embryo–a mechanistic consideration. Anat Rec 1946; 68: 355.
36. Viana R, Batourina E, Huang H, et al. The development of the bladder trigone, the center of the anti-reflux mechanism. Development 2007; 134: 3763–9. [Epub 2007 Sep 19].
37. Cecconi F, Alvarez-Bolado G, Meyer BI, et al. Apaf1 (CED-4 homolog) regulates programmed cell death in mammalian development. Cell 1998; 94: 727–37.
38. Ruano-Gil D, Coca-Payeras A, Tejedo-Mateu A. Obstruction and normal recanalization of the ureter in the human embryo. Its relation to congenital ureteric obstruction. Eur Urol 1975; 1: 287–93.
39. Batourina E, Tsai S, Lambert S, et al. Apoptosis induced by vitamin A signaling is crucial for connecting the ureters to the bladder. Nat Genet 2005; 37: 1082–9. [Epub 2005 Sep 25].
40. Mendelsohn C. Using mouse models to understand normal and abnormal urogenital tract development. Organogenesis 2009; 5: 306–14.
41. Torban E, Dziarmaga A, Iglesias D, et al. PAX2 activates WNT4 expression during mammalian kidney development. J Biol Chem 2006; 281: 12705–12. [Epub 2005 Dec 19].
42. Miyazaki Y, Oshima K, Fogo A, et al. Bone morphogenetic protein 4 regulates the budding site and elongation of the mouse ureter. J Clin Invest 2000; 105: 863–73.
43. Yu OH, Murawski IJ, Myburgh DB, Gupta IR. Overexpression of RET leads to vesicoureteric reflux in mice. Am J Physiol Renal Physiol 2004; 287: F1123–30. [Epub 2004 Aug 24].

44. Ichikawa I, Kuwayama F, Pope JC 4th, et al. Paradigm shift from classic anatomic theories to contemporary cell biological views of CAKUT. Kidney Int 2002; 61: 889–98.
45. Rink RC, Adams MC, Misseri R. A new classification for genital ambiguity and urogenital sinus anomalies. BJU Int 2005; 95: 638–42.
46. Fortunoff S, Lattimer JK, Edson M. Vaginoplasty tque for female pseudohermaphrodites. Surg Gynecol Obstet 1964; 118: 545–8.
47. Pena A. Total urogenital mobilization–an easier way to repair cloacas. J Pediatr Surg 1997; 32: 263–7; discussion 267–8.
48. Ludwikowski B, Oesch Hayward I, Gonzalez R. Total urogenital sinus mobilization: expanded applications. BJU Int 1999; 83: 820–2.
49. Rink RC, Metcalfe PD, Cain MP, et al. Use of the mobilized sinus with total urogenital mobilization. J Urol 2006; 176: 2205–11.
50. Rink RC, Metcalfe PD, Kaefer MA, et al. Partial urogenital mobilization: a limited proximal dissection. J Pediatr Urol 2006; 2: 351–6. [Epub 2006 Jul 10].
51. Domini R, Rossi F, Ceccarelli PL, De Castro, R. Anterior sagittal transanorectal approach to the urogenital sinus in adrenogenital syndrome: preliminary report. J Pediatr Surg 1997; 32: 714–16.
52. Peña A, Filmer B, Bonilla E, et al. Transanorectal approach for the treatment of urogenital sinus: preliminary report. J Pediatr Surg 1992; 27: 681–5.
53. Duhamel B. From the mermaid to anal imperforation: the syndrome of caudal regression. Arch Dis Child 1961; 36: 152–5.
54. Danzer E, Kiddoo D, Redden RA, et al. Structural and functional characterization of bladder smooth muscle in fetal rats with retinoic acid-induced myelomeningocele. Am J Physiol Renal Physiol 2007; 292: F197–206. [Epub 2006 Aug 29].
55. Padmanabhan R, Retinoic acid-induced caudal regression syndrome in the mouse fetus. Reprod Toxicol 1998; 12: 139–51.
56. Mesrobian HG, Sessions RP, Lloyd RA, et al. Cloacal and urogenital abnormalities induced by etretinate in mice. J Urol 1994; 152: 675–8.
57. Govindarajan MJ, Rajan RS, Kalyanpur A, Ravikumar. Magnetic resonance imaging diagnosis of Mayer-Rokitansky-Kuster-Hauser syndrome. J Hum Reprod Sci 2008; 1: 83–5.
58. Ahmed S, Barker A. Single-system ectopic ureters: a review of 12 cases. J Pediatr Surg 1992; 27: 491–6.
59. Fernbach SK, Feinstein KA, Spencer K, Lindstrom CA. Ureteral duplication and its complications. Radiographics 1997; 17: 109–27.
60. Avni FE, Nicaise N, Hall M, et al. The role of MR imaging for the assessment of complicated duplex kidneys in children: preliminary report. Pediatr Radiol 2001; 31: 215–23.
61. Matsumoto S, Kogan BA, Levin RM, et al. Response of the fetal sheep bladder to urinary diversion. J Urol 2003; 169: 735–9.
62. Chwalla R. Eine bemerkenswerte Anomalie der Harnblase bei einem menschlichen Embryo von 32,5mm St.Sch.L. Virchows Archiv 1927; 263: 632–48.
63. Coplen DE, Duckett JW. The modern approach to ureteroceles. J Urol 1995; 153: 166–71.
64. Gonzales E. Clinical pediatric urology. In: Kelalis P KL, Belman AB, ed. Anomalies of Renal Pelvis and Ureter, 3rd edn. Philadelphia: Saunders, 1992.
65. Barthold JS. Individualized approach to the prenatally diagnosed ureterocele. [comment]. J Urol 1998; 159: 1011–12.
66. Upadhyay J, Bolduc S, Braga L, et al. Impact of prenatal diagnosis on the morbidity associated with ureterocele management. J Urol 2002; 167: 2560–5.
67. Merlini E, Lelli Chiesa P. Obstructive ureterocele-an ongoing challenge. World J Urol 2004; 22: 107–14.
68. Shekarriz B, Upadhyay J, Fleming P, et al. Long-term outcome based on the initial surgical approach to ureterocele. J Urol 1999; 162: 1072–6.
69. Chertin B, et al. Endoscopic puncture of ureterocele as a minimally invasive and effective long-term procedure in children. Eur Urol 2001; 39: 332–6.
70. Chertin B, de Caluwe D, Puri P. Is primary endoscopic puncture of ureterocele a long-term effective procedure? J Pediatr Surg 2003; 38: 116–99; discussion 116–19.
71. Cooper CS, Passerini-Glazel G, Hutcheson JC, et al. Long-term followup of endoscopic incision of ureteroceles: intravesical versus extravesical. J Urol 2000; 164: 1097–100.
72. Husmann DA, Strand B, Ewalt D, et al. Management of ectopic ureterocele associated with renal duplication: a comparison of partial nephrectomy and endoscopic decompression. J Urol 1999; 162: 1406–9.
73. Husmann DA, Ewalt DH, Glenski WJ, Bernier PA. Ureterocele associated with ureteral duplication and a nonfunctioning upper pole segment: management by partial nephroureterectomy alone. J Urol 1995; 154: 723–6.
74. Abrahamsson K, Hansson E, Sillén U, et al. Bladder dysfunction: an integral part of the ectopic ureterocele complex. J Urol 1998; 160: 1468–70.

22 Tissue Engineering and Regenerative Medicine for the Female Genitourinary System

Anthony Atala

INTRODUCTION

The use of one body part for another or the exchange of parts from one person to another was mentioned in the medical literature even in antiquity. This concept has captured the imagination of many over time. However, even three decades ago, the technology required to put these techniques into clinical practice did not exist. As technology evolved, however, synthetic materials were introduced to replace or rebuild diseased tissues in the human body. The advent of new manmade materials such as tetrafluoroethylene (Teflon) silicone created a new field that included a wide array of devices that could be applied for human use. However, although these devices could provide structural support, the functional component of the original tissue could not be replicated.

Simultaneously, knowledge of the biologic sciences (cell biology, molecular biology, and biochemistry) increased rapidly, and new techniques for cell harvesting, culture, and expansion were developed. The concept of cell transplantation was developed and culminated with the first human bone marrow cell transplant in the 1970s. At this time, researchers began to combine the scientific fields of devices and materials sciences with cell biology, and in effect started a new field called "tissue engineering." Tissue engineering was defined as "a field which applies the principles of engineering and life sciences towards the development of biological substitutes that restore or improve tissue function" (1). The first use of the term "tissue engineering" in the literature can be traced to a reference dealing with corneal tissue in 1985 (2).

The stem cell field also received a large boost in the early 1980s with the discovery of mouse embryonic stem (ES) cells (3) and later, with the description of human ES (hES) cells in 1998 (4). In 1997, the creation of the first cloned mammal, a sheep named Dolly (5), was announced. In 1999, the term "regenerative medicine" was coined (6) to describe the unifying goal of cell transplantation, tissue engineering, and nuclear transfer—the regeneration of living tissues and organs.

In the last two decades, scientists have attempted to create treatment modalities using regenerative medicine techniques for virtually every tissue of the human body. This chapter reviews some of the progress that has been achieved in the field of female genitourinary regenerative medicine.

Regenerative medicine strategies usually fall into one of three categories: (*i*) cell-based therapies, (*ii*) the use of biomaterials (scaffolds) or inductive agents to activate the body's natural ability to regenerate and to orient or direct new tissue growth, and (*iii*) the use of biomaterials seeded with cells and/or inductive agents to create tissue substitutes.

SOURCES OF CELLS FOR USE IN CELL-BASED THERAPIES

Stem Cells

The cells used for regenerative medicine can be autologous or heterologous, and from either native or stem cell sources. In general, there are three broad categories of stem cells obtained from living tissue that are used for cell therapies. ES cells are obtained through the aspiration of the inner cell mass of a blastocyst or, more recently, a single cell from this mass. Fetal and neonatal amniotic fluid and placenta may contain multipotent cells that may be useful in cell therapy applications. Adult stem cells are usually isolated from organ or bone marrow biopsies. Stem cells are defined as having three important properties: (*i*) the ability to self-renew, (*ii*) the ability to differentiate into a number of different cell types, (*iii*) and the ability to easily form clonal populations (populations of cells derived from a single stem cell). Many techniques for obtaining stem cells have been studied over the past few decades. Some of these techniques have yielded promising results, but others require further research. The main techniques are discussed in detail below, and their advantages and limitations are summarized in Table 22.1.

Embryonic Stem Cells

Given that some cells cannot be expanded ex vivo, ES cells could be an ideal resource for regenerative medicine because of their fundamental properties: the ability to self-renew indefinitely and the ability to differentiate into cells from all three embryonic germ layers. Skin and neurons have been formed, indicating ectodermal differentiation (7–9). Blood, cardiac cells, cartilage, endothelial cells, and muscle have been formed, indicating mesodermal differentiation (10–12). Finally, pancreatic cells have been formed, indicating endodermal differentiation (13). In addition, as further evidence of their pluripotency, ES cells can form embryoid bodies, which are cell aggregations that contain all three embryonic germ layers, while in culture, and they can form teratomas in vivo (14). These cells have demonstrated longevity in culture and can maintain their undifferentiated state for at least 80 passages when grown using current published protocols (4,15).

In addition to the potential for formation of teratomas and teratocarcinomas, the clinical use of ES cells is limited because they represent an allogenic resource and thus have the potential to evoke an immune response. New stem cell technologies [such as somatic cell nuclear transfer (SCNT) and reprogramming] may overcome the rejection challenges. Ethical concerns surrounding the destruction of embryos to obtain human ES cells also limit their clinical utility at this time. A method of

Table 22.1 Summary of Alternate Methods for Generating Pluripotent Stem Cells

Method	Advantages	Limitations
Somatic cell nuclear transfer	Customized stem cells	Requires oocytes
	Has been shown to work in non-human primates	Has not been shown to work in humans
Single cell embryo biopsy	Patient-specific to embryo	Allogeneic cell types
	Does not destroy or create embryos	Is not known if single cells are totipotent
	Has been done in humans	Requires coculturing with a previously established human embryonic stem cell line
Arrested embryos	Cells obtained from discarded embryos	Allogeneic cell types
	Has been done in humans	Quality of cell lines might be questionable
Altered nuclear transfer	Customized stem cells	Ethical issues surround embryos with no potential
		Modified genome
		Has not been done with human cells
Reprogramming	Customized stem cells	Retroviral transduction
	No embryos or oocytes needed	Oncogenes
	Has been done with human cells	

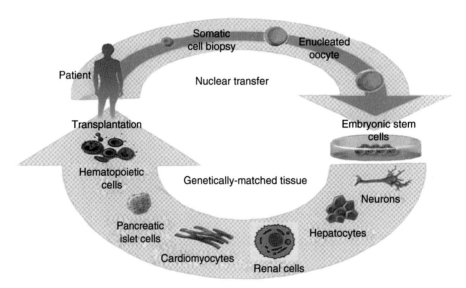

Figure 22.1 Therapeutic cloning strategy and its application to the engineering of tissues and organs.

isolating hES cells without destroying the embryo was described in 2006 (16), based on a technique used to obtain a single cell embryo biopsy for preimplantation genetic diagnosis. Cells were taken from eight-cell blastomeres rather than from blastocysts. The cells differentiated into derivatives of all three embryonic germ layers in vitro and as well as into teratomas in vivo.

Human embryonic stem cell lines can also be derived from arrested embryos (17). During in vitro fertilization, only a small proportion of zygotes produced will develop successfully to the morula and blastocyst stages. Over half the embryos stop dividing and are, therefore, considered dead embryos (18). Such embryos have unequal or fragmented cells and are usually discarded. However, these arrested embryos do contain some normal cells.

Therapeutic Cloning (SCNT)
SCNT, or therapeutic cloning, involves the removal of an oocyte nucleus in culture, followed by its replacement with a

nucleus derived from a somatic cell obtained from a patient. Activation with chemicals or electricity stimulates cell division up to the blastocyst stage. This process is outlined in Figure 22.1.

It is important to differentiate between the two types of cloning that exist—reproductive cloning and therapeutic cloning. Both involve the insertion of donor DNA into an enucleated oocyte to generate an embryo that has identical genetic material to its DNA source. However, in reproductive cloning, the embryo is then implanted into the uterus of a pseudopregnant female to produce an infant that is a clone of the donor (e.g., the birth of Dolly in 1997). There are many ethical concerns surrounding this practice and, as a result, reproductive cloning has been banned in most countries.

While therapeutic cloning also produces an embryo that is genetically identical to the donor, this process is used to generate blastocysts that are explanted and grown in culture, not in utero. The inner cell mass is isolated and cultured, resulting in ES cells that are genetically identical to the patient. Although

ES cells derived from SCNT contain the nuclear genome of the donor cells, there was a question whether mitochondrial DNA (mtDNA) contained in the oocyte could lead to immunogenicity after transplantation. To assess the histocompatibility of tissue generated using SCNT, Lanza et al. microinjected the nucleus of a bovine skin fibroblast into an enucleated oocyte (19). Although the blastocyst was implanted (reproductive cloning), the purpose was to generate renal, cardiac, and skeletal muscle cells, which were then harvested, expanded in vitro, and seeded onto biodegradable scaffolds. These scaffolds were then implanted into the donor steer from which the cells were cloned to determine if cells were histocompatible. Analysis revealed that cloned renal cells showed no evidence of T-cell response, suggesting that rejection will not necessarily occur in the presence of oocyte-derived mtDNA. This finding represents a step forward in overcoming the histocompatibility problem of stem cell therapy.

Non-human primate ES cell lines have been generated by SCNT of nuclei from adult skin fibroblasts (20,21). The low efficiency of SNCT (0.7%) and the inadequate supply of human oocytes currently hinder the therapeutic potential of this technique.

Altered Nuclear Transfer

Altered nuclear transfer is a variation of SCNT in which a genetically modified nucleus from a somatic cell is transferred into a human oocyte. This embryo, which contains a deliberate genetic defect, is capable of developing into a blastocyst, but the induced defect prevents the blastocyst from implanting in the uterus. This process has the potential to generate customized hES cells from the blastocyst stage (22). Human embryos with this genetic defect might lack the capacity to develop into viable fetuses, as a result of their inability to implant, thus providing a source of stem cells without destroying viable embryos. Proof of concept was obtained in mice (23) in 2006 using embryos lacking the *Cdx2* homeobox gene.

Reprogramming (Induced Pluripotent Stem Cells)

Reports of the successful transformation of adult cells into pluripotent stem cells through a type of genetic "reprogramming" have been published. Reprogramming is a technique that involves de-differentiation of adult somatic cells to produce patient-specific pluripotent stem cells, eliminating the need to create embryos. Cells generated by reprogramming would be genetically identical to the somatic cells (and thus, the patient who donated these cells) and would not be rejected. Yamanaka was the first to discover that mouse embryonic fibroblasts and adult mouse fibroblasts could be reprogrammed into an "induced pluripotent state (iPS)" (24). These iPS cells possessed the immortal growth characteristics of self-renewing ES cells, expressed genes specific for ES cells, and generated embryoid bodies in vitro and teratomas in vivo. When iPS cells were injected into mouse blastocysts, they contributed to a variety of cell types. However, although iPS cells selected in this way were pluripotent, they were not identical to ES cells. Unlike ES cells, chimeras made from iPS cells did not result in full-term pregnancies. Gene expression profiles of the iPS cells showed that they possessed a distinct gene expression signature that was different from that of ES cells. In addition, the epigenetic state of the iPS cells was somewhere between that found in somatic cells and that found in ES cells, suggesting that the reprogramming was incomplete.

These results were improved significantly by Wernig and Jaenisch in July 2007 (25). In this study, DNA methylation, gene expression profiles, and the chromatin state of the reprogrammed cells were similar to those of ES cells. Teratomas induced by these cells contained differentiated cell types representing all three embryonic germ layers. Most importantly, the reprogrammed cells from this experiment were able to form viable chimeras and contribute to the germ line like ES cells, suggesting that these iPS cells were completely reprogrammed.

It has recently been shown that reprogramming of human cells is possible (26,27). Yamanaka generated human iPS cells that are similar to hES cells in terms of morphology, proliferation, gene expression, surface markers, and teratoma formation. Thompson's group showed that retroviral transduction of the stem cell markers *OCT4, SOX2, NANOG,* and *LIN28* could generate pluripotent stem cells. However, in both studies, the human iPS cells were similar but not identical to hES cells.

One major obstacle to clinical translation of iPS cell-based therapeutics is the fact that these cells are created using potentially harmful genome-integrating viruses such as retroviruses and lentiviruses. The use of these types of viruses can lead to insertional mutagenesis and carcinogenesis. Thus, cells that contain these potential problems cannot be used clinically, and generation of iPS cells without these integrations would be advantageous. Recently, several groups have described the generation of iPS cells using transient gene expression methods such as adenoviral transfection (28) and nucleofection of a polycistronic gene expression vector (29). Both of these methods were used to transiently express Oct4, Sox2, Klf4, and c-Myc in murine somatic cells, and they resulted in the generation of pluripotent cells, suggesting that the genes for these factors do not need to be inserted into the genome in order to perform reprogramming functions.

Although reprogramming is an exciting phenomenon, our limited understanding of the mechanism underlying it currently limits the clinical applicability of the technique, but the future potential of reprogramming is quite exciting.

Amniotic-Fluid and Placenta-derived Stem (AFPS) Cells

The amniotic fluid and placental membrane contain a heterogeneous population of cell types derived from the developing fetus (30,31). Cells found in this heterogeneous population include mesenchymal stem cells (32,33). In addition, the isolation of multipotent human and mouse AFPS cells that are capable of extensive self-renewal and give rise to cells from all three germ layers was reported in 2007 (34). AFPS cells represent approximately 1% of the cells found in the amniotic fluid and placenta. The undifferentiated stem cells expand extensively without a feeder cell layer and double every 36 hours. Unlike hES cells, the AFPS cells do not form tumors in vivo. Lines maintained for over 250 population doublings retained long telomeres and a normal complement of chromosomes. AFPS cell lines can be induced to differentiate into cells representing each embryonic germ layer. Amniotic fluid-derived stem cells represent a new class of stem cells with properties somewhere between those of embryonic and adult stem cell types. They are probably more agile than adult stem cells, but less so than ES cells. Unlike embryonic and induced pluripotent stem cells, however, AFPS cells do not form teratomas, and if preserved for self-use, the problem of rejection can be avoided. The cells could be obtained either from amniocentesis or chorionic villous sampling in the developing fetus, or from the placenta at the time of birth. They could be preserved for self use or banked. A bank of 100,000 specimens could potentially supply 99% of the U.S. population with a perfect genetic match for transplantation. Such a bank may be easier to create than with other cell sources, since there are approximately 4.5 million births per year in the United States.

Since the description of AFPS cells, other groups have published on the potential of the cells to differentiate to other lineages, such as cartilage (35), kidney (36), and lung (37). Muscle differentiated AFPS cells were also noted to prevent compensatory bladder hypertrophy in a cryo-injured rodent bladder model (38).

Adult Stem Cells
Adult stem cells, especially hematopoietic stem cells, are the best understood cell type in stem cell biology (39). However, adult stem cell research remains an area of intense study, as their potential for therapy may be applicable to a myriad of degenerative disorders. Within the past decade, adult stem cell populations have been found in many adult tissues other than the bone marrow and the gastrointestinal tract, including the brain (40,41), skin (42), and muscle (43). Many other types of adult stem cells have been identified in organs all over the body and are thought to serve as the primary repair entities for their corresponding organs (44). The discovery of such tissue-specific progenitors has opened up new avenues for research.

A notable exception to the tissue-specificity of adult stem cells is the mesenchymal stem cell, also known as the multipotent adult progenitor cell. This cell type is derived from bone marrow stroma (45,46). Such cells can differentiate in vitro into numerous tissue types (47,48) and can also differentiate developmentally if injected into a blastocyst. Multipotent adult progenitor cells can develop into a variety of tissues.

Research into adult stem cells has, however, progressed slowly, mainly because investigators have had great difficulty in maintaining adult non-mesenchymal stem cells in culture. Some cells, such as those of the liver, pancreas, and nerve, have very low proliferative capacity in vitro, and the functionality of some cell types is reduced after the cells are cultivated. Isolation of cells has also been problematic, because stem cells are present in extremely low numbers in adult tissue (49,50). While the clinical utility of adult stem cells is currently limited, great potential exists for future use of such cells in tissue-specific regenerative therapies. The advantage of adult stem cells is that they can be used in autologous therapies, thus avoiding any complications associated with immune rejection.

Native Targeted Progenitor Cells
In the past, one of the limitations of applying cell-based regenerative medicine techniques to organ replacement was the inherent difficulty of growing certain human cell types in large quantities. Native targeted progenitor cells, or native cells, are tissue specific unipotent cells derived from most organs. The advantage of these cells is that they are already programmed to become the cell type needed, without any extra-lineage differentiation. By noting the location of the progenitor cells, as well as by exploring the conditions that promote differentiation and/or self-renewal, it has been possible to overcome some of the obstacles that limit cell expansion in vitro. One example is the urothelial cell. Urothelial cells could be grown in the laboratory setting in the past, but only with limited success. It was believed that urothelial cells had a natural senescence that was hard to overcome. Several protocols have been developed over the last two decades that have improved urothelial growth and expansion (51–54). A system of urothelial cell harvesting was developed that does not use any enzymes or serum and has a large expansion potential. Using these methods of cell culture, it is possible to expand a urothelial strain from a single specimen that initially covers a surface area of 1 cm^2 to one covering a surface area of 4202 m^2 (the equivalent area of one football field) within eight weeks (51).

An additional advantage in using native cells is that they can be obtained from the specific organ to be regenerated, expanded, and used in the same patient without rejection, in an autologous manner (55,56). Bladder, ureter, and renal pelvis cells can be harvested, cultured, and expanded in a similar fashion. Normal human bladder epithelial and muscle cells can be efficiently harvested from surgical material, extensively expanded in culture, and their differentiation characteristics, growth requirements, and other biologic properties can be studied major advances in cell culture techniques have been made within the past two decades, and these techniques make the use of autologous cells possible for clinical application. However, even now, not all human cells can be grown or expanded in vitro. Liver, nerve, and pancreas are examples of human tissues where the technology is not yet advanced to the point where these cells can be grown and expanded from patients.

When cells are used for tissue reconstitution, donor tissue is dissociated into individual cells, and either implanted directly into the host or expanded in culture, attached to a support matrix, and reimplanted after expansion. The implanted tissue can be heterologous, allogeneic, or autologous. Ideally, this approach allows lost tissue function to be restored or replaced into and with limited complications (57). Native cells and tissues are usually preferable for reconstruction. In most cases, the replacement of lost or deficient tissues with functionally equivalent cells and tissues would improve the outcome for these patients. This goal may be attainable with the use of regenerative medicine techniques.

BIOMATERIALS FOR GENITOURINARY REGENERATIVE MEDICINE
Synthetic materials have been used widely for urologic reconstruction. The most common type of synthetic material used

in urologic applications has been silicone. Silicone prostheses have been used for the treatment of urinary incontinence with the artificial urinary sphincter and detachable balloon system, for treatment of vesicoureteral reflux with silicone microparticles, and for impotence with penile prostheses. In some disease states, such as urinary incontinence or vesicoureteral reflux, artificial agents (Teflon paste, glass microparticles) have been used as injectable bulking substances; however, these substances are not entirely biocompatible (58). For regenerative medicine purposes, there are clear advantages in using degradable, biocompatible materials that can function as cell delivery vehicles, and/or provide the structural parameters needed for tissue replacement.

Design and Selection of Biomaterials

The design and selection of the biomaterial is critical in the development of engineered genitourinary tissues. The biomaterial must be capable of controlling the structure and function of the engineered tissue in a predesigned manner by interacting with transplanted cells and/or host cells. Generally, the ideal biomaterial should be biocompatible, promote cellular interaction and tissue development, and possess proper mechanical and physical properties.

The selected biomaterial should be biodegradable and bioresorbable to support the reconstruction of a completely normal tissue without inflammation. Such behavior of the biomaterials avoids the risk of inflammatory or foreign-body responses that may be associated with the permanent presence of a foreign material in the body. The degradation rate and the concentration of degradation products in the tissues surrounding the implant must be at a tolerable level (59).

The biomaterials should provide an appropriate regulation of cell behavior (e.g., adhesion, proliferation, migration, differentiation) in order to promote the development of functional new tissue. Cell behavior in engineered tissues is regulated by multiple interactions with the microenvironment, including interactions with cell-adhesion ligands (60) and with soluble growth factors (61). The biomaterials provide temporary mechanical support sufficient to withstand in vivo forces exerted by the surrounding tissue and maintain a potential space for tissue development. The mechanical support of the biomaterials should be maintained until the engineered tissue has sufficient mechanical integrity to support itself (62). This potentially can be achieved by an appropriate choice of mechanical and degradative properties of the biomaterials (63).

The biomaterials need to be processed into specific configurations. A large ratio of surface area to volume is often desirable to allow the delivery of a high density of cells. A high-porosity, interconnected pore structure with specific pore sizes promotes tissue ingrowth from the surrounding host tissue. Several techniques, such as electrospinning, have been developed that readily control porosity, pore size, and pore structure (64–69).

Types of Biomaterials

Generally, three classes of biomaterials have been used for engineering of genitourinary tissues: naturally derived materials, such as collagen and alginate; acellular tissue matrices, such as bladder submucosa and small-intestinal submucosa; and synthetic polymers, such as polyglycolic acid (PGA), polylactic acid (PLA), and poly(lactic-co-glycolic acid) (PLGA). These classes of biomaterials have been tested in regard to their biocompatibility with primary human urothelial and bladder muscle cells (70). Naturally derived materials and acellular tissue matrices have the potential advantage of biologic recognition. Synthetic polymers can be produced reproducibly on a large scale with controlled properties of strength, degradation rate, and microstructure.

Collagen is the most abundant and ubiquitous structural protein in the body, and it may be readily purified from both animal and human tissues with an enzyme treatment and salt/acid extraction (71). Collagen has long been known to exhibit minimal inflammatory and antigenic responses (72), and it has been approved by the U.S. FDA for many types of medical applications, including wound dressings and artificial skin (73). Intermolecular cross-linking reduces the degradation rate by making the collagen molecules less susceptible to an enzymatic attack. Intermolecular cross-linking can be accomplished by various physical (e.g., ultraviolet radiation, dehydrothermal treatment) or chemical (e.g., glutaraldehyde, formaldehyde, carbodiimides) techniques (71). Collagen contains cell-adhesion domain sequences (e.g., RGD) that exhibit specific cellular interactions. This may help to retain the phenotype and activity of many types of cells, including fibroblasts (74) and chondrocytes (75). This material can be processed into a wide variety of structures such as sponges, fibers, and films (76–78).

Acellular tissue matrices are collagen-rich matrices prepared by removing cellular components from tissues. The matrices are often prepared by mechanical and chemical manipulation of a segment of bladder tissue (79–82). The matrices slowly degrade after implantation and are replaced and remodeled by extracellular matrix proteins synthesized and secreted by transplanted or ingrowing cells. Acellular tissue matrices have been proved to support cell ingrowth and regeneration of genitourinary tissues, including urethra and bladder, with no evidence of immunogenic rejection (82,83). Because the structures of the proteins (e.g., collagen, elastin) in acellular matrices are well conserved and normally arranged, the mechanical properties of the acellular matrices are not significantly different from those of native bladder submucosa (79).

Polyesters of naturally occurring α-hydroxy acids, including PGA, PLA, and PLGA, are widely used in regenerative medicine. These polymers have gained FDA approval for human use in a variety of applications, including sutures (84). The degradation products of PGA, PLA, and PLGA are nontoxic, natural metabolites that are eventually eliminated from the body in the form of carbon dioxide and water (84). Because these polymers are thermoplastics, they can easily be formed into a three-dimensional scaffold with a desired microstructure, gross shape, and dimension by various techniques, including molding, extrusion (85), solvent casting (86), phase separation techniques, and gas foaming techniques (87). More recently, techniques such as electrospinning have been used to quickly create highly porous scaffolds in various conformations (66–68,88).

189

Nanotechnology, which is the ability to use small molecules that have distinct properties in a small scale, has been used to create "smart biomaterials" for regenerative medicine (89,90). Nanoscaffolds have been manufactured specifically for bladder applications (91). The manufacturing of biomaterials can also lead to enhanced cell alignment and tissue formation (66).

REGENERATIVE MEDICINE OF FEMALE GENITOURINARY STRUCTURES
Bladder

Currently, gastrointestinal segments are commonly used as tissues for bladder replacement or repair. However, gastrointestinal tissues are designed to absorb specific solutes, whereas bladder tissue is designed for the excretion of solutes. When gastrointestinal tissue is in contact with the urinary tract, multiple complications may ensue, such as infection, metabolic disturbances, urolithiasis, perforation, increased mucus production, and malignancy (92–95).

Matrices for Bladder Regeneration

Over the last few decades, several bladder wall substitutes have been created with both synthetic and organic materials. Synthetic materials that have been tested in experimental and clinical settings include polyvinyl sponge, Teflon, collagen matrices, Vicryl (PGA) matrices, and silicone. Most of these attempts have failed due to mechanical, structural, functional, or biocompatibility issues. Usually, permanent synthetic materials used for bladder reconstruction succumb to mechanical failure and urinary stone formation, and in contrast, the use of degradable synthetics leads to fibroblast deposition, scarring, graft contracture, and a reduced reservoir volume over time (96,97).

As a result, there has been renewed interest in the use of various natural, collagen-based matrices for tissue regeneration. Allogeneic acellular bladder matrices have served as scaffolds for the ingrowth of host bladder wall components in some studies. These matrices are prepared by mechanically and chemically removing all cellular components from donor bladder tissue (80,81,83,98,99). Cell-seeded allogeneic acellular bladder matrices were used for bladder augmentation in dogs (81), and the regenerated bladder tissues contained a normal cellular organization consisting of urothelium and smooth muscle. They also exhibited a normal compliance. However, biomaterials preloaded with cells before implantation showed better tissue regeneration compared with biomaterials implanted with no cells, in which tissue regeneration depended on ingrowth of the surrounding tissue. As shown in Figure 22.2, the bladders showed a significant increase (100%) in capacity when augmented with scaffolds seeded with cells, compared to scaffolds without cells (30%). Recently, it has been shown that acellular collagen matrices can be enhanced with growth factors to improve bladder regeneration even further (100).

Small intestinal submucosa (SIS), a biodegradable, acellular, xenogeneic collagen-based tissue-matrix graft, was first described by Badylak et al. as a matrix for tissue replacement in vascular applications (101). It has been shown to promote

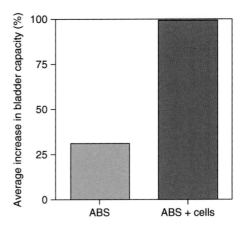

Figure 22.2 Bladders augmented with a collagen matrix derived from bladder submucosa seeded with urothelial and smooth muscle cells [allogenic bladder submucosa (ABS) + cells] showed a 100% increase in capacity compared with bladders augmented with the cell-free ABS, which showed only a 30% increase in capacity within three months after implantation.

regeneration of a variety of host tissues, including blood vessels and ligaments (102). The matrix is derived from pig small intestine. To produce it, the intestinal mucosa is mechanically removed from the inner surface and the serosa and muscular layer are removed from the outer surface of a piece of pig small intestine. Animal studies have indicated that when non-seeded SIS matrix is used for bladder augmentation, it is able to regenerate bladder tissue in vivo (103,104). Histologically, the transitional layer that is formed is the same as that of the native bladder tissue, but, as with other non-seeded collagen matrices used experimentally, the muscle layer does not fully develop. Instead, a large amount of collagen can be found among a smaller number of muscle bundles. A computer-assisted image analysis demonstrated a decreased muscle-to-collagen ratio with loss of the normal architecture in the SIS-regenerated bladders. In vitro contractility studies performed on the SIS-regenerated dog bladders showed a 50% decrease in maximal contractile response when compared to normal bladder tissue. Expression of muscarinic, purinergic, and alpha-adrenergic receptors and functional cholinergic and purinergic innervation were demonstrated (104). Cholinergic and purinergic innervation also occurred in rats (105).

In an important experiment to compare various scaffold materials, bladder augmentation using laparoscopic techniques was performed on minipigs using either porcine bowel acellular tissue matrix, human placental membranes, or porcine SIS. At 12 weeks post-operatively the grafts had contracted to 70%, 65%, and 60% of their original sizes, respectively, and histologically the grafts showed predominantly only mucosal regeneration (106). The same group evaluated the long-term results of laparoscopic hemicystectomy and bladder replacement with SIS with ureteral reimplantation into the SIS material in minipigs. Histopathology studies after one year showed muscle at the graft periphery and center but this muscle tissue consisted only of small fused bundles with significant fibrosis. Nerves were present at the graft periphery and center but they were decreased in number. Compared to primary bladder closure after hemi-cystectomy, no advantage in bladder capacity or compliance was documented (107). More recently, bladder regeneration has been shown to be more reliable when the SIS was derived from the distal ileum (108).

Studies involving acellular matrices that may provide the necessary environment to promote cell migration, growth, and differentiation are being conducted (109). With continued research in this area, these matrices may have a clinical role in bladder replacement in the future.

Regenerative Medicine for Bladder Using Cell Transplantation
Regenerative medicine using selective cell transplantation may provide a novel means to create functional new bladder segments (57). The success of cell transplantation strategies for bladder reconstruction depends on the ability to use donor tissue efficiently and to provide the right conditions for long-term survival, differentiation, and growth. Various cell sources have been explored for bladder regeneration, and native cells are currently preferable as they can be used without rejection (51). It has been shown experimentally that the bladder neck and trigone area have a higher proportion of urothelial progenitor cells (110), and these cells are localized in the basal region (111). Amniotic fluid and bone marrow-derived stem cells can also be used in an autologous manner and have the potential to differentiate into bladder muscle (34,112) and urothelium (113). ES cells also have the potential to differentiate into bladder tissue (114).

Formation of Bladder Tissue
Human urothelial and muscle cells can be expanded in vitro, seeded onto polymer scaffolds, and allowed to attach and form sheets of cells. The cell-polymer scaffold can then be implanted in vivo. Histologic analysis indicated that viable cells were able to self assemble back into their respective tissue types, and would retain their native phenotype (115). These experiments demonstrated, for the first time, that composite layered tissue-engineered structures could be created de novo. Before this study, only non-layered structures had been created in the field of regenerative medicine.

In order to determine the effects of implanting engineered tissues in continuity with the urinary tract, animal models of bladder augmentation were used (81). Partial cystectomies were performed in dogs and the animals were divided into two experimental groups. One group underwent bladder augmentation with a non-seeded bladder-derived collagen matrix, and the second group underwent augmentation with a cell-seeded construct. The bladders augmented with matrices seeded with cells showed a 100% increase in capacity compared with bladders augmented with cell-free matrices, which showed only a 30% increase in capacity.

It has been well established for decades that the bladder is able to regenerate generously over free grafts. Urothelium is associated with a high reparative capacity (116). However, bladder muscle tissue is less likely to regenerate in a normal fashion. Both urothelial and muscle ingrowth are believed to be initiated from the edges of the normal bladder toward the region of the free graft (117,118). Usually, however, contracture or resorption of the graft has been evident. The inflammatory response toward the matrix may contribute to the resorption of the free graft. It was hypothesized that building

the three-dimensional structure constructs in vitro, before implantation, would facilitate the eventual terminal differentiation of the cells after implantation in vivo and would minimize the inflammatory response toward the matrix, thus avoiding graft contracture and shrinkage. The dog study demonstrated a major difference between matrices used with autologous cells (tissue-engineered matrices) and those used without cells (81). Matrices implanted with cells for bladder augmentation retained most of their implanted diameter, as opposed to matrices implanted without cells for bladder augmentation, in which graft contraction and shrinkage occurred. The histomorphology demonstrated a marked paucity of muscle cells and a more aggressive inflammatory reaction in the matrices implanted without cells. Epithelial-mesenchymal signaling is important for the differentiation of bladder smooth muscle (119).

The results of initial studies showed that the creation of artificial bladders may be achieved in vivo; however, it could not be determined whether the functional parameters noted were caused by the augmented segment or by the intact native bladder tissue. To better address the functional parameters of tissue-engineered bladders, an animal model was designed that required a subtotal cystectomy with subsequent replacement with a tissue-engineered organ (120).

Cystectomy-only and non-seeded controls maintained average capacities of 22% and 46% of preoperative values, respectively. An average bladder capacity of 95% of the original precystectomy volume was achieved in the cell-seeded tissue engineered bladder replacements. These findings were confirmed radiographically (Fig. 22.3). The subtotal cystectomy reservoirs that were not reconstructed and the polymer-only reconstructed bladders showed a marked decrease in bladder compliance (10% and 42% total compliance). The compliance of the cell-seeded tissue-engineered bladders showed almost no difference from preoperative values that were measured when the native bladder was present (106%). Histologically, the non-seeded scaffold bladders presented a pattern of normal urothelial cells with a thickened fibrotic submucosa and a thin layer of muscle fibers. The retrieved tissue-engineered bladders showed a normal cellular organization, consisting of a trilayer of urothelium, submucosa, and muscle. Immunocytochemical analyses confirmed the muscle and urothelial phenotype. S-100 staining indicated the presence of neural structures (120). These studies, performed with polyglocolic acid based-scaffolds, have been repeated by other investigators and showed similar results in large numbers of animals long-term (121,122). The strategy of using biodegradable scaffolds with cells can be pursued without concerns for local or systemic toxicity (123). However, not all scaffolds perform well if a large portion of the bladder needs replacement. In a study using SIS for subtotal bladder replacement in dogs, both the unseeded and cell seeded experimental groups showed graft shrinkage and poor results (124). The type of scaffold used is critical for the success of these technologies. The use of bioreactors, wherein mechanical stimulation is started at the time of organ production, has also been proposed as an important parameter for success (125).

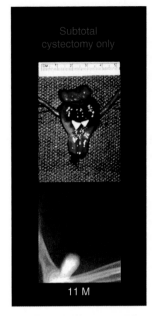
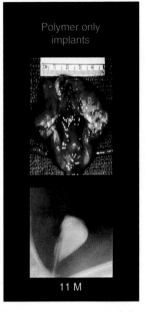
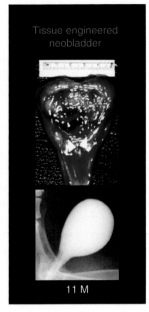

Figure 22.3 Gross specimens and cystograms at 11 months of the cystectomy-only, non-seeded controls, and cell-seeded tissue engineered bladder replacements in dogs. The cystectomy-only bladder had a capacity of 22% of the preoperative value and a decrease in bladder compliance to 10% of the preoperative value. The non-seeded controls showed significant scarring with a capacity of 46% of the preoperative value and a decrease in bladder compliance to 42% of the preoperative value. An average bladder capacity of 95% of the original precystectomy volume was achieved in the cell-seeded tissue engineered bladder replacements and the compliance showed almost no difference from preoperative values that were measured when the native bladder was present (106%).

A clinical experience involving engineered bladder tissue for cystoplasty reconstruction was conducted starting in 1998. A small pilot study of seven patients was reported, using a collagen scaffold seeded with cells either with or without omentum coverage, or a combined PGA-collagen scaffold seeded with cells and omental coverage (Fig. 22.4). The patients reconstructed with the engineered bladder tissue created with the PGA-collagen cell-seeded scaffolds with omental coverage showed increased compliance, decreased end-filling pressures, increased capacities, and longer dry periods over time (126) (Fig. 22.5). It is clear from this experience that the engineered bladders continued their improvement with time, mirroring their continued development. Although the experience is promising in terms of showing that engineered tissues can be implanted safely, it is just a start in terms of accomplishing the goal of engineering fully functional bladders. This was a limited clinical experience, and the technology is not yet ready for wide dissemination, as further experimental and clinical studies are required. FDA Phase 2 studies have now been completed.

An area of concern in the field of tissue engineering in the past was the source of cells for regeneration. The concept of creating engineered constructs involves initially obtaining cells for expansion from the diseased organ. How can one be assured that the cell population that is obtained and being expanded for later autologous implantation is normal and will lead to normal tissue formation? For example, if one is dealing with a patient, will the cells obtained from a neuropathic bladder lead to the engineering of another neuropathic bladder? Cultured neuropathic bladder smooth muscle cells possess and maintain different characteristics than normal smooth muscle cells in vitro, as demonstrated by growth assays, contractility, adherence tests, and microarray analysis (127–129). However, when neuropathic smooth muscle cells were cultured in vitro, and seeded onto matrices and implanted in vivo, the tissue engineered constructs showed the same properties as the tissues engineered with normal cells (130). The progenitor cells, which reside within stem cell niches within each organ, are responsible for new cell differentiation and tissue formation during the normal process of tissue regeneration due to natural turnover, *ageing*, and tissue injury. It is known that genetically normal non-malignant progenitor cells, which are the reservoirs for new cell formation, are programmed to give rise to normal tissue, regardless of whether the niche resides in either normal or diseased tissues (130–132). Therefore, although the mechanisms for tissue self-assembly and regenerative medicine are not fully understood, it is known that the progenitor cells are able to "reset" their program for normal cell differentiation. The stem cell niche and its role in normal tissue regeneration remains a fertile area of ongoing investigation.

From the above studies, it is evident that the use of cell-seeded matrices is superior to the use of non-seeded matrices for the creation of engineered bladder tissues. Although advances have been made with the engineering of bladder tissues, many challenges remain. Current research in many centers is aimed at the development of biologically active and "smart" biomaterials that may improve tissue regeneration.

Vagina

Several pathologic conditions, including congenital malformations and malignancy, can adversely affect normal vaginal development or anatomy. Vaginal reconstruction has traditionally been challenging due to the paucity of available native tissue. Acellular materials have been used experimentally for vaginal reconstruction in rats (133). The feasibility of engineering vaginal tissue with cells in vivo was also investigated (134).

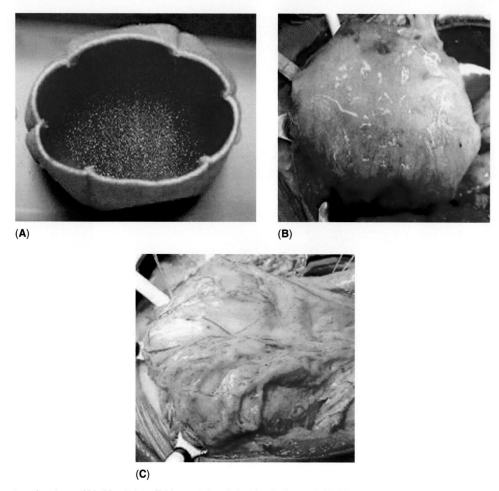

(A) **(B)**

(C)

Figure 22.4 Construction of engineered bladder. (**A**) Scaffold material seeded with cells for use in bladder repair. (**B**) The seeded scaffold is anastamosed to native bladder with running 4-0 polyglycolic sutures. (**C**) Implant covered with fibrin glue and omentum.

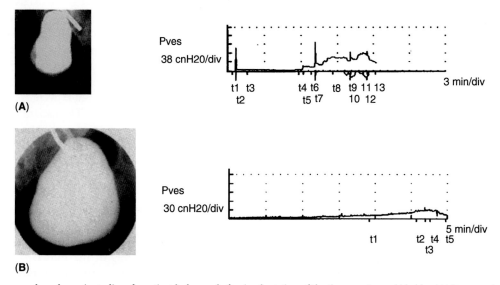

(A)

(B)

Figure 22.5 Cystograms and urodynamic studies of a patient before and after implantation of the tissue engineered bladder. (**A**) Preoperative results indicate an irregular-shaped bladder in the cystogram (*left*) and abnormal bladder pressures as the bladder is filled during urodynamic studies (*right*). (**B**) Postoperatively, findings are significantly improved.

Vaginal epithelial and smooth muscle cells of female rabbits were harvested, grown, and expanded in culture. These cells were seeded onto biodegradable polymer scaffolds, and the cell-seeded constructs were then implanted into mice.

Functional studies in the tissue-engineered constructs showed similar properties to those of normal vaginal tissue. When these constructs were used for autologous total vaginal replacement in a rabbit model, patent functional vaginal structures were

193

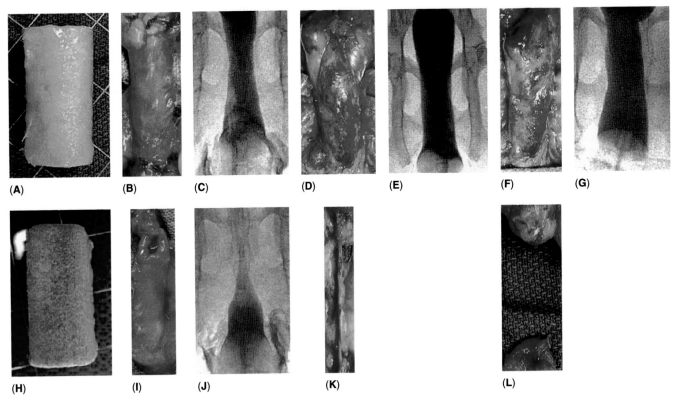

Figure 22.6 Appearance of tissue engineered neo-vaginas. (A) Tubular polymer scaffold after cell seeding and one week in vitro culture, prior to implantation in vivo. (B, D, and F) Gross appearance. (C, E, and G) Vaginography of cell-seeded constructs one, three, and six months, post-implantation, respectively. (H) Unseeded control scaffold prior to implantation. (I, K, and L) Gross appearance of unseeded construct at one, three, and six months post-implantation. (J) Vaginography of unseeded graft at one month.

noted in the tissue-engineered specimens, while the non-cell-seeded structures were noted to be stenotic (135) (Fig. 22.6). These studies indicated that a regenerative medicine approach to clinical vaginal reconstruction would be a realistic possibility. Clinical trials are currently being conducted.

INJECTIBLE THERAPIES IN GENITOURINARY REGENERATIVE MEDICINE

Both urinary incontinence and vesicoureteral reflux are common conditions affecting the genitourinary system for which endoscopic injectable therapy may be useful. There are definite advantages to an endoscopic treatment, as the method is simple and can be completed in less than 15 minutes; it has a low morbidity; and it can be performed on an outpatient basis. The ideal substance for the endoscopic treatment of reflux and incontinence should be injectable, nonantigenic, nonmigratory, volume stable, and safe for human use (136). Toward this goal, long-term animal studies were conducted to determine the effect of injectable chondrocytes in vivo (56). In this study, a biopsy of ear cartilage was taken, followed by chondrocyte processing and endoscopic injection of the autologous chondrocyte suspension for the treatment of incontinence. This system was also adapted for the treatment of reflux in a porcine model (137). Chondrocytes were harvested, injected cystoscopically, and cartilage tissue formed, correcting reflux (137).

The first human application of cell-based regenerative medicine technology for urologic applications occurred with the injection of chondrocytes for the correction of vesicoureteral reflux in children and for urinary incontinence in adults. Two multicenter clinical trials were conducted using the engineered chondrocyte technology. Patients with urinary incontinence secondary to intrinsic sphincter deficiency were treated endoscopically with injected chondrocytes at three different medical centers. Phase 1 trials showed an approximate success rate of 80% at both 3 and 12 months post-operatively (138). Patients with vesicoureteral reflux were treated at 10 centers throughout the United States. The patients had a similar success rate as with other injectable substances in terms of cure. The overall success rate in 29 children (47 ureters) was 86%. At one year follow-up, reflux correction was maintained in 70% of the ureters. Chondrocyte formation was not noted in patients who had treatment failure (139). The success rate was higher with the treatment of incontinence than with reflux, and this was probably because the cells had time to "set" in the sphincter. In contrast, when they are injected into the bladder itself, immediate cycling of the muscle occurs, and the cell mound may be dissipated over a larger surface area.

The use of autologous smooth muscle cells has also been explored for both urinary incontinence and vesicoureteral reflux applications (140). In vivo experiments were conducted in minipigs, and reflux was successfully corrected. The potential use of injectable, cultured myoblasts for the treatment of stress urinary incontinence has also been investigated (141,142). Labeled myoblasts were directly injected into the proximal urethra and lateral bladder walls of nude mice with a micro-syringe in an open surgical procedure. Tissue harvested up to 35 days post injection contained the labeled myoblasts, as well as evidence of differentiation of the labeled myoblasts into regenerative myofibers. The authors reported that a significant portion of the injected myoblast population persisted in vivo. The authors subsequently demonstrated increased leak point pressure and increased sphincter contractility after periurethral injection of muscle-derived stem cells in a rat model of stress urinary incontinence, and in a large animal model (143–145). Similar techniques of sphincteric derived muscle cells have been used for the treatment of urinary incontinence in a pig model (146). The same group showed that urethral closing pressures and treatment efficacy in a porcine model was dose dependent (147).

The use of injectable muscle precursor cells has also been investigated for use in the treatment of urinary incontinence due to irreversible urethral sphincter injury or maldevelopment. Muscle precursor cells are the quiescent satellite cells found in each myofiber that proliferate to form myoblasts and eventually myotubes and new muscle tissue (148). Intrinsic muscle precursor cells have previously been shown to play an active role in the regeneration of injured striated urethral sphincter (149). In a subsequent study, autologous muscle precursor cells were injected into a rat model of urethral sphincter injury, and both replacement of mature myotubes as well as restoration of functional motor units were noted in the regenerating sphincteric muscle tissue (148). This is the first demonstration of the replacement of both sphincter muscle tissue and its innervation by the injection of muscle precursor cells. As a result, muscle precursor cells may be a minimally invasive solution for urinary incontinence in patients with irreversible urinary sphincter muscle insufficiency. A canine model of irreversible urethral sphincter injury was also created to test these technologies (150).

In addition, injectable muscle-based gene therapy and regenerative medicine were combined to improve detrusor function in a bladder injury model, and may potentially be a novel treatment option for urinary incontinence (151). Highly purified muscle-derived cells that display stem cell characteristics were genetically engineered to express the gene encoding B-galactosidase, then injected into the bladder walls of mice. The injectable cells were able to survive in the lower urinary tract and improve the contractility of the bladder following the induced injury, as well as become innervated into the bladder as early as two weeks after injection. Angiogenic gene modification of skeletal muscle cells has also been performed in order to compensate for ageing-induced decline in bioengineered functional muscle tissue (152). These findings may be useful in the setting of urinary incontinence where these muscle-derived cells may help to bulk up the urethral wall, enhance coaptation, and improve the urinary sphincter muscle.

The use of lipoaspirate cells has also been proposed for the treatment on urinary incontinence. The lipoaspirate cells were injected into mouse bladders and urethras, and they produced regenerated muscle tissue (153). The same cells were shown to differentiate into functional smooth muscle cells (154).

Several clinical trials using myoblast injection have been conducted. A group of 42 patients, 29 women and 13 men with urinary stress incontinence, had myoblasts injected into the rhabdosphincter transurethrally and with ultrasound guidance. A cure was reported by 35 patients, and seven had marked improvement (155). The same group reported on an additional clinical trial in women with stress urinary incontinence (156). The authors compared the effectiveness and tolerability of ultrasonography-guided injections of autologous cells with those of endoscopic injections of collagen for stress incontinence in 63 patients, showing improved results for the patients receiving the myoblasts. However, controversy surrounding the trial ensued and the paper was retracted. In another trial, myoblasts isolated from the abdominal wall vasculature were injected in a series of bladder exstrophy patients with urinary incontinence. The authors reported that 88% of patients were socially dry, described as daytime dryness more than three hours. The patients were also on a pelvic floor electrical stimulation and pelvic floor exercise program (157). Another study described the use of autologous muscle-derived stem cell injection to treat stress urinary incontinence. After one year, one of eight women achieved total continence, and five reported improvement (158). Activity has increased in the area of cell therapy for urinary incontinence in the last several years. Further trials and follow-up will be needed in order to determine efficacy long-term.

SUMMARY

Regenerative medicine efforts are currently being undertaken for every type of tissue and organ within the female urogenital system. Most of the efforts expended in the genitourinary field have occurred within the last two decades. Regenerative medicine strategies involve the use of biomaterials alone, biomaterials with cells (currently being tested clinically with bladder and vaginal tissues), and cell therapies alone (clinically for urinary incontinence, initially with chondrocytes, and now with muscle cells). Regenerative medicine is a multidisciplinary field that requires expertise in a wide variety of scientific disciplines, including cell and molecular biology, physiology, pharmacology, chemical engineering, biomaterials, nanotechnology, and clinical sciences. Although modest clinical success has been achieved to date in specific areas, the field is still in its infancy. Long term studies are still essential to assure safety and efficacy before these technologies have widespread clinical application.

REFERENCES

1. Atala A, Lanza R. Preface. In: Atala A, Lanza R, eds. Methods of Tissue Engineering. San Diego: Academic Press, 2001.
2. Wolter JR, Meyer RF. Sessile macrophages forming clear endothelium-like membrane on the inside of successful keratoprosthesis. Graefes Arch Clin Exp Ophthalmol 1985; 222: 109–17.
3. Martin GR. Isolation of a pluripotent cell line from early mouse embryos cultured in medium conditioned by teratocarcinoma stem cells. Proc Natl Acad Sci USA 1981; 78: 7634–8.
4. Thomson JA, Itskovitz-Eldor J, Shapiro SS, et al. Embryonic stem cell lines derived from human blastocysts. Science 1998; 282: 1145–7. [see comment] [erratum appears in Science 1998; 282: 1827].
5. Wilmut I, Schnieke AE, McWhir J, et al. Viable offspring derived from fetal and adult mammalian cells. Nature 1997; 385: 810–13. [see comment] [erratum appears in Nature 1997; 386: 200].
6. Haseltine W. A brave new medicine. A conversation with William Haseltine. Interview by Joe Flower. Health Forum J 1999; 42: 28–30.

7. Reubinoff BE, Itsykson P, Turetsky T, et al. Neural progenitors from human embryonic stem cells. Nat Biotechnol 2001; 19: 1134–40. [see comment].

8. Schuldiner M, Eiges R, Eden A, et al. Induced neuronal differentiation of human embryonic stem cells. Brain Res 2001; 913: 201–5.

9. Zhang SC, Wernig M, Duncan ID, et al. In vitro differentiation of transplantable neural precursors from human embryonic stem cells. Nat Biotechnol 2001; 19: 1129–33. [see comment].

10. Kaufman DS, Hanson ET, Lewis RL, et al. Hematopoietic colony-forming cells derived from human embryonic stem cells. Proc Natl Acad Sci USA 2001; 98: 10716–21.

11. Kehat I, Kenyagin-Karsenti D, Snir M, et al. Human embryonic stem cells can differentiate into myocytes with structural and functional properties of cardiomyocytes. J Clin Invest 2001; 108: 407–14. [see comment].

12. Levenberg S, Golub JS, Amit M, et al. Endothelial cells derived from human embryonic stem cells. Proc Natl Acad Sci USA 2002; 99: 4391–6.

13. Assady S, Maor G, Amit M, et al. Insulin production by human embryonic stem cells. Diabetes 2001; 50: 1691–7.

14. Itskovitz-Eldor J, Schuldiner M, Karsenti D, et al. Differentiation of human embryonic stem cells into embryoid bodies compromising the three embryonic germ layers. Mol Med 2000; 6: 88–95.

15. Reubinoff BE, Pera MF, Fong CY, et al. Embryonic stem cell lines from human blastocysts: somatic differentiation in vitro. Nat Biotechnol 2000; 18: 399–404. [see comment] [erratum appears in Nat Biotechnol 2000 18: 559].

16. Chung Y, Klimanskaya I, Becker S, et al. Embryonic and extraembryonic stem cell lines derived from single mouse blastomeres 3. Nature 2006; 439: 216–19.

17. Zhang X, Stojkovic P, Przyborski S, et al. Derivation of human embryonic stem cells from developing and arrested embryos 1. Stem Cells 2006; 24: 2669–76.

18. Landry DW, Zucker HA. Embryonic death and the creation of human embryonic stem cells 2. J Clin Invest 2004; 114: 1184–6.

19. Lanza RP, Chung HY, Yoo JJ, et al. Generation of histocompatible tissues using nuclear transplantation. Nat Biotechnol 2002; 20: 689–96. [see comment].

20. Byrne J, Pedersen D, Clepper L, et al. Producing primate embryonic stem cells by somatic cell nuclear transfer 1. Nature 2007; 450: 497–502.

21. Mitalipov S. Reprogramming following somatic cell nuclear transfer in primates is dependent upon nuclear remodeling. Hum Reprod 2007; 22: 2232–42.

22. Hurlbut WB. Altered nuclear transfer as a morally acceptable means for the procurement of human embryonic stem cells. Perspect Biol Med 2005; 48: 211–28.

23. Meissner A, Jaenisch R. Generation of nuclear transfer-derived pluripotent ES cells from cloned Cdx2-deficient blastocysts. Nature 2006; 439: 212–15.

24. Takahashi K, Yamanaka S. Induction of pluripotent stem cells from mouse embryonic and adult fibroblast cultures by defined factors. Cell 2006; 126: 663–76.

25. Wernig M, Meissner A, Foreman R, et al. In vitro reprogramming of fibroblasts into a pluripotent ES-cell-like state. Nature 2007; 448: 318–24.

26. Takahashi K, Tanabe K, Ohnuki M, et al. Induction of pluripotent stem cells from adult human fibroblasts by defined factors. Cell 2007; 131: 861–72.

27. Yu J, Vodyanik MA, Smuga-Otto K, et al. Induced pluripotent stem cell lines derived from human somatic cells. Science 2007; 318: 1917–20.

28. Stadtfeld M, Nagaya M, Utikal J, et al. Induced pluripotent stem cells generated without viral integration. Science 2008; 322: 945–9.

29. Gonzalez F, Barragan Monasterio M, Tiscornia G, et al. Generation of mouse-induced pluripotent stem cells by transient expression of a single nonviral polycistronic vector. Proc Natl Acad Sci USA 2009; 106: 8918–22.

30. Polgar K, Adany R, Abel G, et al. Characterization of rapidly adhering amniotic fluid cells by combined immunofluorescence and phagocytosis assays. Am J Hum Genet 1989; 45: 786–92.

31. Priest RE, Marimuthu KM, Priest JH. Origin of cells in human amniotic fluid cultures: ultrastructural features. Lab Invest 1978; 39: 106–9.

32. In 't Anker PS, Scherjon SA, Kleijburg-van der Keur C, et al. Amniotic fluid as a novel source of mesenchymal stem cells for therapeutic transplantation. Blood 2003; 102: 1548–9.

33. Tsai MS, Lee JL, Chang YJ, et al. Isolation of human multipotent mesenchymal stem cells from second-trimester amniotic fluid using a novel two-stage culture protocol 2. Hum Reprod 2004; 19: 1450–6.

34. De Coppi P, Bartsch G Jr, Siddiqui MM, et al. Isolation of amniotic stem cell lines with potential for therapy. Nat Biotechnol 2007; 25: 100–6. [see comment].

35. Kolambkar YM, Peister A, Soker S, et al. Chondrogenic differentiation of amniotic fluid-derived stem cells. J Mol Histol 2007; 38: 405–13.

36. Perin L, Giuliani S, Jin D, et al. Renal differentiation of amniotic fluid stem cells. Cell Prolif 2007; 40: 936–48.

37. Warburton D, Perin L, Defilippo R, et al. Stem/progenitor cells in lung development, injury repair, and regeneration. Proc Am Thorac Soc 2008; 5: 703–6.

38. De Coppi P, Callegari A, Chiavegato A, et al. Amniotic fluid and bone marrow derived mesenchymal stem cells can be converted to smooth muscle cells in the cryo-injured rat bladder and prevent compensatory hypertrophy of surviving smooth muscle cells. J Urol 2007; 177: 369–76.

39. Ballas CB, Zielske SP, Gerson SL. Adult bone marrow stem cells for cell and gene therapies: implications for greater use. J Cell Biochem Suppl 2002; 38: 20–8.

40. Jiao J, Chen DF. Induction of neurogenesis in nonconventional neurogenic regions of the adult central nervous system by niche astrocyte-produced signals. Stem Cells 2008; 26: 1221–30.

41. Taupin P. Therapeutic potential of adult neural stem cells. Recent Patents CNS Drug Discov 2006; 1: 299–303.

42. Jensen UB, Yan X, Triel C, et al. A distinct population of clonogenic and multipotent murine follicular keratinocytes residing in the upper isthmus. J Cell Sci 2008; 121: 609–17.

43. Crisan M, Casteilla L, Lehr L, et al. A reservoir of brown adipocyte progenitors in human skeletal muscle. Stem Cells 2008; 26: 2425–33.

44. Weiner LP. Definitions and criteria for stem cells. Methods Mol Biol 2008; 438: 3–8.

45. Devine SM. Mesenchymal stem cells: will they have a role in the clinic? J Cell Biochem Suppl 2002; 38: 73–9.

46. Jiang Y, Jahagirdar BN, Reinhardt RL, et al. Pluripotency of mesenchymal stem cells derived from adult marrow. Nature 2002; 418: 41–9. [see comment] [erratum appears in Nature 2007; 447: 879–80].

47. Caplan AI. Adult mesenchymal stem cells for tissue engineering versus regenerative medicine. J Cell Physiol 2007; 213: 341–7.

48. da Silva Meirelles L, Caplan AI, Nardi NB. In search of the in vivo identity of mesenchymal stem cells. Stem Cells 2008; 26: 2287–99.

49. Mimeault M, Batra SK. Recent progress on tissue-resident adult stem cell biology and their therapeutic implications. Stem Cell Rev 2008; 4: 27–49.

50. Hristov M, Zernecke A, Schober A, et al. Adult progenitor cells in vascular remodeling during atherosclerosis. Biol Chem 2008; 389: 837–44.

51. Cilento BG, Freeman MR, Schneck FX, et al. Phenotypic and cytogenetic characterization of human bladder urothelia expanded in vitro. J Urol 1994; 152: 665–70.

52. Scriven SD, Booth C, Thomas DF, et al. Reconstitution of human urothelium from monolayer cultures. J Urol 1997; 158: 1147–52.

53. Liebert M, Hubbel A, Chung M, et al. Expression of mal is associated with urothelial differentiation in vitro: identification by differential display reverse-transcriptase polymerase chain reaction. Differentiation 1997; 61: 177–85.

54. Puthenveettil JA, Burger MS, Reznikoff CA. Replicative senescence in human uroepithelial cells. Adv Exp Med Biol 1999; 462: 83–91.

55. Atala A, Vacanti JP, Peters CA, et al. Formation of urothelial structures in vivo from dissociated cells attached to biodegradable polymer scaffolds in vitro. J Urol 1992; 148: 658–62.

56. Atala A, Cima LG, Kim W, et al. Injectable alginate seeded with chondrocytes as a potential treatment for vesicoureteral reflux. J Urol 1993; 150: 745–7.

57. Atala A. Tissue engineering in the genitourinary system. In: Atala A, Mooney DJ, eds. Tissue Engineering. Boston, MA: Birkhauser Press, 1997: 149.

58. Atala A. Use of non-autologous substances in VUR and incontinence treatment. Dial Pediatr Urol 1994; 17: 11–12.

59. Bergsma JE, Rozema FR, Bos RR, et al. In vivo degradation and biocompatibility study of in vitro pre-degraded as-polymerized polyactide particles. Biomaterials 1995; 16: 267–74. [see comment].

60. Hynes RO. Integrins: versatility, modulation, and signaling in cell adhesion. Cell 1992; 69: 11–25.

61. Deuel TF. Growth factors. In: Lanza R, Langer R, Chick WL, eds. Principles of Tissue Engineering. New York, NY: Academic Press, 1997: 133–49.

62. Atala A. Engineering tissues, organs and cells. J Tissue Eng Regen Med 2007; 1: 83–96.

63. Kim BS, Mooney DJ. Development of biocompatible synthetic extracellular matrices for tissue engineering. Trends Biotechnol 1998; 16: 224–30.

64. Yoo JJ, Lee JE, Kim HJ, et al. Comparative in vitro and in vivo studies using a bioactive poly(epsilon-caprolactone)-organosiloxane nanohybrid containing calcium salt. J Biomed Mater Res B Appl Biomat 2007; 83: 189–98.

65. Lee SJ, Van Dyke M, Atala A, et al. Host cell mobilization for in situ tissue regeneration. Rejuvenation Res 2008; 11: 747–56.

66. Choi JS, Lee SJ, Christ GJ, et al. The influence of electrospun aligned poly(epsilon-caprolactone)/collagen nanofiber meshes on the formation of self-aligned skeletal muscle myotubes. Biomaterials 2008; 29: 2899–906.

67. Lee SJ, Liu J, Oh SH, et al. Development of a composite vascular scaffolding system that withstands physiological vascular conditions. Biomaterials 2008; 29: 2891–8.

68. Lee SJ, Oh SH, Liu J, et al. The use of thermal treatments to enhance the mechanical properties of electrospun poly(epsilon-caprolactone) scaffolds. Biomaterials 2008; 29: 1422–30.

69. Lee SJ, Yoo JJ, Lim GJ, et al. In vitro evaluation of electrospun nanofiber scaffolds for vascular graft application. J Biomed Mater Res A 2007; 83: 999–1008.

70. Pariente JL, Kim BS, Atala A. In vitro biocompatibility assessment of naturally derived and synthetic biomaterials using normal human urothelial cells. J Biomed Mater Res 2001; 55: 33–9.

71. Li ST. Biologic biomaterials: tissue derived biomaterials (collagen). In: Bronzino JD, ed. The Biomedical Engineering Handbook. Boca Raton, FL: CRS Press, 1995: 627–47.

72. Furthmayr H, Timpl R. Immunochemistry of collagens and procollagens. Intern Rev Connect Tissue Res 1976; 7: 61–99.

73. Cen L, Liu W, Cui L, et al. Collagen tissue engineering: development of novel biomaterials and applications. Pediatr Res 2008; 63: 492–6.

74. Silver FH, Pins G. Cell growth on collagen: a review of tissue engineering using scaffolds containing extracellular matrix. J Long-Term Eff Med Implants 1992; 2: 67–80.

75. Sams AE, Nixon AJ. Chondrocyte-laden collagen scaffolds for resurfacing extensive articular cartilage defects. Osteoarthritis Cartilage 1995; 3: 47–59.

76. Yannas IV, Burke JF, Gordon PL, et al. Design of an artificial skin. II. Control of chemical composition. J Biomed Mater Res 1980; 14: 107–32.

77. Yannas IV, Burke JF. Design of an artificial skin. I. Basic design principles. J Biomed Mater Res 1980; 14: 65–81.

78. Cavallaro JF, Kemp PD, Kraus KH. Collagen fabrics as biomaterials. Biotechnol Bioeng 1994; 43: 781–91.

79. Dahms SE, Piechota HJ, Dahiya R, et al. Composition and biomechanical properties of the bladder acellular matrix graft: comparative analysis in rat, pig and human. Br J Urol 1998; 82: 411–19.

80. Piechota HJ, Dahms SE, Nunes LS, et al. In vitro functional properties of the rat bladder regenerated by the bladder acellular matrix graft. J Urol 1998; 159: 1717–24.

81. Yoo JJ, Meng J, Oberpenning F, et al. Bladder augmentation using allogenic bladder submucosa seeded with cells. Urology 1998; 51: 221–5.

82. Chen F, Yoo JJ, Atala A. Acellular collagen matrix as a possible "off the shelf" biomaterial for urethral repair. Urology 1999; 54: 407–10.

83. Probst M, Dahiya R, Carrier S, et al. Reproduction of functional smooth muscle tissue and partial bladder replacement. Br J Urol 1997; 79: 505–15.

84. Gilding D. Biodegradable polymers. In: Williams D, ed. Biocompatibility of Clinical Implant Materials. Boca Raton, FL: CRC Press, 1981: 209–32.

85. Freed LE, Vunjak-Novakovic G, Biron RJ, et al. Biodegradable polymer scaffolds for tissue engineering. Biotechnology (NY) 1994; 12: 689–93.

86. Mikos AG, Lyman MD, Freed LE, et al. Wetting of poly(L-lactic acid) and poly(DL-lactic-co-glycolic acid) foams for tissue culture. Biomaterials 1994; 15: 55–8.

87. Harris LD, Kim BS, Mooney DJ. Open pore biodegradable matrices formed with gas foaming. J Biomed Mater Res 1998; 42: 396–402.

88. Han D, Gouma PI. Electrospun bioscaffolds that mimic the topology of extracellular matrix. Nanomedicine 2006; 2: 37–41.

89. Boccaccini AR, Blaker JJ. Bioactive composite materials for tissue engineering scaffolds. Expert Rev Med Devices 2005; 2: 303–17.

90. Harrison BS, Atala A. Carbon nanotube applications for tissue engineering. Biomaterials 2007; 28: 344–53.

91. Harrington DA, Cheng EY, Guler MO, et al. Branched peptide-amphiphiles as self-assembling coatings for tissue engineering scaffolds. J Biomed Mater Res A 2006; 78: 157–67.

92. McDougal WS. Metabolic complications of urinary intestinal diversion. J Urol 1992; 147: 1199–208.

93. Atala A, Bauer SB, Hendren WH, et al. The effect of gastric augmentation on bladder function. J Urol 1993; 149: 1099–102.

94. Kaefer M, Hendren WH, Bauer SB, et al. Reservoir calculi: a comparison of reservoirs constructed from stomach and other enteric segments. J Urol 1998; 160: 2187–90. [see comment].

95. Kaefer M, Tobin MS, Hendren WH, et al. Continent urinary diversion: the children's hospital experience. J Urol 1997; 157: 1394–9.

96. Atala A. Commentary on the replacement of urologic associated mucosa. J Urol 1995; 156: 338.

97. Atala A. Autologous cell transplantation for urologic reconstruction. J Urol 1998; 159: 2–3.

98. Sutherland RS, Baskin LS, Hayward SW, et al. Regeneration of bladder urothelium, smooth muscle, blood vessels and nerves into an acellular tissue matrix. J Urol 1996; 156: 571–7.

99. Wefer J, Sievert KD, Schlote N, et al. Time dependent smooth muscle regeneration and maturation in a bladder acellular matrix graft: histological studies and in vivo functional evaluation. J Urol 2001; 165: 1755–9.

100. Kikuno N, Kawamoto K, Hirata H, et al. Nerve growth factor combined with vascular endothelial growth factor enhances regeneration of bladder acellular matrix graft in spinal cord injury-induced neurogenic rat bladder. BJU Int 2008; 103: 1424–8.

101. Badylak SF, Lantz GC, Coffey A, et al. Small intestinal submucosa as a large diameter vascular graft in the dog. J Surg Res 1989; 47: 74–80.

102. Badylak SF. The extracellular matrix as a scaffold for tissue reconstruction. Semin Cell Dev Biol 2002; 13: 377–83.

103. Kropp BP, Rippy MK, Badylak SF, et al. Regenerative urinary bladder augmentation using small intestinal submucosa: urodynamic and histopathologic assessment in long-term canine bladder augmentations. J Urol 1996; 155: 2098–104.

104. Kropp BP, Sawyer BD, Shannon HE, et al. Characterization of small intestinal submucosa regenerated canine detrusor: assessment of reinnervation, in vitro compliance and contractility. J Urol 1996; 156: 599–607.

105. Vaught JD, Kropp BP, Sawyer BD, et al. Detrusor regeneration in the rat using porcine small intestinal submucosal grafts: functional innervation and receptor expression. J Urol 1996; 155: 374–8.

106. Portis AJ, Elbahnasy AM, Shalhav AL, et al. Laparoscopic augmentation cystoplasty with different biodegradable grafts in an animal model. J Urol 2000; 164: 1405–11.

107. Landman J, Olweny E, Sundaram CP, et al. Laparoscopic mid sagittal hemicystectomy and bladder reconstruction with small intestinal submucosa and reimplantation of ureter into small intestinal submucosa: 1-year followup. J Urol 2004; 171: 2450–5.

108. Kropp BP, Cheng EY, Lin HK, et al. Reliable and reproducible bladder regeneration using unseeded distal small intestinal submucosa. J Urol 2004; 172: 1710–13.

109. Chun SY, Lim GJ, Kwon TG, et al. Identification and characterization of bioactive factors in bladder submucosa matrix. Biomaterials 2007; 28: 4251–6.

110. Nguyen MM, Lieu DK, deGraffenried LA, et al. Urothelial progenitor cells: regional differences in the rat bladder. Cell Prolif 2007; 40: 157–65.

111. Kurzrock EA, Lieu DK, Degraffenried LA, et al. Label-retaining cells of the bladder: candidate urothelial stem cells. Am J Physiol Renal Physiol 2008; 294: F1415–21.

112. Shukla D, Box GN, Edwards RA, et al. Bone marrow stem cells for urologic tissue engineering. World J Urol 2008; 26: 341–9.

113. Anumanthan G, Makari JH, Honea L, et al. Directed differentiation of bone marrow derived mesenchymal stem cells into bladder urothelium. J Urol 2008; 180: 1778–83.

114. Oottamasathien S, Wang Y, Williams K, et al. Directed differentiation of embryonic stem cells into bladder tissue. Dev Biol 2007; 304: 556–66.

115. Atala A, Freeman MR, Vacanti JP, et al. Implantation in vivo and retrieval of artificial structures consisting of rabbit and human urothelium and human bladder muscle. J Urol 1993; 150: 608–12.

116. de Boer WI, Schuller AG, Vermey M, et al. Expression of growth factors and receptors during specific phases in regenerating urothelium after acute injury in vivo. Am J Pathol 1994; 145: 1199–207.

117. Baker R, Kelly T, Tehan T, et al. Subtotal cystectomy and total bladder regeneration in treatment of bladder cancer. J Am Med Assoc 1958; 168: 1178–85.

118. Gorham SD, French DA, Shivas AA, et al. Some observations on the regeneration of smooth muscle in the repaired urinary bladder of the rabbit. Eur Urol 1989; 16: 440–3.

119. Master VA, Wei G, Liu W, et al. Urothlelium facilitates the recruitment and trans-differentiation of fibroblasts into smooth muscle in acellular matrix. J Urol 2003; 170: 1628–32.

120. Oberpenning F, Meng J, Yoo JJ, et al. De novo reconstitution of a functional mammalian urinary bladder by tissue engineering. Nat Biotechnol 1999; 17: 149–55. [see comment].

121. Jayo MJ, Jain D, Ludlow JW, et al. Long-term durability, tissue regeneration and neo-organ growth during skeletal maturation with a neo-bladder augmentation construct. Regenerative Med 2008; 3: 671–82.

122. Jayo MJ, Jain D, Wagner BJ, et al. Early cellular and stromal responses in regeneration versus repair of a mammalian bladder using autologous cell and biodegradable scaffold technologies. J Urol 2008; 180: 392–7. [see comment].

123. Kwon TG, Yoo JJ, Atala A. Local and systemic effects of a tissue engineered neobladder in a canine cystoplasty model. J Urol 2008; 179: 2035–41.

124. Zhang Y, Frimberger D, Cheng EY, et al. Challenges in a larger bladder replacement with cell-seeded and unseeded small intestinal submucosa grafts in a subtotal cystectomy model. BJU Int 2006; 98: 1100–5.

125. Farhat WA, Yeger H. Does mechanical stimulation have any role in urinary bladder tissue engineering? World J Urol 2008; 26: 301–5.

126. Atala A, Bauer SB, Soker S, et al. Tissue-engineered autologous bladders for patients needing cystoplasty. Lancet 2006; 367: 1241–6. [see comment].

127. Lin HK, Cowan R, Moore P, et al. Characterization of neuropathic bladder smooth muscle cells in culture. J Urol 2004; 171: 1348–52.

128. Hipp J, Andersson KE, Kwon TG, et al. Microarray analysis of exstrophic human bladder smooth muscle. BJU Int 2008; 101: 100–5.

129. Dozmorov MG, Kropp BP, Hurst RE, et al. Differentially expressed gene networks in cultured smooth muscle cells from normal and neuropathic bladder. J Smooth Muscle Res 2007; 43: 55–72.

130. Lai JY, Yoon CY, Yoo JJ, et al. Phenotypic and functional characterization of in vivo tissue engineered smooth muscle from normal and pathological bladders. J Urol 2002; 168: 1853–7; discussion 8.

131. Faris RA, Konkin T, Halpert G. Liver stem cells: a potential source of hepatocytes for the treatment of human liver disease. Artif Organs 2001; 25: 513–21. [see comment].

132. Haller H, de Groot K, Bahlmann F, et al. Stem cells and progenitor cells in renal disease. Kid Int 2005; 68: 1932–6.

133. Wefer J, Sekido N, Sievert KD, et al. Homologous acellular matrix graft for vaginal repair in rats: a pilot study for a new reconstructive approach. World J Urol 2002; 20: 260–3.

134. De Filippo RE, Yoo JJ, Atala A. Engineering of vaginal tissue in vivo. Tissue Eng 2003; 9: 301–6.

135. De Filippo RE, Bishop CE, Filho LF, et al. Tissue engineering a complete vaginal replacement from a small biopsy of autologous tissue. [erratum appears in Transplantation. 2008; 86: 751. Note: De Philippo, Roger E [corrected to De Filippo, Roger E]]. Transplantation 2008; 86: 208–14.

136. Kershen RT, Atala A. New advances in injectable therapies for the treatment of incontinence and vesicoureteral reflux. Urol Clin North Am 1999; 26: 81–94.

137. Atala A, Kim W, Paige KT, et al. Endoscopic treatment of vesicoureteral reflux with a chondrocyte-alginate suspension. J Urol 1994; 152: 641–3; discussion 4.

138. Bent AE, Tutrone RT, McLennan MT, et al. Treatment of intrinsic sphincter deficiency using autologous ear chondrocytes as a bulking agent. Neurourol Urodyn 2001; 20: 157–65.

139. Diamond DA, Caldamone AA. Endoscopic correction of vesicoureteral reflux in children using autologous chondrocytes: preliminary results. J Urol 1999; 162: 1185–8.

140. Cilento BG, Atala A. Treatment of reflux and incontinence with autologous chondrocytes and bladder muscle cells. Dial Pediatr Urol 1995; 18: 11.

141. Chancellor MB, Yokoyama T, Tirney S, et al. Preliminary results of myoblast injection into the urethra and bladder wall: a possible method for the treatment of stress urinary incontinence and impaired detrusor contractility. Neurourol Urodyn 2000; 19: 279–87.

142. Yokoyama T, Huard J, Chancellor MB. Myoblast therapy for stress urinary incontinence and bladder dysfunction. World J Urol 2000; 18: 56–61.

143. Lee JY, Cannon TW, Pruchnic R, et al. The effects of periurethral muscle-derived stem cell injection on leak point pressure in a rat model of stress urinary incontinence. Int Urogynecol J 2003; 14: 31–7; discussion 7.

144. Cannon TW, Lee JY, Somogyi G, et al. Improved sphincter contractility after allogenic muscle-derived progenitor cell injection into the denervated rat urethra. Urology 2003; 62: 958–63.

145. Kwon D, Kim Y, Pruchnic R, et al. Periurethral cellular injection: comparison of muscle-derived progenitor cells and fibroblasts with regard to efficacy and tissue contractility in an animal model of stress urinary incontinence. Urology 2006; 68: 449–54.

146. Strasser H, Berjukow S, Marksteiner R, et al. Stem cell therapy for urinary stress incontinence. Exp Gerontol 2004; 39: 1259–65.

147. Mitterberger M, Pinggera GM, Marksteiner R, et al. Functional and histological changes after myoblast injections in the porcine rhabdosphincter. Eur Urol 2007; 52: 1736–43. [see comment] [erratum appears in Eur Urol 2008; 54: 1208 Note: Bartsch, Georg [removed]].

148. Yiou R, Yoo JJ, Atala A. Restoration of functional motor units in a rat model of sphincter injury by muscle precursor cell autografts. Transplantation 2003; 76: 1053–60.

149. Yiou R, Lefaucheur JP, Atala A. The regeneration process of the striated urethral sphincter involves activation of intrinsic satellite cells. Anat Embryol 2003; 206: 429–35.

150. Eberli D, Andersson KE, Yoo J, et al. A canine model of irreversible urethral sphincter insufficiency. BJU Int 2008; 103: 248–53.

151. Huard J, Yokoyama T, Pruchnic R, et al. Muscle-derived cell-mediated ex vivo gene therapy for urological dysfunction. Gene Ther 2002; 9: 1617–26.

152. Delo DM, Eberli D, Williams JK, et al. Angiogenic gene modification of skeletal muscle cells to compensate for ageing-induced decline in bioengineered functional muscle tissue. BJU Int 2008; 102: 878–84.

153. Jack GS, Almeida FG, Zhang R, et al. Processed lipoaspirate cells for tissue engineering of the lower urinary tract: implications for the treatment of stress urinary incontinence and bladder reconstruction. J Urol 2005; 174: 2041–5.

154. Rodriguez LV, Alfonso Z, Zhang R, et al. Clonogenic multipotent stem cells in human adipose tissue differentiate into functional smooth muscle cells. Proc Natl Acad Sci USA 2006; 103: 12167–72.

155. Strasser H, Marksteiner R, Margreiter E, et al. Autologous myoblasts and fibroblasts versus collagen for treatment of stress urinary incontinence in women: a randomised controlled trial. Lancet 2007; 369: 2179–86. [see comment][erratum appears in Lancet 2008; 371: 474] [retraction in Kleinert S, Horton R. Lancet 2008; 372: 789–90; PMID: 18774408].

156. Mitterberger M, Marksteiner R, Margreiter E, et al. Autologous myoblasts and fibroblasts for female stress incontinence: a 1-year follow-up in 123 patients. BJU Int 2007; 100: 1081–5.

157. Kajbafzadeh AM, Elmi A, Payabvash S, et al. Transurethral autologous myoblast injection for treatment of urinary incontinence in children with classic bladder exstrophy. J Urol 2008; 180: 1098–105.

158. Carr LK, Steele D, Steele S, et al. 1-year follow-up of autologous muscle-derived stem cell injection pilot study to treat stress urinary incontinence. Int Urogynecol J 2008; 19: 881–3.

23 Physiology of Micturition

Naoki Yoshimura and Michael B Chancellor

To understand the various organs and nerves involved with urinary control, we like to visualize the micturition process as a complex of neural circuits in the brain and spinal cord that coordinate the activity of smooth muscle in the bladder and urethra (1–3). These circuits act as on-off switches to alternate the lower urinary tract between two modes of operation: storage and elimination. Injuries or diseases of the nervous system in adults can disrupt the voluntary control of micturition, causing the re-emergence of reflex micturition and resulting in detrusor overactivity and urge incontinence (Fig. 23.1) (1–4). Because of the complexity of the central nervous control of the lower urinary tract, urgency incontinence can result from a variety of neurologic disorders. In addition, urgency incontinence may be due to intrinsic detrusor myogenic abnormalities, resulting in detrusor overactivity (5).

BLADDER PHYSIOLOGY

The urinary bladder performs several important functions and does it well most of the time. First, it stores a socially adequate volume of urine. The bladder wall is able to stretch and rearrange itself to allow an increase in bladder volume without significant rise in pressure. The bladder wall must be highly compliant. Second, the smooth muscle and intrinsic nerves are protected from exposure to urine by the urothelium, which also readily expands during filling. The blood-bladder barrier is rigorous to prevent uremia. Third, bladder emptying requires synchronous activation of all the smooth muscles. If only part of the wall contracted, the uncontracted compliant areas would stretch and prevent the increase in pressure necessary for urine to be expelled through the urethra.

The individual smooth muscle cells in the bladder wall are small spindle-shaped cells with a central nucleus (6). The bladder muscle has a broad length-tension relationship, allowing tension to be developed over a large range of resting muscle lengths (7). The tissue shows viscoelasticity that influences muscle tension and is manifested as total bladder wall tension (8). Isolated detrusor strips show spontaneous mechanical activity to a variable extent. It is more frequently seen in small mammal bladders (9) but can also be seen in muscle strips from human detrusor. However, spontaneous fused tetanic contractions such as those commonly seen in smooth muscles from the gastrointestinal tract and uterus are almost never seen in normal bladder. The lack of fused tetanic contractions in normal detrusor smooth muscle strips suggests that there is poor electrical coupling between smooth muscle cells (10). Measurements of tissue impedance support that the detrusor is less well coupled electrically than other smooth muscles (11,12). Poor coupling could be a feature of normal detrusor to prevent synchronous activation of the smooth muscle cells during bladder filling. Nevertheless, some degree of coupling

within a muscle bundle clearly does exist because it is possible to measure the length constant of a bundle (13).

There is also evidence for gap junction coupling between detrusor cells in humans and guinea pigs, detected whole-cell patch clamp recordings (14) and Ca^2 imaging (15), respectively. Significant expression of connexins 43 and 45, gap junction proteins, is found in human detrusor muscles (14,16). However, electrical couplings between detrusor cells seem to be reduced during postnatal development because coordinated, large-amplitude, low-frequency contractile activity seen in the neonate rat bladder declines and is replaced by low-amplitude, high-frequency, more irregular activity in older rats, which appears to depend on the disruption of the intercellular smooth muscle communication (17). It has also been suggested that a change in the properties of the cell coupling may underlie the generation of the uninhibited detrusor contractions occurring in the overactive and aging bladders (5,13,18).

Interstitial Cells

Recent evidence suggests that the "normal" bladder may be spontaneously active and that exaggerated spontaneous contractions could contribute to the development of overactive bladder. In a rat model for detrusor overactivity, local areas of the spontaneous contractions are increased and more coordinated in partial outlet-obstructed rat bladders (19). However, it is still not clear which cells generate spontaneous activity in the bladder. Detrusor myocytes could be spontaneously active and electrical coupling through gap junctions could trigger spontaneous contractions (5,18). Alternatively, another population of cells in the bladder known as interstitial cells or myofibroblasts has been proposed for a pacemaking role in spontaneous activity of the bladder (20,21). Interstitial cells have been identified in human and guinea pig ureter, urethra, and bladder body (21–23).

Suburothelial Interstitial Cells

In the human bladder, subepithelial interstitial cells, which are also called myofibroblasts, stain for vimentin and alpha-smooth muscle actin but not for desmin (24). These cells are linked by gap junctions consisting of connexin 43 proteins and make close appositions with C-fiber nerve endings in the submucosal layer of the bladder, suggesting that there is a network of functionally connected interstitial cells immediately below the urothelium that may be modulated by other nerve fibers (24) (Fig. 23.2). ATP can induce inward currents associated with elevated intracellular Ca^2 in isolated suburothelial interstitial cells (23). Immunohistochemical studies show the expression of P2Y receptors, most notably $P2Y_6$ receptors, and M_3 muscarinic receptors in the suburothelial interstitial cells

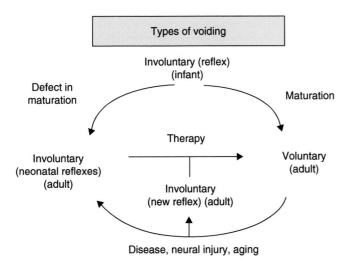

Figure 23.1 Bladder's "circle of life" by influence of maturation, pathologic processes, and aging. In infants, voiding is initiated and coordinated by reflex circuits. After maturation of central neural pathways, voiding is controlled voluntarily by neural circuitry in higher centers in the brain. A defect in neural maturation allows involuntary voiding to persist in adults. Aging, neural injury, or diseases such as benign prostatic hyperplasia can disrupt the central voluntary micturition neural pathways. Pathologic processes can lead to the formation of new reflex circuitry by reemergence of primitive reflex mechanisms that were present in the infant or that appear as the result of synaptic remodeling. The goal of therapy is to reverse the pathologic process and to reestablish normal voluntary control of voiding.

from guinea pigs (23,25). In the human bladder, increased expression of muscarinic M_2 and M_3 receptors in vimentin-stained suburothelial interstitial cells is found and correlated with urgency score in humans with idiopathic detrusor overactivity (26). Because ATP or Ach is known to be released from the urothelium during bladder stretch, suburothelial interstitial cells are in an ideal position between the urothelium and nerve endings to modify a sensory feedback mechanism. Application of nitric oxide (NO) donor sodium nitroprussid (SNP) also attenuates an increase in intracellular Ca^2 and current responses to ATP in guinea pig interstitial cells, suggesting the cGMP-dependent inhibition of cell activity (27).

Intradetrusor Interstitial Cells

Interstitial cells are also found in the detrusor layer and shown to be spontaneously active (21). These cells are stained for c-Kit and located along both boundaries of muscle bundles in the guinea pig bladder (22,28,29). They can fire Ca^2 waves in response to cholinergic stimulation via M_3 muscarinic receptor activation and can be spontaneously active. This suggests they could act as pacemakers or intermediaries in transmission of nerve signals to smooth muscle cells (28,29). However, Hashitani and colleagues (30) have also suggested that interstitial cells in the detrusor may be more important for modulating the transmission of Ca^2 transients originating from smooth muscle cells rather than being the pacemaker of spontaneous

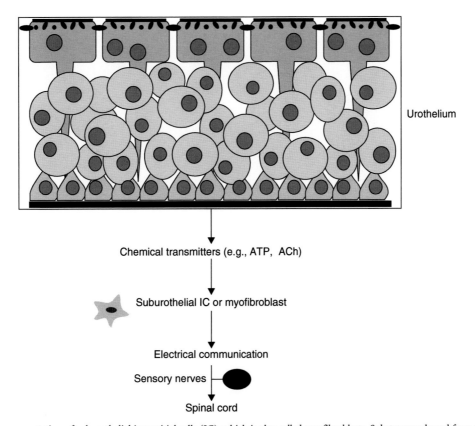

Figure 23.2 Schematic representation of suburothelial interstitial cells (IC), which is also called myofibroblasts. Substances released from the basolateral surface during stretch, such as adenosine triphosphate (ATP) and acetylcholine (ACh), activate afferents in the suburothelial layer through the intermediation of suburothelially located interstitial cells, which express purinergic P2Y receptors, muscarinic M_2 and M_3 receptors or capsacin TRPV1 receptors, and are connected each other by gap junction proteins.

activity because Ca^2 transients occur independently in smooth muscles and interstitial cells. It has also been demonstrated that the c-Kit tyrosine kinase inhibitor Glivec decreased the amplitude of spontaneous contractions in the guinea pig bladder (31,32) and in muscle strips from the overactive human bladder, in which c-Kit-positive cells were increased compared with normal subjects (33). This suggests that targeting these receptors expressed in intradetrusor interstitial cells may provide a new approach for treating overactive bladder. In addition, following application of SNP, an NO donor, interstitial cells throughout the bladder, but not detrusor muscle cells, demonstrate cGMP immunoreactivity (6,34). Thus, increased levels of cGMP in interstitial cells by using phosphodiesterase 5 inhibitors, for example, may diminish synchronicity between detrusor muscle bundles (22). These cells are also a source of prostaglandin E_2 (PGE_2) because of their expression of cyclooxygenase and a reduction in spontaneous activity of bladder muscle strips by PGE_2 receptor (EP) antagonists in rabbits (35).

NEUROPHYSIOLOGY
Urine Storage

During bladder filling there is a low and relatively constant bladder pressure when bladder volume is below the threshold for inducing voiding. The accommodation of the bladder to increasing volumes of urine is primarily a passive phenomenon dependent of intrinsic properties of the vesical smooth muscle and the quiescence of the parasympathetic efferent pathway (1,2,36). The sympathetic reflex also contributes as a negative feedback or urine storage mechanism that promotes closure of the urethral outlet and inhibits neurally mediated contractions of the bladder during bladder filling (37). Reflex

activation of the sympathetic outflow to the lower urinary tract can be triggered by afferent activity induced by distention of the urinary bladder (2,37,38). This reflex response is organized in the lumbosacral spinal cord and persists after transection of the spinal cord at the thoracic levels (Fig. 23.3). However, this bladder to sympathetic mechanism to suppress bladder contractions during urine storage may be weak in humans, given that bilateral retroperitoneal lymph node dissection, in which the sympathetic chains are destroyed, has no discernible alteration of filling or storage function in humans.

During bladder filling, the activity of the sphincter electromyogram also increases (Fig. 23.4), reflecting an increase in efferent firing in the pudendal nerve and an increase in outlet resistance that contributes to the maintenance of urinary continence. Pudendal motoneurons are activated by bladder afferent input (the guarding reflex) (39) whereas during micturition, the motoneurons are reciprocally inhibited (2). External urethral sphincter motoneurons are also activated by urethral or perineal afferents in the pudendal nerve (40). This reflex may represent, in part, a continence mechanism that is activated by proprioceptive afferent input from the urethra or pelvic floor and that induces closure of the urethral outlet. These excitatory sphincter reflexes are organized in the spinal cord. Inhibition of external urethral sphincter reflex activity during micturition is dependent, in part, on supraspinal mechanisms because it is weak or absent in chronic spinal animals and humans, resulting in simultaneous contractions of bladder and sphincter (i.e., detrusor-sphincter dyssynergia) (41,42).

It is well known that stimulation of somatic afferent pathways projecting in the pudendal nerve to the caudal lumbosacral spinal cord can inhibit voiding function. The

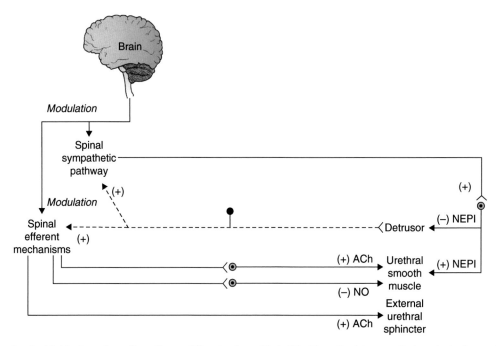

Figure 23.3 Diagram showing bladder to urethra reflex pathways. Afferent pathway *(dashed line)* from the detrusor activates spinal reflex mechanisms that induce firing in somatic cholinergic nerves to the external urethral sphincter, sympathetic adrenergic nerves to the urethral smooth muscle, and cholinergic and nitrergic nerves to the urethral smooth muscle. Bulbospinal pathways from the brain can modulate these spinal reflex mechanisms. *Abbreviations*: ACh, acetylcholine; NEPI, norepinephrine; NO, nitric oxide; excitatory (+) and inhibitory (—) mechanisms.

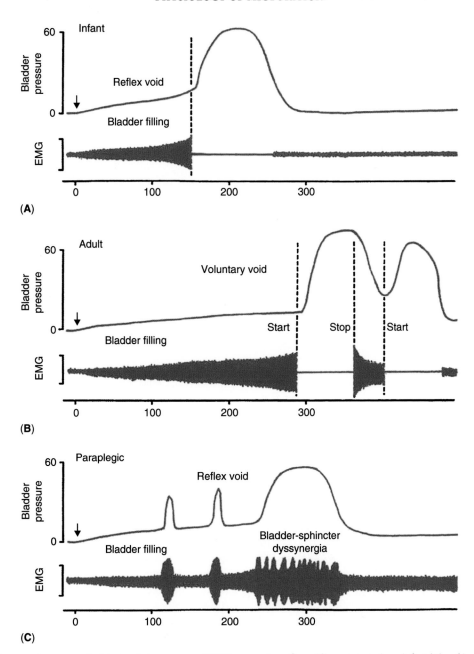

Figure 23.4 Combined cystometrogram and sphincter electromyogram (EMG) comparing reflex voiding responses in an infant (**A**) and in a paraplegic patient (**C**) with a voluntary voiding response in an adult (**B**). The x-axis in all records represents bladder volume in milliliters, and the y-axis represents bladder pressure in centimeters of water and electrical activity of the electromyographic recording. On the left side of each trace, the arrows indicate the start of a slow infusion of fluid into the bladder (bladder filling). Vertical dashed lines indicate the start of sphincter relaxation that precedes by a few seconds the bladder contraction in **A** and **B**. In **B**, note that a voluntary cessation of voiding (stop) is associated with an initial increase in sphincter electromyographic activity followed by a reciprocal relaxation of the bladder. A resumption of voiding is again associated with sphincter relaxation and a delayed increase in bladder pressure. On the other hand, in the paraplegic patient (**C**), the reciprocal relationship between bladder and sphincter is abolished. During bladder filling, transient uninhibited bladder contractions occur in association with sphincter activity. Further filling leads to more prolonged and simultaneous contractions of the bladder and sphincter (bladder-sphincter dyssynergia). Loss of the reciprocal relationship between bladder and sphincter in paraplegic patients interferes with bladder emptying. *Source*: From Ref. 104.

inhibition can be induced by activation of afferent input from various sites including the penis, vagina, rectum, perineum, urethral sphincter, and anal sphincter (2,43,44). Electrophysio-logic studies in cats showed that the inhibition was mediated by suppression of interneuronal pathways in the sacral spinal cord and also by direct inhibitory input to the parasympathetic preganglionic neurons (45). Contractions of the external urethral sphincter and possibly other pelvic floor striated muscles stimulate firing in muscle proprioceptive

afferents, which then activate central inhibitory mechanisms to suppress the micturition reflex (Fig. 23.5). A similar inhibitory mechanism has been identified in monkeys by directly stimulation the anal sphincter muscle (46).

Bladder Emptying
The storage phase of the bladder can be switched to the voiding phase either involuntarily (reflexly) or voluntarily. The former is readily demonstrated in the human infant or in

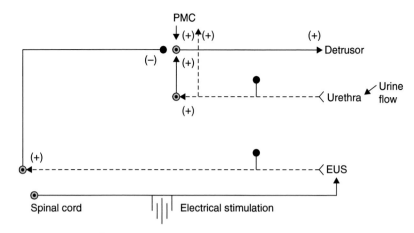

Figure 23.5 Urethra to bladder reflexes. Activity in afferent nerves *(dashed lines)* from the urethra can facilitate parasympathetic efferent outflow to the detrusor by means of a supraspinal pathway passing through the pontine micturition center (PMC) as well as a spinal reflex pathway. Afferent input from the external urethral sphincter (EUS) can inhibit parasympathetic outflow to the detrusor through a spinal reflex circuit. Electrical stimulation of motor axons in the S1 ventral root elicits an EUS contraction and EUS afferent firing that in turn inhibits reflex bladder activity; excitatory (+) and inhibitory (−) mechanisms.

patients with neuropathic bladder when the bladder wall tension due to increased volume of urine exceeds the micturition threshold. At this point, increased afferent firing from tension receptors in the bladder reverses the pattern of efferent outflow, producing firing in the sacral parasympathetic pathways and inhibition of sympathetic and somatic pathways. The expulsion phase consists of an initial relaxation of the urethral sphincter (Fig. 23.4) followed in a few seconds by a contraction of the bladder, an increase in bladder pressure, and the flow of urine. Relaxation of the urethral smooth muscle during micturition is mediated by activation of a parasympathetic pathway to the urethra that triggers the release of NO, an inhibitory transmitter (47,48), and by removal of excitatory inputs to the urethra. Secondary reflexes elicited by flow of urine through the urethra facilitate bladder emptying (1,38,49). These reflexes require the integrative action of neuronal populations at various levels of the neuraxis (Fig. 23.6A). The parasympathetic outflow to the detrusor and urethra has a more complicated central organization involving spinal and spinobulbospinal pathways passing through a micturition center in the pontine micturition center (PMC) (pons) (Fig. 23.6B).

Barrington (50,51) reported that urine flow or mechanical stimulation of the urethra with a catheter could excite afferent nerves that in turn facilitated reflex bladder contractions in the anesthetized cat (Fig. 23.5). He proposed that this facilitatory urethra to bladder reflex could promote complete bladder emptying. Barrington identified two components of this reflex. One component was activated by a somatic afferent pathway in the pudendal nerve and produced facilitation by a supraspinal mechanism involving the PMC (51) (Fig. 23.5). Studies have confirmed the existence of this type of reflex via the pudendal nerve since low-frequency electrical stimulation of afferent axons in the pudendal nerve in humans or the deep perineal nerve, a caudal branch of the pudendal nerve, in cats can initiate reflex bladder contractions and voiding (52,53). The other component was activated by a visceral afferent

pathway in the pelvic nerve and produced facilitation by a spinal reflex mechanism (50).

Studies (49) in the anesthetized rat have also provided additional support for Barrington's findings (54). Measurements of reflex bladder contractions under isovolumetric conditions during continuous urethral perfusion (0.075 mL/min) revealed that the frequency of micturition reflexes was significantly reduced when urethral perfusion was stopped or after infusion of lidocaine (1%) into the urethra. Intraurethral infusion of NO donors (*s*-nitroso-*n*-acetylpenicillamine or nitroprusside, 1–2 mM) markedly decreased urethral perfusion pressure (approximately 30%) and decreased the frequency of reflex bladder contractions (45–75%), but did not change the amplitude of bladder contractions. Desensitization of the urethral afferent with intraurethral capsaicin also dramatically altered the micturition reflex. It was concluded that activation of urethral afferents during urethral perfusion could modulate the micturition reflex in the rat. This may be an explanation of why stress incontinence and urge incontinence often occur together in women. Chancellor speculated that in women with mixed incontinence, leakage of urine into the urethra can stimulate afferents and induce or increase detrusor overactivity. The theory is that stress incontinence can induce urge incontinence (55). Surgical cure of the stress incontinence of women with mixed incontinence has resolved the urge incontinence in up to half of the patients.

Micturition Control Circuitry
Multiple reflex pathways organized in the brain and spinal cord mediate coordination between the urinary bladder and the urethra. The central pathways controlling lower urinary tract function are organized as simple on-off switching circuits (Fig. 23.7) that maintain a reciprocal relationship between the urinary bladder and the urethral outlet (2,56). The principal reflex components of these switching circuits are illustrated in Figure 23.6. Some reflexes promote urine

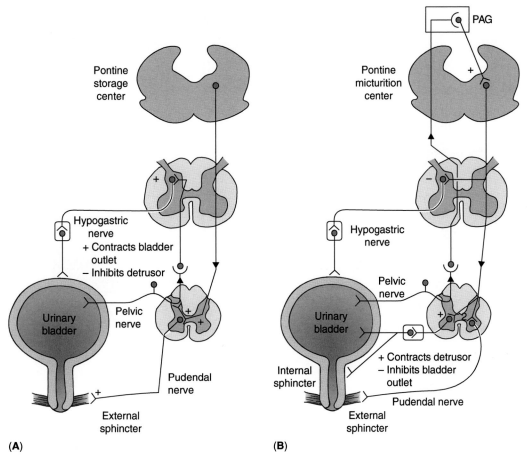

Figure 23.6 Mechanism of storage and voiding reflexes. (**A**), Storage reflexes. During the storage of urine, distention of the bladder produces low-level bladder afferent firing. Afferent firing in turn stimulates the sympathetic outflow to the bladder outlet (base and urethra) and pudendal outflow to the external urethral sphincter. These responses occur by spinal reflex pathways and represent "guarding reflexes," which promote continence. Sympathetic firing also inhibits detrusor muscle and transmission in bladder ganglia. (**B**), Voiding reflexes. At the initiation of micturition, intense vesical afferent activity activates the brainstem micturition center, which inhibits the spinal guarding reflexes (sympathetic and pudendal outflow to the urethra). The pontine micturition center (PMC) also stimulates the parasympathetic outflow to the bladder and internal sphincter smooth muscle. Maintenance of the voiding reflex is through ascending afferent input from the spinal cord, which may pass through the periaqueductal gray matter (PAG) before reaching the PMC.

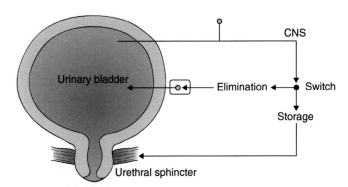

Figure 23.7 Diagram illustrating the anatomy of the lower urinary tract and the "switchlike" function of the micturition reflex pathway. During urine storage, a low level of afferent activity activates efferent input to the urethral sphincter. A high level of afferent activity induced by bladder distention activates the switching circuit in the central nervous system (CNS), producing firing in the efferent pathways to the bladder, inhibition of the efferent outflow to the sphincter, and urine elimination.

storage, whereas others facilitate voiding. It is also possible that individual reflexes might be linked together in a serial manner to create complex feedback mechanisms. For example, the bladder to external urethral sphincter guarding reflex that triggers sphincter contractions during bladder filling could, in turn, activate sphincter muscle afferents that initiate an inhibition of the parasympathetic excitatory pathway to the bladder. Thus, a bladder to sphincter to bladder reflex pathway could in theory contribute to the suppression of bladder activity during urine storage. Alterations in these primitive reflex mechanisms may contribute to neurogenic bladder dysfunction. Direct activation of these reflexes by electrical stimulation of the sacral spinal roots very likely contributes to therapeutic effects of sacral nerve root neuromodulation (57,58).

Peripheral Nervous System

The lower urinary tract is innervated by three sets of peripheral nerves involving the parasympathetic, sympathetic, and somatic nervous systems (Fig. 23.8). Pelvic parasympathetic nerves arise at the sacral level of the spinal cord, excite the bladder, and relax the urethra. Lumbar sympathetic nerves inhibit the bladder body and excite the bladder base and urethra. Pudendal nerves excite the external urethral sphincter. These nerves contain afferent (sensory) as well as efferent axons (2,4,36,59).

205

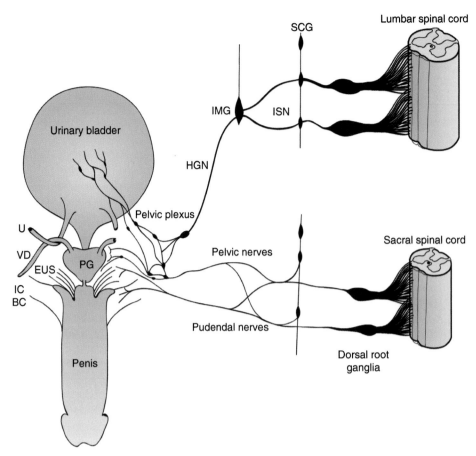

Figure 23.8 Diagram showing the sympathetic, parasympathetic, and somatic innervation of the urogenital tract of the male cat. Sympathetic preganglionic pathways emerge from the lumbar spinal cord and pass to the sympathetic chain ganglia (SCG) and then through the inferior splanchnic nerves (ISN) to the inferior mesenteric ganglia (IMG). Preganglionic and postganglionic sympathetic axons then travel in the hypogastric nerve (HGN) to the pelvic plexus and the urogenital organs. Parasympathetic preganglionic axons that originate in the sacral spinal cord pass in the pelvic nerve to ganglion cells in the pelvic plexus and to distal ganglia in the organs. Sacral somatic pathways are contained in the pudendal nerve, which provides an innervation to the penis and the ischiocavernosus (IC), bulbocavernosus (BC), and external urethral sphincter (EUS) muscles. The pudendal and pelvic nerves also receive postganglionic axons from the caudal sympathetic chain ganglia. These three sets of nerves contain afferent axons from the lumbosacral dorsal root ganglia. *Abbreviations*: PG, prostate gland; U, ureter; VD, vas deferens.

Parasympathetic Pathways

Parasympathetic preganglionic neurons innervating the lower urinary tract are located in the lateral part of the sacral intermediate gray matter in a region termed the sacral parasympathetic nucleus (2,60–63). Parasympathetic preganglionic neurons send axons through the ventral roots to the peripheral ganglia, where they release the excitatory transmitter acetylcholine (38). Parasympathetic postganglionic neurons in humans are located in the detrusor wall layer as well as in the pelvic plexus. This is an important fact to remember because patients with cauda equine or pelvic plexus injury are neurologically decentralized but may not be completely denervated. Cauda equine injury allows possible afferent and efferent neuron interconnection at the level of the intramural ganglia (2,62).

Sympathetic Pathways

Sympathetic outflow from the rostral lumbar spinal cord provides a noradrenergic excitatory and inhibitory input to the bladder and urethra (47). Activation of sympathetic nerves induces relaxation of the bladder body and contraction of the bladder outlet and urethra, which contribute to urine storage in the bladder.

The peripheral sympathetic pathways follow a complex route that passes through the sympathetic chain ganglia to the inferior mesenteric ganglia and then through the hypogastric nerves to the pelvic ganglia (64).

Somatic Pathways

The external urethral sphincter motoneurons are located along the lateral border of the ventral horn, commonly referred to as Onuf's nucleus (Fig. 23.9) (65). Sphincter motoneurons also exhibit transversely oriented dendritic bundles that project laterally in the lateral funiculus, dorsally into the intermediate gray matter, and dorsomedially toward the central canal.

Afferent Pathways

Afferent axons in the pelvic, hypogastric, and pudendal nerves transmit information from the lower urinary tract to the lumbosacral spinal cord (36,66,67). The primary afferent neurons of the pelvic and pudendal nerves are contained in sacral dorsal root ganglia (DRG), whereas afferent innervation in the hypogastric nerves arises in the rostral lumbar DRG. The central axons of the DRG neurons carry the sensory information from the lower urinary tract to second-order neurons in the

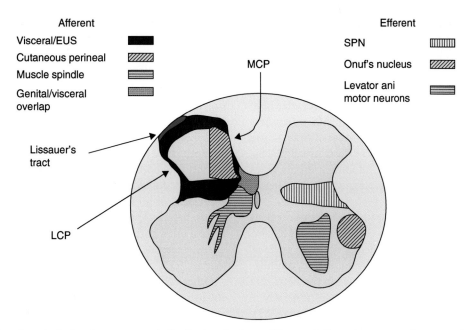

Figure 23.9 Cross section of sacral spinal cord; neuroanatomic distribution of primary afferent and efferent components of storage and micturition reflexes. For purposes of clarity, afferent components are shown only on the left, and efferent components are shown only on the right. Both components are, of course, distributed bilaterally and thus overlap extensively. Visceral afferent components represent bladder, urethral, and genital (glans penis or clitoris) afferent fibers contained in the pelvic and pudendal nerves. Cutaneous perineal afferent components represent afferent fibers that innervate the perineal skin contained in the pudendal nerve. Muscle spindle afferent components represent Ia/b afferent fibers contained in the levator ani nerve that innervate muscle spindles in the levator ani muscle. *Abbreviations*: EUS, external urethral sphincter; LCP, lateral collateral projection; MCP, medial collateral projection; SPN, sacral parasympathetic nucleus.

spinal cord (60,62,65,66) (Fig. 23.9). Visceral afferent fibers of the pelvic (60) and pudendal (65) nerves enter the cord and travel rostrocaudally within Lissauer's tract. Pelvic nerve afferents, which monitor the volume of the bladder and the amplitude of the bladder contraction, consist of myelinated (A) and unmyelinated (C) axons. During neuropathic conditions and possibly inflammatory conditions, there is recruitment of C fibers that from a new functional afferent pathway that can cause urgency incontinence and possibly bladder pain.

Afferent Nerves and Inter-Organ Cross Sensitization
Changes in bladder function after colonic inflammation also appear to be mediated by a change in the cholinergic efferent pathway to the bladder (68). During the active colonic inflammation three days after TNBS instillation into the colon, the bladder was not inflamed but the contractions of bladder strips induced by electrical field stimulation or carbachol, a muscarinic receptor agaonist, were reduced, while the contractions induced by KCl were not changed. During and after recovery of the colonic inflammation (15–30 days) the contractile responses of the bladder returned to normal. It was suggested that bladder dysfunction was mediated by visceral organ cross talk induced by sensitization of a subpopulation of afferents innervating both the bladder and colon.

Spinal and Supraspinal Pathways Involved in the Micturition Reflex
In the spinal cord, afferent pathways terminate on second-order interneurons that relay information to the brain or to other regions of the spinal cord including the preganglionic and motor nuclei. Because disynaptic or polysynaptic pathways

but not menosynaptic pathways mediate bladder, urethral, and sphincter reflex, interneuronal mechanisms play an essential role in the regulation of lower urinary tract function. Electrophysiologic (69,70) and neuroanatomic (59,71–73) techniques have identified lower urinary tract interneurons in the same regions of the cord that receive afferent input from the bladder (Fig. 23.9).

Pharmacologic experiments revealed that glutamic acid is the excitatory transmitter in these pathways (62). The inhibitory neurons release γ-aminobutyric acid (GABA) and glycine. Reflex pathways that control the external sphincter muscles also use glutamatergic excitatory and GABAergic and glycinergic inhibitory interneuronal mechanisms. The micturition reflex can be modulated at the level of the spinal cord by interneuronal mechanisms activated by afferent input from cutaneous and striated muscle targets. Micturition reflex can also be modulated by inputs from visceral organs (1,2,36,56,69,74–77). Stimulation of afferent fibers from various regions (anus, colon-rectum, vagina, uterine cervix, penis, perineum, pudendal nerve) can inhibit the firing of sacral interneurons evoked by bladder distention (69). This inhibition may be a result of presynaptic inhibition at primary afferent terminals or be due to direct postsynaptic inhibition of the second-order neurons. Direct postsynaptic inhibition of bladder preganglionic neurons can also be elicited by stimulation of somatic afferent axons in the pudendal nerve or visceral afferents from the distal bowel (74,78). Suppression of detrusor overactivity in patients by sacral root stimulation may reflect in part activation of the afferent limb of these visceral-bladder and somatic-bladder inhibitory reflexes (58,79,80).

PMC and Brain Stem Modulatory Mechanisms

Various studies indicate that the micturition reflex is normally mediated by a spinobulbospinal reflex pathway passing through relay centers in the brain (1,2,36,56). Studies in animals by use of brain-lesioning techniques revealed that neurons in the brainstem at the level of the inferior colliculus have an essential role in the control of the parasympathetic component of micturition (1–3,36). Removal of areas of brain above the colliculus by intercollicular decerebration usually facilitates micturition by elimination of inhibitory inputs from more rostral centers. However, transections at any point below the colliculi abolish micturition.

In addition to providing axonal inputs to the locus ceruleus and the sacral spinal cord (81–83), neurons in the PMC also send axon collaterals to the paraventricular thalamic nucleus, which is thought to be involved in the limbic system modulation of visceral behavior (82). Some neurons in the PMC also project to the periaqueductal gray region (PAG) (84), which regulates many visceral activities as well as pain pathways (85). Thus, neurons in the PMC communicate with multiple Supraspinal neuronal populations that may coordinate micturition with other functions of the organism. Although the circuitry in humans is uncertain, brain imaging studies have revealed increases in blood flow in this region of the pons during micturition (86). This change presumably reflects increases in neuronal activity. Thus, the PMC appears critical for micturition across species. In the midbrain, there is increasing evidence supporting that the mesencephalic PAG that directly receives information of bladder fullness via ascending spinal tract neurons and sends projections to the PMC seems to play an important role in the integration of the micturition reflex (87–89).

Central Pathways that Modulate the Micturition Reflex

Transneuronal virus tracing methods have identified virus-infected cells in several regions of the hypothalamus and the cerebral cortex after injection of pseudorabies virus into the lower urinary tract in animals (59,72,90). Neurons in the cortex were located primarily in the medial frontal cortex. Tracers injected into the paraventricular nucleus of the hypothalamus labeled terminals in the sacral parasympathetic nucleus as well as the sphincter motor nucleus (88). The influence of the cortex on voiding function could be mediated by a number of pathways, including direct cortical projections from the prefrontal cortex and insular cortex to the PMC, or projections through the hypothalamus and the extrapyramidal system (2). Studies in humans indicate that voluntary control of voiding is dependent on connections between the frontal cortex and the septal-preoptic region of the hypothalamus as well as on connections between the paracentral lobule and the brainstem. Lesions to these areas of cortex appear to directly increase bladder activity by removing cortical inhibitory control (2).

Human Brain Imaging Studies

In the last decade, the areas of the brain involved in the control of micturition have been examined in human brain imaging studies using SPECT, PET, and fMRI (91,92). Some studies evaluated the brain areas responsible for the perception of bladder fullness and the sensation of the desire to void during bladder filling; whereas others examined brain activity during micturition, or voluntary contractions of the pelvic floor during urine withholding or during cold stimulation of the bladder. PET scan studies in normal men and women revealed that during voiding two cortical areas (the dorsolateral prefrontal cortex and anterior cingulated gyrus) were active (i.e., exhibited increased blood flow). The hypothalamus including the preoptic area as well as the pons and the PAG also showed activity in concert with voluntary micturition (84,86). Another PET study during voiding also confirmed that micturition was associated with increased activity in the pons, inferior frontal gyrus, hypothalamus, and PAG, while also showing activity in several other cortical areas (postcentral gyrus, superior frontal gyrus, thalamus, insula, and globus palidus) and the cerebellar vermis (93).

Other PET studies that examined the changes in brain activity during filling of the bladder revealed that increased activity occurred in the PAG, the midline pons, the anterior and mid-cingulate gyrus, anterior insula, and bilaterally in the frontal lobes (94–96). The results were consistent with the notion that the PAG receives information about bladder fullness and then relays this information to other brain areas involved in the control of bladder storage. In fMRI studies in men and women, activation during urinary storage is found in the supplementary motor area, mid-cingulate cortex, insula and right prefrontal cortex, and the right anterior insula and midbrain PAG were more active at higher rather than at lower bladder volumes (97,98). Other fMRI studies also addressed the effect of pelvic floor contraction with a full bladder and reported activation of the parietal cortex, cerebellum, putamen, and supplementary motor area (99) or the frontal cortex, basal ganglia, and cerebellum (100).

Brain imaging studies have also been performed to identify changes in cerebral perception of detrusor overactivity. A PET study in patients with Parkinson's disease reported activation of the PAG, supplementary motor area, basal ganglia, and cerebellum during detrusor overactivity (101). In comparison between healthy control subjects and those with confirmed overactivity using fMRI, infusion in the bladder is associated with activity in the PAG, thalamus, insula, and anterior cingulated gyrus; however, weak responses in the anterior cingulate gyrus at large bladder volumes are observed in urge-incontinent patients (102,103). Based on the results in human imaging studies, Griffiths proposes that: (i) during urine storage in healthy subjects, bladder and urethral afferents received in the PAG and mapped in the insula form normal sensations of desire to void (which is monitored by the anterior cingulated gyrus), and the voiding reflex is continuously inhibited until the decision to void is made in the prefrontal cortex; and (ii) urgency-incontinent subjects have weak responses or deactivation observed in the prefrontal cortex or the limbic system, leading to a defect on supraspinal bladder control that may cause urgency incontinence, and enhanced responses in the anterior cingulaet gyrus, which may be due to abnormal bladder afferents or related to a loss of control in other brain areas and could be correlated with urgency sensations (92). Radiographic imaging of the CNS with control and dysregulation of the lower urinary tract is an exciting area of research but the results are preliminary. Subjects are conscious and thinking about their bladder during the test and may have an indwelling catheter that may alter what parts of the brain are activated naturally or artificially.

CONCLUSIONS

The lower urinary tract has two main functions: storage and periodic elimination of urine. These functions are regulated by unique biomechanics of bladder and urethral muscles as well as by a complex neural control system located in the brain and spinal cord. The neural control system performs like a simple switching circuit to maintain a reciprocal relationship between the reservoir (urinary bladder) and the outlet components (urethra and urethral sphincter) of the urinary tract. The switching circuit is modulated by various neurotransmitters and is sensitive to a variety of drugs. In infants, the switching circuits function in a purely reflex manner to produce involuntary voiding; however, in adults, urine storage and release are subject to voluntary control.

Injuries or diseases of the nervous system can disrupt the voluntary control of micturition, causing the re-emergence of reflex micturition, resulting in detrusor overactivity and incontinence. Because of the complexity of the central nervous control of the lower urinary tract, incontinence can result from a variety of neurologic disorders. Experimental studies indicate that detrusor overactivity occurs after a wide range of neurologic diseases, including interruption of cortical inhibitory circuits, disruption of basal ganglia function in models of Parkinson's disease, damage to pathways from the brain to the spinal cord (multiple sclerosis, spinal cord injury), and sensitization of bladder afferents. Various mechanisms contribute to the emergence of bladder dysfunction including: reorganization of synaptic connections in the spinal cord, changes in the expression of neurotransmitters and receptors, alterations in neural target organ interactions mediated by neurotrophic factors, and changes in smooth muscle function. An understanding of the physiologic events mediating micturition and continence provides a rational basis for the management of lower urinary tract dysfunction.

REFERENCES

1. Torrens M, Morrison JFB. The Physiology of the Lower Urinary Tract. London, New York: Springer-Verlag; 1987.
2. de Groat WC, Booth AM, Yoshimura N. Neurophysiology of micturition and its modification in animal models of human disease. In: Maggi CA, editor. Nervous Control of the Urogenital System. London: Harwood Academic Publishers; 1993: 227–90.
3. Yoshimura N, de Groat WC. Neural control of the lower urinary tract. Int J Urol 1997; 4: 111–25.
4. Wein A. Neuromuscular dysfunction of the lower urinary tract. In: Walsh P, Retik A, Stamey T, Vaughan E, editors. Campbells Urology. 6th ed. Philadelphia: WB Saunders; 1992.
5. Brading AF. A myogenic basis for the overactive bladder. Urology 1997; 50(6A Suppl): 57–67; discussion 8–73.
6. Smet PJ, Jonavicius J, Marshall VR, de Vente J. Distribution of nitric oxide synthase-immunoreactive nerves and identification of the cellular targets of nitric oxide in guinea-pig and human urinary bladder by cGMP immunohistochemistry. Neuroscience 1996; 71: 337–48.
7. Uvelius B, Gabella G. Relation between cell length and force production in urinary bladder smooth muscle. Acta Physiol Scand 1980; 110: 357–65.
8. Venegas JG. Viscoelastic properties of the contracting detrusor. I. Theoretical basis. Am J Physiol 1991; 261: C355–63.
9. Sibley GN. A comparison of spontaneous and nerve-mediated activity in bladder muscle from man, pig and rabbit. J Physiol 1984; 354: 431–43.
10. Uvelius B, Mattiasson A. Detrusor collagen content in the denervated rat urinary bladder. J Urol 1986; 136: 1110–2.
11. Brading AF, Mostwin JL. Electrical and mechanical responses of guinea-pig bladder muscle to nerve stimulation. Br J Pharmacol 1989; 98: 1083–90.
12. Parekh AB, Brading AF, Tomita T. Studies of longitudinal tissue impedance in various smooth muscles. Prog Clin Biol Res 1990; 327: 375–8.
13. Seki N, Karim OM, Mostwin JL. Changes in action potential kinetics following experimental bladder outflow obstruction in the guinea pig. Urol Res 1992; 20: 387–92.
14. Wang HZ, Brink PR, Christ GJ. Gap junction channel activity in short-term cultured human detrusor myocyte cell pairs: gating and unitary conductances. Am J Physiol Cell Physiol 2006; 291: C1366–76.
15. Neuhaus J, Wolburg H, Hermsdorf T, et al. Detrusor smooth muscle cells of the guinea-pig are functionally coupled via gap junctions in situ and in cell culture. Cell Tissue Res 2002; 309: 301–11.
16. John H, Wang X, Wehrli E, et al. Evidence of gap junctions in the stable nonobstructed human bladder. J Urol 2003; 169: 745–9.
17. Szell EA, Somogyi GT, de Groat WC, Szigeti GP. Developmental changes in spontaneous smooth muscle activity in the neonatal rat urinary bladder. American journal of physiology 2003; 285: R809–16.
18. Brading AF. Smooth muscle research: from Edith Bulbring onwards. Trends Pharmacol Sci 2006; 27: 158–65.
19. Drake MJ, Hedlund P, Harvey IJ, et al. Partial outlet obstruction enhances modular autonomous activity in the isolated rat bladder. J Urol 2003; 170: 276–9.
20. Andersson KE, Arner A. Urinary bladder contraction and relaxation: physiology and pathophysiology. Physiol Rev 2004; 84: 935–86.
21. Kumar V, Cross RL, Chess-Williams R, Chapple CR. Recent advances in basic science for overactive bladder. Curr Opin Urol 2005; 15: 222–6.
22. Hashitani H. Interaction between interstitial cells and smooth muscles in the lower urinary tract and penis. J Physiol 2006; 576: 707–14.
23. Fry CH, Sui GP, Kanai AJ, Wu C. The function of suburothelial myofibroblasts in the bladder. Neurourol Urodyn 2007; 26(6 Suppl): 914–9.
24. Fry CH, Ikeda Y, Harvey R, et al. Control of bladder function by peripheral nerves: avenues for novel drug targets. Urology 2004; 63(3 Suppl 1): 24–31.
25. Grol S, Essers PB, van Koeveringe GA, et al. M(3) muscarinic receptor expression on suburothelial interstitial cells. BJU Int 2009; 398–405.
26. Mukerji G, Yiangou Y, Grogono J, et al. Localization of M2 and M3 muscarinic receptors in human bladder disorders and their clinical correlations. J Urol 2006; 176: 367–73.
27. Sui GP, Wu C, Roosen A, et al. Modulation of bladder myofibroblast activity: implications for bladder function. Am J Physiol Renal Physiol 2008; 295: F688–97.
28. McCloskey KD, Gurney AM. Kit positive cells in the guinea pig bladder. J Urol 2002; 168: 832–6.
29. Hashitani H, Yanai Y, Suzuki H. Role of interstitial cells and gap junctions in the transmission of spontaneous Ca2+ signals in detrusor smooth muscles of the guinea-pig urinary bladder. J Physiol 2004; 559: 567–81.
30. Johnston L, Carson C, Lyons AD, et al. Cholinergic-induced Ca2+ signaling in interstitial cells of Cajal from the guinea pig bladder. Am J Physiol Renal Physiol 2008; 294: F645–55.
31. Kubota Y, Biers SM, Kohri K, Brading AF. Effects of imatinib mesylate (Glivec) as a c-kit tyrosine kinase inhibitor in the guinea-pig urinary bladder. Neurourol Urodyn 2006; 25: 205–10.

32. Kubota Y, Kajioka S, Biers SM, et al. Investigation of the effect of the c-kit inhibitor Glivec on isolated guinea-pig detrusor preparations. Auton Neurosci 2004; 115: 64–73.

33. Biers SM, Reynard JM, Doore T, Brading AF. The functional effects of a c-kit tyrosine inhibitor on guinea-pig and human detrusor. BJU Int 2006; 97: 612–6.

34. Gillespie JI, Markerink–van Ittersum M, de Vente J. cGMP-generating cells in the bladder wall: identification of distinct networks of interstitial cells. BJU Int 2004; 94: 1114–24.

35. Collins C, Klausner AP, Herrick B, et al. Potential for Control of Detrusor Smooth Muscle Spontaneous Rhythmic Contraction by Cyclooxygenase Products Released by Interstitial Cells of Cajal. J Cell Mol Med 2009: 3236–50.

36. Yoshimura N, Kaiho Y, Miyazato M, et al. Therapeutic receptor targets for lower urinary tract dysfunction. Naunyn Schmiedebergs Arch Pharmacol 2008; 377: 437–48.

37. de Groat WC, Theobald RJ. Reflex activation of sympathetic pathways to vesical smooth muscle and parasympathetic ganglia by electrical stimulation of vesical afferents. Journal of Physiology (London). 1976; 259: 223–37.

38. de Groat WC, Booth AM. Synaptic transmission in pelvic ganglia. In: Maggi CA, editor. Nervous Control of the Urogenital System, London: Harwood Academic Publishers; 1993: 291–347.

39. Park JM, Bloom DA, McGuire EJ. The guarding reflex revisited. Br J Urol 1997; 80: 940–5.

40. Fedirchuk B, Hochman S, Shefchyk SJ. An intracellular study of perineal and hindlimb afferent inputs onto sphincter motoneurons in the decerebrate cat. Exp Brain Res 1992; 89: 511–6.

41. Rossier AB, Ott R. Bladder and urethral recordings in acute and chronic spinal cord injury patients. Urol Int 1976; 31: 49–59.

42. Blaivas JG. The neurophysiology of micturition: a clinical study of 550 patients. J Urol 1982; 127: 958–63.

43. de Groat WC, Booth AM, Krier J, et al. Neural control of the urinary bladder and large intestine. In: Brooks CM, Koizumi K, Sato A, editors. Integrative functions of the autonomic nervous system. Tokyo: Tokyo Univ. Press; 1979: 50–67.

44. de Groat WC, Fraser MO, Yoshiyama M, et al. Neural control of the urethra. Scand J Urol and Nephrol 2001: 35–43; discussion 106–25.

45. de Groat WC, Booth AM, Milne RJ, Roppolo JR. Parasympathetic preganglionic neurons in the sacral spinal cord. J Autonom Nerv Syst 1982; 5: 23–43.

46. McGuire E, Morrissey S, Zhang S, Horwinski E. Control of reflex detrusor activity in normal and spinal injured non-human primates. J Urol 1983; 129: 197–9.

47. Andersson K-E. Pharmacology of lower urinary tract smooth muscles and penile erectile tissues. [Review]. Pharmacological Reviews. 1993; 45: 253–308.

48. Bennett BC, Kruse MN, Roppolo JR, et al. Neural control of urethral outlet activity in vivo: role of nitric oxide. J Urol 1995; 153: 2004–9.

49. Jung SY, Fraser MO, Ozawa H, et al. Urethral afferent nerve activity affects the micturition reflex; implication for the relationship between stress incontinence and detrusor instability. J Urol 1999; 162: 204–12.

50. Barrington FJF. The component reflexes of micturition in the cat. Part III. Brain 1941; 64: 239–43.

51. Barrington FJF. The component reflexes of micturition in the cat. Parts I and II. Brain 1931; 54: 177–88.

52. Shefchyk S, Buss R. Urethral pudendal afferent-evoked bladder and sphincter reflexes in decerebrate and acute spinal cats. Neurosci Lett 1998; 244: 137–140.

53. Boggs JW, Wenzel BJ, Gustafson KJ, Grill WM. Spinal micturition reflex mediated by afferents in the deep perineal nerve. J Neurophysiol 2005; 93: 2688–97.

54. Dokita S, Morgan WR, Wheeler MA, et al. NG-nitro-L-arginine inhibits non-adrenergic, non-cholinergic relaxation in rabbit urethral smooth muscle. Life Sci 1991; 48: 2429–36.

55. Lavelle JP, Meyers SA, Ruiz WG, et al. Urothelial pathophysiological changes in feline interstitial cystitis: a human model. Am J Physiol Renal Physiol 2000; 278: F540–53.

56. de Groat WC. Nervous control of the urinary bladder of the cat. Brain Research 1975; 87: 201–11.

57. Dijkema HE, Weil EH, Mijs PT, Janknegt RA. Neuromodulation of sacral nerves for incontinence and voiding dysfunctions. Clinical results and complications. Eur Urol 1993; 24: 72–6.

58. Chancellor M, Chartier-Kastler E. Principles of sacral nerve stimulation (SNS) for the treatment of bladder and urethral sphincter dysfunctions. Neuromodulation 2000; 3: 16–26.

59. Sugaya K, Roppolo JR, Yoshimura N, et al. The central neural pathways involved in micturition in the neonatal rat as revealed by the injection of pseudorabies virus into the urinary bladder. Neurosci Lett 1997; 223: 197–200.

60. Morgan C, Nadelhaft I, de Groat WC. The distribution of visceral primary afferents from the pelvic nerve to Lissauer's tract and the spinal gray matter and its relationship to the sacral parasympathetic nucleus. J Comp Neurol 1981; 201: 415–40.

61. Morgan CW, de Groat WC, Felkins LA, Zhang SJ. Intracellular injection of neurobiotin or horseradish peroxidase reveals separate types of preganglionic neurons in the sacral parasympathetic nucleus of the cat. J Comp Neurol 1993; 331: 161–82.

62. deGroat WC, Vizzard MA, Araki I, Roppolo J. Spinal interneurons and preganglionic neurons in sacral autonomic reflex pathways. Prog Brain Res 1996; 107: 97–111.

63. Nadelhaft I, Degroat WC, Morgan C. Location and morphology of parasympathetic preganglionic neurons in the sacral spinal cord of the cat revealed by retrograde axonal transport of horseradish peroxidase. J Comp Neurol 1980; 193: 265–81.

64. Kihara K, de Groat WC. Sympathetic efferent pathways projecting to the bladder neck and proximal urethra in the rat. J Autonom Nerv Syst 1997; 62: 134–42.

65. Thor KB, Morgan C, Nadelhaft I, et al. Organization of afferent and efferent pathways in the pudendal nerve of the female cat. J Comp Neurol 1989; 288: 263–79.

66. de Groat WC. Spinal cord projections and neuropeptides in visceral afferent neurons. Prog Brain Res 1986; 67: 165–87.

67. Janig W, Morrison JF. Functional properties of spinal visceral afferents supplying abdominal and pelvic organs, with special emphasis on visceral nociception. Prog Brain Res 1986; 67: 87–114.

68. Noronha R, Akbarali H, Malykhina A, et al. Changes in urinary bladder smooth muscle function in response to colonic inflammation. Am J Physiol Renal Physiol 2007; 293: F1461–7.

69. de Groat WC, Nadelhaft I, Milne RJ, et al. Organization of the sacral parasympathetic reflex pathways to the urinary bladder and large intestine. J Autonom Nerv Syst 1981; 3: 135–60.

70. Araki I, de Groat WC. Developmental synaptic depression underlying reorganization of visceral reflex pathways in the spinal cord. J Neurosci 1997; 17: 8402–7.

71. Birder LA, de Groat WC. Induction of c-fos expression in spinal neurons by nociceptive and nonnociceptive stimulation of LUT. Am J Physiol 1993; 265: R326–33.

72. Vizzard MA, Erickson VL, Card JP, et al. Transneuronal labeling of neurons in the adult rat brainstem and spinal cord after injection of pseudorabies virus into the urethra. J Comp Neurol 1995; 355: 629–40.

73. Nadelhaft I, Vera PL. Neurons in the rat brain and spinal cord labeled after pseudorabies virus injected into the external urethral sphincter. J Comp Neurol 1996; 375: 502–17.

74. de Groat WC. Inhibitory mechanisms in the sacral reflex pathways to the urinary bladder. In: Ryall RW, Kelly JS, editors. Iontophoresis and transmitter mechanisms in the mammalian central nervous system. Amsterdam, Holland: Elsevier; 1978: 366–8.

75. McGuire E. Experimental observations on the integration of bladder and urethral function. Trans Am Assoc Genitourin Surg 1977: 68: 38.

76. McMahon SB, Morrison JF. Spinal neurones with long projections activated from the abdominal viscera of the cat. J Physiol 1982; 322: 1–20.

77. Morrison JF, Sato A, Sato Y, Yamanishi T. The influence of afferent inputs from skin and viscera on the activity of the bladder and the skeletal muscle surrounding the urethra in the rat. Neurosci Res 1995; 23: 195–205.

78. de Groat WC, Ryall RW. Reflexes to sacral parasympathetic neurones concerned with micturition in the cat. J Physiol (London) 1969; 200: 87–108.

79. Wheeler JS, Jr., Walter JS, Zaszczurynski PJ. Bladder inhibition by penile nerve stimulation in spinal cord injury patients. J Urol 1992; 147: 100–3.

80. Bosch JL, Groen J. Sacral (S3) segmental nerve stimulation as a treatment for urge incontinence in patients with detrusor instability: results of chronic electrical stimulation using an implantable neural prosthesis. J Urol 1995; 154: 504–7.

81. Ding YQ, Takada M, Tokuno H, Mizuno N. Direct projections from the dorsolateral pontine tegmentum to pudendal motoneurons innervating the external urethral sphincter muscle in the rat. J Comp Neurol 1995; 357: 318–30.

82. Otake K, Nakamura Y. Single neurons in Barrington's nucleus projecting to both the paraventricular thalamic nucleus and the spinal cord by way of axon collaterals: a double labeling study in the rat. Neurosci Lett 1996; 209: 97–100.

83. Valentino RJ, Chen S, Zhu Y, Aston-Jones G. Evidence for divergent projections to the brain noradrenergic system and the spinal parasympathetic system from Barrington's nucleus. Brain Res 1996; 732: 1–15.

84. Blok BF, van Maarseveen JT, Holstege G. Electrical stimulation of the sacral dorsal gray commissure evokes relaxation of the external urethral sphincter in the cat. Neurosci Lett 1998; 249: 68–70.

85. Valentino RJ, Pavcovich LA, Hirata H. Evidence for corticotropin-releasing hormone projections from Barrington's nucleus to the periaqueductal gray and dorsal motor nucleus of the vagus in the rat. J Comp Neurol 1995; 363: 402–22.

86. Blok BF, Willemsen AT, Holstege G. A PET study on brain control of micturition in humans. Brain 1997; 120: 111–21.

87. Blok BF. Central pathways controlling micturition and urinary continence. Urology 2002; 59: 13–7.

88. Holstege G, Mouton LJ. Central nervous system control of micturition. Int Rev Neurobiol 2003; 56: 123–45.

89. Holstege G. Micturition and the soul. J Comp Neurol 2005; 493: 15–20.

90. Nadelhaft I, Vera PL. Reduced urinary bladder afferent conduction velocities in streptozotocin-diabetic rats. Neuroscience Letters 1992; 135: 276–8.

91. Ranan DasGupta, Kavia RB, Fowler CJ. Cerebral mechanisms and voiding function. BJU International 2007; 99: 731–4.

92. Griffiths D, Tadic SD. Bladder control, urgency, and urge incontinence: evidence from functional brain imaging. Neurourol Urodyn 2008; 27: 466–74.

93. Nour S, Svarer C, Kristensen JK, et al. Cerebral activation during micturition in normal men. Brain 2000; 123: 781–9.

94. Athwal B, Berkley K, Brennan A, et al. Brain activity associated with the urge to void and bladder fill volume in normal men: preliminary data from a PET study. BJU Int 1999; 84: 148–9.

95. Athwal BS, Berkley KJ, Hussain I, et al. Brain responses to changes in bladder volume and urge to void in healthy men. Brain: J Neurol 2001; 124: 369–77.

96. Matsuura S, Kakizaki H, Mitsui T, et al. Human brain region response to distention or cold stimulation of the bladder: a positron emission tomography study. J Urol 2002; 168: 2035–9.

97. Kuhtz-Buschbeck JP, Gilster R, van der Horst C, et al. Control of bladder sensations: an fMRI study of brain activity and effective connectivity. NeuroImage 2009; 47: 18–27.

98. Kuhtz-Buschbeck JP, van der Horst C, Pott C, et al. Cortical representation of the urge to void: a functional magnetic resonance imaging study. J Urol 2005; 174: 1477–81.

99. Zhang H, Reitz A, Kollias S, et al. An fMRI study of the role of suprapontine brain structures in the voluntary voiding control induced by pelvic floor contraction. NeuroImage 2005; 24: 174–80.

100. Seseke S, Baudewig J, Kallenberg K, et al. Voluntary pelvic floor muscle control—an fMRI study. NeuroImage 2006; 31: 1399–407.

101. Kitta T, Kakizaki H, Furuno T, et al. Brain activation during detrusor overactivity in patients with Parkinson's disease: a positron emission tomography study. J Urol 2006; 175: 994–8.

102. Griffiths D, Tadic SD, Schaefer W, Resnick NM. Cerebral control of the bladder in normal and urge-incontinent women. NeuroImage 2007; 37: 1–7.

103. Griffiths D, Derbyshire S, Stenger A, Resnick N. Brain control of normal and overactive bladder. J Urol 2005; 174: 1862–7.

104. de Groat WC. Basic neurophysiology and neuropharmacology. In: Abrams P, Khoury S, Wein A, eds. Incontinence. Plymouth, UK: Health Publications, 1999: 112.

24 Pharmacology of the Bladder
Karl-Erik Andersson

INTRODUCTION

The lower urinary tract (LUT) is controlled by a complex interplay between the central and peripheral nervous systems and local regulatory factors (1). Malfunction at various levels may result in micturition disorders, which roughly can be classified as disturbances of storage or emptying. Failure to store urine may lead to various forms of incontinence (mainly urgency and stress incontinence), and failure to empty to urinary retention. LUT symptoms (LUTS) include storage, voiding, and postmicturition symptoms. Storage symptoms (urgency, frequency with and without incontinence, nocturia) form the overactive bladder (OAB) syndrome, which may or may not be associated with involuntary detrusor contractions demonstrated by cystometry [detrusor overactivity (DO)]. Pharmacologic treatment of urinary incontinence is a main option, and several drugs with different modes and sites of action have been tried (2–4). However, to be able to optimize existing therapies, and to identify suitable new targets for treatment, knowledge about the mechanisms of micturition is necessary.

Below, a brief review is given of the normal nervous control of the LUT and of some therapeutic principles used for treatment of urinary incontinence.

NERVOUS MECHANISMS FOR BLADDER EMPTYING AND URINE STORAGE

The nervous mechanisms for bladder emptying and urine storage involve a complex pattern of afferent and efferent signaling in *parasympathetic*, *sympathetic*, and *somatic* nerves. These nerves constitute reflex pathways, which either maintain the bladder in a relaxed state, enabling urine storage at low intravesical pressure, or which initiate micturition by relaxing the outflow region and contracting the bladder smooth muscle. Under normal conditions, there is a reciprocal relationship between the activity in the detrusor and the activity in the outlet region. During voiding, contraction of the detrusor muscle is preceded by a relaxation of the outlet region, thereby facilitating the bladder emptying (5–7). On the contrary, during the storage phase, the detrusor muscle is relaxed, and the outlet region is contracted to maintain continence.

Contraction of the detrusor smooth muscle and relaxation of the outflow region result from activation of *parasympathetic* neurons located to the sacral parasympathetic nucleus in the sacral spinal cord at the level of S2–S4 (8). The axons pass through the pelvic nerve and synapse with the postganglionic nerves in either the pelvic plexus, in ganglia on the surface of the bladder (vesical ganglia), or within the walls of the bladder and urethra (intramural ganglia) (9). The preganglionic neurotransmission is predominantly mediated by acetylcholine (ACh) acting on nicotinic receptors, although the

transmission can be modulated by adrenergic, muscarinic, purinergic, and peptidergic presynaptic receptors (10). The postganglionic neurons in the pelvic nerve mediate the excitatory input to the normal human detrusor smooth muscle by releasing ACh acting on muscarinic receptors. However, an atropine-resistant [non-adrenergic, non-cholinergic (NANC)] contractile component is regularly found in the bladders of most animal species (11,12). Such a component can also be demonstrated in functionally and morphologically altered human bladder tissue (13–15), but contributes only to a few percent to normal detrusor contraction (1). ATP is one important mediator of the NANC contraction (16) although the involvement of other transmitters cannot be ruled out (1,17). The pelvic nerve also conveys parasympathetic nerves to the outflow region and the urethra. These nerves exert an inhibitory effect on the smooth muscle by releasing nitric oxide (18) and other transmitters (19–21).

Most of the *sympathetic* innervation of the bladder and urethra originates from the intermediolateral nuclei in the thoraco-lumbar region (T10-L2) of the spinal cord. The axons leave the spinal cord via the splanchnic nerves and travel either through the inferior mesenteric ganglia (IMF) and the hypogastric nerve, or pass through the paravertebral chain to the lumbosacral sympathetic chain ganglia and enter the pelvic nerve. Thus, sympathetic signals are conveyed in both the hypogastric nerve and the pelvic nerve (9). The preganglionic sympathetic transmission is, like the parasympathetic preganglionic transmission, predominantly mediated by ACh acting on nicotinic receptors. Some preganglionic terminals synapse with the postganglionic cells in the paravertebral ganglia or in the IMF, while other synapse closer to the pelvic organs, and short postganglionic neurons innervate the target organs. Thus, the hypogastric and pelvic nerves contain both pre- and postganglionic fibers (9). The predominant effect of the sympathetic innervation is to contract the bladder base and the urethra. In addition, the sympathetic innervation inhibits the parasympathetic pathways at spinal and ganglionic levels. In humans, noradrenaline is released in response to electrical stimulation in vitro (22), and the normal response to released noradrenaline is relaxation (23,24). However, the importance of the sympathetic innervation for relaxation of the human detrusor has never been established. In contrast, in several animal species the adrenergic innervation has been demonstrated to mediate relaxation of the detrusor during filling.

Most of the *sensory* nerves to the bladder and urethra originate in the dorsal root ganglia at the lumbosacral level of the spinal cord and travel via the pelvic nerve to the periphery. In addition, some afferents originate in dorsal root ganglia at the thoracolumbar level and travel in the hypogastric nerve. The sensory nerves to the striated muscle of the external urethral sphincter travel in the pudendal nerve to the sacral region of the spinal cord (9). The most important afferents for the micturition process are myelinated Aδ-fibers and unmyelinated C-fibers traveling in the pelvic nerve to the sacral spinal cord (25,26), conveying information from receptors in the bladder wall. The Aδ-fibers respond to passive distension and active contraction, thus conveying information about bladder filling (27). The activation threshold for Aδ-fibers are 5 to 15 mm H$_2$O. This is the intravesical pressure at which humans report the first sensation of bladder filling (10). C-fibers have a high mechanical threshold and respond primarily to chemical irritation of the bladder urothelium/suburothelium (28) or cold (29). Following chemical irritation, the C-fiber afferents exhibit spontaneous firing when the bladder is empty and increased firing during bladder distension (28). These fibers are normally inactive and are therefore termed "silent fibers."

The *somatic* innervation of the urethral rhabdosphincter and of some perineal muscles (for example, compressor urethrae and urethrovaginal sphincter), is provided by the pudendal nerve. These fibers originate from sphincter motor neurons located in the ventral horn of the sacral spinal cord (levels S2–S4) in a region called Onuf's (Onufrowicz's) nucleus (30).

The Storage Phase

During the storage phase the bladder has to relax in order to maintain a low intravesical pressure. Urine storage is regulated by two separate storage reflexes, of which one is sympathetic (autonomic) and the other is somatic (30). The sympathetic storage reflex (pelvic-to-hypogastric reflex) is initiated as the bladder distends (myelinated Aδ-fibers) and the generated afferent activity travels in the pelvic nerves to the spinal cord. Within the spinal cord, sympathetic firing from the lumbar region (L1–L3) is initiated, which, by effects at the ganglionic level decreases excitatory parasympathetic inputs to the bladder, but also through postganglionic neurons releases noradrenaline, which facilitates urine storage by stimulating mainly β$_3$ adrenoceptors (ARs) in the detrusor smooth muscle (see below). As mentioned previously, there is little evidence for a functionally important sympathetic innervation of the human detrusor, which is in contrast to what has been found in several animal species. The sympathetic innervation of the human bladder is found mainly in the outlet region, where it mediates contraction. During micturition, this sympathetic reflex pathway is markedly inhibited via supraspinal mechanisms to allow the bladder to contract and the urethra to relax. Thus, the Aδ afferents and the sympathetic efferent fibers constitute a vesico-spinal-vesical storage reflex which maintains the bladder in a relaxed mode while the proximal urethra and bladder neck are contracted.

In response to a sudden increase in bladder pressure, such as during a cough, laugh, or sneeze, a more rapid somatic storage reflex (pelvic-to-pudendal reflex), also called the guarding or continence reflex, is initiated. The evoked afferent activity travels along myelinated Aδ afferent nerve fibers in the pelvic nerve to the sacral spinal cord, where efferent somatic urethral motor neurons, located in the nucleus of Onuf, are activated. Afferent information is also conveyed to the periaqueductal grey (PAG) and to the pontine storage center (the L-region).

Axons from these motor neurons of the nucleus of Onuf travel in the pudendal nerve and release ACh, which activates nicotinic cholinergic receptors on the rhabdosphincter, which contracts. This pathway is tonically active during urine storage. During sudden abdominal pressure increases, however, it becomes dynamically active to contract the rhabdosphincter. During micturition this reflex is strongly inhibited via spinal and supraspinal mechanisms to allow the rhabdosphincter to relax and permit urine passage through the urethra. In addition to this spinal somatic storage reflex, there is also supraspinal input from the pons, which projects directly to the nucleus of Onuf and is importance for volitional control of the rhabdosphincter (31).

The Emptying Phase
Vesico-Bulbo-Vesical Micturition Reflex
Electrophysiological experiments in cats and rats provide evidence for a voiding reflex mediated through a vesico-bulbo-vesical pathway involving neural circuits in the pons, which constitute the pontine micturition center (PMC). Other regions in the brain, important for micturition, include the hypothalamus and cerebral cortex (10,32,33). Bladder filling leads to increased activation of tension receptors within the bladder wall and thus to increased afferent activity in Aδ-fibers. These fibers project on spinal tract neurons mediating increased sympathetic firing to maintain continence as discussed above (storage reflex). In addition, the spinal tract neurons convey the afferent activity to more rostral areas of the spinal cord and the brain. One important receiver of the afferent information from the bladder is the PAG in the rostral brainstem. The PAG receives information from both afferent neurons in the bladder and from more rostral areas in the brain, i.e., cerebral cortex and hypothalamus. This information is integrated in the PAG and the medial part of the PMC (the M-region), which also control the descending pathways in the micturition reflex. Thus, PMC can be seen as a switch in the micturition reflex, inhibiting parasympathetic activity in the descending pathways when there is low activity in the afferent fibers, and activating the parasympathetic pathways when the afferent activity reaches a certain threshold (10,33). The threshold is believed to be set by the inputs from more rostral regions in the brain. In cats, lesioning of regions above the inferior colliculus usually facilitates micturition by elimination of inhibitory inputs from more rostral areas of the brain. On the other hand, transections at a lower level inhibit micturition. Thus, the PMC seems to be under a tonic inhibitory control. A variation of the inhibitory input to PMC results in a variation of bladder capacity. Experiments on rats have shown that the micturition threshold is regulated by, e.g., γ-aminobutyric acid (GABA)-ergic inhibitory mechanisms in the PMC neurons (34).

Vesico-Spinal-Vesical Micturition Reflex
Spinal lesion rostral to the lumbo-sacral level interrupt the vesico-bulbo-vesical pathway and abolish the supra spinal and voluntary control of micturition. This results initially in an areflexic bladder accompanied by urinary retention (10). An automatic vesico-spinal-vesical micturition reflex develops

slowly, although voiding is generally insufficient due to bladder-sphincter dyssynergia, i.e., simultaneous contraction of bladder and urethra. It has been demonstrated in chronic spinal cats that the afferent limb of this reflex is conveyed through unmyelinated C-fibers which usually do not respond to bladder distension (28), suggesting changed properties of the afferent receptors in the bladder. Accordingly, the micturition reflex in chronic spinal cats is blocked by capsaicin, a neurotoxin which is believed to block C-fiber mediated neurotransmission (35,36).

TARGETS FOR PHARMACOLOGIC INTERVENTION
Central Nervous System (CNS) Targets
Anatomically, several CNS regions may be involved in micturition control: supraspinal structures, such as the cortex and diencephalon, midbrain, and medulla, but also spinal structures (32,33,37–40). Several transmitters and their receptors are involved in the reflexes and sites described above and may be targets for drugs aimed for control of micturition. Although few drugs with a CNS site of action have been developed, several agents acting on the CNS may have effects on micturition.

Opioid Receptors
Endogenous opioid peptides and corresponding receptors are widely distributed in many regions in the CNS of importance for micturition control, e.g., the PAG, the PMC, the spinal parasympathetic nucleus, and the nucleus of Onuf (41–44).

It has been well established that morphine, given by various routes of administration to animals and humans, can increase bladder capacity and eventually cause urinary retention. Given intrathecally (IT) to anesthetized rats and intravenously (IV) to humans, the μ-opioid receptor antagonist, naloxone, has been shown to stimulate micturition (44,45), suggesting that a tonic activation of μ-opioid receptors has a depressant effect on the micturition reflex.

Morphine given IT was effective in patients with DO due to spinal cord lesions (46), but was associated with side-effects, such as nausea and pruritus. Further side-effects of opioid receptor agonists comprise respiratory depression, constipation, and abuse. Attempts have been made to reduce these side-effects by increasing selectivity towards one of the different opioid receptor types (47). At least three different opioid receptors—2, μ, δ, and κ—bind stereospecifically with morphine, and have been shown to interfere with voiding mechanisms. Theoretically, selective receptor actions, or modifications of effects mediated by specific opioid receptors, may have useful therapeutic effects for micturition control.

Tramadol is a well-known analgesic drug (48). By itself, it is a weak μ-receptor agonist, but it is metabolized to several different compounds, some of them almost as effective as morphine at the μ-receptor. However, the drug (metabolites) also inhibits serotonin [5-hydroxytryptamine (5-HT)] and noradrenaline reuptake (48). This profile is of particular interest, since both μ-receptor agonism and amine reuptake inhibition may be useful principles for treatment of OAB/DO, as shown in a placebo controlled study with duloxetine (49).

In rats, tramadol abolished experimentally induced DO caused by cerebral infarction (50). Tramadol also inhibited

DO induced by apomorphine in rats (51)— a crude model of bladder dysfunction in Parkinson's disease. Singh et al. gave tramadol epidurally and found the drug to increase bladder capacity and compliance, and to delay filling sensations without ill effects on voiding (52). Safarinejad and Hosseini evaluated in a double-blind, placebo-controlled, randomized study, the efficacy, and safety of tramadol in patients with idiopathic DO (53). A total of 76 patients 18 years or older were given 100 mg tramadol sustained release every 12 hours for 12 weeks. Clinical evaluation was performed at baseline and every two weeks during treatment. Tramadol significantly reduced the number of incontinence periods and induced significant improvements in urodynamic parameters. The main adverse event was nausea. It was concluded that in patients with non-neurogenic DO, tramadol provided beneficial clinical and urodynamic effects. Even if tramadol may not be the best suitable drug for treatment of LUTS/OAB/DO due to side effects (nausea, constipation, dependency), the study proofs the principle of modulating micturition via the μ-receptor.

Central stimulation of δ-opioid receptors in anaesthetized cats and rats inhibited micturition (54,55) and inhibited parasympathetic neurotransmission in cat bladder gangliae (56). In humans, nalbuphine, a μ-receptor antagonist and κ-receptor agonist, increased bladder capacity (57), buprenorphine (a partial μ-receptor agonist and κ-receptor antagonist) decreased micturition pressure and increased bladder capacity more than morphine (57). These effects should be considered when the drugs are used, for example, pain control. In addition, further exploration of these non μ-opioid receptor mediated actions on micturition seems motivated.

Serotonin (5-HT) Mechanisms
It is well established that the lumbosacral autonomic, as well as the somatic motor nuclei (Onuf's nuclei), receive a dense serotonergic input from the raphe nuclei, an innervation which is not subjected to the general decline in lumbosacral spinal innervation found with increasing age (58). Multiple 5-HT receptors have been found at sites where processing of afferent and efferent impulses from and to the LUT take place (59). Although, as pointed out by de Groat, there is some evidence in the rat for serotonergic facilitation of voiding, the descending pathway is essentially an inhibitory circuit, with 5-HT as a key neurotransmitter (60). Thus, electrical stimulation of 5-HT-containing neurons in the caudal raphe nucleus causes inhibition of bladder contractions (61,62). Most experiments in rats and cats indicate that activation of the central serotonergic system by 5-HT reuptake inhibitors, as well as by 5-HT_{1A} and 5-HT_2 receptor agonists, depresses reflex bladder contractions, and increases the bladder volume threshold for inducing micturition (60). 5-HT_{1A} receptors are involved in multiple inhibitory mechanisms controlling the spinobulbospinal micturition reflex pathway. The regulation of the frequency of bladder reflexes is presumably mediated by a suppression of afferent input to the micturition switching circuitry in the pons, whereas the regulation of bladder contraction amplitude may be related to an inhibition of the output from the pons to the parasympathetic nuclei in the spinal cord.

It has been discussed whether or not there is a deficiency in serotonin behind both depression and OAB (63–65). If there is, the question is if selective serotonin reuptake inhibitors (SSRIs) are effective for micturition control only in depressed patients, or if selective serotonin uptake inhibition is a general principle that can be used for treatment of OAB. There are no randomized controlled clinical trials (RCTs) showing that SSRIs are useful for the treatment of OAB/DO (4). In contrast, there are reports suggesting that the SSRIs in patients without incontinence actually can cause incontinence, particularly in the elderly. Patients exposed to serotonin uptake inhibitors had an increased risk (15 out of 1000 patients) for developing urinary incontinence (66). This causes doubts over the anecdotal reports that SSRIs may be used as a general treatment for OAB. On the other hand, in an RCT, the combined serotonin and noradrenaline reuptake inhibitor, duloxetine, was shown to be effective in patients with OAB (49).

γ-Amino Butyric Acid Mechanisms

GABA has been identified as a main inhibitory transmitter in the brain and spinal cord. GABA functions appear to be triggered by binding of GABA to its ionotropic receptors, $GABA_A$ and $GABA_C$, which are ligand-gated chloride channels, and its metabotropic receptor, $GABA_B$ (67). Since blockade of $GABA_A$ and $GABA_B$ receptors in the spinal cord (68,69) and brain (69,70) stimulated rat micturition, an endogenous activation of $GABA_{A + B}$ receptors may be responsible for continuous inhibition of the micturition reflex within the CNS. In the spinal cord $GABA_A$ receptors are more numerous than $GABA_B$ receptors, except for the dorsal horn where $GABA_B$ receptors predominate (71,72).

Experiments using conscious and anesthetized rats demonstrated that exogenous GABA, muscimol ($GABA_A$ receptor agonist) and baclofen ($GABA_B$ receptor agonist) given IV, IT, or intracerebroventricularly (ICV) inhibit micturition (69,73). Similar effects were obtained in non-anesthetized mice (74). Baclofen given IT attenuated oxyhemoglobin induced DO in rats, suggesting that the inhibitory actions of $GABA_B$ receptor agonists in the spinal cord may be useful for controlling micturition disorders caused by C-fiber activation in the urothelium and/or suburothelium (69). In mice, where DO was produced by intravesical citric acid, baclofen given subcutaneously, had an inhibitory effect which was blocked by the selective $GABA_B$ receptor antagonist CGP55845 (74). Beneficial effects of baclofen have also been documented in humans with DO (75).

Stimulation of the PMC results in an immediate relaxation of the external striated sphincter and a contraction of the detrusor muscle of the bladder. Blok et al. demonstrated in cats a direct pathway from the PMC to the dorsal gray commissure of the sacral cord (31). It was suggested that the pathway produced relaxation of the external striated sphincter during micturition via inhibitory modulation by GABA neurons of the motoneurons in the sphincter of Onuf. In rats, IT baclofen and muscimol ultimately produced dribbling urinary incontinence (68,69), and this was also found in conscious mice given muscimol and diazepam subcutaneously (74). Thus, normal relaxation of the striated urethral sphincter is probably mediated

via $GABA_A$ receptors (69), $GABA_B$ receptors having a minor influence on motoneuron excitability (76).

Gabapentin

Gabapentin was originally designed as an anticonvulsant GABA mimetic capable of crossing the blood–brain barrier (77). However, its effects do not appear to be mediated through interaction with GABA receptors, and its mechanism of action is still controversial (77). Gabapentin is also widely used not only for seizures and neuropathic pain, but for many other indications such as anxiety and sleep disorders due to its apparent lack of toxicity.

In a pilot study, Carbone et al. reported on the effect of gabapentin on neurogenic detrusor activity (78). They found a positive effect on symptoms and a significant improvement of urodynamic parameters after treatment, and suggested that the effects of the drug should be explored in further controlled studies in both neurogenic and non-neurogenic DO (NDO). Kim et al. found that 14 of 31 patients with (OAB) and nocturia, refractory to antimuscarinic treatment, improved with oral gabapentin (79). The drug was generally well tolerated and was considered to be an option in selective patients when conventional treatment modalities have failed.

Noradrenaline and α-ARS

Noradrenergic neurons in the brainstem project to the sympathetic, parasympathetic, and somatic nuclei in the lumbosacral spinal cord. Bladder activation through these bulbospinal noradrenergic pathways may involve excitatory $α_1$-ARs. In rats undergoing continuous cystometry, doxazosin, given IT, decreased micturition pressure, both in normal rats and in animals with post-obstruction bladder hypertrophy (80). The effect was much more pronounced in the animals with hypertrophied/OABs. Doxazosin given IT, but not intra-arterially, to spontaneously hypertensive rats exhibiting bladder overactivity, normalized bladder activity (81). It was suggested that doxazosin has a site of action at the level of the spinal cord and ganglia. However, there are no RCTs documenting positive effects of α-AR antagonists in OAB/DO (4).

Neurokinin 1 (NK1)-Receptor Antagonists

The main endogenous tachykinins, substance P (SP), NKA, and NKB, and their preferred receptors, NK1, NK2, and NK3, respectively, have been demonstrated in various CNS regions, including those involved in micturition control (82–84). NK1 receptor expressing neurons in the dorsal horn of the spinal cord may play an important role in DO, and tachykinin involvement via NK1 receptors in the micturition reflex induced by bladder filling has been demonstrated (85) in normal, and more clearly, rats with bladder hypertrophy secondary to bladder outlet obstruction (BOO). Capsaicin-induced DO was reduced by blocking NK1 receptor-expressing neurons in the spinal cord, using IT administered SP-saponin conjugate (86). Furthermore, blockade of spinal NK1 receptor could suppress detrusor activity induced by dopamine receptor (L-DOPA) stimulation (87).

In conscious rats undergoing continuous cystometry, antagonists of both NK1 and NK2 receptors inhibited micturition, decreasing micturition pressure and increasing bladder capacity at low doses, and inducing dribbling incontinence at high doses. This was most conspicuous in animals with outflow obstruction (88). ICV administration of NK1 and NK2 receptor antagonists to awake rats suppressed detrusor activity induced by dopamine receptor (L-DOPA) stimulation (89). Taken together, available information suggests that spinal and supraspinal NK1 and NK2 receptors may be involved in micturition control.

Aprepitant, an NK-1 receptor antagonist used for treatment of chemotherapy-induced nausea and vomiting (90), significantly improved symptoms of OAB in postmenopausal women with a history of urgency incontinence or mixed incontinence (with predominantly urgency urinary incontinence), as shown in a well designed pilot RCT (91). The primary end point was percent change from baseline in average daily micturitions assessed by a voiding diary. Secondary end points included average daily total urinary incontinence and urgency incontinence episodes, and urgency episodes. Aprepitant significantly decreased the average daily number of micturitions compared with placebo at eight weeks. The average daily number of urgency episodes was also significantly reduced compared to placebo, and so were the average daily number of urgency incontinence and total urinary incontinence episodes, although the difference was not statistically significant. Aprepitant was generally well tolerated and the incidence of side effects, including dry mouth, was low. The results of this initial proof of concept study suggest that NK-1 receptor antagonism holds promise as a potential treatment approach for OAB.

Dopamine and Dopamine Receptors
Many patients with Parkinson's disease have NDO (detrusor hyperreflexia) (92), possibly as a consequence of nigrostriatal dopamine depletion and failure to activate inhibitory D1 receptors (93). However, other dopaminergic systems may activate D2 receptors, facilitating the micturition reflex. Sillén et al. showed that apomorphine, which activates both D1 and D2 receptors, induced bladder overactivity in anesthetized rats via stimulation of central dopaminergic receptors (94). The effects were abolished by infracollicular transection of the brain, and by prior intra-peritoneal administration of the centrally acting dopamine receptor blocker, spiroperidol. Kontani et al. suggested that the bladder overactivity induced by apomorphine in anesthetized rats resulted from synchronous stimulation of the micturition centers in the brain stem and spinal cord, and that the response was elicited by stimulation of both dopamine D1 and D2 receptors (95,96). Blockade of central dopamine receptors may be expected to influence voiding; however, the therapeutic potential of drugs having this action has not been established. On the other hand, the effects on micturition of various dopamine receptor active drugs used, for example, different psychiatric conditions, should not be neglected.

Peripheral Targets
Possible peripheral targets for pharmacologic intervention may be (*i*) the efferent neurotransmission, (*ii*) the smooth muscle itself, including ion-channels and intracellular second messenger systems, and (*iii*) the afferent neurotransmission. Although many effective drugs are available for these target systems, most of them are less useful in the clinical situation due to the lack of selectivity for the LUT, which may result in intolerable side effects. Thus, a main task is to find systems or receptors, more or less specific for the LUT, which can be manipulated without disturbing other systems in the body, or alternatively, to design drugs in a way that results in higher tissue concentrations in the LUT than elsewhere in the body.

Muscarinic Receptors
Muscarinic receptors comprise five subtypes, encoded by five distinct genes (97). The five gene products correspond to pharmacologically defined receptors, and M_1–M_5 is used to describe both the molecular and pharmacological subtypes. In the human bladder, the mRNAs for all muscarinic receptor subtypes have been demonstrated (98,99), with a predominance of mRNAs encoding M_2 and M_3 receptors (98,100). These receptors are also functionally coupled to G-proteins, but the signal transduction systems vary (101–104).

Detrusor smooth muscle contains muscarinic receptors of mainly the M_2 and M_3 subtypes (101–105). The M_3 receptors in the human bladder are believed to be the most important for detrusor contraction. Jezior et al. suggested that muscarinic receptor activation of detrusor muscle includes both non-selective cation channels and activation of Rho-kinase (106). Supporting a role of Rho-kinase in the regulation of rat detrusor contraction and tone, Wibberley et al. found that Rho-kinase inhibitors (Y-27632, HA 1077) inhibited contractions evoked by carbachol without affecting the contraction response to KCl (107). They also demonstrated high levels of Rho-kinase isoforms (I and II) in the bladder. Schneider et al. (2004) concluded that carbachol-induced contraction of human urinary bladder is mediated via M_3 receptors and largely depends on Ca^{2+} entry through nifedipine-sensitive channels and activation of the Rho-kinase pathway (105). Thus, the main pathway for muscarinic receptor activation of the detrusor via M_3 receptors may be calcium influx via L-type calcium channels, and increased sensitivity to calcium of the contractile machinery produced via inhibition of myosin light chain phosphatase through activation of Rho-kinase (108).

The functional role for the M_2 receptors has not been clarified, but it has been suggested that M_2 receptors may oppose sympathetically mediated smooth muscle relaxation, mediated by β-ARs (109). M_2 receptor stimulation may also activate non-specific cation channels (110) and inhibit K_{ATP} channels through activation of protein kinase C (111,112). In certain disease states, M_2 receptors may contribute to contraction of the bladder. Thus, in the denervated rat bladder, M_2 receptors, or a combination of M_2 and M_3, mediated contractile responses and the two types of receptor seemed to act in a facilitatory manner to mediate contraction (113–115). In obstructed, hypertrophied rat bladders, there was an increase in total and M_2 receptor density, whereas there was a reduction in M_3 receptor density (116). The functional significance of this change for voiding function has not been established. Pontari et al. analyzed bladder muscle specimens from patients with neurogenic bladder dysfunction to determine whether the muscarinic receptor subtype mediating contraction shifts from M_3 to the M_2 receptor subtype, as found in the denervated, hypertrophied rat bladder (117). They concluded that whereas normal detrusor contractions are mediated by the M_3 receptor subtype, in patients with neurogenic bladder dysfunction, contractions can be mediated by the M_2 receptors.

Muscarinic receptors may also be located on the presynaptic nerve terminals and participate in the regulation of transmitter release. The inhibitory pre-junctional muscarinic receptors have been classified as M_4 in the human bladder (118). Pre-junctional facilitatory muscarinic receptors appear to be of the M_1 (119). The muscarinic facilitatory mechanism seems to be upregulated in hyperactive bladders from chronic spinal cord transected rats. The facilitation in these preparations is primarily mediated by M_3 muscarinic receptors (119,120).

Muscarinic receptors have also been demonstrated on the urothelium/suburothelium. The porcine urothelium was found to expresses a high density of muscarinic receptors, even higher than the bladder smooth muscle (121), and, in the rat and human urothelium, the receptor proteins, and mRNAs, respectively, for all muscarinic receptor subtypes (M1–M5) were demonstrated (122). However, the expression pattern of the different subtypes in the human urothelium was reported to differ: the M_1 receptors on basal cells, M_2 on umbrella cells, M_3 and M_4 homogenously, and M_5 with a decreasing gradient from luminal to basal cells (99). Mansfield et al. found, using reverse transcription-polymerase chain reaction analysis, an abundant expression of muscarinic M_2 receptors in the human bladder mucosa (123). These receptors may occur at other locations than the urothelium, e.g., on suburothelial interstitial cells (124,125).

The suburothelial nerve plexus is close to the urothelium (126–128). The urothelium, as mentioned previously, has been suggested to work as a mechanosensory conductor, and in response to distension, it releases ATP affecting underlying afferent nerve fibers via purinoceptors (129,130). This may consequently modify the afferent response of the bladder (131,132). ACh is produced in the urothelium, but the mechanism behind its release does not seem to involve vesicular exocytosis (133,134). The organic cation transporter three subtype has been demonstrated in and suggested to be involved in the non-neuronal release from rat urothelium (134).

Adrenergic Receptors
α-Adrenoceptors

α-ARs may have effects on different locations in the bladder: the detrusor smooth muscle, the detrusor vasculature, the afferent and efferent nerve terminal, and intramural ganglia. For some of these possible sites only fragmentary information is available. Most investigators agree on that there is a low expression of these receptors in the derusor muscle (135–137). In the human bladder studies Malloy et al. found that two-third of the α_1-AR mRNA expressed was α_{1D}, there was no α_{1B}, and one-third was α_{1A} (135).

Nomiya and Yamaguchi confirmed the low expression of α_1-AR mRNA in normal human bladder, and further demonstrated that there was no upregulation of any of the adrenergic

receptors with obstruction (138). In addition, in functional experiments they found a small response to phenylephrine at high drug concentrations with no difference between normal and obstructed bladders. Thus, in the obstructed human bladder, there seemed to be no evidence for α_1-AR upregulation. This finding was challenged by Bouchelouche et al. who found an increased response to α_1-AR stimulation in obstructed human bladders (139). If there is a change of sensitivity to α_1-AR stimulation in the obstructed bladder of clinical importance (influencing the response to α_1-AR blockers) remains to be established.

All subtypes of α_1-ARs can be found in different parts of the human vascular tree, and they all mediate contraction. The expression varies with vessel bed and increases with age. In the bladder, the function of the detrusor muscle is dependent on the vasculature and the perfusion. Hypoxia induced by partial outlet obstruction is believed to play a major role in both the hypertrophic and degenerative effects of partial outlet obstruction. Das et al. investigated in rats whether doxazosin affected blood flow to the bladder and reduced the level of bladder dysfunction induced by partial outlet obstruction (140). They found that four weeks treatment with doxazosin increased bladder blood flow in both control and obstructed rats. Furthermore, doxazosin treatment reduced the severity of the detrusor response to partial outlet obstruction. Thus, doxazosin could reduce the increase in bladder weight in obstructed animals which could be one of the mechanisms that contributed to a positive effect on DO caused by the obstruction.

β-Adrenoceptors

It has been known for a long time that isoprenaline, a non subtype selective β-AR agonist, can relax bladder smooth muscle (17). Even if the importance of β-ARs for human bladder function still remains to be established (141), this does not exclude that they can be useful therapeutic targets. All three subtypes of β-ARs (β_1, β_2, and β_3) can be found in the detrusor muscle of most species, including humans (136,141), and also in the human urothelium (142). However, the expression of β_3-AR mRNA (136,138) and functional evidence indicate a predominant role for this receptor in both normal and neurogenic bladders (136,143,144). The human detrusor also contains β_2-ARs, and most probably both receptors are involved in the physiological effects (relaxation) of noradrenaline in the bladder (136,141). β_3-AR agonists have a pronounced effect on spontaneous contractions of isolated detrusor muscle (145), which may be the basis for their therapeutic effects in OAB/DO.

It is generally accepted that β-AR-induced detrusor relaxation is mediated by activation of adenylyl cyclase with the subsequent formation of cAMP (146). However, there is evidence suggesting that in the bladder K^+ channels, particularly BK_{ca} channels, may be involved in β-AR mediated relaxation independent of cAMP (147–150).

The in vivo effects of β_3-AR agonists on bladder function have been studied in several animal models. It has been shown that β_3-AR agonists increase bladder capacity with no change in micturition pressure and residual volume (151–154). For example, Hicks et al. studied the effects of the selective β_3-AR agonist, GW427353, in the anesthetized dog and found that the drug evoked an increase in bladder capacity under conditions of acid evoked bladder hyperactivity, without affecting voiding (155).

β_3-AR selective agonists are currently being evaluated as potential treatment for OAB/DO in humans (156). One of these, mirabegron (YM187), which mediated muscle relaxation in human bladder strips (157), was given to patients with OAB in a controlled clinical trial (158). The primary efficacy analysis showed a statistically significant reduction in mean micturition frequency, compared to placebo, and with respect to secondary variables, mirabegron was significantly superior to placebo concerning mean volume voided per micturition, mean number of incontinence episodes, nocturia episodes, urgency incontinence episodes, and urgency episodes per 24 hours. The drug was well tolerated, and the most commonly reported side effects were headache and gastrointestinal adverse effects. The results of this proof of concept study showed that the principle of β_3-AR agonism may be useful for treatment of patients with OAB/DO.

Phosphodiesterase (PDE) Inhibitors
Drugs stimulating the generation of cAMP are known to relax smooth muscles, including the detrusor (141,146). It is also well established that drugs acting through the NO/cGMP system can relax the smooth muscle of the bladder outflow region (141). Use of PDE inhibitors to enhance the presumed cAMP- and cGMP-mediated relaxation of LUT smooth muscles (detrusor prostate, urethra) should then be a logical approach (159). There are presently 11 families of PDEs, some of which preferentially hydrolyse either cAMP or cGMP (159).

As a basis for PDE inhibitor treatment of LUTS, Uckert et al. investigated human bladder tissue, revealing messenger RNA for PDEs 1A, 1B, 2A, 4A, 4B, 5A, 7A, 8A, and 9A; most of these PDEs preferably inhibit the breakdown of cAMP (160). In vitro, human detrusor muscle responded poorly to sodium nitroprusside, and to agents acting via the cGMP system (161). However, significant relaxation of human detrusor muscle, paralleled by increases in cyclic nucleotide levels, was induced by papaverine, vinpocetine (a low affinity inhibitor of PDE 1), and forskolin (stimulating the generation of cAMP), suggesting that the cAMP pathway and PDE 1 may be important in regulation of detrusor smooth muscle tone (162). Significant dose-dependent relaxations were also induced by human cAMP analogs (162). With these studies as a background, Truss et al. presented preliminary clinical data with vinpocetine in patients with urgency/urgency incontinence or low compliance bladders, and not responding to standard antimuscarinic therapy (163). This initial open pilot study suggested a possible role for vinpocetine in the treatment of OAB. However, the results of a larger RCT in patients with DO showed that vinpocetine only showed statistically significant results for one parameter (164). Studies with other PDE 1 inhibitors than vinpocetin (which may not be an optimal drug for elucidation the principle) do not seem to have been performed.

PDE 4 (which also preferably hydrolyses cAMP) has been implicated in the control of bladder smooth muscle tone. PDE 4 inhibitors reduced the in vitro contractile response of guinea pig (165) and rat (166,167) bladder strips, and also suppressed rhythmic bladder contractions of the isolated guinea pig bladder (168). Previous experiences with selective PDE 4 inhibitors showed emesis to be a dose-limiting effect (169). If this side action can be avoided, PDE 4 inhibition seems to be a promising approach.

NO has been demonstrated to be an important inhibitory neurotransmitter in the smooth muscle of the urethra and its relaxant effect is associated with increased levels of cyclic GMP (1). However, few investigations have addressed the cAMP- and cGMP-mediated signal transduction pathways and its key enzymes in the mammalian urethra. Morita et al. examined the effects of isoproterenol, prostaglandin E_1 and E_2, and SNP on the contractile force and tissue content of cAMP and cGMP in the rabbit urethra (170). They concluded that both cyclic nucleotides can produce relaxation of the urethra. Werkstrom et al. characterized the distribution of PDE 5, cGMP, and PKG1 in female pig and human urethra, and evaluated the effect of pharmacological inhibition of PDE-5 in isolated smooth muscle preparations (171). After stimulation with the NO donor, DETA NONO-ate, the cGMP-immunoreactivity (IR) in urethral and vascular smooth muscles increased. There was a wide distribution of cGMP- and vimentin-positive interstitial cells between pig urethral smooth muscle bundles. PDE-5 IR could be demonstrated within the urethral and vascular smooth muscle cells, but also in vascular endothelial cells that expressed cGMP-IR. Nerve-induced relaxations of urethral preparations were enhanced at low concentrations of sildenafil, vardenafil, and tadalafil, whereas there were direct smooth muscle relaxant actions of the PDE-5 inhibitors at high concentrations.

The distribution of PDEs in the male urethral structures does not seem to have been studied.

The observation that patients treated for erectile dysfunction with PDE 5 inhibitors had an improvement of their LUTS, has sparked a new interest in using these drugs also for treatment of LUTS and OAB. After the report in an open study (172) that treatment with sildenafil appeared to improve urinary symptom scores in men with ED and LUTS, this observation has been confirmed in several well designed and conducted RCTs (173–175).

The mechanism behind the beneficial effect of the PDE inhibitors on LUTS/OAB and their site(s) of action largely remain to be elucidated. If the site of action was the smooth muscles of the outflow region (and the effect relaxation), an increase in flow rate should be expected. In none of the trials referred to such an effect was found. However, there are several other structures in the LUT that may be involved, including those in the urothelial signaling pathway (urothelium, interstitial cells, and suburothelial afferent nerves).

Ion-Channels
Ion-channels are important regulators of the cell function. Located within the plasma membrane, they control the permeability of different ions. The two most thoroughly investigated classes of ion-channels are calcium channels and potassium channels (141).

Calcium Channels

Calcium is a key component for cell function in many cells. In smooth muscle, increased intracellular calcium concentrations activate the contractile mechanisms, and in nerve terminals, calcium influx in response to action potentials is an important mechanism for neurotransmitter release. Calcium channels can be divided into at least four different subtypes: L, N, P, and Q-channels. The calcium channels present in smooth muscles are L-type (dihydropyridine sensitive) calcium channels and seem to be involved in contraction of the human bladder irrespective of the mode of activation (176). A decrease of the membrane potential (depolarization) increases the open probability for calcium channels, thereby increasing the calcium influx. Thus, the channels dependent on the membrane potential and are termed voltage-operated calcium channels (VOCC). Elevated intracellular calcium levels are also believed to initiate release of calcium from intracellular stores, a mechanism called calcium-induced calcium release (177,178). Thus, regulation of the intracellular calcium concentration in smooth muscle cells is one conceivable way to modulate bladder contraction. Dihydropyridines, e.g., nifedipine, have a potent inhibitory effect on isolated detrusor muscle. Inhibitory effects have also been demonstrated on experimentally induced contractions under in vivo conditions in rats, and clinically in patients with DO (17). However, therapeutically, there is no evidence that calcium antagonists have any useful effects in the treatment of OAB/DO (4).

Potassium Channels

Potassium channels represent another mechanism to modulate the excitability of the smooth muscle cells. Under normal conditions, the resting membrane potential in smooth muscle cells is determined predominantly by the membrane conductivity for potassium ions. Increased potassium conductivity will lower the membrane potential by increasing the potassium efflux. As a consequence, this will increase the threshold for opening of VOCC and initiation of contraction. There are several different types of K^+-channels and at least two subtypes have been found in the human detrusor, ATP-sensitive K^+-channels (K_{ATP}) and large conductance calcium-activated K^+-channels (BK_{Ca}). Studies on isolated human detrusor muscle and on bladder tissue from several animal species have demonstrated that K^+-channel openers reduce spontaneous contractions as well as contractions induced by carbachol and electrical stimulation (141). However, the lack of selectivity of presently available K^+-channel blockers for the bladder versus the vasculature has thus far limited the use of these drugs. No effects of cromakalim or pinacidil on the bladder were found in studies on patients with spinal cord lesions or detrusor instability secondary to outflow obstruction (179,180). Some new K channel openers have been developed and claimed to have selectivity towards the bladder (141). However, so far there is no evidence that K^+ channels openers is an option for treatment of OAB/DO (4).

Afferent Signaling Mechanisms
Urothelium

Recent evidence suggests that the urothelium may serve as a mechanosensor which, by producing NO, ATP, ACh, and other mediators, can control the activity in afferent nerves, and thereby the initiation of the micturition reflex (181,182). Low pH, high K^+, increased osmolality, and low temperatures can all influence afferent nerves, possibly via effects on the "vanilloid" [transient receptor potential vanilloid 1 (TRPV1] receptor, which is expressed both in afferent nerve terminals and in the epithelial cells that line the bladder lumen (183,184). A network of interstitial cells [interstitial cells of cajal (ICC)], extensively linked by Cx43-containing gap junctions, was found to be located beneath the urothelium in the human bladder (185,186). This interstitial cellular network was suggested to operate as a functional syncytium, integrating signals, and responses in the bladder wall. The firing of suburothelial afferent nerves and the threshold for bladder activation may be modified by both inhibitory (e.g., NO) and stimulatory (e.g., ATP, ACh, tachykinins, prostanoids) mediators. ATP, generated by the urothelium, has been suggested as an important mediator of urothelial signaling (181,182). Supporting such a view, intravesical ATP induces DO in conscious rats (187). Furthermore, mice lacking the $P2X_3$ receptor were shown to have hypoactive bladders (130,188).

There seem to be other, thus far unidentified, factors in the urothelium that could influence bladder function (1). Fovaeus et al. found a previously unrecognized nonadrenergic, nonnitrergic, non-prostanoid inhibitory mediator is released from the rat urinary bladder by muscarinic receptor stimulation (189). However, it was not clear whether this factor came from the detrusor muscle or from both the bladder and the urothelium. Hawthorn et al. presented data suggesting the presence of a diffusable, urothelium-derived inhibitory factor, which could not be identified, but appeared to be neither nitric oxide, a cyclooxygenase product, a catecholamine, adenosine, GABA, nor any substance sensitive to apamin (121). The identity and possible physiologic role of the unknown factor remains to be established and should offer an interesting field for further research. These mechanisms can be involved in the pathophysiology of the OAB syndrome and DO and thus seem to be interesting targets for pharmacologic intervention.

Myocytes

Myogenic activity can be defined as the ability of a smooth muscle cell to generate mechanical activity independent of external stimuli (141). In the individual myocyte, contractile activity is preceded and initiated by an action potential, which is calcium driven (190). It has been suggested that the detrusor muscle is arranged into units (modules), which are circumscribed areas of muscle (191). These modules show contractile activity during the filling phase of the micturition cycle and might be controlled by several factors including a peripheral myovesical plexus, consisting of intramural ganglia and ICC (192,193). Intercellular connections may contribute to module control, but also locally generated mediators. Kinder and Mundy found that spontaneous contractile activity developed more often in muscle strips from overactive than normal bladders (194), a finding underlined by Brading (195), and confirmed by Mills et al. (196). Turner and Brading discussed the occurrence of "patchy denervation" in cases of DO with subsequent changes of the smooth muscle cells, e.g., supersensitivity to ACh (197). Such an increased sensitivity has been demonstrated in smooth muscle preparations from patients with idiopathic and neurogenic DO (198). It has been reported that suburothelial ICC respond to purinergic stimulation by firing Ca^{2+} transients (199). Interestingly, these suburothelial ICC may be able to affect the activity of the detrusor myocytes (200–202). The frequency of the spontaneous rhythmic contractions of isolated detrusor smooth muscle preparations seems to vary between species, and is probably also dependent on experimental factors (141,192). Characteristically, these contractions are resistant to the Na-channel blocker (tetrodotoxin) and cannot be blocked by hexamethonium, atropine, α-AR blockers, β-AR blockers, or suramin, apparently excluding direct involvement of nerves and nerve-released transmitters (141). Contractions can be effectively inhibited by L-type Ca^{2+} channel blockers and K^+ channel openers, supporting the important role of L-type Ca^{2+} channels for the activity. It cannot be excluded that these spontaneous contractions generates part of the afferent activity ("afferent noise") during filling of the bladder (163).

Sensory Nerves and Vanilloid Receptors

Intravesical administration of capsaicin or resiniferatoxin (RTX) has been shown to increase bladder capacity and decrease urge incontinence in patients with neurogenic, as well as nonneurogenic forms of DO (4,164). Vanilloids are exogenous ligands of vanilloid receptor type 1 (TRPV1 or VR1), an ion channel present in the membrane of type C primary afferent nerve fibers innervating the bladder wall and the periurethral zone of the prostate gland (203). This receptor, which plays a key role in inflammatory pain perception and control of the micturition reflex (203,204), may be upregulated by nerve growth factor (NGF), a neurotrophic molecule detected in high concentrations in overactive detrusors generated by chronic BOO (205). Vanilloids, by reducing uptake of NGF through sensory neurons, may counteract TRPV1 upregulation. In addition, vanilloids decrease the response of already expressed TRPV1 receptors (desensitization) (204).

Important sensory information from the prostate and bladder is conveyed by C fibers. Local anaesthesia of the prostatic urethra was shown to increase bladder volume to first sensation to urinate and maximal bladder capacity, and also to reduce or abolish DO, in patients with benign prostatic enlargement (206). Likewise, intravesical lidocaine was shown to reduce involuntary detrusor contractions in patients with DO (207). Lidocaine is more effective to anesthetize C- than Aδ-fibers supporting the contribution of prostate and bladder C-fiber input to abnormal detrusor activity.

The ice water test triggers a capsaicin-sensitive spinal micturition reflex mediated by unmyelinated C fibers in the bladder and urethra (208). Chai et al. demonstrated a positive ice water test in 71% of subjects with BOO (12 of 17), which was significantly higher than the 7% positive ice water test rate in nonobstructed subjects (3 of 44) (209). The authors suggested this to be caused by an enhanced spinal micturition reflex, possibly due to plasticity of bladder afferents after BOO. If this is the case, intravesical treatment of patients with LUTS associated with BOO with intravesical vanilloids, by desensitizing

C-fibers would be an interesting approach. Two preliminary studies with intravesical RTX suggested that this may be the case (210,211). In a controlled study on neurogenic DO, Silva et al. (2005) concluded that the drug was effective for treatment of this disorder (212). Several other studies have arrived at divergent results, some claiming good effects and others not demonstrating any superiority of RTX over placebo (4).

Despite some evidence of efficacy in LUTS/OAB/DO, capsaicin and RTX are no longer widely used (4). Side effects (pain) and lack of stable RTX preparations, available for easy bladder instillation, will make further investigation of the compound difficult. Different origins of the vanilloid and different ways for preparation and storage of the solutions might have caused substantial differences in the amount of active compound effectively administered to the patients. In addition, RTX adheres to plastics, another reason to the discrepancies that have been observed among RTX studies.

Botulinum Toxin (BoNT)

BoNT is a neurotoxin produced by *Clostridium botulinum*. Of the seven subtypes of BoNT, sub-type A (BoNT-A) is the most relevant clinically. Most of the intravesical experience reported on BoNT-A deals with Botox®.

BoNT consists of a heavy and a light chain linked by a disulphide bond. In the synaptic cleft the toxin binds to synaptic vesicle protein or SV2 through its heavy chain and is internalized by the nerve terminal (213). Upon cleavage, the light chain is released in the cytosol, where it impedes binding of neurotransmitter-containing synaptic vesicles to the plasma membrane. The rationale for using botulinum toxin to treat human DO is based on the assumption that effects of the toxin on skeletal muscle would be replicated in bladder smooth muscle (214,215), and that detrusor muscle paralysis would reduce the symptoms of bladder overactivity (216). Botulinum toxin has been currently developed as a second-line treatment option (following failure of, or intolerance to, appropriate antimuscarinic therapy) for patients with NDO with urinary incontinence or other neurogenic OAB symptoms, and who are able and willing to perform clean intermittent catheterization (CIC).

The first report of the application of BoNT-A in NDO appeared in 2000 (215). Since then, the efficacy of BoNT-A injection into the detrusor muscle in adult patients with NDO refractory to, and/or intolerant of, antimuscarinic agents has been confirmed in a number of studies which have been the subject of systematic review (4,217,218). The analysis by Karsenty et al. evaluated 18 trials with BOTOX® BoNT-A, involving a total of 698 patients, of whom 83% had NDO with urinary incontinence (217). Significant benefits were seen in clinical variables (micturition frequency and number of incontinence episodes) as well as urodynamic variables (maximum detrusor pressure, maximum cystometric capacity). Complete continence was achieved in 40% to 80% of patients.

Efficacy has also been demonstrated in spinal cord injury patients with detrusor-sphincter dyssynergia (219–221). A significant response to BoNT-A is seen as early as one week following treatment, however maximum effects were seen between one and four weeks. The efficacy of BoNT-A appears

to persist for at least three to four months and up to one year, but does decline over time (222), meaning that repeat injections are required for continued therapeutic effect. Repeat injections have been shown to be effective and well tolerated (222–224), and there is no reported evidence of a reduction in response over time, after two to nine repeat injections. The beneficial clinical and urological effects of BoNT-A in adults with NDO are accompanied by improvement in patients' quality of life (225,226).

BoNT-A is generally well tolerated. Data from a systematic review of the role of BoNT-A in NDO indicated that the most frequent adverse events are injection site pain, procedure-related urinary tract infection, and mild hematuria (217). A potential adverse effect resulting from the use of botulinum toxin in patients not using CIC is an increase in postvoid residual volume that may result in de novo CIC (6–88% of patients), with associated impact on quality of life (217,227). Systemic side effects, although rare, could be very disabling for patients with spinal cord injury (228).

Important factors to consider in relation to the risk of adverse events during urological use of BoNT-A are the drug dosage, the formulation used, and injection technique. Available data indicate that Dysport® may be associated with a higher risk of side effects related to drug migration (e.g., muscle weakness) than Botox® (229). It should be noted that the doses typically evaluated in clinical trials in urologic indications differ between the commercially available formulations of BoNT-A. It should also be noted that systemic adverse reactions, including respiratory compromise and death, have been reported following the use of BoNT-A and BoNT-B for both FDA-approved and unapproved uses (229). The most serious cases involved treatment of children for cerebral palsy-associated limb spasticity, and the FDA is currently reviewing safety data relating to marketed botulinum toxin products.

CONCLUSION

To effectively control bladder activity, and to treat urinary incontinence caused by DO, identification of suitable targets for pharmacological intervention is necessary. Such targets may be found in the CNS or peripherally. Drugs, specifically directed for control of bladder activity are under development and will hopefully lead to improved treatment of urinary incontinence.

REFERENCES

1. Andersson KE, Wein AJ. Pharmacology of the lower urinary tract: basis for current and future treatments of urinary incontinence. Pharmacol Rev 2004; 56: 581–631.
2. Ouslander JG. Management of overactive bladder. N Engl J Med 2004; 350: 786–99.
3. Zinner NR, Koke SC, Viktrup L. Pharmacotherapy for stress urinary incontinence: present and future options. Drugs 2004; 64: 1503–16.
4. Andersson K-E, Chapple CR, Cardozo L, et al. Pharmacological treatment of urinary incontinence. In: Abrams P, Cardozo L, Khoury S, Wein A, eds. Incontinence, 4th International Consultation on Incontinence. UK, Plymouth: Plymouth, Plymbridge Distributors Ltd., 2009: 631–99.
5. Tanagho EA, Miller ER. Initiation of voiding. Br J Urol 1970; 42: 175–183.
6. Asmussen M, Ulmsten U. Simultaneous urethrocystometry with a new technique. Scand J Urol Nephrol 1976; 10: 7–11.
7. Low JA. Urethral behaviour during the involuntary detrusor contraction. Am J Obstet Gynecol 1977; 128: 32–42.
8. Fletcher TF, Bradley WE. Neuroanatomy of the bladder—urethra. J Urol 1978; 119: 153–160.
9. Lincoln J, Burnstock G. Autonomic innervation of the urinary bladder and urethra. In: Maggi CA, ed. The Autonomic Nervous System. Vol. 6, Chapter 2, Nervous Control of the Urogenital System. London: Harwood Academic Publisher, 1993: 33–68.
10. De Groat WC, Booth AM, Yoshimura N. Neurophysiology of micturition and its modification in animal models of human disease. In: Maggi CA, ed. Nervous Control of the Urogenital System. London: Harwood Academic, 1993: 227–90.
11. Ambache H, Zar MA. Non-cholinergic transmission by postganglionic motor neurons in the mammalian bladder. J Physiol (Lond) 1970; 210: 761–83.
12. Burnstock G, Dumsday B, Smythe A. Atropine resistant excitation of the urinary bladder: the possibility of transmission via nerves releasing a purine nucleotide. Br J Pharmacol 1972; 44: 451–61.
13. Sjogren C, Andersson KE, Husted S, Mattiasson A, Moller-Madsen B. Atropine resistance of transmurally stimulated isolated human bladder muscle. J Urol 1982; 128: 1368–71.
14. Bayliss M, Wu C, Newgreen D, Mundy AR, Fry CH. A quantitative study of atropine-resistant contractile responses in human detrusor smooth muscle, from stable, unstable and obstructed bladders. J Urol 1999; 162: 1833–9.
15. O'Reilly BA, Kosaka AH, Knight GF, et al. P2X receptors and their role in female idiopathic detrusor instability. J Urol 2002; 167: 157–64.
16. Burnstock G. Purinergic signalling in lower urinary tract. In: Abbracchio MP, Williams M, eds. Purinergic and Pyrimidinergic Signalling I Molecular, Nervous and Urogenitary System Function. Berlin: Springer Verlag, 2001: 151, 423–515.
17. Andersson K-E. Pharmacology of lower urinary tract smooth muscles and penile erectile tissues. Pharmacol Rev 1993; 45: 253–308.
18. Andersson K-E, Persson K. The L-arginine/nitric oxide pathway and non-adrenergic, non-cholinergic relaxation of the lower urinary tract. Gen Pharmacol 1993; 24: 833–9.
19. Bridgewater M, Brading AF. Evidence for a non-nitrergic inhibitory innervation in the pig urethra. Neurourol Urodyn 1993; 12: 357–8.
20. Hashimoto S, Kigoshi S, Muramatsu I. Nitric oxide-dependent and -independent neurogenic relaxation of isolated dog urethra. Eur J Pharmacol 1993; 231: 209–14.
21. Werkstrom V, Persson K, Ny L, et al. Factors involved in the relaxation of female pig urethra evoked by electrical field stimulation. Br J Pharmacol 1995; 116: 1599–604.
22. Mattiasson A, Andersson KE, Elbadawi A, et al. Interaction between adrenergic and cholinergic nerve terminals in the urinary bladder of rabbit, cat and man. J Urol 1987; 137: 1017–19.
23. Åmark P, Nergardh A, Kinn AC. The effect of noradrenaline on the contractile response of the urinary bladder. An in vitro study in man and cat. Scand J Urol Nephrol 1986; 20: 203–7.
24. Perlberg S, Caine M. Adrenergic response of bladder muscle in prostatic obstruction. Its relation to detrusor instability. Urology 1982; 20: 524–7.
25. Kuru M. Nervous control of micturition. Physiol Rev 1965; 45: 425–94.
26. de Groat WC, Yoshimura N. Afferent nerve regulation of bladder function in health and disease. Handb Exp Pharmacol. 2009; (194): 91–138.
27. Janig W, Morrison JF. Functional properties of spinal visceral afferents supplying abdominal and pelvic organs, with special emphasis on visceral nociception. Prog Brain Res 1986; 67: 87–114.
28. Habler HJ, Janig W, Koltzenburg M. Activation of unmyelinated afferent fibres by mechanical stimuli and inflammation of the urinary bladder in the cat. J Physiol 1990; 425: 545–62.
29. Fall M, Lindstrom S, Mazieres L. A bladder-to-bladder cooling reflex in the cat. J Physiol 1990; 427: 281–300.
30. Thor KB, Donatucci C. Central nervous system control of the lower urinary tract: new pharmacological approaches to stress urinary incontinence in women. J Urol 2004; 172: 27–33.

31. Blok BF, de Weerd H, Holstege G. The pontine micturition center projects to sacral cord GABA immunoreactive neurons in the cat. Neurosci Lett 1997; 233: 109–12.

32. Griffiths DJ. Cerebral control of bladder function. Curr Urol Rep 2004; 5: 348–52.

33. Fowler CJ, Griffiths D, de Groat WC. The neural control of micturition. Nat Rev Neurosci 2008; 9: 453–66.

34. Mallory BS, Roppolo JR, de Groat WC. Pharmacological modulation of the pontine micturition center. Brain Res 1991; 546: 310–32.

35. de Groat WC, Nadelhaft I, Milne RJ, et al. Organization of the sacral parasympathetic reflex pathways to the urinary bladder and large intestine. J Auton Nerv Syst 1981; 3: 135–60.

36. Maggi CA. The dual sensory and 'efferent' function of the capsaicin-sensitive primary sensory neurons in the urinary bladder and urethra. In: Maggi CA, ed. Nervous Control of the Urogenital System. London: Harwood Academic, 1993: 383–422.

37. Blok BF, Sturms LM, Holstege G. Brain activation during micturition in women. Brain 1998; 121(Pt 11): 2033–42.

38. Griffiths D. Clinical studies of cerebral and urinary tract function in elderly people with urinary incontinence. Behav Brain Res 1998; 92: 151–5.

39. Nour S, Svarer C, Kristensen JK, Paulson OB, Law I. Cerebral activation during micturition in normal men. Brain 2000; 123(Pt 4): 781–9.

40. Athwal BS, Berkley KJ, Hussain I, et al. Brain responses to changes in bladder volume and urge to void in healthy men. Brain 2001; 124(Pt 2): 369–77.

41. Kuhar MJ, Pert CB, Snyder SH. Regional distribution of opiate receptor binding in monkey and human brain. Nature 1973; 245: 447–50.

42. Mansour A, Fox CA, Akil H, Watson SJ. Opioid-receptor mRNA expression in the rat CNS: anatomical and functional implications. Trends Neurosci 1995; 18: 22–9.

43. de Groat WC, Yoshimura N. Pharmacology of the lower urinary tract. Annu Rev Pharmacol Toxicol 2001; 41: 691–721.

44. Murray KH, Feneley RC. Endorphins—a role in lower urinary tract function? The effect of opioid blockade on the detrusor and urethral sphincter mechanisms. Br J Urol 1982; 54: 638–40.

45. Dray A, Nunan L, Wire W. Naloxonazine and opioid-induced inhibition of reflex urinary bladder contractions. Neuropharmacology 1987; 26: 67–74.

46. Herman RM, Wainberg MC, delGiudice PF, Willscher MK. The effect of a low dose of intrathecal morphine on impaired micturition reflexes in human subjects with spinal cord lesions. Anesthesiology 1988; 69: 313–18.

47. Kieffer BL. Opioids: first lessons from knockout mice. Trends Pharmacol Sci 1999; 20: 19–26.

48. Grond S, Sablotzki A. Clinical pharmacology of tramadol. Clin Pharmacokinet 2004; 43: 879–923.

49. Steers WD, Herschorn S, Kreder KJ, et al. Duloxetine compared with placebo for treating women with symptoms of overactive bladder. BJU Int 2007; 100: 337.

50. Pehrson R, Stenman E, Andersson KE. Effects of tramadol on rat detrusor overactivity induced by experimental cerebral infarction. Eur Urol 2003; 44: 495–9.

51. Pehrson R, Andersson KE. Tramadol inhibits rat detrusor overactivity caused by dopamine receptor stimulation. J Urol 2003; 170: 272–5.

52. Singh SK, Agarwal MM, Batra YK, Kishore AV, Mandal AK. Effect of lumbar-epidural administration of tramadol on lower urinary tract function. Neurourol Urodyn 2008; 27: 65–70.

53. Safarinejad MR, Hosseini SY. Safety and efficacy of tramadol in the treatment of idiopathic detrusor overactivity: a double-blind, placebo-controlled, randomized study. Br J Clin Pharmacol 2006; 61: 456–63.

54. Hisamitsu T, de Groat WC. The inhibitory effect of opioid peptides and morphine applied intrathecally and intracerebroventricularly on the micturition reflex in the cat. Brain Res 1984; 298: 51–65.

55. Dray A, Nunan L, Wire W. Central delta-opioid receptor interactions and the inhibition of reflex urinary bladder contractions in the rat. Br J Pharmacol 1985; 85: 717–26.

56. de Groat WC, Kawatani M. Enkephalinergic inhibition in parasympathetic ganglia of the urinary bladder of the cat. J Physiol 1989; 413: 13–29.

57. Malinovsky JM, Le Normand L, Lepage JY, et al. The urodynamic effects of intravenous opioids and ketoprofen in humans. Anesth Analg 1998; 87: 456–61.

58. Ranson RN, Dodds AL, Smith MJ, Santer RM, Watson AH. Age-associated changes in the monoaminergic innervation of rat lumbosacral spinal cord. Brain Res 2003; 972: 149–58.

59. Thor KB, Blitz-Siebert A, Helke CJ. Autoradiographic localization of 5hydroxytryptamine1A, 5-hydroxytryptamine1B and 5-hydroxytryptamine1C/2 binding sites in the rat spinal cord. Neuroscience 1993; 55: 235–52.

60. de Groat WC. Influence of central serotonergic mechanisms on lower urinary tract function. Urology 2002; 59(5 Suppl 1): 30–6.

61. McMahon SB, Spillane K. Brain stem influences on the parasympathetic supply to the urinary bladder of the cat. Brain Res 1982; 234: 237–49.

62. Sugaya K, Ogawa Y, Hatano T, et al. Evidence for involvement of the subcoeruleus nucleus and nucleus raphe magnus in urine storage and penile erection in decerebrate rats. J Urol 1998; 159: 2172–6.

63. Zorn BH, Montgomery H, Pieper K, Gray M, Steers WD. Urinary incontinence and depression. J Urol 1999; 162: 82–4.

64. Steers WD, Lee KS. Depression and incontinence. World J Urol 2001; 19: 351–7.

65. Littlejohn JO Jr, Kaplan SA. An unexpected association between urinary incontinence, depression and sexual dysfunction. Drugs Today (Barc) 2002; 38: 777–82.

66. Movig KL, Leufkens HG, Belitser SV, Lenderink AW, Egberts AC. Selective serotonin reuptake inhibitor-induced urinary incontinence. Pharmacoepidemiol Drug Saf 2002; 11: 271–9.

67. Chebib M, Johnston GAR. The 'ABC' of GABA receptors: a brief review. Clin Exp Pharmacol Physiol 1999; 26: 937–40.

68. Igawa Y, Mattiasson A, Andersson KE. Effects of GABA-receptor stimulation and blockade on micturition in normal rats and rats with bladder outflow obstruction. J Urol 1993; 150(2 Pt 1): 537–42.

69. Pehrson R, Lehmann A, Andersson KE. Effects of gamma-aminobutyrate B receptor modulation on normal micturition and oxyhemoglobin induced detrusor overactivity in female rats. J Urol 2002; 168: 2700–5.

70. Maggi CA, Furio M, Santicioli P, Conte B, Meli A. Spinal and supraspinal components of GABAergic inhibition of the micturition reflex in rats. J Pharm Exp Ther 1987; 240: 998–1005.

71. Coggeshall RE, Carlton SM. Receptor localization in the mammalian dorsal horn and primary afferent neurons. Brain Res Brain Res Rev 1997; 24: 28–66.

72. Malcangio M, Bowery NG. GABA and its receptors in the spinal cord. Trends Pharm Sci 1996; 17: 457–62.

73. Maggi CA, Santicioli P, Giuliani S, et al. The effects of baclofen on spinal and supraspinal micturition reflexes in rats. Naunyn Schmiedebergs Arch Pharmacol 1987; 336: 197–203.

74. Zhu Q-M, Hu D-Q, Tsung S, Blue DR, Ford AP. Differential effects of GABA$_A$ and GABA$_B$ receptor agonists on cystometry in conscious mice. J Urol 167; 4(Suppl): 39–40. (Abstract 157)

75. Taylor MC, Bates CP. A double-blind crossover trial of baclofen—a new treatment for the unstable bladder syndrome. Br J Urol 1979; 51: 504–5.

76. Rekling JC, Funk GD, Bayliss DA, Dong XW, Feldman JL. Synaptic control of motoneuronal excitability. Physiol Rev 2000; 80: 767–852.

77. Maneuf YP, Gonzalez MI, Sutton KS, et al. Cellular and molecular action of the putative GABA-mimetic, gabapentin. Cell Mol Life Sci 2003; 60: 742–50.

78. Carbone A, Tubaro A, Morello P, et al. The effect of gabapentin on neurogenic detrusor overactivity, a pilot study. Eur Urol Suppl 2:141, 2003 (abstract 555)

79. Kim YT, Kwon DD, Kim J, et al. Gabapentin for overactive bladder and nocturia after anticholinergic failure. Int Braz J Urol 2004; 30: 275–8.

80. Ishizuka O, Persson K, Mattiasson A, et al. Micturition in conscious rats with and without bladder outlet obstruction – role of spinal alpha(1)-adrenoceptors. Br J Pharmacol 1996; 117: 962–6.

81. Persson K, Pandita RK, Spitsbergen JM, et al. Spinal and peripheral mechanisms contributing to hyperactive voiding in spontaneously hypertensive rats. Am J Physiol 1998; 275: R1366–73.

82. Lecci A, Maggi CA. Tachykinins as modulators of the micturition reflex in the central and peripheral nervous system. Regul Pept 2001; 101: 1–18.

83. Saffroy M, Torrens Y, Glowinski J, Beaujouan JC. Autoradiographic distribution of tachykinin NK2 binding sites in the rat brain: comparison with NK1 and NK3 binding sites. Neuroscience 2003; 116: 761–73.

84. Coveñas R, Martin F, Belda M, et al. Mapping of neurokinin-like immunoreactivity in the human brainstem. BMC Neurosci 2003; 4: 3.

85. Ishizuka O, Igawa Y, Lecci A, et al. Role of intrathecal tachykinins for micturition in unanaesthetized rats with and without bladder outlet obstruction. Br J Pharmacol 1994; 113: 111–16.

86. Seki S, Erickson KA, Seki M, et al. Elimination of rat spinal neurons expressing neurokinin 1 receptors reduces bladder overactivity and spinal c-fos expression induced by bladder irritation. Am J Physiol Renal Physiol 2005; 288: F466–73.

87. Ishizuka O, Mattiasson A, Andersson KE. Effects of neurokinin receptor antagonists on L-dopa induced bladder hyperactivity in normal conscious rats. J Urol 1995; 154: 1548–51.

88. Gu BJ, Ishizuka O, Igawa Y, Nishizawa O, Andersson KE. Role of supraspinal tachykinins for micturition in conscious rats with and without bladder outlet obstruction. Naunyn Schmiedebergs Arch Pharmacol 2000; 361: 543–8.

89. Ishizuka O, Igawa Y, Nishizawa O, Andersson KE. Role of supraspinal tachykinins for volume- and L-dopa-induced bladder activity in normal conscious rats. Neurourol Urodyn 2000; 19: 101–9.

90. Massaro AM, Lenz KL. Aprepitant: a novel antiemetic for chemotherapy-induced nausea and vomiting. Ann Pharmacother 2005; 39: 77–85.

91. Green SA, Alon A, Ianus J, et al. Efficacy and safety of a neurokinin-1 receptor antagonist in postmenopausal women with overactive bladder with urge urinary incontinence. J Urol 2006; 176(6 Pt 1): 2535–40.

92. Berger Y, Blaivas JG, DeLaRocha ER, Salinas JM. Urodynamic findings in Parkinson's disease. J Urol 1987; 138: 836–8.

93. Yoshimura N, Mizuta E, Kuno S, et al. The dopamine D1 receptor agonist SKF 38393 suppresses detrusor hyperreflexia in the monkey with parkinsonism induced by 1-methyl-4 phenyl-1,2,3,6-tetrahydropyridine (MPTP). Neuropharmacology 1993; 32: 315–21.

94. Sillén U, Rubenson A, Hjalmas K. On the localization and mediation of the centrally induced hyperactive urinary bladder response to l-dopa in the rat. Acta Physiol Scand 1981; 112: 137–40.

95. Kontani H, Inoue T, Sakai T. Dopamine receptor subtypes that induce hyperactive urinary bladder response in anesthetized rats. Jpn J Pharmacol 1990a; 54: 482–6.

96. Kontani H, Inoue T, Sakai T. Effects of apomorphine on urinary bladder motility in anesthetized rats. Jpn J Pharmacol 1990b; 52: 59–67.

97. Caulfield MP, Birdsall NJM. International Union of Pharmacology: XVII. Classification of muscarinic acetylcholine receptors. Pharmacol Rev 1998; 50: 279–90.

98. Sigala S, Mirabella G, Peroni A, et al. Differential gene expression of cholinergic muscarinic receptor subtypes in male and female normal human urinary bladder. Urology 2002; 60: 719–25.

99. Bschleipfer T, Schukowski K, Weidner W, et al. Expression and distribution of cholinergic receptors in the human urothelium. Life Sci 2007; 80: 2303–7.

100. Yamaguchi O, Shishido K, Tamura K, et al. Evaluation of mRNAs encoding muscarinic receptor subtypes in human detrusor muscle. J Urol 1996; 156: 1208–13.

101. Eglen RM, Hegde SS, Watson N. Muscarinic receptor subtypes and smooth muscle function. Pharmacol Rev 1996; 48: 531–65.

102. Hegde SS, Eglen RM. Muscarinic receptor subtypes modulating smooth muscle contractility in the urinary bladder. Life Sci 1999; 64: 419–28.

103. Chess-Williams R. Muscarinic receptors of the urinary bladder: detrusor, urothelial and prejunctional. Auton Autacoid Pharmacol 2002; 22: 133–45.

104. Giglio D, Tobin G. Muscarinic receptor subtypes in the lower urinary tract. Pharmacology 2009; 83: 259–69.

105. Schneider T, Fetscher C, Krege S, Michel MC. Signal transduction underlying carbachol-induced contraction of human urinary bladder. J Pharmacol Exp Ther 2004; 309: 1148–53.

106. Jezior JR, Brady JD, Rosenstein DI, et al. Dependency of detrusor contractions on calcium sensitization and calcium entry through LOE-908-sensitive channels. Br J Pharmacol 2001; 134: 78–87.

107. Wibberley A, Chen Z, Hu E, Hieble JP, Westfall TD. Expression and functional role of Rho-kinase in rat urinary bladder smooth muscle. Br J Pharmacol 2003; 138: 757–66.

108. Andersson K-E. Detrusor contraction—focus on muscarinic receptors. Scand J Urol Nephrol Suppl 2004; 215: 54–7.

109. Hegde SS, Choppin A, Bonhaus D, et al. Functional role of M-2 and M-3 muscarinic receptors in the urinary bladder of rats in vitro and in vivo. Br J Pharmacol 1997; 120: 1409–18.

110. Kotlikoff MI, Dhulipala P, Wang YX. M2 signaling in smooth muscle cells. Life Sci 1999; 64: 437–42.

111. Bonev AD, Nelson MT. Muscarinic inhibition of ATP-sensitive K$^+$ channels by protein kinase C in urinary bladder smooth muscle. Am J Physiol 1993; 265(6 Pt 1): C1723–8.

112. Nakamura T, Kimura J, Yamaguchi O. Muscarinic M2 receptors inhibit Ca^{2+}-activated K$^+$ channels in rat bladder smooth muscle. Int J Urol 2002; 9: 689–96.

113. Braverman AS, Luthin GR, Ruggieri MR. M2 muscarinic receptor contributes to contraction of the denervated rat urinary bladder. Am J Physiol 1998; 275: R1654–60.

114. Braverman A, Legos J, Young W, Luthin G, Ruggieri M. M2 receptors in genito-urinary smooth muscle pathology. Life Sci 1999; 64: 429–36.

115. Braverman AS, Tallarida RJ, Ruggieri MR Sr. Interaction between muscarinic receptor subtype signal transduction pathways mediating bladder contraction. Am J Physiol Regul Integr Comp Physiol 2002; 283: R663–8.

116. Braverman AS, Ruggieri MR Sr. Hypertrophy changes the muscarinic receptor subtype mediating bladder contraction from M3 toward M2. Am J Physiol Regul Integr Comp Physiol 2003; 285: R701–8.

117. Pontari MA, Braverman AS, Ruggieri MR Sr. The M2 muscarinic receptor mediates in vitro bladder contractions from patients with neurogenic bladder dysfunction. Am J Physiol Regul Integr Comp Physiol 2004; 286: R874–80.

118. D'Agostino G, Bolognesi ML, Lucchelli A, et al. Prejunctional muscarinic inhibitory control of acetylcholine release in the human isolated detrusor: involvement of the M4 receptor subtype. Br J Pharmacol 2000; 129: 493–500.

119. Somogyi GT, de Groat WC. Function, signal transduction mechanisms and plasticity of presynaptic muscarinic receptors in the urinary bladder. Life Sci 1999; 64: 411–18.

120. Somogyi GT, Zernova GV, Yoshiyama M, et al. Change in muscarinic modulation of transmitter release in the rat urinary bladder after spinal cord injury. Neurochem Int 2003; 43: 73–7.

121. Hawthorn MH, Chapple CR, Cock M, Chess-Williams R. Urothelium-derived inhibitory factor(s) influences on detrusor muscle contractility in vitro. Br J Pharmacol 2000; 129: 416–19.

122. Tyagi S, Tyagi P, Van-le S, et al. Qualitative and quantitative expression profile of muscarinic receptors in human urothelium and detrusor. J Urol 2006; 176(4 Pt 1): 1673–8.

123. Mansfield KJ, Liu L, Mitchelson FJ, et al. Muscarinic receptor subtypes in human bladder detrusor and mucosa, studied by radioligand binding and quantitative competitive RT-PCR: changes in ageing. Br J Pharmacol 2005; 144: 1089–99.

124. Mukerji G, Yiangou Y, Grogono J, et al. Localization of M2 and M3 muscarinic receptors in human bladder disorders and their clinical correlations. J Urol 2006; 176: 367–73.

125. Grol S, Essers PB, van Koeveringe GA, et al. M(3) muscarinic receptor expression on suburothelial interstitial cells. BJU Int 2009. [Epub ahead of print].

126. Wakabayashi Y, Tomoyoshi T, Fujimiya M, Arai R, Maeda T. Substance P-containing axon terminals in the mucosa of the human urinary bladder: pre-embedding immunohistochemistry using cryostat sections for electron microscopy. Histochemistry 1993; 100: 401–7.

127. Persson K, Alm P, Johansson K, Larsson B, Andersson KE. Co-existence of nitrergic, peptidergic and acetylcholine esterase-positive nerves in the pig lower urinary tract. J Auton Nerv Syst 1995; 52: 225–36.

128. Gabella G, Davis C. Distribution of afferent axons in the bladder of rats. J Neurocytol 1998; 27: 141–55.

129. Ferguson DR, Kennedy I, Burton TJ. ATP is released from rabbit urinary bladder epithelial cells by hydrostatic pressure changes—a possible sensory mechanism? J Physiol 1997; 505(Pt 2): 503–11.

130. Vlaskovska M, Kasakov L, Rong W, et al. P2X3 knock-out mice reveal a major sensory role for urothelially released ATP. J Neurosci 2001; 21: 5670–7.

131. Birder LA, Barrick SR, Roppolo JR, et al. Feline interstitial cystitis results in mechanical hypersensitivity and altered ATP release from bladder urothelium. Am J Physiol Renal Physiol 2003; 285: F423–9.

132. Kullmann FA, Artim DE, Birder LA, de Groat WC. Activation of muscarinic receptors in rat bladder sensory pathways alters reflex bladder activity. J Neurosci 2008; 28: 1977–87.

133. Yoshida M, Inadome A, Maeda Y, et al. Non-neuronal cholinergic system in human bladder urothelium. Urology 2006; 67: 425–30.

134. Hanna-Mitchell AT, Beckel JM, Barbadora S, et al. Non-neuronal acetylcholine and urinary bladder urothelium. Life Sci 2007; 80: 2298–302.

135. Malloy BJ, Price DT, Price RR, et al. Alpha1-adrenergic receptor subtypes in human detrusor. J Urol 1998; 160: 937–43.

136. Michel MC, Vrydag W. Alpha1-, alpha2- and beta-adrenoceptors in the urinary bladder, urethra and prostate. Br J Pharmacol 2006; 147(Suppl 2): S88–119.

137. Andersson KE, Gratzke C. Pharmacology of alpha1-adrenoceptor antagonists in the lower urinary tract and central nervous system. Nat Clin Pract Urol 2007; 4: 368–78.

138. Nomiya M, Yamaguchi O. A quantitative analysis of mRNA expression of alpha 1 and beta-adrenoceptor subtypes and their functional roles in human normal and obstructed bladders. J Urol 2003; 170(2 Pt 1): 649–53.

139. Bouchelouche K, Andersen L, Alvarez S, Nordling J, Bouchelouche P. Increased contractile response to phenylephrine in detrusor of patients with bladder outlet obstruction: effect of the alpha1A and alpha1D-adrenergic receptor antagonist tamsulosin. J Urol 2005; 173: 657–61.

140. Das AK, Leggett RE, Whitbeck C, et al. Effect of doxazosin on rat urinary bladder function after partial outlet obstruction. Neurourol Urodyn 2002; 21: 160–6.

141. Andersson KE, Arner A. Urinary bladder contraction and relaxation: physiology and pathophysiology. Physiol Rev 2004; 84: 935–86.

142. Otsuka A, Shinbo H, Matsumoto R, Kurita Y, Ozono S. Expression and functional role of beta-adrenoceptors in the human urinary bladder urothelium. Naunyn Schmiedebergs Arch Pharmacol 2008; 377: 473–81.

143. Badawi JK, Seja T, Uecelehan H, et al. Relaxation of human detrusor muscle by selective beta-2 and beta-3 agonists and endogenous catecholamines. Urology 2007; 69: 785–90.

144. Leon LA, Hoffman BE, Gardner SD, et al. Effects of the beta 3-adrenergic receptor agonist disodium 5-[(2R)-2-[[(2R)-2-(3-chlorophenyl)-2-hydroxyethyl]amino]propyl]-1,3-benzodioxole-2,2-dicarboxylate (CL-316243) on bladder micturition reflex in spontaneously hypertensive rats. J Pharmacol Exp Ther 2008; 326: 178–85.

145. Biers SM, Reynard JM, Brading AF. The effects of a new selective beta3-adrenoceptor agonist (GW427353) on spontaneous activity and detrusor relaxation in human bladder. BJU Int 2006; 98: 1310–14.

146. Andersson K-E. Pathways for relaxation of detrusor smooth muscle. In: Baskin LS, Hayward SW, eds. Advances in Bladder Research. New York: Kluwer Academic/Plenum Publishers, 1999: 241–52.

147. Uchida H, Shishido K, Nomiya M, Yamaguchi O. Involvement of cyclic AMP-dependent and -independent mechanisms in the relaxation of rat detrusor muscle via beta-adrenoceptors. Eur J Pharmacol 2005; 518: 195–202.

148. Frazier EP, Peters SL, Braverman AS, Ruggieri MR Sr, Michel MC. Signal transduction underlying the control of urinary bladder smooth muscle tone by muscarinic receptors and beta-adrenoceptors. Naunyn Schmiedebergs Arch Pharmacol 2008; 377: 449–62.

149. Takemoto J, Masumiya H, Nunoki K, et al. Potentiation of potassium currents by beta-adrenoceptor agonists in human urinary bladder smooth muscle cells: a possible electrical mechanism of relaxation. Pharmacology 2008; 81: 251–8.

150. Hristov KL, Cui X, Brown SM, et al. Stimulation of beta3-adrenoceptors relaxes rat urinary bladder smooth muscle via activation of the large-conductance Ca^{2+}-activated K^+ channels. Am J Physiol Cell Physiol 2008; 295: C1344–53. [Epub 2008 Sep 17].

151. Fujimura T, Tamura K, Tsutsumi T, et al. Expression and possible functional role of the beta3-adrenoceptor in human and rat detrusor muscle. J Urol 1999; 161: 680–5.

152. Woods M, Carson N, Norton NW, Sheldon JH, Argentieri TM. Efficacy of the beta3-adrenergic receptor agonist CL-316243 on experimental bladder hyperreflexia and detrusor instability in the rat. J Urol 2001; 166: 1142–7.

153. Takeda H, Yamazaki Y, Igawa Y, et al. Effects of beta(3)-adrenoceptor stimulation on prostaglandin E(2)-induced bladder hyperactivity and on the cardiovascular system in conscious rats. Neurourol Urodyn 2002; 21: 558–65.

154. Kaidoh K, Igawa Y, Takeda H, et al. Effects of selective beta2 and beta3-adrenoceptor agonists on detrusor hyperreflexia in conscious cerebral infarcted rats. J Urol 2002; 168: 1247–52.

155. Hicks A, McCafferty GP, Riedel E, et al. GW427353 (solabegron), a novel, selective beta3-adrenergic receptor agonist, evokes bladder relaxation and increases micturition reflex threshold in the dog. J Pharmacol Exp Ther 2007; 323: 202–9.

156. Colli E, Digesu GA, Olivieri L. Overactive bladder treatments in early phase clinical trials. Expert Opin Investig Drugs 2007; 16: 999–1007.

157. Takasu T, Ukai M, Sato S, et al. Effect of (R)-2-(2-aminothiazol-4-yl)-4â²-{2-[(2-hydroxy-2-phenylethyl)amino]ethyl} acetanilide (YM178), a novel selective beta3-adrenoceptor agonist, on bladder function. J Pharmacol Exp Ther 2007; 321: 642–7. [Epub 2007 Feb 9].

158. Chapple CR, Yamaguchi O, Ridder A, et al. Clinical proof of concept study (Blossom) shows novel B3 adrenoceptor agonist YM178 is effective and well tolerated in the treatment of symptoms of overactive bladder. Eur Urol Suppl 2008; 7: 239 (abstract 674).

159. Andersson KE, Uckert S, Stief C, Hedlund P. Phosphodiesterases (PDEs) and PDE inhibitors for treatment of LUTS. Neurourol Urodyn 2007; 26(6 Suppl): 928–33.

160. Uckert S, Kuthe A, Jonas U, Stief CG. Characterization and functional relevance of cyclic nucleotide phosphodiesterase isoenzymes of the human prostate. J Urol 2001; 166: 2484–90.

161. Truss MC, Stief CG, Uckert S, et al. Initial clinical experience with the selective phosphodiesterase-I isoenzyme inhibitor vinpocetine in the treatment of urge incontinence and low compliance bladder. World J Urol 2000; 18: 439–43.

162. Truss MC, Stief CG, Uckert S, et al. Phosphodiesterase 1 inhibition in the treatment of lower urinary tract dysfunction: from bench to bedside. World J Urol 2001; 19: 344–50.

163. Gillespie JI, van Koeveringe GA, de Wachter SG, de Vente J. On the origins of the sensory output from the bladder: the concept of afferent noise. BJU Int 2009; 1: 1324–33.

164. Cruz F, Dinis P. Resiniferatoxin and botulinum toxin type A for treatment of lower urinary tract symptoms. Neurourol Urodyn 2007; 26(6 Suppl): 920.

165. Longhurst PA, Briscoe JA, Rosenberg DJ, Leggett RE. The role of cyclic nucleotides in guinea-pig bladder contractility. Br J Pharmacol 1997; 121: 1665–72.

166. Nishiguchi J, Kwon DD, Kaiho Y, et al. Suppression of detrusor overactivity in rats with bladder outlet obstruction by a type 4 phosphodiesterase inhibitor. BJU Int 2007; 99: 680–6.

167. Kaiho Y, Nishiguchi J, Kwon DD, et al. The effects of a type 4 phosphodiesterase inhibitor and the muscarinic cholinergic antagonist tolterodine tartrate on detrusor overactivity in female rats with bladder outlet obstruction. BJU Int 2008; 101: 615–20.

168. Gillespie JL. Phosphodiesterase-linked inhibition of nonmicturition activity in the isolated bladder. BJU Int 2004; 93: 1325–32.

169. Giembycz MA. Life after PDE4: overcoming adverse events with dual-specificity phosphodiesterase inhibitors. Curr Opin Pharmacol 2005; 5: 238–44.

170. Morita T, Ando M, Kihara K, et al. Effects of prostaglandins E1, E2 and F2 alpha on contractility and cAMP and cGMP contents in lower urinary tract smooth muscle. Urol Int 1994; 52: 200–3.

171. Werkström V, Svensson A, Andersson KE, Hedlund P. Phosphodiesterase 5 in the female pig and human urethra: morphological and functional aspects. BJU Int 2006; 98: 414–23.

172. Sairam K, Kulinskaya E, McNicholas TA, Boustead GB, Hanbury DC. Sildenafil influences lower urinary tract symptoms. BJU Int 2002; 90: 836–9.

173. McVary KT, Roehrborn CG, Kaminetsky JC, et al. Tadalafil relieves lower urinary tract symptoms secondary to benign prostatic hyperplasia. J Urol 2007a; 177: 1401–7.

174. McVary KT, Monnig W, Camps JL Jr, et al. Sildenafil citrate improves erectile function and urinary symptoms in men with erectile dysfunction and lower urinary tract symptoms associated with benign prostatic hyperplasia: a randomized, double-blind trial. J Urol 2007b; 177: 1071–7.

175. Stief CG, Porst H, Neuser D, Beneke M, Ulbrich E. A randomised, placebo-controlled study to assess the efficacy of twice-daily vardenafil in the treatment of lower urinary tract symptoms secondary to benign prostatic hyperplasia. Eur Urol 2008; 53: 1236–44.

176. Forman A, Andersson KE, Henriksson L, et al. Effects of nifedipine on the smooth muscle of the human urinary tract in vitro and in vivo. Acta Pharmacol Toxicol 1978; 43: 111–18.

177. Ganitkevich VY, Isenberg G. Contribution of Ca(2+)-induced Ca2+ release to the [Ca2+]i transients in myocytes from guinea-pig urinary bladder. J Physiol (Lond) 1992; 458: 119–37.

178. Isenberg G, Wendt-Gallitelli MF, Ganitkevich V. Contribution of Ca(2+)-induced Ca2+ release to depolarization-induced Ca2+ transients of myocytes from guinea-pig urinary bladder myocytes. Jpn J Pharmacol 1992; 58: 81P–86P.

179. Hedlund H, Mattiasson A, Andersson K-E. Effects of pinacidil on detrusor instability in men with bladder outlet obstruction. J Urol 1991; 146: 1345–47.

180. Komersova K, Rogerson JW, Conway EL, et al. The effect of levcromakalim (BRL 38227) on bladder function in patients with high spinal cord lesions. Br J Clin Pharmacol 1995; 39: 207–9.

181. Andersson K-E. Bladder activation: afferent mechanisms. Urology 2002; 59(5 Suppl 1): 43–50.

182. Birder LA, de Groat WC. Mechanisms of disease: involvement of the urothelium in bladder dysfunction. Nat Clin Pract Urol 2007; 4: 46–54.

183. Birder LA, Kanai AJ, de Groat WC, et al. Vanilloid receptor expression suggests a sensory role for urinary bladder epithelial cells. Proc Natl Acad Sci USA 2001; 98: 13396–401.

184. Birder LA, Nakamura Y, Kiss S, et al. Altered urinary bladder function in mice lacking the vanilloid receptor TRPV1. Nat Neurosci 2002; 5: 856–60.

185. Sui GP, Rothery S, Dupont E, Fry CH, Severs NJ. Gap junctions and connexin expression in human suburothelial interstitial cells. BJU Int 2002; 90: 118–29.

186. Sui GP, Wu C, Fry CH. Electrical characteristics of suburothelial cells isolated from the human bladder. J Urol 2004; 171(2 Pt 1): 938–43.

187. Pandita RK, Andersson KE. Intravesical adenosine triphosphate stimulates the micturition reflex in awake, freely moving rats. J Urol 2002; 168: 1230–4.

188. Cockayne DA, Hamilton SG, Zhu QM, et al. Urinary bladder hyporeflexia and reduced pain-related behaviour in P2X3-deficient mice. Nature 2000; 407: 1011–15.

189. Fovaeus M, Fujiwara M, Hogestatt ED, Persson K, Andersson KE. A non-nitrergic smooth muscle relaxant factor released from rat urinary bladder by muscarinic receptor stimulation. J Urol 1999; 161: 649–53.

190. Hashitani H, Brading AF, Suzuki H. Correlation between spontaneous electrical, calcium and mechanical activity in detrusor smooth muscle of the guinea-pig bladder. Br J Pharmacol 2004; 141: 183–93.

191. Drake MJ, Mills IW, Gillespie JI. Model of peripheral autonomous modules and a myovesical plexus in normal and overactive bladder function. Lancet 2001; 358: 401–3.

192. Gillespie JI. The autonomous bladder: a view of the origin of bladder overactivity and sensory urge. BJU Int 2004; 93: 478–83.

193. Gillespie JI. A developing view of the origins of urgency: the importance of animal models. BJU Int 2005; 96(Suppl 1): 22–8.

194. Kinder RB, Mundy AR. Pathophysiology of idiopathic detrusor instability and detrusor hyper-reflexia. An in vitro study of human detrusor muscle. Br J Urol 1987; 60: 509–15.

195. Brading AF. A myogenic basis for the overactive bladder. Urology 1997; 50(6A Suppl): 57–67; discussion 68–73.

196. Mills IW, Greenland JE, McMurray G, et al. Studies of the pathophysiology of idiopathic detrusor instability: the physiological properties of the detrusor smooth muscle and its pattern of innervation. J Urol 2000; 163: 646–51.

197. Turner WH, Brading AF. Smooth muscle of the bladder in the normal and the diseased state: pathophysiology, diagnosis and treatment. Pharmacol Ther 1997; 75: 77–110.

198. Stevens LA, Chapple CR, Chess-Williams R. Human idiopathic and neurogenic overactive bladders and the role of M2 muscarinic receptors in contraction. Eur Urol 2007; 52: 531–8.

199. Wu C, Sui GP, Fry CH. Purinergic regulation of guinea pig suburothelial myofibroblasts. J Physiol 2004; 559(Pt 1): 231–43.

200. Fry CH, Sui GP, Kanai AJ, Wu C. The function of suburothelial myofibroblasts in the bladder. Neurourol Urodyn 2007; 26(6 Suppl): 914–19.

201. Ikeda Y, Kanai A. Urotheliogenic modulation of intrinsic activity in spinal cord-transected rat bladders: role of mucosal muscarinic receptors. Am J Physiol Renal Physiol 2008; 295: F454–61.

202. Sui GP, Wu C, Roosen A, et al. Modulation of bladder myofibroblast activity: implications for bladder function. Am J Physiol Renal Physiol 2008; 295: F688–97.

203. Dinis P, Charrua A, Avelino A, et al. The distribution of sensory fibers immunoreactive for the TRPV1 (capsaicin) receptor in the human prostate. Eur Urol 2005; 48: 162–7.

204. Messeguer A, Planells-Cases R, Ferrer-Montiel A. Physiology and pharmacology of the vanilloid receptor. Curr Neuropharmacol 2006; 4: 1–15.

205. Steers WD, Tuttle JB. Mechanisms of disease: the role of nerve growth factor in the pathophysiology of bladder disorders. Nat Clin Pract Urol 2006; 3: 101–10.

206. Chalfin SA, Bradley WE. The etiology of detrusor hyperreflexia in patients with infravesical obstruction. J Urol 1982; 127: 938–42.

207. Yokoyama O, Komatsu K, Kodama K, et al. Diagnostic value of intravesical lidocaine for overactive bladder. J Urol 2000; 164: 340–3.

208. Geirsson G, Fall M. Reflex interaction between the proximal urethra and the bladder. A clinical experimental study. Scand J Urol Nephrol 1999; 33: 24–6.

209. Chai TC, Gray ML, Steers WD. The incidence of a positive ice water test in bladder outlet obstructed patients: evidence for bladder neural plasticity. J Urol 1998; 160: 34–8.

210. Dinis P, Silva J, Ribeiro MJ, et al. Bladder C-fiber desensitization induces a long-lasting improvement of BPH-associated storage LUTS: a pilot study. Eur Urol 2004; 46: 88–93; discussion 93–4.

211. Kuo HC. Multiple intravesical instillation of low-dose resiniferatoxin is effective in the treatment of detrusor overactivity refractory to anticholinergics. BJU Int 2005; 95: 1023–7.

212. Silva C, Silva J, Ribeiro MJ, Avelino A, Cruz F. Urodynamic effect of intravesical resiniferatoxin in patients with neurogenic detrusor overactivity of spinal origin: results of a double-blind randomized placebo-controlled trial. Eur Urol 2005; 48: 650–5.

213. Dong M, Yeh F, Tepp WH, et al. SV2 is the protein receptor for botulinum neurotoxin A. Science 2006; 312: 592.

214. Schurch B, Schmid DM, Stöhrer M. Treatment of neurogenic incontinence with botulinum toxin A. N Engl J Med 2000a; 342: 665.

215. Schurch B, Stöhrer M, Kramer G, et al: Botulinum A toxin for treating detrusor hyperreflexia in spinal cord—injured patients: a new alternative to anticholinergic drugs? Preliminary results. J Urol 2000b; 164: 692–7.

216. Duthie J, Wilson DI, Herbison GP, Wilson D. Botulinum toxin injections for adults with overactive bladder syndrome. Cochrane Database Syst Rev 2007; 3: CD005493.

217. Karsenty G, Denys P, Amarenco G, et al. Botulinum toxin A (Botox) intradetrusor injections in adults with neurogenic detrusor overactivity/neurogenic overactive bladder: a systematic literature review. Eur Urol 2008; 53: 275.

218. Apostolidis A, Dasgupta P, Denys P, et al. Recommendations on the use of botulinum toxin in the treatment of lower urinary tract disorders and pelvic floor dysfunctions: a European Consensus Report. Eur Urol 2008. [Epub ahead of print].

219. Dykstra DD, Sidi AA. Treatment of detrusor-striated sphincter dyssynergia with botulinum A toxin. J Urol 1990; 138: 1155–60.

220. Dykstra DD, Sidi AA, Scott AB, et al. Effects of botulinum A toxin on detrusor-sphincter dyssynergia in spinal cord injury patients. J Urol 1998; 139: 919–22.

221. Schurch B, Hauri D, Rodic B, et al: Botulinum-A toxin as treatment of detrusor sphincter dyssynergia: a prospective study in 24 spinal cord injury patients. J Urol 1996; 155: 1023–9.

222. Grosse J, Kramer G, Stohrer M. Success of repeat detrusor injections of botulinum a toxin in patients with severe neurogenic detrusor overactivity and incontinence. Eur Urol 2005; 47: 653–9.

223. Karsenty G, Reitz A, Lindemann G, Boy S, Schurch B. Persistence of therapeutic effect After repeated injections of botulinum toxin type A to treat incontinence due to neurogenic detrusor overactivity. Urology 2006; 68: 1193–7.

224. Giannantoni A, Mearini E, Del Zingaro M, Porena M. Six-year follow-up of botulinum toxin A intradetrusorial injections in patients with refractory neurogenic detrusor overactivity: clinical and urodynamic results. Eur Urol 2008. [Epub ahead of print].

225. Kalsi V, Apostolidis A, Popat R, et al. Quality of life changes in patients with neurogenic versus idiopathic detrusor overactivity after intradetrusor injections of botulinum neurotoxin type A and correlations with lower urinary tract symptoms and urodynamic changes. Eur Urol 2006; 49: 528–35.

226. Schurch B, Denys P, Kozma CM, et al. Botulinum toxin A improves the quality of life of patients with neurogenic urinary incontinence. Eur Urol 2007; 52: 850–8.

227. Shaban AM, Drake MJ. Botulinum toxin treatment for overactive bladder: risk of urinary retention. Curr Urol Rep 2008; 9: 445–51.

228. De Laet K, Wyndaele JJ. Adverse events after botulinum A toxin injection for neurogenic voiding disorders. Spinal Cord 2005; 43: 397–9.

229. Dmochowski R, Sand PK. Botulinum toxin A in the overactive bladder: current status and future directions. BJU Int 2007; 99: 247–62.

25 Classification of Lower Urinary Tract Dysfunction in the Female Patient
David R Staskin and Alan J Wein

INTRODUCTION
Devising a Classification System
The purpose of a classification system is communication. The value of grouping and interrelating concepts and facts into an organizational structure can be measured by the ability of the final product to provide a logical framework for introducing new theories, scientific findings, and clinical observations into the existing knowledge. In addition, the system should act as a useful clinical tool for diagnosing and treating disease. Rather than create new areas of contention, a classification system that is proposed for general use should ideally incorporate ideas and resolve conflicts. The attempt to devise an all inclusive system that completely describes lower urinary tract (LUT) function and dysfunction and the decision to adopt this single classification system would certainly be ideal, but is confounded by difficulties in agreement concerning construct and the standardization of terminology.

Complex interrelationships create difficulty in maintaining the simplicity of such systems. Filling (storage) and voiding (emptying) dysfunction may be classified by multiple methods. Classification can be done by symptoms (patient interview eliciting LUT symptoms), the precipitating LUT activity from those symptoms and the anticipated condition as in Table 25.1; by bladder activity or outlet activity (overactive or underactive) as in Table 25.2; by neurological activity (neurogenic) as in Table 25.3; by objective LUT testing (urodynamic studies) as in Table 25.4; or descriptively in a more complex system which combines the aspects of structure (anatomy) function (physiology), disease states (clinical diagnosis and the expected effect on LUT function), and observed LUT behavior (LUT dysfunction associated with a specific lesion or disease) as in Table 25.5.

The standardization of terminology is vital to insure that the meaning of a "common language" employed by the users of the system reflects the same symptoms and signs and methods and measurements. The reader is directed to the ICS Standardization of Terminology (Appendices I–V) for a review of ICS "standards" (1–5). As with classification systems that must undergo constant evolution, the ICS terminology has been revised and terms have been added, modified, and even subtracted without substitution (6,7). When devising and presenting these classification systems, ICS terminology has been has been generally been preserved, but the reader will note some differences between the ICS terms and the utilization of descriptors in the expanded descriptive classification (e.g., "sensory" terminology) included in Table 25.5.

The following classification systems are oriented to LUT symptoms with or without incontinence. In the case of incontinence the presumption is that the "wetness" experienced by the patient is urine and that the source of egress is the urethra. The clinical assessment should rule out wetness secondary to perspiration, inflammation or discharge, or from vaginal and/or rectal sources. For example, specific to the differential diagnosis of "wetness" is the importance of ruling out vesicovaginal or uretero-vaginal fistula. The extended-descriptive classification attempts to provide a complex but illustrative functional model.

This chapter does not include an in depth review of LUT pathophysiology, diagnosis, or therapy, but these are reviewed exhaustively elsewhere within this textbook. In addition, this chapter is not intended to be a review of the historical development of the various methods of classification, although prior historical models are selectively referenced. However, the readers are strongly encouraged to utilize these models to "organize their thoughts" and facilitate the development of a logical approach to care.

Proposing Simple and more Complex Classification Systems: Symptomatic and Functional Classifications
A symptomatic classification system is presented in Table 25.1. It is based on the concept that symptoms may suggest inclusively the underlying abnormal activity, pathophysiology, and condition. Since the patient's symptoms may be extremely useful or misleading due to overlapping findings in LUT conditions (8–10), an illustrative differential diagnosis of common conditions is also presented.

A classification system that is specifically oriented towards the description of LUT function and activity should divide the LUT into its two anatomical areas—the "bladder" (detrusor) and "bladder outlet" (sphincter) during the physiological functions of "storage" (filling) and "emptying" (voiding). A simple functional classification is presented in Table 25.2. The bladder or outlet activity is described as "overactive," "normal," or "underactive." An OAB represents an unwanted increase in detrusor activity ("pressure"–episode(s) of undesired contractility or a decrease in bladder compliance or the "sensation of filing"–an increase in afferent acitivty) during urinary storage, an underactive bladder represents insufficient detrusor activity/pressure during bladder emptying (absent or poorly sustained contraction). An overactive outlet describes increased activity or resistance/obstruction during emptying (anatomic blockage, deficient voluntary sphincter coordination, neurogenic sphincter dyssynergia), and an underactive outlet represents insufficient activity/resistance during storage (inadequate intrinsic function or altered anatomical support relationships). These abnormalities in function/activity can occur alone, or in combination (11–17).

The classification of neurogenic voiding dysfunction may also be adapted to a similar functional system based

Table 25.1 Classification by Symptoms

Stress urinary incontinence (SUI)

- *Symptom*—the involuntary loss of urine on effort or exertion (lift, strain, cough, sneeze).
- *Activity*—underactive outlet.
- *Condition*—urodynamic stress incontinence—the involuntary loss of urine resulting from an increase in intra-abdominal pressure which overcomes the resistance of the bladder outlet in the absence of a true bladder contraction. The decrease in bladder outlet or urethral resistance may result from poor anatomical support of the bladder neck (urethral hypermobility/SUI-A) or a loss of urethral function (intrinsic sphincter deficiency SUI-ISD) or, most commonly a mixture.
- *Clinical confusion*—the patient describes the symptom of urinary loss with "activity" but the etiology of involuntary leakage is actually an uninhibited bladder contraction–SUI should have urinary loss synchronous with "effort"; similarly, many patients will describe SUI as a sensation, which is confused with "urgency"; finally, stress and urgency incontinence may coexist.

Urgency urinary incontinence (UUI)

- *Symptom*—the loss of urine with the sensation of urgency, voiding before the ability to toilet.
- *Activity*— overactive bladder (OAB-wet)–detrusor overactivity.
- *Condition*—Urinary urgency incontinence (urodynamic)–the involuntary loss of urine resulting from an increase in bladder pressure secondary to detrusor overactivity (an uninhibited bladder contraction or unstable bladder). Detrusor overactivity may be the result of a suprasacral spinal or intracranial neurological lesion that results in uncontrolled reflex contractions (detrusor hyperreflexia) or may be idiopathic. Patients may demonstrate other symptoms associated with "urgency" (frequency, urgency, nocturia) without urinary loss (OAB-dry).
- *Clinical confusion*—the patient has decreased sensation, and loses urine from motor activity of the detrusor without the feeling of "urgency". OAB is a syndrome consisting of the symptoms "urgency, with or without urgency incontinence, usually with frequency and nocturia" suggestive of urodynamic bladder overactivity but inclusive of "urgency and frequency without incontinence" OAB-dry (vida infra) or the sensation of urgency (desire to void in the absence of a detectable rise in detrusor pressure–sensory urgency).

Mixed urinary incontinence

- *Symptom*—mixed symptoms of UUI and SUI, urinary loss with effort and with urgency.
- *Activity*—OAB-wet detrusor overactivity and underactive sphincter.
- *Condition*—a mixture of the conditions described above as SUI and UUI.
- *Clinical Confusion*—urinary loss may be from SUI or UUI but the predominance and bother resulting from one condition or the other may not be discernable from the history and physical exam alone, thus creating difficulty in choosing treatment for the "primary" symptom.

Urgency and frequency without incontinence

- *Symptom*—urgency and frequency without urinary loss.
- *Activity*—detrusor overactivity with compensatory sphincter activity or no detrusor activity or abnormal afferent activity or processing (sensory).
- *Condition*—Urgency is the complaint of a sudden compelling desire to pass urine which is difficult to defer, and frequency is the complaint by the patient who considers that she voids too often by day or at night (going to bed and arising), whereas nocturia is waking at night one or more times to void preceded by and followed by sleep). "Sensory urgency" a term which has been removed from the ICS lexicon, and was used to describe the sensation of urinary urgency without a detectable rise in detrusor pressure.
- *Clinical confusion*—the classification of a moderate or strong "desire to void" without true "urgency" is unresolved. "Sensory urgency–desire to void" is not in the current ICS lexicon.

Overflow incontinence

- *Symptom*—the involuntary loss of urine resulting from urinary retention with bladder overdistention. The retention (failure to empty) may result from inadequate bladder contractility or outlet obstruction (or both).
- *Activity*—underactive bladder (retention)/overactive outlet (obstruction).
- *Condition*—Urinary loss occurs when the intravesical pressure overcomes the urethral resistance as a result of bladder contractility, increases in intra-abdominal pressure and/or urethral relaxation.
- *Clinical confusion*—the symptoms that are described may be a mixture of stress (SUI) and urgency (OAB) complaints.

Altered bladder sensation and pain

- *Symptom*—frequent voiding with or without pain–conversely a loss of sensation.
- *Activity*—no detrusor contraction/alteration in afferent input or processing.
- *Condition*—Bladder pain, discomfort, and pressure can be characterized by type, frequency, duration, location, and precipitating and relieving factors. Bladder sensation can be described as increased, normal, reduced, absent, or non-specific (neurologic). Increased or decreased voiding may be correlated with the sensation.
- *Clinical confusion*—Urinary urgency and frequency without incontinence may be a product of abnormal sensation or bladder contractile activity. The source of pelvic pain may not be the lower urinary tract. Interstitial cystitis or chronic urethritis remain diagnoses of exclusion.

Functional incontinence

- *Symptom*—the involuntary loss of urine resulting from a deficit in the ability to perform toileting functions secondary to physical or mental limitations.
- *Activity*—abnormal lower urinary tract function usually co-exists with functional issues.
- *Clinical confusion*—the underlying pathophysiology of stress, urge or overflow incontinence may coexist, as well as difficulty in eliciting an accurate history. The patient's primary "functional" issue may be dementia, delirium, or other forms of altered cognition; physical disability preventing easy and rapid toilet access. These conditions often exist alone or in combination with lower urinary tract dysfunction.

on the nature of the lesion, the expected behavior of detrusor and sphincter, and similarly can be correlated with symptoms as in Table 25.3 (18–23). The neurological terms of detrusor hyperreflexia, normoreflexia, and areflexia, and the outlet descriptive of dyssynergic, normal, or denervated are utilized and correlate with the type of function/activity.

The interrelationship between the LUT and the outlet, including the pelvic floor, requires a classification system that recognizes the individual contributions and the combined effects of the efferent systems (anatomy and function/acitvity), and the afferent systems from the bladder musculature and mucosa, the bladder neck, urethral mechanisms, and the pelvic floor structures (24–29). It is simplistic to combine the effects of the bladder musculature and mucosa, the outlet-sphincter, and the levator complex on bladder activity without acknowledging the complex integration and interrelationship of these areas on LUT behavior. In addition, combining them into one functional area should not limit investigation into their individual contributions. The complex interrelationship of the bladder outlet and pelvic floor structures with voiding behavior are apparent in several common clinical conditions. For example, in the case of "urodynamic stress incontinence" or stress urinary incontinence (SUI), the ability to preserve or augment urethral basal tone, urethral sphincter function and anatomical support from levator anatomy or contraction is critical for understanding the ability to maintain continence during "effort" (30–37). Conversely, the initiation of voiding requires both pelvic floor and urethral sphincter relaxation in the absence of anatomical obstruction

(23–28). Conversely, symptoms of decreased emptying or urinary retention may result from the inhibition of detrusor contractility, secondary to increased pelvic floor or sphincter afferents, decreased afferent detrusor muscular or mucosal input, or by voluntary contraction of the striated sphincter (psuedo-dyssynergia) during voiding. Similarly, an understanding of urgency incontinence and OAB syndrome symptoms require an appreciation of the relationship between afferent and efferent neurological pathways to the LUT the bladder neck, and the pelvic floor on the detrusor, although definitive reflex arcs in the human may not have been identified (38–43).

Table 25.4 **Classification by Urodynamics (Bladder and Outlet)**

	Storage	Emptying
Bladder	[a]Cystometrogram–F [b]DLPP	[f]Cystometrogram–V [g]Pdet-flow [h]Residual urine
Outlet	[c]UPP [d]VLPP [e]Fluoroscopy	[i]Pdet-flow [j]EMG [k]MUPP [l]Fluoroscopy [m]Residual urine

[a]Filling cystometrogram (filling pressure)
[b]Detrusor leak point pressure (bladder compliance)
[c]Urethral pressure profile (urethral closure)
[d]Valsalva leak point pressure (pressure to leak)
[e]Fluoroscopy (anatomy of outlet closure mechanism)
[f]Voiding cystometrogram (emptying pressure)
[g]Pressure flow (detrusor contractility/flow/calculated resistance)
[h]Residual urine (after void)
[i]-Pressure flow (detrusor contractility/flow/calculated resistance)
[j]Electromyography (striated sphincter activity)
[k]Micturition urethral pressure profile (localized urethral pressure)
[l]Fluoroscopy (anatomy of outlet opening)
[m]Residual urine (after void).
Source: Adapted from Ref. 17.

Table 25.2 **Classification by Bladder and Outlet Activity***

Bladder	Outlet
Overactive (urgency)	Overactive (obstruction)
Normoactive	Normoactive
Underactive (retention)	Underactive (stress incontinence)

*Symptoms in parentheses.

Table 25.3 **Classification by Neurological Activity**

(a) *Neurogenic classification**

Bladder/detrusor	Outlet/sphincter
Hyperreflexic (overactive—*urgency*)	Uncoordinated (overactive—*obstruction*)
	Coordinated
Normoreflexic	Denervated (underactive—*stress inc.*)
Areflexic (underactive—*retention*)	

(b) *Expected behavior of the bladder, internal sphincter, and external sphincter based on location of the lesion*

	Bladder	Internal (smooth muscle) sphincter	External (skeletal) sphincter
Peripheral	Hypo-areflexic, underactive	Dernevated (+/–)	Denervated (+/–)
Infrasacral	Areflexic, underactive	Innervated	Denervated, underactive
Spinal	Hyperreflexic, overactive	Uncoordinated if T6 or above	Dyssynergic, overactive
Suprapontine	Hyperreflexic	Coordinated	Coordinated

*Underlining denotes function; italic type denotes symptoms.
Source: Adapted from Refs. 22 and 23.

Table 25.5 Expanded Functional Classification of Voiding Dysfunction Including Bladder Afferents and Pelvic Floor Activity

I. Outlet dysfunction: bladder outlet and pelvic floor

A. *Underactive outlet (decreased urethral resistance)*

Symptomatic: SUI

1. Anatomical support defects (SUI-A) (types I and II SUI):Pathophysiology: anatomical motion creates inequities in transmission pressures to bladder and outlet, overcoming urethral resistance, and/or and conformational changes caused by vaginal wall motion disrupt outlet integrity.
    (a) Anatomical defects of fascia, muscles, ligaments, and bony pelvis.
    (b) Functioning support: muscular contraction—denervation or loss of identification, strength or coordination of levator musculature.
    (c) A degree of ISD (see 2) that in combination with SUI-A I or II contributes to critical decreases in resistance during effort to permit urinary leakage.
2. ISD (SUI-ISD) (type III) (LUCP)
   Pathophysiology: deficiency of the urethral closure mechanism secondary to decreased innervation, vascularization or trauma to mucosa, submucosa or smooth, non-striated skeletal or skeletal musculature of urethra–intrinsic deficiency of the closure mechanism.
    (a) Proximal urethral sphincter: bladder neck (smooth muscle) and proximal urethra (SUI-ISD-p).
    (b) External sphincter: denervation or loss of resting tone, voluntary or reflex contraction (SUI-ISD-d).
    (c) Combined or total proximal and external sphincter deficiency (SUI-ISD-t).
3. Combined SUI (SUI-A-ISD)
   Pathophysiology: a degree of both anatomical motion and sphincter dysfunction.
    (a) Leakage from ISD may exist without hypermobility.
    (b) Hypermobility alone without a degree of ISD is not be sufficient to result in urinary loss.
4. *Failure to inhibit the detrusor: decreased pelvic floor inhibitory activity of bladder (etiology for OAB–see C).*
   Pathophysiology: failure to contract pelvic floor releases detrusor reflex and decreases ability to inhibit active contraction.
    (a) Neurological: (infrasacral) denervation (areflexia of pelvic floor).
    (b) Behavioral: failure to contract pelvic floor (lack of identification/strength/coordination).
    (c) Mechanical: damage to pelvic floor structures with intact innervation.

B. *Overactive outlet (increased urethral resistance)*

Symptomatic: overflow incontinence/retention; frequency–urgency.

1. Anatomical obstruction (physical blockage)Pathophysiology: increased outlet resistance secondary to compression or narrowing.
    (a) Iatrogenic: surgical (e.g., for urinary incontinence).
    (b) Other: congenital, inflammatory, neoplastic, traumatic.
2. Functional obstruction (failure of relaxation)
   Pathophysiology: increased outlet resistance–inappropriate contraction or failure of normal relaxation.
    (a) Neurogenic: detrusor sphincter dyssynergia (skeletal musculature).
    (b) Behavioral: failure to relax pelvic floor musculature or external sphincter.
3. Combined anatomical and functional obstruction
4. *Inhibition of detrusor activity: increased pelvic floor activity*
   Pathophysiology: failure to relax pelvic floor inhibits initiation of detrusor activity and inhibits ability to develop or continue a sustained detrusor contraction.
    (a) Neurological: (suprasacral) overactivity/hyperreflexia (dyssynergic pelvic floor activity).
    (b) Behavioral: failure to relax pelvic floor (learned, acquired, maladaptive, psychogenic).
    (c) Situational: "voluntary" inhibition secondary to environment or pain.

II. Bladder dysfunction

A. *Detrusor overacitivity (increased intravesical pressure)*

Symptomatic: urgency incontinence (with or without sensation)– (OAB) wet (OAB-wet).

1. Involuntary detrusor contractions: detrusor overacitivty (motor urgency).Pathophysiology: increased detrusor (intravesical) pressure overcomes urethral resistance or causes sensation of urinary urgency.
    (a) Detrusor overactivity (DO):primary = idiopathic, subclinical neurological, or symptomatic phasic detrusor activity; secondary = obstruction, reflex urethral relaxation, increased detrusor/mucosal afferent activity.(OAB)-urgency, with (OAB-wet) or without (OAB-dry) incontinence, usually with frequency and nocturia (absence of other pathology).
    (b) Detrusor overacitvity (hyperreflexia):suprapontine (intracranial) neurological lesion (with or without sphincter control); spinal (suprascral) neurological lesion (with or without sphincteric dyssynergia).
2. Decreased compliance
   Pathophysiology: increased intravesical pressure secondary to decreased accommodation of detrusor.
    (a) Fibrosis: radiation, inflammation, immune response.
    (b) Neurological: loss/reversal of accommodation refle—conus medullaris or peripheral.
3. Combined detrusor contractions and decreased compliance
4. *Pelvic floor underactivity (see I.A.4 above– decrease pelvic floor inhibition*

(Continued)

Table 25.5 Expanded Functional Classification of Voiding Dysfunction Including Bladder Afferents and Pelvic Floor Activity (*Continued*)

B. *Underactive bladder (decreased intravescial pressure)*
Symptomatic: overflow incontinence/retention

    1. Peripheral denervation or neuropathy.Pathophysiology: decreased contractility-neural efferent or myogenic/decreased afferent stimulation.
        (a) Congenital, inflammatory, neoplastic or trauma lesion to peripheral nerves.
        (b) Diabetes or other metabolic cause.
    2. Detrusor myopathy
        Pathophysiology: decreased contractility secondary to smooth muscle damage.
        (a) Fibrosis/collagen deposition.
        (b) Inflammation/obstruction/overdistension.
    3. Pharmacological inhibition
        Pathophysiology: decreased contractility secondary to receptor blockade of neural efferents or afferents.
        (a) Antimuscarinics.
        (b) Smooth muscle relaxants/spasmolytics/membrane stabilizers.
    4. *Pelvic floor overactivity (see I.B.4 above)*

III. Combined outlet and bladder dysfunction (I and II)

IV. Disorders of sensation

A. *Decreased sensation*

    1. Decreased bladder sensationPathophysiology: denervation, myopathy, behavioral, pharmacological.
        (a) Decreased sense of fullness and normal urge response.
        (b) Loss of sense of fullness/urge warning only with active contraction.
        (c) Loss of sense of fullness/urge incontinence without appreciation of "desire to void".
        (d) Urinary retention without appreciation of distension.
    2. Decreased bladder outlet and pelvic floor sensation
        Pathophysiology: denervation, myopathy, behavioral, pharmacological causing decreased ability to identify/contract/coordinate.
        (a) Bladder overactivity (I.A.4): failure to inhibit?
        (b) Bladder underactivity (myogenic or mucosal) (II.B.4): failure to initiate?
        (c) Contributory to decreased bladder sensation? (IV.A.1.a–d).
        (d) Sexual dysfunction—anorgasmia.

B. *Increased sensation*

    1. Increased sensation of the bladder/bladder outletPathophysiology: neuropathic, inflammatory, mucosal permeability defect, psychogenic, afferent amplification.
        (a) Frequency–urgency symptoms.
        (b) Suprapubic and pelvic pain syndromes.
    2. *Increased sensation of the pelvic floor/bladder outlet*
        Pathophysiology: neuromuscular myalgia, neuropathic, inflammatory, psychogenic.
        (a) Levator myalgia.
        (b) Frequency–urgency and pelvic pain syndromes.
    3. Combined deficit

Abbreviations: LUCP = low urethral closure pressure; ISD = intrinsic sphincter deficiency; OAB = overactive bladder; *Pelvic floor activity–in italics*; SUI = stress urinary incontinence.

EXPANDED CLASSIFICATION OF VOIDING DYSFUNCTION–INCLUDING PELVIC FLOOR ACTIVITY

Outlet Dysfunction: Bladder Outlet and Pelvic Floor

The underactive outlet–The bladder outlet (sphincteric mechanism) is responsible for "outlet resistance" during urinary storage. The bladder outlet remains closed at rest. Resistance to leakage is provided by the intrinsic closure pressure along the length of the urethra. The urethra can be divided into two functional areas: these are (a) the "proximal" sphincteric mechanism—a product of mucosa, submucosa, and smooth muscle incorporating the bladder neck and proximal urethra—and (b) the distal mechanism or "external" sphincteric mechanism located in the middle of the "anatomical urethra" and intimately related anatomically and physiologically to the levator ani complex. Anatomical support facilitates transmission of intra-abdominal pressure to both areas and is provided by both the anterior vaginal wall and its attachments to the pelvis, and by the constant tone (slow-twitch fibers). Active contraction (fast-twitch fibers) of the levator complex can increase this support, but is usually seen only after pelvic muscle training, and is not a "normal" reflex.

SUI is the involuntary loss of urine per urethra—which occurs when intravesical pressure overcomes the urethral resistance owing to an increase in intra-abdominal pressure in the absence of a true bladder contraction. Urethral closure pressure is maintained by preserving or augmenting anatomical support and by increasing the intrinsic activity of the external sphincter complex. The preservation or enhancement of the anatomical backboard facilitates pressure transmission in the proximal and distal sphincteric mechanism, and preserves the anatomical relationships of the sphincteric components to maintain or increase closure pressure. Proper anatomical support provides an obvious mechanical advantage and, just as importantly, allows efficient action of the individual structures. Type I or type II SUI is classified as "poor anatomical support," associated with bladder-neck and urethral motion. However, an understanding of the contribution of pelvic floor activity and dysfunction allows one to appreciate that the etiology of urinary leakage is probably multi-factorial. Classically, an important event in maintaining continence is the preservation of intra-abdominal pressure transmission to the bladder neck and proximal urethra with respect to the bladder during stress maneuvers. In addition, inhibiting the rotational motion of the urethra prevents a relative differential in the movement of the posterior urethra with relation to the anterior urethra, and the development of a shearing force between the anterior and posterior urethral walls which decreases urethral coaptation and compression. The most fixed point, and the area of maximal pressure transmission during increases in intra-abdominal pressure, is the external sphincter—levator complex in the mid-anatomical urethra. Transmission forces as well as active sphincteric contraction provide urethral resistance during stress maneuvers.

The combination of defects at many levels of the sphincteric mechanism may combine to decrease urethral resistance. Type III SUI, intrinsic sphincter deficiency or low urethral closure pressure, describe a deficiency in any of the intrinsic urethral functions through atrophy, denervation, devascularization, or scarring, as detailed above. The degree of pudendal nerve denervation during childbirth may contribute to deficiencies in anatomical support both by affecting levator support and by decreasing intrinsic sphincter function.

It is reasonable to assume that the complex etiology of SUI is a mixture of anatomical support abnormalities and intrinsic sphincter abnormalities. The pathophysiology is related to the relative loss of mechanical (ligament) support of functioning (innervated) intrinsic (urethral) and extrinsic musculature (slow- and fast-twitch fibers of the levator complex). Therapy may be directed at correcting the defect, or compensating for the deficiency, by increasing the function of another component that contributes to urethral resistance. In fact, the most common operation for SUI is a mid-urethral sling. The mechanism of action has been described as a "kinking" or "backboard" effect which in fact does not correct the common finding of bladder neck hypermobility but does increase urethral resistance to leakage and compensate for defects in anatomical support and intrinsic urethral deficiency.

The overactive outlet–Failure to empty the bladder may be due to elevated outlet resistance or to impaired contractility of the bladder. The most commonly observed clinical etiology of elevated outlet resistance is iatrogenic, obstruction following incontinence surgery. Other forms of anatomic urethral

obstruction are less common. Neurogenic outlet obstruction, commonly seen following injury to the suprasacral spinal cord, is due to a loss of coordination between the bladder and sphincter (detrusor sphincter dyssynergia). The paradoxical failure of the outlet to relax during voiding may result in anatomical obstruction to flow or to inhibition of the initiation or completion of the detrusor contraction. Contraction of the pelvic floor or sphincter is a normal response for bladder inhibition, but when pathological may be classified as psuedo-dyssynergia (voluntary or behavioral) or true dyssynergia (neurogenic). The relaxation of the urethral sphincter during voiding and dyssynergic activity in spinal cord injury has been documented. It is not known whether the specific anatomical areas of the urethra or pelvic floor (sphincter urethra, compressor urethra, urethrovaginal sphincter, bulbocavernosus, anal sphincter, levator complex) act in unison, individually, or at all in detrusor inhibition in normal subjects.

The OAB–The symptoms of OAB syndrome are urgency, with or without urge incontinence, usually with frequency and nocturia. Multiple etiologies have been proposed, including reduced suprapontine inhibition, damaged axonal paths in spinal cord, increased LUT afferent input, loss of peripheral inhibition, and enhancement of excitatory neurotransmission in the micturition reflex pathway. Therefore, the central and peripheral nervous systems mediate bladder control through complex voluntary pathways and reflex arcs. Central efferent control of the bladder smooth musculature is mediated by afferent activity from the detrusor musculature and bladder mucosa (facilatory) and the reflex and voluntary contractions of the pelvic floor and sphincter musculature (inhibitory).

The underactive bladder–During the initial phase of bladder emptying, the pelvic floor and external sphincter relax in order to decrease urethral resistance and facilitate low pressure flow. In addition, this relaxation decreases the reflex inhibition of bladder contractility. Relaxation is followed by a detrusor contraction, which continues until voiding is completed. When emptying failure is secondary to bladder dysfunction, it may be a result of either detrusor smooth muscle pathology or insufficient neural stimulation of the detrusor. Insufficient neural stimulation may occur at the neuromuscular level (pharmacological), with nerve impairment (neuropathy), or with alterations in central control of micturition (conus medullaris, spinal column, or brain). The impairment of detrusor contractility by the absence of pelvic floor relaxation is evident in spinal cord disease (failure to empty following adequate sphincterotomy in the spinal cord patient due to incomplete detrusor contractions) and Parkinsonism (failure to empty secondary to pelvic floor bradykinesia).

Mixed-Combined disorders–Disorders of the bladder and outlet during storage and emptying may occur alone and in combination. The most common in the female patient is underactive outlet (SUI) and OAB. In addition, in the elderly female or in patients with neurological disease may demonstrate detrusor overactivity (hyperreflexia) with impaired contractility (poorly sustained contraction).

Sensory disorders–Afferent neurons from the bladder and urethra are of major importance during both the storage and emptying phases, both initiating the voiding reflex and sustaining the voiding drive during bladder emptying. Somatic activity may inhibit the emptying reflex by voluntary contraction of the external sphincter or pelvic floor—and although not established in humans, may provide inhibitory activity during bladder filling. Traditional classification systems have focused on motor rather than sensory activity. Disorders of bladder and bladder outlet sensation may result from central or peripheral denervation, from psychological causes, or from pharmacological agents such as pain medications. The role of decreased sensation in the function of the pelvic floor and the interaction between the pelvic floor and bladder with relation to the sensory pathway on the micturition reflexes await further investigation. The pudendal nerve is responsible for the innervation of pelvic floor structures as well as of the genital skin, urethral mucosa, and anal canal. Proprioceptive information of the periurethral musculature and sensory innervation of the levator ani muscles are also mediated by the pudendal branches. Increased sensation or pain attributed to the bladder is a major clinical challenge.

The symptoms of urinary frequency, urgency and suprapubic pressure often result in diagnostic evaluations and therapy for bladder disorders, even in the absence of definitive findings of mucosal or smooth muscle abnormality. Pain that may originate from fascial, muscular, or neurological etiologies within the pelvic floor should be included in the differential diagnosis of the patient with urethral or bladder syndromes. In addition, pelvic floor or bladder pain and OAB should not be considered mutually exclusive in spite of the fact that each is usually exclusion criteria when studying the other during studies involving pharmacotherapy.

Summary–The classification of voiding dysfunction has been presented with the major focus incorporating the division of the LUT into the bladder and the bladder outlet and the "activity" during storage/filling and emptying/voiding. These systems can be clearly illustrated with the functional areas of the bladder and outlet on the vertical and axis the functions of filling/storage and voiding/emptying on the horizontal. These graphic representations can be utilized to correlate functional anatomy, LUT function, urodynamic testing, etiology, and therapy.

Classification systems will continue to evolve as our understanding of LUT functions expands and our understanding of the complex interactions of storage/filling and emptying, efferent/motor and afferent/sensory, bladder and outlet, LUT and surrounding pelvic floor structures must assimilate this knowledge into the categorical constructs. The reader is encouraged to incorporate these systems into their own clinical algorithms and critique and modify them based on additional evidence or "opinion."

REFERENCES

1. Bates P, Bradley WE, Glen E, et al. The standardization of terminology of lower urinary tract function. Eur Urol 1976; 2: 274–6.
2. Abrams P, Blaivas JG, Stanton S, Andersen JT. ICS standardisation of terminology of lower urinary tract function. Scand J Urol Nephrol 1988; Supp 114: 5–19.
3. Abrams P, Blaivas JG, Stanton SL, Andersen J. ICS 6th report on the standardisation of terminology of lower urinary tract function. Neurourol Urodyn 1992; 11: 593–603.
4. Stohrer M, Goepel M, Kondo A, et al. ICS report on the standardisation of terminology in neurogenic lower urinary tract dysfunction. Neurourol Urodyn 1999; 18: 139–58.
5. Abrams P, Cardozo L, Fall M, et al. Standardisation Sub-committee of the International Continence Society. The standardisation of terminology of lower urinary tract function: report from the standardisation sub-committee of the international continence society. Neurourol Urodyn 2002; 21: 167–78.
6. Sand P, Dmochowski R. Analysis of the standardisation of terminology of lower urinary tract dysfunction: Report from the Standardisation Sub-Committee of the International Continence Society. Neurourol Urodyn 2002; 21: 167–78.
7. Homma Y. Lower urinary tract symptomatology: its definition and confusion. Int J Urol 2008; 15: 35–43.
8. Bergman A, Bader K. Reliability of the patient's history in the diagnosis of urinary incontinence. Int J Gyneacol Obstet 1990; 32: 255.
9. Versi E, Cardozo L, Anand D, Cooper D. Symptoms analysis for the diagnosis of genuine stress incontinence. Br J Obstet Gynaecol 1991; 98: 815.
10. Holroyd-Leduc J, Tannenbaum C, Thorpe H, et al. What type of urinary incontinence does this woman have? JAMA 2008; 299: 1446–56.
11. Wein AJ. Classification of neurogenic voiding dysfunction. J Urol 1981; 125: 605.
12. Staskin DR, Wein AJ, Andersson KE. Urinary incontinence: classification and pharmacological therapy. Ciba Found Symp 1990; 151: 289–306; discussion 306–17.
13. Wein AJ. Pathophysiology and categorization of voiding dysfunction. In: Walsh PC, Retik AB, Vaughn ED Jr., eds. Campbell's Urology, 8th edn. Philadelphia: Elsevier Science (Saunders), 1998: 917–26.
14. Staskin DR. Classification of voiding dysfunction. In: Cardozo and Staskin, eds. Textbook of Female Urology and Urogynecology, 1st edn. London UK: Isis Medical Media, 2001: 83–90.
15. Wein AJ. Pathophysiology and categorization of voiding dysfunction. In: Walsh PC, Retik AB, Vaughn ED Jr., eds. Campbell's Urology, 8th edn. Philadelphia: Elsevier Science (Saunders), 2002: 887–99.
16. Staskin DR, Wein AJ. Classification of voiding dysfunction in the female patient. In: Cardozo and Staskin, eds. Textbook of Female Urology and Urogynecology, 2nd edn. UK: Informa Healthcare Oxon, 2006: 173–84.
17. Wein AJ. Pathophysiology and classification of voiding dysfunction. In: Wein AJ, Kavoussi LR, Novick AC, Partin AW, Peters CA, eds. Campbell-Walsh Urology, 9th edn. Philadelphia: Elsevier Science (Saunders), 2007: 1973–85.
18. Lapides J. Neuromuscular, vesical and uretreral dysfunction. In: Campbell MF, Harrison JGH, eds. Urology. Philadelphia: WB Saunders, 1970: 1343–279.
19. Hald T, Bradley WE. The Urinary Bladder: Neurology and Dynamics, Baltimore: Williams and Wilkins, 1982: 278–88.
20. Krane RJ, Siroky MB. Classification of voiding dysfunction: Value of classification systems. In: Barrett and Wein, eds. Controversies in Neuro-Urology. New York: Churchill Livingston, 1984: 223–38.
21. de Groat WC. A neurologic basis for the overactive bladder. Urology 1997; 50(Suppl 6A): 36–52.
22. Krane RJ, Siroky MB. Classification of neuro-urologic disorders. In: Krane and Siroky, eds. Clinical Neuro-Urology. Boston: Little Brown, 1979: 419–21.
23. Staskin D. Classification of voiding dysfunction. In: Krane R, Siroky MB, eds. Clinical Neurourology, 2nd edn. Boston: Little Brown, 1991: 411–26.
24. Haeusler G, Sam C, Chiari A, Tempfer C, Hanzal E, Koelbl H. Effect of spinal anaesthesia on the lower urinary tract in continent women. Br J Obstet Gynaecol 1998; 105: 103–6.
25. Bo K, Stien R. Pelvic floor muscle function and urethral closure mechanism in young nullipara subjects with and without stress incontinence symptoms. Neurourol Urodyn 1994; 13: 35–41.
26. Deindl F, Vodusek DB, Hesse U, Schussler B. Activity patterns of pubococcygeal muscles in nulliparous continent women. A kinesiological EMG study. Brit J Urol 1994; 73: 413.
27. Gunnarsson M, Mattiasson A. Female stress, urge, and mixed urinary incontinence are associated with a chronic and progressive pelvic floor/vaginal neuromuscular disorder: An investigation of 317 healthy and incontinent women using vaginal surface electromyography. Neurourol Urodyn 1999; 18: 613–21.
28. Bø K. Pelvic floor muscle training is effective in treatment of female stress urinary incontinence, but how does it work? Int Urogynecol J Pelvic Floor Dysfunct 2004; 15: 76–84. Review

29. Messelink B, Benson T, Berghmans B, et al. Standardization of terminology of pelvic floor muscle function and dysfunction: report from the pelvic floor clinical assessment group of the International Continence Society. Neurourol Urodyn 2005; 24: 374–80.

30. Enhorning G. Simultaneous recording of intravesical and intraurethral pressure. Acta Chir Scand 1961: 276(Suppl): 1–68.

31. Petros PE, Ulmsten UI. An integral theory and its method for the diagnosis and management of female urinary incontinence. Scand J Urol Nephrol Suppl 1993; 153: 1–93.

32. Papa Petros PE, Ulmsten U. An anatomical classification–a new paradigm for management of urinary dysfunction in the female. Int Urogynecol J Pelvic Floor Dysfunct 1999; 10: 29–35.

33. Staskin DR, Zimmern PE, Hadley HR, Raz S. The pathophysiology of stress incontinence. Urol Clin North Am 1985; 12: 271–8.

34. Constantinou CE. Resting and stress urethral pressures as a clinical guide to the mechanism of continence in the female patient. Urol Clin North Am 1985; 12: 247–58.

35. DeLancey JO. Structural support of the urethra as it relates to stress urinary incontinence: the hammock hypothesis. Am J Obstet Gynecol 1994: 170: 1713–7.

36. Plzak L 3rd, Staskin D. Genuine stress incontinence theories of etiology and surgical correction. Urol Clin North Am 2002; 29: 527–35.

37. DeLancey JO, Trowbridge ER, Miller JM, et al. Stress urinary incontinence: relative importance of urethral support and urethral closure pressure. J Urol 2008; 179: 2286–9.

38. Andersson K-E. Antimuscarinics for treatment of overactive bladder. Lancet Neurol 2004; 3: 46–53.

39. Birder LA. More than just a barrier: urothelium as a drug target for urinary bladder pain. Am J Physiol Renal Physiol 2005; 289: F489–95. Review

40. Yoshimura N. Lower urinary tract symptoms (LUTS) and bladder afferent activity. Neurourol Urodyn 2007; 26(6 Suppl): 908–13. Review

41. Wyndaele JJ, De Wachter S. The sensory bladder (1): an update on the different sensations described in the lower urinary tract and the physiological mechanisms behind them. Neurourol Urodyn 2008; 27: 274–8. Review

42. Andersson KE, Fullhase C, Soler R. Urothelial effects of oral agents for overactive bladder. Curr Urol Rep 2008; 9: 459–64. Review

43. Birder L, Drake M, De Groat et al. Neural control. In: Abrams, Cardozo, Khoury, Wein, eds. Incontinence, 4th edn–4th International Consultation on Incontinence. Paris Fr: Health Publications, Editions 21, 2009: 167–254. Committee 3.

26 History and Examination

Vik Khullar and Demetri C Panayi

INTRODUCTION

A precise history and examination are integral to the management of women with pelvic floor dysfunction. An accurate history is required to determine a patient's symptoms; a thorough exam ascertains the patient's signs. Whilst this chapter deals with salient aspects of history and examination, it should be remembered that this information alone is not sufficient in the assessment of a patient. Other tools are employed to supplement the information obtained from taking a history and examining a patient. These include bladder diary and questionnaires to determine the impact of a patient's symptoms on her quality of life, expectations, and goals.

The most recent standardization document produced jointly by the International Continence Society (ICS) and International Urogynaecology Association (IUGA) defines symptoms as any morbid phenomenon or departure from the normal in structure, function, or sensation, experienced by the woman and indicative of disease or a health problem. Symptoms are either volunteered by, or elicited from the individual, or may be described by the individual's caregiver. The environment and a woman's ability to cope with her disease can profoundly alter her quality of life. A woman who is always close to a toilet may not notice her urinary frequency but the same woman with no access to a toilet will have urinary incontinence, wear protective pads, and be severely incapacitated.

Can the severity of urinary symptoms be modified by behavior? Lifestyle changes are first line treatments in the management of women with lower urinary tract symptoms. Reduction of fluid intake improves symptoms of urgency and frequency (1). Women with severe detrusor overactivity may restrict their fluid intake to less than 200 ml per day. On direct questioning the urinary problem may not appear severe, with a normal diurnal urinary frequency, and it is only with a frequency volume chart that a complete picture of the severity of the detrusor overactivity can be determined. The volume of urine excreted relies not only on fluid intake but also on the secretion of antidiuretic hormone which is impaired in diabetes insipidus. The circadian secretion of this hormone is reversed in women suffering nocturia and nocturnal polyuria (2). The most recently published ICS standardization report on lower urinary tract terminology was published in 2002 (3) and the definitions used in this chapter are according to the terminology used in the report. This standardization document has recently been updated in a joint ICS/IUGA report and is due to be published imminently.

History

History taking must take place using the patient's own words. Patients often fail to understand terms such as stress incontinence with a majority thinking that this relates to being stressed and leaking (4). This is then clarified into an easily understandable list of graded symptoms using a standard questionnaire (Fig. 26.1). A review of studies in the English language revealed an overall worldwide prevalence of urinary incontinence of approximately 28% with the commonest cause of urinary incontinence being stress urinary incontinence (50%), then mixed urinary incontinence (32%), and urge urinary incontinence (14%) (5). In the United States using national health and nutrition examination survey 2001 to 2002 data, 49% women reported some degree of urinary incontinence and the overall prevalence of stress, urge, mixed was 23.7%, 9.9%, 14.5% respectively (6).

When comparing the symptoms and final urodynamic diagnosis, there is a marked overlap between diagnostic groups. A diagnosis based on history corresponds to urodynamic diagnosis in only up to 55% of women (7). Symptom complexes have been used in an attempt to improve diagnostic accuracy. The use of bladder diary to enable patients to record fluid intake, output, and incontinence episodes has also shown discrepancy between patient reporting of their symptoms and findings of the bladder diary (8,9). However the use of a self completed symptom questionnaire does produce a better relationship between urinary symptoms and urodynamic diagnosis (10).

If symptoms are not of diagnostic value, why record them? Symptoms are valuable as a guide in determining treatment. In addition, symptoms should be taken into consideration during the urodynamic test as the provocative maneuvers should mimic conditions encountered by the woman in her normal daily activities and lead to her urinary symptoms. A 90-year-old woman with urgency and no stress incontinence is an inappropriate candidate for performing "star jumps" with a full bladder!

When questioning women complaining of urinary symptoms, all symptoms complained of should be explained in a woman's own words. Stress incontinence is the term used to describe urinary leakage which occurs with a cough or sneeze or follows it by a few seconds, even when considerable urgency is associated with the leakage.

The severity of each symptom and its effect on the woman's quality of life are noted, as cure can be achieved through directing treatment to relieve the troublesome symptoms. The length of time that the symptoms have been present discriminates between transient and established incontinence and whether this has changed over time. General enquiry should be made of all urinary symptoms as the woman may not be able to describe them or may be too embarrassed to mention them. For this reason a questionnaire is a useful guide as it ensures that all symptoms are enquired about.

Urinary symptoms–direct questioning
to be completed with the doctor

Daytime frequency ☐   Night-time ☐
Volume range

Incontinence symptoms

Stress incontinence	☐	Urgency	☐
Urge incontinence	☐	Wet at rest	☐
Wet on standing	☐	Wet at night	☐
Unaware of wetness	☐	Pads/pants	☐

Voiding characteristics

Poor stream	☐	Unable to interrupt flow	☐
Postmicturition dribble	☐	Strain to void	☐
Incomplete emptying	☐		☐

Other symptoms

Cough	☐	Constipation	☐
Leg weakness	☐	Rectal soiling	☐
Perineal discomfort	☐	Enuresis after school age	☐
Pain on micturition	☐	Pain on intercourse	☐
		Leakage on intercourse	☐

0 = no problem, 1 = occasionally, 2 = frequently
Pain on micturition 0 = nil, 1 = urethral, 2 = perineal,
3 = suprapubic, 4 = loin
Pain on intercourse 0 = no pain, 1 = superficial, 2 = deep

Figure 26.1 Standard questionnaire for urinary symptoms.

Table 26.1 Classification of Symptoms into Groups

Abnormal storage
- Incontinence: urge, stress
- Frequency/nocturia
- Nocturnal enuresis

Abnormal voiding
- Straining to void
- Hesitancy
- Incomplete emptying
- Poor stream
- Postmicturition dribble

Abnormal sensation
- Urgency
- Dysuria
- Absent sensation
- Painful bladder

The questionnaire should be validated in the language in which it is to be used and often the symptom questionnaire will be attached to a quality of life questionnaire (11,12). The method used to obtain the symptoms will alter the answers. Questionnaires postally administered appear to produce higher severity responses from patients than the same questions used in an interview (13).

Symptoms can be grouped into storage problems, voiding disorders, and sensory problems (Table 26.1). This classification of symptoms does not help in diagnosis as overflow incontinence can produce symptoms similar to those of detrusor overactivity: urinary frequency in overflow incontinence is caused by incomplete bladder emptying resulting in a reduced bladder capacity; detrusor overactivity causes urinary frequency due to an over active detrusor—the same symptom is produced by the different mechanisms.

URINARY SYMPTOMS
Urinary Incontinence
Urinary incontinence is a failure of urinary storage and requires careful evaluation. This is defined as the complaint of any involuntary loss of urine (3). Loss of urine through channels other than the urethra is extraurethral incontinence (3). It is important that incontinence is regarded as a symptom or a sign and not a diagnosis. Severe urinary incontinence of any origin has overlapping symptoms associated with urethral sphincter incompetence and detrusor overactivity. There are many causes of urinary incontinence (Table 26.2). It is important to determine whether the urine loss is continuous or intermittent.

Continuous urine loss is rare. It is usually seen when there is an ectopic ureter or fistula, and the woman will often complain of nocturnal incontinence as opposed to nocturnal enuresis. This occurs most often following pelvic surgery or as a result of malignancy, following surgery or radiotherapy. Obstetric fistulae are more commonly seen in developing countries. Some women complain that they are "never dry," and suffer from severe intermittent urinary incontinence, rather than a continuous loss of urine. This occurs in women who have had multiple previous operations and have a fixed and fibrosed "drainpipe" (type 3) urethra (14). Otherwise women who complain of urinary loss "all the time" have severe detrusor overactivity.

The pattern of intermittent urinary incontinence should be linked with associated activity such as physical exercise, laughing, putting the key in the front door, sexual intercourse, or orgasm. The severity of the incontinence can be quantified not only by volume but also by the type and number of pads or changes of underwear required in 24 hours and the magnitude of the provoking stimulus. There is often little relationship between the findings of urodynamic tests and the symptoms described by the woman in her daily life, and this may reflect modifications in behavior and lifestyle that she has made to ameliorate the effect of lower urinary tract dysfunction. It does not, however, reduce the importance of the urinary symptoms as they may still be impairing her quality of life. Often women will not admit to urinary incontinence but state that they leak when a history is taken.

Table 26.2 Causes of Urinary Incontinence

Urethral sphincter incompetence
- Sphincter dysfunction
- Abnormal bladder neck support

Detrusor overactivity
- Idiopathic detrusor overactivity
- Neurogenic detrusor overactivity (e.g., multiple sclerosis, spinal trauma)

Mixed incontinence
Urethral diverticulae
Congenital abnormalities (e.g., epispadias, ectopic ureter, bladder exstrophy, spina bifida occulta)
Transient incontinence
- Urinary tract infection
- Restricted mobility
- Constipation
- Excessive urine production
  - a. Diuretic therapy
  - b. Diabetes mellitus
  - c. Diabetes insipidus
  - d. Cardiac failure
  - e. Hypercalcemia
- Confusion (e.g., dementia, acute illness)
- Atrophic urethritis and vaginitis

Pharmacologic causes (e.g., diuretics, tranquilizers, cholinergic agents, prazosin)
Fistulae (e.g., urethral, vesical, ureteral)
Overflow incontinence
- Hypotonic detrusor
- Rarely urethral obstruction

Urethral instability
Functional

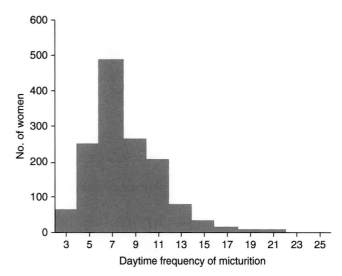

Figure 26.2 Daytime frequency of micturition in a symptomatic population.

Urge and Urge Urinary Incontinence

Urgency is the sudden compelling desire to pass urine that is difficult to defer (3). If this symptom is recorded more often than once a week it may be considered abnormal. Urge urinary incontinence is the involuntary leakage of urine that is accompanied by, or immediately preceded by urgency (3). Often women will describe getting the sensation of the desire to void and not getting to the toilet in time. The quantity of urine lost can be anything from a few drops on lowering the undergarments prior to voiding to quite a large volume, and it is not uncommon for the patient to describe at least one occasion where the urine has poured down both legs uncontrollably.

This may be triggered by changes in temperature, opening the front door, hearing running water, and occasionally during sexual intercourse at orgasm. As the main coping strategy for this symptom is increasing voiding frequency, pad usage or incontinent episodes are not useful in assessing the severity of the condition.

The overactive bladder syndrome is defined as urgency with or without urge urinary incontinence usually associated with frequency and nocturia (3).

Frequency

Daytime frequency is the number of times a woman voids during waking hours; normal diurnal frequency is considered to be between four to seven voids per day. In a symptomatic population the range may be greater (Fig. 26.2). Increased daytime frequency is defined as the complaint by the patient that she voids too often during the day (3), therefore this is a subjective definition dependent on each individual rather than a numerical cut off. Frequency is not diagnostic for detrusor overactivity or for urodynamic stress incontinence although women with detrusor overactivity do void more frequently. Clustering of voids during the day may suggest a cause such as diuretics prescribed for congestive cardiac failure, drinking large volumes of fluid, or bad habit. Urinary frequency may occur for a number of reasons (Table 26.3). Women who void infrequently are at increased risk of developing voiding difficulties. The diurnal frequency does not increase with age in the symptomatic population seen in a urodynamic clinic (Table 26.4). The 95% upper limit of normal for urinary frequency in an asymptomatic population has recently been reported as being 13 voids per day and this suggests a wide variation in the normal population as the median and mean values in this test–retest study was eight and seven, respectively (15).

Nocturia

Nocturia is defined as the complaint that the patient has to wake one or more times during the night to void (3). It is important to discriminate between this and a woman voiding because she is awake. It is difficult to be precise about the prevalence of nocturia, but approximately one-third of adults reported waking once at night and one-sixth twice at night (16). Nocturia can be extremely disruptive and affect quality of life as well as being associated with other co-morbidities such as hip fractures in the elderly (17). The normal upper limit to the number of voids alters with age (Table 26.5). If a woman passes urine more than once a night up to the age of 70 years this is abnormal; voiding at night increases on average once every decade after the age of 70 in normal women. This change is probably due to changing sleep patterns in the elderly and to postural effects due to daytime pooling of extracellular

Table 26.3 Causes of Abnormal Urinary Frequency

Increased fluid intake and urine output; normal bladder capacity
- Osmotic diuresis (e.g., diabetes mellitus)
- Abnormal antidiuretic hormone production (e.g., diabetes insipidus)
- Polydipsia; often the woman enjoys drinking a favorite beverage and only rarely is the behavior psychotic

Reduced functional bladder capacity
- Inflamed bladder, increasing bladder sensation (e.g., acute bacterial cystitis, interstitial cystitis)
- Detrusor overactivity
- Habit or fear of urinary incontinence
- Urinary residual secondary to detrusor hypotonia or outlet obstruction (rare)
- Increased bladder sensation, normal bladder (e.g., anxiety)

Reduced structural bladder capacity
- Fibrosis after infection (e.g., tuberculosis)
- Non-infective cystitis (e.g., interstitial cystitis, carcinoma)
- Irradiation fibrosis (e.g., for bladder or cervical carcinoma)
- Postsurgery (e.g., partial cystectomy)
- Detrusor hypertrophy

Decreased urinary frequency
- Detrusor hypotonia
- Impaired bladder sensation (e.g., diabetic neuropathy)
- Reduced fluid intake

Table 26.4 Diurnal Frequency in a Symptomatic Population[a]

Age (yrs)	Mean frequency	n
5–14	6.00	5
15–24	4.48	41
25–34	5.47	176
35–44	6.31	364
45–54	6.05	513
55–64	5.87	361
65–74	5.63	263
75–84	5.04	137
85–94	5.93	33
		Total 1893

[a]Patients seen in the urodynamic clinic, King's college hospital, London, between January 1993 and September 1994.

Table 26.5 Nocturnal Voids and Nocturia with Age[a]

Age (yrs)	Mean voids per night	Nocturia (%)	n
5–14	0.8	0	5
15–24	1.24	17	41
25–34	1.79	27	176
35–44	1.83	38	364
45–54	1.53	30	513
55–64	1.94	31	361
65–74	2.20	47	263
75–84	2.55	46	137
85–94	2.69	58	33

[a]Patients seen in the urodynamic clinic, King's college hospital, London, between January 1993 and September 1994.

fluid in the lower limbs returning to the vascular compartment at night, as a result of subclinical heart failure.

It is important to discriminate between the woman who is awake and therefore voids and the woman who is woken by the desire to void; the first group of women often have no increase in their diurnal urinary frequency.

Nocturnal Enuresis
Nocturnal enuresis is the complaint of loss of urine occurring during sleep. It is important to differentiate between this complaint and waking with urgency and then leaking before arriving at the toilet, which is urge urinary incontinence.

Nocturnal enuresis can be primary or secondary. Primary nocturnal enuresis starts in childhood and can persist into adulthood, the woman never having consistently been dry at night. Secondary nocturnal enuresis is when the incontinence restarts in adulthood following a period of night-time continence, even if it resolved as a child.

The causes of nocturnal enuresis can be abnormal circadian secretion of antidiuretic hormone, detrusor overactivity or abnormal control of the micturition reflex, or abnormal sleep pattern. A family history should be sought and the presence of diurnal symptoms noted.

Nocturnal Urine Volume
This is defined as the total volume of urine passed between the time the individual goes to bed with the intention of sleeping and the time of waking with the intention of rising. Therefore, it excludes the last void before going to bed but includes the first void after rising in the morning.

Nocturnal Polyuria
Nocturnal polyuria is present when an increased proportion of the 24-hour output occurs at night (normally during the eight hours while the patient is in bed). The normal range of nocturnal urine production differs with age and normal ranges have not been defined. Generally, nocturnal polyuria is present when more than 20% (young adults) to 33% (greater than 65 years) is produced at night.

Stress Urinary Incontinence
Stress urinary incontinence is defined as the involuntary loss of urine with exertion or effort or with coughing and sneezing. It is assciated with activities involving a rise in intra-abdominal pressure without associated urgency and must be differentiated from urge urinary incontinence when obtaining a history. The accuracy of diagnosing urodynamic stress incontinence based on the pure symptom of stress urinary incontinence (even with a normal frequency volume chart) is poor, with 8% of incontinence in this group being due to detrusor overactivity or other causes (18).

Mixed Urinary Incontinence
Women with mixed urinary incontinence satisfy the definitions for having both stress urinary incontinence and urge urinary incontinence. The prevalence of mixed urinary incontinence is variable but can account for approximately 40% of western women who present with symptoms of urinary

incontinence (19). Women with mixed urinary incontinence are a challenge to manage and have an associated worse outcome after continence surgery than women with pure stress urinary incontinence (20).

Coital Incontinence

The latest definition of coital incontinence produced by the joint report of IUGA/ICS describes coital incontinence as the complaint of involuntary loss of urine associated with coitus which may be further subdivided into with penetration or with orgasm. Urinary leakage on penetration is more likely to occur in women with urethral sphincter incompetence and with a cystocele. This type of urinary incontinence is not associated with urgency. Urinary incontinence can also occur with orgasm. The leakage may be associated with urgency and is thought to be related to detrusor overactivity (21).

Insensible Incontinence

This is a new definition produced by the recent joint report of IUGA/ICS due for publication. It defines insensible incontinence as the complaint of urinary incontinence where the woman is unaware of how it occurred. Women may describe discovering urine in their underwear or on a pad that they wear at the end of the day because of the involuntary leakage of which they were unaware.

VOIDING SYMPTOMS

Voiding difficulties may present with a variety of symptoms. Voiding symptoms are symptoms experienced during the voiding phase (3).

Hesitancy

Hesitancy is defined as the description by an individual of having difficulty in initiating micturition resulting in a delay of the onset of voiding after she is ready to pass urine (3). It is not common in women but when described the volume voided on these occasions should be noted, as small volumes (less than 100 ml) are difficult to void in normal women. However, hesitancy when voiding a full bladder may be an indication that: (*i*) the urethral sphincter is not relaxing when the detrusor contracts (voiding dysfunction or detrusor sphincter dyssnergia); (*ii*) the detrusor muscle is not contracting effectively during voiding; or (*iii*) psychological inhibition of bladder contraction, which occurs in women who can only void when alone. This symptom does not discriminate between these problems. Women with detrusor overactivity may complain of hesitancy and poor stream but this probably relates to the small volumes of urine passed by them in response to urgency.

Straining to Void

Straining to void describes the muscular effort used to initiate, maintain, or improve the urinary stream (3). The intraabdominal pressure is increased during a Valsalva maneuver, which increases the intravesical pressure and this can improve bladder emptying. The urinary stream is impaired and may be intermittent, each transient increase in flow associated with an increase in intra-abdominal pressure. In the longer term, this method of voiding can lead to the development of urogenital prolapse.

Incomplete Emptying

Feeling of incomplete emptying is a self-explanatory term for a feeling experienced by the individual after passing urine (3). The sensation can be due to fluid remaining in the bladder, can be secondary to an abnormality of sensation or due to aftercontractions in women with detrusor overactivity. These women rarely have increased postmicturition urinary residual volumes.

Women with prolapse can develop a functional obstruction of the urethra due to external compression and may have urinary residuals. A cystocele can act as a sump and a rectocele can press anteriorly on the urethra in women who void by straining, preventing complete emptying. Urinary retention is now defined as the inability to pass urine despite persistent effort. This may be also caused by urinary tract infection, presence of an intrabdominal mass such as fibroid uterus, or gravid uterus, and be a consequence of neurological compromise such as women who suffer stroke, spinal cord injury, or multiple sclerosis.

Postmicturition Dribble

Postmicturition dribble is the term used when an individual describes the involuntary loss of urine immediately after she has finished passing urine (3), usually after leaving the toilet in men, or after rising from the toilet in women. This symptom may be related to a urethral diverticulum, a cystourethrocele or detrusor overactivity. Where detrusor contractions occur after the completion of voiding, urgency will often accompany the urinary leakage. Postmicturition dribble should be distinguished from terminal dribble which is the term used when an individual describes a prolonged final part of micturition when the flow has slowed to a trickle or dribble (3).

Slow Stream

Slow stream is reported by the individual as a perception of reduced urine flow (3), usually compared to previous performance or in comparison to others. Decreased urinary stream is often described as "decreased force." Urine flow rate is dependent on the volume of urine passed; if it is less than 150 ml this should be assessed with reference to a frequency/volume chart. A reduced urine flow can be due to reduced voided volumes, bladder outflow obstruction (rare in women), or decreased bladder contractility. This can be neuropathic (lower motor neuron lesion) or myopathic.

Position Dependent Micturition

This new definition describes the complaint of having to adopt specific positions to be able to micturate spontaneously or improve bladder emptying. Women may describe squatting, sitting forwards on the toilet, or leaning backwards in order to succesfully void.

Bladder/Urethral Pain

Pain, discomfort, and pressure are part of a spectrum of abnormal sensations felt by the individual. Pain produces the greatest impact on the patient and may be related to bladder filling or voiding, may be felt after micturition, or be continuous. Pain should also be characterized by type, frequency, duration,

239

precipitating and relieving factors, and by location such as bladder, urethral, vulval, vaginal, and perineal pain. Dysuria, strangury, and bladder spasm are not recommended terms as these symptoms are difficult to define.

Urethral Pain
This is felt in the urethra and the individual indicates the urethra as the site (3). It is often described as "burning on passing urine" and can be aggravated by sexual intercourse. As an isolated symptom it is associated with urinary tract infections or urethritis.

Bladder Pain
Bladder pain is felt suprapubically or retropubically, and usually increases with bladder filling (3); it may also persist after voiding. Bladder pain is associated with inflammation of the bladder, bladder stones, or tumor. The pain more commonly occurs after micturition as the bladder mucosa closes down. Some women complain of pain after voiding and have detrusor overactivity. The pain has been found to coincide with contractions.

The presence of bladder pain is an indication for cystoscopy and occasionally bladder biopsy. Suprapubic pain may also be associated with pathology outside the bladder but within the pelvis and thus would be called pelvic pain. Endometriosis on the bladder may cause urethral pain which is present at certain times in the menstrual cycle. Pelvic inflammatory disease may cause urethral pain; however, the woman will have symptoms of vaginal discharge and pyrexia.

Loin Pain
This pain originates in the flank and radiates to the groin of the ipsilateral side. The pain is referred from the sensory nerves innervating the kidney and ureter, for which there are many causes (Table 26.6). Acute or chronic obstruction of the urinary tract can cause pain. This becomes more acute as the pressure generated within the urinary tract is higher. Women

with detrusor overactivity may complain of loin pain associated with urgency; this may indicate vesicoureteric reflux.

Dyspareunia
This is the symptom of pain during sexual intercourse. This can be sub-divided into superficial and deep dyspareunia. Superficial dyspareunia may be associated with vaginal dryness or following episiotomy or vaginal wall repair. Dyspareunia associated with the anterior vaginal wall may reflect bladder or urethral pain syndromes. Perineal pain is felt between the posterior fourchette and the anus and may be persistent or recurrent episodic. It may be related to the micturition cycle or associated with symptoms suggestive of urinary tract or sexual dysfunction (3).

Prolapse Symptoms
Pelvic organ prolapse often co-exists and may contribute to lower urinary tract symptoms. Women may describe the feeling of a lump, heaviness, a dragging senstion in the vagina, or lower back pain. They may also describe the learned behavior of using their fingers to reduce the bulge in order to succesfully micturate or defecate which is referred to as digitation. As vaginal prolapse alters the range of treatments for urinary incontinence, enquiries about symptoms of vaginal prolapse and prolapse affecting micturition and defecation should be made. The feeling of a lump at or beyond the vaginal introitus, low back ache, heaviness, dragging sensation, or the need to digitally replace or support the prolapse in order to defecate or micturate, are among the symptoms that may be described. Over 40% of women with urethral sphincter incompetence will also have significant cystoceles, making this an important symptom affecting management of a woman's urinary incontinence. As vaginal prolapse can mask urethral sphincter incompetence, it is important to identify the prolapse before a urodynamic test, so that a vaginal ring can be inserted during the provocative phase of urodynamics to expose any underlying urethral incompetence (22). This is referred to as occult incontinence.

Hematuria
Blood in the urine should always be investigated and never be ignored. This would involve imaging of the entire urinary tract with ultrasound, cytological analysis of a urine sample, as well a cystoscopy, and possbly a biopsy.

NEUROLOGIC HISTORY
Women should be questioned about any alteration in sensation and motor power in the legs or perineum. The latter may be described as altered sensation during sexual intercourse or an inability to feel their urinary stream during micturition. Fecal incontinence is described as diarrhea which causes staining of underwear or urgency to defecate. Worsening symptoms of back pain with urinary and neurologic symptoms must be treated rapidly and seriously as these may indicate a worsening central intervertebral disk prolapse. Neurologic symptoms can also be a result of peripheral neuropathy associated with diabetes mellitus, cerebrovascular accidents, Parkinson's disease, or multiple sclerosis.

Table 26.6 Causes of Loin Pain

Vesicoureteric reflux
Renal trauma
Acute ureteric obstruction
  • Stone
  • Blood clot
  • Papillary necrosis
Chronic ureteric obstruction
  • Tumor (e.g., transitional cell carcinoma, renal cell carcinoma, Wilms' tumor)
  • Ureteric stricture
  • Retroperitoneal fibrosis
  • Stone
  • Congenital anomaly
Renal inflammation
  • Pyelonephritis
  • Perinephric abscess
Renal infarction

GYNECOLOGICAL SYMPTOMS

The lower urinary tract has estrogen receptors (23). Thus it is important to enquire about changes in urinary symptoms during the menstrual cycle and note the woman's menopausal state.

Previous continence operations have an important influence on the future success of continence surgery, as the urethral sphincter may be altered by scarring and damage to sphincter innervation by previous vaginal surgery, as well as distortion and narrowing of the bladder neck. Operations on the uterus may interfere with the innervation of the bladder, particularly after radical hysterectomy for carcinoma and radiotherapy.

PAST MEDICAL HISTORY

It is important to record all past major abdominal and pelvic surgery, and urinary complications as a result of the surgery should be noted. The postoperative course can often be revealing, particularly when women have been unable to void spontaneously and required catheterization. This could indicate prolonged overdistension which can lead to voiding difficulties due to detrusor hypotonia. Surgery to the spine and neurologic impairment after this must be recorded, particularly in relation to any possible nerve damage. Operations on the large bowel, especially those involving dissection at the side wall of the pelvis, may result in denervation, such as abdominoperineal resection of the rectum.

Conditions increasing abdominal pressure, such as chronic cough or constipation, can produce the symptom of stress incontinence and make a minor problem more severe. Cardiac and renal failure can produce frequency and nocturia through polyuria. Endocrine disorders such as diabetes mellitus or diabetes insipidus may lead to polyuria and polydipsia. Chronic diabetes mellitus can produce frequency as a result of overflow incontinence secondary to a hypotonic detrusor and impaired bladder sensation.

There does appear to be an association between schizophrenia and detrusor overactivity (24). Additionally, women suffering from dementia may not empty their bladders frequently and may not be aware of the need to void.

The number of proven urinary tract infections during the past two years should be recorded. Childhood enuresis is particularly important as often these patients have detrusor overactivity.

The obstetric history should include parity, length of labor, mode of delivery, and weight of the largest infant; however, such information has not been shown to be very useful as the details of labor are not recalled accurately. Cesarean section or epidural block during labor and the retention of urine post partum are possible progenitors of voiding difficulties (25,26).

DRUG HISTORY

Many drugs affect the lower urinary tract. Diuretics can produce urgency, frequency, and urge urinary incontinence. Benzodiazepines sedate and may cause confusion and secondary incontinence, particularly in elderly patients (27). Alcohol impairs mobility, produces a diuresis, and can impair the woman's perception of bladder filling. Anticholinergic drugs impair detrusor contractility and may cause urinary retention with secondary overflow incontinence. These include antipsychotic drugs, antidepressants, opiates, antispasmodics, and antiparkinsonian drugs. Drugs that improve bladder storage are shown in Table 26.7.

Sympathomimetic drugs, often found in cold remedies, can increase the urethral sphincter resistance and produce voiding difficulty. α-adrenergic blockers such as doxazosin used to treat hypertension, have may cause bladder smooth muscle or urethral relaxation and resultant stress urinary incontinence (27,28). Cystitis is a common complication of chemotherapy treatment with hemorrhagic cystitis a direct result of antineoplastic treatment. Chemotherapy-induced cystitis can arise from agents directly instilled into the bladder as part of a

---

Table 26.7 Drugs that Improve Urine Storage

Anticholinergic drugs
- Propantheline bromide
- Emepronium bromide/carrageenate
- Tolterodine
- Darafenacin
- Solifenacin

Musculotrophic drugs
- Oxybutynin chloride
- Dicycloverine chloride
- Flavoxate hydrochloride

Calcium antagonists
- Nifedipine
- Flunarizine

Tricyclic antidepressants
- Imipramine
- Doxepin

β-Adrenoceptor agonists
- Terbutaline
- Salbutamol
- Isoprenaline

α-Adrenoceptor antagonists
- Phenoxybenzamine
- Prazosin

Prostaglandin synthetase inhibitors
- Flurbiprofen
- Indometacin

Neurotoxins
- Capsaicin
- Resiniferatoxin

Drugs reducing urine production
- Desmopressin

Drugs increasing outlet resistance
- α-Adrenergic agonists
  a. Phenylpropanolamine hydrochloride
  b. Midodrine
- Serotonin noradrenaline reuptake inhibitors
  a. Duloxetine
- β-Adrenergic antagonist
  a. Propranolol

Estrogens

Table 26.8 Drugs that Improve Bladder Emptying

Increased detrusor contractility

Cholinergic agents
- Carbachol
- Bethanecol

Anticholinesterase
- Distigmine

Prostaglandins
- E2$_\alpha$
- F2$_\alpha$

Decreased outlet resistance

α-Sympathetic blocking agents
- Phenoxybenzamine
- Phentolamine
- Prazosin

Striated muscle relaxants
- Baclofen
- Dantrolene
- Lisidonal
- Diazepam

treatment program for superficial cancer of the bladder or from toxic metabolites of renally excreted anti-neoplastic agents which come in contact with the bladder. Drugs that improve bladder emptying are shown in Table 26.8.

EXAMINATION

Before examining the woman it is important to reassure her about the possibility of urinary leakage and explain that she should not be embarrassed as a result of this. The woman's mobility and mental state play a role in her ability to react to her incontinence problem and may influence management. A mini-mental state examination can be performed, as well an assessment of the woman's motivation and manual dexterity, as these may influence her compliance with possible treatments and follow-up.

Abdominal examination precedes vaginal assessment. Inspection will reveal evidence of previous abdominal surgery, and palpation may demonstrate the presence of a full or distended bladder as well as other abdominal or pelvic masses or elicit pain.

It is important to perform a screening neurologic examination testing the tone, strength, and movement of the lower limbs. It is particularly useful to test the abduction and spreading of toes as the innervation for the lateral abductors comes from S3. The anal tone should be assessed and gentle tapping of the clitoris will produce a reflex contraction of the anal sphincter (bulbocavernosus reflex). Additionally, a voluntary cough should cause a reflex contraction of the anal sphincter. An intact sacral reflex can be tested by stroking the skin lateral to the anus, which should elicit a contraction of the external anal sphincter.

GYNECOLOGIC EXAMINATION

The condition of the vulval skin is important as there may be signs of excoriation, edema, or erythema due to exposure of the skin to urine on the vulva for prolonged periods of time

and concomitant candidiasis. Vaginal atrophy, particularly in women more than 10 years after the menopause, may be seen.

Genital prolapse can now be assessed using the methods produced by the ICS and IUGA most recent report on the standardization of terminology. It suggests that women should be assessed with an empty bladder and ideally an empty rectum because an increased bladder volume can restrict the degree of descent of the vaginal prolapse. Any cystocele, rectocele, uterine, or vault descent can be best assessed in the Sims' (left lateral) position on coughing and straining using a Sims' speculum. Alternatively, examination may also be made in lithotomy using the lower blade of a Graves' speculum to assist in assessing the opposite vaginal wall (29). Women may also be examined standing and this may be the only way for the prolapse to be demonstrated successfully (30). After examination for pelvic organ prolapse, the clinician should report the degree of prolapse in terms of the descent of the anterior and posterior vaginal walls, as well as the cervix, or in the case of a woman who has had a hysterectomy, the vaginal vault. Various staging or grading methods have been described and the level of the hymen is usually used. The pelvic organ prolapse quantification system is a validated method which involves using a measuring device marked in centimeters to measure specific points on the anterior and posterior vaginal wall as well as the descent of the cervix or vaginal cuff allowing quantification of the degree of vaginal prolapse (31). This method allows staging of the prolapse from 0 to IV where 0 is no prolapse and stages I to III are increased descent of the prolapse through the vagina and stage IV is complete eversion of the total length of the genital tract. Women can be reproducibly examined in the left lateral and supine positions (31). The vagina should also be examined for evidence of atrophy, inflammation, pain, or scarring from previous surgical procedures.

Other aspects of pelvic examination include examination of the urethra where urethral mucosal prolapse or caruncle may be seen. A urethral diverticulum may present with a midline anterior vaginal wall swelling or with tenderness over the length of the urethra. Vaginal cysts such as gardners duct cyst may present with similar findings.

If a woman is complaining of a discharge, or has had a recent onset of symptoms of urgency and frequency, it may be useful to obtain swabs to culture for Chlamydia and gonococcus. A bimanual examination should be performed to exclude abnormal pelvic organs, masses, or uterine impaction, and can exclude a large postmicturition urinary residual. Pelvic masses such as ovarian cysts and uterine enlargement greater than 12 weeks' size can cause pressure symptoms resulting in frequency; often the symptoms resolve once the mass has been removed.

Pelvic floor muscle examination may be appropriate which assesses tone at rest, and strength with voluntary and reflex contraction. This may be assessed by simple observation and with digital palpation circumferentially. The ICS has produced a standardized document which details pelvic floor muscle assessment (32). If pelvic pain is a problem it is important by digital examination to assess where the pain originates in particular trigger points in the levator ani but also tenderness on palpating the pelvic organs adjacent to the vagina. Finally, rectal examination is particularly important in the elderly to exclude fecal impaction, which can aggravate urinary incontinence.

CONCLUSION

History and examination alone cannot diagnose female urinary disorders but can guide future investigation and management. In some cases a very obvious cause can be found and dealt with, thus avoiding the need for further investigations which may be embarrassing, expensive, and invasive.

REFERENCES

1. Swithinbank L, Hashim H, Abrams P. The effect of fluid intake on urinary symptoms in women. J Urol 2005; 174: 187–9.
2. Asplund R. Diuresis pattern, plasma vasopressin and blood pressure in healthy elderly persons with nocturia and nocturnal polyuria. Neth J Med 2002; 60: 276–80.
3. Abrams P, Cardozo L, Fall M, et al. The standardisation of terminology of lower urinary tract function: report from the Standardisation Subcommittee of the International Continence Society. Am J Obstet Gynecol 2002; 187: 116–26.
4. Digesu GA, Khullar V, Panayi D, et al. Should we explain lower urinary tract symptoms to patients? Neurourol Urodyn 2008; 27: 368–71.
5. Minassian VA, Drutz HP, Al-Badr A. Urinary incontinence as a worldwide problem. Int J Gynaecol Obstet 2003; 82: 327–38.
6. Minassian VA, Stewart WF, Wood GC. Urinary incontinence in women: variation in prevalence estimates and risk factors. Obstet Gynecol 2008; 111(2 Pt 1): 324–31.
7. Digesu GA, Khullar V, Cardozo L, et al. Overactive bladder symptoms: do we need urodynamics? Neurourol Urodyn 2003; 22: 105–8.
8. Stav K, Dwyer PL, Rosamilia A. Women overestimate daytime urinary frequency: the importance of the bladder diary. J Urol 2009; 181: 2176–80.
9. Kenton K, Fitzgerald MP, Brubaker L. What is a clinician to do-believe the patient or her urinary diary? J Urol 2006; 176: 633–5.
10. Khan MS, Chaliha C, Leskova L, et al. The relationship between urinary symptom questionnaires and urodynamic diagnoses: an analysis of two methods of questionnaire administration. BJOG 2004; 111: 468–74.
11. Avery K, Donovan J, Peters TJ, et al. ICIQ: a brief and robust measure for evaluating the symptoms and impact of urinary incontinence. Neurourol Urodyn 2004; 23: 322–30.
12. Reese PR, Pleil AM, Okano GJ, et al. Multinational study of reliability and validity of the King's Health Questionnaire in patients with overactive bladder. Qual Life Res 2003; 12: 427–42.
13. Khan MS, Chaliha C, Leskova L, et al. A randomized crossover trial to examine administration techniques related to the Bristol female lower urinary tract symptom (BFLUTS) questionnaire. Neurourol Urodyn 2005; 24: 211–14.
14. Blaivas JG, Appell RA, Fantl JA, et al. Definition and classification of urinary incontinence: recommendations of the urodynamic society. Neurourol Urodyn 1997; 16: 149–51.
15. Fitzgerald MP, Brubaker L. Variability of 24-hour voiding diary variables among asymptomatic women. J Urol 2003; 169: 207–9.
16. Appell RA, Sand PK. Nocturia: etiology, diagnosis, and treatment. Neurourol Urodyn 2008; 27: 34–9.
17. Asplund R. Hip fractures, nocturia, and nocturnal polyuria in the elderly. Arch Gerontol Geriatr 2006; 43: 319–26.
18. Digesu GA, Hendricken C, Fernando R, et al. Do women with pure stress urinary incontinence need urodynamics? Urology 2009; 74: 278–81.
19. Lasserre A, Pelat C, Gueroult V, et al. Urinary incontinence in French women: prevalence, risk factors, and impact on quality of life. Eur Urol 2009; 56: 177–83.
20. Kulseng-Hanssen S, Husby H, Schiotz HA. The tension free vaginal tape operation for women with mixed incontinence: do preoperative variables predict the outcome? Neurourol Urodyn 2007; 26: 115–21.
21. Serati M, Salvatore S, Uccella S, et al. Urinary incontinence at orgasm: relation to detrusor overactivity and treatment efficacy. Eur Urol 2008; 54: 911–15.
22. Araki I, Haneda Y, Mikami Y, et al. Incontinence and detrusor dysfunction associated with pelvic organ prolapse: clinical value of preoperative urodynamic evaluation. Int Urogynecol J Pelvic Floor Dysfunct 2009; 20: 1301–6.
23. Iosif CS, Batra S, Ek A, et al. Estrogen receptors in the human female lower urinary tract. Am J Obstet Gynecol 1981; 141: 817–20.
24. Bonney WW, Gupta S, Hunter DR, et al. Bladder dysfunction in schizophrenia. Schizophr Res 1997; 25: 243–9.
25. Guiheneuf A, Weyl B. Postpartum-urinary retention. A report of two cases and a review of literature. J Gynecol Obstet Biol Reprod (Paris) 2008; 37: 614–17.
26. Simmons SW, Cyna AM, Dennis AT, et al. Combined spinal-epidural versus epidural analgesia in labour. Cochrane Database Syst Rev 2007; (3): CD003401.
27. Tsakiris P, Oelke M, Michel MC. Drug-induced urinary incontinence. Drugs Aging 2008; 25: 541–9.
28. Furuta A, Asano K, Egawa S, et al. Role of alpha2-adrenoceptors and glutamate mechanisms in the external urethral sphincter continence reflex in rats. J Urol 2009; 181: 1467–73.
29. Baden WF, Walker TA. Physical diagnosis in the evaluation of vaginal relaxation. Clin Obstet Gynecol 1972; 15: 1055–69.
30. Digesu GA, Khullar V, Cardozo L, et al. Inter-observer reliability of digital vaginal examination using a four-grade scale in different patient positions. Int Urogynecol J Pelvic Floor Dysfunct 2008; 19: 1303–7.
31. Digesu GA, Athanasiou S, Cardozo L, et al. Validation of the pelvic organ prolapse quantification (POP-Q) system in left lateral position. Int Urogynecol J Pelvic Floor Dysfunct 2009; 20: 979–83.
32. Messelink B, Benson T, Berghmans B, et al. Standardization of terminology of pelvic floor muscle function and dysfunction: report from the pelvic floor clinical assessment group of the International Continence Society. Neurourol Urodyn 2005; 24: 374–80.

27 Voiding Diary
Matthew Parsons

INTRODUCTION

The voiding diary is an important tool in the investigation of patients with lower urinary tract symptoms (LUTS) and voiding dysfunction (1). The chart is variously known as a frequency-volume (FV) chart, bladder diary, or voiding diary, and is completed daily by the patient over a number of days prior to the visit to the doctor. They may range in complexity, from the simple records of intake and output to more complex diaries including symptoms and incontinence episodes, and pad use, to facilitate history-taking about the degree of frequency, nocturia, and volumes voided at each episode. They are useful in the following circumstances:

- Fluid intake—compulsive or excessive fluid consumption is easily identified. Metabolic disorders such as diabetes may be identified in this way.
- Normal fluid volumes consumed at inappropriate times (e.g., bedtime) may cause nocturia.
- Excessive intake of alcohol or caffeine causing exacerbation of symptoms.
- Learned or habitual frequency may be semi-objectively assessed.

On the basis of findings in the FV chart, simple instruction and behavioral modification, can be recommended immediately allowing treatment to commence without recourse to more complex and expensive modalities.

FV charts have developed in design and content over the last 20 years although there has been little systematic work developing the FV chart as a clinical, rather than a research, tool, and it remains one of the most neglected diagnostic instruments (2).

COMPONENTS OF THE DIARY
Diary

Most institutions use a paper diary that is easily posted out in advance or handed directly to the patient. They are easy to produce, cheap to post, and easily and safely stored.

The FV chart should have space to record fluid intake, with at least a recording of the volume and time of consumption. There should also be room to record the volume and timing of urine passed, and a recording of any relevant LUTS, especially incontinence (Fig. 27.1).

Instructions

Culture- and age-specific instructions should be included, explaining what information is to be collected and the relevance for the woman attending for investigation. In a four-week audit of completion of bladder diaries prior to attending our one-stop clinic, of the 68 women attending who received the diary, only 22 (32%) had completed it (3). Interestingly, the addition of an explanatory letter describing the importance of the diary in the overall assessment increased the compliance to 75.5%, when the audit cycle was closed. Non-Caucasian races, and pelvic organ prolapse as the primary clinical complaint, are significantly correlated with non-completion of a bladder diary (4), although this was a poor predictor of an absence of urinary symptoms.

In a paper looking specifically at instruction prior to completion of a FV chart (5), 278 women involved in one of three other trials completed a seven-day minimal instruction diary prior to clinical evaluation, and a seven-day intensive instruction diary afterwards. The diaries were compared for the number of episodes of voluntary diurnal and nocturnal voids, and incontinence episodes. Correlation co-efficients ranged from 0.67 to 0.78 for each of the symptoms, although intra-subject analysis revealed a decline in reported nocturnal voids, which were not explained by urodynamic or demographic findings. This may be most likely explained by "diary fatigue," which is seen to occur with longer diaries. However, the study does suggest that minimal paper instructions sent out in advance are sufficient in order to gain the maximum benefit from the diary for each woman.

Validity and Reliability

The FV chart has been shown to be a valuable, reliable tool for the assessment of micturition patterns (6), as there is poor correlation between subjective and charted estimates of diurnal and nocturnal urinary frequency (7). FV charts have been shown to be both valid, useful. In a study comprising 18 patients (mean age 63 years, range 20–80 years) completing a three-day diary and recording fluid intake and voided volumes, a 24-hour urine collection was undertaken in addition. Median difference between recorded volume and volume collected was 100 ml/24 hr (0–1450 ml/24 hr) and 10 ml/void (0–117 ml/void) (8), which was not significant.

Furthermore, when 63 patients were recruited to complete two diaries of three days duration more than a week apart, 51 managed to finish the study. There was excellent correlation for both mean voided volume (r = 0.86) and 24-hour frequency (r = 0.9) (9), suggesting intra-individual reliability of the diary over time. Individual variation was greater for urinary frequency; this natural variation may invalidate apparently successful treatment outcomes, and the authors recommended use of mean voided volume in the assessment of treatment outcomes.

Maximum voided volume is usually taken to represent functional capacity. Significant positive correlation has been shown between cystometric bladder capacity and maximum voided volume on the diary (r = 0.4938, p < 0.01), establishing the validity of a home diary in clinical

Birmingham Women's NHS

NHS Foundation Trust

Frequency Volume Chart

Time	Day 1			Day 2			Day 3		
	In	Out	Wet	In	Out	Wet	In	Out	Wet
7 am		340						260	
8 am	300			400	330		350		
9 am		200						170	
10 am	200	150		150	200		200		
11 am			W		175			150	
12 pm		200		150				50	
1 pm	150			150	200	W			
2 pm		175					320	200	
3 pm				200				200	
4 pm	450	150			220				W
5 pm		100					150		
6 pm		100	W	300			150	175	
7 pm	250	175		500	200 150				
8 pm	200	50		400	150 150	W	450	100	
9 pm	100				50	W		100	W
10 pm	350	180	860	150			400	200	
11 pm					210	860		210	860
12 am									
1 am		270					200		
2 am	100					W			
3 am		300							
4 am					210				
5 am									
6 am									

Figure 27.1 Three-day diary as used at Birmingham Women's Hospital.

practice (10). As a tool to assess bladder sensation, bladder diary has been assessed by comparison with sensation during filling cystometry (11). On charts, 65% of all voids were made without sensation to void; urgent desire was not noted unless voluntary delay of voiding occurred. High grades of perception of fullness were associated with higher voided volumes, and mean volumes for different sensations on the charts were not significantly different from volumes at similar sensations during cystometry. FV charts may therefore provide a reliable and non-invasive method of assessing bladder sensation.

Bladder diaries are less effective at charting quantity of urine lost during incontinence episodes (12). In a study of 51 women with mild to moderate urinary incontinence, no significant correlations existed between a pad test and a questionnaire reporting volume of urine loss. There was a weak but significant correlation between a questionnaire regarding incontinence episode frequency and a six-day urinary diary result ($r = 0.33$, $p = 0.045$). The correlation between six-day urinary diary and questionnaire was stronger for urinary frequency ($r = 0.65$, $p = 0.000$). There is therefore only a weak correlation between subjective and objective measures of urinary loss.

Test-retest reliability studies show high intra-class correlation coefficients of 0.81 to 0.86 for symptoms of strong urge, diurnal and nocturnal micturitions, total incontinence- and urge-incontinence episodes (13). Moderate correlations with global questions on urge-incontinence and urinary frequency supported the validity of the diary.

The ability of the diary to differentiate between normal and affected individuals (14) is of potential clinical importance. Larsson et al. (6,15,16) reported on the reliability of the voiding diary in differentiating those with detrusor over-activity (DO) (15), or urodynamic stress incontinence (USI) (16), from normal subjects and concluded that the overlap between normal patients and patients with DO was great for all parameters. He reached the same conclusion regarding patients with USI. Accordingly, the diary is not a reliable test for diagnostic discrimination between either condition and normal bladder function.

Duration

Optimal duration has not been standardized. Some support the use of a seven day diary, to encompass the entire week, incorporating both work and leisure time (17). Patient compliance, however, decreases with increasing length of the diary (5) in addition to other clinical correlates. A 48-hour diary has been shown to significantly correlate with a seven-day diary (6), and in another study, the first three days' results correlated well with the results of the last four days (18). Test-retest reliability of voiding diaries and pad tests in women referred for LUTS was assessed by Lin's concordance correlation coefficient (CCC) (with a cut-off value of 0.7 indicating test-retest reliability), using 24-, 48-, and 72-hour diaries. For the 24-hour diary the total number of incontinence episodes measured was reliable, while the number of voiding episodes was marginally reliable (mean CCC 0.785 and 0.689, respectively); for the 48-hour diary the number of incontinence episodes and total number of voiding episodes were reliable (mean CCC 0.78 and 0.83, respectively); for the 72-hour diary each parameter was highly reliable (CCC 0.86 and 0.826, respectively). It was, however, noted that the increased duration diaries had a lower patient compliance (19). A recent paper has reported the concept of diary despair (20)—a seven-day diary had more errors than a three-day diary, even in the first three days.

In order for a FV chart to have value, it must be completed correctly. If the length of diary is too great, then compliance is likely to be poor. Increasing bias from day to day variability may compromise reduced length diaries of one or two days, and so a three-day diary has been suggested as optimal (8).

PAPER AND ELECTRONIC DIARIES

If information were readily available in the clinic setting, the consultation would most likely be facilitated. The problem with paper charts (Fig. 27.1), however, is that they still need to be manually calculated, which may be time consuming in a busy clinic, and inaccuracies may occur when pressed for time. Although this is very difficult to quantify, in a trial comparing electronic and paper diaries, there were no data calculation errors in the electronic diaries, allowing rapid review in clinical

and research settings (21). Hand-held computerized diaries have been developed to overcome the lack of patient compliance that has been noted in many studies (22). Matched patients and controls completed a seven-day paper diary and a seven-day computerized diary. Patients felt that their symptoms were more properly reflected by the computerized version, felt more motivated to provide the data, and found it easier to remember. The two methods were not comparable, however, as the computerized diary prompted more data entry (urgency, urgency with leak, intake) than the written diary, where patients were only asked to mark the time of a normal void and intake, with no space for any other information. It is interesting to note that, despite the skeletal nature of the conventional diary, patients still found it easier to comply with the computerized diary. Naturally, a computer diary in a clinical setting would cost considerably more than a paper diary, for completion by every patient in a reasonably sized unit.

Intelligent Character Recognition

A character-recognition program with appropriate hardware might combine the cheaper cost of the paper diary with the rapid and accurate data manipulation of the computer system, and make possible more quantitative clinical measures than are currently feasible. (Fig. 27.2).

Sensation-Related Bladder Diary (SR-BD)

Increased bladder sensation is one of the most troubling aspects of overactive bladder syndrome, but this is difficult to evaluate non-invasively. It is relatively easy to demonstrate sensation thresholds at cystometry, but this is invasive and laboratory-bound for the most part.

Some groups have started to record sensation in the bladder diaries. De Wachter and Wyndaele (23) have demonstrated that it is possible to record bladder sensation in daily life using a perception of fullness scale. This would therefore help identify women who are "convenience-voiders" (24), which has a significant impact on some diaries. A difference between three-day SR-BD from healthy volunteers and women with urinary incontinence has been demonstrated (25); further, in a study comparing SR-BD between women with a urodynamic diagnosis and those who remain un-categorized, more disturbed bladder sensation was present in those with DO (urge urinary incontinence) and to a lesser degree those with mixed urinary incontinence (26). This enhances the possibility of raising the clinical suspicion of DO from a diary.

NORMATIVE VALUES IN A HEALTHY POPULATION

There are very few data available about the voiding habits of asymptomatic women, although this has recently been addressed by a number of groups (27–30). (Table 27.1).

Normal urinary habits have been studied in a limited sample over 24 hours but more age and race-matched data are needed (31). In a 24-hour diary study of asymptomatic women, the use of eight voids per 24 hours was questioned as defining "frequency" (32). Thirteen or more voids per 24 hours were found to represent the upper range in the normal distribution. A small study has published a comparison of pre-, peri-, and

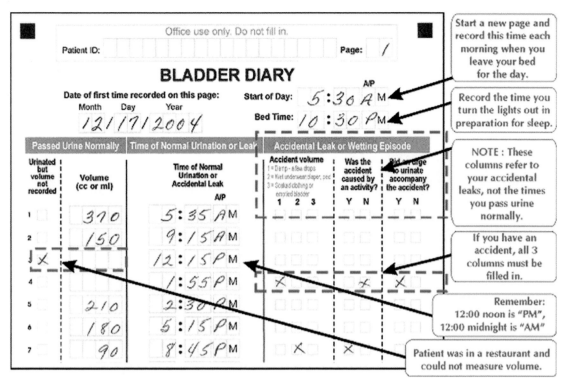

Figure 27.2 Intelligent character recognition form with patient instructions. (LifeTech Inc).

Table 27.1 Bladder Diary Measurements in an Asymptomatic Population (30)

Variable	Mean (SD)	Range	Median (5th–95th centile)	Skewness
24-hr volume (V_{24}) mls	1730 (721)	437–3861	1576 (734–3150)	0.80
24-hr frequency (F_{24})	7.1 (1.9)	2.0–13.0	7.0 (4.4–10.4)	0.22
Min volume/void (V_{min}) mls	81 (47)	10–300	75 (25–172)	1.36
Max volume/void (V_{max}) mls	514 (190)	150–1000	480 (250–775)	0.70
Average volume/void (V_{avg}) mls	245 (91)	93–519	237 (119–406)	0.56

All are quite variable. For example, V_{24} ranges from 400 ml to almost 4000 ml; F_{24} ranges from 2 to 13, and Vmax ranges from 150 to 1000 ml. Table 27.1 also shows that the frequency distributions of all of the bladder diary measurements are skewed to the right (positive skewness). *Abbreviation:* SD, standard deviation.

post-menopausal women's bladder diary parameters (27). There was no significant difference between the age groups for daytime or night time urine output, nor daytime frequency. The nocturnal proportion of 24-hour volume approached significance (p = 0.09) whereas the night time frequency was significantly higher in the postmenopausal group (1.2 vs. 0; p = 0.05). A direct link between the number of voids per liter intake and the degree of bother with urinary frequency has been expressed (28).

Recent independent studies by van Haarst et al. (29) and Amundsen et al. (30) (592 and 161 asymptomatic females respectively) found that volume per void (volume/void) decreases, and frequency increases, with age, and that both frequency and volume/void increase with increasing 24-hour volume (Figs. 27.3 and 27.4). The robust relationship between 24-hour volume and volume/void runs counter to the widely held assumption that "bladder capacity" remains relatively constant, regardless of total urine output, and that an increase in voiding frequency is the primary response to increased urine production.

The data show that although frequency does increase with increasing 24-hour volume, the concomitant increase in volume/void limits the frequency increase. Thus, the van Haarst and Amundsen studies (29,30) show that a 70-year-old asymptomatic woman is likely to have a higher frequency and smaller volume/void than a 20-year-old asymptomatic woman. Similarly, a woman who voids 3000 ml in 24 hours is likely to have a higher frequency and larger volume/void than a woman of similar age who voids only 1000 ml in 24 hours.

Since "normal" volume/void and frequency are influenced by age and 24-hour volume, "normal limits" of these voiding diary measurements should be adjusted for these parameters. Table 27.2, which was obtained by regression analysis, shows confidence limits of frequency and volume/void that are adjusted for age and 24-hour-volume (29).

CONCLUSION

Although there are limits as to the ability of the FV chart to differentiate between normal and abnormal voiding patterns,

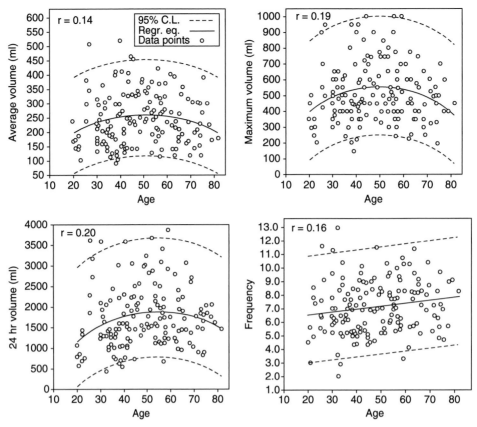

Figure 27.3 Regression analyses of the relationships between age and functional bladder capacity (average and maximum volumes), 24-hour volume and 24-hour frequency. *Abbreviations*: C.L., confidence limits; r, correlation coefficient; Regr. Eq., regression equation.

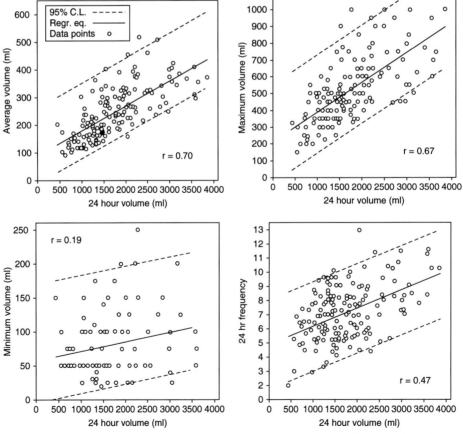

Figure 27.4 Scatter plots and regression analyses of volume-per-void measurements (minimum, maximum, and average volumes), and 24- hour frequency versus 24-hour volume. Dashed lines show 95% confidence limits of the data points (adjusted for skew). The degree-of freedom adjusted correlation coefficient (r) is shown on each chart. *Abbreviations*: C.L., confidence limits; Regr. Eq., regression equation.

Table 27.2 Normal Limits as Published in Asymptomatic Women (30)

Age	\multicolumn{6}{c}{24-hr volume (ml)}					
	1000	1500	2000	2500	3000	3500
24-hr frequency—95th percentiles						
20	8.7	9.3	9.9	10.5	11.2	11.8
30	8.8	9.4	10.1	10.7	11.3	11.9
40	9.0	9.6	10.2	10.8	11.5	12.1
50	9.1	9.7	10.4	11.0	11.6	12.2
60	9.3	9.9	10.5	11.1	11.8	12.4
70	9.4	10.0	10.7	11.3	11.9	12.5
80	9.6	10.2	10.8	11.4	12.1	12.7
Average voided volume (ml)—5th percentiles						
20	107	152	197	242	288	333
30	103	148	194	239	284	329
40	100	145	190	235	281	326
50	96	141	187	232	277	322
60	93	138	183	228	274	319
70	89	134	180	225	270	315
80	86	131	176	221	266	312
Maximum voided volume (ml)—5th percentiles						
20	223	312	402	491	581	670
30	214	303	393	482	572	661
40	226	295	384	474	563	653
50	205	286	375	465	554	644
60	196	277	367	456	546	635
70	188	268	358	447	537	626
80	179	260	349	439	528	618

Table 27.2 presents "normal limits" of bladder diary measurements—defining "normal limit" to include 5% of the reference population (i.e., the 5% or 95% confidence limit). As shown, the lower 5% confidence limit for functional bladder capacity (as measured by V_{avg} and V_{max}) decreases with increasing age and increases with increasing volume, and the upper 95% limit for F_{24} increases with both age and V_{24}. Abbreviations: V_{avg}, average volume/void; V_{max}, max volume/void; F_{24}, 24-hour frequency; V_{24}, 24-hour volume.

it remains integral in the assessment of women with LUTS, and valid for the assessment of urinary frequency and functional capacity. It is easy to complete with even basic instruction to facilitate history taking.

The assessment of computerized diaries has shown promise, but data are still limited. Cost is a serious limiting issue. Intelligent character recognition combines the speed and accuracy of computerized analysis while limiting the cost to a single desktop PC and paper forms.

REFERENCES

1. Abrams P, Fenely R, Torrens M. Patient assessment. In: Abrams P, Fenely R, Torrens M, eds. Urodynamics, 1st edn. New York: Springer, 1983: 6–27.
2. Fink D, Perucchini D, Schaer GN, Haller U. The role of the frequency-volume chart in the differential diagnostic of female urinary incontinence. Acta Obstet Gynecol Scand 1999; 78: 254–7.
3. Parsons M, Dixon A, Thomas M, Cardozo L. An audit of completion of a bladder diary prior to urodynamic studies. King's College Hospital Audit Meeting, July 2004.
4. Heit M, Brubaker L. Clinical correlates in patients not completing a voiding diary. Int Urogynecol J 1996; 7: 256–9.
5. Robinson D, McClish DK, Wyman JF, et al. Comparison between urinary diaries completed with and without intensive patient instructions. Neurourol Urodyn 1996; 15: 143–8.
6. Larsson G, Victor A. Micturition patterns in a healthy female population, studied with a frequency-volume chart. Scand J Urol Nephrol Suppl 1988; 114: 53–7.
7. McCormack M, Infante-Rivard C, Schick E. Agreement between clinical methods of measurement of urinary frequency and functional bladder capacity. Br J Urol 1992; 9: 17–21.
8. Palnæs Hansen C, Klarskov P. The accuracy of the frequency-volume chart: comparison of self-reported and measured volumes. Br J Urol 1998; 81: 709–11.
9. Bryan NP, Chapple CR. Frequency volume charts in the assessment and evaluation of treatment: how should we use them? Eur Urol 2004; 46: 636–40.
10. Diokno AC, Wells TJ, Brink CA. Comparison of self-reported voided volume with cystometric bladder capacity. J Urol 1987; 137: 698–700.
11. de Wachter S, Wyndaele J-J. Frequency-volume charts: a tool to evaluate bladder sensation. Neurourol Urodyn 2003; 22: 638–42.
12. Miller JM, Ashton-Miller JA, Carchidi LT, DeLancey JO. On the lack of correlation between self-report and urine loss measured with standing provocation test in older stress-incontinent women. J Womens Health 1999; 8: 157–62.
13. Brown JS, McNaughton KS, Wyman JF, et al. Measurement characteristics of a voiding diary for use by men and women with overactive bladder. Urology 2003; 61: 802–9.
14. Kahn KS, Chien PFW, Honest MR, Norman GR. Evaluation measurement variability in clinical investigations: the case of ultrasonic estimation of urinary bladder volume. Br J Obstet Gynaecol 1997; 104: 1036–42.
15. Larsson G, Abrams P, Victor A. The frequency/volume chart in detrusor instability. Neurourol Urodyn 1991; 10: 533–43.
16. Larsson G, Victor A. The frequency/volume chart in genuine stress incontinent women. Neurourol Urodyn 1992; 11: 23–31.
17. Abrams P, Klevmark B. Frequency volume charts: an indispensable part of the lower urinary tract assessment. Scand J Urol Nephrol Suppl 1996; 179: 47–53.
18. Nygaard I, Holcomb R. Reproducibility of the seven-day voiding diary in women with stress urinary incontinence. Int Urogynaecol J 2000; 11: 15–17.
19. Groutz A, Blaivas JG, Chaikin DC, et al. Noninvasive outcome measures of urinary incontinence and lower urinary tract symptoms: a multicenter study of micturition diary and pad tests. J Urol 2000; 164(3 Pt 1): 698–701.
20. Tincello DG, Williams KS, Joshi M, Assassa RP, Abrams KR. Urinary diaries: a comparison of data collected for three days versus seven days. Obstet Gynecol 2007; 109(2 Pt 1): 277–80.
21. Quinn P, Goka J, Richardson H. Assessment of an electronic daily diary in patients with overactive bladder. BJU International 2003; 91: 647–52.
22. Rabin JM, McNett J, Badlani GH. Computerised voiding diary. Neurourol Urodyn 1993; 12: 541–54.
23. De Wachter S, Wyndaele JJ. Frequency-volume charts: a tool to evaluate bladder sensation. Neurourol Urodyn 2003; 22: 638–42.
24. Darling R, Neilson D. Convenience voids: an important new factor in urinary frequency volume chart analysis. J Urol 2005; 173: 487–9.
25. Naoemova I, De Wachter S, Wyndaele JJ. Comparison of sensation-related voiding patterns between continent and incontinent women: a study with a 3-day sensation-related bladder diary (SR-BD). Neurourol Urodyn 2008; 27: 511–14.
26. Naoemova I, De Wachter S, Wuyts FL, Wyndaele JJ. Do sensation-related bladder diaries differ between patients with urodynamically confirmed and non-objectivised urinary incontinence? Int Urogynecol J Pelvic Floor Dysfunct 2008; 19: 213–16.
27. Pfisterer MH, Griffiths D, Rosenberg L, Schaefer W, Resnick N. Parameters of bladder function in pre-, peri-, and post-menopausal continent women without detrusor overactivity. Neurourol Urodyn 2007; 26: 356–61.
28. Fitzgerald MP, Butler N, Shott S, Brubaker L. Bother arising from urinary frequency in women. Neurourol Urodyn 2002; 21: 36–41.
29. Van Haarst EP, Heldeweg EA, Newling DW, Schlatmann TJ. The 24-h frequency–volume chart in adults reporting no voiding complaints: defining reference values and analysing variables. BJU Int 2004; 93: 1257–61.
30. Amundsen CL, Parsons M, Tissot B, et al. Bladder diary measurements in asymptomatic females: functional bladder capacity, frequency and 24 hour volume. Neurourol Urodyn 2007; 26: 341–9.
31. Fitzgerald MP, Brubaker L. Variability of 24-hour voiding diary variables among asymptomatic women. J Urol 2003; 169: 207–9.
32. Fitzgerald MP, Stablein U, Brubaker L. Urinary habits among asymptomatic women. Am J Obstet Gynecol 2002; 187: 1384–8.

28 Pad Tests
Marie-Andrée Harvey

HISTORICAL ASPECTS

In 1971 James et al. first described the quantification of urine loss to determine response before and after treatment (1). This was achieved using a pair of elongated electrodes embedded within the absorbent layer of a diaper, which contained dry electrolytes. Following urine loss, the moisture between electrodes resulted in a change in electrical conductivity that could be detected and recorded. It was marketed under the name of Urilos (N. H. Eastwood & Son, Ltd, London, England) (2). However, the equipment was rather cumbersome and never caught on.

The pad test, as we know it today, was originally simultaneously described by Sutherst et al. and by Walsh and Mills in 1981 (3,4). It consists of the use of a perineal pad to document urinary incontinence and to quantify its severity quantitatively, under natural conditions. The amount of loss is calculated by subtracting the weight of the pad before the test, from its weight after the end of the test. A standardized one-hour pad test (Table 28.1) was then proposed in 1983 (5), and endorsed by the International Continence Society (ICS) in 1988 (6).

Other innovative methods were developed, going from the distal urethral electrical conductance (DUEC) test (7,8) to the temperature sensitive device (9). The DUEC involves a 7 Fr catheter placed in the distal urethra, on which two rings, mounted 1mm apart, register the electric potential change occurring when fluid gets into contact with the electrodes. The temperature sensitive device uses a diode temperature sensor imbedded in the outermost layer of a pad, which records a change in voltage across the diode when urine (warmer than the perineum) is lost. These two methods are devised to detect urine leakage during ambulatory urodynamic studies (UDS) without the bulk of the Urilos, but are unable to quantify loss.

The clinical use of these devices has never been evaluated and their accuracy was disputed. The Urilos was said to be able to detect volumes from <1 ml to approximately 100 ml, with a variation of up to 20% when repeated. In subsequent reliability studies the difference in volume recorded between different nappies varied between 13% (2) and 25% (10). When comparing nappies from different boxes, the variation between them was as much as 68% (10). Furthermore, the Urilos was noted to be more uncomfortable, and to not absorb large volumes of fluid (11). Consequently, the Urilos nappy never gained widespread popularity. The DUEC test has experienced a similar fate. In a small study comparing the ICS pad test to the DUEC, the DUEC showed no benefit over the one-hour ICS pad test, with a greater complexity involved (12). A recent study (13) evaluated its role in the diagnosis of women with symptoms of stress urinary incontinence (SUI) but without demonstrable leak on urodynamics or cough stress test (in which a leak is observed when coughing with a comfortably full bladder).

While it detected SUI in 28% of symptomatic women with negative UDS, the DUEC test failed to detect stress incontinence in 33% of symptomatic women with demonstrable stress incontinence during standard UDS.

INDICATIONS

A pad test can thus be used in two manners: as an objective mean of detection of urine leakage when clinical testing is otherwise negative, or to quantify urine loss prospectively. The objective demonstration of urinary incontinence is of importance in its diagnosis and should be part of the clinical assessment of all patients with incontinence (14) and adding a pad test likely improves the identification of women with SUI (15). It is of particular value during research studies for the objective evaluation of treatment response (16). Neither the patient's perception of incontinence (2) nor her perception of its severity (17) are well correlated with urodynamic measures.

Pad tests are generally divided into short (<1 hour, 1 hour, 2 hours), or long (24 hours, 48 hours). Standardization only exists for the ICS one-hour pad test (6). Short pad test are easily performed in an outpatient clinical setting (18). Long-term protocols have, as yet, not been subject to standardization. A pad test should not be done during menstruation.

RELIABILITY AND VALIDITY

"Before one can obtain evidence that an instrument is measuring what is it intended, it is first necessary to gather evidence that [it] is measuring something in a reproducible fashion; it says nothing about what is being measured. To determine that the test is measuring what was intended requires some evidence of 'validity.'" (19) "Validity expresses the relation between observed measurements and the true state of the entity being studied" (20).

Reliability can be defined broadly by two characteristics: internal consistency and stability (19). Internal consistency represents the average of the correlations among all items in the instrument, using different calculations (e.g., Cronbach's alpha). This applies to an instrument with multiple items, such as a questionnaire. In the case of the pad test, reliability is best demonstrated through its stability, i.e., the degree of agreement between different observers (inter-observer reliability), between observations made by the same observer on two different occasions (intra-observer reliability) or observation on the same patient on two distinct occasions, separated by a time-interval (test-retest reliability).

The second dimension that is important in an instrument is its validity. Validity seeks to determine that the tool is measuring what it is intended to measure (urine loss) and does so by comparing the performance of a new tool against that of a known tool, a "gold standard." When such standard is

Table 28.1 Standardized one-hour Pad Test

0 min
    Apply pre-weighed pad
    Drink 500 cc sodium-free liquid
    Sit and rest
30 mins
    Walk and stairs climbing
45 mins
    Activities
        Sit/stand × 10
        Cough × 10
        Run in place × 1 min
        Pick up objects from floor
        Wash hands under running water × 1 min
60 mins
    Collect and weigh pad
    Patient voids, volume measured

Source: Adapted from Ref. 6.

inexistent, validity can be compared or "constructed." In the former situation, the current tool is compared to other tools testing the same or similar condition. This is usually referred to as *criterion, convergent,* or *concurrent validity* and in the case of pad test, can be achieved by comparing pad tests to symptom questionnaires, UDS or other validated pad tests. *Construct validity* is achieved by studying two or more different (e.g., continent vs. incontinent) or similar populations in which it is expected to find a difference, or similarity respectively, between test results. Validity of the pad test can further be revealed by the accuracy of the measured volume lost and its sensitivity in detecting such a loss. If the sensitivity is poor, the test will at times not detect the true state of the entity, namely the presence of incontinence. However, as there is currently no means of detecting the true amount of urine leak with each incontinence episode, the validity of the pad test will be reflected in its ability to demonstrate incontinence in a patient who complains of urinary incontinence, and a lack of urine loss in patients who report continence.

SHORT PAD TESTS

This category includes the following tests: standardized ICS one-hour pad test; modified version of the ICS one-hour test, usually incorporating different exercise intensity; and pad tests <1 hour, using a fixed bladder volume, with retrograde filling.

The type of activity leading to urine loss and the impact of voiding during the test period has been evaluated (21). Irrespective of urodynamic diagnosis, activities leading to leakage in all women included (in increasing order of urine loss) walking around/bed making (3–4 g), climbing stairs up and down with or without heavy pack (5–6 g), picking objects on the floor (6 g), and spending several minutes hand washing (10 g). Voiding during the test had no effect of the result, with a similar proportion being dry on the pad test whether they voided or not.

Some studies have evaluated the feasibility of a home short pad test, where a subject would be given pre-weighted pads

and return the pads in a sealed plastic envelop (22,23). Mailing delays were not shown to significantly alter the measurement of pad weight.

Detection Limit

Increased weight of the pad test may be due to urine, but also to vaginal discharge, sweating, or menstruation. Comparing 50 continent women to 100 incontinent women, a maximum pad weight gain of 1 g was measured in all continent patients versus a mean of 12.2 g in incontinent women (3). Walsh (4) tested six healthy continent volunteers for three consecutive days from 9 am to 9 pm, during which pads were changed every two hours and reported a 1.2 g/2 hr weight gain due to perspiration. Versi and Cardozo (24) compared the one-hour pad test to video-UDS (v-UDS) in 90 continent and 99 UDS-confirmed stress incontinent women. In continent women with normal v-UDS, the mean pad weight gain was 0.4 g, with a 99% upper confidence limit of 1.4 g.

ICS One-hour Pad Test

The ICS one -hour pad test was developed to define a standardized objective measure, which would facilitate comparison between studies. The ICS fixed the threshold for negative pad test at <2 g. However, despite earlier favorable reports, the ICS one-hour has been subsequently shown to have insufficient reliability (25–27), except in one study (28). However, better reproducibility was noted (25) when bladder volume at the start of the test was taken into account. Inter-observer (29) and test-retest (27) reliabilities studies were found to be poor, as show by wide limits of agreement.

It is important to note that a correlation coefficient merely quantifies *association* between two test results. If the two tests compared are the same test, evidently they will be associated, but high association does not necessarily translate in high agreement. The limit of agreement using the Bland and Altman method (30) is a better statistical analysis in describing *agreement* between two tests measuring the same outcome.

Construct validity testing showed that the ICS one-hour pad test correctly identifies continent subjects, but has a substantial false-negative rate in incontinent women (6–32%), when compared to UDS (24,26), except in one study (31), where all 42 women were correctly identified. Versi et al. studied 311 additional women presenting with urinary complaints and failed to show that the test could screen for the pathology found on v-UDS, as the sensitivity was poor (68%) (32). The measure of agreement (kappa's coefficient) between the pad test and the presence of pathology on UDS denoted a moderate agreement (33).

Convergent validity of the ICS one hour pad test has been tested against many symptoms and quality of life questionnaire: the international consultation on incontinence questionnaire (ICIQ-SF) (34), urogenital distress inventory (UDI-6) (34), incontinence impact questionnaire (IIQ-6) (34), the Stamey grading scale (34), the King's health questionnaire (35), the symptom impact index and symptom severity index (36), the UDI and the IIQ (37,38), the patient's perception of incontinence severity (35,39), and the frequency of incontinence episodes on diary (40) with often significant but weak correlations.

Similarly, convergent validity was also tested against UDS. Studies evaluating the relationship between the ICS one-hour pad test and urodynamic measures of urethral integrity reported a weak but significant negative correlation between the urine loss on pad test and the Valsalva leak point pressure (VLPP) in some studies (41,42) but not others (43) and a correlation with maximal urethral pressure (MUCP) (37). That is, with increasing urine loss on pad testing, the VLPP decreased and MUCP decreased. The correlation with MUCP was weak and not found in other studies. The urodynamic diagnosis has a variable effect on pad weight. In one study, women with urodynamic stress incontinence have greater leakage on one hour pad test than those with detrusor overactivity; however, the amount of loss was not discriminatory of the urodynamic diagnosis (40). The opposite was noted elsewhere (44).

Assuming that UDS would represent the gold standard, the pad test seems to be able to discriminate between continent and incontinent women (construct validity) most of the time; a positive test correctly identify incontinent patient, but a negative test may be found in women demonstrated to be incontinent on UDS. It is unable to discriminate among the different types of incontinence pathology found on UDS, or to consistently determine incontinence severity (24,32).

Pad tests can help predict surgical outcome: women with more severe SUI as judged by on one hour pad test weight gain were shown to respond more poorly to surgical repair (42,45). The importance of a negative pad test as an outcome measure following therapy varies considerably between patients, nurses, and physicians, patients being the group for whom cure on pad testing was scored at 67/100 on visual analogue scale (46). The role of pad tests in outcomes research remains to be determined (47).

A suggested classification of the degree of incontinence was suggested by Klarskov and Hald (28): slight to moderate (1–10 ml), severe (10–50), and very severe (>50). This classification has never been validated against other measures of severity.

In light of its limited reliability, it may not come as a surprise that, although endorsed by the ICS, the ICS one-hour pad test is only rarely (33%) followed in outcomes research (48). Surprisingly, despite reports of its poor reproducibility, high urine loss detected on the pad test nevertheless influences clinicians in selecting a surgical treatment option rather than conservative management (49). Furthermore, when used in the research setting, women tend to be less compliant with the study protocol when follow up involves a pad test and a diary (50).

Modified One-hour Pad Tests

Consequently, some have sought to improve the reliability of one-hour pad test, through increasing exercise intensity or controlling the bladder volume.

There is insufficient data to stipulate that an aggressive protocol adds any reliability or sensitivity to the current one-hour test. Subjects were asked to drink 1 L of water in 15 minutes. One hour after starting drinking, they were asked to drink an additional 500 ml (51). The pad test was started as soon as subject felt a full bladder. Fourteen different vigorous exercises

were performed. At the end of the test, voided volume was measured. Exercises included, but were not limited to, star jumps, sprinting, vacuuming, lifting, carrying and putting down a 10 kg box, pulling on an elastic band in addition to standard exercises as included in the ICS one-hour pad test. None of the 18 controls reported or demonstrated any leakage on the pad test. Among the 25 women with symptoms of urinary incontinence tested, eight (32%) had a negative test. Test-retest was obtained in 16 of the 25 women with a correlation of 0.73.

Studies have demonstrated an improved correlation with fixed bladder volume. Subjects have significantly more urine loss with increased bladder volume (25,52). Using a fixed 250 cc bladder volume, a 20 minute pad test is more sensitive than the ICS one hour pad test (53). Performing the pad test once a strong desire (mean 292 ml) is reached further improves sensitivity of the short pad test (54). At 200 cc, a modified one hour pad test did not correlate with leak point pressure (38).

Test-retest reliability of a fixed-bladder volume short pad test showed a substantial difference in the test and retest pad weight, and thus reliability remains limited. Correlations between tests were generally good (44), but such measure of agreement is generally a poor choice when the two tests compared are the same (see above). The limit of agreement (30) showed considerable variability (+24–30 g) with authors, admitting that sensitivity was "hardly much better" than the ICS one-hour (55). However, the difference in mean pad weight was significantly different between the test and the retest (9 g), thus limiting the test reliability. A similar result was reported when bladder was filled at 75% capacity (56), and at 50% capacity (55,57), and at 300 cc (58).

A study of the short pad test with standard volume evaluated the correlation with symptoms (recall of number of clothing changes) (59), which was weak.

The committee on imaging and other investigations from the second International Consultation on Incontinence (60) concluded that the one-hour pad test was not accurate, unless done at fixed bladder volume; the sequence of exercises did not affect the result; and a positive pad test was one weighting >1 g. They suggested that 20 minutes to one-hour ward test with fixed bladder volume be used if a short pad test was done.

Pyridium Test

Phenazopyridine hydrochloride (Pyridium, Parke-Davis) ingestion results in the dye being excreted by the kidney with consequent coloring (orange) of the urine. It has been used by clinicians to detect incontinence due to the compound's property of coloring urine orange. Wall et al. (31) reported the sensitivity and specificity of pyridium as a qualitative test in incontinent patients. While very sensitive, the addition of pyridium was not specific. The poor specificity was due to a high false-positive rate in asymptomatic patients. This may be explained by staining of the perineum at the time of a prior void, resulting in tinting of a subsequent pad on vulvar contact or by a minimal, non-clinically significant, loss of urine in normal women. These results were subsequently confirmed in a study testing continent (self-reported) women, during exercise (61), in which pyridium staining in nearly 100% of

subjects after physical activity, with a mean pad weight of 4.59 + 3.55 g (outdoor exercise) or 1.33 + 0.97 g (indoor exercise). Pyridium staining was minimal, with a mean stained area of 2.66 mm (range 0–11 mm). No cut off limit in the pad weight has been previously established to define a normal pad test during exercise given that there would be a greater weight gain due to perspiration alone.

In the light of these report, the use of pyridium in detecting urethral incontinence can be perceived as unreliable and non-specific. Nonetheless, it remains useful in the diagnosis of extra-urethral urine loss (e.g., fistulae).

LONG PAD TEST

The one-hour pad test has been criticized because of its artificial setting and short duration. A longer duration pad test was first described by Sutherst's group, in an abstract (62). But the aim of the study then was to determine if the one-hour pad test was representative of urine loss experienced during regular activity, not to assess if it was better in detecting and quantifying incontinence than its shorter counterpart. It was suggested by Lose et al. performing a test during regular daily activities would be more sensitive than during a single one-hour test (63).

Typically, a long pad test is performed at home, during a typical day's activities. The subject is given a number of pre-weighed pads, placed in individual sealed envelope. She is instructed to wear the pad consecutively for a given period (12, 24, 48, or 72 hours) and to return the pads in their sealed envelope for weighing. The 24 hour pad test showed only limited diagnostic value for self-reporting of incontinence in pregnancy or postpartum (64).

Detection Limit

Lose et al. first established a detection limit by studying 23 asymptomatic female subjects (63). They noted that the median weight obtained for the 24-hour pad test was 4.0 g, with a 99% upper limit of 8 g for the 24 hour period. Ryhammer et al. (65) studied 78 self-reported continent women. Their mean loss was 3.1 g (range 0–9 g) during a 24-hour pad test. Versi et al. (66) studied 24 young continent women during a 48-hour pad test and reported a mean loss of 7.1 g, with a 95% upper confidence limit of 14.5 g. Mouritsen et al. (67) reported a detection limit in normal subjects, for a 24 hour pad test of a mean 2.6 g, 95% upper confidence limit of 5.5 g. In a more recent study, an upper limit of 1.3 g/24 hr was noted (68). Although supported by only the later study, the committee on imaging and other investigations from the second International Consultation on Incontinence (60) recommended that a pad gain of ≥1.3 g during a 24-hour pad test be considered as positive.

Reliability and Validity

The long pad tests have a good test-retest reliability as shown by the correlation obtained, keeping in mind the limitations of the ability of this measure of association in determining agreement. Victor et al. were the first to compare test-retest of the 24-hour pad test (69). Fifteen women performed a 48-hour pad test and repeated it one week later. When comparing the

first 24 hours of the two 48-hour pad tests, correlation was significant (r = 0.66). Lose et al. (63) performed test-retest evaluation of the 24-hour home pad test in 31 women referred for incontinence. A significant correlation (r = 0.82) was noted between the two tests. The limit of agreement was approximately +100 g, which means that the second test done could yield greater or lesser results the second time by as much a 100 g. This represents a large variability of results. Rasmussen et al. (70) evaluated 14 women for test-retest reliability of the 24-hour pad test. They failed to find a linear correlation between the two tests. The second test could be anywhere between a third less to three times more than the first 24-hour period tested. Versi et al. (66) looked at the reproducibility of the first 24 hours from a 48 hour pad test, compared to the first 24 hours of a second 48 hour pad test in 140 symptomatic patients. They noted a strong correlation (0.9) and a difference between the two tests of 7%. When looking at the test-retest done during the first 24 hours of a 72 hour pad test done twice in 106 women, Groutz et al. (71) used another statistical marker of reliability [Lin's concordance correlation coefficient (CCC) (72), in which reliability was defined as a coefficient >0.7]. The coefficient obtained was 0.72. More recently, Karantanis et al. (73) assessed the repeatability of seven consecutive 24 hour pad tests on 108 women using repeated measure analysis of variance (ANOVA). No difference in mean pad test among the seven days was detected, suggesting repeatability.

Similarly, the test-retest reliability of the 48-hour and 72-hour pad test has been reported to be very good, although the statistic used (correlation) is of limited strength to measure association. Victor et al. (69) reported a correlation coefficient of 0.9 between two tests performed at least one week apart. Versi et al. (66) reported similar correlation, with a difference in weight between the two tests of only 1.6%. Groutz et al. (71), when comparing the first two days of a 72 hour pad test done on two different occasions, found a Lin's CCC of 0.88. The test-retest correlation (using Lin's CCC) was greatest for the 72-hour pad test (CCC = 0.94). The first 24 hours of a 48 hour pad test has been compared to the full 48 hour test and the two tests have been shown to highly correlate (r = 0.92), suggesting that the 48 hours did not add much to a 24 hour test (74). More recently, Karantanis et al. (73) reported high correlation (r = 0.88) between the first 24 hour pad test and the seven day average of seven consecutive 24 hour pad tests.

Attempts at categorizing the severity of incontinence according to weight gain on long pad test was done by applying the percentage of the data which was classified as mild, moderate or severe on the one-hour tests. Leakage of <20 g on a 24 hour pad test was classified as mild, 20 to 74 g as moderate and ≥75 g as severe (75). Here also, no validity study has been done to assess agreement of this categorization with other measures of incontinence severity.

A balance between response rate desired and accuracy of the method must be struck, as the need to perform a 24-hour pad test had been shown to deter patients' participation in trials (50). Consequently, the committee on imaging and other investigations from the second International Consultation on Incontinence (60) concluded that the 24-hour pad test was reproducible and recommended that a test lasting more than

24 hours had little advantage. It has been suggested that the 24 hour pad test be used as a composite outcome measures in research, as it was noted to reflect surgical results more accurately (76).

The construct and convergent validity of the home pad test, i.e., its ability to not record weight gain in continent women and its ability to detect urine loss in patients with established urinary incontinence on UDS has been reported. Using continent volunteers, Molloy et al. (77) noted that the weight loss or gain of pads pre-infused with precise volume did not show clinically relevant differences, albeit a statistical significance of up to +1.3 cc was noted for each 12 hour periods. One study failed to confirm construct validity, with continent and incontinent women showing no difference in pad weight gain (65). Convergent validity showed weak correlation between a 24 hour pad test and the severity index (78), the quality of life questionnaire (IIQ) or the symptom questionnaire (UDI) but high correlation with the number of incontinence frequency as recorded on diary (79,80), and on ICIQ-SF questionnaire (80). No correlation with Stamey grade was noted (80). The 48 hour pad test correlated moderately with the urinary incontinence severity score and strongly with a visual analogue scale quantifying bothersomeness of current incontinence (81).

Convergent validity with UDS was assessed in numerous studies. Some concluded that the 24 hour test was perhaps more sensitive than Video-UDS (66,82). The false negativity of the 24 hour pad test has been estimated to be around 8% (66). These earlier studies suggest a reasonably low false-negative 24-hour pad test compared to UDS and an improved detection of urinary incontinence in symptomatic subjects with negative UDS. This is in contrast with a later study in which 33% of women with urodynamic stress incontinence, 43% of those with detrusor overactivity and 37% of women with missed UDS diagnoses were dry on the 24 hour pad test (40). The amount lost on 24 hour pad test is not discriminatory of the urodynamic diagnosis (40). Furthermore, the 24 hour pad correlates negatively only very weakly with the VLPP (79).

SHORT VS. LONG PAD TEST
Overall, the home pad tests (24- or 48-hours) poorly correlate with one-hour pad tests and are more sensitive than the shorter one-hour pad test.

Ali et al. (62) first compared in an abstract, the 1-hour to a 12-hour pad test, and they noted a "close correlation." In another study (63,83), 31 women with urinary incontinence who had a one-hour pad test (standard volume of 200–300 ml) and a 24-hour pad test were studied. Of these, 13 had a negative one-hour pad test, of which however, 10 had a positive 24-hour pad test, giving a false negative rate of 39% for the one-hour pad test, compared to the 24-hour. No correlation was found between the 1-hour and the 24-hour. This report was echoed by others (69,74,82). More recent studies have found a moderate to strong correlation between the 24-hour and the 1-hour tests, in addition to reporting that the one-hour detected more incontinent women than the 24-hour (38,40).

Both tests lack the ability to discriminate between UDS diagnoses as there is considerable overlap between pad loss across UDS diagnoses (40).

PAPER TOWEL TEST
Most of the methods objectively quantifying urine loss preclude detection of small volumes, as these may overlap with perspiration and vaginal secretions. A simple non-invasive test was developed to detect losses associated with stress incontinence (84). While a tri-fold brown paper towel is held under the perineum, the patient is asked to cough three times consecutively. The surface of the wetted area is calculated using the ellipse formula (ϖxy), x and y being the orthogonal axes of the area, and then converted to volume of urine lost (using a standard curve). The relationship between the measured area and a known fluid volume was found to have a very strong correlation ($r = 0.998$). In a test-retest evaluation within the same visit and between visits the authors also showed a high correlation coefficient and concluded that the quantitative paper towel test was accurate and reliable in detecting small losses of urine due to stress incontinence. The paper towel test has not been found to correlate with self-reported severity of incontinence (85). Test-retest reproducibility was within 1 cc (86). This test has not been validated against a gold standard diagnostic method such as multichannel video-urodynamics.

SUMMARY
To date, the objective urine loss test most useful in clinical practice remains the perineal pad test. A short version has been standardized to a certain degree by the ICS, rendering its use more uniform for research data collection. However, the bladder volume at the beginning of the one-hour test should be standardized. The one-hour pad test has not been found to have good reproducibility, although it is improved with standardized bladder volume. The short-term pad test was found to be valid in differentiating normal from abnormal continence mechanisms; however, its validity is somewhat limited as it has a significant false-negative rate. Finally, the ability of the short-term pad test (≤1 hour) to categorize severity of incontinence was noted to be poor.

The long-term pad test (≥24 hours), on the other hand, was found to be valid in detecting incontinence, with a good sensitivity and a lower false negatives rate. The reproducibility was similarly noted to be good for both a 48 hour and a 24 hour test period. Hence, a 24 hour home pad test represents a good tool in detecting and quantifying incontinence. Neither test can distinguish between different types of urodynamic diagnoses.

ACKNOWLEDGMENT
I would like to acknowledge the contribution from Dr. Eboo Versi, co-author in the first edition of this chapter.

REFERENCES
1. James ED, Flack FC, Caldwell KP, Martin MR. Continuous measurement of urine loss and frequency in incontinent patients. Preliminary report. Br J Urol 1971; 43: 233–7.
2. Stanton SL. Urilos: the practical detection of urine loss. Am J Obstet Gynecol 1977; 128: 461–3.

3. Sutherst J, Brown M, Shawer M. Assessing the severity of urinary incontinence in women by weighing perineal pads. Lancet 1981; 1: 1128–30.

4. Walsh JB, Mills GL. Measurement of urinary loss in elderly incontinent patients. A simple and accurate method. Lancet 1981; 1: 1130–1.

5. Bates P, Bradley W, Glen E, et al. Fifth report on the standardization of terminology of lower urinary tract function. Bristol International Society Committee on Standardisation of Terminology, 1983.

6. Abrams P, Blaivas JG, Stanton SL, Andersen JT. The standardisation of terminology of lower urinary tract function. The international continence society committee on standardisation of terminology. Scand J Urol Nephrol Suppl 1988; 114: 5–19.

7. Plevnik S, Vrtacnik P, Janez J. Detection of fluid entry into the urethra by electric impedance measurement: electric fluid bridge test. Clin Phys Physiol Meas 1983; 4: 309–13.

8. Plevnik S, Brown M, Sutherst JR, Vrtacnik P. Tracking of fluid in urethra by simultaneous electric impedance measurement at three sites. Urol Int 1983; 38: 29–32.

9. Eckford SD, Finney R, Jackson SR, Abrams P. Detection of urinary incontinence during ambulatory monitoring of bladder function by a temperature-sensitive device. Br J Urol 1996; 77: 194–7.

10. Wilson PD, Al Samarrai MT, Brown AD. Quantifying female incontinence with particular reference to the Urilos system. Urol Int 1980; 35: 298–302.

11. Eadie A, Glen E, Rowan D. Assessment of urinary loss over a two-hour test period: a comparison between the Urilos recording nappy system and the weighed perineal pad method. Proceedings of the 14th Annual Scientific Meeting of the International Continence Society. Innsbruck, 1984: 94–5.

12. Holmes D, Plevnik S, Stanton SL. Distal urethral electric conductance (DUEC) test for the detection of urinary leakage. Proceedings of the 15th Annual Meeting of the International Continence Society. London, 1985: 94–5.

13. Adekanmi OA, Freeman RM, Reed H, Bombieri L. Improving the diagnosis of genuine stress incontinence in symptomatic women with negative cough stress test: the Distal Urethral Electrical Conductance test (DUEC) revisited. Int Urogynecol J 2003; 14: 9–12.

14. Abrams P, Cardozo L, Fall M, et al. The standardisation of terminology of lower urinary tract function: report from the Standardisation Sub-committee of the International Continence Society. Neurourol Urodyn 2002; 21: 167–78.

15. Martin JL, Williams KS, Abrams KR, et al. Systematic review and evaluation of methods of assessing urinary incontinence. Health Technol Assess (Winchester, England) 2006; 10: 1–132, iii–iv.

16. Payne C, Blaivas JG, Brown J, et al. Research methodology. In: Abrams P, Cardozo L, Khoury S, Wein A, eds. Incontinence. West Caldwell: Health Publication, 2005: 97–148.

17. Frazer MI, Haylen BT, Sutherst JR. The severity of urinary incontinence in women. Comparison of subjective and objective tests. Br J Urol 1989; 63: 14–15.

18. Batista Miranda JE, Da SV, Granda CM, et al. Quantification of urine leaks: standardized one-hour pad test. Actas Urol Esp 1997; 21: 111–16.

19. Streiner D, Norman G. Basic concepts. In: Health Measurements Scales: A practical Guide to Their Development and Use, 2nd edn. Oxford: Oxford University Press, 1995.

20. Khan KS, Chien PF, Honest MR, Norman GR. Evaluating measurement variability in clinical investigations: the case of ultrasonic estimation of urinary bladder volume. BJOG 1997; 104: 1036–42.

21. Sutherst JR, Brown MC, Richmond D. Analysis of the pattern of urine loss in women with incontinence as measured by weighing perineal pads. Br J Urol 1986; 58: 273–8.

22. Wilson PD, Mason MV, Herbison GP, Sutherst JR. Evaluation of the home pad test for quantifying incontinence. Br J Urol 1989; 64: 155–7.

23. Flisser AJ, Figueroa J, Bleustein CB, Panagopoulos G, Blaivas JG. Pad test by mail for home evaluation of urinary incontinence. Neurourol Urodyn 2004; 23: 127–9.

24. Versi E, Cardozo LD. Perineal pad weighing versus videographic analysis in genuine stress incontinence. Br J Obstet Gynecol 1986; 93: 364–6.

25. Lose G, Gammelgaard J, Jorgensen TJ. The one-hour pad-weighing test: Reproducibility and the correlation between the test result, the start volume in the bladder, and the diuresis. Neurourol Urodyn 1986; 5: 17–21.

26. Jørgensen L, Lose G, Andersen JT. One-hour pad-weighing test for objective assessment of female urinary incontinence. Obstet Gynecol 1987; 69: 39–42.

27. Simons AM, Yoong WC, Buckland S, Moore KH. Inadequate repeatability of the one-hour pad test: the need for a new incontinence outcome measure. BJOG 2001; 108: 315–19.

28. Klarskov P, Hald T. Reproducibility and reliability of urinary incontinence assessment with a 60 min test. Scand J Urol Nephrol 1984; 18: 293–8.

29. Christensen SJ, Colstrup H, Hertz JB. Inter- and intra-departmental variations of the perineal pad weighing test. Neurourol Urodyn 1986; 5: 23–8.

30. Bland JM, Altman DG. Statistical methods for assessing agreement between two methods of clinical measurement. Lancet 1986; 1: 307–10. [see comment].

31. Wall LL, Wang K, Robson I, Stanton SL. The pyridium pad test for diagnosing urinary incontinence: a comparative study of asymptomatic and incontinent women. J Reprod Med 1990; 35: 682–4.

32. Versi E, Cardozo L, Anand D. The use of pad tests in the investigation of female urinary incontinence. J Obstet Gynaecol 1988; 8: 270–3.

33. Groen J, Bosch JLHR. Agreement between cystometry and noninvasive incontinence tests in stress incontinent females. Urodinamica 2002; 12: 4–9.

34. Franco AV, Lee F, Fynes MM. Is there an alternative to pad tests? Correlation of subjective variables of severity of urinary loss to the 1-h pad test in women with stress urinary incontinence. BJU Int 2008; 102(5):586-90.

35. Abdel-fattah M, Barrington JW, Youssef M. The standard 1-hour pad test: does it have any value in clinical practice? Euro Urol 2004; 46: 377–80.

36. Aslan E, Beji NK, Coskun A, Yalcin O. An assessment of the importance of pad testing in stress urinary incontinence and the effects of incontinence on the life quality of women. Int Urogynecol J Pelvic Floor Dysfunct 2003; 14: 316–19.

37. Costantini E, Lazzeri M, Bini V, et al. Sensitivity and specificity of one-hour pad test as a predictive value for female urinary incontinence. Urol Int 2008; 81: 153–9.

38. Peterson AC, Amundsen CL, Webster GD. The 1-hour pad test is a valuable tool in the initial evaluation of women with urinary incontinence. Journal of Pelvic Medicine and Surgery 2005; 11: 251–6.

39. Oh SJ, Ku JH, Hong SK, et al. Factors influencing self-perceived disease severity in women with stress urinary incontinence combined with or without urge incontinence. Neurourol Urodyn 2005; 24: 341–7.

40. Matharu GS, Assassa RP, Williams KS, et al. Objective assessment of urinary incontinence in women: comparison of the one-hour and 24-hour pad tests. Eur Urol 2004; 45: 208–12.

41. Ku JH, Shin JW, Oh SJ, Kim SW, Paick JS. Clinical and urodynamic features according to subjective symptom severity in female urinary incontinence. Neurourol Urodyn 2006; 25: 215–20.

42. Paick JS, Ku JH, Shin JW, et al. Significance of pad test loss for the evaluation of women with urinary incontinence. Neurourol Urodyn 2005; 24: 39–43.

43. Lee SU, Lee SH, Kim H. The comparison of the abdominal leak point pressure and the 1-hour pad test in patients with stress urinary incontinence. [Korean]. Korean J Urol 2006; 47: 847–51.

44. Fantl JA, Harkins SW, Wyman JF, Choi SC, Taylor JR. Fluid loss quantiation test in women with urinary incontinence: a test-retest analysis. Obstet Gynecol 1987; 70: 739–43.

45. O'Sullivan R, Simons A, Prashar S, et al. Is objective cure of mild undifferentiated incontinence more readily achieved than that of moderate incontinence? Costs and 2-year outcome. Int Urogynecol J Pelvic Floor Dysfunct 2003; 14: 193–8.

46. Tincello DG, Alfirevic Z. Important clinical outcomes in urogynecology: views of patients, nurses and medical staff. Int Urogynecol J 2002; 13: 96–8.

47. Weber AM, Abrams P, Brubaker L, et al. The standardization of terminology for researchers in female pelvic floor disorders. Int Urogynecol J 2001; 12: 178–86.

48. Soroka D, Drutz HP, Glazener CM, Hay-Smith EJ, Ross S. Perineal pad test in evaluating outcome of treatments for female incontinence: a systematic review. Int Urogynecol J Pelvic Floor Dysfunct 2002; 13: 165–75.

49. Thomson AJ, Tincello DG. The influence of pad test loss on management of women with urodynamic stress incontinence. BJOG 2003; 110: 771–3.

255

50. Singh M, Bushman W, Clemens JQ. Do pad tests and voiding diaries affect patient willingness to participate in studies of incontinence treatment outcomes? J Urol 2004; 171: 316–18.

51. Devreese AM, De Weerdt WJ, Feys HM, et al. Functional assessment of urinary incontinence: the perineal pad test. Clin Rehabil 1996; 10: 210–15.

52. Jakobsen H, Kromann-Andersen B, Nielsen KK, Maegaard E. Pad weighing tests with 50% or 75% bladder filling. Does it matter? Acta Obstet Gynecol Scand 1993; 72: 377–81.

53. Wu WY, Sheu BC, Lin HH. Comparison of 20-minute pad test versus 1-hour pad test in women with stress urinary incontinence. Urology 2006; 68: 764–8.

54. Wu WY, Sheu BC, Lin HH. Twenty-minute pad test: comparison of infusion of 250 ml of water with strong-desire amount in the bladder in women with stress urinary incontinence. Eur J Obstet Gynecol Reprod Biol 2008; 136: 121–5.

55. Lose G, Rosenkilde P, Gammelgaard J, Schroeder T. Pad-weighing test performed with standardized bladder volume. Urology 1988; 32: 78–80.

56. Kinn A-C, Larsson B. Pad test with fixed bladder volume in urinary stress incontinence. Acta Obstet Gynecol Scand 1987; 66: 369–71.

57. Hahn I, Fall M. Objective quantification of stress urinary incontinence: a short, reproducible, provocative pad-test. Neurourol Urodyn 1991; 10: 475–81.

58. Persson J, Bergqvist CE, Wolner-Hanssen P. An ultra-short perineal pad-test for evaluation of female stress urinary incontinence treatment. Neurourol Urodyn 2001; 20: 277–85.

59. Elser DM, Fantl JA, Mcclish DK. Comparison of "subjective" and "objective" measures of severity of urinary incontinence in women. Program for Women Research Group. Neurourol Urodyn 1995; 14: 311–16.

60. Artibani W, Andersen JT, Gajewski JB, et al. Imaging and other investigations. In: Abrams P, Cardozo L, Khoury S, Wein A, eds. Incontinence. Health Publication Ltd, 2002: 425–77.

61. Nygaard I, Zmolek G. Exercise pad testing in continent exercisers: reproducibility and correlation with voided volume, pyridium staining, and type of exercise. Neurourol Urodyn 1995; 14: 125–9.

62. Ali K, Murray A, Sutherst J, Brown. Perineal pad weighing test: comparison of one hour ward pad test with twelve hours home pad test. Proceedings of the 13th Annual Meeting of the International Continence Society. Aachen, 1983: 380–2.

63. Lose G, Jorgensen L, Thunedborg P. 24-hour home pad weighing test versus 1-hour ward test in the assessment of mild stress incontinence. Acta Obstet Gynecol Scand 1989; 68: 211–15.

64. Wijma J, Weis Potters AE, Tinga DJ, Aarnoudse JG. The diagnostic strength of the 24-h pad test for self-reported symptoms of urinary incontinence in pregnancy and after childbirth. Int Urogynecol J Pelvic Floor Dysfunct 2008; 19: 525–30.

65. Ryhammer AM, Laurberg S, Djurhuus JC, Hermann AP. No relationship between subjective assessment of urinary incontinence and pad test weight gain in a random population sample of menopausal women. J Urol 1998; 159: 800–3.

66. Versi E, Orrego G, Hardy E, et al. Evaluation of the home pad test in the investigation of female urinary incontinence. Br J Obstet Gynecol 1996; 103: 162–7. [see comment].

67. Mouritsen L, Berlid G, Hertz J. Comparison of different methods for quantification of urinary leakage in incontinent women. Neurourol Urodyn 1989; 8: 579–87.

68. Karantanis E, O'Sullivan R, Moore KH. The 24-hour pad test in continent women and men: normal values and cyclical alterations. BJOG 2003; 110: 567–71.

69. Victor A, Larsson G, Asbrink AS. A simple patient-administered test for objective quantitation of the symptom of urinary incontinence. Scand J Urol Nephrol 1987; 21: 277–9.

70. Rasmussen A, Mouritsen L, Dalgaard A, Frimodt-Moller C. Twenty-four hour pad weighing test: reproducibility and dependency of activity level and fluid intake. Neurourol Urodyn 1994; 13: 261–5.

71. Groutz A, Blaivas JG, Chaikin DC, et al. Noninvasive outcome measures of urinary incontinence and lower urinary tract symptoms: a multicenter study of micturition diary and pad tests. J Urol 2000; 164(3 Pt 1): 698–701.

72. Lin LI. A concordance correlation coefficient to evaluate reproducibility. Biometrics 1989; 45: 255–68.

73. Karantanis E, Allen W, Stevermuer TL, et al. The repeatability of the 24-hour pad test. Int Urogynecol J Pelvic Floor Dysfunct 2005; 16: 63–8.

74. Thind P, Gerstenberg TC. One-hour ward test vs. 24-hour home pad weighing test in the diagnosis of urinary incontinence. Neurourol Urodyn 1991; 10: 241–5.

75. O'Sullivan R, Karantanis E, Stevermuer TL, Allen W, Moore KH. Definition of mild, moderate and severe incontinence on the 24-hour pad test. BJOG 2004; 111: 859–62.

76. Groutz A, Blaivas JG, Rosenthal JE. A simplified urinary incontinence score for the evaluation of treatment outcomes. Neurourol Urodyn 2000; 19: 127–35. [see comment] [comment].

77. Molloy SS, Nichols TR, Sexton WL, Murahata RI. Validity and reliability of a pad test model using a simulated urine leak and healthy continent females. Urol Nurs 2007; 27: 300–4.

78. Sandvik H, Seim A, Vanvik A, Hunskaar S. A severity index for epidemiological surveys of female urinary incontinence: comparison with 48-hour pad-weighing tests. Neurourol Urodyn 2000; 19: 137–45.

79. Albo M, Wruck L, Baker J, et al. The relationships among measures of incontinence severity in women undergoing surgery for stress urinary incontinence. Journal of Urology 2007; 177: 1810–4.

80. Karantanis E, Fynes M, Moore KH, Stanton SL. Comparison of the ICIQ-SF and 24-hour pad test with other measures for evaluating the severity of urodynamic stress incontinence. Int Urogynecol J Pelvic Floor Dysfunct 2004; 15: 111–16.

81. Stach-Lempinen B, Kirkinen P, Laippala P, Metsanoja R, Kujansuu E. Do objective urodynamic or clinical findings determine impact of urinary incontinence or its treatment on quality of life? Urology 2004; 63: 67–71.

82. Griffiths DJ, McCRacken PN, Harrison GM. Incontinence in the elderly: objective demonstration and quantitative assessment. Br J Urol 1991; 67: 467–71.

83. Jørgensen L, Steen A, Bagger P, Fisher-Rasmussen W. The one-hour pad-weighing test for assessment of the result of female incontinence surgery. Proceedings of the 15th annual meeting of the international continence society. London, 1985: 392–3.

84. Miller JM, Ashton-Miller JA, Delancey JOL. Quantification of cough-related urine loss using the paper towel test. Obstet Gynecol 1998; 91: 705–9.

85. Miller JM, Ashton-Miller JA, Carchidi LT, Delancey JOL. On the lack of correlation between self-report and urine loss measured with standing provocation test in older stress-incontinent women. J Womens Health 1999; 8: 157–62.

86. Neumann P, Blizzard L, Grimmer K, Grant R. Expanded paper towel test: an objective test of urine loss for stress incontinence. Neurourol Urodyn 2004; 23: 649–55.

29 Uroflowmetry
Matthias Oelke and Jean-Jacques Wyndaele

INTRODUCTION

Urodynamic observations (e.g., measurement of urinary flow) have been defined by the International Continence Society (ICS) as observations made during urodynamic studies (1). A particular urodynamic observation (e.g., decreased urinary flow rate) may have a variety of underlying causes and, therefore, may not be sufficient to make a definitive diagnosis of a disease or condition. Hence, uroflowmetry should never be used as a single test but always combined with clinical information (e.g., history, physical examination, voiding chart, or pad-test) and other tests (e.g., measurement of postvoid residual urine, ultrasound assessment of the lower or upper urinary tract) to draw useful conclusions with regard to diagnosis or treatment benefit. Urodynamic observations may occur in the presence or absence of symptoms and signs.

Abrams regarded uroflowmetry as a screening test that should be performed as an essential examination prior to all other urodynamic testing and as a routine examination for the pre- and post-operative assessment of lower urinary tract dysfunction (LUTD) (2). The report of the ICS Standardization Committee on Good Urodynamic Practices confirms this postulate (3). The French Committee of Female Urology and Urogynecology recommends evaluation of bladder emptying by uroflowmetry and measurement of postvoid residual urine in all patients prior to surgery (4). In women with urinary incontinence, the current version of the European Association of Urology Guidelines on urinary incontinence suggests that uroflowmetry should be performed especially in those individuals who have "complicated" incontinence which includes, next to others, recurrent urinary tract infections, reported voiding dysfunction, significant pelvic organ prolapse, failed previous incontinence surgery, and after radiotherapy or pelvic surgery (5).

This chapter deals with the urodynamic observation of urinary flow. Such measurement objectively determines the volume of urine expelled from the bladder per time sequence and quantifies voiding. Moreover, if this volume-time equation is drawn as a curve, the measurement of urinary flow also gives information on how urine evacuation exactly proceeds. Objective and quantitative data, which primarily help in the understanding of voiding symptoms, are provided by measurement of urinary flow. As with all investigations, the diagnostic value of uroflowmetry depends on the way the test is performed, quality of the measuring equipment, and knowledge of the individual who interprets the measurement. This chapter provides information accordingly.

SYMPTOMS RELATED TO FLOW

Uroflowmetry aims to reproduce, qualify, and quantify urinary symptoms which have brought the patient to consultation or the patient reported about during systematic initial assessment. However, uroflowmetry can only objectively investigate symptoms related to flow but cannot determine symptoms related to urine storage. In daily life, the patient is usually the only observer of her urinary flow, and the interpretation of subjective observations may need to be objectively confirmed and quantified by flow measurements. There might be a discrepancy between subjective reporting and objective measurement of flow. Long standing uroflow abnormalities might not be perceived as abnormal because a comparison with normal voiding is lacking in those individuals. Furthermore, most women void in privacy and have little opportunity to compare voiding patterns (6).

The following urinary symptoms are related to voiding and defined by the ICS Standardization Committee on Terminology of Lower Urinary Tract Function (1):

- *Hesitancy* is the term used when an individual describes difficulty in initiating micturition resulting in a delay in the onset of voiding after the individual is ready to pass urine.
- *Straining* to void describes the muscular effort used to initiate, maintain, or improve the urinary stream.
- *Slow stream* is reported by the individual as her perception of reduced urine flow, usually compared to previous performance or in comparison to others.
- *Splitting* or *spraying* of the urine stream is the term used when urine flows to different directions.
- *Intermittency* (or *intermittent stream*) describes urine flow that stops and starts during micturition. In contrast, continuous flow is when the individual reports emptying the bladder without pauses during a single voiding attempt.
- *Terminal dribble* is the term used when an individual describes a prolonged final part of micturition, when the flow has slowed to a trickle or dribble. In contrast, postmicturition dribbling is the term used when the individual describes the involuntary loss of urine immediately after she has finished voluntary voiding, usually after rising up from the toilet.

UROFLOWMETRY EQUIPMENT

The first documented urine flow measurement was performed by Eugen Rehfisch in Berlin, Germany in 1897 using a flowmeter based on air displacement (7). Historically, many different types of uroflowmeters have been proposed. Some were based on the principle of voiding distance (8,9), audio (10), weight (11), variations of a constant magnetic field (12), rotating disk, measurement of size and velocity of drops (13), and air displacement (14). Susset et al. (15) compared weight, rotating disk, and air displacement techniques, and found all of them to have certain values and limitations. The ICS Working Party on Urodynamic Equipment described the most commonly used uroflowmeters employing one of the following methods (16):

- *The gravimetric method*: This technique operates by measuring the weight of the collected fluid or hydrostatic pressure at the base of the collecting cylinder. In both cases, the output signal is proportional to the collected fluid mass. Gravimetric meters therefore measure accumulated mass, and mass flow rate is obtained by differentiation. Nowadays, most of the uroflowmeters use this principle of uroflow measurement which is considered the most precise measurement technique.
- *The electronic dip-stick method*: The electrical capacitance of a dip-stick mounted in the collecting chamber changes as the urine accumulates. The output signal is proportional to the accumulated volume and the volumetric flow rate is obtained by differentiation.
- *The rotating disk method*: The voided fluid is directed onto a rotating disk, thereby increasing the inertia of the disk. The power required to keep the disk rotating at a constant speed is proportional to the mass flow rate of the fluid. The accumulated mass is obtained by integration.

The accuracy of uroflowmeters was discussed in the ICS Good Urodynamic Practices report (3). There are differences in accuracy and precision of the flow rate signals that depend on the type of uroflowmeter, internal signal processing, and the proper use as well as calibration of the flowmeter. The desired and actual accuracy of uroflowmetry should be assessed in relation to the potential information that could be obtained from the urinary stream compared to the information actually abstracted for clinical and research purposes. Some relevant aspects of the physiologic and physical information contained in the urinary stream are outlined in the report (3).

The desired clinical accuracy may differ from the technical accuracy. The ICS report (3,10) recommends as standards a range of 0 to 50 ml/sec for maximum urinary flow rate (Q_{max}), 0 to 1000 ml for voided volume, maximum time constant of 0.75 seconds, and an accuracy of $\pm 5\%$ relative to full scale. As most flowmeters are mass flowmeters using the gravimetric method, variations in the specific gravity of the fluid will have a direct influence on the measured flow rate. For example, urine of high concentration increase apparent flow rate by up to 3%. With X-ray medium, the flow rate may be overestimated by as much as 10%. Correction by calibration software is possible but seldom performed.

Since the overall accuracy of flow rate signals is not better than $\pm 5\%$, it is not important to report Q_{max} to a resolution better than a full milliliter per second. A better resolution is possible under carefully controlled research conditions but such advanced measurement accuracy is usually not required in daily clinical practice, especially when screening of LUTD.

UROFLOW MEASUREMENT

Normal voiding occurs when the bladder outlet (internal and external urethral sphincters) completely relaxes and the detrusor actively contracts. The mechanical properties of a relaxed bladder outlet are usually constant, and the properties can be defined by the relationship between the cross-sectional area of the urethral lumen and the intraurethral pressure at the flow controlling zone. Below the minimum urethral opening pressure the urethral lumen is closed and the urine remains in the bladder; the lumen then widely opens with little additional pressure increase and urinary flow starts to emerge. The interpretation of uroflow curves can be performed by measuring several parameters and by gross interpretation of the flow curve itself.

Parameters of Uroflowmetry (1) (Figs. 29.1a and b)

- *Flow time* is the time over which measurable flow actually occurs. Flow time is expressed in seconds (sec).
- *Voiding time* is the total duration of micturition, including interruptions. When voiding is completed without interruption, voiding time is equal to flow time. Voiding time is expressed in seconds.
- *Voided volume* is the total expelled volume via the urethra and expressed in milliliters (ml).
- *Flow rate* is defined as the volume of expelled fluid via the urethra per time unit and expressed in milliliters per second (ml/sec).
- *Maximum flow rate (Q_{max})* is the maximum measured value of the flow rate after correction for artifacts and expressed in milliliters per second.
- *Time to maximum flow* is the elapsed time from onset of flow to Q_{max} and expressed in seconds.
- *Average flow rate (Q_{ave})* is voided volume divided by flow time, expressed in milliliters per second. The average flow should be interpreted with caution if the flow is interrupted or there is terminal dribbling.

Shape of the Flow Curve

The shape of the flow curve is determined by the contractile properties of the detrusor, the ability to relax the bladder outlet, and by the presence or absence of abdominal straining during voiding (1). The ICS good urodynamic practices guidelines (3) state that an easily distensible, relaxed bladder outlet together with a normal detrusor contraction will result in a smooth, arc-shaped curve with high amplitude (Fig. 29.2). When the bladder outlet is completely relaxed and the woman voids without straining, the shape of the curve is only determined by the kinetics of the detrusor contraction which reflects the properties of slowly contracting detrusor smooth muscle cells; therefore, flow rate should not have rapid variations. The continuous flow curve is defined either as a smooth arc-shaped curve or as fluctuating when there are multiple peaks during a period of continuous urine flow (Fig. 29.3). It is a widespread assumption that normal micturition is always associated with a normal flow pattern. However, this would also mean that a

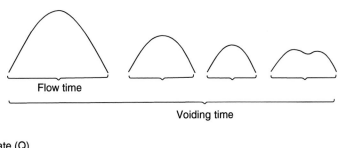

(A)

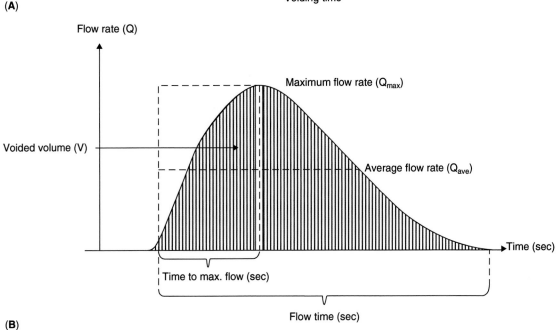

(B)

Figure 29.1 (**A**) Difference between flow time and voiding time (1). (**B**) Schematic explanation of uroflow recording, with nomenclature and units recommended by the International Continence Society (1).

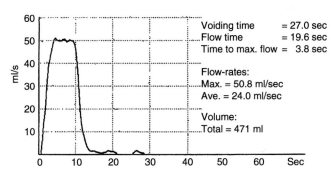

Voiding time = 27.0 sec
Flow time = 19.6 sec
Time to max. flow = 3.8 sec

Flow-rates:
Max. = 50.8 ml/sec
Ave. = 24.0 ml/sec

Volume:
Total = 471 ml

Figure 29.2 Bell-shaped uroflow with normal flow values.

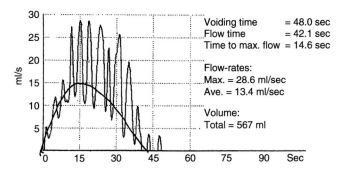

Voiding time = 48.0 sec
Flow time = 42.1 sec
Time to max. flow = 14.6 sec

Flow-rates:
Max. = 28.6 ml/sec
Ave. = 13.4 ml/sec

Volume:
Total = 567 ml

Figure 29.3 Fluctuating flow curve with multiple peaks, prolonged flow time, and normal maximum flow rate (Q_{max}) during automatic evaluation but decreased Q_{max} after correction (straight arc drawn in flow recording). Flow curve possibly due to straining.

normal flow curve would correspond with normal voiding and would even permit the exclusion of LUTD. Pauwels et al. (17) demonstrated that a "normal" bell-shaped flow curve does not exclude female voiding dysfunction by investigating the value of a normal flow pattern in four different groups: women with stress urinary incontinence (SUI), detrusor over-activity, healthy middle-aged volunteers, and healthy young students. These women voided with a bell-shaped flow curve in 50%, 65%, 57%, and 50%, respectively. Women who strained during voiding (a major component of dysfunctional voiding) managed to void a bell-shaped flow curve in 46%, 60%, 70%, and 100%, respectively.

Other shapes of flow curves, such as flat (Fig. 29.4), asymmetric, or multiple interrupted curves (Fig. 29.5), are indicative of abnormal voiding but not specific for a certain disease or condition. Impairment of detrusor power (detrusor under-activity) and/or increased urethral pressure will both result in decreased Q_{max} and Q_{ave} as well as a smooth, flat curve. Constrictive obstruction (e.g., due to urethral strictures or perforated vaginal tapes) is caused by a reduced size of the urethral lumen and results in a plateau-like curve (Fig. 29.4). The magnitude of Q_{max} is determined by the residual ure-thral diameter at the level of obstruction. However, the same pattern may also originate from detrusor underactivity in ageing females.

Fluctuations in detrusor contractility, straining, or inter-mittent sphincter activity during voiding may result in com-

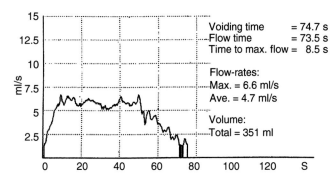

Figure 29.4 Flat flow curve with decreased maximum flow rate (Q_{max}) and increased flow time, suspicious of bladder outlet obstruction, detrusor underactivity, or dysfunctional voiding.

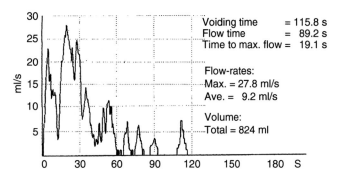

Figure 29.5 Multiple interrupted flow curve (staccatos) with abnormal maximum flow rate (Q_{max}), possibly due to straining, detrusor-sphincter dysfunction, or voiding next to the collecting device.

plex flow patterns (Figs. 29.3 and 29.5). Rapid changes in flow rate may be due to sphincter/pelvic floor contractions, mechanical compression of the urethral lumen or interference at the meatus, or to changes in the driving energy as with straining. Rapid changes may also be due to artifacts caused by interference between the stream and the collecting device, movement of the stream across the surface of the funnel or patient movements. If fast variations of urinary flow have been observed, patients should be asked if this voiding pattern reflects normal voiding at home, they have strained, or emptied their bladder next to the collecting device. A visual control with regard to urine remnants next to the flowmeter might be useful in cases of suspected voiding next to the uroflowmeter.

INTERPRETATON OF UROFLOW VALUES AND CURVES (3)

As already mentioned, uroflow values and the shape of the flow curve might suggest LUTD but reliable, specific, and detailed information about the exact cause for abnormal voiding cannot be derived from a flow curve alone (18). Only measurement of the pressure–flow relationship by computerurodynamic investigation can clarify the exact pathophysiology. Urine flow measurements are influenced by several factors which have to be taken into consideration during flow evaluation and interpretation. Not all relationships between voiding

and specific conditions have been equally investigated in both men and women but they are assumed to be similar in the context of this chapter:

- *Detrusor contractility*: For stable outlet conditions and voiding without straining, all variations in flow rate are related only to changes of detrusor activity and power. Detrusor contraction strength can decrease in patients with neurogenic, myogenic, and combined diseases.
- *Bladder outflow resistance*: With changes of outflow resistance, for example due to voluntary or involuntary sphincter contractions during voiding or due to bladder outlet obstruction, flow rate will change if detrusor contractility is constant. Q_{max} <15 ml/sec and/or postvoid residual urine volume >50 ml with a minimum total bladder volume of 150 ml before voiding (volume voided + residual) as well as the 10th percentile curve of the Liverpool Nomogram for Q_{max} both correlate well with bladder outlet obstruction in women (Fig. 29.6) (19).
- All *intra-abdominal modulations* of the flow rate are physiologic artifacts and should be minimized, for example, by asking the patient to relax and not to strain.
- *Patient age*: Healthy female volunteers aged between 16 and 64 years showed no statistically significant variation in urine flow rate with regard to age, parity, or first versus repeated voiding (20). In female patients aged 40 years or older, Madersbacher et al. (21) described decreasing urine flow rates (Q_{max}, Q_{ave}) and increasing post-void residuals with ageing indicating that older individuals have reduced bladder contractility (detrusor underactivity) and/or a less compliant urethras. Additionally, bladder capacity, voided volume, functional urethral length, and maximum urethral closure pressure significantly decrease with increasing age.
- The *influence of urethral manipulation* on uroflowmetry results remains controversial. One study in women showed no difference between pre- and post-catheterization flow rates (22). However, catheterization to fill the bladder in order to perform quick uroflowmetry can alter the following flow parameters: Q_{max} and Q_{ave} can decrease and time to maximum flow as well as duration of flow can increase (23–25). Catheters with a diameter of seven French or more are likely to alter urine flow (26). Although the effect of cystoscopy on urine flow parameters was only evaluated in men Issa et al. (27) demonstrated that Q_{max} significantly decreased by 27% after instrumentation. Therefore, urethral manipulation should be avoided prior to uroflowmetry whenever possible.
- Oral or intravenous *diuretics* as well as increased fluid intake significantly reduce waiting time for flow measurement but do not significantly alter uroflow parameters such as Q_{max} or voided volume (28–30).

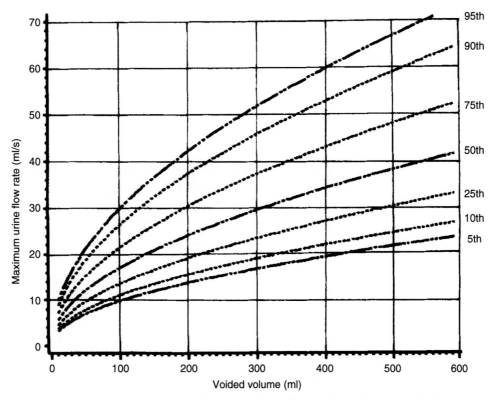

Figure 29.6 Liverpool Nomogram for the judgment of maximum flow rate (Q_{max}) relative to voided volume (38).

Although uroflowmetry is a non-invasive test excessive fluid intake may rarely be associated with water intoxication resulting in hyponatremia and seizure (31).

- *Patient behavior*: Nervousness during flow testing in the hospital may lead to incomplete sphincter relaxation and decreased urinary flow rate or even intermittent flow.
- *Circadian rhythm*: It was shown in men that urine flow varies during the 24 hour period with higher Q_{max} values, smaller voided volumes, and reduced flow time in the early afternoon when compared with the late evening, early morning, and the midnight to morning periods (32).
- *Influence of posture*: Devreese et al. (33) investigated the influence of three different postures on urine flow parameters in 21 healthy volunteers. Sitting in anteversion, retroversion, or forward bending, all without straining, showed no significant differences for Q_{max}, Q_{ave}, and total flow time. However, intermittent flow (staccatos) was less frequently seen in the forward-bending position suggesting that this position permits optimal relaxation of the pelvic floor muscles and, therefore, is the preferable voiding position. Non-adapted height of the toilet seat preventing the feet from resting on the floor or crouching over the toilet is associated with postvoid residual urine.
- *Influence of straining*: A considerable number of healthy women strain to initiate or maintain voiding;

in a prospective study of healthy, asymptomatic women 42% strained during voiding (34). Independent of the posture on the toilet, straining has been shown to increase Q_{max} and Q_{ave} and decrease total voiding time (33). This reinforcement of flow occurs only when the urethra is completely relaxed and the flow controlling zone of the urethra is not under the influence of the abdominal pressure. Needle or surface electrodes did not show relevant sphincter activity in healthy women who strained during voiding (34,35). As discussed previously, straining can also produce a bell-shaped flow curve (17).

- *Bladder volume*: Q_{max} and Q_{ave} are physiologically dependent on bladder volume. A positive correlation has been found between bladder filling volume and Q_{max}/Q_{ave} (Figs. 29.6 and 29.7) (20,36–38). As the bladder volume increases and the detrusor muscle progressively stretches, the potential bladder power and work associated with contraction will also increase. This is most pronounced in the range from an empty bladder up to approximately 200 ml of bladder filling. At bladder filling volumes higher than 400 to 500 ml, the detrusor becomes overstretched and contractility may decrease again; however, there are large inter-individual differences. The flow–bladder volume relationship also varies with the type and degree of pathology as, for example, in constrictive obstruction where Q_{max} is almost independent of bladder volume.

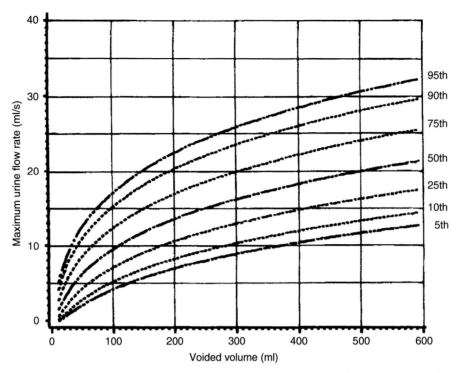

Figure 29.7 Liverpool Nomogram for the judgment of average flow rate (Q_{ave}) relative to voided volume (38).

- *Nomograms:* These have been developed to correctly judge the relationship between voided volume and Q_{max} or Q_{ave} (37,38). (Liverpool Nomogram, Figs. 29.6 and 29.7).
- *Free uroflowmetry versus flow recording during pressure-flow studies:* It is necessary to insert a catheter into the bladder for pressure recording; however, a transurethral catheter might interfere with voiding. Flow time is significantly increased and flow rates are significantly decreased in women with urethral catheters compared to those without catheters indicating that invasive uroflowmetry does not reflect physiologic urination (25,26,39). In women with invasive flow measurement, there were no differences between 4.5 and 6 F catheters but significant differences were shown between 4.5 and 7 F catheters. Furthermore, intermittent flow is more common with inserted catheters (25).
- *Intraobserver variability of measurements:* Variability in interpretation was seen when done by four physicians with a minimum of six months experience in urogynecology and with an eight-week interval between both evaluations (18). The difference was not large in the study by Jorgensen et al. (40) when the evaluation showed that visually read values were significantly lower than the mechanically determined ones, especially for Q_{max} in abnormal curves. The authors concluded that automatic computerized evaluation of uroflow curves may be misleading and cannot replace visual evaluation.
- *Interobserver variability of flow curve assessment:* Visual assessment of uroflow curves by urodynamists

demonstrated a substantial agreement of Q_{max}, Q_{ave}, flow time, voiding time, and the judgment of the curve as being "normal" or "abnormal" (41). These results were independent of physicians' age or experience with uroflowmetry (less than 5, 5–10, or more than 10 yrs). Interestingly, there was a higher agreement between physicians who dedicated an appropriate amount of their time to uroflowmetry compared to those who spent less than 5% of their time to urodynamic practices. Computerized artifact detection and correction eliminates a relevant fraction of the variability of uroflow (Q_{max}) and decreases intra- and inter-observer variability (42,43).

- *Home uroflowmetry* by means of a portable device proved to be a more accurate because it facilitates multiple measurements in a normal environment (44,45). A close relationship between Q_{max} at home and in the hospital was found but voided volume and voiding time were significantly larger in the hospital (44). However, these variations between home and office flows appear to be irrelevant for screening of LUTD.

RECOMMENDATIONS FOR UROFLOW MEASUREMENT (3,4,46)

1. The flowmeter should be regularly calibrated and the calibration documented.
2. Patients should void with a "comfortably full bladder." Since this might be difficult to arrange in a hospital, patients should have the opportunity to drink fluids and void several times during one consultation.

3. Provide a separate room with clean material but without stimuli that might interfere with voiding (e.g., noise, music, disturbance, smell, dark atmosphere, or insufficient light). The flow curve should be recorded outside the flow room using electronic data transfer in order to avoid distraction during uroflow performance.

4. Offer a toilet seat that allows the feet resting on the floor.

5. After voiding, patients should be asked if the void was representative of their usual voiding pattern at home. Additionally, patients should be asked if they strained during uroflowmetry.

6. Compare the results of uroflowmetry with data obtained by the patient's own recording on a frequency-volume chart.

7. For graphic depiction of the flow curve, the x-axis represents time and 1 mm should equal one second. The y-axis represents the flow rate and 1 mm should equal 1 ml/sec and 10 ml voided volume.

8. A sliding average over two seconds should be used to remove positive and negative spike artifacts in order to make electronically recorded Q_{max} values more reliable, comparable, and clinically useful.

9. Flow traces and the computer output derived form should be carefully scrutinized for artifacts and corrected, if necessary.

10. Only flow rate values smoothed either electronically or manually should be reported (40). When reading Q_{max} graphically, the line should be smoothed by the eye into a continuous curve so that, in each period of two seconds, there are no rapid changes.

11. Q_{max} should be rounded to the nearest whole number (e.g., a recorded value of 10.25 ml/sec should be reported as 10 ml/sec).

12. Voided volume and post-void residual urine should be rounded to the nearest 10 ml (e.g., a recorded value of 322 ml should be reported as 320 ml).

13. Q_{max} should always be documented together with voided volume and post-void residual urine volume.

14. If a flow-volume nomogram is used, this should be stated and referenced (e.g., Liverpool Nomogram, Figs. 29.6 and 29.7).

15. Do more than one test, especially when the first flow does not permit a clear interpretation, has shown pathological values or a pathological flow curve, or was reported not to be representative of home flows.

16. Measurement of post-void residual urine improves interpretation of the test.

UROFLOWMETRY IN HEALTHY VOLUNTEERS

For correct assessment of measured values and curves and for adequate interpretation of the results of uroflowmetry, it is important to have data of age-matched healthy individuals. This normative data should derive from groups of healthy, asymptomatic, and disease-free volunteers. Table 29.1 lists free uroflowmetry data of volunteers who voided with full bladder (34,47,48). Normal Q_{max} depends on the voided volume and

Table 29.1 Normal Values of Free Uroflowmetry in Healthy, Symptom- and Disease Free Women Who Voided with Full Bladder

Population	Wyndaele (47) 10 healthy women	Pauwels et al. (34) 32 healthy women	Oelke et al. (48) 30 healthy women
Age (yrs) (range)	24 (19–28)	49 ± 6 (38–60)	26.2 ± 7.3 (16–40)
Voided volume (ml)	337.5 ± 234.2	340 ± 165	492 ± 175
Q_{max} (ml/sec)	30.5 ± 10.8	29.3 ± 11.8	33 ± 12
Q_{ave} (ml/sec)	21.5 ± 13.7	17.5 ± 8.1	19 ± 9.3
Time to Q_{max} (sec)	8.3 ± 8.1	7 ± 3	10 ± 5
Voiding time (sec)	27.6 ± 22	23 ± 12	32 ± 15
Flow time (sec)	26 ± 20	20 ± 9	30 ± 17

ranges between 12 and 40 ml/sec (49). Normal Q_{ave} values vary from 6 to 25 ml/sec with a substantial overlap between normal and abnormal individuals. Voiding time varies from 10 to 20 seconds at a volume of 100 ml to 25–35 seconds for a volume of 400 ml (50).

Arbitrary criteria have been proposed by a number of authors to diagnose LUTD. For bladder outlet obstruction, the equation of Q_{max} <15 ml/sec and/or postvoid residual urine volume >50 ml in a bladder filled with a minimum of 150 ml before voiding (volume voided + post-void residual) was suggested (19,51). Costantini et al. (19) showed that these criteria correlated well with results of the Liverpool Nomogram when voided volumes <15 and >600 ml were excluded. It was concluded that values below the 10th percentile are abnormal (Fig. 29.6).

Wyndaele (47) compared the uroflow curve in 10 young female volunteers and found seven to have a bell-shaped curve on free flow, one voiding in two separate curves, and two presenting a continuous but undulating curve during the entire flow. If compared to the curve pattern obtained during a subsequent pressure-flow study seven had the same pattern but three, with bell-shaped flow during free flow, had an irregular or interrupted flow pattern. Pauwels et al. (17) found that during free uroflowmetry only 83% of middle-aged healthy women and only 75% of young and healthy individuals voided with a normal voiding pattern. In uroflowmetry recorded during pressure-flow analysis, only half of the healthy women voided with a normal flow pattern. The flow patterns during free flow and pressure-flow recording corresponded in 47% to 75%, respectively, depending on patients' symptoms. Free flow and pressure flow patterns matched better in healthy women than in patients.

Miyata et al. (52) analyzed voiding parameters in 36 healthy adult females and found voiding time to be a useful parameter that was independent of the voided volume between 100 and 400 ml and never exceeded 21 seconds in all voiding attempts. Voiding time was shorter in healthy volunteers than in 84% of neurogenic patients and 67% of patients with chronic cystitis.

UROFLOWMETRY IN FEMALE PATIENTS

Several conditions might have an influence on uroflowmetry and should be taken into consideration before flow measurement and during interpretation of the flow curve. Voiding difficulties, defined as abnormally slow and incomplete voiding, are often not reported by the affected women and only diagnosed during systematic evaluation of voiding function. Therefore, a detailed voiding history and screening uroflowmetry are recommended in women at risk:

- *Pregnancy and puerperium*: A significant increase in flow rate was only seen in the second trimester of pregnancy (53). A significant decrease in flow rate was documented during intravenous tocolysis with α-adrenoceptor agonists. Urinary flow rates were worse after forceps delivery but better after spontaneous delivery compared to controls. However, all flow rates remained within the normal range.

- *Delivery*: Comparison of urinary flow curves between primaparas and nulliparas showed no differences in Q_{max}, Q_{ave}, voided volume, voiding time, and time to peak flow (33). However, cesarean section seems to be more frequently associated with postvoid dribbling.

- *Menstrual cycle*: No difference was seen in any measured uroflowmetry parameter when comparing similar voids between different phases of the menstrual cycle. Therefore, when evaluating premenopausal patients, uroflowmetry may be scheduled and performed during either phase of the menstrual cycle (24).

- *SUI*. Conflicting data has been published with regard to Q_{max} in women with SUI. Bottaccini et al. (54) contended that stress incontinent women void with a lower flow rate than healthy women because the distal urethral cross-sectional area appears to be incapable of opening as widely as the distal urethra of normal women. However, other studies have demonstrated the opposite: SUI women void with higher flow rates because of lower bladder outlet resistance (55). Free flow appears to have a low positive predictive value for indicating abnormal pressure-flow studies in SUI women with or without previous surgery (56,57).

- *Genital prolapse*: Q_{max}, Q_{ave}, and voided volume have been described to be significantly lower than in healthy controls (45). Cystocele appears significantly more frequent in patients with voiding difficulties and, vice versa, the frequency of cystocele and voiding dysfunctions was shown to be significantly higher in women with abnormal uroflowmetry (19). Valentini et al. (58) demonstrated a constrictive effect on the bladder outflow in women with various degrees of cystocele. Poor flow rates and elevated postvoid residual urine appears to be associated with higher grades of cystoceles (59).

- *Large uterine fibroids*: One study reported that Q_{max}, Q_{ave}, and voided volume are significantly lower in diseased than in healthy controls (45).

- *Uroflowmetry in women before and after SUI surgery*: Normal or abnormal uroflow parameters, including Q_{max} of free flow, do not predict urinary retention after SUI surgery (60,61). There is, however, some evidence that poor bladder emptying, defined as low flow rates and/or postvoid residual urine, may predict voiding difficulties after surgery for SUI (62,63). Free uroflow at a follow-up of one year after tension-free vaginal tape (TVT) implantation was compared to preoperative values and demonstrated a statistically significant decrease in Q_{max} and increase in postvoid residual urine (64). By applying modeling of free uroflow, Fritel et al. (65) showed development of compressive obstruction in 34 of 50 patients (68%) after the TVT-procedure. The counter-pressure of the tape on the urethra results in continence. During voiding, this effect can be unmasked if women strain, resulting in lower flow rate. The hypothesis of constrictive obstruction with reduction of the cross-section of the urethra of about 60% was proposed for 27 patients.

- *Radical hysterectomy for cervical cancer*: Compared to the preoperative situation, increased postvoid residual urine volumes and decreased flow rates were detected in women after radical hysterectomy (66). Bladder dysfunction was attributed to a significant reduction in detrusor contractility with concomitant abdominal straining due to impaired parasympathetic motor innervation (67). However, the values improved from baseline to six months after surgery.

CONCLUSIONS

Uroflowmetry is a valuable, inexpensive, non-invasive, and fairly reliable screening test for women with suspected LUTD. Practical application and interpretation have to follow strict rules. Uroflowmetry should always be combined with other clinical tests for assessment of bladder function or screening for treatment. In patients with a pathological outlet, additional pressure-flow studies are recommended to evaluate the exact cause of LUTD.

REFERENCES

1. Abrams P, Cardozo L, Fall M, et al. The standardisation of terminology of lower urinary tract function: report from the Standardisation Subcommittee of the International Continence Society. Neurourol Urodyn 2002; 21: 167–78.
2. Abrams P. The practice of urodynamics. In: Mundy AR, Stephenson TP, Wein AJ, eds. Urodynamics. Principles, Practice and Application. Edinburgh: Churchill Livingstone, 1984: 76–92.
3. Schäfer W, Abrams P, Liao L, et al. Good urodynamic practices: uroflowmetry, filling cystometry, and pressure-flow studies. Neurourol Urodyn 2002; 21: 261–74.
4. Hermieu JF; Comité d'Urologie et de Pelvi-périneologie de la Femme Association Frannaise de'Urologie. Recommendations for the urodynamic examination in the investigation of non-neurological female urinary incontinence. Prog Urol 2007; 17(6 Suppl 2): 1264–84.
5. Schröder A, Abrams P, Andersson KE, et al. Guidelines on urinary incontinence. In: European Association of Urology Pocket Guidelines. Arnhem: EAU Guidelines Office, 2009: 138–49.
6. Nitti VW, Tu LM, Gitlin J. Diagnosing bladder outlet obstruction in women. J Urol 1999; 161: 1535–40.

7. Ryall RL, Marshall VR. Measurement of urinary flow rate. Urology 1983; 22: 556–64.

8. Schwartz O, Brenner A. Untersuchung über die Physiologie und Pathologie der Blasenfunktion. VIII: Die Dynamik der Blase. Z Urol Chir 1922; 8: 32.

9. Ballenger EG, Elder OF, McDonald HP. Voiding distance decrease as important symptom of prostatic obstruction. South Med J 1932; 25: 863.

10. Keitzer WA, Huffman GC. The voiding audiograph: a new voiding test. J Urol 1966; 96: 404–10.

11. Drake WM Jr. The uroflowmeter in the study of bladder neck obstructions. J Am Med Assoc 1954; 156: 1079–80.

12. Cardus D, Quesada EM, Scott FB. Use of an electromagnetic flowmeter for urine flow measurements. J Appl Physiol 1963; 18: 845–7.

13. Zinner NR, Ritter RC, Sterling AM, et al. Drop spectro-meter: a non-obstructive, non-interfering instrument for analyzing hydrodynamic properties of human urination. J Urol 1969; 101: 914–8.

14. Palm L, Nielsen OH. Evaluation of bladder function in children. J Pediatr Surg 1967; 2: 529–35.

15. Susset JG, Picker P, Kretz M, et al. Critical evaluation of uroflowmeters and analysis of normal curves. J Urol 1973; 109: 874–8.

16. Rowan D, James ED, Kramer AE, et al. Urodynamic equipment: technical aspects. produced by the International Continence Society Working Party on Urodynamic Equipment. J Med Eng Technol 1987; 11: 57–64.

17. Pauwels E, De Wachter S, Wyndaele JJ. A normal flow pattern in women does not exclude voiding pathology. Int Urogynecol J Pelvic Floor Dysfunct 2005; 16: 104–8.

18. Chou TP, Gorton E, Stanton SL, et al. Can uroflowmetry patterns in women be reliably interpreted? Int Urogynecol J Pelvic Floor Dysfunct 2000; 11: 142–7.

19. Costantini E, Mearini E, Pajoncini C, et al. Uroflowmetry in female voiding disturbances. Neurourol Urodyn 2003; 22: 569–73.

20. Sjöberg B, Nyman CR. Hydrodynamics of micturition in healthy females: pressure and flow at different micturition volumes. Urol Int 1981; 36: 23–34.

21. Madersbacher S, Pycha A, Schatzl G, et al. The aging lower urinary tract: a comparative urodynamic study of men and women. Urology 1998; 51: 206–12.

22. Bergman A, Bhatia NN. Uroflowmetry: spontaneous versus instrumented. Am J Obstet Gynecol 1984; 150: 788–90.

23. Tessier J, Schick E. Does urethral instrumentation affect uroflowmetry measurements? Br J Urol 1990; 65: 261–3.

24. Visco AG, Cholhan HJ, O'Toole L, et al. Effects of menstrual cycle and urinary tract instrumentation on uroflowmetry. Neurourol Urodyn 2000; 19: 147–52.

25. Groutz A, Blaivas JG, Sassone AM. Detrusor pressure uroflowmetry studies in women: effect of a 7Fr transurethral catheter. J Urol 2000; 164: 109–14.

26. Sorensen S, Jonler M, Knudsen UB, et al. The influence of a urethral catheter and age on recorded urinary flow rates in healthy women. Scand J Urol Nephrol 1989; 23: 261–6.

27. Issa MM, Chun T, Thwaites D, et al. The effect of urethral instrumentation on uroflowmetry. BJU Int 2003; 92: 426–8.

28. Gurevitch EJ, Kella N, Gapin T, Roehrborn CG. Urinary flow rate recording: the impact of a single dose of a diuretic on clinic logistics and flow rate parameters. J Urol 1999; 161: 1509–12.

29. Oztürk B, Cetinkaya M, Oztekin V, et al. Effects of forced diuresis archieved by oral hydration and oral diuretic administration on uroflowmetric parameters and clinical waiting time of patients with lower urinary tract symptoms. Urol Int 2003; 71: 22–5.

30. Allen DJ, Ewe SH, Kucheria R, et al. Impact of intravenous furosemide on flow rate characteristics and clinic waiting times. Int J Urol 2008; 15: 344–5.

31. Issa MM, Pruthi RS, Vial C, et al. An unusual complication following uroflowmetry: water intoxication resulting in hyponatremia and seizure. Urol Int 1997; 59: 129–30.

32. Witjes WP, Wijkstra H, Debryne FM, de la Rosette JJ. Quantitative assessment of uroflow: is there a circadian rhythm? Urology 1997; 50: 221–8.

33. Devreese AM, Nuyens G, Staes F, et al. Do posture and straining influence urinary-flow parameters in normal women? Neurourol Urodyn 2000; 19: 3–8.

34. Pauwels E, De Laet K, De Wachter S, Wyndaele JJ. Healthy, middle-aged, history-free, continent women—do they strain to void? J Urol 2006; 175: 1403–7.

35. Bo K, Stein R. Needle EMG registration of striated urethral wall and pelvic floor muscle activity patterns during cough, Valsalva, abdominal contractions. Neurourol Urodyn 1994; 13: 35–41.

36. Rollema HJ, Griffiths DJ, van Duyl WA, et al. Flow rate versus bladder volume. An alternative way of presenting some features of the micturition of healthy males. Urol Int 1977; 32: 401–12.

37. Siroky MB, Olsson CA, Krane RJ. The flow rate nomogram: I. Development. J Urol 1979; 122: 665–8.

38. Haylen BT, Ashby D, Sutherst JR. Maximum and average urine flow rates in normal male and female populations—the Liverpool nomograms. Br J Urol 1989; 64: 30–8.

39. Scaldazza CV, Morosetti C. Effect of different sized transurethral catheters on pressure-flow studies in women with lower urinary tract symptoms. Urol Int 2005; 75: 21–5.

40. Jorgensen JB, Mortensen T, Hummelmose T, et al. Mechanical versus visual evaluation of urinary flow curves and patterns. Urol Int 1993; 51: 15–8.

41. Gacci M, Del Popolo G, Artibani W, et al. Visual assessment of uroflowmetry curves: description and interpretation by urodynamists. World J Urol 2007; 25: 333–7.

42. Witjes WP, de la Rosette JJ, Zerbib M, et al. Computerized artifact detection and correction of uroflow curves: towards a more consistent quantitative assessment of maximum flow. Eur Urol 1998; 33: 54–63.

43. Witjes WP, de la Rosette JJ, van den Berg-Segers A, et al. Computerized assessment of maximum flow: an efficient, consistent and valid approach. Eur Urol 2002; 41: 206–13.

44. Boci R, Fall M, Walden M, et al. Home uroflowmetry: improved accuracy in outflow measurement. Neurourol Urodyn 1999; 18: 25–32.

45. Porru D, Scarpa RM, Onnis P, et al. Urinary symptoms in women with gynecological disorders: the role of symptom evaluation and home uroflowmetry. Arch Esp Urol 1998; 51: 843–8.

46. Homma Y, Batista J, Bauer S, et al. Urodynamics. In: Abrams P, Cardozo L, Khoury S, Wein A, eds. Incontinence. Plymouth: Health Publication, 2002:318–72.

47. Wyndaele JJ. Normality in urodynamics studied in healthy adults. J Urol 1999; 161: 899–902.

48. Oelke M, Höfner K, Jonas U, et al. Ultrasound measurement of detrusor wall thickness in healthy adults. Neurourol Urodyn 2006; 25: 308–17.

49. Blaivas JG. Techniques of evaluation. In: Yalla SV, McGuire EJ, Elbadawi A, Blaivas JG, eds. Neurourology and Urodynamics. Principles and Practice. New York: Macmillan, 1988: 155–98.

50. Kondo A, Mitsuya H, Torii H. Computer analysis of micturition parameters and accuracy of uroflowmeter. Urol Int 1978; 33: 337–44.

51. Romanzi LJ, Chaikin DC, Blaivas JG. The effect of genital prolapse on voiding. J Urol 1999; 161: 581–6.

52. Miyata M, Mizunaga M, Saga Y, et al. Micturition and uroflowmetric analysis of adult females. Nippon Hinyokika Gakkai Zasshi 1990; 81: 1071–8.

53. Fischer W, Kittel K. Urine flow measurement in pregnancy and the puerperium. Zentralbl Gynakol 1990; 112: 593–9.

54. Bottaccini MR, Gleason DM. Urodynamic norms in women. I. Normals versus stress incontinents. J Urol 1980; 124: 659–62.

55. Lemack GE, Baseman AG, Zimmern PE. Voiding dynamics in women: a comparison of pressure-flow studies between asymptomatic and incontinent women. Urology 2002; 59: 42–6.

56. Defreitas GA, Lemack GE, Zimmern PE. Nonintubated uroflowmetry as a predictor of normal pressure flow study in women with stress urinary incontinence. Urology 2003; 62: 905–8.

57. Gravina GL, Costa AM, Galatioto GP, et al. Urodynamic obstruction in women with stress urinary incontinence—do nonintubated uroflowmetry and symptoms aid diagnosis? J Urol 2007; 178: 959–63.

58. Valentini FA, Besson GR, Nelson PP, et al. A mathematical micturition model to restore simple flow recordings in healthy and symptomatic individuals and enhance uroflow interpretation. Neurourol Urodyn 2000; 19: 153–76.

59. Coates KW, Harris RL, Cundiff GW, et al. Uroflowmetry in women with urinary incontinence and pelvic organ prolapse. Br J Urol 1997; 80: 217–21.

60. Miller EA, Amundsen CL, Toh KL, et al. Preoperative urodynamic evaluation may predict voiding dysfunction in women undergoing pubovaginal sling. J Urol 2003; 169: 2234–7.

61. Lemack GE, Krauss S, Litman H, FitzGerarld MP, et al. Normal preoperative urodynamic testing does not predict voiding dysfunction after Burch colposuspension versus pubovaginal sling. J Urol 2008; 180: 2076–80.

62. McLennan MT, Melick CF, Bent AE. Clinical and urodynamic predictors of delayed voiding after fascia lata sub-urethral sling. Obstet Gynecol 1998; 92: 608–12.

63. Thompson PK, Duff DS, Thayer PS. Stress incontinence in women under 50: does urodynamics improve surgical outcome? Int Urogynecol J Pelvic Floor Dysfunct 2000; 11: 285–9.

64. Al-Badr A, Ross S, Soroka D, et al. Voiding patterns and urodynamics after a tension-free vaginal tape procedure. J Obstet Gynaecol Can 2003; 25: 725–30.

65. Fritel X, Valentini F, Nelson P, et al. Contribution of modeling to the analysis of mictional modifications caused by TVT: study of free uroflows. Prog Urol 2004; 14: 197–202.

66. Chuang TY, Yu KJ, Penn IW, et al. Neurourological changes before and after radical hysterectomy in patients with cervical cancer. Acta Obstet Gynecol Scand 2003; 82: 954–9.

67. Scotti RJ, Bergman A, Bhatia NN, et al. Urodynamic changes in urethrovesical function after radical hysterectomy. Obstet Gynecol 1986; 68: 111–20.

30 Cystometry

Hashim Hashim and Paul Abrams

DEFINITION

Cystometry, part of urodynamic studies, is the measurement of relevant physiologic parameters taken during the filling and voiding phases of micturition, allowing direct assessment of lower urinary tract function (1). It can be divided into two parts:

1. *Filling cystometry*: the method by which the relationship of pressure and volume in the bladder is measured during bladder filling.
2. *Pressure-flow studies of voiding*: the method by which the relationship of pressure in the bladder and urine flow rate is measured during bladder emptying.

AIMS

Cystometry is performed clinically as part of urodynamic investigations in patients complaining of lower urinary tract symptoms (LUTS) to help make a diagnosis and hence plan a suitable treatment or further appropriate investigations.

Cystometry aims to evaluate detrusor and urethral function during the storage (filling) and voiding phases of micturition. It is essential that diagnoses made at the time of cystometry are related to the patient's signs and symptoms, and the physical findings at the time of examination. The aim is to reproduce the patient's symptoms and to quantify the pathophysiological processes, thus providing an explanation of the patient's problems and an understanding of their implications.

Cystometry can also be used for research purposes or to provide objective measurements following particular treatments.

INDICATIONS

Ideally, all patients with LUTS suggesting a bladder or urethral disorder should undergo urodynamic studies. The bladder is known to be an "unreliable witness:" urinary symptoms alone do not always allow the correct diagnosis to be made and inappropriate treatment may be given (2–6). However, with limited health-care resources and access to such a service, patients with "clear-cut" symptoms can initially be managed empirically, e.g., by pelvic floor exercises or with duloxetine (serotonin nor-epinephrine re-uptake inhibitor), available in some parts of the world for suspected stress urinary incontinence, and by bladder training and antimuscarinic medication for overactive bladder syndrome and suspected detrusor overactivity (DO).

Urodynamics should not be performed without clear indications and a proposed "urodynamics question" that will be answered by the investigation (7). Cystometry should be preceded by the completion of a frequency/volume chart and multiple free uroflowmetry (8).

Urodynamics tests should be considered in women:

- with mixed LUTS in whom surgery is contemplated (e.g., urgency/urgency incontinence and stress urinary incontinence);
- with a suspected voiding disorder;
- being considered for bladder neck surgery;
- with previous unsuccessful incontinence surgery;
- with neurogenic bladder disorders;
- in whom conservative and pharmacologic measures have failed (e.g., physiotherapy for symptoms of stress urinary incontinence, and antimuscarinic drug treatment and bladder training for symptoms of overactive bladder syndrome).

PREPARING FOR CYSTOMETRY
Quality Control During Cystometry

Quality control is vital to allow accurate, reproducible, and interpretable pressure readings and to allow identification of artifacts. The International Continence Society (ICS) has defined these steps in the 2002 Good Urodynamic Practices report (7):

- *Flushing*: The manometer tubing connecting the transducers must be flushed before setting zero to remove any air bubbles that could give low false pressure readings.
- *Setting zero at atmospheric pressure*: This can be done either prior to inserting the catheters into the patient or after insertion as long as the transducers are open *only* to atmosphere. Zero pressure is the value recorded when an external transducer is open only to the environment (the other two sides of a three-way tap are closed) or when the open end of a connected, fluid-filled tube is at the same vertical level as the transducer before insertion into the patient (Fig. 30.1).
- *Calibrating the transducers*: They should be calibrated at 0 and +100 cmH$_2$O; the bladder (vesical) pressure (p$_{ves}$) and rectal or vaginal intra-abdominal pressure (p$_{abd}$) lines should be in the positive range +5 to +50 cmH$_2$O (depending on body position, lying or standing, and body habitus). The detrusor pressure (p$_{det}$) should be between 0 and +10 cmH$_2$O; however, in clinical practice it can usually range from −5 to +10 cmH$_2$O (9).
- *Establishing a reference level for pressure*: The superior border of the symphysis pubis is the fixed reference level for external and fluid-filled catheter systems; the transducers should be levelled to this horizontal plane so that all measurements have the same hydrostatic component.

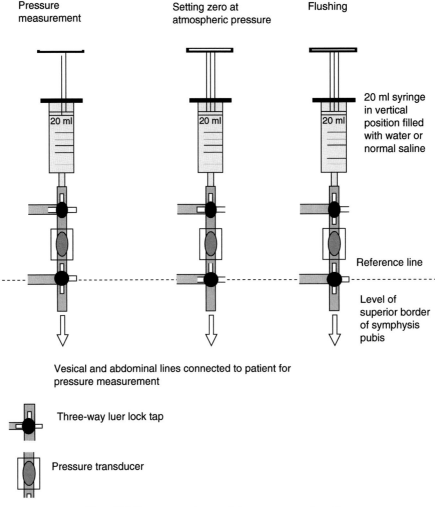

Pressure
measurement

Setting zero at
atmospheric pressure

Flushing

20 ml syringe
in vertical
position filled
with water or
normal saline

Reference line

Level of
superior border
of symphysis
pubis

Vesical and abdominal lines connected to patient for
pressure measurement

Three-way luer lock tap

Pressure transducer

Figure 30.1 Pressure transducer and three-way tap configurations.

It is easier to add two three-way taps to the pressure transducers, so that all procedures can be done by turning the valves alone without disconnecting any tubing and using syringes in a vertical position, maintaining connections, to eliminate all air bubbles, and to avoid any new air bubbles (Fig. 30.1).

During the investigation, quality control is ensured by asking the patient to cough at regular (e.g., one minute) intervals (Fig. 30.2). Before recording is started, the patient is asked to cough and the p_{ves} and p_{abd} traces are observed. The two cough spikes should show an equal rise in the two pressure lines (p_{ves} and p_{abd}) and a complete subtraction of these two pressures should result in no change of the p_{det} line. Sometimes a small artifactual biphasic blip (Fig. 30.2) is seen on p_{det}, but this also indicates acceptable subtraction. The biphasic blip occurs due to different speeds of transmission of the pressure waves from the bladder and rectum/vagina to the two transducers and is seen mainly in older urodynamic systems. The two blips of the biphasic wave should be equal in size; if they are not equal in height this can indicate poor quality. The patient should cough before and after voiding to reconfirm quality control and that no displacement of catheters has occurred. During filling, the p_{ves} and p_{abd} lines should not decline.

Patient Position

For convenience, the catheters are put in position with the patient supine after the physical examination (Fig. 30.3). Cystometry should then be done in the upright (sitting) position because: (*i*) this is the physiologic position in which women spend most of their time when awake; (*ii*) the majority of women complain of symptoms when upright and active, and (*iii*) at least 30% of DO will be missed if the patient is filled supine, resulting in sub-optimal treatment decisions (10). It is expedient to ask the patient to sit on a commode with a flowmeter situated below it to measure any leakage of urine during the test, and also because most women void when sitting down. Some women complain of leakage when changing position (e.g., on bending over or getting up from the sitting position); these changes in posture can be mimicked during the test to try to reflect everyday stresses on the bladder and to reproduce leakage. Whenever the patient's position is altered, the position of the transducer must be readjusted to the pressure reference level of the upper border of the symphysis pubis.

With the catheters in position, the filling catheter is connected to a bag of suitable filling medium (see below). The rest of the equipment should be close to the patient for

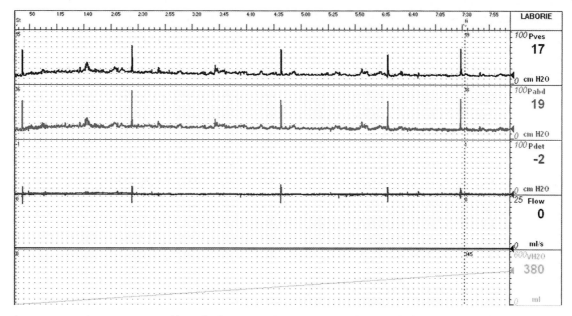

Figure 30.2 Normal cystometrogram with coughs showing equal rises on intravesical pressure (p~ves~) and intra-abdominal pressure (p~abd~).

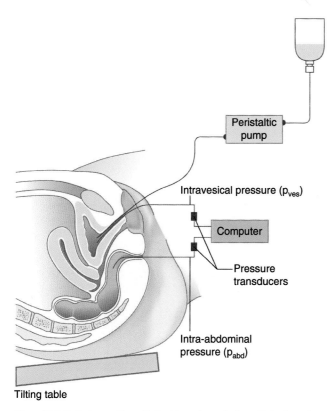

Figure 30.3 Catheter positions. Patient is supine only for catheter insertion.

convenience and, if a computer screen is available, this should be in a position viewable by the patient so that explanations can be given during the test.

If there is severe DO that prevents adequate filling, even at a reduced rate (10–20 ml/min), then filling in the supine position may be required in order for any useful information to be gathered from cystometry.

Reduced mobility or severe disablement of patients (e.g., by neurologic disease) may necessitate cystometry in the supine position.

Filling Medium

Water and 0.9% (normal) saline are the fluids most frequently used, as they are cheap, convenient, and mimic urine. The fluid is commonly used at room temperature (22°C); however, body temperature (37°C) may be more physiological. Cystometry has been performed with the filling medium warmed to body temperature with no observable difference in results (11); however, this has not yet been scientifically investigated and standardization is required. It is known that ice-cold infusion fluid can stimulate bladder contraction at low bladder volumes (12) and therefore should not be used in routine cystometry.

In the past, carbon dioxide has been used in gas cystometry (13), but is no longer recommended as it is not a physiologic medium for the bladder. It dissolves in urine to form irritant carbonic acid, and it can cause pain in "hypersensitive" bladders; furthermore, capacity measurement is inaccurate as the gas is both compressible and soluble in urine (14). In addition, it is not possible to obtain a pressure–flow analysis of the voiding phase of micturition after gas cystometry.

Filling Rates

Previously, three filling rates were defined by the ICS (15):

1. Slow-fill cystometry up to 10 ml/min
2. Medium-fill cystometry between 10 and 100 ml/min
3. Fast-fill cystometry when the rate is >100 ml/min

In the latest standardization report (1), the ICS no longer divides filling rates into slow, medium, or fast. Currently, the term "non-physiologic filling rate" is being used, and the precise filling rate should be stated. We recommend a filling rate of 50 ml/min, which, although convenient in the setting of a busy urodynamic unit, is not so fast as to be grossly non-physiological; it also allows time to discuss symptoms with the patient and to assess whether those symptoms have been successfully reproduced. In a patient with very marked DO, the rate should be reduced to 30 ml/min or lower.

Slower filling rates are indicated in patients with neurogenic bladders. There is little point in more rapid filling, which is rarely used, although some believe it to be a further provocative test for DO.

Equipment

Multi-channel cystometry requires a urine flowmeter, two (or three) transducers, an electronic subtraction unit to derive p_{det} ($p_{ves} - p_{abd}$), a recorder with a printout, and an amplifying unit (Fig. 30.4). All measurements are made in centimeters of water.

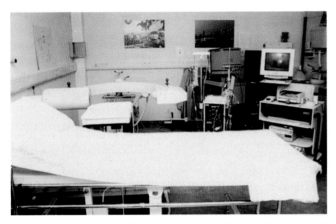

Figure 30.4 Equipment: couch, cystometry unit, patient unit, flowmeter, and image intensifier used in video-urodynamics.

The bladder pressure is measured using either:

- a fluid-filled line (a double-lumen or single-lumen epidural catheter is inserted into the bladder and connected to an external pressure transducer; Fig. 30.5A & B), or
- a solid micro-tip pressure transducer (a transducer is mounted on the tip of a solid 7 Fr catheter and hence is an internal pressure transducer system; Fig. 30.6).

This catheter-mounted transducer eliminates artifacts arising from the fluid-filled system, which needs to be connected to an external transducer.

Abdominal pressure is measured with a rectal (or occasionally vaginal) (16) catheter (6 Fr manometer tubing covered with a fingerstall obtained from a non-sterile surgical rubber glove to prevent blockage by feces) which is inserted into the rectum to a distance approximately 10 cm above the anal margin. If the patient has no rectum or vagina but has a colostomy, then that can be used for the abdominal pressure measurement. It is important to make sure that a small cut is made in the fingerstall to allow expulsion of fluid during flushing. If a hole is not made in the glove, then the pressure measured will be that of the water-filled balloon and not true rectal pressure. This line is taped to the patient's buttock close to the anal verge to prevent any slippage during the test. The tubing must be flushed from the transducer end before recording is commenced. This is a very economical way of making rectal catheters; however, some companies make their own, more

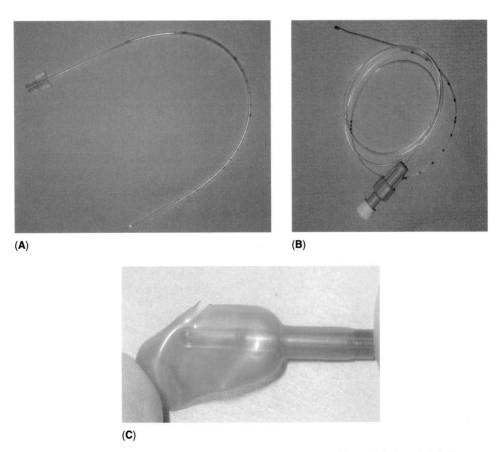

(A)   (B)

(C)

Figure 30.5 (**A**) Filling catheter (8Fr), (**B**) epidural catheter (16G), (**C**) rectal line with hole made in balloon.

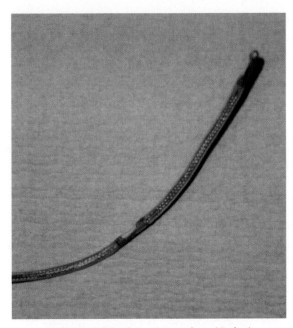

Figure 30.6 Solid catheter-tip transducer (Gaeltec).

expensive, rectal catheters. It is important to remember that some of these commercial rectal catheters do not have a hole and thus if you keep on flushing, the balloon continues to expand, resulting in false rectal pressures. It is therefore advisable to make a small cut in the rectal balloon even if you are using a commercial rectal catheter (Fig. 30.5C). Making a hole in the rectal balloon is not in the ICS Good Urodynamic Practices report (7) and the report suggests filling the balloon to 10% to 20% of it capacity however this is often difficult to gauge and the balloon could easily be filled more than that, causing error in measurement.

The reference height for all measurements is taken as being level with the upper edge of the symphysis pubis and the transducers are zeroed to atmospheric pressure. A double-lumen filling catheter (6 Fr) is inserted into the bladder via the urethra (or, occasionally, by the suprapubic route). Sometimes a single-lumen (8 Fr) filling catheter with a 16G epidural catheter (for pressure measurement) inserted alongside it can be used instead of the double-lumen. Double-lumen catheters are expensive and thus the two-catheter combination is a cheaper alternative that gives similar results. The single-lumen filling catheter is pulled out just before voiding and the epidural catheter is left in the bladder and used to measure pressure. The advantage of the double-lumen catheter is that the patient's bladder can be filled and refilled multiple times should the test require it, and the post-void residual (if any) can easily be drained and measured through it; however, it is more expensive to use. The catheters are fixed in place by tape close to the external urethral meatus on the medial aspect of the thigh.

MEASUREMENTS
The following measurements are made (Fig. 30.2):

1. p_{ves} is measured via a urethral or suprapubic catheter connected to the bladder transducer

2. p_{abd} is the pressure outside and around the bladder and measured in the rectum (or vagina) with a rectal catheter
3. p_{det} is obtained by subtracting the abdominal from the intravesical pressure ($p_{det} = p_{ves} - p_{abd}$) and represents the pressure generated by the bladder wall, usually as detrusor contractions
4. The volume infused into the bladder is recorded
5. The urine flow rate, as leakage during filling and flow during voiding, is recorded

Measuring bladder and intra-abdominal pressure simultaneously ensures that any pressure changes observed can be interpreted correctly. A rise in the vesical pressure could be due to either DO or abdominal straining being transmitted to the bladder. The electronic subtraction allows detrusor pressure to be measured and any change in pressure seen on the traces to be attributed appropriately.

Detrusor function is assessed directly from observation of the pressure changes. Urethral function must be inferred from the pressure changes within the bladder, and by measuring any leakage during filling and urine flow during voiding.

METHOD
The basic details of the test and the most frequent side effects (e.g., risk of urinary tract infection) should be fully explained to the patient and, in particular, the importance of indicating any bladder sensations during the test, as they happen, should be emphasized. The symptoms can then be used to annotate the cystometry trace and help with interpretation.

Urinalysis and free uroflowmetry should be performed before embarking on cystometry to exclude any abnormality that may preclude proceeding with the test or may need extra-precautions to be taken during the test such as a urinary tract infection. Any residual urine on subsequent catheterization is then measured. We normally empty the bladder of any residual urine in non-neurogenic bladders, as this allows us to assess bladder function when the bladder is empty which may be important if treatment involves emptying the bladder, such as when using intermittent self-catheterization.

Filling Cystometry
The filling phase starts when filling commences and ends when the patient is given permission to void by the urodynamicist. Bladder sensation, detrusor activity, bladder compliance, bladder capacity, and urethral function should all be assessed during this procedure. Bladder capacity should be correlated with the results of the frequency–volume chart.

Bladder Sensation
During the filling phase the patient is asked to indicate when and if the following occur:

- First sensation of bladder filling (1): This is the feeling of first becoming aware of bladder filling. This sensation may not be truly representative, owing to the interfering presence of the catheter.

- First desire to void (FDV) (1): This is the feeling that would lead to passing urine at the next convenient moment, but voiding can be delayed if necessary. Essentially this is the normal desire to void in the old ICS terminology (15).
- Strong desire to void (SDV) (1): This is the persistent desire to void, without the fear of leakage.
- Urgency (1): This is the complaint of a sudden compelling desire to void, which is difficult to defer.

The volumes should be noted. The above terminology has been defined by the ICS (1). Other terms that are also used during filling cystometry and related to bladder sensation include first sensation of bladder filling, and bladder pain, and bladder sensation which can be categorized as increased, normal, reduced, absent, or non-specific (seen mainly in neurologic patients).

Bladder hypersensitivity is a term that has been used in the past and found to be helpful (11). It is defined as a condition where there is an early FDV at <100 ml and this persists and worsens, limiting the bladder cystometric capacity to 250 ml. This term has now been replaced with the term "increased bladder sensation," which is an early first sensation of bladder filling (or an early desire to void) and/or an early SDV, which occurs at low bladder volume and which persists. The new term is subjective and thus it is not possible to quantify volumes.

Detrusor Activity
Detrusor activity, during filling, is described as either "normal" or "overactive." A normal detrusor allows bladder filling with little or no change in pressure, and with no involuntary phasic contractions occurring during cystometry, despite provocation (1).

The presence of involuntary phasic detrusor contractions, occurring throughout filling, is diagnosed by a rise in the detrusor pressure line (there is no lower limit for the amplitude of an involuntary detrusor contraction) with a similar rise in the vesical line, but no rise in the abdominal line, during filling cystometry (Fig. 30.7). The patient should be asked whether there is any associated sensation (urgency) and if the sensation mimics the one that is normally experienced and causes problems. Provocative factors such as coughing or running water maybe used to provoke symptoms, such as stress incontinence or urgency due to DO and should be noted.

If the bladder is shown during cystometry to contract spontaneously or with provocation, then it is said to have phasic DO. Some women will not experience any symptoms at the time of these contractions, in which case the significance of DO is unknown. If a single involuntary detrusor contraction occurs at the end of filling, resulting in incontinence, with no overactivity during filling, then this is known as terminal DO.

When there is a known neurologic condition (e.g., multiple sclerosis), any DO observed is termed neurogenic DO (this replaces the older term of detrusor hyperreflexia). DO is idiopathic if there is no identified cause.

Bladder Compliance
The term bladder compliance describes the relationship between change in bladder volume and detrusor pressure ($\Delta V / \Delta p_{det}$) and is measured in milliliter per centimeters of water. Normal compliance is at least 40 ml/cmH$_2$O. As a normal bladder fills there is very little or no change in the pressure (i.e., the bladder is a high-compliance system). As filling rates can alter bladder compliance, the filling rate of cystometry must always be documented. In neurologically normal women, reduced compliance is usually artifactual owing to the bladder being filled excessively fast. Should

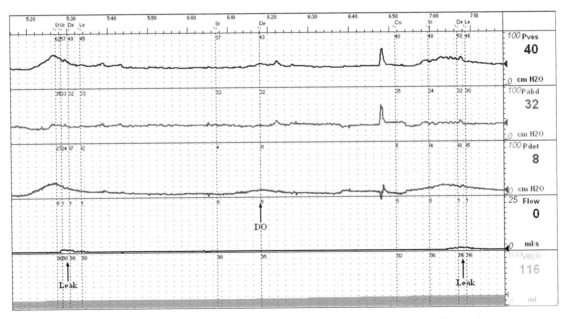

Figure 30.7 Cystometrogram showing detrusor overactivity (DO) and detrusor overactivity incontinence (leak). *Abbreviations:* p$_{det}$, detrusor pressure; p$_{abd}$, intra-abdominal pressure; p$_{ves}$, vesical pressure; flow rate in milliliters per second; V$_{H2O}$, volume of filling-medium infused.

compliance start to rise during filling, the filling should be stopped for approximately one minute to see if the compliance returns to normal: if compliance returns to normal, the increase is artifactual and secondary to fast filling; if compliance does not return to normal, then it is secondary to a pathologic condition. Continued filling should be at a slower rate of not more than 20 ml/min.

Urethral Function
During the filling phase, in normal women, the urethral closure pressure ($p_{ura} - p_{ves}$) remains positive (i.e., urethral pressure is greater than the vesical pressure), even at times of increased abdominal pressure; hence, continence is maintained. To allow voiding, closure pressure falls to zero as the urethra relaxes. If involuntary loss of urine is observed without detrusor activity, then the urethral closure mechanism is said to be incompetent.

A diagnosis of urodynamic stress incontinence (USI) can be made if leakage is associated with an increase in intraabdominal pressure that causes the vesical pressure to exceed the urethral pressure in the absence of a detrusor contraction (Fig. 30.8). When filling volume reaches 200 ml, the patient is asked to strain and then to cough to observe any leakage during these two maneuvers which tend to increase abdominal pressure above urethral pressure in women with the symptom of stress urinary incontinence. The intravesical pressure at which urine leakage occurs due to increased abdominal pressure in the absence of a detrusor contraction is known as the abdominal leak point pressure (1).

Voiding Cystometry
At the end of filling, the bladder-filling catheter is removed (only if filling and epidural catheters are used instead of a double-lumen catheter) to avoid any artifacts during voiding as a result of urethral obstruction. If leakage has not been noted during the filling phase, the patient is asked to cough a few times. If leakage is still not noted at this time, the patient is asked to stand and is given provocative instructions to try to induce leakage. Provocative maneuvers for DO incontinence include standing with the legs apart and running water from the taps and/or hand washing whereas coughing, jumping (star jumps), and squatting are tests for USI.

The patient, now back on the commode with the vesical and rectal pressure catheters still in situ, is instructed to void and the detrusor pressure and urine flow rate are recorded simultaneously. Detrusor pressure at maximum flow ($p_{det}Q_{max}$) and flow rate are recorded.

Voluntary initiation of a detrusor contraction is usually required for normal micturition and this is normally sustained until the bladder is empty, although some women can void by just relaxing their pelvic floor. The pressure rise is dependent on the outlet resistance and on the contraction of the detrusor itself (Table 30.1): If the detrusor pressure is low with low flow rates, the detrusor is defined as underactive; if the pressure is high with low or normal flow rates, this may be indicative of bladder outlet obstruction. If the detrusor muscle is functioning normally, then abdominal straining should not be required for bladder emptying. Many nomograms have been suggested as being able to diagnose bladder outlet obstruction and detrusor underactivity in women; however, neither the ICS nor the international consultation on incontinence has yet adopted a nomogram for women and none has been widely used or universally accepted.

A further rise in detrusor pressure after the completion of voiding, known as an "after-contraction," is sometimes seen at the end of a completed void, in patients with DO; however, the

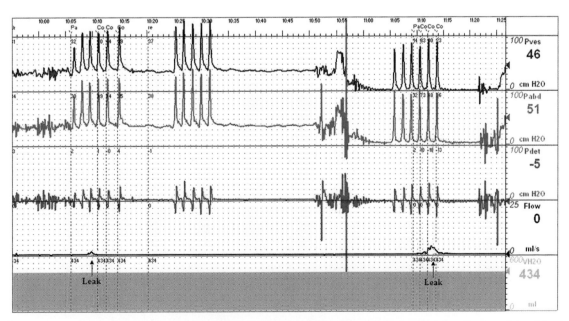

Figure 30.8 Cystometrogram showing urodynamic stress incontinence (leak) with coughing. *Abbreviations*: p_{det}, detrusor pressure; p_{abd}, intra-abdominal pressure; p_{ves}, vesical pressure; flow rate in milliliters per second; V_{H2O}, volume of filling-medium infused.

significance of this finding is unknown. The patient is asked to cough at the end of voiding to check for quality control, and to ensure that the p_{ves} measuring catheter has not moved out of the bladder during voiding. If it has, then the p_{ves} data for voiding should be regarded as unreliable and consideration given to repeating the voiding phase if the required information cannot be extracted.

Table 30.1 Lower Urinary Tract Function According to Clinical Diagnosis, and Detrusor and Urethral Function During the Filling and Voiding Cycles of Micturition with Possible Urodynamic Diagnosis

Clinical diagnosis	Detrusor function	Urethral function	Urodynamic diagnosis
Filling phase			
Normal	Normal	Competent	Normal
SUI	Normal	Incompetent	USI
OAB "dry"	Overactive	Competent	DO
OAB "wet"	Overactive	Competent	DOI
OAB "dry" + SUI	Overactive	Incompetent	DO + USI
OAB "wet" + SUI (mixed incontinence)	Overactive	Incompetent	DOI + USI
Voiding phase			
Normal	Normal	Relaxed	Normal
POP	Normal	Obstructed	High pressure/ low flow (BOO)
Difficulty voiding	Underactive	Relaxed	Low flow/low pressure

Abbreviations: SUI, stress urinary incontinence; OAB, overactive bladder; USI, urodynamic stress incontinence; DO, detrusor overactivity; DOI, detrusor overactivity incontinence; POP, pelvic organ prolapse; BOO, bladder outlet obstruction.

PITFALLS OF CYSTOMETRY

To ensure accurate measurements, the bladder line, rectal line, and all tubing should be flushed to ensure that all air bubbles have been removed before recording begins. In addition, all connections should be tight, as any leak will cause errors in the pressure measurements recorded. Pressure values will tend to be lower, and recorded with a delay, if there are bubbles or leaks in the pressure system.

Rectal contractions can sometimes be seen on the recording trace (Fig. 30.9) and may be misinterpreted as DO; it is, therefore, important to be aware of rectal activity. If possible, the patient should have an empty rectum for the test. If the rectal line slips slowly during the recording, the p_{abd} line will be seen to drift downwards, which could be incorrectly interpreted as a rise in the detrusor pressure and reduced compliance: careful examination of the vesical line shows the bladder pressure to be constant and should allow this artefact to be noticed, and corrected.

Quality control at the start of each cystometrogram is vital, and should be repeated at regular intervals during the test and again at the end of the test to ensure that good pressure transmission is continuing. This is done by asking the patient to cough and seeing an equal rise in the cough spikes in both the abdominal and vesical line with no rise (other than a small biphasic deflection in a fluid-filled system) on the detrusor line.

NORMAL CYSTOMETRY

Cystometry of a normal bladder shows the following:

1. residual urine of <50 ml;
2. FDV between 150 and 250 ml;
3. capacity (taken as SDV) between 400 and 600 ml;
4. little or no detrusor pressure rise on filling (Fig. 30.10);
5. absence of detrusor contractions during the filling phase;

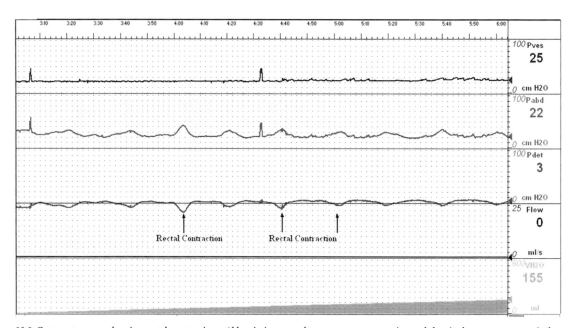

Figure 30.9 Cystometrogram showing rectal contractions. *Abbreviations*: p_{det}, detrusor pressure; p_{abd}, intra-abdominal pressure; p_{ves}, vesical pressure.

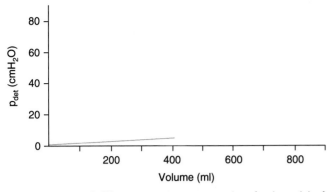

Figure 30.10 Normal filling cystometrogram annotation showing minimal increase in detrusor pressure (p_{det}). The filling speed is 50 ml/min, the patient is seated, the bladder capacity is 403 ml, and the first desire to void is at 160 ml.

6. no leakage on coughing;
7. no detrusor contraction provoked by coughing or running water (precipitating factors); and
8. a maximum voiding detrusor pressure of <50 cmH$_2$O, with a maximum flow rate >15 ml/sec for a volume >150 ml.

If cystometry has been performed for storage symptoms, then at the end of the test the question that has to be answered is: "Did the cystometry succeed, partially succeed, or fail to reproduce the patient's symptoms?"

Cystometry is a component of urodynamics studies used to investigate lower urinary tract dysfunction. It is vital that women are assessed with a proper history and examination, and the results of the cystometric findings evaluated in light of the signs and symptoms with the aid of voiding diaries. The majority of women will have their symptoms explained during urodynamics, and/or further management decisions can be made from conventional cystometry. Further, cystometry can be performed using ambulatory monitoring over a longer period of time and in more natural circumstances, or together with video cystourethrography when a simultaneous assessment of the anatomy is desirable.

REFERENCES

1. Abrams P, Cardozo L, Fall M, et al. The standardisation of terminology of lower urinary tract function: report from the Standardisation Subcommittee of the International Continence Society. Neurourol Urodyn 2002; 21: 167–78.
2. Hashim H, Abrams P. Is the bladder a reliable witness for predicting detrusor overactivity? J Urol 2006; 175: 191–5.
3. Cardozo LD, Stanton SL. Genuine stress incontinence and detrusor instability—a review of 200 patients. Br J Obstet Gynaecol 1980; 87: 184–90.
4. Shepherd AM, Powell PH, Ball AJ. The place of urodynamic studies in the investigation and treatment of female urinary tract symptoms. J Obstet Gynecol 1982; 3: 123–5.
5. Largo-Janssen AL, Debruyne FM, van Weel C. Value of the patient's case history in diagnosing urinary incontinence in general practice. Br J Urol 1991; 67: 569–72.
6. Jarvis GJ, Hall S, Stamp S, et al. An assessment of urodynamic examination in incontinent women. Br J Obstet Gynaecol 1980; 87: 893–6.
7. Schäfer W, Abrams P, Liao L, et al. Good urodynamic practices: uroflowmetry, filling cystometry and pressure flow studies. Neurourol Urodyn 2002; 21: 261–74.
8. Reynard JM, Peters TJ, Lim C, Abrams P. The value of multiple free-flow studies in men with lower urinary tract symptoms. Br J Urol 1996; 77: 813–18.
9. Sullivan J, Lewis P, Howell S, et al. Quality control in urodynamics: a review of urodynamic traces from one centre. BJU Int 2003; 91: 201–7.
10. Al-Hayek S, Belal M, Abrams P. Does the patient's position influence the detection of detrusor overactivity? Neurourol Urodyn 2008; 27: 279–86.
11. Abrams P. Urodynamic techniques—cystometry. Urodynamics, 3rd edn. London: Springer, 2006: 64.
12. Hellström PA, Tammela TL, Kontturi MJ, Lukkarinen OA. The bladder cooling test for urodynamic assessment: analysis of 400 examinations. Br J Urol 1991; 67: 275–9.
13. Torrens MJ. A comparative evaluation of carbon dioxide and water cystometry and sphincterometry. Proceedings of the International Continence Society 7th Annual Meeting. Portoroz, Slovenia, 1977: 103–104 [abstract 46].
14. Wein AJ, Hanno PM, Dixon DO, et al. The reproducibility and interpretation of carbon dioxidecystometry. J Urol 1978; 120: 205–6.
15. Abrams P, Blaivas JG, Stanton SL, et al. The standardisation of terminology of lower urinary tract function. The International Continence Society Committee on Standardisation of Terminology. Scand J Urol Nephrol Suppl 1988; 114: 5–19.
16. James ED, Niblett PG, MacNaughton JA, et al. The vagina as an alternative to the rectum in measuring abdominal pressure during urodynamic investigations. Br J Urol 1987; 60: 212–16.

31 Pressure–Flow Plot in the Evaluation of Female Incontinence and Postoperative Obstruction

Rashel Haverkorn, Jason Gilleran, and Philippe Zimmern

INTRODUCTION

The definition of bladder outlet obstruction (BOO) in women remains controversial since it is a much less frequent condition than in men, and the leading etiologies resulting in BOO are more complex and not just limited to prostatic conditions. For men with lower urinary tract symptoms (LUTS) secondary to benign prostatic enlargement, several nomograms are available, but it is now accepted that these cannot be applied to obstruction in women. Because the definition is uncertain, the prevalence of BOO is unknown and has been estimated to be between 2.7% and 8% of women in large urodynamic database studies (1,2). In its purest form, the only means of defining BOO is by the pressure–flow study (PFS) portion of the urodynamic study (UDS). After briefly exploring limitations of the PFS, this chapter will focus on PFS interpretation and its role in the evaluation of female incontinence and in patients with voiding complaints in whom obstruction is clinically suspected.

BIOMECHANICS OF THE LOWER URINARY TRACT

Voiding is governed by the bladder (which facilitates storage of urine and, in most cases, provides the driving force behind emptying) and by the urethra (which acts not only as a major continence mechanism but also as a point of outlet resistance in a variety of pathologic states). To aid understanding of the clinical aspects of the PFS, we will review the physiology of the "pump" (bladder) and the "pipe" (urethra) and attempt to understand their relationship.

The Bladder

The mechanical properties of smooth muscle, such as the detrusor, have not been explored as thoroughly as those of striated muscle, but the general principles relevant to striated muscle provide a valid approximation (3). In addition, these tissue properties appear to be organ-specific and not gender-specific.

Muscle contraction is dependent upon the tension and the speed at which the muscle can shorten. The maximum isometric force (when there is no shortening allowed) is dependent primarily upon the velocity of shortening of the muscle in a manner similar to that described by Hill (4) for striated muscle. The equation that describes this relationship is:

$$(F/F_{iso} + a/F_{iso})(u + b) = (1 + a/F_{iso})b$$

where b and a/F_{iso} are constants independent of the degree of extension, F_{iso} is the isometric force of the bladder, F/F_{iso} is the ratio of observed force of contraction to isometric force and u is the speed of shortening.

Griffiths adapted the Hill equation to the bladder and described the bladder output relation relating detrusor pressure (p_{det}) to urinary flow (5). This adaptation was achieved by mathematically relating the changes in a single strip of bladder to the changes occurring in the whole bladder. If the bladder is treated as a simple sphere of radius R, then p_{det} is given by:

$$p_{det} = T/\pi R^2$$

where T is the total tension across the bladder circumference and R is the radius of the sphere. This relates p_{det}, measured clinically, to the tension measured in muscle strips in laboratory experiments (6). Likewise, a relationship between linear speed of shortening of a bladder strip and flow rate from the bladder may be derived:

$$(p_{det}/p_{det,iso} + a/F_{iso})(Q + Q*) = (1 + a/F_{iso})Q*$$

where Q is the flow rate from the bladder and Q* is a volume-dependent measure of the speed of shortening of the bladder muscle (7). p_{det} is dependent upon both the volume of urine within the bladder and the outlet resistance, with an optimal pressure–flow relationship obtained during the plateau phase of voiding. The isovolumetric p_{det} is largely volume independent and may be used to assess the contractile function of the bladder. The stop test—voluntary cessation of voiding—may be performed to determine a value for isometric pressure ($p_{det,iso}$). Using the values on the pressure–flow plot just before and just after the stop test, a straight line may be plotted to give an approximate value for Q*, which is reasonably accurate provided that p_{det} during flow is more than half of $p_{det,iso}$. Because of the volume dependence of Q*, the bladder volume should be above 200 ml. In practice, assessment of detrusor contractile function is difficult: the shape of the relationship, the dependence on bladder volume, and variations during voiding all complicate the process. "Watts factor," which represents the power of the bladder during contraction, may be calculated from p_{det}, flow rate, and bladder volume at any point during a void, but has not yet found much clinical relevance (8).

The hydrodynamic findings thus far described reflect "normal" bladder function. Prolonged obstruction has been shown to impair detrusor contractile function that may persist even after the relief of obstruction. Based on studies in the male rabbit, the initial stages of obstruction (approximately 2 weeks) are characterized by focal hypoxia, increased bladder mass secondary to increased vascularization (angiogenesis), and blood flow (9). The point at which the bladder enters a "decompensation" stage—which features decreased blood flow, altered compliance, and contractile responses to electrical stimulation, as well as increased deposition of connective tissue elements—depends on the severity and duration of obstruction. Bladder wall ischemia is at least partially contributory to these changes (9). Age at which obstruction occurs also appears to have an impact. Although the physiologic alterations as a response to partial outlet obstruction are similar, more extensive histologic damage has been observed in younger rabbits compared to adult counterparts (10).

How much of these findings in male animal models apply to BOO in women is unknown. Additionally, obstruction in the animal model is created acutely whereas the clinical setting of obstruction in women can be both acute (obstruction from a sling) or chronic (large cystocele or urethral pathology).

The Urethra

The properties of the urethra interact with the contracting detrusor throughout voiding. Thus, the urethral outlet resistance modulates the performance of the bladder and influences what may be measured clinically. A prior edition of this book covered urethral properties influencing flow in men, treating the urethra as an elastic, distensible tube, the properties of which change throughout voiding (11). In women, much less is known regarding urethral resistance and the flow-controlling zone, other than what has been measured by urodynamic testing in controls. Note that patients with stress incontinence cannot serve as controls since it was found that

they have a lower urethral resistance compared to age-matched controls (12,13). Certainly, urethral resistance in neurologically intact women plays a lesser role than in men. A good example of a unique voiding mechanism in women is urethral relaxation with no demonstrable rise in p_{det} and a normal flow.

RECORDING THE PRESSURE–FLOW PLOT

The PFS represents a graphic record of the relationship between the detrusor contraction and the flow rate over time. Detrusor pressure (p_{det}) is measured by subtraction cystometry using vesical and rectal catheters which read the intravesical pressures (p_{ves}) and p_{abd}, respectively, and is expressed in centimeters of water (cmH_2O). The flow is measured by a number of methods—rotating disc, air displacement, etc., (14)—and expressed in milliliters per second (ml/sec). These two measurements, alone or combined, provide some information on the voiding function; however, these findings can be affected by several factors (Table 31.1). After briefly reviewing the parameters affecting the PFS, we will discuss its interpretation and its role in female incontinence and postoperative obstruction.

Factors Affecting the PFS

Catheter Effects

As in men (15), the presence of a catheter alone can affect flow rates. In one study that examined flow rates in 20 healthy

Table 31.1 "Troubleshooting" the Pressure–Flow Study in Women

"Action"	Effect on PFS	"Reaction"
Pre-void		
Positional change: standing to sitting	Change in pressure readings in relation to position of transducers	Adjust transducers to upper edge of symphysis pubis. Annotate tracing "sit," then "transducers adjusted"
Poor recording from one or both catheters prior to voiding study	Inability to detect changes in p_{abd} or p_{ves} makes the p_{det} measurement invalid	Confirm recording with pre-void cough and verify pressure agreement between p_{ves} and p_{abd}
During void		
Expulsion of bladder or rectal catheter	Loss of tracing for either p_{abd} or p_{ves} renders p_{det} uninterpretable	Reinsert catheter, secure properly. Refill to capacity, and repeat PFS
Drop in p_{abd} secondary to pelvic floor relaxation	Decrease in p_{abd} artificially raises the p_{det} (by subtraction)	Measure Δp_{ves} (change from p_{ves} at baseline to p_{ves} at Q_{max}) to determine true detrusor contraction
Patient unable to void	No flow generated; difficult to interpret true obstruction vs. catheter effect	Give patient privacy and time to relax. May stimulate patient with sound of running water. Otherwise, may need to rely on NIF only
Straining during voiding (Valsalva voiding)	Elevation of p_{abd} may artificially lower the p_{det}, or no p_{det} is recorded when $p_{abd} = p_{ves}$ (both pressure lines mirror each other)	Possible catheter artifact. Repeat PFS and/or NIF to confirm same voiding pattern
Post-void		
Poor recording from one or both catheters during voiding study	Inability to detect changes in p_{abd} or p_{ves} makes the p_{det} measurement invalid	Confirm recording with cough at end of void to verify pressure agreement between p_{ves} and p_{abd}. (Note: vesical recording may be blunted or absent if bladder is empty)

Abbreviations: NIF, non-intubated flow; p_{abd}, intra-abdominal pressure; p_{det}, detrusor pressure; PFS, pressure–flow study, p_{ves}, intravesical pressure, Q_{max}, maximum flow rate.

female volunteers with and without a 6 Fr double-lumen urethral catheter in place, a significant difference in mean maximum flow rate (Q_{max}) values (22.65 vs. 16.25 ml/sec, p = 0.0006) was observed (16). Similar findings were noted in another study which compared the free-flow Q_{max} values in 100 women to PFS with a 7 Fr catheter in place, excluding those in whom the non-intubated flow (NIF) voided volumes differed by >20% from the PFS voided volume (17). The mean Q_{max} was significantly higher in free compared to intubated flow (26.9 vs. 13.9 ml/sec, p < 0.001) and a higher percentage of patients had an intermittent, interrupted flow curve during PFS. Placing two catheters during filling cystometrogram, with removal of the larger filling catheter prior to voiding, is another option that has been studied. A study of 33 women with a variety of LUTS used a 12 Fr catheter for filling (18). This large catheter was then removed, leaving only a 4 Fr urethral pressure catheter for pressure–flow recording. No significant difference was between free Q_{max} and intubated Q_{max} across different categories of voided volumes (101–250 ml, 251–500 ml, and >500 ml).

More recently, the effect of catheter diameter during PFS was investigated. A prospective study randomized 239 women to a 7 or 9 Fr catheter for PFS. Regardless of catheter size, a significantly lower level of Q_{max} was noted compared to free flow in each subset of volume voided from 150 to 400 ml and over (19). Catheter size was not shown to have an impact on diagnosing BOO when using the criteria $Q_{max} \leq 15$ ml/sec and detrusor pressure at peak flow (PFP or $p_{det}Q_{max}$) ≥ 20 cmH$_2$O.

Prolapse Reduction
Significant pelvic organ prolapse, particularly cystocele, can mechanically obstruct the bladder neck by creating an angulation at the urethrovesical junction. This finding may be more pronounced after a prior anti-incontinence procedure if this particular procedure also added an element of outlet obstruction. Reducing the cystocele may relieve obstruction (Fig. 31.1). Urinary retention, defined as post-void residual (PVR) ≥ 100 ml, was eliminated in 18/24 (75%) of women who underwent reduction of stage three and four anterior vaginal wall prolapse with a pessary prior to repair (20). This "pessary test" involved an outpatient trial of pessary reduction followed by preoperative UDS and PVR by in–out catheterization, and was predictive of a low PVR after prolapse repair. Using alternative methods of reduction (speculum, swab, or physician's fingers), another study also demonstrated normalization of PVR after surgical correction and found these methods predicted postoperative voiding function if the preoperative study was normal (21). Among the cystocele reduction methods, a vaginal pack has been recommended as a less operator-dependent and interfering method during UDS. However, conceivably such a pack could be too tight and artificially obstruct the bladder neck. A recent study noted a low incidence of pack-induced obstruction and a high frequency of BOO resolution during PFS with the pack in place (22). Prolapse reduction methods during UDS were examined in a sub-analysis of the colpopexy and urinary reduction efforts trial (CARE). A variety of techniques were studied, including manual reduction with fingers, pessary placement, swab insertion, forceps, and speculum.

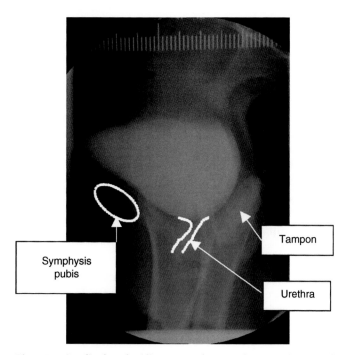

Figure 31.1 Standing lateral voiding cystourethrogram demonstrating normal bladder and urethral position in a woman with a large cystocele on physical examination reduced by a tampon in place (arrow) which is visible due to absorption of voided contrast. The bladder neck and urethra, as well as the symphysis pubis, are outlined in this voiding view (*dashed lines*).

The goal was to determine which was the most successful and effective means of prolapse reduction during the UDS evaluation to elicit stress incontinence. The swab was the method that most closely predicted the presence of stress incontinence, though each method was relatively similar in terms of sensitivity and specificity (23).

Patient Position During Voiding
The effect of position on voiding is very important for obstructed patients. Maneuvers such as bending forward, tilting sideways, half-standing, or leaning back are often reported by these patients and can favorably influence the test results. Most published data are on non-invasive flow (24) and sometimes relate to cultural differences (squatting vs. sitting) (25). Reporting on patient positioning during PFS is critical to a proper interpretation of the study, and should be clearly annotated on the PFS tracing.

Filling Medium
Saline, sterile water, or iodinated contrast can be used as the filling fluid depending on whether conventional or videourodynamics is being performed. The higher specific gravity of contrast may falsely elevate the Q_{max} by as much as 10% (as compared to water, saline, or urine of normal concentration) when the flow is measured by weight transduction (26).

PFS INTERPRETATION
Firstly, a brief review of how an ideal PFS tracing should look in order to be considered valid and interpretable is warranted. A representative tracing is depicted in Figure 31.2. Before the study, the transducers are opened to air and "zeroed" to

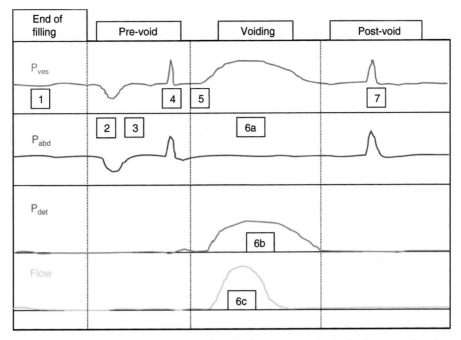

Figure 31.2 An ideal pressure–flow study (PFS) with key components highlighted. All these steps need to be clearly annotated on the tracing. (1) At end of filling, maximum cystometric capacity is reached. (2) There is a normal drop in vesical and abdominal pressures with change from standing to sitting position. (3) This is followed by an adjustment of transducers to the upper edge of the symphysis pubis. (4) Pre-void cough test confirms agreement in pressure recording from both catheters. (5) Before the void starts, and just after the cough, it is important to have a short section of tracing to determine the PFS baseline. Ideally, detrusor pressure (p_{det}) at baseline should be between 0 and +5 cmH$_2$O. (6) A parallel rise in (a) intravesical pressure (p_{ves}) and (b) p_{det} with no change in intra-abdominal pressure (p_{abd}) is indicative of a normal detrusor contraction (amplitude and duration), accompanied by (c) a normal, "bell-shaped" flow curve. (7) At completion of the detrusor contraction, a post-void cough test is performed to confirm that both catheters functioned properly during voiding.

atmosphere according to good urodynamic practices (26). The bladder is filled to maximum cystometric capacity (MCC). In some studies, the patient remains sitting throughout; in others the patient may be standing for the filling cystometry. It is important, in this situation, to annotate when the patient sits to void and when the transducers are readjusted to the upper edge of the symphysis pubis. A cough confirms agreement of pressure transmission from both catheters and a PFS baseline is established as a reference point before the start of voiding. During voiding, a parallel rise in p_{ves} and p_{det}, with minimal or no change in p_{abd}, is observed, indicating a detrusor contraction of normal amplitude and duration accompanied by a normal, "bell-shaped" flow curve. At completion of the detrusor contraction, a post-void cough is performed to confirm that both catheters functioned adequately during voiding. Alterations in the p_{det} curve can be due to artifact (Fig. 31.3) or variable voiding patterns that may be considered "normal" in some women (Fig. 31.4).

Following these guidelines is expected but not always realized in real-life practice. A recent "quality control" review of 100 male PFS tracings at one center focused on frequency of cough annotations before and after voiding and on pressure concordance between p_{abd} and p_{ves} during each cough. A grading system was recommended, with the best cough having a 70% to 100% concordance (grade A) which occurred in 86% of cases (27). Furthermore, an ideal tracing, even in a normal subject, is not always easily obtainable due to several artifacts, which must be recognized and corrected during the test. Simple adjustments to obtain a valid and interpretable PFS tracing

are suggested in Table 31.1. In cases where the tracing is severely altered and cannot be interpreted, the test should be repeated until a valid and plausible tracing is obtained.

Recognizing variability amongst technique, the Urodynamic Study Work Group of the Urinary Incontinence Treatment Network (UITN) worked on developing a standardized UDS protocol for use across all participating treatment sites to improve study performance and interpretation reliability. This effort was carried out for the stress incontinence surgical treatment efficacy randomized (SISTEr) trial and then continued with slight modifications for subsequent trials such as trial of mid-urethral slings (TOMUS). Consideration was made to providing realistic guidelines in performing UDS which could be generalizable to the community as well as the researcher (28).

Electromyography (EMG)

One simple method to document pelvic floor relaxation during voiding employs surface patch EMG. Needle electrodes have also been recommended to document urethral relaxation (29). EMG amplitude at rest with an empty bladder is usually 20 to 100 mV, and activity will typically increase as the bladder is filled and with coughing or straining (30).

During normal voiding, pelvic floor relaxation is reflected in the silencing or minimal activity on the EMG tracing. Inability of the pelvic floor to relax may be seen in conditions such as dysfunctional voiding and detrusor–sphincter dyssynergia, but may also appear as an artifact from straining to initiate the void or towards its end.

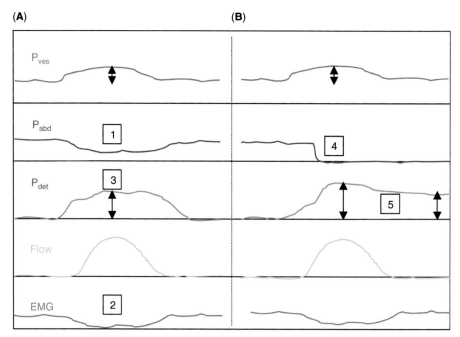

Figure 31.3 Representative examples of abnormalities in the pressure–flow study tracing that artificially elevate the detrusor pressure (p_{det}). Tracing (**A**): a mild drop in abdominal pressure (1) is common due to pelvic floor relaxation (2), resulting in an artificially elevated p_{det}. Tracing (**B**): expulsion of the rectal catheter is reflected in the sharp drop in intra-abdominal pressure (p_{abd}) to a zero level (4), which also results in an artificially elevated p_{det} (5) which remains elevated. Note that the rise in intravesical pressure (p_{ves}) during each void is identical, but does not correlate with the corresponding rise in p_{det} (arrows). *Abbreviation*: EMG, electromyography.

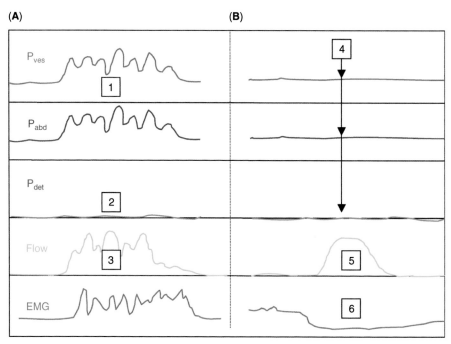

Figure 31.4 Representative examples of voiding patterns in which no rise in detrusor pressure (p_{det}) is observed. Tracing (**A**): straining pattern as demonstrated by irregular, fluctuating pressure curve similar for intra-abdominal pressure (p_{abd}) and intravesical pressure (p_{ves}) (1), resulting in minimal or no change in p_{det} (2) and a corresponding irregular flow curve (3). Tracing (**B**): No discernible change in p_{ves}, p_{abd} or p_{det} (4), with a normal flow curve (5) due to voiding by urethral relaxation, as reflected by the silent EMG during voiding (6). *Abbreviation*: EMG, electromyography.

URODYNAMIC DEFINITION OF BOO

In men, a number of nomograms exist to define and quantify BOO secondary to benign prostatic enlargement, including the Abrams–Griffith, Schäfer, and the linear passive urethral resistance, all of which are readily available and used in clinical practice. Not only is BOO less prevalent in women than in men, but anatomic differences, aging changes, duration of obstruction, and the various etiologies for BOO render the extension of male BOO nomograms to women somewhat irrelevant. Historically, the first attempts at defining obstruction were based on arbitrary values and observations in women who had a history suggestive of obstruction. Parameters included free flow rate, $p_{det}Q_{max}$, PVR, and urethral resistance, the last defined as pressure/flow^2 (P/F^2) with an abnormal value <0.2 (1). However, limitations recognized early included the facts that only 40% of these "obstructed" women complained of the classic storage symptoms (hesitancy, poor flow, and incomplete emptying), and that a number of normal women void by urethral relaxation or with a low-pressure detrusor contraction (31).

Once it became clear that such arbitrary values for diagnosing obstruction were not particularly accurate, receiver operator characteristics (ROC) were used to determine cut-off values for BOO in women and attain the optimal sensitivity and specificity for combining Q_{max} and $p_{det}Q_{max}$ values. One study reported using cut-off values of $Q_{max} \leq 15$ ml/sec and $p_{det}Q_{max} \geq 20$ cmH$_2$O to define obstruction, and found a sensitivity and specificity of 74.3% and 91.1%, respectively (32). These values were then applied to an expanded group of 87 women with clinical obstruction (women in urinary retention and those who strained during voiding were not included in the analysis), and referenced to 124 stress-incontinent controls (33). Optimal values to define BOO in this study were $Q_{max} \leq 11$ ml/sec and $p_{det}Q_{max} \geq 21$ cmH$_2$O. Several years later, the same group of researchers published details of their growing experience with 169 women with clinical BOO compared to PFS data in 20 healthy volunteers with no urologic complaints by urogenital distress inventory (UDI-6) questionnaire (12). Using a minimum specificity of 60% with the highest sensitivity, the authors determined that a $Q_{max} \leq 12$ ml/sec and $p_{det}Q_{max} \geq 25$ cmH$_2$O was the most accurate cut-off criteria in defining BOO (Fig. 31.5).

Another approach to the diagnosis of BOO sought to combine PFS data with bladder neck and urethral imaging by fluoroscopy (videourodynamics) or voiding cystourethrogram (VCUG). In one study, women with radiographic evidence of obstruction on videourodynamics and a sustained detrusor contraction during PFS were compared to those with no obstruction on imaging and were found to have a lower Q_{max} (9 vs. 20.2 ml/sec), a higher $p_{det}Q_{max}$ (42.8 vs. 22.1 cmH$_2$O), and a higher PVR (157 vs. 33 ml) (34). Contrary to videourodynamics, VCUG is a readily available tool that carries a low radiation risk (35). In addition, it can provide high-resolution lateral views of the urethra during voiding (34), which may help in determining the site of obstruction, as detailed in Figure 31.6.

To reduce the effect of a urethral catheter during PFS, one study defined BOO by plotting the non-intubated Q_{max} on one hand, and the maximum p_{det} ($p_{det-max}$) generated during a separate PFS on the other (2). Their definition—free flow $Q_{max} \leq 12$ ml/sec and a $p_{det-max} \geq 20$ cmH$_2$O—did not rely solely on PFS parameters; it was further expanded to include those who were unable to generate a flow by using radiographic evidence of obstruction during videourodynamics with a sustained detrusor contraction ≥20 cmH$_2$O. Of 50 women who met these obstruction criteria, two were in retention, and five were unable to void with the catheter in place. The NIF-Q_{max} was plotted against the $p_{det-max}$ and a four-zone nomogram (zones 0, I, II, and III) was constructed, similar to the Abrams–Griffith nomogram in men. However, since the free Q_{max} and $p_{det-max}$ were obtained during different voids, this nomogram failed to account for differences in voided volume and the presence of straining during the PFS or NIF. In addition, 10/50 (20%) clinically unobstructed women had plotted values consistent with mild or borderline mild obstruction. A recent prospective study applied this nomogram to 109 women with urinary incontinence and found 68.7% were obstructed (57.8% mild, 11% moderate, 0.9% severe) (36), a much higher percentage than the reported prevalence of 6.5% on the initial application of these criteria to a urodynamic database of 587 consecutive women (37).

In search for a better definition of BOO, a method to calculate the area under the p_{det} curve (AUC$_{det}$) for a given Q_{max} and voided volume was recently reported (38). The AUC$_{det}$ is a product of $p_{det} \times$ time (dt) and reflects the whole bladder contraction during voiding, using the formula $\int_0^t (p_{det} \times dt)$, and is expressed as cmH$_2$O/sec/ml (Fig. 31.7). In the initial report, these calculated values were applied to 85 women categorized as obstructed, unobstructed, or equivocal by two urologists blinded to each other's findings. Criteria traditionally used to diagnose obstruction—storage symptoms within three months after anti-incontinence surgery, conditions associated with obstruction (urethral stenosis, stage III–IV prolapse, and primary bladder neck obstruction), $Q_{max} < 12$ ml/sec on NIF, and PVR > 150 ml—were compared to the AUC$_{det}$ data. Linear discriminant analysis classified an AUC$_{det}$ value >5.83 cmH$_2$O/sec/ml as obstructed, 2.56 to 5.83 as equivocal, and <2.56 as unobstructed. These AUC$_{det}$ values have not yet been applied to unobstructed controls, and have not been tested by other investigators.

Computerized mathematical micturition models have been introduced for men. One of them, the VBN, which derives pressure within the urethra and counter-pressure outside the urethra, as well as detrusor function during voiding (13), has been applied to women. The effect of prolapse reduction of a grade IV cystocele was studied with the VBN model and demonstrated an improvement in urethral parameters in 10/14 patients, but no change in detrusor function (39). The same model was applied to 50 continent women after a tension-free vaginal tape (TVT) procedure and determined that a compressive obstruction could explain the continence mechanism in 34 (68%) of the women (40).

Each of the aforementioned series, summarized in Table 31.2, has contributed valuable insights into the urodynamic criteria necessary to define BOO in women. However, none of them can be applied rigidly to all women, but rather should take into consideration clinical data (from history, physical examination, cystourethroscopy, and imaging methods) and act as an adjunct in confirming a diagnosis of obstruction.

Therefore, reflecting on the challenges posed by a urodynamic definition of obstruction, it is apparent that a number of obstacles must be overcome to create a valid obstruction nomogram for women. First and foremost is defining "a normal PFS" in age-matched controls. Even when asymptomatic candidates are willing to undergo an invasive test such as a PFS, not all are truly asymptomatic. Of 59 community-dwelling adult women recruited to undergo PFS, 39 were

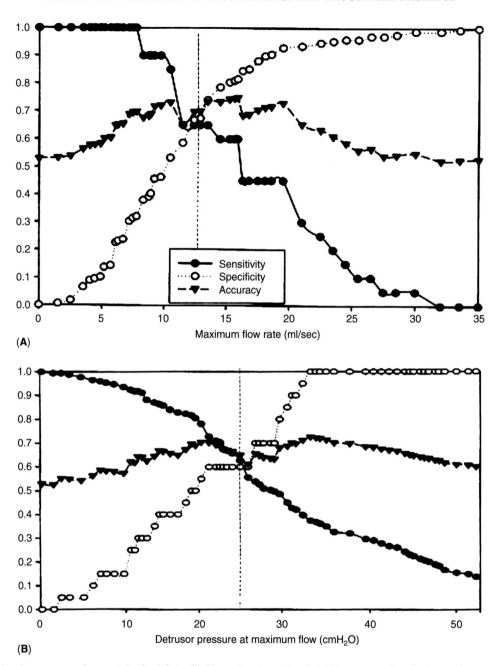

Figure 31.5 (**A, B**) Receiver–operator characteristics for defining bladder outlet obstruction (BOO) in women using the Q_{max} and corresponding $p_{det}Q_{max}$. The dashed vertical line in each graph represents the best sensitivity, specificity, and accuracy. Optimal cut-off values in 169 women with clinical BOO compared to 20 controls were found at $Q_{max} \leq 12$ ml/sec and $p_{det}Q_{max} \geq 25$ cmH$_2$O. *Abbreviations*: $p_{det}Q_{max}$, detrusor pressure at peak flow; Q_{max}, maximum flow rate. *Source*: Reproduced from Ref. 12.

excluded due to abnormal UDI questionnaire answers, prior bladder surgery, or withdrawal from the study (41). Clinically obstructed women for the most part tend to be older, and normative data for PFS have not been published in this age group in whom a high prevalence of mild voiding urinary symptoms (frequency and urgency) exists at baseline (42–45). Moreover, the voiding pattern and PFS parameters of normal volunteers are not necessarily consistent over time. In a study investigating PFS findings in 10 young, asymptomatic nulliparous women, a disparity of normative values was observed, many of which would really be considered pathologic, including a low Q_{max} (46).

The use of non-neurogenic women with pure stress urinary incontinence (SUI) as controls was common in earlier studies (33,34,47,48). These women have since been found to void with relatively low p_{det}, thought in part to be due to decreased urethral resistance (49). Comparing 20 asymptomatic volunteers with 40 stress-incontinent women, a significantly higher Q_{max} and lower $p_{det}Q_{max}$ was observed in the stress-incontinent population stratified for age, menopausal status, and parity (41). Furthermore, the presence of SUI does not necessarily exclude concomitant obstruction (50). These findings strongly argue that women with SUI should not serve as controls to establish PFS criteria for obstruction.

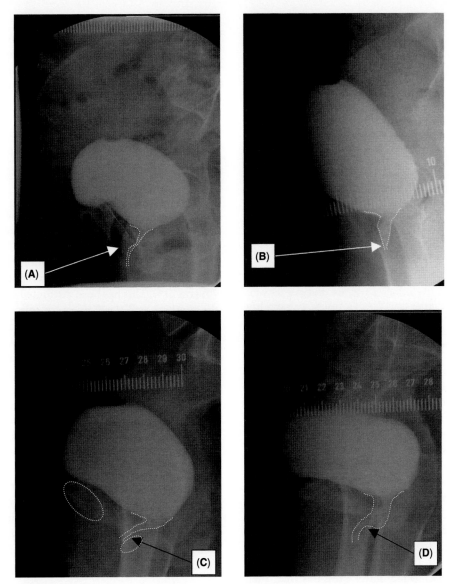

Figure 31.6 Representative examples of urethral obstruction on lateral voiding views from differing etiologies. All patients were obstructed clinically with abnormal pressure–flow studies. Periurethral fibrosis causes obstruction throughout the entire length of the urethra (**A**) or distally with proximal dilation (**B**). (**C**) Extrinsic compression is seen underneath the urethra in a woman with an unsuspected urethral diverticulum (oval with arrow). Mid-urethral obstruction with proximal dilation (**D**) in a woman after transvaginal tape placement requiring urethrolysis.

Beyond establishing normative age-matched values for the pressure–flow plot, study technique should be uniform to eliminate inconsistencies and artifacts. Minimizing catheter interference by using the smallest size catheter—preferably 7 Fr or less—is recommended; a smaller size catheter (e.g., 4 Fr) would be optimal but filling the bladder with smaller catheters is time-consuming and the filled volume is not reliable. To compare patients, voided volume categories may be necessary since volume and flow are interrelated (51). A number of other technical issues have been raised earlier in this chapter (voiding position, prolapse reduction, documentation of pelvic floor relaxation by EMG, etc.) and will require further study before the PFS procedure can be better standardized.

Assuming a valid and plausible PFS tracing with clear annotations, the interpretation of the tracing must follow guidelines that should be validated both between observers (interobserver) and by the same observer at different times

(intraobserver). In a single-center study on PFS tracings in 621 women, good intra- and interobserver agreement was noted for all parameters, with the exception of intraobserver agreement on $p_{det}Q_{max}$ (52). In the SISTEr trial completed by the UITN, interpretation guidelines had to be developed to enhance the interrater reliability between local and central reviewers (53). As a subanalysis in the SISTEr trial, urodynamic evaluations of all participants were reviewed and reference values were extracted in this cohort of 655 predominantly stress incontinent women. The urodynamic findings of this normative study for women with symptomatic SUI can be useful to the practitioner involved with urodynamic interpretation and surgical decision making. The key points are summarized as follows: (*i*) baseline bladder and abdominal pressures were between 12 and 60 cm of water; (*ii*) first desire to void should be expected at one-third of maximum bladder capacity while strong desire to void is usually near two-thirds

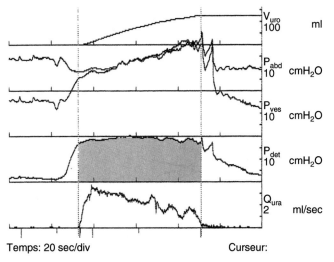

Temps: 20 sec/div   Curseur:

Figure 31.7 Pressure–flow plot in an obstructed patient with the calculated area under detrusor pressure curve in shading. Note that changes in the intra-abdominal pressure (p_{abd}) occurring throughout the voiding study may have an effect on the detrusor pressure (p_{det}) curve and in turn on this method's accuracy. *Abbreviations*: p_{ves}, intravesical pressure; Q_{ura}, flow rate in ml/sec; V_{uro}, voided volume. *Source*: Reproduced from Ref. 38.

of maximum bladder capacity; (*iii*) change in p_{det} during the filling phase of UDS should be <16 cmH$_2$O, (*iv*) 10% of women with positive cough stress test during physical exam did not display evidence of stress incontinence during the UDS; (*v*) <10% of participants demonstrated detrusor overactivity (DO), confirming that screening for DO in SUI predominant patients prior to surgery may be low yield; (*vi*) the median Q_{max} on PFS was 20 ml/sec, which was significantly less than the median value of 23.6 ml/sec for the NIF obtained during free uroflowmetry; and (*vii*) the average p_{det} at maximum flow was 19 cmH$_2$O as compared to 47 to 58 cmH$_2$O in the male population as reported in the literature, reinforcing the idea that women void at significantly lower pressures than their male counterparts (54).

Overall, there is a recognized need to further our understanding of voiding mechanisms in women. As discussed in the next section, several procedures to correct incontinence may result in various degrees of outlet obstruction. Some believe it is a necessary result to achieve continence (55), whereas others worry about the long-term effect of raising urethral outlet resistance on detrusor function (56). This debate can only be solved if a consensus can be reached on the urodynamic definition of BOO.

INCONTINENCE SURGERY AND THE PRESSURE–FLOW PLOT

When UDS is performed before deciding on an anti-incontinence procedure, its first aim is to document the presence of SUI and assess its severity by determining the leak point pressure. Possibly more important, its second aim should be to gain some baseline knowledge on voiding detrusor function. Altered voiding dynamics is often reflected by changes in PFS parameters following anti-incontinence surgery. In this final section, we will review the PFS data following anti-incontinence procedures in the recent literature.

Anti-Incontinence Surgery

Bladder neck suspension (BNS), pubovaginal sling (PVS), and mid-urethral sling procedures all aim to correct SUI by restoring support to the bladder neck and urethra with minimal tension. Nevertheless, the risk of inadvertently creating obstruction exists with each procedure. Postoperative voiding changes can occur across a broad spectrum, ranging from minor changes with no significant clinical relevance to frank obstruction and/or urinary retention requiring surgical intervention.

Bladder Neck Suspension

Whether or not the mechanism by which various transvaginal and retropubic BNS techniques restore continence is based on creating obstruction has long been debated. Obstruction following a retropubic Marshall–Marchetti–Kranz (MMK) procedure has been reported as being between 7% and 21%. This has been attributed to suture placement in the urethral wall itself, or more commonly to periurethral scarring (57), but little is known about PFS parameters in asymptomatic continent women after MMK. Pre- and post-operative urodynamic parameters (maximum voiding pressures, urethral resistance) were compared in 20 continent women after a modified Pereyra BNS and no significant changes were observed, suggesting that this procedure did not cause outflow obstruction (58). On the contrary, changes in urethral resistance at one year postoperatively (52) and long term (59), and significant differences in pressure–flow parameters, have been reported after retropubic colposuspension (60). These studies differed in concluding that a retropubic suspension returns voiding parameters to a "normal" level versus an "storage" state. Interestingly, some have suggested that the superior outcome of the retropubic suspensions over needle suspensions (61) is due to the more "storage" nature of the former procedures.

Pubovaginal and Midurethral Sling

The incidence of urethral obstruction after placement of a PVS, regardless of the material used, has been reported in approximately 8% of cases (61), and is thought to be due to excessive tensioning. In one study comparing preoperative videourodynamic findings to those three months after rectus fascia PVS in 85 women, a statistically significant increase in the mean $p_{det}Q_{max}$ and a decrease in Q_{max} was noted (62). Conversely, a comparative videourodynamic study examined 50 women who underwent PVS—24 using rectus fascia, 26 using polypropylene mesh—and noted a non-significant decrease in Q_{max} at 7 to 14 days postoperatively which returned to baseline upon reassessment at three to six months (63). Similarly, a short-term outcome study examined PFS findings at three to six months in 48 women with successful outcomes after a modified vaginal wall sling procedure, and reported no significant difference in any pressure–flow or urethral pressure profile parameter (64).

Although the TVT and transobturator tape (TOT) procedures have success rates comparable to more established anti-incontinence procedures, voiding dysfunction, and urinary retention occur in 1.4% to 9% of patients postoperatively (65).

Table 31.2 Published Series on Definitions of Female Obstruction

Author (yr)	n (mean age in yrs) BOO	Controls	Etiology of BOO	Control population	Catheter size	Definition of obstruction
Massey and Abrams (1988) (1)	163 (NR)	None	Extramural (39), intramural (120), intraluminal (4)	N/A	NR	Q_{max} < 12 ml/sec, $p_{det}Q_{max}$ > 50 cmH$_2$O, urethral resistance > 0.2, PVR > 100 ml
Chassagne et al. (1998) (32)	35 (NR)	124 (NR)	Prior BNS (13), prolapse (11), other (6)[a]	SUI, no prior pelvic surgery, no cystocele or urethral pathology on VCUG	6 Fr	Q_{max} < 15 ml/sec, $p_{det}Q_{max}$ >20 cmH$_2$O ROC curve (sensitivity 74.3%, specificity 91.1%)
Nitti et al. (1999) (34)	76 (57.5)	184 (55)	DV (25), POP (24), PBNO (12), AIS (11), US (3), UD(1)	Women with LUTS who did not meet the specified criteria	7 Fr	Radiographic evidence of BOO with a sustained detrusor contraction of any magnitude on videourodynamics
Blaivas and Groutz (2000) (2)	50 (64.4)	50 (64.8)	AIS (10), POP (8), US (9), PBNO (3), UD (3), DV (2), DSD (2), idiopathic (11)	20 with LUTS and "normal" UDS, 30 with sphincteric incontinence	7 Fr	Free Q_{max} < 12 ml/sec and $p_{det\text{-}max}$ > 20 cmH$_2$O; or evidence of obstruction on fluoroscopy with detrusor contraction >20 cmH$_2$O
Lemack and Zimmern (2000) (33)	87 (NR)	124 (NR)	Cystocele (33), prior BNS (25), other[a] (29)	SUI, no prior pelvic surgery, no storage complaints, no cystocele or urethral pathology on VCUG	6 Fr	Q_{max} < 11 ml/sec, $p_{det}Q_{max}$ > 21 cmH$_2$O ROC curve (sensitivity 73.6%, specificity 91.5%)
Cormier et al. (2002) (38)	85 (55)	None	Prior BNS (7), US (5), PBNO (1), POP (1), idiopathic (7)	"Traditional" diagnosis of BOO	6 Fr	Area under detrusor pressure curve (AUC$_{det}$)/voided volume >5.83 cmH$_2$O per ml/sec
Defreitas et al. (2004) (12)	169 (60)	20 (42)	Cystocele (53), AIS (48), distal urethral fibrosis (68)	Normal UDI-6, no history of prior pelvic surgery	6 Fr	Q_{max} < 12 ml/sec, $p_{det}Q_{max}$ > 25 cmH$_2$O ROC curve (accuracy 68%)
Di Grazia et al. (2004) (48)	43 (55[b])	136 (55[b])	Advanced POP (20), prior BNS (6), DV (6), PBNO (2), US (1), idiopathic (8)	UI, no prior AIS, POP <grade 1 (B-W), no urethral pathology on cystoscopy or VCUG	12 Fr + 4 Fr (filling) 4 Fr only (voiding)	Q_{max} < 13 ml/sec, $p_{det\text{-}max}$ > 22 cmH$_2$O ROC curve (sensitivity 55.8%, specificity 96.3%)

[a]Periurethral fibrosis (21), retroverted uterus (4), excessive collagen (1), UD (1).
[b]Mean age reported only for all patients in study.
Abbreviations: AIS, anti-incontinence surgery; BNS, bladder neck suspension; BOO, bladder outlet obstruction; B-W, Baden–Walker halfway classification system; DSD, detrusor–sphincter dyssynergia; DV, dysfunctional voiding; LUTS, lower urinary tract symptoms; N/A, not applicable; NR, not reported; PBNO, primary bladder neck obstruction; POP, pelvic organ prolapse; PVR, post-void residual; ROC, receiver operator characteristics; SUI, stress urinary incontinence; UD, urethral diverticulum; UDI-6, Urogenital Distress Inventory; UDS, urodynamic study; UI, urinary incontinence; US, urethral stricture/stenosis; VCUG, voiding cystourethrogram, $p_{det}Q_{max}$, detrusor pressure at peak flow; AUC$_{det}$, area under the detrusor pressure curve.

Preoperative and one-year postoperative PFS data were reported in 65 patients who underwent TVT sling placement with a 25% decrease in flow rate and a 21% increase in $p_{det}Q_{max}$ (p < 0.001 and 0.02, respectively) (66). Other pressure–flow parameters as well as the non-intubated Q_{max} were also negatively affected; short-term (median duration 4 days) urinary retention occurred in 36% of patients, with 8% ultimately requiring sling release. A recent study in which 38 women undergoing TVT were examined pre-operatively with UDS, with 29 of those patients having routine repeat uroflowmetry evaluations at 1 and 3.5 years after surgery, noted that there were statistically significant changes in voiding parameters at one year after surgery, particularly a decrease in Q_{max} and an increase in PVR compared to preoperative baseline values.

These changes were relatively stable at 3.5 years, with no clinically or statistically significant differences compared to changes seen at one year after surgery. Complete pressure flow data (baseline, 1 year post-sling, and 3.5 years post-sling) was available for a limited number of patients, but demonstrated that post-operative pressure flow parameters were unchanged between the studies at the different time points (67).

In a randomized trial comparing the suprapubic arc (SPARC) sling to TVT, no significant difference in flow rates during PFS was noted (68), whereas a case-control series reported contrasting results, observing a significantly lower free Q_{max} at a mean follow-up of seven months in 69 and 37 women who underwent TVT or SPARC, respectively (69). Preoperative and one-year postoperative PFS were performed in a multicenter randomized trial comparing TVT (n = 30) to TOT (n = 31) and reported no significant difference in the rate of BOO between the two procedures (70).

Outcomes of TVT versus PVS using rectus fascia were examined in a randomized surgical trial at an average follow-up time of 38 and 40 months respectively. There was no difference in subjective or objective cure rates between the techniques. Comparison of pre-operative and post-operative uroflow parameters noted a decrease in Q_{max} in both groups by approximately 4 ml/sec (71).

It has been suggested that in some patients with mixed urinary incontinence the treatment of SUI with a PVS can improve urgency and urge urinary incontinence (UUI) symptoms. An NIH funded trial that aimed to address this question in a randomized fashion between a surgical and a medical arm was terminated early due to low enrollment numbers. However, a small study employing pre-operative PFS to predict resolution of DO after TVT was performed which determined that OAB symptoms resolved in 51% of patients after TVT. Of those patients in which urgency and UUI persisted, there was noted to be a significant decrease in Q_{max} and increase in p_{det} during voiding (72).

All these data suggest that altered voiding dynamics following each of the above anti-incontinence procedures can occur to varying degrees. Long-term data on these procedures with pressure–flow information will be needed to test their long-term effect on detrusor function

PREDICTIVE VALUE OF THE PRESSURE–FLOW PLOT

Thus far we have discussed the PFS as a means of documenting pre- and postoperative changes after anti-incontinence surgery. The predictive merit of PFS in the preoperative evaluation of incontinence has also been investigated. Impaired detrusor function on preoperative PFS appears to have some value in predicting voiding dysfunction after anti-incontinence procedures. One report examining preoperative voiding patterns in 30 women undergoing Burch colposuspension revealed that women who voided by Valsalva maneuver and urethral relaxation were 12 times more likely to require postoperative catheterization >7 days (73). Using time to resume normal voiding postoperatively, findings in two studies differed with regard to the predictive value of abdominal straining on preoperative PFS prior to Burch colposuspension (74,75). Accelerated flow rate (AFR)—which reflects the speed of detrusor contraction and opening of the bladder neck and is defined as the Q_{max} divided by the time to reach maximum flow during PFS—was investigated in 209 women with stress incontinence who underwent a Burch colposuspension (76). The AFR, which is independent of voided volume, was useful in predicting the outcome of continence surgery and the occurrence of de novo DO in 18% of women at one year.

Pubovaginal Sling

Clinical obstruction may occur more frequently after PVS in those patients with an abnormal preoperative PFS. The presence of a Valsalva-only voiding mechanism on preoperative PFS was associated with a longer duration of postoperative catheterization and objective failure after rectus fascia sling

placement in 50 women (77). Although Valsalva voiding did not correlate with urinary retention in 73 women followed after allograft fascia lata sling placement, another study found that no woman with a detrusor contraction >12 cmH$_2$O on preoperative PFS developed urinary retention, while 23% of those who voided without a detrusor contraction developed urinary retention (78). Conversely, preoperative urodynamic investigation poorly predicted the necessity of long-term catheterization after rectus fascia sling in 58 non-neurogenic women using the contraction parameters power factor WF and bladder contractility index (79).

A small study of 29 women undergoing PVS using autologous rectus fascia in Japan compared pre-operative and post-operative urodynamic parameters including PFS data and found that the Q_{max} was decreased in these patients by approximately 11 ml/sec. Detrusor voiding pressures were increased by an average of 11 cmH$_2$O and PVR was also increased by nearly 50 ml post-operatively, findings attributed to an increase in urethral resistance after surgery. The authors determined that predictors of voiding dysfunction defined as patients requiring long-term catheterization (>1 month) were preoperative PVR of >100 ml and/or Q_{max} on free uroflowmetry of 20 ml/sec or less (80).

Furthermore, in a sub-analysis of data collected from the SISTEr trial, pre-operative urodynamics parameters where evaluated to predict the outcomes of Burch colposuspension and the autologous PVS. Of 655 women who participated in the study, eight women in the Burch arm developed voiding dysfunction (defined as the need for catheterization beyond six weeks post-operatively or the need for post-operative surgical intervention due to perceived voiding difficulties) as compared to 49 women in the PVS group. Of the 57 women developing voiding dysfunction, 19 required surgical intervention, all of whom were in the sling arm. Data analysis determined that no pre-operative urodynamic parameter predicted voiding dysfunction in either group, and that pressure flow data was similar for patients who developed voiding difficulties and those who had no voiding complaints after initial surgery (81).

Finally, a recently completed surgical trial in which patients were randomized to TVT or TOT (TOMUS) incorporated a unique UDS design in that the patient and the surgeon were blinded to the urodynamic findings. Even though the study was not powered to investigate the role of pre-operative urodynamics, it should provide an interesting perspective on the relationship between baseline UDS and surgical outcome that might become useful to the practitioner (82). A specific randomized controlled trial focusing on the merit of pre-operative urodynamic testing in women with stress predominant urinary incontinence is underway and should provide more definitive answers to this scientific dilemma (www.UITN.net).

Mid-Urethral Slings

Data regarding the predictive role of the preoperative pressure–flow plot on voiding function after TVT or other mid-urethral slings is limited. Attempts to do so using linear regression analysis have been unable to find a correlation between PFS and outcomes such as postoperative voiding dysfunction (83), time to voiding, or urinary retention (66,84). Although the existing literature has focused on short-term changes, these often do not reflect the voiding status at intermediate and long-term follow-up.

URETHROLYSIS AND THE PRESSURE–FLOW PLOT

Conservative measures for relieving iatrogenic BOO have been described—including pharmacotherapy, urethral dilation, sling stretching, and/or incision—but the definitive intervention has been urethrolysis. Originally described by Richardson and Stonington in 1969 to treat "urethral syndrome" in a young woman (85), the technique was later reported by Leach and Raz in 1984 to manage obstruction after anti-incontinence surgery (86). The procedure is most commonly performed transvaginally, but has been described using a suprameatal or a retropubic approach.

PFS may assist in documenting obstruction prior to transvaginal urethrolysis (TVU), especially when there is no clear temporal relationship between the anti-incontinence procedure and onset of BOO symptoms. The "classic" findings of high p_{det} with low flow suggestive of obstruction are not always observed, and have been reported as being between 33% and 61%, even when clinical obstruction is suspected (87,88). The predictive role of PFS with regard to outcome after urethrolysis has been somewhat disappointing. A study involving 41 patients who underwent TVU found that the strength of detrusor contraction and the PFS did not predict the clinical outcome (88). Similar findings were described in a series of 32 women who underwent suprameatal TVU (89). Obstruction was defined as $p_{det}Q_{max} > 20$ ml/sec with a $Q_{max} < 12$ ml/sec, but the success rate after urethrolysis in patients who met these criteria was no different from those who underwent TVU based on physical examination and clinical judgment.

In a small population of women with bladder or urethral erosion of mesh mid-urethral slings, symptom presentation varied from pain and infection to voiding dysfunction. Abnormality on UDS was noted pre-operatively in 69% of patients with only one-thirteenth demonstrating the typical parameters of high p_{det} and low urinary flow rate indicative of BOO. Following mesh removal, voiding symptoms resolved in 21% of patients, with recurrent SUI noted in 42% of patients (90).

CONCLUSION

The PFS is a valuable tool in the evaluation of incontinence and obstruction in women. It remains the most challenging step in a UDS, not only because of numerous technical issues, but also because of current limitations in defining normative values and the lack of universally agreed-upon interpretation guidelines. These shortcomings currently limit its clinical usefulness as a stand-alone test, thus forcing the clinician to use the PFS information judiciously in combination with other clinical elements.

REFERENCES

1. Massey JA, Abrams PH. Obstructed voiding in the female. Br J Urol 1988; 61: 36–9.
2. Blaivas JG, Groutz A. Bladder outlet obstruction nomogram for women with lower urinary tract symptomatology. Neurourol Urodyn 2000; 19: 553–64.
3. Vowles JE, Wagg AS. The pressure-flow plot in the evaluation of female incontinence. BJU Int 1999; 84: 948–52.
4. Hill AV. The heat of shortening and the dynamic constants of muscle. Proc R Soc Lond B Biol Sci 1938; 126: 136–95.
5. Griffiths DJ. The Mechanics and Hydrodynamics of the Lower Urinary Tract. Medical Physics Handbooks, 4th edn. Bristol: Adam Hilger: 1980.
6. Griffiths DJ. Proceedings: Urethral resistance to flow: the urethral resistance relation. Abbreviated report. Urol Int 1975; 30: 28.
7. van Mastrigt R, Griffiths DJ. Clinical comparison of bladder contractility parameters calculated from isometric contractions and pressure-flow studies. Urology 1987; 29: 102–6.
8. Schafer W. The contribution of the bladder outlet to the relation between pressure and flow rate during micturition. In: Hinman FJ, ed. Benign Prostatic Hypertrophy. New York: Springer-Verlag; 1983: 470–96.
9. Buttyan R, Chen MW, Levin RM. Animal models of bladder outlet obstruction and molecular insights into the basis for the development of bladder dysfunction. Eur Urol 1997; 32(Suppl 1): 32–9.
10. Agartan CA, Whitbeck C, Chichester P, Kogan BA, Levin RM. Effect of age on rabbit bladder function and structure following partial outlet obstruction. J Urol 2005; 173: 1400–5.
11. Wagg A. The pressure-flow plot in the evaluation of female incontinence. In: Cardozo L, Staskin D, eds. Textbook of Female Urology and Urogynecology. London: Taylor and Francis; 2001.
12. Defreitas GA, Zimmern PE, Lemack GE, Shariat SF. Refining diagnosis of anatomic female bladder outlet obstruction: comparison of pressure-flow study parameters in clinically obstructed women with those of normal controls. Urology 2004; 64: 675–9; discussion 679–81.
13. Valentini FA, Besson GR, Nelson PP, Zimmern PE. A mathematical micturition model to restore simple flow recordings in healthy and symptomatic individuals and enhance uroflow interpretation. Neurourol Urodyn 2000; 19: 153–76.
14. Susset JG, Picker P, Kretz M, Jorest R. Critical evaluation of uroflowmeters and analysis of normal curves. J Urol 1973; 109: 874–8.
15. Ryall RL, Marshall VR. The effect of a urethral catheter on the measurement of maximum urinary flow rate. J Urol 1982; 128: 429–32.
16. Baseman AG, Baseman JG, Zimmern PE, Lemack GE. Effect of 6F urethral catheterization on urinary flow rates during repeated pressure-flow studies in healthy female volunteers. Urology 2002; 59: 843–6.
17. Groutz A, Blaivas JG, Sassone AM. Detrusor pressure uroflowmetry studies in women: effect of a 7Fr transurethral catheter. J Urol 2000; 164: 109–14.
18. Di Grazia E, Bartolotta S, Nicolosi F, Nicolosi D. Detrusor pressure uroflowmetry studies in women: effect of 4 Fr transurethral. Arch Ital Urol Androl 2002; 74: 134–7.
19. Costantini E, Mearini L, Biscotto S, et al. Impact of different sized catheters on pressure-flow studies in women with lower urinary tract symptoms. Neurourol Urodyn 2005; 24: 106–10.
20. Lazarou G, Scotti RJ, Mikhail MS, Zhou HS, Powers K. Pessary reduction and postoperative cure of retention in women with anterior vaginal wall prolapse. Int Urogynecol J Pelvic Floor Dysfunct 2004; 15: 175–8.
21. Fitzgerald MP, Kulkarni N, Fenner D. Postoperative resolution of urinary retention in patients with advanced pelvic organ prolapse. Am J Obstet Gynecol 2000; 183: 1361–3; discussion 1363–4.
22. Gilleran JP, Lemack G, Zimmern PE, eds. Impact of a vaginal pack in reducing cystocele during preoperative urodynamic studies. International Continence Society (ICS) Annual Meeting. Montreal, CA: ICS; 2005.
23. Visco AG, Brubaker L, Nygaard I, et al. The role of preoperative urodynamic testing in stress-continent women undergoing sacrocolpopexy: the colpopexy and urinary reduction efforts (CARE) randomized surgical trial. Int Urogynecol J Pelvic Floor Dysfunct 2008; 19: 607–14.
24. Devreese AM, Nuyens G, Staes F, et al. Do posture and straining influence urinary-flow parameters in normal women? Neurourol Urodyn 2000; 19: 3–8.
25. Moore KH, Richmond DH, Sutherst JR, Imrie AH, Hutton JL. Crouching over the toilet seat: prevalence among British gynaecological outpatients and its effect upon micturition. Br J Obstet Gynaecol 1991; 98: 569–72.
26. Schafer W, Abrams P, Liao L, et al. Good urodynamic practices: uroflowmetry, filling cystometry, and pressure-flow studies. Neurourol Urodyn 2002; 21: 261–74.

27. Sullivan J, Lewis P, Howell S, et al. Quality control in urodynamics: a review of urodynamic traces from one centre. BJU Int 2003; 91: 201–7.

28. Nager CW, Albo ME, Fitzgerald MP, et al. Process for development of multicenter urodynamic studies. Urology 2007; 69: 63–7; discussion 67–8.

29. FitzGerald MP, Brubaker L. The etiology of urinary retention after surgery for genuine stress incontinence. Neurourol Urodyn 2001; 20: 13–21.

30. O'Donnell P. Electromyography. In: Nitti V, ed. Practical Urodynamics. Philadelphia: WB Saunders, 1998: 65–71.

31. Tanagho EA. Vesico-urethral dynamics. In: Lutzyer W, Melchior H, eds. Urodynamics. Berlin: Springer-Verlag, 1973: 215.

32. Chassagne S, Bernier PA, Haab F, et al. Proposed cutoff values to define bladder outlet obstruction in women. Urology 1998; 51: 408–11.

33. Lemack GE, Zimmern PE. Pressure flow analysis may aid in identifying women with outflow obstruction. J Urol 2000; 163: 1823–8.

34. Nitti VW, Tu LM, Gitlin J. Diagnosing bladder outlet obstruction in women. J Urol 1999; 161: 1535–40.

35. Arbique GM, Gilleran JP, Guild JB, et al. Radiation exposure during standing voiding cystourethrography in women. Urology 2006; 67: 269–74.

36. Massolt E, Groen J, Vierhout M. Application of the Blaivas-Groutz bladder outlet obstruction nomogram in women with urinary incontinence. Neurourol Urodyn 2005; 24: 1–6.

37. Groutz A, Blaivas JG, Chaikin DC. Bladder outlet obstruction in women: definition and characteristics. Neurourol Urodyn 2000; 19: 213–20.

38. Cormier L, Ferchaud J, Galas JM, Guillemin F, Mangin P. Diagnosis of female bladder outlet obstruction and relevance of the parameter area under the curve of detrusor pressure during voiding: preliminary results. J Urol 2002; 167: 2083–7.

39. Valentini F, Zimmern PE, Besson G, Nelson P. Modelled analysis of the effect of cystocele reduction with vaginal pack on miction in women with grade IV cystocele. Prog Urol 2000; 10: 432–7.

40. Fritel X, Valentini F, Nelson P, Besson G. Contribution of modeling to the analysis of mictional modifications caused by TVT: study of free uroflows. Prog Urol 2004; 14: 197–202; discussion 202.

41. Lemack GE, Baseman AG, Zimmern PE. Voiding dynamics in women: a comparison of pressure-flow studies between asymptomatic and incontinent women. Urology 2002; 59: 42–6.

42. Madersbacher S, Pycha A, Schatzl G, et al. The aging lower urinary tract: a comparative urodynamic study of men and women. Urology 1998; 51: 206–12.

43. Desgrandchamps F, Cortesse A, Rousseau T, Teillac P, Duc AL. Normal voiding behaviour in women. Study of the I-PSS in an unselected population of women in general practice. Eur Urol 1996; 30: 18–23.

44. Terai A, Matsui Y, Ichioka K, et al. Comparative analysis of lower urinary tract symptoms and bother in both sexes. Urology 2004; 63: 487–91.

45. Svatek R, Roche V, Thornberg J, Zimmern P. Normative values for the American urological association symptom index (AUA-7) and short form urogenital distress inventory (UDI-6) in patients 65 and older presenting for non-urological care. Neurourol Urodyn 2005; 24: 606–10.

46. Wyndaele JJ. Normality in urodynamics studied in healthy adults. J Urol 1999; 161: 899–902.

47. Lemack G, Zimmern P. Voiding cystourethrography and magnetic resonance imaging of the lower urinary tract. In: Corcos J, Schnick E, eds. The Urinary Sphincter. New York: Marcel Dekker, 2001: 407–21.

48. Di Grazia E, Troyo Sanroman R, Aceves JG. Proposed urodynamic pressure-flow nomogram to diagnose female bladder outlet obstruction. Arch Ital Urol Androl 2004; 76: 59–65.

49. Karram MM, Partoll L, Bilotta V, Angel O. Factors affecting detrusor contraction strength during voiding in women. Obstet Gynecol 1997; 90: 723–6.

50. Bradley CS, Rovner ES. Urodynamically defined stress urinary incontinence and bladder outlet obstruction coexist in women. J Urol 2004; 171(2 Pt 1): 757–60; discussion 760–1.

51. Haylen BT, Ashby D, Sutherst JR, Frazer MI, West CR. Maximum and average urine flow rates in normal male and female populations—the Liverpool nomograms. Br J Urol 1989; 64: 30–8.

52. Digesu GA, Hutchings A, Salvatore S, Selvaggi L, Khullar V. Reproducibility and reliability of pressure flow parameters in women. BJOG 2003; 110: 774–6.

53. Nager CW, Albo ME, FitzGerald MP, Network eaftUIT. Quality control of multicenter urodynamic studes. Neurourol Urodyn 2005; in press.

54. Nager CW, Albo ME, Fitzgerald MP, et al. Reference urodynamic values for stress incontinent women. Neurourol Urodyn 2007; 26: 333–40.

55. Klutke JJ, Klutke CG, Bergman J, Elia G. Bladder neck suspension for stress urinary incontinence: how does it work? Neurourol Urodyn 1999; 18: 623–7.

56. Zimmern PE. Vaginal surgery for stress urinary incontinence: beyond horizon 2000. In: Stanton SL, Zimmern PE, eds. Female Pelvic Reconstructive Surgery. Berlin: Springer-Verlag, 2002: 360–3.

57. Zimmern PE, Hadley HR, Leach GE, Raz S. Female urethral obstruction after Marshall–Marchetti–Krantz operation. J Urol 1987; 138: 517–20.

58. Leach GE, Yip CM, Donovan BJ. Mechanism of continence after modified Pereyra bladder neck suspension. Prospective urodynamic study. Urology 1987; 29: 328–31.

59. Herbertsson G, Iosif CS. Surgical results and urodynamic studies 10 years after retropubic colpourethrocystopexy. Acta Obstet Gynecol Scand 1993; 72: 298–301.

60. Belair G, Tessier J, Bertrand PE, Schick E. Retropubic cystourethropexy: is it an obstructive procedure? J Urol 1997; 158: 533–8.

61. Leach GE, Dmochowski RR, Appell RA, et al. Female stress urinary incontinence clinical guidelines panel summary report on surgical management of female stress urinary incontinence. The American Urological Association. J Urol 1997; 158(3 Pt 1): 875–80.

62. Fulford SC, Flynn R, Barrington J, Appanna T, Stephenson TP. An assessment of the surgical outcome and urodynamic effects of the pubovaginal sling for stress incontinence and the associated urge syndrome. J Urol 1999; 162: 135–7.

63. Kuo HC. Comparison of video urodynamic results after the pubovaginal sling procedure using rectus fascia and polypropylene mesh for stress urinary incontinence. J Urol 2001; 165: 163–8.

64. Mikhail MS, Rosa H, Palan P, Anderson P. Comparison of preoperative and postoperative pressure transmission ratio and urethral pressure profilometry in patients with successful outcome following the vaginal wall patch sling technique. Neurourol Urodyn 2005; 24: 31–4.

65. Sander P, Moller LM, Rudnicki PM, Lose G. Does the tension-free vaginal tape procedure affect the voiding phase? Pressure-flow studies before and 1 year after surgery. BJU Int 2002; 89: 694–8.

66. Lukacz ES, Luber KM, Nager CW. The effects of the tension-free vaginal tape on voiding function: a prospective evaluation. Int Urogynecol J Pelvic Floor Dysfunct 2004; 15: 32–8; discussion 38.

67. Sander P, Sorensen F, Lose G. Does the tension-free vaginal tape procedure (TVT) affect the voiding function over time? Pressure-flow studies 1 year and 3(1/2) years after TVT. Neurourol Urodyn 2007; 26: 995–7.

68. Tseng LH, Wang AC, Lin YH, Li SJ, Ko YJ. Randomized comparison of the suprapubic arc sling procedure vs tension-free vaginal taping for stress incontinent women. Int Urogynecol J Pelvic Floor Dysfunct 2005; 16: 230–5.

69. Dietz HP, Foote AJ, Mak HL, Wilson PD. TVT and sparc suburethral slings: a case-control series. Int Urogynecol J Pelvic Floor Dysfunct 2004; 15: 129–31; discussion 131.

70. deTayrac R, Deffieux X, Droupy S, et al. A prospective randomized trial comparing tension-free vaginal tape and transobturator suburethral tape for surgical treatment of stress urinary incontinence. Am J Obstet Gynecol 2004; 190: 602–8.

71. Sharifiaghdas F, Mortazavi N. Tension-free vaginal tape and autologous rectus fascia pubovaginal sling for the treatment of urinary stress incontinence: a medium-term follow-up. Med Princ Pract 2008; 17: 209–14.

72. Duckett JR, Basu M. The predictive value of preoperative pressure-flow studies in the resolution of detrusor overactivity and overactive bladder after tension-free vaginal tape insertion. BJU Int 2007; 99: 1439–42.

73. Bhatia NN, Bergman A. Urodynamic predictability of voiding following incontinence surgery. Obstet Gynecol 1984; 63: 85–91.

74. Sze EH, Miklos JR, Karram MM. Voiding after Burch colposuspension and effects of concomitant pelvic surgery: correlation with preoperative voiding mechanism. Obstet Gynecol 1996; 88(4 Pt 1): 564–7.

75. Kobak WH, Walters MD, Piedmonte MR. Determinants of voiding after three types of incontinence surgery: a multivariable analysis. Obstet Gynecol 2001; 97: 86–91.

76. Digesu GA, Khullar V, Cardozo L, Sethna F, Salvatore S. Preoperative pressure-flow studies: useful variables to predict the outcome of continence surgery. BJU Int 2004; 94: 1296–9.

77. Iglesia CB, Shott S, Fenner DE, Brubaker L. Effect of preoperative voiding mechanism on success rate of autologous rectus fascia suburethral sling procedure. Obstet Gynecol 1998; 91: 577–81.

78. Miller EA, Amundsen CL, Toh KL, Flynn BJ, Webster GD. Preoperative urodynamic evaluation may predict voiding dysfunction in women undergoing pubovaginal sling. J Urol 2003; 169: 2234–7.

79. Groen J, Bosch JL. Bladder contraction strength parameters poorly predict the necessity of long-term catheterization after a pubovaginal rectus fascial sling procedure. J Urol 2004; 172: 1006–9.

80. Mitsui T, Tanaka H, Moriya K, Kakizaki H, Nonomura K. Clinical and urodynamic outcomes of pubovaginal sling procedure with autologous rectus fascia for stress urinary incontinence. Int J Urol 2007; 14: 1076–9.

81. Lemack GE, Krauss S, Litman H, et al. Normal preoperative urodynamic testing does not predict voiding dysfunction after Burch colposuspension versus pubovaginal sling. J Urol 2008; 180: 2076–80.

82. Albo M, (UITN) eaftUITN. The trial of mid-urethral slings (TOMUS): design and methodology. Th J Appl Res 2008; 8: 1–13.

83. Al-Badr A, Ross S, Soroka D, et al. Voiding patterns and urodynamics after a tension-free vaginal tape procedure. J Obstet Gynaecol Can 2003; 25: 725–30.

84. Sokol AI, Jelovsek JE, Walters MD, Paraiso MF, Barber MD. Incidence and predictors of prolonged urinary retention after TVT with and without concurrent prolapse surgery. Am J Obstet Gynecol 2005; 192: 1537–43.

85. Richardson FH, Stonington OG. Urethrolysis and external urethroplasty in the female. Surg Clin North Am 1969; 49: 1201–8.

86. Leach GE, Raz S. Modified Pereyra bladder neck suspension after previously failed anti-incontinence surgery. Surgical technique and results with long-term follow-up. Urology 1984; 23: 359–62.

87. Webster GD, Kreder KJ. Voiding dysfunction following cystourethropexy: its evaluation and management. J Urol 1990; 144: 670–3.

88. Nitti VW, Raz S. Obstruction following anti-incontinence procedures: diagnosis and treatment with transvaginal urethrolysis. J Urol 1994; 152: 93–8.

89. Petrou SP, Brown JA, Blaivas JG. Suprameatal transvaginal urethrolysis. J Urol 1999; 161: 1268–71.

90. Starkman JS, Wolter C, Gomelsky A, Scarpero HM, Dmochowski RR. Voiding dysfunction following removal of eroded synthetic mid urethral slings. J Urol 2006; 176: 1040–4.

32 Tests of Urethral Function

Ahmet Bedestani, Christopher J Chermansky, Mohamed Ghafar and J Christian Winters

URETHRAL ANATOMY AND MECHANISMS OF URETHRAL CONTINENCE

Adequate bladder outlet resistance is essential in order to maintain urinary continence in women, particularly during periods of increased intra-abdominal pressure. Thus, the anatomy and function of the urethra are important determinants of continence. The female urethra throughout its length has a complex luminal architecture, which serves a dual function as conduit as well as a barrier protecting the underlying stroma from urinary irritants. This muscular lumen passes from retropubic space and ends in the vestibule. The distance between the bladder neck and external urethral meatus determines the anatomic length of the urethra. The urethra mucosa is a transitional epithelium, which contains many infoldings and is supported by loose elastic connective tissue, containing bundles of collagen fibers. This promotes excellent distention during voiding as well as coaptation (or urethral seal effect) during storage. The mucosa, submucosal tissues, and the periurethral fascia connective tissues promote urethral closure and the urethral seal effect. The urethra contains a complex of smooth and striated muscles, which contribute to the sphincteric mechanism. A relatively thick layer of inner longitudinal smooth muscle continues from the bladder to the external meatus to insert into periurethral fatty and fibrous tissue. A rather thin layer of circular smooth muscle envelops the longitudinal fibers throughout the length of the urethra. It is thought that the longitudinal smooth muscle of the urethra contracts coordinately with the detrusor during micturition to shorten and widen the urethra (1). The urethral smooth muscle composed of circular and longitudinal muscle both join the detrusor muscle in the base of the bladder and form the intrinsic sphincter mechanism, with predominant function in the proximal urethra (2). The striated urethral sphincter invests the distal two-thirds of the female urethra (3). It is composed exclusively of delicate type I (slow-twitch) fibers surrounded by abundant collagen. Proximally, near the mid-urethra, it forms a complete ring around the urethra that corresponds to the zone of highest urethral closure pressure. This striated muscular complex adds resting tone to the urethra, further enhancing urethral closure. DeLancey et al. (2,4,5) have provided a comprehensive description of urethral support. The pubocervical and periurethral fascia support the bladder base and proximal urethra respectively in a sling like fashion, which is attached bilaterally to the arcus tendineus fascia. In addition, the pubourethral ligament complex provides stability to the midurethra. During periods of increased intra-abdominal pressure, the urethra is closed by the hammock of support created by the periurethral fascia, and by contraction of the pubococcygeus muscles (levator ani) which close the urethra against the pubourethral ligaments. Discrete defects in the pubocervical or periurethral fascia or detachment of these structures from the arcus promotes a loss of bladder neck and proximal urethral support, creating "urethral hypermobility." This loss of urethral support prevents the hammock effect of urethral closure or compression of the urethra against the pubourethral ligaments (6). Thus, defects in anatomic support of the female urethra can disrupt urethral and pelvic floor function, which maintain continence during periods of increased intra-abdominal pressure (Fig. 32.1).

Assessment of Urethral Anatomy

Physical Examination

An examination of the external genitalia and anterior vaginal wall will provide substantial information regarding urethral anatomy. Urethral caruncles, urethral prolapse, and Skene's gland obstruction or inflammation are easily detected. The presence of urethral scarring or induration may also suggest post-operative or alternative conditions, which could adversely affect urethral function. Vaginal wall thinning or a pale appearance to the urethra implies vaginal atrophy, which can predispose to certain urologic conditions. Lastly, a bulging or purulent expressate is suspicious for urethral diverticulum, and this could predispose to leakage, infection and rarely obstruction. A loss of urethral support can be assessed using a half-speculum, and examining the anterior vaginal wall in the resting and straining state. Urethral hypermobility is usually easily discernable on examination by the classic rotational appearance of the urethra. In most instances, a visual assessment is enough to confirm the presence of urethral hypermobility. In select instances, a Q-Tip test may be used. This test has demonstrated good interobserver reliability (7,8). The Q-tip test is performed by inserting a sterile lubricated Q-tip into the bladder, and gently withdrawing it until resistance is felt insuring proper positioning at urethrovesical junction. The angle of deflection with straining should be measured with goniometer. Urethral hypermobility is defined as maximal straining angle of more than 30° from horizontal (9) or from resting angle. In most cases, this test is unnecessary and may be uncomfortable, so its use should be limited to those cases where it will change the course of treatment.

Ultrasound

Different ultrasound techniques have been used to quantify bladder neck mobility, including transrectal, transvaginal (10), perineal (11), and introital. The transperineal approach is the most commonly used. The bladder neck is identified, and by performing systematic measurements of descent with relation

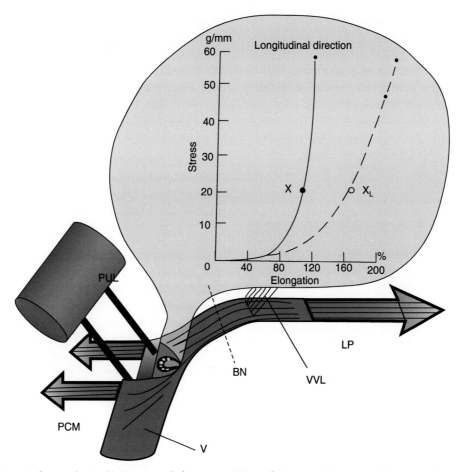

Figure 32.1 Urethral anatomy: Influence of vaginal laxity on muscle force transmission and urinary continence. *Inset,* Stress extension curve of vagina. BN, bladder neck; LP, levator plate; PCM, pubococcygeus muscle; PUL, pubourethral ligament; V, vaginal hammock; VVL, vaginal attachment to the bladder base; X, normal elasticity; XL, vaginal laxity. The authors propose that an increase in urethral pressure before cough transmission proves that an active continence mechanism is involved in preventing stress urinary incontinence. *Source:* Reproduced from Ref. 6 with permission.

to the symphysis pubis, normal values of descent have been reported with good interobserver reliability (12). This modality of ultrasound assessment is expensive and requires specific training in order to develop proficiency. In addition, the precise role of ultrasound imaging has not been determined.

FLOUROSCOPY (VIDEOURODYNAMICS)
Urodynamics is a provocative test of vesicourethral function. Videourodynamics (VUDS) is the synchronous measurement and display of urodynamic parameters with radiographic visualization of the lower urinary tract. During VUDS, the clinician can better appreciate the interrelationships between the various urodynamic parameters with the periodic sampling of fluoroscopic images during filling, voiding, and provocative maneuvers such as leak point pressure (LPP) measurement. The addition of concomitant cystourethrography to urodynamics does allow the clinician to better evaluate the state of the bladder neck and the site of urethral obstruction. VUDS is a useful test in the diagnosis of detrusor sphincter dyssnergia, acquired voiding dysfunction, and anatomic urethral obstruction.

Detrusor External Sphincter Dyssnergia (DESD)
DESD is characterized by involuntary contractions of the striated musculature of the urethral sphincter during an involuntary detrusor contraction. It represents inappropriate sphincter

activity during voiding, and it is functional obstruction of the urethra. This condition is seen after suprasacral spinal cord injury, multiple sclerosis, myelodysplasia, and transverse myelitis (13). True DESD may only exist in the presence of a neurologic lesion that lies between the brain stem and the sacral spinal cord. In DESD, the contraction of the external sphincter [and increase in electromyography (EMG) activity] always occurs prior to the onset of the detrusor contraction. The classic appearance of DESD with VUDS shows a dilated proximal urethra and a narrowed distal urethra associated with increased EMG activity and an involuntary detrusor contraction (Fig. 32.2).

Acquired Voiding Dysfunction (AVD)—Hinman's Syndrome
With AVD the patient involuntarily (and subconsciously) contracts the external urethral sphincter (14). The images of these contractions are identical to those seen in DESD since both cause functional urethral obstruction (Fig. 32.3). Yet, in DESD the contraction of the external sphincter always occurs prior to the onset of the detrusor contraction. In contrast, in AVD the detrusor contraction occurs prior to the subconscious contraction of the external sphincter. Concentric needle electrode provides a superior signal source compared with the surface electrode in the evaluation of AVD.

There are several theories as to why adults develop AVD. The most plausible theory is that it develops as a learned behavior in response to an adverse event, such as infection, inflammation, irritation, or trauma. McGuire et al. attributed AVD to detrusor overactivity with the sphincter response developing as a result of a sudden unanticipated detrusor contraction (15). The pelvic floor sphincter complex normally contracts to control sudden urgency, and this will cause reflex inhibition of the detrusor. When this action becomes habitual with time, it can lead to such voiding symptoms as intermittent stream and incomplete bladder emptying. Carlson et al. retrospectively

studied 26 women with AVD (16). Storage symptoms were more common than voiding symptoms in their study group. Detrusor overactivity and sensory urgency was seen in 42% of the patients. Urological history and VUDS prompted neurological investigation, which identified neurological disease in five cases that were then reclassified as DESD. The authors concluded that occult neurological disease should be suspected in all patients with AVD.

Anatomic Urethral Obstruction

Urethral obstruction in women is defined as Pdet @ Qmax > 20 cmH$_2$O and Qmax < 12 ml/sec (17). Nitti et al. proposed that urethral obstruction be defined as radiographic evidence of obstruction between the bladder neck and the distal urethra in the presence of a sustained detrusor contraction (18). The symptoms of urethral obstruction in women include storage symptoms (urinary frequency, urgency, and urge incontinence) and voiding symptoms (weak stream, hesitancy, dysuria, and post-void dribbling). The two most common causes of anatomic urethral obstruction in women are pelvic organ prolapse (POP) and complications after anti-incontinence surgery. With the use of VUDS, the site of obstruction is defined as the narrowest point in the urethra during voiding cystourethrography.

In patients with high grade POP, the descent may create urethral kinking and urethral compression (19). Documenting the presence of stress urinary incontinence (SUI) in patients with the prolapse reduced is helpful in the preoperative management of women with high-grade POP. SUI occurring in presumably continent women after prolapse correction is known as occult SUI. It is essential for women with high-grade POP to undergo an evaluation with the prolapse reduced in order to identify if they are at risk for occult SUI. To diagnose occult SUI, the prolapse may be reduced with vaginal packing, rectal swabs, a speculum blade, or pessary. VUDS is helpful in showing both urethral obstruction and occult SUI (20) (Figs. 32.4 and 32.5).

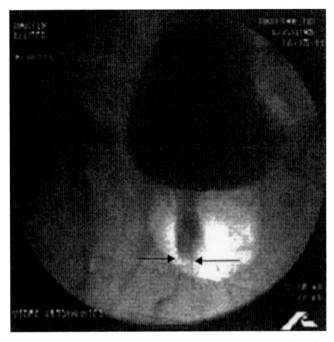

Figure 32.2 X-ray obtained at Pdet @ Qmax in patient with DESD shows the classic picture of complete obstruction at the membranous urethra (arrows) and a "Christmas tree" shaped bladder *Source:* Reproduced from Ref. 81 with permission. *Abbreviation:* DESD, detrusor external sphincter dyssnergia.

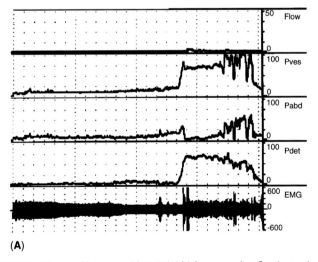

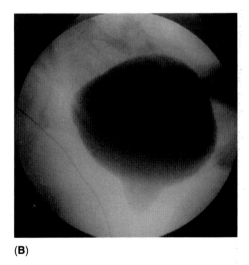

(A) (B)

Figure 32.3 VUDS in 33-year-old woman with AVD (A) high pressure, low flow is associated with increased EMG activity (B) fluoroscopic visualization of urethra during voiding shows dilated proximal urethra with point of obstruction at external sphincter *Source:* Reproduced from Ref. 16 with permission. *Abbreviations:* AVD, acquired voiding dysfunction; EMG, electromyography; Pves, intravesical pressure; Pabd, abdominal pressure; Pdet, detrusor pressure; VUDS, videourodynamics.

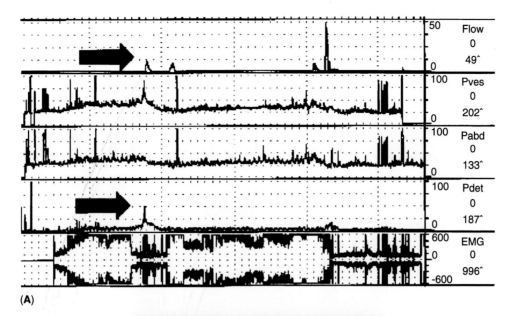

(A)

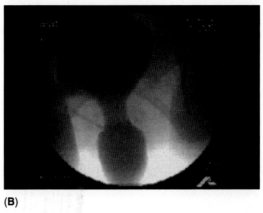

(B)

Figure 32.4 VUDS in 65-year-old woman with grade 4 anterior compartment prolapse (**A**) at the arrows she voids with detrusor pressure (Pdet) of 50 cmH$_2$O and a flow of 6 ml/sec, indicating urethral obstruction (**B**) voiding cystogram taken at the arrow shows a large cystocele obscuring the urethra and causing urethral obstruction *Source*: Reproduced from Ref. 20 with permission. *Abbreviations*: EMG, electromyography; Pves, intravesical pressure; Pabd, abdominal pressure; VUDS, videourodynamics.

In their database of 587 consecutive women undergoing evaluation with VUDS, Groutz et al. diagnosed anatomic urethral obstruction in 38 patients (6.5%) (21). Of those 38 patients, 10 (26%) had urethral obstruction from previous anti-incontinence surgery (Fig. 32.6). The predominant symptomatology was a mix of voiding (obstructive) and storage (irritative) symptoms, with the most common symptom being weak stream. Klutke et al. reported urethral obstruction in 17 of 600 patients (2.8%) that underwent tension-free vaginal tape (TVT) surgery (22). The patients presented with symptoms of urinary retention, poor flow, or urgency. All of the 17 patients voided within 24 hours of sling incision or loosening.

While urethral function can be inferred from physical examination, radiographic tests, and cystometry, more accurate assessments of urethral function are commonly needed. Urethral function may be better characterized in a number of ways: LPP measurement, urethral pressure profilometry (UPP), retrograde urethral perfusion pressure, and EMG. A description of these techniques is included.

ABDOMINAL LEAK POINT PRESSURE (ALPP)

Another way to examine urethral function is with the assessment of LPPs. There are two methods of LPP assessment that analyze different functional areas of the lower urinary tract. The detrusor leak point pressure (DLPP), as defined by the International Continence Society (ICS), is the lowest detrusor pressure (Pdet) at which urine leakage occurs in the absence of either a detrusor contraction or increased abdominal pressure (23). It is not a test of urethral function but rather a test of bladder storage function. In contrast, the ALPP or valsalva leak point pressure (VLPP) is a measure of urethral function. The ALPP, as defined by the ICS, is the lowest intravesical pressure (Pves) at which urine leakage occurs because of increased abdominal pressure in the absence of a detrusor contraction (23).

McGuire et al. introduced the concept of ALPP in 1993 as a means of differentiating urinary incontinence due to either urethral hypermobility or intrinsic sphincter deficiency (ISD) (24). This measurement is used to quantify the *stress competence* of the urethra or the ability of the urethra to maintain continence during increased periods of intra-abdominal pressure. McGuire

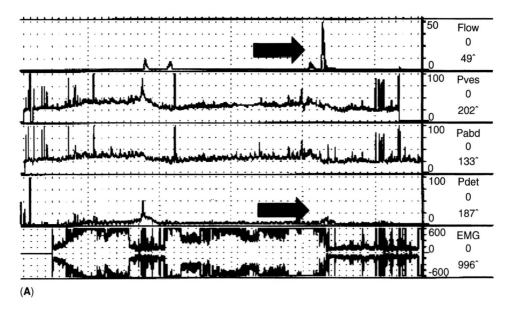

(A)

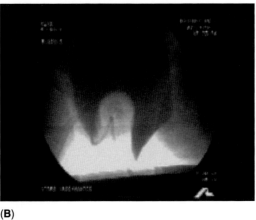

(B)

Figure 32.5 The same 65-year-old woman as in Figure 32.4 with her POP reduced (**A**) at the arrows she voids with a detrusor pressure (Pdet) of <10 cmH$_2$O and a flow of 49 ml/sec. VLPP was about 90 cmH$_2$O (**B**) voiding cystogram taken at the arrow shows high flow and low pressure *Source:* Reproduced from Ref. 20 with permission. *Abbreviations:* EMG, electromyography; Pves, intravesical pressure; Pabd, abdominal pressure; POP, pelvic organ prolapse; VLPP, valsalva leak point pressure; VUDS, videourodynamics.

proposed that ALPP is a measure of sphincter strength. Increased abdominal pressure does not open a normally positioned and closed urethral sphincter. Urine leakage can be caused only by an increase in abdominal pressure when the urethra is abnormal. Thus, ALPP cannot be quantified if the subject does not demonstrate SUI during urodynamic testing. In addition, the Pdet at the time of ALPP testing must be low. High Pdet (due to poor bladder compliance) at the time of ALPP testing will result in the false impression that urethral function is impaired (25). In this scenario, it would be DLPP being measured.

Technique of ALPP

An acceptable technique to measure ALPP involves first placing a six French dual-lumen urodynamic catheter into the bladder. Cystometry then proceeds until the bladder has been filled to 200 cc. The patient is then asked to perform a valsalva maneuver by gradually increasing his/her intra-abdominal pressure until he or she leaks (Fig. 32.7). The lowest bladder pressure at which leakage occurs is defined the ALPP. If there is no urine leakage

with a bladder volume of 200 ml, the test is repeated with a bladder volume of 300 ml. If ALPP testing is negative at this volume, filling continues with repeat testing performed at 50 ml increments until maximum cystometric capacity is reached.

If the patient is not able to generate a valsalva pressure sufficient enough to produce leakage, then the patient is asked to cough several times with increasing strength until leakage occurs. Compared to the straining performed with a valsalva maneuver, coughing generates faster intra-abdominal pressures. As such, precise measurements are more difficult to obtain with coughing. Once leakage has been observed, the force of the cough is reduced until it generates the minimal amount of abdominal pressure required to produce leakage.

Patient position is important. If patients only leak standing, then the test may need to be done in the standing position. Also, it has been reported that the urethral catheter may need to be removed, as this may mask leakage in certain situations. In this situation the pressure measurements can be made from the rectal pressure catheter (or Pves). Measurements at capacity may only be recorded if there is no spontaneous detrusor activity.

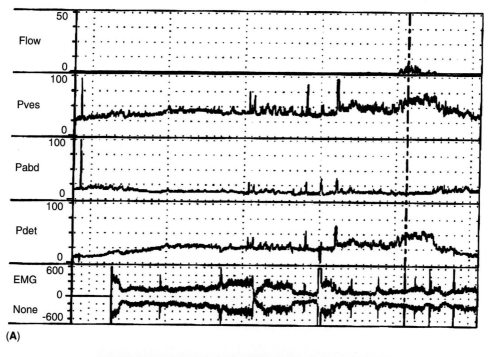

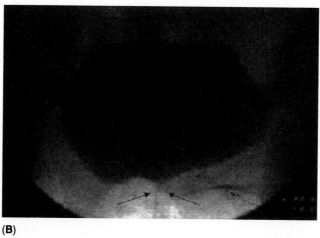

(B)

Figure 32.6 Urethral obstruction five years status post autologous fascial pubovaginal sling (**A**) Urodynamic tracing. Pdet @ Qmax = 50 cmH$_2$O and Qmax = 6 ml/sec (vertical dashed line). (**B**) X-ray exposed at Qmax shows a narrow urethra just distal to the vesical neck (arrows) *Source*: Reproduced from Ref. 81 with permission. *Abbreviations*: EMG, electromyography; Pves, intravesical pressure; Pabd, abdominal pressure; Pdet, detrusor pressure.

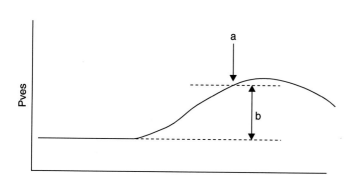

Figure 32.7 Measurement of VLPP: Patient is asked to bear down progressively while holding breath. Leakage is recorded (*arrow* at a) at the precise moment that fluid is observed at urethral meatus. The rise on Pves over baseline (b) represent VLPP. *Source*: Reproduced from Ref. 31 with permission. *Abbreviations*: Pves, intravesical pressure; VLPP, valsalva leak point pressure.

Bladder Volume and ALPP

ALPP testing has been correlated with bladder volume in the majority of clinical studies. Theofrastous et al. performed a study of 120 women with SUI who underwent VLPP testing at bladder volumes of 100 ml, 200 ml, 300 ml, and at maximum cystometric capacity (26). With a bladder volume of 100 ml and positioned sitting in the 45° upright position, 33 women leaked during VLPP testing with a volume of 100 ml compared to only 19 women leaking with a volume of 300 ml. In addition, the authors found that women who leaked with valsalva maneuvers at lower bladder volumes had worse measures of incontinence (# of incontinent episodes/week and # of pads/week) compared with women who leaked at higher volumes. Also, they found that the mean VLPP was higher at lower bladder volumes compared to VLPP at maximum cystometric capacity. The authors concluded that VLPP in women with SUI decreases significantly with bladder filling.

295

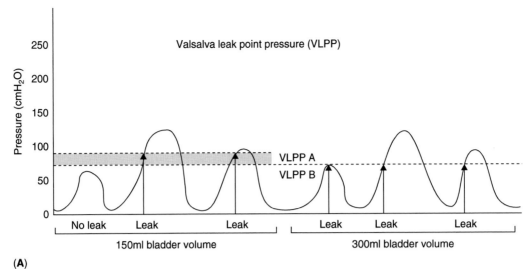

(A)

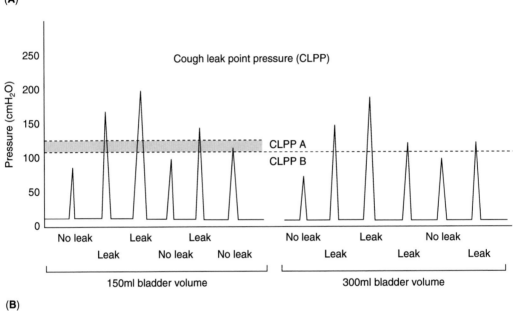

(B)

Figure 32.8 Effect of bladder volume on VLPP and CLPP *Source:* Reproduced from Ref. 73 with permission.

Faerber et al. also found that VLPP decreased significantly with increasing bladder volumes (27). Using VUDS, they found that a bladder volume of 250 to 300 cc allowed for the most appropriate classification of patients. Miklos et al. sought out to assess whether ALPP is affected by the method of provocation, the presence of an intravesical catheter, and bladder volume (28). With respect to bladder volume, they too noted a decrease in ALPP with increasing bladder volume (Fig. 32.8). With valsalva testing, the ALPP decreased by 19 cmH_2O as the bladder volume rose from 150 cc to >400 cc. With coughing, the ALPP decreased by 35 cmH_2O as the bladder volume rose from 150 cc to >400 cc. In contrast, Petrou et al. found no significant difference in VLPP at various bladder volumes (29). They concluded that the volume in the bladder does not alter the category of SUI or statistically change the VLPP determination.

Cough vs. Valsalva to Measure ALPP
Several authors have concluded that coughing and valsalva maneuvers result in different classifications of SUI. In their evaluation of 59 women with SUI, Peschers et al. found the

ALPP to be higher with coughing than with valsalva maneuvers (112.5 ± 46.9 cmH_2O versus 58.9 ± 27.6 cmH_2O, p < 0.0001) (30). In addition, the ALPP was negative in only two women with coughing compared to it being negative in 24 women with valsalva maneuvers. Defining ISD as an ALPP of <65 cmH_2O, the authors found ISD in 16.9% of the women using coughing to measure ALPP compared to 35.6% of the women using valsalva maneuvers to measure ALPP. Miklos et al. also found that cough LPP (CLPP) were higher than VLPP at all bladder capacities in those patients that demonstrated urine loss by both provocation methods (28). In their study of 60 women with genuine SUI, Bump et al. found CLPP to be significantly higher than VLPP, regardless of urodynamic catheter size (31). They postulated that the CLPP was higher because of reflex contraction of the pelvic floor.

Urodynamic Catheter Size and Location
Bump et al. also studied the effect of urodynamic catheter size on VLPP (31). Using an 8 Fr urodynamic catheter, they found the VLPP was 9.2 cmH_2O higher than when using a 3 Fr

urodynamic catheter, p = 0.01. In addition, the same authors found that LPPs were higher with transurethral catheters (regardless of size) compared to intravaginal catheters. Miklos et al. also noted a significant decrease in both CLPP and VLPP at all bladder capacities when removing the transurethral catheter and using only an intravaginal catheter (28).

Test-Retest Reliability

Bump et al. found the average pressure differences between the first and second VLPP to be clinically and statistically insignificant, regardless of urodynamic catheter size (31). The pressure difference between the two consecutive VLPPs was 2.2 cmH$_2$O using the 8 Fr urodynamic catheter and 1.5 cmH$_2$O using the 3 Fr urodynamic catheter. Nager et al. published reference urodynamic values for the 655 stress incontinence women that comprised the stress incontinence surgical treatment efficacy trial (SISTEr) (32). All filling cystometrograms were performed with subjects in the standing position. All vesical pressures were measured with a urodynamic catheter 8 Fr or smaller in size. Each of the 428 patients with measurable VLPPs had reproducible values. For 50% of the women, the VLPP intra-patient range was ≤15 cmH$_2$O. On average, there was only a 10 cmH$_2$O difference between the mean VLPP (117 cmH$_2$O) and the minimum VLPP (107 cmH$_2$O).

Factors Associated with ALPP

Fleischmann et al. studied the relationships between VLPP, urethral hypermobility, and incontinence severity in 65 women with SUI (33). A linear regression model showed no correlation of VLPP with urethral hypermobility in women with SUI. In addition, no significant difference in incontinence episodes or pad weight was seen in women with urethral hypermobility and a VLPP <60 cmH$_2$O and women with no urethral hypermobility and a VLPP <60 cmH$_2$O. Lemack et al. sought to determine which clinical and demographic factors were associated with the women undergoing either Burch colposuspension or autologous rectus fascial sling as part of the SISTEr trial (34). A multivariate analysis showed that older age, lower body mass index (BMI), smaller bladder capacity, higher maximum flow rate, and lower voiding pressures were all independently associated with lower VLPP. Each one year increase in age resulted in a decrease in VLPP of 0.77 cmH$_2$O. Each one-unit increase in BMI value resulted in an increase in VLPP of 0.66 cmH$_2$O. Urethral hypermobility, as assessed by Q-tip testing, did not achieve a significant association with VLPP when controlling for POP-Q stage. The authors concluded that Q-tip testing had no role in predicting VLPP in women with urethral hypermobility and SUI.

Effect of POP on ALPP

POP often artificially elevates VLPP because the prolapse provides a sink that dissipates the effect of the increased abdominal pressure on the urethra (25). As such, they recommended that VLPP testing be performed with and without prolapse reduction to identify if they are at risk for occult SUI. Romanzi et al. studied the effect of genital prolapse on voiding in 60 women (35). All of the women with grade 3 or 4 cystocele who had SUI (either symptomatic or occult) also had ALPP

<60 cmH$_2$O, which they defined as ISD. Gallentine et al. prospectively evaluated 24 patients with high-grade POP to determine the change in ALPP with reduction of the POP (19). The prolapse reduction was performed using gauze packing and a speculum blade. The mean decrease in ALPP was 59 cmH$_2$O after prolapse reduction. The decrease in ALPP with prolapse reduction was much greater in patients with vaginal vault prolapse than in patients with cystocele alone. Gilleran at el. evaluated the effect of cystocele reduction by a vaginal gauze pack on urodynamic studies (UDS) (36). Occult SUI was seen in 6% of women, and the mean VLPP of 54 cmH$_2$O in these women suggested ISD.

Relationship of ALPP to Incontinence Severity

Early studies reported significant correlation between VLPP and measures of incontinence severity. Nitti et al. evaluated 64 women with SUI using stress, emptying, anatomy, protection, and instability (SEAPI) grade (37). Using VUDS, the authors found that a VLPP of 90 cmH$_2$O or less did correlate highly with more severe symptoms of SUI. Also, Nager et al. demonstrated significant decreases in VLPP with increasing severity of incontinence as determined by stamey grade (p < 0.01) (38). However, they found no correlation between VLPP and pad weight or the 16-question quality of life (QOL) questionnaire from the 'Q' section of the SEAPI. More recently, Albo et al. sought to examine the relationship between severity measures of urinary incontinence in women undergoing either Burch colposuspension or autologous rectus fascial sling as part of the SISTEr trial (39). Weak to moderate correlations were observed between medical, epidemiological and social aspects of aging, incontinence episode frequency, pad weight, incontinence impact questionnaire , and urogenital distress inventory . However, VLPP correlated poorly with all incontinence severity measures. The authors concluded that VLPP is not associated with symptom severity, quantity of urine loss, or QOL impairment. They stated that VLPP neither reflects the bother from incontinence nor takes into account lifestyle activity.

Relationship of ALPP and Stress Continence Outcomes

Rodriguez et al. evaluated the role of prospective VLPP in predicting the outcome of distal urethral polypropylene sling (DUPS) surgery (40). They divided 174 patients into four groups based on VLPP: no leakage, VLPP >80 cmH$_2$O, VLPP 30 to 80 cmH$_2$O, and VLPP <30 cmH$_2$O. The groups were matched with respect to age, number of previous surgeries, and severity of SUI symptoms. When evaluating outcomes based on both daily pad use and patient driven questionnaires, all groups reported similar success 14 months after DUPS regardless of pre-operative VLPP. The authors concluded that VLPP is more likely a measure of incontinence severity than a test defining the mechanism of incontinence. Nager et al. sought out to determine the prognostic value of preoperative urodynamic results in women with SUI as part of the SISTEr trial (41). Women were eligible for the study if they had predominant SUI symptoms, a positive cough stress test, a bladder capacity >200 ml, and urethral hypermobility. The association of VLPP and success, controlling for the treatment group, was compared using the analysis of variance. Women who failed either Burch colposuspension or autologous rectus fascial sling did not have a lower mean VLPP compared to those that achieved success at the 24 month stress specific outcome assessment (Table 32.1). Note that overall treatment success required a negative pad test, no urinary incontinence on a three-day diary, a negative stress test, no self-reported SUI symptoms, and no re-treatment for SUI. The authors concluded that the level of VLPP did not predict the success of outcomes after either burch colposuspension or autologous rectus fascial sling procedures in women with pure or predominant SUI.

UPP

The urethral pressure (Pura) profile is commonly measured during normal bladder storage, and provides information regarding the functional status of the urethra. Most commonly, these measurements are obtained under non-voiding conditions with the urethra at rest, which is sometimes referred to as the resting Pura profile. However dynamic measurements may also be obtained during coughing (stress Pura profile) and voiding (micturitional Pura profile) to obtain functional information regarding the urethra during these conditions. Due to the multifactorial nature of this test, it is best to recognize the standardized terminology as it relates to the techniques of UPP being discussed, and the terminology that has been recommended by the ICS is listed in (Table 32.2) (42).

Technique of Pura Profile

The most commonly utilized methods of Pura measurements are derived from the techniques introduced by Brown and Wickham (43). This technique is the most commonly utilized to measure Pura. The basic principle of this technique is the measurement of pressure needed to perfuse a pressure-sensing catheter at a constant rate. Thus, this technique measures the occlusive pressure of the urethral walls by recording the fluid pressure required to "lift" the urethra off the catheter. The catheters are optimally less than 10 Fr in size and contain two-opposing side holes, which are some distance from the catheter tip. This requires a double or triple lumen catheter with separate bladder and Pura lumens that can simultaneously measure bladder and Pura. The urethral port of the catheter is connected to a pressure measuring transducer and a motorized syringe pump (usually via a "Y" connector). Constant perfusion at a rate of 2 to 5 ml/min is maintained. The catheter is then withdrawn at a rate of <5 mm/sec in order to achieve satisfactory measurements. This may be accomplished manually or more precisely by a mechanical "puller" device. (Fig. 32.9) Other catheter types can be utilized to measure Pura at rest. Microtransducer tip catheters may be employed. These catheters have the advantage of better resolution and accuracy when compared to perfusion catheters. However, these catheters are expensive, require sterilization and, most importantly, are prone to rotation artifacts within the urethra. The position of the transducer in the urethral lumen greatly affects the Pura measurements. Balloon catheters have also been utilized. These catheters consist of fluid filled balloons over the side holes, and the Pura represent the average pressure measured over the length of the entire balloon. This design leads to many

Table 32.1 VLPP does not Predict Success of Either Burch or Pubovaginal Sling

	Burch	Pubovaginal sling
Mean cmH$_2$O (SD)/No.	Overall outcome	
Success	115 (40)/57	117 (33)/71
Failure	115 (37)/104	121 (39)/105
Mean cmH$_2$O (SD)/No.	Stress specific outcome	
Success	116 (40)/80	117 (34)/109
Failure	114 (37)/87	125 (41)/72

Source: Reproduced from Ref. 41.
Abbreviations: VLPP, valsalva leak point pressure; SD, standard deviation.

Table 32.2 ICS Terminology for UPP Testing

Urethral pressure measurements
Urethral pressure: The fluid pressure needed to just open a closed urethra
Urethral pressure profile: A graph indicating the intraluminal pressure along the length of the urethra
Urethral closure pressure profile: The subtraction of intravesical pressure from urethral pressure
Maximum urethral pressure: The maximum pressure of the measured profile
Maximum urethral closure pressure: The maximum difference between the urethral pressure and the intravesical pressure
Functional profile length: The length of the urethra along which the urethral pressure exceeds intravesical pressure in women
Pressure transmission ratio: The increment in urethral pressure on stress as a percentage of the simultaneously recorded increment in intravesical pressure

Abbreviations: ICS, International Continence Society; UPP, urethral pressure profilometry.

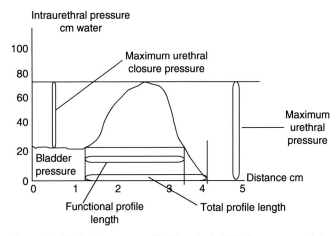

Figure 32.9 Urethral pressure profile: Note the individual parameters of the urethral pressure profile, and the relationship to intravesical pressure. *Source*: Reproduced from Ref. 82 with permission.

distortions in pressure measurement. When a catheter holding a transducer is within the urethra, it is reading the force generated by the walls of urethra, which are not equal in the 360° of the long axis. It has been found that pressures can range from the uppermost range to the lowest by changing the direction of the micro transducer from anterior to posterior. Catheter sizes between 8 and 12 French have been shown not to affect study parameters. This is not the case for bladder volume and patient position, as the pressure within the urethra goes up with increasing volume within the bladder, and a more upright stance. A comparison of air-charged and microtransducer catheters in the evaluation of urethral function showed high concordance for maximum urethral closure pressure (MUCP) and VLPP, but not for functional urethral length (44).

The resting Pura profile is usually performed supine. The bladder contains at least 50 ml, and the baseline bladder pressure is recorded. The catheter is then withdrawn at a constant rate (<5 mm/sec) and the catheter is perfused at 2 ml/min. Continuous Pura measurement occurs as the catheter is withdrawn, and these measurements should be made with the bladder at resting pressure (45). The resting Pura profile will produce a characteristic curve. In addition, the Pura measurements can be taken at a fixed site in the urethra by securing the catheter with the Pura sensors in the desired location. This is done fluoroscopically, or by using the measuring landmarks on the catheter. The stress urethral profile is performed in a similar manner. However, during the stress UPP the patient is asked to cough at regular intervals during catheter withdrawal. Alternatively, one may position the catheter at fixed sites along the urethra (0.5 cm intervals) while the patient coughs or performs a valsalva maneuver. This method of Pura measurement purportedly records the efficiency of pressure transmission into the proximal urethra.

The catheter withdrawal technique as described generates an infusion profile curve representative of the UPP (Fig. 32.10). The parameters obtained are defined by the ICS as: Pves, which is the pressure measurement within the bladder; maximum Pura, which is the highest pressure obtained during catheter withdrawal; UCPmax, which is the difference in pressure obtained when Pves is subtracted from Pura, which represents the pressure gradient from the urethra to the Pves; the functional urethral length is the urethral length where the intraurethral pressure exceeds the bladder pressure; and the total urethral length is the entire length of the urethra as measured using the withdrawal technique. Thus urethral length has two aspects, an anatomical one where it is the complete length of the urethra, and the functional length, which is distance of the urethra where Pura exceeds the pressure found within the bladder (46).

Interpretation of Pura Profile

In most continent women, the functional urethral length is approximately 3 cm and the MUCP is 40 to 60 cmH_2O, but there exists considerable variability between studies (47). It has been suggested that UPP can be helpful in women undergoing stress incontinence surgery. Through the early works of McGuire and Sand, patients with UCPs <20 cm water were noted to have higher failure rates of their incontinence repairs (48,49). These findings have been supported by other studies showing that a low MUCP is a predictor of poor outcomes for retropubic suspension surgery (50,51). These findings have prompted many surgeons to utilize sling procedures as the anti-incontinence procedure of choice for patients with low UCP (52,53). This change in practice must be taken in the context of a strong trend toward sling procedures [particulary midurethral slings (MUS)] for all cases of stress incontinence, with or without low Pura, which makes the UPP increasingly irrelevant to the choice of surgical procedure (54). Weber demonstrated the inherent problems in utilizing UPP measurements in the diagnosis and management of SUI. In this very detailed meta-analysis, she pointed out the significant variability within the reported values of Pura measurements (55). Differences in pressure measurements were seen with different types of catheters, varying positions of the catheter within the urethra, patient position, bladder volume, and the

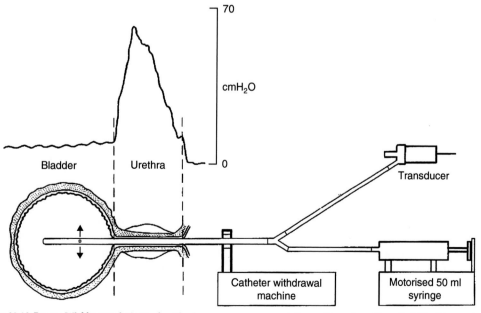

Figure 32.10 Brown-Wickham technique of urethral pressure measurement. *Source*: Reproduced from Ref. 83 with permission.

presence of POP. In addition, detrusor overactivity can affect urethral function resulting in decreases in functional urethral length and pressure transmission ratio with bladder filling (56). Although the investigator can control technical factors, there are still substantial differences in inter-operator and per patient reproducibility. These factors account for widespread differences in reported values across urodynamics laboratories. As one examines the reported values of Pura among investigators, there is considerable variability between investigators with the MUCP varying from 36 to 101 in nonstress incontinent patients. In addition, there are large standard deviations of reported data, suggesting significant variability within the reported values (55). Despite these differences, however, there is a trend among studies that the UCPs are lower in stress incontinent women. However, in many of these studies, the differences are not significantly different statistically and the overlap is so great that it is impossible to select a cut-off value that discriminates continent from incontinent patients (55).

If the urethra and the bladder were thought of as a continuous system free of the muscular activity that surrounds it, then the pressure transmission ratio (PTR) can be thought of as the sequential increase in Pura during a concurrent increase in bladder pressure (47). This proportion can exist at a solitary point, or several can be determined at distinct points to produce a pressure transmission profile. Although it has been reported that stress incontinent women with urethral hypermobility generally have lower PTRs than stress continent women (57), other studies have questioned its validity and the value of this test has been called into question (58). The PTR also cannot discriminate between stress incontinent patients and controls (59). As a result of such divergent data the ICS has stated the clinical utility of Pura measurement is unclear (60). Given the fact that UPP deals with urethra in a nonphysiologic state of rest, it provides little information regarding incontinence as a result of anatomic derangement. Furthermore, no single parameter of the UPP is useful in diagnosing stress incontinence (61). These reports have prompted the International Consultation on Incontinence Committee on Dynamic testing to make the following recommendations regarding UPP (62): First, investigators and clinicians should recognize the poor sensitivity and specificity of Pura measurements and their normal test-retest variation. In addition, the committee does not recommend Pura measurements as the only urodynamic test of incontinence. If performed, these measurements should be judged in relationship to other elements of the examination.

In conclusion the clinical role of Pura and the UCP is questionable as there is no Pura measurement that can discriminate urethral incompetence from other disorders, provide a measure of the severity of the condition, or provide a reliable indicator of surgical success after intervention (60). Although attempts have been made to correlate a low MUCP with the presence of stress incontinence and with the presence of ISD (MUCP <20 cmH_2O), the test proves to lack both sensitivity and specificity, and there are many continent women with low MUCPs and vice versa (63).

RETROGRADE PURA PROFILE

The urethral retro-resistance pressure (URP) was first described by Slack et al. in the literature in 2004 (64). The URP is obtained using the Gynecare MoniTorr (ETHICON, Inc., Somerville, NJ), and it is defined as the pressure required to achieve and maintain an open sphincter. The URP measurement is obtained by placing a cone-shaped plug 5 mm into the external urethral meatus to create a seal. The device infuses fluid at a rate of 1 ml/sec, and the device then displays the URP as the pressure at which the graph plateaus. Because the device does not involve placing a catheter per urethra, the authors state that URP provides a more physiologic testing condition.

URP values were defined in a multicenter trial of women with and without symptoms of SUI (65). The mean URP of asymptomatic women was 112.6 ± 39.2 cmH_2O. This was significantly different from the mean URP of 69.9 cmH_2O in symptomatic women (p < 0.0001). Good test-retest correlation was seen within the same subjects. In a separate study of 258 patients, the same authors compared URP to urodynamic measures (MUCP and VLPP) and to incontinence severity (24-hour pad test, I-QOL, and urinary incontinence severity score) (64). The correlations between URP and both MUCP and LPP were weak. In contrast, URP had a consistent relationship with incontinence severity. Specifically, the URP decreased with increasing incontinence severity. Unfortunately, the authors made no mention of technical difficulties during the study (fluid leaking around the plug or the pressure required to keep the plug in place), nor did they address how these difficulties could influence the URP measurement.

A recent non-industry study evaluated the role of preoperative URP in predicting incontinence severity (24-hour pad test, I-QOL, King's health questionnaire, and three-day voiding diary) (66). In addition, the change in URP after MUS was also examined. A total of 100 women were examined and randomized to either TVT (n = 54) or TVT-O (n = 46). These patients were evaluated prior to and three months after MUS. The mean preoperative URP bore no relationship to the severity of urine loss assessed by 24-hour pad test. Also, there was no correlation between URP and the other measures of incontinence severity. In addition, preoperative and postoperative URP values were not significantly different (62.7 ± 19.4 cmH_2O versus 61.2 ± 20.4 cmH_2O, p = 0.57). The authors concluded that URP is not a useful measure of urethral function. Thus, it seems clear that the full clinical utility of URP remains to be defined.

EMG

Electric activity produced within a cell is a result of the interaction of various ions of opposing charge separated by a lipoprotein bilayer. Unequal distributions of ions on either side of the bilayer cause a gradient that leads to a difference in electric potential across the membrane. Before moving forward in the discussion of neurophysiology one must consider the model of the motor unit comprised of an anterior horn cell, its axon, and terminal branches (all of which make up the motor neuron), the neuromuscular junction, and all the individual muscle fibers it innervates. The size of the motor unit, that is the number of muscle fibers innervated by a single anterior horn cell, varies with each muscle. In general, muscles exhibiting fine motor control have low innervation ratios (e.g., 10 to 20:1 in the extraocular muscles), whereas big, bulk-supporting muscles have high innervation ratios (e.g., 1500 to 2000:1 in the gastrocnemius muscle) (67). When an anterior horn cell is activated all muscle fibers belonging to that motor unit are depolarized, the electrical activity from these muscle fibers summate to generate a motor unit action potential (MUAP) (68) that is first detected by an electrode that's placed close to the origin of the signal. Such activity produces a characteristic triphasic wave with distinct components. There is a positive (downward) deflection as the electrical impulse moves along the muscle fiber membrane towards the extracellular recording electrode, which is then followed by a negative (upward) deflection when the impulse reaches the electrode, and finally another positive (downward) deflection as the impulse moves away from the electrode. (Fig. 32.11) Potentials are detected by electrodes, which make them integral to the technique of EMG. There are numerous types of electrodes but can be broken down into two distinct groups; surface and needle electrodes. All of them have their positive attributes as well as negative characteristics.

Skin patch electrodes are usually self-adhesive and have the benefit of being essentially non-invasive, with a patch being placed on the perineum. However, some contend that

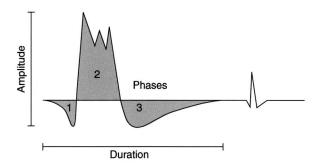

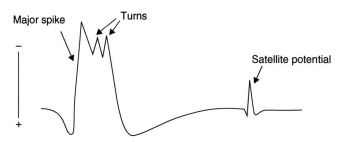

Figure 32.11 Duration is measured as the time from the initial deflection of the MUAP from baseline to its final return to baseline. It is the parameter that best reflects the number of muscle fibers in the motor unit. Amplitude reflects only muscle fibers very close to the needle and is measured peak to peak. Phases (shaded areas) can be determined by counting the number of baseline crossings and adding 1. MUAPs are generally triphasic. Serrations (also called turns) are changes in direction of the potential that do not cross the baseline. The major spike is the largest positive-to-negative deflection, usually occurring after the first positive peak. Satellite, or linked, potentials occur after the main potential and usually represent early reinnervation of muscle fibers. *Source:* Reproduced from Ref. 84 with permission.

the signal source may be inferior (69). In preparation for a study using such electrodes it should be noted that the skin should be shaved and prepared with alcohol to reduce surface resistance and the electrode placed directly on the skin overlying the muscle of interest (70). With surface electrodes, EMG pattern recordings depict the net electrical activity occurring in the muscle. Surface electrodes therefore demonstrate an electronically generated summation of muscular electrical activity but are incapable of distinguishing individual motor unit potentials. This can be seen in the area of the striated urethral sphincter and levator ani, which are located in close proximity, but anatomically and neurologically discontinuous (71). Thus, such perineal surface measurements may not reflect the true unilateral striated sphincter activity, but rather compounding of motor unit signals from all the muscles of the pelvic floor. A recent study evaluating patch versus needle electrodes during pressure flow studies found that needle electrode EMG was more often interpretable and showed motor unit quiescence of the external sphincter more often, suggesting that the signal obtained from the pelvic floor musculature in the region may mass the actual signal obtained from the external sphincter (72). These surface adhesive patch electrodes as stated can be compared to the information that is provided by various needle electrode types. Needle electrodes are able to isolate electrical activity from specific muscle fibers within a .5 mm radius of the tip (72). Such accurate information of course does come with a drawback of being much more invasive and restrictive to patients. Such needle electrodes can be either monopolar, concentric or single fiber in type varying in dimensions and the type of metal that is used.

Monopolar electrodes are thin needles coated with an insulating material that do have an exposed tip. A reference electrode such as a surface stick or subcutaneous needle attached to the skin near the muscle being examined is needed. Concentric electrodes have a hollow cannula which serves as the reference electrode. Extending down the shaft to the tip is an insulated fine wire with a beveled tip, which is the active electrode. The advantage of these concentric electrodes is its more predictable surface area, which produces more reliable measurements of MUAPs (73).

To obtain representative EMG studies of the perineal floor, electrodes may be placed into the bulbocavernosus muscle through the perineum in men, and the superficial anal sphincter in women. In women the superficial anal sphincter is obtained with an electrode placed through the perineum at the twelve o'clock position. This is advanced just under the skin at the mucocutaneous junction to obtain EMG signal (74). To obtain activity of the external urethral sphincter in women using these types of electrodes a needle is placed lateral to the urethral meatus and advanced parallel to the urethra a distance of about 1 to 2 cm. This of course may be difficult and painful for women, and meticulous attention to detail is required. The technical acuity of precise needle placement is quite important in order to accurately record the activity within the true urethral sphincteric complex. If localized properly, "noise" from the adjacent pelvic floor can

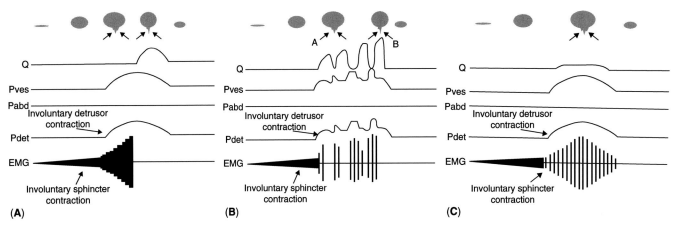

Figure 32.12 Three types of DESD (**A**) Type 1 DESD—sphincter relaxes at peak of detrusor contraction. (**B**) Type 2 DESD—sporadic sphincter contractions throughout detrusor contraction (**C**) Type 3 DESD—crescendo-decrescendo pattern of sphincter contraction. *Source*: Reproduced from Ref. 85 with permission. *Abbreviations*: DESD, detrusor external sphincter dyssnergia; EMG, electromyography; Pves, intravesical pressure; Pabd, abdominal pressure; Pdet, detrusor pressure.

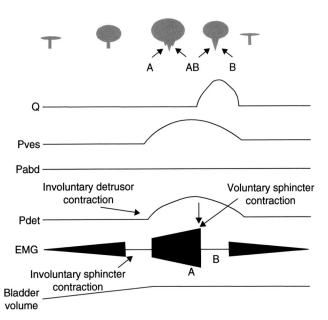

Figure 32.13 Acquired voiding dysfunction (AVD). An involuntary detrusor contraction is heralded by complete relaxation of the sphincter EMG. As the patient senses the detrusor contraction, she contracts her sphincter (increased EMG activity) in an attempt to prevent incontinence (arrows A). Once the sphincter fatigues, the urethra opens and incontinence ensues (arrows B). *Source*: Reproduced from Ref. 85 with permission. *Abbreviations*: EMG, electromyography; Pves, intravesical pressure; Pabd, abdominal pressure; Pdet, detrusor pressure.

be eliminated resulting in a true measurement of isolated sphincter function.

Normal EMG findings imply a lack of neurologic basis for a patients voiding dysfunction; whereas an abnormal EMG study indicates a need for further work-up. Findings must be taken in relation to the subject's concurrent action. In patients free of pathology, the EMG activity is low at rest, and it increases in amplitude and frequency with increases in pressure of the abdomen, such as with coughing and laughing, and with bladder filling (69).

Due to the complex neurophysiological process of micturition there exists a coordinated effort between the urethral sphincter mechanism and bladder. During voiding, the urethra should be relaxed so as to permit the passage of urine. Focused EMG studies utilizing surface or needle electrodes can be carried out on the distal sphincter of the urethra. During a void the urethra should be in a relaxed state, which would correspond to silence on the EMG, whereas during filling a increase in electrical activity should be observed (75). The goal of EMG during a urodynamic study is to determine whether the external urethral sphincter complex is coordinated or uncoordinated with the bladder during voiding (76). During the study the absence of urethral relaxation during a void may signify an abnormality in urethral function. Such an abnormality in the context of a known neurologic condition in the presence of detrusor overactivity is termed DESD (77). Constant urethral tension during voluntary micturition in the presence of no known neurologic pathology is known as dysfunctional voiding, and it may represent a learned behavior (16).

EMG: Clinical Interpretation

Urethral sphincter EMG is used to make the diagnosis of DESD, and it is used to distinguish the three types of DESD (Fig. 32.12) (81). In type one DESD there is a sudden and complete relaxation of the striated sphincter at the peak of the detrusor contraction, and unobstructed voiding occurs. Type two DESD is characterized by sporadic involuntary contractions of the striated sphincter throughout the detrusor contraction. Voiding occurs in bursts during sphincter relaxation. With type three DESD there is a crescendo-decrescendo pattern of sphincter contraction which results in urethral obstruction throughout the entire detrusor contraction. In all three types of DESD, the involuntary sphincter contraction precedes the involuntary detrusor contraction. In contrast, with AVD the sphincter EMG activity diminishes just prior to the detrusor contraction, then sporadically increases as the patient contracts and relaxes the striated sphincter (Fig. 32.13) (81).

Fowler syndrome was first described in 1985 in young women with urinary retention (78). The sphincter EMG signal in these women contains repetitive discharges and decelerating bursts. This impairs sphincter relaxation and leads to obstructed voiding and either incomplete or complete retention. The development of the sphincter abnormality may be under the influence of estrogens, as suggested by the high association of polycystic ovaries in these women (79). Sacral neuromodulation has a rapid effect in restoring voiding function in these women, suggesting that it works by reversing the inhibitory effect of the sphincter contraction. The abnormalities of sphincter function (abnormal EMG activity and high MUCP) are not reversed with neuromodulation (80).

REFERENCES

1. Gosling J. The structure of the bladder and urethra in relation to function. Urol Clin North Am 1979; 6: 31–8.
2. DeLancey JO. Correlative study of paraurethral anatomy. Obstet Gynecol 1986; 68: 91–7.
3. Oelrich TM. The striated urogenital sphincter muscle in the female. Anat Rec 1983; 205: 223–32.
4. DeLancey JO. Structural aspects of the extrinsic continence mechanism. Obstet Gynecol 1988; 72(3 Pt 1): 296–301.
5. DeLancey JO. Anatomy of the female bladder and urethra. In: Ostergaard DR, Bent AE, eds. Urogynecology and Urodynamics. Baltimore, MD: Williams Wilkins 1991: 3–18.
6. Petros PE, Ulmsten UI. An integral theory and its method for the diagnosis and management of female urinary incontinence. Scand J Urol Nephrol Suppl 1993; 27(Suppl 153): 1–93.
7. Thorp JM, Jones LH, Wells E, Ananth CV. Assessment of pelvic floor function: a series of simple tests in nulliparous women. Int Urogynecol J Pelvic Floor Dysfunct 1996; 7: 94–7.
8. Crystle CD, Charme LS, Copeland WE. Q-tip test in stress urinary incontinence. Obstet Gynecol 1971 38: 313–5.
9. Fantl JA, Hurt WG, Bump RC, Dunn LJ, Choi SC. Urethral axis and sphincteric function. Am J Obstet Gynecol 1986; 155: 554–8.
10. Quinn MJ, Beynon J, Mortensen NJ, Smith PJ. Transvaginal endosonography: a new method to study the anatomy of the lower urinary tract in urinary stress incontinence. Br J Urol 1988; 62: 414–8.
11. Kohorn EI, Scioscia AL, Jeanty P, Hobbins JC. Ultrasound cystourethrography by perineal scanning for the assessment of female stress urinary incontinence. Obstet Gynecol 1986; 68: 269–72.
12. Schaer GN, Koechli OR, Schuessler B, Haller U. Perineal ultrasound for evaluating the bladder neck in urinary stress incontinence. Obstet Gynecol 1995; 85: 220–4.
13. Blaivas JG, Sinha HP, Zayed AA, Labib KB. Detrusor-external sphincter dyssynergia. J Urol 1981; 125: 542–4.
14. Groutz A, Blaivas JG, Pies C, Sassone AM. Learned voiding dysfunction (non-neurogenic, neurogenic bladder) among adults. Neurourol Urodyn 2001; 20: 259–68.
15. McGuire EJ, Savastano JA. Urodynamic studies in enuresis and the nonneurogenic neurogenic bladder. J Urol 1984; 132: 299–302.
16. Carlson KV, Rome S, Nitti VW. Dysfunctional voiding in women. J Urol 2001; 165: 143–7; discussion 147–8.
17. Blaivas JG, Groutz A. Bladder outlet obstruction nomogram for women with lower urinary tract symptomatology. Neurourol Urodyn 2000; 19: 553–64.
18. Nitti VW, Tu LM, Gitlin J. Diagnosing bladder outlet obstruction in women. J Urol 1999; 161: 1535–40.
19. Gallentine ML, Cespedes RD. Occult stress urinary incontinence and the effect of vaginal vault prolapse on abdominal leak point pressures. Urology 2001; 57: 40–4.
20. Flisser AJ, Blaivas JG. Evaluating incontinence in women. Urol Clin North Am 2002; 29: 515–26.
21. Groutz A, Blaivas JG, Chaikin DC. Bladder outlet obstruction in women: definition and characteristics. Neurourol Urodyn 2000; 19: 213–20.
22. Klutke C, Siegel S, Carlin B, et al. Urinary retention after tension-free vaginal tape procedure: incidence and treatment. Urology 2001; 58: 697–701.
23. Abrams P, Cardozo L, Fall M, et al. The standardisation of terminology of lower urinary tract function: report from the Standardisation Sub-committee of the International Continence Society. Neurourol Urodyn 2002; 21: 167–78.
24. McGuire EJ, Fitzpatrick CC, Wan J, et al. Clinical assessment of urethral sphincter function. J Urol 1993; 150(5 Pt 1): 1452–4.
25. McGuire EJ, Cespedes RD, O'Connell HE. Leak-point pressures. Urol Clin North Am 1996; 23: 253–62.
26. Theofrastous JP, Cundiff GW, Harris RL, Bump RC. The effect of vesical volume on valsalva leak-point pressures in women with genuine stress urinary incontinence. Obstet Gynecol 1996; 87(5 Pt 1): 711–4.
27. Faerber GJ, Vashi AR. Variations in valsalva leak point pressure with increasing vesical volume. J Urol 1998; 159: 1909–11.
28. Miklos JR, Sze EH, Karram MM. A critical appraisal of the methods of measuring leak-point pressures in women with stress incontinence. Obstet Gynecol 1995; 86: 349–52.
29. Petrou SP, Kollmorgen TA. Valsalva leak point pressure and bladder volume. Neurourol Urodyn 1998; 17: 3–7.
30. Peschers UM, Jundt K, Dimpfl T. Differences between cough and valsalva leak-point pressure in stress incontinent women. Neurourol Urodyn 2000; 19: 677–81.
31. Bump RC, Elser DM, Theofrastous JP, McClish DK. Valsalva leak point pressures in women with genuine stress incontinence: reproducibility, effect of catheter caliber, and correlations with other measures of urethral resistance. Continence Program For Women Research Group. Am J Obstet Gynecol 1995; 173: 551–7.
32. Nager CW, Albo ME, Fitzgerald MP, et al. Reference urodynamic values for stress incontinent women. Neurourol Urodyn 2007; 26: 333–40.
33. Fleischmann N, Flisser AJ, Blaivas JG, Panagopoulos G. Sphincteric urinary incontinence: relationship of vesical leak point pressure, urethral mobility and severity of incontinence. J Urol 2003; 169: 999–1002.
34. Lemack GE, Xu Y, Brubaker L, et al. Clinical and demographic factors associated with valsalva leak point pressure among women undergoing burch bladder neck suspension or autologous rectus fascial sling procedures. Neurourol Urodyn 2007; 26: 392–6.
35. Romanzi LJ, Chaikin DC, Blaivas JG. The effect of genital prolapse on voiding. J Urol 1999; 161: 581–6.
36. Gilleran JP, Lemack GE, Zimmern PE. Reduction of moderate-to-large cystocele during urodynamic evaluation using a vaginal gauze pack: 8-year experience. BJU Int 2006; 97: 292–5.
37. Nitti VW, Combs AJ. Correlation of valsalva leak point pressure with subjective degree of stress urinary incontinence in women. J Urol 1996; 155: 281–5.
38. Nager CW, Schulz JA, Stanton SL, Monga A. Correlation of urethral closure pressure, leak-point pressure and incontinence severity measures. Int Urogynecol J Pelvic Floor Dysfunct 2001; 12: 395–400.
39. Albo M, Wruck L, Baker J, et al. The relationships among measures of incontinence severity in women undergoing surgery for stress urinary incontinence. J Urol 2007; 177: 1810–4.
40. Rodriguez LV, de Almeida F, Dorey F, Raz S. Does valsalva leak point pressure predict outcome after the distal urethral polypropylene sling? Role of urodynamics in the sling era. J Urol 2004; 172: 210–4.
41. Nager CW, FitzGerald M, Kraus SR, et al. Urodynamic measures do not predict stress continence outcomes after surgery for stress urinary incontinence in selected women. J Urol 2008; 179: 1470–4.
42. Abrams P, Cardozo L, Fall M, et al. The standardisation of terminology in lower urinary tract function: report from the Standardisation Sub-committee of the International Continence Society. Urology 2003; 61: 37–49.
43. Brown M, Wickham JE. The urethral pressure profile. Br J Urol 1969; 41: 211–7.
44. Pollak JT, Neimark M, Connor JT, Davila GW. Air-charged and microtransducer urodynamic catheters in the evaluation of urethral function. Int Urogynecol J Pelvic Floor Dysfunct 2004; 15: 124–8; discussion 128.
45. Hilton P, Stanton SL. A clinical and urodynamic assessment of the burch colposuspension for genuine stress incontinence. Br J Obstet Gynaecol 1983; 90: 934–9.
46. Robinson DNP. Diagnosis and management of urinary incontinence. In: Stovall TG, Mann WJ, eds. Gynecologic Surgery. New York, NY: Churchill Livingstone 1996: 704.
47. Steele GS SM, Yalla SV. Urethral pressure profilometry: Vesicourethral pressure measurements under resting and voiding conditions. In: Nitti VW, eds. Practical Urodynamcs. Philadelphia, PA: Saunders 1998: 108–30.

48. McGuire EJ. Urodynamic findings in patients after failure of stress incontinence operations. Prog Clin Biol Res 1981; 78: 351–60.

49. Sand PK, Bowen LW, Panganiban R, Ostergard DR. The low pressure urethra as a factor in failed retropubic urethropexy. Obstet Gynecol 1987; 69(3 Pt 1): 399–402.

50. Koonings PP, Bergman A, Ballard CA. Low urethral pressure and stress urinary incontinence in women: risk factor for failed retropubic surgical procedure. Urology 1990; 36: 245–8.

51. Bowen LW, Sand PK, Ostergard DR, Franti CE. Unsuccessful Burch retropubic urethropexy: a case-controlled urodynamic study. Am J Obstet Gynecol 1989; 160: 452–8.

52. Horbach NS, Blanco JS, Ostergard DR, Bent AE, Cornella JL. A suburethral sling procedure with polytetrafluoroethylene for the treatment of genuine stress incontinence in patients with low urethral closure pressure. Obstet Gynecol 1988; 71: 648–52.

53. Rezapour M, Falconer C, Ulmsten U. Tension-free vaginal tape (TVT) in stress incontinent women with intrinsic sphincter deficiency (ISD)–a long-term follow-up. Int Urogynecol J Pelvic Floor Dysfunct 2001; 12(Suppl 2): S12–4.

54. Appell RA. Primary slings for everyone with genuine stress incontinence? The argument for. Int Urogynecol J Pelvic Floor Dysfunct 1998; 9: 249–51.

55. Weber AM. Is urethral pressure profilometry a useful diagnostic test for stress urinary incontinence? Obstet Gynecol Surv 2001; 56: 720–35.

56. Chaliha C, Digesu GA, Hutchings A, Khullar V. Changes in urethral function with bladder filling in the presence of urodynamic stress incontinence and detrusor overactivity. Am J Obstet Gynecol 2005; 192: 60–5.

57. Bump RC, Copeland WE, Jr., Hurt WG, Fantl JA. Dynamic urethral pressure/profilometry pressure transmission ratio determinations in stress-incontinent and stress-continent subjects. Am J Obstet Gynecol 1988; 159: 749–55.

58. Richardson DA. Value of the cough pressure profile in the evaluation of patients with stress incontinence. Am J Obstet Gynecol 1986; 155: 808–11.

59. Rosenzweig BA, Bhatia NN, Nelson AL. Dynamic urethral pressure profilometry pressure transmission ratio: what do the numbers really mean? Obstet Gynecol 1991; 77: 586–90.

60. Lose G, Griffiths D, Hosker G, et al. Standardisation of urethral pressure measurement: report from the Standardisation Sub-committee of the International Continence Society. Neurourol Urodyn 2002; 21: 258–60.

61. Versi E. Discriminant analysis of urethral pressure profilometry data for the diagnosis of genuine stress incontinence. Br J Obstet Gynaecol 1990; 97: 251–9.

62. Hosker G RP, Gajewski J, et al. 4th international consultation on incontinence committee on dynamic testing. In: Abrams P, Cardozo L, Khoury S, Wein A, eds. Incontinence. 2009: Paris, France: Health Publication Ltd 413–522.

63. McGuire EJ. Diagnosis and treatment of intrinsic sphincter deficiency. Int J Urol 1995; 2(Suppl 1): 7–10; discussion 16–18.

64. Slack M, Culligan P, Tracey M, et al. Relationship of urethral retro-resistance pressure to urodynamic measurements and incontinence severity. Neurourol Urodyn 2004; 23: 109–14.

65. Slack M, Tracey M, Hunsicker K, et al. Urethral retro-resistance pressure: a new clinical measure of urethral function. Neurourol Urodyn 2004; 23: 656–61.

66. Roderick T, Paul M, Christopher M, Douglas T. Urethral retro-resistance pressure: association with established measures of incontinence severity and change after midurethral tape insertion. Neurourol Urodyn 2009; 28: 86–9.

67. Feinstein B, Lindegard B, Nyman E, Wohlfart G. Morphologic studies of motor units in normal human muscles. Acta Anat (Basel) 1955; 23: 127–42.

68. Dumitru D. Physiologic basis of potentials recorded in electromyography. Muscle Nerve 2000; 23: 1667–85.

69. O'Donnell P. Electromyography. In: Nitti VW, eds. Practical Urodynamics. Philadelphia, PA: WB Saunders 1998: 65–71.

70. Barrett DM. Disposable (infant) surface electrocardiogram electrodes in urodynamics: a simultaneous comparative study of electrodes. J Urol 1980; 124: 663–5.

71. Brostrom S, Jennum P, Lose G. Motor evoked potentials from the striated urethral sphincter and puborectal muscle: normative values. Neurourol Urodyn 2003; 22: 306–13.

72. Mahajan ST, Fitzgerald MP, Kenton K, Shott S, Brubaker L. Concentric needle electrodes are superior to perineal surface-patch electrodes for electromyographic documentation of urethral sphincter relaxation during voiding. BJU Int 2006; 97: 117–20.

73. Benson J. Electrophysiologic testing. In: Walters M, Karram M, eds. Urogynecology and Reconstructive Pelvic Surgery, 2nd edn. St. Louis, MO: CV Mosby 1999: 100.

74. Siroky MB. Electromyography of the perineal floor. Urol Clin North Am 1996; 23: 299–307.

75. Rovner E, Wein AJ. Practical Urodynamics. AUA Update Series. 2002: 21(19–20).

76. Peterson A, Webster G: The neurourologic evaluation. In: Walsh PC, Retik AB, Vaughan Ed, et al., eds. Campbell's Urology, 8th edn. Philadelphia, PA: WB Saunders Company 2002: 905–28.

77. Kelly C, Nitti VW. Evaluation of neurogenic bladder dysfunction: basic urodynamics. In: Corcos J, Schick E, eds. Textbook of the Neurogenic Bladder. Abington, Oxfordshire, UK: Taylor and Francis Group 2004: 415–23.

78. Fowler CJ, Kirby RS. Abnormal electromyographic activity (decelerating burst and complex repetitive discharges) in the striated muscle of the urethral sphincter in 5 women with persisting urinary retention. Br J Urol 1985; 57: 67–70.

79. Fowler CJ, Christmas TJ, Chapple CR, et al. Abnormal electromyographic activity of the urethral sphincter, voiding dysfunction, and polycystic ovaries: a new syndrome? BMJ 1988; 297: 1436–8.

80. DasGupta R, Fowler CJ. Urodynamic study of women in urinary retention treated with sacral neuromodulation. J Urol 2004; 171: 1161–4.

81. Blaivas Jerry, Chancellor Michael, Weiss Jeffrey, Verhaaren Michael, eds. Atlas of Urodynamics, 2nd edn. United Kingdom: Blackwell Publishing, Oxford, 2007: 81, 127, 148, 150, and 151.

82. Winters JC, Appell RA. Practical urodynamics. In: O'Donnell PD, eds. Urinary Incontinence. New York, NY: Mosby Year Book. 1997: 181–9.

83. Abrams P, eds. Urodynamics, 3rd edn. London: Springer-Verlag, 2006: 98–110.

84. Preston DC, Shapiro BE. Electromyography and Neuromuscular Disorders. Boston: Butterworth-Heinemann, 1998: 541–60.

33 Clinical Neurophysiologic Testing
David B Vodušek and Clare J Fowler

INTRODUCTION

Recordings of bioelectrical activity from muscles and the nervous system have been found clinically useful and named "clinical neurophysiologic tests." (Sometimes tests of nervous function other than electrophysiologic are listed as "neurophysiologic," but these other tests will not be described in this chapter.)

Clinical neurophysiologic tests are many and are grouped together into subcategories according to different criteria. It is practical to distinguish recordings from muscle [electromyography (EMG)] and tests of nerve and nervous pathways function (conduction studies). Typically, the different tests are referred to with disconcerting capital letter abbreviations, and even professionals close to the field have some difficulty in understanding the terminology, complex physiological, and technical background of the methods, and distinguishing the different types of information provided by different tests. This chapter aims at clarifying these issues.

Recording Electrical Muscle Activity—EMG

EMG is the extracellular recording of bioelectrical activity generated by muscle fibers. Modern EMG started with the introduction of the concentric needle electrode (CNE) in 1929 (1), the design of which has endured ever since, almost unchanged (Fig. 33.1) (2). Clinical EMG studies of the pelvic floor were sparse till the 1970s (3); since then EMG has been used increasingly in urogynecology, neurourology, and proctology research. Nowadays it is used as a routine diagnostic investigation.

EMG may be performed for two quite distinct although complementary purposes. On the one hand, it can reveal the "behavior" (i.e., patterns of activity) of a particular muscle; on the other, it can be used to demonstrate whether a muscle is normal, myopathic, or denervated/reinnervated. The former can be called "kinesiologic EMG" and the latter "motor unit (MU)" EMG, but usually this division is not specified and both types of examination are just called "EMG," which can confuse the uninitiated. There are of course anatomical, physiological, and practical specificities of pelvic floor and perineal EMG, but the techniques are intrinsically same for all striated muscles.

Testing Conduction of Nerves and Nervous Pathways

Conduction studies examine the capacity of a nerve (or nervous pathway) to transmit along its length a test volley of depolarization elicited by a stimulus. Tests have been as a rule introduced for limb nerves (and their central connections), and only later modified by workers in pelvic (uro-) neurophysiology (4).

Conduction along a nerve (or central nervous system pathway) depends on anatomic integrity of the structure. In finer detail, the velocity of conduction depends on thickness of constituent axons and their myelin sheath. All these may be altered by pathology, and reflected as changes in either latency of the recorded response (or velocity of conduction), or the amplitude (and configuration). It needs to be appreciated that "pure" conduction via nervous pathways is only measured where there is no synapse between the stimulated and the recorded site (such as for instance in stimulating a nerve and recording from the same nerve). The "conduction" across several synapses (as for instance in recording a reflex response) is not only "longer" because of synapses, but variable (dependent on various additional factors, not only anatomical integrity and myelination).

Testing a nerve with a motor function, its responsiveness can be measured by electrical stimulation of the nerve and recording the elicited muscle response (Fig. 33.2). Both the time taken to muscle activation (latency) as well as the amplitude of the muscle response [known as the *compound muscle action potential* or *"M" response* (5)] can be measured. The latter depends on the number of intact individual motor fibers, whereas measures of *motor latency* (i.e., time to onset of response) and *motor conduction velocity* reflect the conduction speed of the fastest nerve fibers. For this reason, measures of latency are a poor guide to integrity of innervation. The amplitude of the evoked muscle response gives a better guide, but because this measurement depends so heavily on the configuration of the electrodes employed, amplitude is not as valuable as might have been expected on a theoretical basis. Ideally, to measure compound muscle action potential amplitude, the reference electrode should be placed over the tendon and the active recording reference over the motor end plate (i.e., point of entry of nerve into muscle). For a strap-shaped muscle this can be identified as midway along its anatomic length, but in more anatomically complex muscles such as exist in the pelvis, the motor end plate region has not been identified and recording well-formed compound muscle action potentials is difficult.

The nerve roots carrying nerve fibers for particular muscles can be stimulated over the spinal column, thus testing the conduction over the whole length of the peripheral motor axons. Stimulation of the motor cortex area for particular muscle groups can be achieved from the scalp, thus testing the whole motor pathway (both central and peripheral). The muscle responses obtained by such stimulation are called "motor evoked potentials (MEPs)."

If the peripheral nerve being tested is accessible over sufficient length so that stimulating and recording electrodes can be placed at some distance from each other (at least 10 cm is recommended to lessen stimulus artifact), it may be possible to record nerve activity directly. This response is called a

Needle recording electrode	Needle tip and recording surface	Pick-up	Needle diameter	Filter settings	Activity recorded
Concentric needle electrode: central insulated platinum wire inside a steel cannula	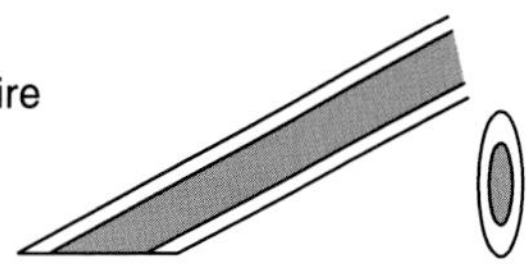	Hemisphere radius 0.5 mm	0.3–0.65 mm	5–10 kHz	Motor units
Single-fiber needle electrode: fine platinum wire (25 μm diameter) inside steel cannula which records from a side aperture	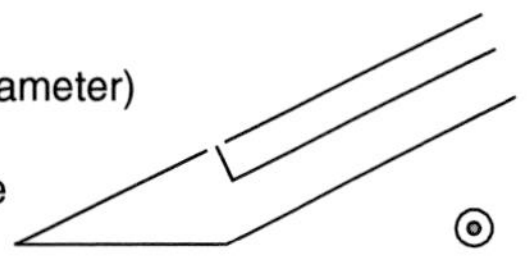	Hemisphere radius 250–300 μm	0.5–0.6 mm	500–10 kHz	Individual muscle fibers of motor units. In health the potentials are either singles or pairs: after reinnervation the potentials have multiple components

Figure 33.1 The concentric needle electrode and the single fiber needle electrode, their physical characteristics, the filter settings required for use, and the nature of the activity that each records. *Source:* Modified from Ref. 2.

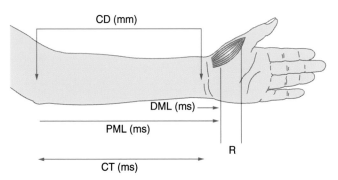

Figure 33.2 Measurements to be made in calculating motor conduction velocity (CV) CV = CD/CT. *Abbreviations:* CD, conduction distance; CT, conduction time; DML, distal motor latency; PML, proximal motor latency; R, recording electrodes.

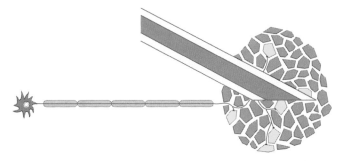

Figure 33.3 Diagram of a motor unit showing the motor neuron which is located in the anterior horn of the spinal cord, Onuf's nucleus in the case of the sphincters, the motor axon which travels in the peripheral nerve to the muscle. Here it divides, innervating a number of muscle fibers, most of which are not adjacent. *Source:* Modified from Ref. 2.

"compound nerve action potential." The amplitude of a compound nerve action potential is related to the number of nerve fibers being depolarized by the stimulating impulse and is a good measure of the number of active nerve fibers.

If the stimulated nerve is purely sensory, as may be the case for some peripheral cutaneous branches, the compound nerve action potential is called the "sensory neurogram (sensory nerve action potential)." Such recordings are not routinely practical in the pelvis for anatomic reasons.

On stimulation of sensory nerves or innervated skin or mucosa an "electrical" response from the central nervous system (i.e., from the spinal cord and the brain) can be recorded. The recorded potentials are called "somatosensory evoked potentials (SEPs)."

On stimulation of sensory receptors in skin or mucosa, or stimulation of sensory nerves, reflex responses are also elicited, and can be recorded (e.g., the *bulbocavernosus reflex*).

THE MOTOR UNIT
Knowledge of the structure and function of the MU is fundamental to understanding the application of EMG methods.

"Muscle electrical activity" is generated by depolarization of single muscle fibers (i.e., consisting of muscle fiber action potentials). But the innervation of muscle is such that a single muscle fiber does not contract on its own but rather in concert

with other muscle fibers which are part of the same MU, i.e., innervated by the same motor neuron.

Motor neurons that innervate striated muscle lie in the anterior horn of the spinal cord. Their cell bodies are relatively large and their axonal processes correspondingly of large diameter and myelinated to allow rapid conduction of impulses, although the neurons which innervate the sphincters are relatively smaller than those innervating skeletal limb and trunk muscles. Within the muscle, the motor axon tapers and then branches to innervate muscle fibers which are scattered throughout the muscle (Fig. 33.3). The innervation of muscle is such that it is unlikely that fibers that are part of the same MU will be adjacent to one another. The number of muscle fibers innervated by an axon is known as the "innervation ratio." There is no simple neurophysiologic method for estimating this parameter and the number of MUs per muscle is also difficult to estimate by clinical neurophysiologic means.

The contraction properties of a MU depend on the nature of its constituent muscle fibers. Muscle fibers can be classified according to their twitch tension, speed of contraction, and histochemical staining properties. The fatigue-resistant type 1 fibers constitute MUs which fire for prolonged periods of time at lower firing frequencies, i.e., "tonically" (see below). Type 2 fibers make up MUs which fire briefly and rapidly in bursts, i.e., "phasically." Unfortunately, there is no clinical electrophysiologic method which can estimate the proportion of MUs of different muscle fiber types. In the pelvic floor and sphincters the majority of muscle fibers are type 1 (with some regional variation).

ELECTROMYOGRAPHIC METHODS
Kinesiologic EMG
Method

By prolonged recording of bioelectrical activity of a muscle, a qualitative and quantitative description of its activity over time is obtained. Such techniques are used in rehabilitation and sports medicine to study movement. Meaningful kinesiologic EMG can, of course, only be performed from an innervated muscle. If the lower motor neuron integrity of a particular muscle is questioned, "MU" EMG analysis (see below) has to be performed first.

The choice of muscle for EMG examination depends on the aims of the investigation. Routine EMG as part of urodynamic testing usually employs a single channel for recording from the urethral or anal sphincter muscle. The sphincters being small circular muscles, it is assumed that the two sides react in a similar fashion, although this may not always be the case, as was shown for the levator ani (6).

When we are interested in the pattern of activity of an individual muscle, the technique should ideally provide a selective recording, uncontaminated by neighboring muscles, and a faithful detection of any activity within the source muscle. Unfortunately, both objectives are difficult to achieve simultaneously and the purpose of the investigation will suggest an acceptable compromise. Overall detection from the bulk of a muscle can only be achieved with non-selective electrodes; selective recordings from small muscles can only be made with intramuscular electrodes with small detection surfaces. Non-selective recordings carry the risk of contamination with activity from other muscles; selective recordings may fail to detect activity in all parts of the source muscle. Meaningful recordings from deep muscles can only be accomplished by invasive techniques.

Considering the above, truly selective recording from sphincter muscles can probably only be obtained by intramuscular electrodes; in clinical routine, often the CNE is used. This electrode has the advantage of being widely available, easy to introduce, and adjust in position, and has a standardized active surface. It is, however, painful to have inserted and subsequent movement of the source muscle can be uncomfortable and the needle then easily dislodged. Instead, two thin isolated/bare tip wires (with a hook at the end) can be introduced into the muscle with a cannula; the latter is then withdrawn, and the wires stay in place. The advantage of this type of recording is good positional stability and painlessness once the wires are inserted, although their position cannot be much adjusted.

To make EMG recording less invasive, various types of surface electrode have been devised, also for intravaginal placement (7), anal plug electrodes, and catheter-mounted ring electrodes (8) to record from the urethral sphincter (Fig. 33.4).

Recordings with surface electrodes are more artifact prone and, furthermore, the artifacts may be less easily identified.

Critical on-line assessment of the "quality of the EMG signal" is mandatory in kinesiologic EMG, and this requires either auditory or oscilloscope monitoring of the raw signal. Integration of high quality EMG signals may help in quantification of results, as can automatic analysis of the interference pattern (IP) (9).

Findings in Normal and Abnormal Conditions

The normal kinesiologic sphincter EMG shows some continuous activity at rest (which may be increased voluntarily or reflexly) (Fig. 33.5); such activity could be recorded for up to two hours, and even after a subject has fallen asleep during the examination (3,10). This physiologic spontaneous activity may be called "tonic." It consists of prolonged firing of tonic MUs, not rapidly interchanging activation and inactivation of different MUs (10).

The "amount" of recorded activity depends on the uptake area of the electrode (Fig. 33.1). Using a CNE, activity from

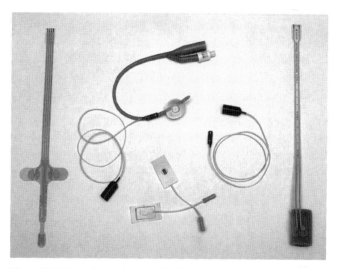

Figure 33.4 Electrodes used to record sphincter activity. *Source:* Reproduced from Ref. 2.

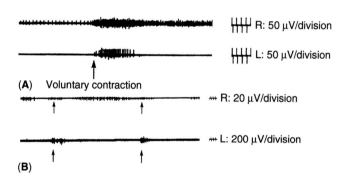

Figure 33.5 Kinesiologic EMG recordings from the pubococcygeus muscles (recording with intramuscular wires: *right*, upper traces; *left*, lower traces). (**A**) Recordings from a 33-year-old nulliparous woman. Continuous firing of motor unit potentials is seen on the right with a gradual recruitment on voluntary contraction. On the left, no ongoing activity is present. Symmetrical recruitment on voluntary contraction is present. (**B**) Recordings from a 52-year-old stress urinary incontinent woman. Some ongoing muscle activity can be seen in both pubococcygeal muscles. On voluntary contraction, recruitment can only be seen on the left. On the right, there is actually a decrease in firing of motor units on "voluntary contraction."

one to five MUs is usually recorded per detection site in the anal sphincter at rest. "Tonic" activity is encountered in many but not all detection sites of the levator ani muscle (11). Typically, it consists of low amplitude MU potentials (MUPs) that fire fairly regularly at low frequencies. In a study of 39 such MUs from the anal sphincter in 17 subjects (inclusion criterion was rhythmic spontaneous firing for two minutes before onset of measurement), the range of discharge rates was found to be 2.5 to 9.4 Hz (mean ± SD 5.3 ± 1.8 Hz) (12). Any reflex or voluntary activation procedure is mirrored first by an increase in the firing frequency of the MUs; then, with any stronger activation or increase in abdominal pressure, now so-called "phasic" MUs are recruited (Fig. 33.5). These are usually of higher amplitude and their discharge rates are higher and irregular. A small percentage of MUs with an "intermediate" activation pattern can also be encountered (12). Both the urethral and anal sphincter show short-lasting voluntary activation times (typically below one minute), which is also the case for pubococcygeus muscles (11).

On voiding, all EMG activity in the urethral sphincter ceases prior to a detrusor contraction. Coordinated detrusor/sphincter activity is lost with lesions between the lower sacral segments and the upper pons (the pontine micturition center); detrusor contractions are then accompanied by an increase in sphincter EMG activity (13). This pattern of activity is called "detrusor sphincter dyssynergia." On the basis of the temporal relationship between urethral sphincter and detrusor contractions, three types of dyssynergia have been described (14). This neurogenic uncoordinated sphincter behavior has to be differentiated from "voluntary" contractions that may occur in the so-called "non-neuropathic voiding disorders" that may be a learned abnormality of behavior (15), and may be encountered in women with dysfunctional voiding (16).

Urethral sphincter contraction, or at least failure of relaxation during involuntary detrusor contractions, has also been reported in patients with Parkinson's disease (17). Normal physiologic behavior of the striated anal sphincter is characterized by its relaxation with defecation (18); a paradoxical sphincter activation during defecation has been described in Parkinson's disease, so-called "anismus" (19).

The pubococcygeus in the healthy female reveals patterns of activity similar to those found in the urethral and anal sphincters at most detection sites, i.e., continuous activity at rest, some increase in activity during bladder filling, and a reflex increase in activity during any activation maneuver such as talking, deep breathing, and coughing. It relaxes during voiding and in health the muscles on both sides act in concert (11). Timely activation of the levator ani muscle has been demonstrated to be an important aspect of stable bladder neck support; its activation precedes activity of other muscles in the cough reflex (20). In stress-incontinent women, the physiologic patterns of activation, as well as the coordination between the two sides, may be lost (6) (Fig. 33.5). A delay in muscle activation on coughing has also been demonstrated, as compared to continent women (19).

Little is known about the normal complexity of activity patterns of different pelvic floor muscles (i.e., urethral sphincter, urethrovaginal sphincter, anal sphincter muscle, different parts of the levator ani), but it is generally assumed that they act as one, in a coordinated fashion. Differences have, however, been demonstrated even between the intra- and periurethral sphincter (21). Coordinated behavior is often lost in disease states, as has been shown, for example, for the levator ani and the urethral and anal sphincters (22). Disturbances of pelvic floor muscles activity have been modified by using the kinesiologic EMG recording as a biofeedback signal (23).

Diagnostic Usefulness of Kinesiologic EMG

The demonstration of voluntary and reflex activation of pelvic floor muscles is indirect proof of the integrity of respective neural pathways. Kinesiologic EMG recordings of sphincter muscles, either urethral or anal, are obtained in selected patients in urodynamic laboratories to ascertain sphincter behavior during bladder filling and voiding. Such simultaneous studies of detrusor and sphincter activity are, as a rule, obtained only in patients with suspected detrusor–sphincter dyssynergia. External anal sphincter (EAS) EMG is recorded in some laboratories in the assessment of anorectal dysfunction (18).

Other than the polygraphic urodynamic recordings to diagnose detrusor–sphincter dyssynergia, the diagnostic contribution of kinesiologic EMG is yet to be established.

EMG METHODS TO DIFFERENTIATE NORMAL FROM PATHOLOGIC MUSCLE

Needle EMG may help to differentiate between normal, denervated, reinnervated, and myopathic muscle. Such EMG has also been called "MU" EMG to distinguish it from "kinesiologic" EMG.

The needle electrode needs to be placed appropriately in the target muscle. The levator ani muscle can be located by transrectal or transvaginal palpation and reached transcutaneously. The anal sphincter is easily located. The urethral sphincter is anatomically separate from the pelvic floor musculature (24) and can be approached either perineally with a needle insertion 0.5 cm laterally to the urethral orifice (the authors suggest one single skin insertion per side) or it can be reached transvaginally using a Sims speculum to retract the posterior vaginal wall. The latter approach has been estimated as less uncomfortable (25), but is not used by many. The position of the needle should be adjusted in a systematic way so that the same muscle area is not repeatedly sampled.

Normal Findings Using a CN EMG Electrode

The needle electrode most commonly used in EMG is the single use disposable CNE; it consists of a central insulated platinum wire encased within a steel cannula and the tip ground to give an elliptical area of 580×150 μm (Fig. 33.1). This type of electrode has the recording characteristics necessary to record spike or near activity from about 20 muscle fibers. The number of MUs recorded therefore depends both upon the local arrangement of muscle fibers within the MU and the level of contraction of the muscle (2).

CNE EMG can provide information on insertion activity, abnormal spontaneous activity, MUPs, and IP (2).

In healthy skeletal muscle, initial placement of the needle elicits a short burst of "insertion activity" which is due to mechanical stimulation of excitable membranes. This phenomenon may also be seen in the sphincters; however, because of the reflex, pain-induced burst of MUs which occurs, insertion activity may be difficult to discern. Insertion activity is recorded at a sensitivity setting of 50 μV/division, which is also the gain used to record spontaneous activity. Absence of insertion activity with an appropriately placed needle electrode usually indicates a complete denervation atrophy of the examined muscle.

At rest, tonic MUPs are the only normal activity recorded. In partially denervated sphincter muscle there is—by definition—a loss of MUs. The number of continuously active MUPs during relaxation can be estimated by counting the number of continuously firing low-threshold MUPs. In patients with cauda equina or conus medullaris lesions, fewer MUPs fire continuously during relaxation, probably due to partial axonal loss. In addition to continuously firing low-threshold ("tonic") MUs, new MUPs are recruited voluntarily and reflexly in the sphincters. It has been shown that the two MUP populations differ in their characteristics, reflexly or voluntarily activated high-threshold MUPs being larger than continuously active "low-threshold MUPs." As a consequence, a standardized level of activity at which a template-based multi-MUP analysis obtains between three and five MUPs on a single muscle site was suggested (26). The main obstacle to qualified assessment of a reduced number of activated MUs, and activation of MUs at increased firing rates (as occurs in limb muscles), is a lack of concomitant measurement of the level of contraction of the examined muscle (this can be readily assessed when studying limb muscles).

Phasic (high threshold) MUPs can be activated reflexly or voluntarily. Normally, MUPs should inter-mingle to produce an "interference" pattern on the oscilloscope during muscle contraction, and during a strong cough.

MUPs should be analyzed at a sensitivity setting which allows their full display. The commonly used time scale is 5 or 10 ms/division, with an amplitude gain of 50 to 500 μV/division (Fig. 33.6). The commonly used amplifier filter settings for CN EMG are 10 to 10,000 Hz. The amplitude of a MUP is largely determined by the activity of those muscle fibers closest to the recording electrode. Other fibers within a 0.5 mm radius of the recording electrode contribute little to the amplitude but in a normal MU there are unlikely to be more than two or three fibers belonging to the same MU. Amplitude is highly sensitive to needle position and very minor adjustments of the electrode will result in major changes, i.e., a change in position by 0.5 mm alters the amplitude 10- to 100-fold (2).

The duration of a MU is the time between the first deflection and the point when the waveform finally returns to the baseline. This will depend on the number of muscle fibers within the MU and is little affected by the proximity of the recording electrode to the nearest fiber. The difficulty with this measurement is defining the exact point of return to the baseline. The phases of a MUP are defined by the number of times the potential crosses the baseline. A unit that has four phases or more is said to be polyphasic. A related parameter is a "turn" which is defined as a shift in direction of a potential of greater than a specified amplitude.

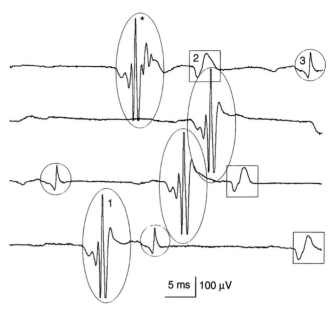

Figure 33.6 Concentric needle EMG recording of motor unit potentials from the urethral sphincter of a 35-year-old stress incontinent female, several years after second vaginal delivery. At this detection site three motor unit potentials are firing continuously, and can be analyzed. It can be seen that the motor unit potential (MUP) with the asterisk is different from the others of similar overall shape. Further analysis of such a signal is needed to ascertain whether it is a superimposition of two individual MUPs or an instability within a complex of MUPs. The use of trigger and delay facility is advantageous to solve such questions (Fig. 33.7).

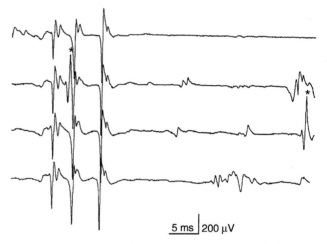

Figure 33.7 A concentric needle EMG recording from the urethral sphincter of an 18-year-old nulliparous female four years after a partial cauda equina injury. A trigger and delay facility is used. A complex motor unit potential (MUP) with prolonged duration is shown. Superimposition of another individual MUP (asterisk) may be falsely interpreted as instability of the potential.

Using the standard recording facilities available on all modern EMG machines, individual MUPs can be captured and their amplitude and duration measured. To allow identification of MUPs, and to be certain the late components of complex potentials are not due to superimposition of several MUPs, it is necessary to capture the same potential repeatedly (Fig. 33.7). MUPs are mostly below 1 mV in the normal urethral sphincter and below 2 mV in the normal anal sphincter.

Most are <7 ms, and few (<15%) are above 10 ms in duration. Additionally, most are bi- and triphasic, but up to 15% to 33% may be polyphasic. Normal MUPs are stable—their shape on repetitive recording does not change (21,27,28).

There are two approaches to analyzing the bioelectrical activity of MUs quantitatively: either individual MUPs are analyzed, or the overall activity of intermingled MUPs (the "IP") is analyzed. Generally, three techniques of MUP analysis ("manual-MUP," "single-MUP," and "multi-MUP") and one technique of IP analysis [turn/amplitude (T/A)] are available on advanced EMG systems. By either method a relevant sample of EMG activity needs to be analyzed for the test to be valid. In the small half of the sphincter muscle collecting 10 different MUPs has been accepted as the minimal requirement for using single-MUP analysis.

Using manual-MUP and multi-MUP techniques, sampling of 20 MUPs (standard number in limb muscles) from each EAS presents no difficulty in healthy controls and most patients. Normative data obtained from the EAS muscle by standardized EMG technique using all three MUP analysis techniques (manual-MUP, single-MUP, multi-MUP) have been published (29,30). The technical differences in the methods are many and no in-depth description is attempted here. The more technical issues of quantitative EMG, the relevance and usefulness of various parameters, etc., is discussed in neurophysiological sources.

MUPs are identified either using a trigger and delay line ("single-MUP") or appearing repeatedly in a prolonged recording of EMG activity ("manual-MUP"). Both approaches favor identification of relatively larger MUPs and become less reliable on stronger activation of muscle. Both methods are relatively slow and subject to examiner bias. The template-based multi-MUP analysis and the T/A analysis of IP (both run by automated computer analysis) are fast (5–10 and 2–3 minutes per muscle, respectively), easy to apply, and allow little opportunity for examiner bias (30). Use of quantitative MUP and IP analyses of the EAS is facilitated by the availability of normative values that can be introduced into the EMG system's software. It has been shown that normative data are not significantly affected by age, gender, number of uncomplicated vaginal deliveries, mild chronic constipation, and the part of the EAS muscle (i.e., subcutaneous or deeper) examined (31–33). This makes quantitative analysis much simpler and results from different laboratories easily comparable.

The main draw back of the multi-MUP method is its tendency to chop up long polyphasic MUPs (such as occur in anal sphincter of MSA patients) into "components," thus "missing" these highly abnormal MUPS. If the electromyographer checks the native EMG and observes such MUPs, the "collected MUPs" should be carefully scrutinized, and possibly a "manual MUP" analysis performed for a quality check.

Similar in-depth analyzed normative data from standardized techniques for other pelvic floor and perineal muscles are not yet available, but individual laboratories use their own normative data.

Single Fiber EMG (SFEMG)

SFEMG is used in general clinical neurophysiologic laboratories to diagnose disturbed neuromuscular transmission (as in

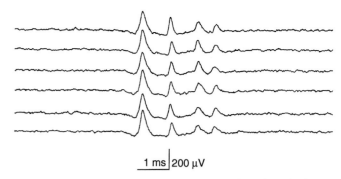

1 ms | 200 µV

Figure 33.8 Single fiber electromyography recording from the anal sphincter of a 51-year-old nulliparous female with an extrapyramidal syndrome and recent development of poor bladder emptying accompanied by stress incontinence. The fiber density in the anal sphincter was found to be 3.7 and a diagnosis of possible multiple system atrophy was suggested. Further development of the clinical picture supported the diagnosis.

Myasthenia gravis). The original recording needles are specially constructed (with a small recording area oriented "sideways" on the thin cannula—Fig. 33.1), very expensive, and disposable versions are not available. An adapted method using disposable CNEs is being used in many laboratories, as it is becoming unacceptable not to use disposable needles. When recording SFEMG, the amplifier filters are set so that low frequency activity is eliminated (500 to 10 kHz). Thus the contribution of each muscle fiber appears as a biphasic positive–negative action potential.

In the past SFEMG has been used not only to record the neuromuscular "jitter" (a measure of neuromuscular transmission), but also "fiber density" (FD), which is the mean number of muscle fibers belonging to an individual MU per detection site (a parameter that reflects MU morphology). To measure FD, recordings from 20 different detection sites are necessary (Fig. 33.8) and the number of component potentials to each MU recorded and averaged (34). The normal FD for the anal sphincter is below 2.0 (35–37). Small changes with age have been reported; women have significantly greater FD than men (37).

Due to its technical characteristics, a SFEMG electrode is able to record even small changes that occur in MUs due to reinnervation, but is less suitable to detect changes due to denervation itself, i.e., abnormal insertion and spontaneous activity. SFEMG has indeed never been used in "routine uro-neurophysiological diagnostics," only in research.

EMG Findings due to Denervation and Reinnervation

After complete denervation, all MU activity ceases and there may be electrical silence for several days. Between 10 and 20 days after a denervating injury, "insertion activity" becomes more prolonged and abnormal spontaneous activity in the form of short biphasic spikes ("fibrillation potentials") and biphasic potentials with prominent positive deflections ("positive sharp waves") appear (38). In perineal muscles, complete denervation can be observed after traumatic lesions to the lumbosacral spine and damage to the cauda equina. Most lesions will, however, cause only partial denervation. In partially denervated muscle, some MUPs remain and mingle eventually with abnormal spontaneous activity. As the MUPs in sphincter muscles are also short and mostly bi- or triphasic, it requires considerable EMG experience to recognize abnormal spontaneous activity in the presence of surviving MUs. In longstanding partially denervated muscle a peculiar abnormal insertion activity appears, so-called "repetitive discharges." These are made up of repetitively firing groups of potentials with so little jitter between the potentials that it is assumed the activity must be due to ephaptic or direct transmission of impulses between muscle fibers (39). However, this activity may be found in the striated muscle of the urethral sphincter without any other evidence of neuromuscular disease and it has been hypothesized that it causes impaired relaxation of the muscle when spontaneous and profuse (40).

Abnormal spontaneous activity has also been described as a marker for degeneration of Onuf's nucleus occurring in patients with multiple system atrophy (MSA) (41).

After complete denervation, axonal reinnervation may occur and MUPs appear again; first short bi- and triphasic, soon becoming polyphasic, serrated, and of prolonged duration (38).

In partially denervated muscle, there is a certain loss of the number of MUs; some MUPs remain, however, the amount is difficult to estimate as the amount of MU activity recorded depends on needle position and voluntary activation. In partially denervated muscle, collateral reinnervation takes place; surviving motor axons will sprout and grow out to reinnervate those muscle fibers which have lost their nerve supply, resulting in a change in the arrangement of muscle fibers within the unit. Whereas in healthy muscle it is unusual for two adjacent muscle fibers to be part of the same MU, following reinnervation several muscle fibers all belonging to the same MU come to be adjacent to one another. Early in the process of reinnervation the newly outgrown motor sprouts are thin and therefore conduct slowly so that the time taken for excitatory impulses to spread through the axonal tree is abnormally prolonged. This is reflected by prolongation of the waveform of the MUP which may have small, late components (Fig. 33.7). Neuromuscular transmission in these newly grown sprouts may also be insecure so that the MU may show "instability." In skeletal muscle, with time and provided there is no further deterioration in innervation, the reinnervating axonal sprouts increase in diameter, and thus increase their conduction velocity so that activation of all parts of the reinnervated MU become more synchronous. This has the effect of increasing the amplitude and reducing towards normal the duration of the MUPs measured with a CNE. This phenomenon may be different in the sphincter muscles where long duration MUs seem to remain a prominent feature of reinnervated MUs (42).

There are several conditions in which gross changes of reinnervation may be detected in MUs of the pelvic floor. Typically, after a nerve—or nerve root lesion such as a lesion to cauda equina—the MUPs are likely to be prolonged and polyphasic (43). Marked changes of this type are seen in patients with lumbosacral myelomeningoceles, and also patients with MSA (42). MSA is a progressive neurodegenerative disease which often, particularly in its early stages, is mistaken for Parkinson's disease but is poorly responsive to antiparkinsonian treatment. Autonomic failure causing postural hypotension, and cerebellar ataxia causing unsteadiness, and clumsiness,

may be additional features. Urinary incontinence in both women and men occurs early in this condition, often some years before the onset of obvious neurologic features (44). As part of the neurodegenerative process, loss of MUs occurs in Onuf's nucleus so that partial but progressive denervation of the sphincter occurs and recorded MUs show changes of reinnervation, becoming markedly prolonged. Sphincter EMG has been demonstrated to be of value in distinguishing between idiopathic Parkinson's disease and MSA (42,45), but may not be obvious in the early phase of disease (46). Similar changes of chronic reinnervation may be found in other parkinsonian syndromes such as progressive supranuclear palsy (47).

EMG Changes After Vaginal Delivery—EMG in Idiopathic Incontinence

Electrophysiological methods have played a major role in establishing the neuromuscular lesion due to vaginal delivery as a risk factor for incontinence and pelvic organ prolapse (in addition to histopathological findings) (48). Studies using computer-assisted quantified and less operator-biased techniques have confirmed older findings (49,50) of at least subtle neurogenic pelvic floor muscle changes in parous women (32,51).

It is a common experience that EMG changes are more pronounced in the urethral sphincter, and in women with complicated vaginal deliveries. The finding of decreased intramuscular nerve density in the female urethral sphincter, which correlates with decreased muscular tissue, provides validation for the reported EMG abnormalities (52). The abnormalities demonstrated in EAS and pudendal nerves have been suggested to be of pathogenetic significance also for idiopathic fecal incontinence (53). The development of imaging techniques has improved the diagnosis of postpartum structural (anatomical) damage to pelvic floor structures (including sphincters), which has put the importance of the postpartum neurogenic electrophysiological changes in perspective, which, when minor, may have little functional consequences.

The neurogenic damage caused by vaginal delivery is acknowledged to be, to a large extent, repaired by regenerative processes, but may then recur in the long run (53). Repetitive straining at stool due to constipation has been the main implicated pathogenetic mechanism for such chronic progression of the neuromuscular lesion. Indeed, prolongation of pudendal nerve terminal latency has been demonstrated after one minute of hard straining (54). Cumulative damage to the pudendal nerve may occur in severe chronic constipation. Our study in patients with mild chronic constipation failed, however, to reveal any neurogenic anal sphincter changes, as compared to non-constipated controls (55).

On the other hand, myogenic changes in pelvic floor muscles after vaginal delivery were also reported (56).

The usefulness of EMG in individual patients with idiopathic incontinence is limited, as its predictive value for treatment outcome has not been established. In routine diagnostics, CN EMG of pelvic floor muscles in women after vaginal delivery and/or with undefined urinary incontinence should be restricted to the rare cases in whom a substantial pudendal nerve or sacral plexus involvement is suspected (57).

EMG Changes in Women with Urinary Retention and Obstructed Voiding

For many years it was said that isolated urinary retention in young women was due either to psychogenic factors or was the first symptom of onset of multiple sclerosis (58). However, CN EMG in this group has demonstrated that many such patients have profuse complex repetitive discharges (CRDs) and decelerating burst (DB) activity in the urethral sphincter muscle (59). The CRDs have a very characteristic sound quality over the loudspeaker on the EMG machine, similar to a helicopter or motorcycle engine. It is the DBs which produce the myotonic-like sound which has been likened to underwater recordings of whales. The jitter between the CRD potentials is very small (39).

It was proposed that this pathologic spontaneous activity leads to sphincter contraction, which endures during micturition and causes obstruction to flow. Positive proof of this has been demonstrated by combined CN EMG and kinesiologic EMG analysis of a group of females with dysfunctional voiding (16).

The syndrome described by one of the authors is associated with polycystic ovaries (Fowler's syndrome) (59). There may be some (as yet unidentified) hormonal susceptibility of the female striated urethral sphincter which causes a loss of stability of the muscle membrane and permits ephaptic transmission to develop, manifest as CRDs. The current hypothesis is that it is the sustained contraction of the urethral sphincter that has an inhibitory effect on bladder afferents and efferents resulting in loss of bladder sensation and urinary retention.

Although urethral sphincter EMG may indicate the presence of an abnormality, it is inevitably only a sample and it is difficult to know whether the abnormality is sufficient to account for the clinical finding of complete or partial urinary retention. The investigations that have proved to be useful as adjuncts to the EMG are measurement of the urethral pressure profile (UPP) and volume of the sphincter muscle estimated with ultrasound (60). Young women with urinary retention due to the sphincter abnormality regularly have UPPs in excess of 100 cmH$_2$O.

The typical clinical presentation of this syndrome is of a young woman with either spontaneous onset of urinary retention or retention following some sort of operative intervention. The mean age of a series of women with this problem was 27 years; spontaneous onset appears to be more common in women under 30 (60). Characteristically, the women present with a bladder capacity in excess of 1 L and, although this may cause painful distension, they lack any expected sensations of urinary urgency. There may or may not be a history of infrequent voiding prior to the onset of urinary retention. These women are taught to do clean intermittent self-catheterization and commonly experience difficulties with this technique, in particular pain and difficulty in removing the catheter. Patients with Fowler's syndrome respond well to sacral neuromodulation (61). The stimulation does not, however, cause a cessation of the abnormal EMG activity (62).

Because CN EMG will detect changes of both denervation and reinnervation as occur with a cauda equina lesion, as well as abnormal spontaneous activity, it has been argued that this test is mandatory in women with urinary retention (63). It should certainly be carried out before stigmatizing a woman as having "psychogenic urinary retention."

EMG Changes in Primary Muscle Disease

CN EMG changes reflect pathologic changes in the structure of the MU, but also changes due to disease of the muscle fibers. With degeneration of muscle fibers, the MUs loose them; the number of MUs, however, may not change. The "typical" CN EMG features of myopathy of skeletal muscle are abundant small, low amplitude polyphasic units recruited at mild effort. Such changes have not been reported in the pelvic floor, even in patients known to have generalized myopathy (64). Pelvic floor muscle involvement in limb-girdle muscular dystrophy in a nulliparous female has been reported, but CN EMG of her urethral sphincter was reported as normal (65). Myopathic changes were observed in the puborectalis and the EAS in patients with myotonic dystrophy.

Little is currently known about what might be expected of an EMG recording from traumatized muscle which has been subject to a severe stretch injury—as occurs during childbirth—but there may well be changes reflecting rupture of individual muscle fibers and injury to small intramuscular nerves.

Diagnostic Usefulness of EMG Methods

Both CN EMG and SFEMG have been employed in neurourologic, urogynecologic, and proctologic research. In routine diagnostics, using CN EMG, an experienced examiner can quickly come to a conclusion regarding normality or abnormality of the muscle examined simply by "observing" the abnormal spontaneous activity, and the MU activity on the oscilloscope screen. This is one reason why quantified determination of MUP parameters by CN EMG is not as widely used as would be expected. If quantification is desirable, quantified CN EMG does provide the same information on reinnervation changes in muscle as the SFEMG parameter of "FD" (10,66). An ideal quantitative EMG method has not been found yet, however, and expertise is required from the electromyographer to allow good quality control.

CN EMG is the electrophysiologic method of choice in routine examination of skeletal muscle. It should be logical to extend an "EMG examination" from, for example, lumbar and upper sacral myotomes to the lower sacral myotomes in a child with myelomeningocele or an adult after a cauda equina lesion. Furthermore, the concentric electrode can be employed at the same diagnostic session for recording motor evoked responses and/or reflex responses (26).

CONDUCTION STUDIES OF THE SACRAL MOTOR SYSTEM

Measurement of motor conduction velocity is routinely carried out to evaluate limb motor nerves. However, the technique requires access to stimulation of the nerve at two separated points and measurement of the distance between them (4) (Fig. 33.3)—a requirement which cannot be practically met in the pelvis. An electrophysiologic parameter that requires a shorter length of motor nerve to be accessible is measurement of the terminal motor latency of a muscle response (2).

Terminal motor latency of the pudendal nerve can be measured by recording with a CNE from the bulbocavernosus, anal, or urethral sphincter muscles in response to bipolar stimulation placed on the perianal or perineal surface. The latencies of MEPs from the perineal muscles obtained by this means are between 4.7 and 5.1 ms; (67) similar latencies have been obtained for the same method of stimulation and recording from the anal sphincter (68,69).

The more widely employed technique of obtaining the pudendal terminal motor latency relies on stimulation with a special "surface electrode assembly" fixed on a gloved index finger (70), often referred to as the "St. Mark's" device. It consists of a bipolar stimulating electrode fixed to the tip of the gloved finger with the recording electrode pair placed 5 cm proximally on the base of the finger. The finger is inserted into the rectum or vagina and stimulation is performed close to the ischial spine. A "rounded" response is recorded from the surface electrodes at the base of the finger (which is claimed to be the M wave from the EAS) with a typical latency around 2 ms. This test is usually referred to as the "pudendal nerve terminal motor latency (PNTML)" test. If a catheter-mounted electrode is used, responses from the urethral sphincter can also be obtained. In studies, as a rule only latencies have been studied as amplitudes of the "M wave" response have not proved contributory. From studies using this test it was concluded that occult damage to the pudendal innervation of the EAS occurs after vaginal delivery, and the conditions worsens over many years by abnormal straining patterns of defecation (53). It was said to be of pathogenetic importance for idiopathic stress urinary incontinence, fecal incontinence, and pelvic floor prolapse (49). Sultan et al. (71) also demonstrated a small but statistically significant increase in pudendal nerve latency following vaginal delivery. More importantly, they demonstrated a defect of either the internal or EAS, or both, in 35% of women after vaginal delivery using anal endosonography, and a strong association between these defects and the development of bowel symptoms. The prolonged latency and the muscle defect were thought to reflect a common traumatic cause.

Although no correlation of PNTML to parity was found in some studies (72), the term "pudendal neuropathy" has become established in the literature for a while, and authors less familiar with clinical neurophysiology theory tended to equate a prolongation of pudendal motor latency with pelvic floor denervation. This however, is mistaken, as prolongation of latency is a poor measure of denervation. In fact, experts now mostly doubt the validity of the test. A lack of correlation to sphincter pressure measurements has been demonstrated: In one study, approximately 50% of patients with PNTML had normal anal canal squeeze pressures (73). In contrast to earlier studies, more recent work suggests the test does not predict improvement, or the lack of improvement, after surgical repair of anal sphincter defects (74). A prospective evaluation of anorectal physiologic tests in 90 patients with fecal incontinence did not find that pudendal terminal latency test results changed treatment decisions (75). Indeed, the American Gastroenterological Association statement indicated that "pudendal terminal latency cannot be recommended for evaluation of patients with fecal incontinence" (76). Currently, measuring pudendal nerve latencies in incontinence is not recommended (77).

A selective needle recording of a (sphincter or pelvic floor) muscle reponse (M wave) on appropriate electrical stimulation may be informative in selected patients with suspected "lower motor neuron type" lesions.

Anterior Sacral Root (Cauda Equina) Stimulation

Transcutaneous stimulation of deeply situated nervous tissue became possible with the development of special electrical (78) and magnetic (79) stimulators. When applied over the spine these stimulators stimulate mainly the roots at the exit from the vertebral canal (80). There have been reports of these techniques applied to the sacral roots (81). Parasympathetic efferents most probably cannot be stimulated using magnetic stimulation. While it has been claimed that MEPs from detrusor can be produced following magnetic stimulation of the cauda equina (82), others have demonstrated inhibition of detrusor hyperreflexia following sacral root stimulation (83), which is expected after depolarization of perineal afferents.

Needle EMG electrodes rather than non-selective surface electrodes should be used to record MEPs to electrical or magnetic stimulation because both depolarize underlying neural structures in a non-selective fashion and there may be activation of several muscles innervated by lumbosacral segments. It has been shown that responses from gluteal muscles may contaminate attempts to record from the sphincters and lead to error (84).

Recording of MEPs with magnetic stimulation has been less successful, at least with standard coils (85,86), than with electrical stimulation, and there is often large stimulus artifact. Positioning of the ground electrode between the recording electrodes and the stimulating coil should decrease the artifact (Fig. 33.9). Stimulation of the roots may be used to obtain a peripheral conduction time so that a central conduction time (see next section) can be calculated (85).

Demonstrating the presence of a perineal MEP on stimulation over the lumbosacral spine and recording this with a CN

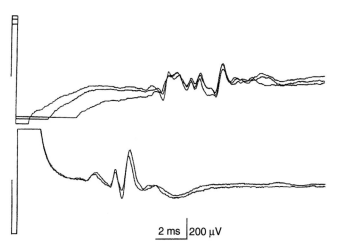

2 ms | 200 μV

Figure 33.9 Concentric needle electromyography recording from the anal sphincter showing responses on "strong" electrical stimulation with surface electrodes over the back (upper trace at level L1; lower trace at level S3). Digitimer stimulator: stimulus duration 50 μs, stimulus amplitude 50%. Three and two consecutive responses are superimposed, respectively.

EMG electrode may occasionally be helpful; however, an absent response has to be evaluated with caution and the clinical value of the test has yet to be established.

Assessment of Central Motor Pathways

Using the same magnetic or electrical stimulation as mentioned above, it is possible to stimulate the motor cortex and record a response from the pelvic floor. Magnetic stimulation is less unpleasant; electrical cortical stimulation is nowadays only used intraoperatively in anesthetized patients.

By electrical stimulation over the motor cortex of healthy subjects, MEPs in anal and urethral sphincters, and in the bulbocavernosus (84) muscles were reported. The mean latencies were between 30 and 35 ms if no "facilitatory maneuver" was used. If, however, stimulation was performed during a period of slight voluntary contraction of the muscle, the latencies of MEPs shortened significantly (for up to 8 ms) (Fig. 33.10).

By applying stimulation both over the scalp and in the back (at level L1), and subtracting the latency of the respective MEPs, a "central conduction time" can be obtained. Central conduction times of approximately 22 ms without, and about 15 ms with, the facilitation (i.e., slight voluntary contraction) have been reported (85).

Substantially longer central conduction time in patients with multiple sclerosis and spinal cord lesions as compared to healthy controls have been found (86), but all those patients had clinically recognizable cord disease.

Normative values for the urethral sphincter and the puborectal muscle in adult women have been reported for transcranial magnetic stimulation (87,88). The necessity to use concentric needle EMG for recording has been reconfirmed (89).

MEP have opened an avenue of research on excitability of motor cortex. It has been demonstrated that in comparison to the motor area for hand muscles the anal sphincter motor cortex has less intracortical inhibition (90).

Because of the significant influence of voluntary contraction there is a possibility of variability of both total conduction times and central conduction times. A well-formed sphincter

MEP with a normal latency in a patient with a functional disorder or a medico legal case may on occasion be helpful.

CONDUCTION STUDIES OF THE SACRAL SENSORY SYSTEM

Cerebral Somatosensory Evoked Potentials

The pudendal evoked response is easily recorded following electrical stimulation of the clitoral nerve (85,91–93). This SEP is of highest amplitudes at the central recording site [(Cz −2 cm: Fz) of the international 10 to 20 electroencephalogram system] (94) and is highly reproducible. Amplitudes of the P40 measure between 0.5 and 12 μV. The first positive peak at 41 ± 2.3 ms (called P1 or P40) is usually clearly defined in healthy subjects using a stimulus two to four times the sensory threshold current strength (91) (Fig. 33.11). Later negative (at around 55 ms) and then further positive waves are interindividually quite variable in amplitude and expression, and furthermore have little known clinical relevance.

Pudendal SEP recordings have been widely employed in patients with neurogenic bladder dysfunction due to multiple sclerosis (86), but it has since been shown that the tibial cerebral SEPs are more often abnormal than the pudendal SEP, and only in exceptional cases is the pudendal SEP abnormal but the tibials normal, pointing to an isolated conus involvement (95). Cerebral SEPs on clitoral stimulation were reported as a possibly valuable intraoperative monitoring method in patients with cauda equina or conus at risk of a surgical procedure (96,97).

Special techniques of stimulation isolate each dorsal clitoral nerve and may be more sensitive at locating the precise site of pathology (98). Following spinal cord injury, tibial, and pudendal SEPs have been claimed to predict recovery in bladder control (99). Pudendal SEPs were used to study the mechanism of sacral neuromodulation (100).

A study which looked at the value of the pudendal evoked potential when investigating urogenital symptoms for detecting relevant neurologic disease found it to be of lesser value than a clinical examination looking for signs of spinal cord disease in the lower limbs, i.e., lower limb hyperreflexia and

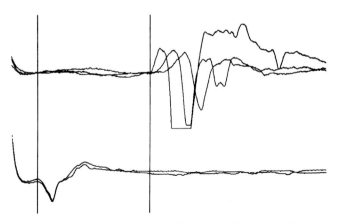

Figure 33.10 Recording from the urethral sphincter with a concentric needle electrode in response to magnetic stimulation of the lower lumbar spine (lower trace; latency 6.5 ms) and the motor cortex (upper trace; latency 25.4 ms). The effect of "facilitation" (i.e., a slight voluntary contraction) on shortening the latency of the response following cortical stimulation is evident.

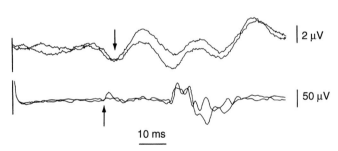

Figure 33.11 Cerebral somatosensory evoked potential (SEP) (*above*) and bulbocavernosus reflex (*below*) on dorsal clitoral nerve stimulation (rectangular pulses, 0.2 ms long at 1 Hz) in a 37-year-old woman with a compressive fracture of L1, complaining of difficulties in initiation of micturition. SEP is recorded with surface electrodes (Cz −2 cm: Fz); the bulbocavernosus reflex is recorded from the anal sphincter with surface electrodes. Two consecutive averages of 128 responses are superimposed. The P40 of the SEP and the first component of the bulbocavernosus reflex are indicated. The first reflex component is spurious at the applied stimulation strength, which was two-times sensory threshold; the second (late) reflex component is obvious.

extensor plantar responses (101). There may, however, be circumstances in routine diagnostics—such as when a patient is complaining of loss of bladder or vaginal sensation—that it is reassuring to be able to record a normal pudendal evoked response.

Electrical Stimulation of Urethra, Bladder, and Anal Canal

Cerebral SEPs can also be obtained on stimulation of the bladder urothelium (102). When making such measurements, it is of utmost importance to use bipolar stimulation in the bladder or proximal urethra, otherwise somatic afferents will be depolarized (103,104). These cerebral SEPs have been shown to have a maximum amplitude over the mid-line (Cz –2 cm: Fz) (104); but the potential is of low amplitude (1 μV or less) and of variable configuration, and may be difficult to identify in some control subjects (104,105). The typical latency of the most prominent negative potential (N 1) is approximately 100 ms (104,105). The responses were claimed to be of more relevance to neurogenic bladder dysfunction than the pudendal SEP, as the Aδ delta sensory afferents from bladder and proximal urethra accompany the autonomic fibers in the pelvic nerves (104).

Another stimulation site in the perineal region is the anal canal, following which cerebral SEPs with a slightly longer latency than those obtained following stimulation of the clitoris have been reported, but it is not possible to record this response from all control subjects. The rectum and sigmoid colon have also been stimulated, and cerebral SEPs of two types recorded. One was similar in shape and latency to pudendal SEP, and the other to SEP recorded on stimulation of bladder/posterior urethra (106).

SACRAL REFLEXES
Physiologic Background, Methods, and Terminology

"Sacral reflexes" refer to electrophysiologically recordable responses of perineal/pelvic floor muscles to (electrical) stimulation in the urogenitoanal region. There are two reflexes—the anal and the bulbocavernosus—which are commonly clinically elicited in the lower sacral segments; both have the afferent and efferent limb of their reflex arc in the pudendal nerve, and are centrally integrated at the S2–S4 cord levels (Fig. 33.11). Electrophysiologic correlates of these reflexes have been described. EMG recording of the sacral reflex has been shown to be more reliable than the clinically assessed response (e.g., observing and palpating the contraction) in males and particularly in females (107).

It is possible to use electrical (67), mechanical (108), or magnetic stimulation. Electrical stimulation can also be applied perianally (67). The pudendal nerve itself may be stimulated by applying needle electrodes transperineally (109) or by using "St. Mark's electrode" (110). As a rule, reflex responses are recorded as EMG activation of target muscles, but responses of the external urethral sphincter have also been recorded with a micro-tip transducer catheter as pressure rises, with latencies between 27 and 41 ms (111).

Bladder neck/proximal urethra can be stimulated using a catheter-mounted ring electrode (103) and reflex responses obtained from perineal muscles. These reflexes have been referred to as "vesicourethral" and "vesicoanal" (112), depending from which muscle the reflex response is recorded. With visceral denervation (e.g., following radical hysterectomy) the viscerosomatic reflexes (from both bladder and urethral stimulation) may be lost while the bulbocavernosus reflex is preserved. Loss of bladder–urethral reflex with preservation of bladder–anal reflex has been described with urethral afferent injury after recurrent urethral surgeries (113).

Reports of sacral reflexes obtained following electrical stimulation of clitoral nerve give consistent mean latencies of between 31 and 38.5 ms (67,93). Sacral reflex responses obtained on perianal or bladder neck/proximal urethra stimulation have latencies between 50 and 65 ms (67). This more prolonged response is thought to be due to the afferent limb of the reflex being conveyed by thinner myelinated nerves with slower conduction velocities than the thicker myelinated pudendal afferents. The longer latency "anal reflex"—the contraction of the anal sphincter on stimulation of the perianal region—may also have thinner myelinated fibers in its afferent limb as it is produced by a nociceptive stimulus. On stimulation perianally, a short latency potential can also be recorded as a result of depolarization of motor branches to the anal sphincter (67,68) (being a "M wave").

Sacral Reflex on Electrical Stimulation of Penis or Clitoris

The sacral reflex evoked on dorsal penile or clitoral nerve stimulation is most commonly called the "bulbocavernosus reflex," but several different names have been proposed, the most logical being the alternative that defines the site of stimulation and the site of recording (i.e., "clitoro-anal" reflex). There is, however, as yet no consensus on terminology. This reflex was shown to be a complex response, often formed by two components (67,114). The first component (with typical latency of about 33 ms) is the response that has been most often called the bulbocavernosus reflex. It is stable, does not habituate, and is thought to be an oligosynaptic reflex response, as the variability of single motor neuron discharges within this reflex is similar to that of the first component of the blink reflex (114). The second component has a similar latency to the sacral reflexes evoked by stimulation perianally or from the proximal urethra. The variability of single motor neuron responses within this component is much larger, as is typical for a polysynaptic reflex (114). The second component is not always demonstrable as a discreet response. The two components of the reflex may behave somewhat differently in control subjects and in patients. Whereas in normal subjects it is usually the first component that has a lower threshold, in patients with partially denervated pelvic floor muscles the first reflex component cannot be obtained with single stimuli, but on strong stimulation the later reflex component does occur. This can cause confusion, and very "delayed" reflex responses may be recorded in patients without recognizing the possibility that it is not a delayed first component but an isolated second component of the reflex. The situation can be clarified by using double stimuli that facilitate the reflex response, and may reveal the first component, which was not obvious on stimulation with single stimuli (115).

Sacral reflex responses recorded with needle or wire electrodes can be analyzed separately for each side of the anal sphincter; this is important because unilateral or asymmetrical lesions are common. Special techniques of stimulation isolate each dorsal clitoral nerve and may be more sensitive for identifying pathology (98). Using unilateral dorsal penile nerve blocks, the existence of two unilateral bulbocavernosus reflex arcs has been demonstrated (116,117). Thus, by detection from the left and right bulbocavernosus (and probably also the EAS) muscles, separate testing of right and left reflex arcs can be performed. In cases of unilateral (sacral plexopathy, pudendal neuropathy) or asymmetrical lesions (cauda equina), a healthy reflex arc may obscure a pathologic one.

Sacral reflex responses on stimulation of the clitoral nerve have been proposed as being valuable in patients with cauda equina and lower motor neuron lesions; however, a reflex with a normal latency does not exclude the possibility of an axonal lesion in its reflex arc. Although most reports deal with abnormally prolonged sacral reflex latencies, it was suggested that a very short reflex latency may indicate the possibility of a tethered cord (118), the shorter latency being attributed particularly to the low location of conus. Shorter latencies of sacral reflexes in patients with suprasacral cord lesions were also reported. Continuous intraoperative recording of sacral reflex responses on clitoris stimulation is feasible if double pulses (119,120) or a train of stimuli are used.

Sacral Reflex on Mechanical Stimulation

Mechanical stimulation has been used to elicit the bulbocavernosus reflex in both sexes (121), but there is as yet little experience with female patients. Either a standard commercially available reflex hammer or a customized electromechanical hammer can be used (105). Such stimulation is painless and can be used in children or patients with pacemakers in whom electrical stimulation is contraindicated.

Diagnostic Usefulness of Sacral Reflex Testing

Sacral reflex testing should be a part of the "diagnostic battery" of which concentric needle EMG exploration of the pelvic floor muscles is the most important part (26). Measurement of sacral reflexes is established and carried out in laboratories worldwide and is—apart from EMG—the most time-honored uroneurophysiologic diagnostic procedure. However, the expectation of some authors that, with measurement of sacral reflexes, a single, easily learned test could distinguish between neurogenic and non-neurogenic sacral dysfunction was unrealistic. Although testing reflex responses is a valid and useful method to assess integrity of reflex arcs, and electrophysiologic assessment of sacral reflexes is a more quantitative, sensitive, and reproducible way of assessing the S2–S4 reflex arcs than any of the clinical methods, uncritical interpretation of results should be discouraged.

AUTONOMIC NERVOUS SYSTEM

The uroneurophysiologic methods discussed so far assess only the myelinated fibers, whereas it is the autonomic nervous system, and the parasympathetic component in particular, that is most relevant for sacral organ function. It has been argued

that local involvement of the sacral nervous system (such as trauma, compression, etc.) will usually involve somatic and autonomic fibers simultaneously. However, as there are some local pathologic conditions (such as mesorectal excision of carcinoma or radical hysterectomy) which can cause a pure autonomic lesion, methods by which the parasympathetic and sympathetic nervous systems innervating the pelvic viscera could be assessed directly would be very helpful. Information on parasympathetic bladder innervation can, to some extent, be obtained by cystometry, but direct electrophysiologic testing would be desirable. In cases where a general involvement of thin fibers is expected, an indirect way to examine autonomic fibers is to assess thin sensory fiber function. As unmyelinated afferent fibers transmit temperature sensation and pain, unmyelinated fiber neuropathy can be identified by testing thermal sensitivity. Thin (visceral sensory) fibers are tested by stimulating the proximal urethra or bladder, and recording sacral reflex responses or cerebral SEPs.

Sympathetic Skin Response

The sympathetic nervous system mediates sweat gland activity in the skin, and changes in this activity lead to changes in skin resistance. On "stressful stimulation," a potential shift can be recorded with surface electrodes from the skin of palms and soles, and has been reported to be a useful parameter in assessment of neuropathy involving unmyelinated nerve fibers (122). The response [sympathetic skin response (SSR)] can also be recorded from perineal skin (123). The SSR is a reflex which consists of myelinated sensory fibers, a complex central integrative mechanism, and a sympathetic efferent limb (with postganglionic non-myelinated C-fibers).

The stimulus used in clinical practice is usually an electric pulse delivered to the upper or lower limb (to mixed nerves), but the genital organs can also be stimulated (123). The responses are easily habituated, and depend on a number of endogenous and exogenous factors including skin temperature, which should be at least above 28°C. The latencies of SSR on the penis following stimulation of a median nerve at the wrist could be obtained in all normal subjects (123). No equivalent control data exist in women as yet.

Limited literature exists regarding the relationship between SSR results and bladder dysfunction. One study reports that diabetic cystopathy was associated with autonomic neuropathy as detected by SSR (124). A correlation has been shown between the absence of the SSR response in foot and bladder neck dyssynergia following spinal cord injury (125). Recording from the perineal region increases the diagnostic sensitivity for assessing sympathetic nerve function within the thoracolumbar cord (126).

The test is not sensitive for partial lesions as only complete absence of response has been regarded as abnormal. Its utility in evaluating bladder and urethral dysfunction is not yet established.

CONCLUSIONS

In routine diagnostics uroneurophysiological testing is becoming established in patients with (suspected) peripheral nervous system lesions, where particularly (quantitative) concentric needle EMG and recording the bulbocavernosus reflex is recommended as standard (and standardized) procedure in selected patients, particularly if they are candidates for invasive therapeutic procedures (26,127). It has been demonstrated that both techniques are indeed complementary, and have—performed in the same patient—a higher sensitivity than each test on its own (i.e., 96%) (128).

Uroneurophysiologic techniques continue to be useful in research, and may become more relevant in the future for intraoperative identification and monitoring of nervous structures.

REFERENCES

1. Adrian ED, Bronck DW. The discharge of impulses in motor nerve fibres. Part II. The frequency of discharge in reflex and voluntary contractions. J Physiol (Lond) 1929; 67: 119–51.
2. Fowler CJ, Tedman BM. Electromyography: normal and pathological findings. In: Binnie CD, Cooper R, Mauguiere F, et al., eds. Clinical Neurophysiology: EMG, Nerve Conduction and Evoked Potentials, Vol. 1 (revised and enlarged edition). Amsterdam: Elsevier, 2004: 77–105.
3. Jesel M, Isch-Treussard C, Isch F. Electromyography of striated muscle of anal and urethral sphincters. In: Desmedt JE, ed. New Developments in Electromyography and Clinical Neurophysiology. Basel: Karger, 1973: 406.
4. Chantraine A, Leval J, Onkelinx A. Motor conduction velocity in the internal pudendal nerves. In: Desmedt JE, ed. New Developments in Electromyography and Clinical Neurophysiology. Basel: Karger, 1973: 433–8.
5. Fowler CJ, Tedman BM. Clinical measurements of nerve conduction. In: Binnie CD, Cooper R, Mauguiere F, et al., eds. Clinical Neurophysiology: EMG, Nerve Conduction and Evoked Potentials, Vol. 1 (revised and enlarged edition). Amsterdam: Elsevier, 2004: 59–75.
6. Deindl FM, Vodusek DB, Hesse U, Schüssler B. Pelvic floor activity patterns: comparison of nulliparous continent and parous urinary stress incontinent women. A kinesiological EMG study. Br J Urol 1994; 73: 413–17.
7. Lose G, Tanko A, Colstrup H, Andersen JT. Urethral sphincter electromyography with vaginal surface electrodes: a comparison with sphincter electromyography recorded via periurethral coaxial, anal sphincter needle and perianal surface electrodes. J Urol 1985; 133: 815–18.
8. Nordling J, Meyhoff HH, Walter S, Andersen JT. Urethral electromyography using a new ring electrode. J Urol 1978; 120: 571–3.
9. Aanestad O, Flink R, Stalberg E. Interference pattern in perineal muscles: I. A quantitative electromyographic study in normal subjects. Neurourol Urodyn 1989; 8: 1–9.
10. Vodusek DB. Neural control of pelvic floor muscle. In: Baesler K, Schuessler B, Burgio KL, et al., eds. Pelvic Floor Re-education: Principles and Practice, 2nd edn. London: Springer-Verlag, 2008: 22–35.
11. Deindl FM, Vodusek DB, Hesse U, Schussler B. Activity patterns of pubococcygeal muscles in nulliparous continent women. Br J Urol 1993; 72: 46–51.
12. Vodusek DB. Neurophysiological study of bulbocavernosus reflex in man [in Slovene]. Ljubljana: University of Ljubljana, 1988: 1–129.
13. Blaivas JG, Sinha HP, Zayed AA, Labib KB. Detrusor–external sphincter dyssynergia. J Urol 1981; 125: 542–4.
14. Chancellor MB, Kaplan SA, Blaivas JG. Detrusor–external sphincter dyssynergia. Ciba Found Symp 1990; 151: 195–206; discussion 207–13.
15. Rudy DC, Woodside JR. Non-neurogenic neurogenic bladder: the relationship between intravesical pressure and the external sphincter electromyogram. Neurourol Urodyn 1991; 10: 169–76.
16. Deindl FM, Vodusek DB, Bischoff C, Hoffmann R, Hartung R. Voiding in women: which muscles are responsible? Br J Urol 1998; 82: 814–19.
17. Pavlakis AJ, Siroky MB, Goldstein I, et al. Neurourologic findings in Parkinson's disease. J Urol 1983; 129: 80–3.
18. Read NW. Functional assessment of the anorectum in faecal incontinence. In: Bock G, Wheelan J, eds. Neurobiology of Incontinence (Ciba Foundation Symposium 151). Chichester: Wiley, 1990: 119.
19. Mathers SE, Kempster PA, Law PJ, et al. Anal sphincter dysfunction in Parkinson's disease. Arch Neurol 1989; 46: 1061–4.
20. Barbič M, Kralj B, Cör A. Compliance of the bladder neck supporting structures: Importance of activity pattern of levator ani muscle and content of elastic fibers of endopelvic fascia. Neurourol Urodyn 2003; 22: 269–76.
21. Chantraine A, de Leval J, Depireux P. Adult female intra- and periurethral sphincter–electromyographic study. Neurourol Urodyn 1990; 9: 139–44.
22. Nordling J, Meyhoff HH. Dissociation of urethral and anal sphincter activity in neurogenic bladder dysfunction. J Urol 1979; 122: 352–6.
23. O'Donnell PD, Doyle R. Biofeedback therapy technique for treatment of urinary incontinence. Urology 1991; 37: 432–6.
24. Gosling JA, Dixon JS, Humperson JR. Functional Anatomy of the Urinary Tract, vol. 1, Ch. 5. London: Churchill Livingstone, 1983.
25. Lowe EM, Fowler CJ, Osborne JL, et al. Improved method for needle electromyography of the urethral sphincter in women. Neurourol Urodyn 1994; 13: 29–33.
26. Podnar S, Vodušek DB. Protocol for clinical neurophysiologic examination of the pelvic floor. Neurourol Urodyn 2001; 20: 669–82.
27. Vodusek DB, Light JK. The motor nerve supply of the external urethral sphincter muscles. Neurourol Urodyn 1983; 2: 193–200.
28. Fowler CJ, Kirby RS, Harrison MJG, et al. Individual motor unit analysis in the diagnosis of disorders of urethral sphincter innervation. J Neurol Neurosurg Psychiatry 1984; 47: 637–41.
29. Podnar S, Vodušek DB, Stålberg E. Standardization of anal sphincter electromyography: normative data. Clin Neurophysiol 2000; 111: 2200–7.
30. Podnar S, Vodušek DB, Stålberg E. Standardization of anal sphincter electromyography: comparison of quantitative techniques of anal sphincter electromyography. Muscle Nerve 2002; 25: 83–92.
31. Podnar S, Vodušek DB. Standardization of anal sphincter electromyography: uniformity of the muscle. Muscle Nerve 2000; 23: 122–5.
32. Podnar S, Lukanovič A, Vodušek DB. Anal sphincter electromyography after vaginal delivery: neuropathic insufficiency or normal wear and tear? Neurourol Urodynam 2000; 19: 249–57.
33. Podnar S, Vodušek DB. Standardization of anal sphincter electromyography: effect of chronic constipation. Muscle Nerve 2000; 23: 1748–51.
34. Stalberg E, Trontelj JV. Single Fiber Electromyography: Studies in Healthy and Diseased Muscle, 2nd edn. New York: Raven Press, 1994.
35. Neill ME, Swash M. Increased motor unit fibre density in the external anal sphincter muscle in ano-rectal incontinence: a single fibre EMG study. J Neurol Neurosurg Psychiatry 1980; 43: 343–7.
36. Vodusek DB, Janko M. SFEMG in striated sphincter muscles [abstract]. Muscle Nerve 1981; 4: 252.
37. Jameson JS, Chia YW, Kamm MA, et al. Effect of age, sex and parity on anorectal function. Br J Surg 1994; 81: 1689–92.
38. Brown WF. The Physiological and Technical Basis of Electromyography. London: Butterworth, 1984.
39. Trontelj J, Stalberg E. Bizarre repetitive discharges recorded with single fibre EMG. J Neurol Neurosurg Psychiatry 1983; 46: 310–16.
40. Fowler CJ, Kirby RS, Harrison MJ. Decelerating burst and complex repetitive discharges in the striated muscle of the urethral sphincter, associated with urinary retention in women. J Neurol Neurosurg Psychiatry 1985; 48: 1004–9.
41. Schwarz J, Kornhuber M, Bischoff C, Straube A. Electromyography of the external anal sphincter in patients with Parkinson's disease and multiple system atrophy: frequency of abnormal spontaneous activity and polyphasic motor unit potentials. Muscle Nerve 1997; 20: 1167–72.
42. Palace J, Chandiramani VA, Fowler CJ. Value of sphincter electromyography in the diagnosis of multiple system atrophy. Muscle Nerve 1997; 20: 1396–403.
43. Podnar S, Oblak C, Vodušek DB. Sexual function in men with cauda equina lesions: a clinical & electromyographic study. J Neurol Neurosurg Psychiatry 2002; 73: 715–20.
44. Beck RO, Betts CD, Fowler CJ. Genitourinary dysfunction in multiple system atrophy: clinical features and treatment in 62 cases. J Urol 1994; 151: 1336–41.

45. Eardley I, Quinn NP, Fowler CJ, et al. The value of urethral sphincter electromyography in the differential diagnosis of parkinsonism. Br J Urol 1989; 64: 360–2.

46. Stocchi F, Carbone A, Inghilleri M, et al. Urodynamic and neurophysiological evaluation in Parkinson's disease and multiple system atrophy. J Neurol Neurosurg Psychiatry 1997; 62:507–11.

47. Valldeoriola F, Valls Sole J, Tolosa ES, et al. Striated anal sphincter denervation in patients with progressive supranuclear palsy. Mov Disord 1995; 10: 550–5.

48. Gilpin SA, Gosling JA, Smith AR, Warrell DW. The pathogenesis of genitourinary prolapse and stress incontinence of urine. A histological and histochemical study. Br J Obstet Gynaecol 1989; 96: 15–23.

49. Smith ARB, Hosker GL, Warrell DW. The role of partial denervation of the pelvic floor in aetiology of genitourinary prolapse and stress incontinence of urine. A europhysiological study. Brit J Obstetr Gynaecol 1989; 96: 24–28.

50. Allen R, Hosker G, Smith A, Warrell D. Pelvic floor damage and childbirth: a neurophysiological study. Brit J Obstet Gynaecol 1990; 97: 770–9.

51. Weidner AC, Barber MD, Visco AG, Bump RC, Sander DB. Pelvic muscle electromyography of levator ani and external anal sphincter in nulliparous women and women with pelvic floor dysfunction. Am J Obstet Gynecol 2000; 183: 1390–401.

52. Pandit M, DeLancey JOL, Ashton-Miller JA, et al. Quantification of intramuscular nerves within the female striated urogenital sphincter muscle. Obstet Gynecol 2000; 95: 797–800.

53. Snooks SJ, Swash M, Mathers SE, Henry MM. Effect of vaginal delivery in the pelvic floor: a 5-year follow-up. Br J Surg 1990; 77: 1358–60.

54. Engel AF, Kamm MA. The acute effect of straining on pelvic floor neurological function. Int J Colorect Dis 1994; 9: 8–12.

55. Podnar S, Vodušek DB. Standardization of anal sphincter electromyography: effect of chronic constipation. Muscle Nerve 2000; 23: 1748–51.

56. Takahashi S, Homma Y, Fujishiro T, et al. Electromyographic study of the striated urethral sphincter in type 3 stress incontinence: evidence of myogenic-dominant damages. Urology 2000; 56: 946–50.

57. Vodušek DB. The role of electrophysiology in the evaluation of incontinence and prolapse. Curr Opin Obstet Gyn 2002; 14: 509–14.

58. Siroky MB, Krane RJ. Functional voiding disorders in women. In: Krane RJ, Siroky MB, eds. Clinical Neuro-urology. Boston: Little, Brown, 1991: 445–57.

59. Fowler CJ, Christmas TJ, Chapple CR, et al. Abnormal electromyographic activity of the urethral sphincter, voiding dysfunction, and polycystic ovaries: a new syndrome? Br Med J 1988; 297: 1436–8.

60. Swinn MJ, Wiseman OJ, Lowe E, et al. The cause and natural history of isolated urinary retention in young women. J Urol 2002; 167: 151–6.

61. Swinn MJ, Kitchen ND, Goodwin RJ, et al. Sacral neuromodulation for women with Fowler's syndrome. Eur Urol 2000; 38: 439–43.

62. DasGupta R, Fowler CJ. Urodynamic study of women in urinary retention treated with sacral neuromodulation. J Urol 2004; 171: 1161–4.

63. Fowler CJ, Kirby RS. Electromyography of urethral sphincter in women with urinary retention. Lancet 1986; 1: 1455–7.

64. Caress JB, Kothari MJ, Bauer SB, Shefner JM. Urinary dysfunction in Duchenne muscular dystrophy. Muscle Nerve 1996; 19: 819–22.

65. Dixon PJ, Christmas TJ, Chapple CR. Stress incontinence due to pelvic floor muscle involvement in limb-girdle muscular dystrophy. Br J Urol 1990; 65: 653–4.

66. Rodi Z, Denišlič M, Vodušek DB. External anal sphincter electromyography in the differential diagnosis of parkinsonism. (Letter to the Editor). J Neurol Neurosurg Psychiatry 1996; 60: 460–1.

67. Vodusek DB, Janko M, Lokar J. Direct and reflex responses in perineal muscles on electrical stimulation. J Neurol Neurosurg Psychiatry 1983; 46: 67–71.

68. Bartolo DC, Jarratt JA, Read NW. The cutaneo-anal reflex: a useful index of neuropathy? Br J Surg 1983; 70: 660–3.

69. Pedersen E, Klemar B, Schroder J, et al. Anal sphincter responses after perianal electrical stimulation. J Neurol Neurosurg Psychiatry 1982; 45: 770–3.

70. Kiff ES, Swash M. Normal proximal and delayed distal conduction in the pudendal nerves of patients with idiopathic (neurogenic) faecal incontinence. J Neurol Neurosurg Psychiatry 1984; 47: 820–3.

71. Sultan AH, Kamm MA, Hudson CN, et al. Anal-sphincter disruption during vaginal delivery. N Engl J Med 1993; 329: 1905–11.

72. Jameson JS, Chia YW, Kamm MA, et al. Effect of age, sex and parity on anorectal function. Br J Surg 1994; 81: 1689–92.

73. Wexner SD, Marchetti F, Salanga VD, et al. Neurophysiologic assessment of the anal sphincters. Dis Colon Rectum 1991; 34: 606–12.

74. Malouf AJ, Morton CS, Engel AF, et al. Long-term results of overlapping anterior anal-sphincter repair for obstetric trauma. Lancet 2000; 355: 260–5.

75. Liberman H, Faria J, Ternent CA, et al. A prospective evaluation of the value of anorectal physiology in the management of fecal incontinence. Dis Colon Rectum 2001; 44: 1567–74.

76. Barnett JL, Hasler WL, Camilleri M. American Gastroenterological Association medical position statement on anorectal testing techniques. Gastroenterology 1999; 116: 732–60.

77. Abrams P, Cardozo L, Khoury S, Wein A, eds. Incontinence; 4th International Consultation on Incontinence. Health Publication Ltd., 2009 (in press).

78. Merton PA, Morton HB. Stimulation of the cerebral cortex in the intact human subject. Nature 1980; 285: 227.

79. Barker AT, Jalinous R, Freeston IL. Non-invasive magnetic stimulation of human motor cortex. Lancet 1985; 1: 1106–7.

80. Mills KR, Murray NM. Electrical stimulation over the human vertebral column: which neural elements are excited? Electroencephalogr Clin Neurophysiol 1986; 63: 582–9.

81. Swash M, Snooks SJ. Slowed motor conduction in lumbosacral nerve roots in cauda equina lesions: a new diagnostic technique. J Neurol Neurosurg Psychiatry 1986; 49: 808–16.

82. Bemelmans BLH, van Kerrebroeck EV, Debruyne FMJ. Motor bladder responses after magnetic stimulation of the cauda equina. Neurourol Urodyn 1991; 10: 380–1.

83. Sheriff MK, Shah PJ, Fowler C, et al. Neuromodulation of detrusor hyper-reflexia by functional magnetic stimulation of the sacral roots. Br J Urol 1996; 78: 39–46.

84. Vodusek DB, Zidar J. Perineal motor evoked responses. Neurourol Urodyn 1988; 7: 236–7.

85. Opsomer RJ, Caramia MD, Zarola F, Pesce F, Rossini PM. Neurophysiological evaluation of central–peripheral sensory and motor pudendal fibres. Electroencephalogr Clin Neurophysiol 1989; 74: 260–70.

86. Eardley I, Nagendran K, Lecky B, et al. Neurophysiology of the striated urethral sphincter in multiple sclerosis. Br J Urol 1991; 68: 81–8.

87. Brostrom S, Jennum P, Lose G. Motor evoked potentials from the striated urethral sphincter and puborectal muscle: normative values. Neurourol Urodyn 2003; 22: 306–13.

88. Brostrom S. Motor evoked potentials from the pelvic floor. Neurourol Urodyn 2003; 22: 620–37.

89. Brostrom S, Jennum P, Lose G. Motor evoked potentials from the striated urethral sphincter: a comparison of concentric needle and surface electrodes. Neurourol Urodyn 2003; 22: 123–9.

90. Lefaucheur J-P. Excitability of the motor cortical representation of the external anal sphincter. Exp Brain Res 2005; 160: 268–72.

91. Vodusek DB. Pudendal SEP and bulbocavernosus reflex in women. Electroencephalogr Clin Neurophysiol 1990; 77: 134–6.

92. Haldeman S, Bradley W, Bhatia N, et al. Cortical evoked potentials on stimulation of pudendal nerve in women. Urology 1983; 21: 590–3.

93. Vodusek DB. Pudendal somatosensory evoked potentials. Neurologija 1990; 39(Suppl 1): 149–55.

94. Guerit J, Opsomer R. Bit-mapped imagine of somatosensory evoked potentials after stimulation of the posterior tibial nerves and dorsal nerve of the penis/clitoris. Electroencephalogr Clin Neurophysiol 1991; 80: 228–37.

95. Rodi Z, Vodusek DB, Denislic M. Clinical uro-neurophysiological investigation in multiple sclerosis. Eur J Neurol 1996; 3: 574–80.

96. Vodusek DB, Deletis V, Abbott, R, et al. Prevention of iatrogenic micturition disorders through intraoperative monitoring. Neurourol Urodyn 1990; 9: 444–5.

97. Cohen BA, Major MR, Huizenga BA. Pudendal nerve evoked potential monitoring in procedures involving low sacral fixation. Spine 1991; 16(Suppl 8): S375–8.

98. Yang CC, Bowen JR, Kraft GH. Cortical evoked potentials of the dorsal nerve of the clitoris and female sexual dysfunction in multiple sclerosis. J Urol 2000; 164: 2010–13.

99. Curt A, Rodic B, Schurch B, Dietz V. Recovery of bladder function in patients with acute spinal cord injury: significance of ASIA scores and somatosensory evoked potentials. Spinal Cord 1997; 35: 368–73.

100. Malaguti S, Spinelli M, Giardiello G, et al. Neurophysiological evidence may predict the outcome of sacral neuromodulation. J Urol 2003; 170(6 Pt 1): 2323–6.

101. Delodovici ML, Fowler CJ. Clinical value of the pudendal somatosensory evoked potential. Electroencephalogr Clin Neurophysiol 1995; 96: 509–15.

102. Badr G, Fall M, Carlsson CA, et al. Cortical evoked potentials following stimulation of the urinary bladder in man. Electroencephalogr Clin Neurophysiol 1982; 54: 494–8.

103. Sarica Y, Karacan I. Bulbocavernosus reflex to somatic and visceral nerve stimulation in normal subjects and in diabetics with erectile impotence. J Urol 1987; 138: 55–8.

104. Hansen MV, Ertekin C, Larsson LE. Cerebral evoked potentials after stimulation of the posterior urethra in man. Electroencephalogr Clin Neurophysiol 1990; 77: 52–8.

105. Gaenzer H, Madersbacher H, Rumpl E. Cortical evoked potentials by stimulation of the vesicourethral junction: clinical value and neurophysiological considerations. J Urol 1991; 146: 118–23.

106. Loening-Baucke V, Read NW, Yamada T. Further evaluation of the afferent nervous pathways from the rectum. Am J Physiol 1992; 262(5 Pt 1): G927–33.

107. Wester C, FitzGerald MP, Brubaker L, Welgoss J, Benson JT. Validation of the clinical bulbocavernosus reflex. Neurourol Urodynam 2003; 22: 589–92.

108. Podnar S, Vodušek DB, Tršinar B, Rodi Z. A method of uroneurophysiological investigation in children. Electroenceph Clin Neurophysiol 1997; 104: 389–92.

109. Vodusek DB, Plevnik S, Vrtačnik P, Janež J. Detrusor inhibition on selective pudendal nerve stimulation in the perineum. Neurourol Urodyn 1988; 6: 389–93.

110. Contreras Ortiz O, Bertotti AC, Rodriguez Nunez JD. Pudendal reflexes in women with pelvic floor disorders. Zentralbl Gynaekol 1994; 116: 561–5.

111. Reitz A, Schmid DM, Curt A, Knapp PA, Schurch B. Afferent fibers of the pudendal nerve modulate sympathetic neurons controlling the bladder neck. Neurourol Urodyn 2003; 22: 597–601.

112. Fowler CJ, Betts CD. Clinical value of electrophysiological investigations of patients with urinary symptoms. In: Mundy AR, Stephenson TP, Wein AJ, eds. Urodynamics: Principles, Practice and Application, 2nd edn. Edinburgh: Churchill Livingstone, 1994: 165–81.

113. Benson JT. Clinical neurophysiologic techniques in urinary and fecal incontinence. In: Bent AE, ed. Ostergaard's Urogynecology and Pelvic Floor Dysfunction. Philadelphia: Lippincott Williams and Wilkins, 2003: 155–84.

114. Vodusek DB, Janko M. The bulbocavernosus reflex. A single motor neuron study. Brain 1990; 113(Pt 3): 813–20.

115. Rodi Z, Vodusek DB. The sacral reflex studies: single versus double pulse stimulation. Neurourol Urodyn 1995; 14: 496–7.

116. Rechthand E. Bilateral bulbocavernosus reflexes: crossing of nerve pathways or artifact? Muscle Nerve 1997; 20: 616–18.

117. Amarenco G, Kerdraon J. Clinical value of ipsi- and contralateral sacral reflex latency measurement: a normative data study in man. Neurourol Urodyn 2000; 19: 565–76.

118. Hanson P, Rigaux P, Gillard C, Biset E. Sacral reflex latencies in tethered cord syndrome. Am J Phys Med Rehabil 1993; 72: 39–43.

119. Vodušek DB, Deletis V, Abbott R, et al. Intraoperative monitoring of pudendal nerve function. In: Rother M, Zwiener U eds. Quantitative EEG analysis - clinical utility and new methods. Jena: Universitätsverlag Jena, 1993: 309–12.

120. Deletis V, Vodusek DB. Intraoperative recording of the bulbocavernosus reflex. Neurosurgery 1997; 40: 88–92; discussion 92–3.

121. Dykstra D, Sidi A, Cameron J, et al. The use of mechanical stimulation to obtain the sacral reflex latency: a new technique. J Urol 1987; 137: 77–9.

122. Shahani BT, Halperin JJ, Boulu P, Cohen J. Sympathetic skin response—a method of assessing unmyelinated axon dysfunction in peripheral neuropathies. J Neurol Neurosurg Psychiatry 1984; 47: 536–42.

123. Opsomer RJ, Pesce F, Abi-Aad A, et al. Electrophysiologic testing of motor sympathetic pathways: normative data and clinical contribution in neurourological disorders. Neurourol Urodyn 1993; 12: 336–8.

124. Ueda T, Yoshimura N, Yoshida O. Diabetic cystopathy: relationship to autonomic neuropathy detected by sympathetic skin response. J Urol 1997; 157: 580–4.

125. Schurch B, Curt A, Rossier AB. The value of sympathetic skin response recordings in the assessment of the vesicourethral autonomic nervous dysfunction in spinal cord injured patients. J Urol 1997; 157: 2230–3.

126. Rodic B, Curt A, Dietz V, Schurch B. Bladder neck incompetence in patients with spinal cord injury: significance of sympathetic skin response. J Urol 2000; 163: 1223–7.

127. Vodušek DB, Amarenco G, Batra A, et al. Committee 8: clinical neurophysiology. In: Abrams P, Cardozo L, Khoury S, Wein A, eds. Incontinence, Vol. 1. Basics & Evaluation, chapter 12. 3rd International Consultation on Incontinence, June 26–29, 2004. Health Publication Ltd., 2005: 675–706.

128. Podnar S. Sphincter electromyography and the penilo-cavernosus reflex: are both necessary? Neurourol Urodyn 2008; 27: 813–18.

34 Videourodynamics

Sender Herschorn and Blayne Welk

INTRODUCTION

Videourodynamics is a diagnostic tool that incorporates urodynamics with simultaneous imaging of the lower urinary tract. The incorporation of radiologic visualization of the lower urinary tract during bladder filling and voiding is useful for determining the site of bladder outlet obstruction, the integrity of the sphincter mechanism, and the presence of vesicoureteral reflux, bladder diverticula, fistulae, and trabeculation (1). Urodynamics was first synchronized with cineradiography in the early 1950s through the pioneering efforts of ER Miller (2–3). The initial goal was to minimize the radiation exposure to the patient during cystourethrography. Originally, patient exposure to radiation was high when movies were taken, but with the advent of image intensifiers, video transduction, and later videotape recording, the patient exposure was reduced. This permitted bursts of continuous activity to be recorded during critical phases of lower urinary tract activity without overexposing the patient. Today most studies can be done with less than one minute of fluoroscopy time (4). These developments have contributed to the wealth of information about lower urinary tract function and dysfunction. Modern videourodynamic techniques incorporate fluoroscopy with the evolution of the urodynamic machine from a strip chart recorder to a microcomputer.

Videourodynamic studies are not necessary in every patient and simpler studies frequently provide enough information to adequately delineate and treat the dysfunction. Videourodynamic studies are beneficial when simultaneous evaluation of function and anatomy are needed to provide detailed information about the whole or parts of the storage and emptying phases. Common indications well suited for videourodynamic evaluation include complex incontinence, where the history does not fit with the findings on preliminary investigations; incontinence when there has been previous anti-incontinence surgery; and incontinence in the face of a neurologic abnormality. Videourodynamic can help characterize the degree of hypermobility in women with stress incontinence and identify the level of outlet obstruction in both men and woman.

Aside from the minimal radiation exposure to the patient, the only disadvantage of videourodynamics is its cost. This is a result of the time and effort of the personnel required and the expense of the equipment which may limit its utility to larger centers with larger patient populations. The cost can, however, be justified by its utility in solving complicated problems. The patient generally tolerates the study well, and videourodynamic studies are associated with only minimal to moderate anxiety, pain, and embarrassment (5). In this chapter the procedures are outlined, examples of the applications are provided and the limitations discussed.

COMPONENTS OF VIDEOURODYNAMICS

A typical arrangement for videourodynamic studies includes a multichannel recorder, a flouroscopy unit with a table that can be positioned in the supine and upright position, and a flow meter (Fig. 34.1). A commode seat attachment facilitates fluoroscopic screening of voiding in the seated position, which is ideal for women. Most modern systems are computer based, which allows for complex analysis to be performed. A schematic diagram of the setup is in Figure 34.2.

Multichannel Recorder

As the procedure involves measuring simultaneous pressures during both phases of lower urinary tract function and flow during the voiding phase, a multichannel recorder is necessary (Fig. 34.3). Many systems are available (6), most of which have dispensed with a strip chart output in favor of television monitor display of the procedure.

The choice of components of the study is up to the individual clinician. Figure 34.2 illustrates possible inclusions. The channels demonstrating volume of fluid instilled and volume voided are helpful but not essential, as these can be measured manually. The sphincter electromyography (EMG) channel is not necessary for routine clinical practice but can be helpful in patients with neurologic disease; its inclusion introduces another level of complexity and sophistication.

Controversy exists regarding the use of subtracted detrusor pressure (Pdet) versus intravesical pressure (Pves), although most reports at present use the subtracted pressures (Pves minus the intra-abdominal pressure). Bladder pressures can only be recorded using a pressure line in the bladder. This pressure is affected by intra-abdominal pressure, which can be measured separately by a rectal catheter. Increases in intra-abdominal pressure can result from straining, the upright position, and other provocative activities such as coughing, jumping, and heel jouncing. In order to get an accurate recording of bladder pressure and to eliminate the effect of intra-abdominal pressure, Bates et al. (7) emphasized the value of electronically subtracting the intra-abdominal pressure from the Pves. However, even with the patient quiescent and totally co-operative, artifacts may be produced by intrinsic rectal contractions (4) since the bladder pressure is derived from the electronic subtraction. On the other hand, McGuire et al. (8) did not measure rectal or abdominal pressure (Pabd) with a separate catheter. They monitored urethral pressure along with bladder pressure via two lumens of the same catheter. They stated that urethral pressure reflects rectal or Pabd allowing them to differentiate bladder contractions from abdominal straining. In our unit, we use subtracted Pdets.

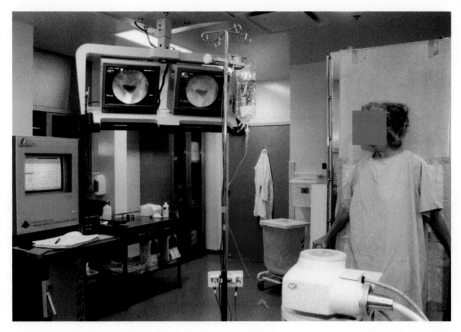

Figure 34.1 A videourodynamic suite. The patient's bladder has been filled and she is in the upright position after the filling catheter has been removed. She will be asked to cough and strain to demonstrate stress incontinence and then to void. The study will be stored on the multichannel recorder.

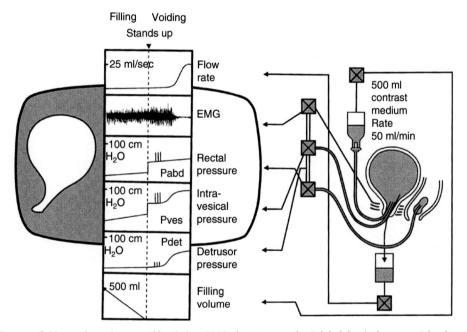

Figure 34.2 Schematic diagram of videourodynamic setup. *Abbreviations:* EMG, electromyography; Pabd, abdominal pressure; Pdet, detrusor pressure; Pves, intravesical pressure.

Urine Flow Meters

Flow meters are commonly of one of three types: weight, electronic dip-stick, or rotating disc (9). The first measures the weight of the collected urine; the second measures the changes in electrical capacitance of a dip-stick mounted in the collecting chamber; and the third measures the power required to keep a rotating disc rotating at a constant speed while the urine, which tends to slow it down, is directed towards it. A commode chair with uroflow is in Figure 34.4. All three can provide sensitive and reproducible data. The voided volume

should not be <150 ml, and the bladder should not be overly distended, as either of these conditions will make the flow rate difficult to interpret without a nomogram (10).

Fluoroscopy

A good quality fluoroscopy unit with a high resolution image intensifier and a table that can function in both the supine and erect positions is required. Fluoroscopic images are obtained selectively during the filling and voiding study and are either superimposed on the pressure-flow tracing or displayed on a

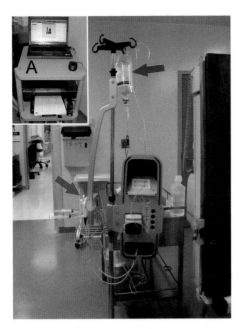

Figure 34.3 Multichannel urodynamic recorder. Pressures are measured with external pressure transducers (red arrow) monitoring rectal abdominal pressure (Pabd) and total abdominal or intravesical pressure (Pves). Bladder filling is through a separate catheter from the IV bag (blue arrow). The results are transmitted to a computer and printed (inset A).

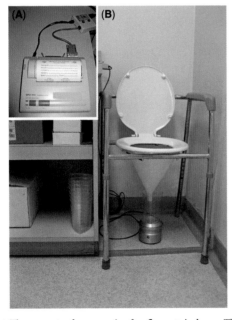

Figure 34.4 The apparatus for measuring free flow rate is shown. The recorder that measures the flow rate and computes the various parameters of the flow is shown in (**A**). The patient sits or stands to void into the machine (**B**). The urine goes through the funnel into the collection beaker. The change in weight in the load cell is measured and converted to urine flow rate, volume, and other parameters which are printed out automatically.

separate screen. The fluoroscopic images can be stored and reproduced individually or as continuous clips during key parts of the study. A recording of the procedure can be made for subsequent review.

Since the contrast medium instilled into bladder is unlikely to be absorbed we generally use the less expensive high osmolality contrast media. A dilute solution of one liter of hypaque is prepared by the pharmacy and supplied in sterile intravenous bags.

VIDEOURODYNAMIC TECHNIQUE

The patient reports for the study with a full bladder and a flow rate is obtained. The equipment is zeroed and the transducer is placed at a height adjacent to the upper edge of the patient's symphysis pubis. Either a double lumen catheter or two 8 F feeding tubes (one for filling which is removed prior to the voiding study and one for pressure measurements) are inserted into the bladder. Residual urine is measured. The 42 cm, 14 Fr rectal catheter has a balloon over the tip. If desired, EMG recording devices may be applied to the patient.

The study is conducted by a urodynamics specialist who is present in the room, communicating with the patient throughout the procedure, and records the findings manually and electronically. A supine or semi-oblique filling study is carried out and various measurements are taken during the study and responses to actions such as credé, cough, and valsalva are recorded. The filling rate is no longer divided into slow, medium, or fast; rather, it is described as physiologic or non-physiologic (11). In practice, most clinicians use a medium fill rate of 50 to 75 cc per minute (12). The bladder is filled, emptied, and then refilled in the patient's usual voiding position (lying, sitting, or standing). Two bladder fillings are usually done since decreased compliance may be a result of the medium filling (13) and a second test verifies it. The upright position of the second filling is also a provocative test for overactivity (12). Additional responses to credé, cough, and valsalva are again recorded. Another commonly used method is to fill the bladder only once supine and stand the patient up for provocative manoeuvres.

During the study, recordings are made of bladder images in the filling phase in the supine and/or in the upright positions (Fig. 34.3). Antero-posterior (AP) and oblique views are obtained. The AP position permits documentation of reflux and its extent, and in the oblique position the course of the urethra can be seen separate from a cystocele. Vesicoureteral reflux may be a primary issue, or secondary to bladder dysfunction. If it is present at low filling volumes it suggests the ureter and renal pelvis may be acting as a "pelvic organ prolapse (POP) off valve" and compensating for a poorly compliant bladder. This means the urodynamic study will record a falsely low Pdet and increase the measured "bladder" capacity.

Note is made of the bladder outline, the appearance of the bladder neck at rest, and its position relative to the inferior margin of the symphysis at rest and with straining and coughing. Leakage of urine with overactivity, decreased compliance, or with various stress maneuvers is recorded. In the upright position, the presence of a cystocele and its relationship to the urethra are also noted. If the patient is able to void in front of the camera, the voiding phase (or parts of it) are recorded along with the pressures and flow tracings. If the patient is unable to void with the catheters in place, they are removed and a flow rate and a voided volume are measured. Total fluoroscopy time is usually less than one minute.

The recorded study provides an opportunity for the case to be reviewed and discussed. All of the events of the study are recorded and displayed on the monitor during the study. The urodynamic machine is usually equipped with the capability of compressing the study so that it can be viewed on an ordinary letter size sheet of paper.

TESTS PERFORMED
Urinary Flow Rate

A urinary flow rate is a simple urodynamic test that can provide objective and quantitative measures on both storage and voiding symptoms (14). An abnormal pattern is generated in the presence of a weak detrusor, abdominal straining, or bladder outlet obstruction. Although the urodynamic catheters have less effect on voiding patterns in females than males, it is still useful to obtain a urinary flow rate on arrival that may be compared with the flow data generated during the urodynamic study.

The flow rate has not been well studied or standardized in females. In addition, varying degrees of prolapse of the bladder base can influence the urine's velocity. While a peak urine flow rate >30 ml/sec can rule out urodynamic bladder outlet obstruction, a reduced urine flow does not always correlate with urodynamic bladder outlet obstruction (15).

After the initial flow is completed, a post void residual (PVR) can be determined on introduction of the urodynamic catheters. A high PVR raises the possibility of bladder dysfunction. In the female urinary incontinence population, 16% of women had a PVR >100 ml (16).

Cystometry

The first part of the filling study is cystometry, the method by which the pressure-volume relationship of the bladder is measured (11). It is used to assess sensation, detrusor overactivity, compliance, and capacity. The Pdet is calculated by subtraction of the Pabd, as measured by a balloon in the rectum, vagina, or bowel stoma, from the total Pves, as measured by the intravesical catheter. The subtracted Pdet reflects the activity and pressures generated by the detrusor muscle alone. Artifacts in the Pdet may be produced by intrinsic rectal contractions, movement of the cathéters, or the patient (12).

Sensation during cystometry is variable, and is influenced by the fill rate, fluid temperature, and patient position and anxiety. The terminology to describe detrusor activity has been standardized by the International Continence Society (11). *Detrusor overactivity* is characterized by spontaneous or provoked involuntary detrusor contractions during filling. Although an involuntary contraction was originally defined as a minimum pressure rise of 15 cm water (17), there is presently no lower limit for the amplitude of an involuntary contraction (11). When leakage is detected in association with an involuntary detrusor contraction, it is termed *detrusor overactivity incontinence*. *Detrusor overactivity* can be further characterized into *idiopathic* and *neurogenic detrusor overactivity*. *Idiopathic detrusor overactivity* describes involuntary detrusor contractions of unknown etiology and has replaced the term *detrusor instability*. An involunatary detrusor contraction secondary to an underlying neurologic condition is *neurogenic detrusor overactivity*, which has replaced *detrusor hyperreflexia* (11).

The finding of detrusor overactivity on cystometry is important if it correlates with the clinical condition of the patient. Idiopathic detrusor overactivity has been reported in 30% to 35% of patients with stress incontinence undergoing surgery. It resolves in the majority following repairs and does not have a significant impact on outcomes (18–19). Alternatively, if the patient's symptoms are primarily from bladder overactivity or other factors predisposing to abnormal bladder behavior are present the cystometric findings will influence treatment. These include a history of radiation, chronic bladder inflammation, indwelling catheter, chronic infection, chemotherapy, voiding dysfunction following pelvic surgery, or other neurological conditions.

Another type of overactive bladder dysfunction is reduced compliance. *Bladder compliance* is defined as the change in pressure for a given change in volume. It is calculated by dividing the volume change by the change in Pdet during that change in bladder volume, and is expressed as ml per cmH_2O (11). Normal bladder compliance is high and in the laboratory the normal pressure rise is <6 to 10 cm water (4). Low bladder compliance implies a poorly distensible bladder. The actual numeric values to indicate normal, high, or low compliance have yet to be defined (11). Bladder capacity can refer to several different measurements. Functional bladder capacity refers to the maximal volume voided on a voiding diary. Urodynamic capacity refers to the maximum capacity during filling cystography beyond which the patient can no longer postpone voiding. Maximum anesthetic capacity refers to the bladder capacity when filled to a standard pressure under general anesthesia.

Leak Point Pressures

The valsalva or abdominal leak point pressure (VLPP or ALPP) is the Pves that exceeds the continence mechanism resulting in a leakage of urine in the absence of a detrusor contraction (11). This is performed by a progressive valsalva maneuver (producing a smooth pressure rise) or cough (producing a sharp pressure rise) (20). In our center we perform both of these maneuvers at maximal cystometric capacity; urodynamic reproduction of incontinence may be better with valsalva for women with detrusor overactivity, and cough for women with stress urinary incontinence (SUI) (21). VLPP tests the strength of the urethra. The study is performed in the sitting or standing position with at least 150 to 200 ml of fluid in the bladder. Historically, a VLPP of <60 cmH_2O was evidence of significant intrinsic sphincter deficiency (ISD), between 60 and 90 cmH_2O suggested a component of ISD, and >90 cmH_2O suggested minimal ISD with leakage mainly due to hypermobility (4). Currently, no prospective studies have shown that VLPP <60 can accurately diagnose ISD. The VLPP has been shown to be reproducible (22) but has not yet been standardized.

There are limitations to a VLPP. If the patient's valsalva effort is inadequate, or there is an abdominal hernia urinary leakage may not be seen and thus a VLPP cannot be determined. A cystocele may produce inferior pressure on an incompetent urethra that will prevent incontinence or falsely

323

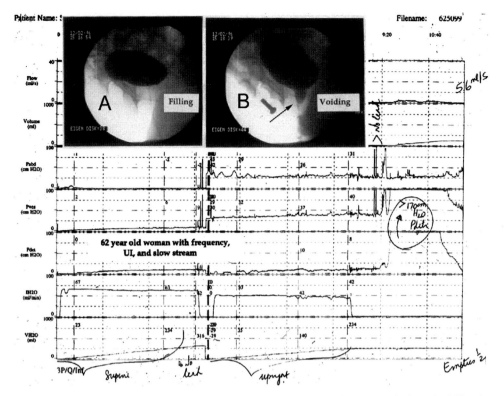

Figure 34.5 Videourodynamic study of a 62-year-old woman with urgency, frequency, and slow stream following multiple urethral dilatations. The study shows no detrusor overactivity on filling. Her voiding pressure exceeds 170 cmH$_2$O and her flow rate is low. There is a urethral stricture visible (arrow in B) with proximal urethral dilatation. *Abbreviatons*: Pabd, abdominal pressure; Pdet, detrusor pressure; Pves, intravesical pressure, UI, urinary incontinence; IH$_2$O, infused rate of water pumped into the bladder; VH$_2$O, volume of water infused.

elevate the VLPP. When a cystocele is present the VLPP should be repeated with the prolapse reduced by insertion of a vaginal pack or pessary.

The detrusor or bladder leak point pressure (DLPP) is the Pdet at which urinary leakage occurs during bladder filling on cystometry. This parameter is used to investigate and follow patients with neurogenic and low compliant bladders. In general, patients with a DLPP greater than approximately 25 to 40 cmH$_2$O are at risk for upper tract deterioration from reflux or obstruction (23–24). In these patients it is necessary to assess compliance as well. A high DLPP indicates poor compliance with urethral obstruction whereas a low DLPP is seen in patients with incompetent urethras. In order to demonstrate poor compliance in these patients filling may be done with a Foley catheter to obstruct the outlet (25).

Pressure-Flow Studies

Pressure-flow studies are designed to provide dynamic information on the emptying phase of lower urinary tract function. Obstruction is not common in females (26) but may be found after surgical correction of SUI and less commonly with detrusor sphincter dyssynergia in patients with a neurological lesion, pseudodyssynergia (related to dysfunctional voiding) (27), primary bladder neck obstruction, and rarely stricture disease. Primary bladder neck dysfunction can be diagnosed with the presence of cystographic obstruction at the bladder neck during voiding, and a maximal flow rate <15 ml/sec with a Pdet at maximal flow >20 cmH$_2$O (28). Interference with voiding may also be associated with POP. Although there are no established nomograms to depict pressure/flow in women as

there are in men, the pattern of high Pdet and low urinary flow indicates obstruction (Fig. 34.5).

Pdet during voiding is characteristically low in females. A preoperative study that demonstrates a low Pdet with a low flow rate may aid in counseling the patient about postoperative urinary retention after stress incontinence surgery.

EMG

Sphincter EMG during videourodynamics is used to examine striated sphincter activity during filling and voiding. These are termed kinesiologic studies and can be performed with surface electrodes, vaginal or anal probes, and needles. Normal sphincter EMG activity has characteristic audio quality that may be monitored simultaneously. Its most important role is the identification of abnormal sphincter activity in patients with neurogenic bladder dysfunction and in those with behavioral voiding dysfunction (29). The fluoroscopy component however can demonstrate detrusor external sphincter dyssynergia in patients with suprasacral lesions and can show urethral obstruction in patients with dysfunctional voiding. EMG recordings are not usually necessary in routine videourodynamics for incontinence in females who have no neurologic abnormalities. Artifacts can be secondary to room appliances, fluorescent lights, defective insulation, and patient movement (4).

INDICATIONS WITH EXAMPLES
Urinary Incontinence
The main advantage of fluoroscopic imaging during the urodynamic study is to obtain an anatomic view of the function or dysfunction. The technique is ideally suited to evaluation of

Table 34.1 Radiologic Type of Stress Incontinence (30)

Type 0	Vesical neck and proximal urethra closed at rest and situated at or above the lower end of the symphysis pubis. They descend during stress but incontinence is not seen
Type I	Vesical neck closed at rest and is well above the inferior margin of the symphysis. During stress the vesical neck and proximal urethra open and descend <2 cm. Incontinence is seen
Type IIa	Vesical neck closed at rest and is above the inferior margin of the symphysis. During stress the vesical neck and proximal urethra open and descend >2 cm. Incontinence is seen
Type IIb	Vesical neck closed at rest and is at or below the inferior margin of the symphysis. During stress there may or may not be further descent but as the proximal urethra opens incontinence is seen
Type III	Vesical neck and proximal urethra are open at rest. The proximal urethra no longer functions as a sphincter. There is obvious urinary leakage with minimal increases in intravesical pressure

incontinence. A useful anatomic/radiologic classification of female incontinence, devised by Blaivas (30), is described in Table 34.1 and illustrated in Figure 34.6. We have used this classification to determine the radiologic abnormality and add to it the information from the VLPP and the position of the urethra in relation to the cystocele to describe the functional problem. Each of the following urodynamic tracings in the figures is shown in full with annotations made during the study. The video recordings depicting parts of the studies were obtained from video printer connected to the fluoroscopy. Although the classification is used less frequently now it may still be useful to assess the degree of hypermobility associated with stress incontinence.

Mild hypermobility (type I abnormality) is illustrated in Figure 34.7 where the patient has a VLPP of 62 cmH$_2$O and minimal hypermobility. The patient in Figure 34.8 has a VLPP of >120 cmH$_2$O on straining during upright filling. At the end of filling a cough caused a large leak without much hypermobility and appears to be accompanied by a small bladder contraction. This indicates that she has stress incontinence as well as cough induced overactivity.

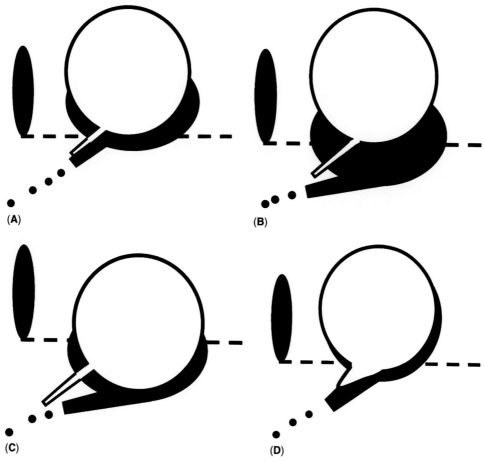

(A) **(B)**

(C) **(D)**

Figure 34.6 Radiologic images of the various types of female stress urinary incontinence. (**A**) Type I. The bladder neck is closed at rest and is well above the inferior margin of the symphysis. During stress, the bladder neck and proximal urethra open and descend <2 cm and incontinence is seen. (**B**) Type IIa. The bladder neck is closed at rest and is above the inferior margin of the symphysis. During stress the bladder neck and proximal urethra open and descend >2 cm. Incontinence is seen. (**C**) Type IIb. The bladder neck is closed at rest and is at or below the inferior margin of the symphysis. During stress there may or may not be further descent but as the proximal urethra opens, incontinence is seen. (**D**) Type III. The bladder neck and proximal urethra are open at rest. The proximal urethra no longer functions as a sphincter. There is obvious urinary leakage with minimal increases in intravesical pressure.

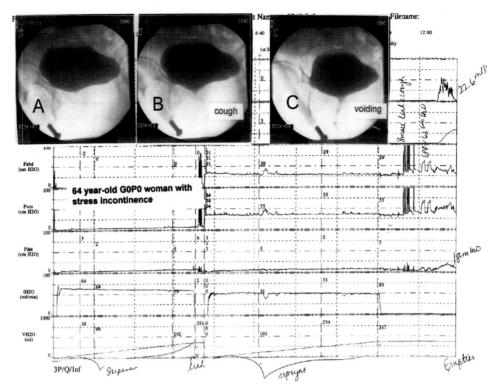

Figure 34.7 Videourodynamic study of a 64-year-old G4P4 woman with stress incontinence and a mild degree of hypermobility (type I). She has a bladder capacity of >300 cc. The bladder neck is slightly open at rest (A). With coughing there is a small amount of descent and her VLPP is 62 cmH$_2$O (**B**). She has no apparent cystocele and her voiding phase is normal (**C**). *Abbreviatons*: Pabd, abdominal pressure; Pdet, detrusor pressure; Pves, intravesical pressure, VLPP, valsalva leak point pressure; IH$_2$O, infused rate of water pumped into the bladder; VH$_2$O, volume of water infused.

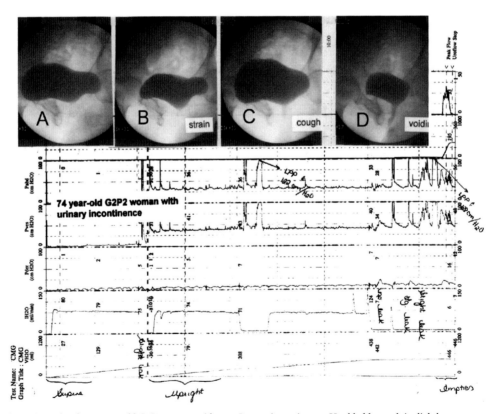

Figure 34.8 Videourodynamic study of a 74-year-old G2P2 woman with type I stress incontinence. Her bladder neck is slightly open at rest (**A**). In the upright position (**B**) she leaks with straining and a VLPP of 122 cmH$_2$O. She also leaks with coughing (**C**). Her voiding is normal (**D**). *Abbreviatons*: Pabd, abdominal pressure; Pdet, detrusor pressure; Pves, intravesical pressure, VLPP, valsalva leak point pressure; IH$_2$O, infused rate of water pumped into the bladder; VH$_2$O, volume of water infused.

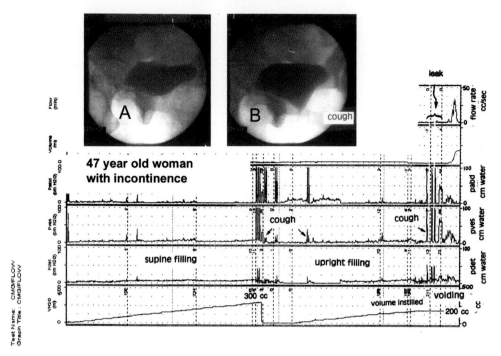

Figure 34.9 Videourodynamic study of a 47-year-old G1P1 woman with stress incontinence and moderate hypermobility (type IIa). Her bladder neck is open at rest (**A**). Leakage and hypermobility is seen with coughing (**B**). *Abbreviatons*: Pabd, abdominal pressure; Pdet, detrusor pressure; Pves, intravesical pressure; IH$_2$O, infused rate of water pumped into the bladder; VH$_2$O, volume of water infused.

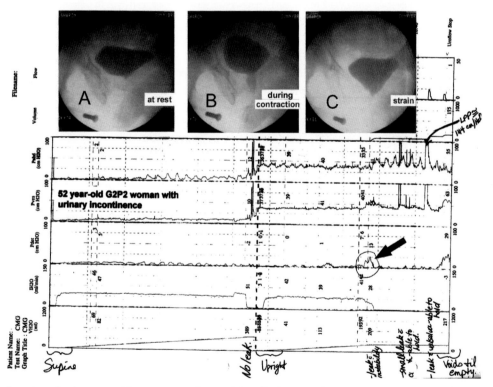

Figure 34.10 Videourodynamic study of a 52-year-old G2P2 woman who complains of both stress and urgency incontinence. The bladder neck is slightly open at rest (**A**). She has an uninhibited contraction (arrow) on upright filling that results in incontinence (**B**). With straining she leaks with a VLPP of >140 cmH$_2$O (**C**) and has moderate hypermobility (type IIa). *Abbreviatons*: Pabd, abdominal pressure; Pdet, detrusor pressure; Pves, intravesical pressure, VLPP, valsalva leak point pressure; IH$_2$O, infused rate of water pumped into the bladder; VH$_2$O, volume of water infused.

Figures 34.9 to 34.11 demonstrate moderate hypermobility (type IIa abnormalities). The patient in Figure 34.9 has a high VLPP without any appreciable cystocele. In Figure 34.10, the patient has an involuntary detrusor contraction with incontinence in the upright position and a high VLPP. The patient shown in Figure 34.11 has a grade II cystocele that appears with straining. She probably has mainly a lateral defect.

327

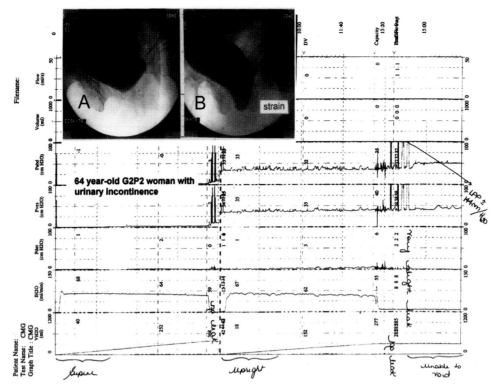

Figure 34.11 Videourodynamic study of a 64-year-old G2P2 woman with stress incontinence. Her bladder neck is above the lower margin of the symphysis on upright filling (A) and with straining (B) she leaks with a VLPP of 144 cmH$_2$O and a cystocele is demonstrated (type IIa). She most likely has mainly a lateral defect. *Abbreviatons*: Pabd, abdominal pressure; Pdet, detrusor pressure; Pves, intravesical pressure, VLPP, valsalva leak point pressure; IH$_2$O, infused rate of water pumped into the bladder; VH$_2$O, volume of water infused.

A different kind of hypermobility in which the bladder neck is positioned below the lower margin of the symphysis (type IIb) is shown in Figures 34.12 to 34.14. The bladder neck in Figure 34.12 is seen well below the lower margin of the symphysis and is associated with a grade II cystocele. Since the bladder neck is above the base of the cystocele, but below the lower margin of the symphysis, the patient most likely has a combined central and lateral defect. In Figure 34.13, the large cystocele is not associated with demonstrable stress incontinence, despite coughing and straining pressures of >100 cmH$_2$O. It appears to be primarily a central defect. Clinical examination must include reducing the cystocele and checking for stress incontinence. The patient in Figure 34.14 has a combined central and lateral defect. She has marked detrusor overactivity with leakage but stress incontinence is not demonstrated most likely because of the compressive effect of the cystocele.

SUI without hypermobility (type III) or that strongly associated with ISD is demonstrated by the patient in Figure 34.15. Her bladder neck is open at rest, no appreciable descent is seen with coughing or straining and her VLPP is low at 59 cmH$_2$O.

The clinical utility of the Blaivas Classification (30) is now less in the era of mid-urethral slings. A simpler approach is to classify patients on the presence or absence of hypermobility. The degree of hypermobility can still be ascertained with videourodynamics as illustrated with the case examples.

Neurogenic Bladder Dysfunction
Videourodynamics can be helpful in assessing bladder dysfunction patients with neurologic disorders. Since incontinence

and upper tract dilatation can be prevented and treated by achieving low-pressure bladder storage and emptying (19,26), the urodynamic study provides a framework for treatment. Anatomic abnormalities can also be correlated with pressure changes.

Examples of neurogenic problems are shown in Figures 34.16 to 34.18. Since the flow rate is not measured in Figures 34.16 and 34.17 fewer channels are used during the study.

The patient in Figure 34.16 has a small capacity overactive but compliant bladder with grade I left vesicoureteral reflux. Her main problem was incontinence between catheterizations and she was treated with anticholinergics and upper tract monitoring. The patient in Figure 34.17 has a markedly trabeculated overactive bladder with filling pressures of >100 cmH$_2$O. The study demonstrates detrusor external sphincter dyssynergia with an open bladder neck and tight sphincter. She also had bilateral hydronephrosis on upper tract imaging and required an augmentation cystoplasty for management. Since she was quadriplegic a continent abdominal stoma was brought from the augmentation to the umbilicus to permit self-intermittent catheterization.

The patient in Figure 34.18 developed increasing hydronephrosis and elevated creatinine after insertion of an artificial sphincter for urinary incontinence. She had previously undergone multiple bilateral ureteral reimplants for reflux. The study shows a bladder with poor compliance and gross bilateral reflux. The refluxing ureters probably dampen the bladder pressure thus improving the appearance of the compliance curve. She was treated with an augmentation cystoplasty.

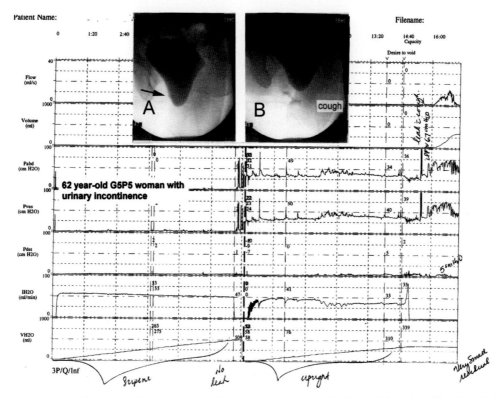

Figure 34.12 Videourodynamic study of a 62-year-old G5P5 woman with stress incontinence. Her bladder neck (arrow) on filling (**A**) is below the lower margin of the inferior symphysis and a cystocele is seen (type IIb). She most likely has a combined central and lateral defect. She has leakage with coughing (**B**) and a VLPP of 62 cmH2O on straining. *Abbreviatons*: Pabd, abdominal pressure; Pdet, detrusor pressure; Pves, intravesical pressure, VLPP, valsalva leak point pressure; IH$_2$O, infused rate of water pumped into the bladder; VH$_2$O, volume of water infused.

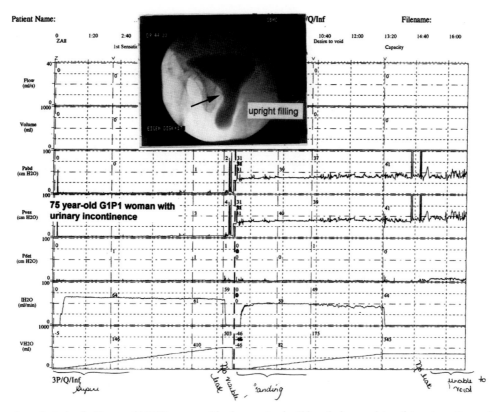

Figure 34.13 Videourodynamic study of a 75-year-old G1P1 woman with a large cystocele. Although she complains of stress incontinence it is not visible on this study. Her bladder neck (arrow) is at the lower margin of the symphysis. The cystocele appears primarily to be a central defect. Clinical evaluation must include reducing the cystocele and testing for stress incontinence. *Abbreviatons*: Pabd, abdominal pressure; Pdet, detrusor pressure; Pves, intravesical pressure; IH$_2$O, infused rate of water pumped into the bladder; VH$_2$O, volume of water infused.

329

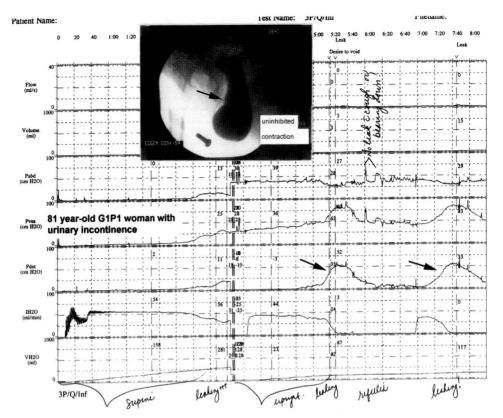

Figure 34.14 Videourodynamic study of an 81-year-old G1P1 woman with a central and lateral defect. The bladder neck is below the symphysis (arrow). She has marked detrusor overactivity on supine and upright filling (arrows). Although she complains of stress, in addition to urge incontinence, it is not demonstrated on this study. *Abbreviatons*: Pabd, abdominal pressure; Pdet, detrusor pressure; Pves, intravesical pressure; IH₂O, infused rate of water pumped into the bladder; VH₂O, volume of water infused.

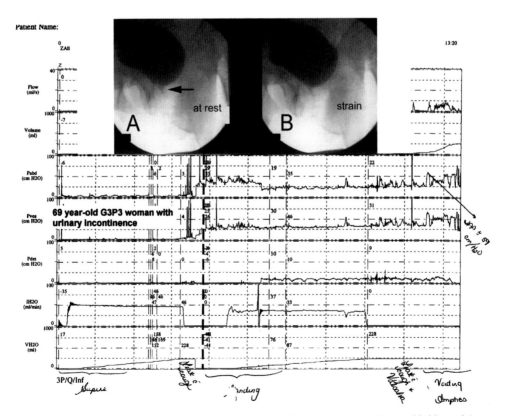

Figure 34.15 Videourodynamic study of a 69-year-old G3P3 woman stress incontinence after two previous repairs. Her bladder neck is open at rest (arrow in **A**). On straining (**B**) there is almost no urethral movement on straining and her VLPP is 59 cmH₂O (type III). *Abbreviatons*: Pabd, abdominal pressure; Pdet, detrusor pressure; Pves, intravesical pressure, VLPP, valsalva leak point pressure; IH₂O, infused rate of water pumped into the bladder; VH₂O, volume of water infused.

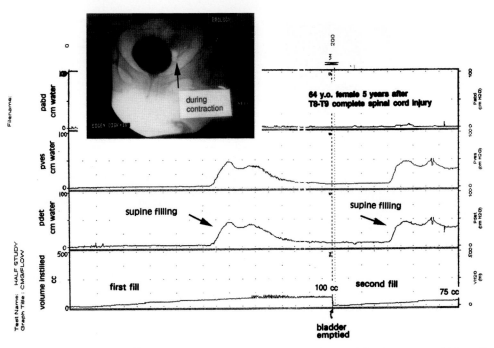

Figure 34.16 Videourodynamic study of a 64-year-old woman five years after a T8–9 spinal cord injury following a motor vehicle accident. She has left vesicoureteral reflux (arrow) seen during an involuntary detrusor contraction (arrows). *Abbreviatons*: Pabd, abdominal pressure; Pdet, detrusor pressure; Pves, intravesical pressure; VH₂O, volume of water infused.

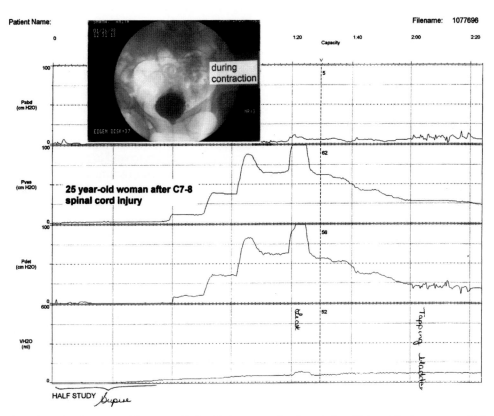

Figure 34.17 Videourodynamic study of a 25-year-old woman with C7–8 lesion 16 months after spinal cord injury following a motor vehicle accident. She needed an indwelling catheter for repeated attacks of autonomic dysreflexia and her upper tracts showed marked bilateral hydronephrosis. Her bladder is markedly trabeculated and during contractions of >75 to 100 cmH2O her external sphincter remains tight consistent with detrusor sphincter dyssynergia. She was subsequently treated with an ileal augmentation cystoplasty and a continent abdominal stoma. *Abbreviatons*: Pabd, abdominal pressure; Pdet, detrusor pressure; Pves, intravesical pressure; VH₂O, volume of water infused.

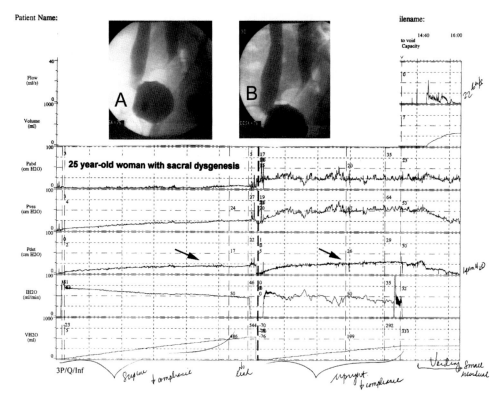

Figure 34.18 Videourodynamic study of a 25-year-old woman with sacral dysgenesis. She had an artificial sphincter inserted for urinary incontinence at age 14 and then developed bilateral vesicoureteral reflux unresponsive to multiple ureteral reimplantations. The study shows decreased bladder compliance on filling (arrows). She has gross bilateral reflux and a small capacity bladder. The reflux most likely dampens the poor compliance measurement. She subsequently underwent augmentation ileal cystoplasty and bilateral reimplants. *Abbreviatons*: Pabd, abdominal pressure; Pdet, detrusor pressure; Pves, intravesical pressure; IH$_2$O, infused rate of water pumped into the bladder; VH$_2$O, volume of water infused.

Obstruction

Although outflow obstruction is uncommon in females (27), it is occasionally seen. The patient in Figure 34.4 had an iatrogenic and functionally significant urethral obstruction that was treated with a visual internal urethrotomy and subsequent long-term self-dilation.

Complex Problems

Videourodynamics allows for the identification and characterization of a pathologic process that can be associated with complex voiding dysfunction, including reflux, diverticula, fistulas, and stones (4). The patient in Figure 34.19 had a fistula at the anastomosis between an ileal neobladder and the urethra after a cystectomy for bladder cancer. The study was done with a catheter obstructing the bladder neck to test the compliance. The neobladder itself was compliant, had no overactivity, and was not contributing to the incontinence. No urethral leakage was seen with stress. All of the contrast emanated through the vagina. She was successfully treated with a transvaginal fistula repair with an interposition labial fat pad flap.

PITFALLS OF VIDEOURODYNAMICS

Patient co-operation, comfort, and compliance are necessary in order to obtain a meaningful and relevant study. Occasionally apprehensive patients will have a vasovagal reflex and faint when the table is moved from the supine to the upright position and the study cannot be completed.

Stress incontinence may not be demonstrated due to the patient's anxiety, the urethral catheter, or the abnormal environment Of 2259 studies that we reviewed in our laboratory for neurologically normal women whose chief complaint was stress incontinence, we were unable to demonstrate stress incontinence on fluoroscopy in 630 (28%). It is also difficult for many patients to void in front of the camera with catheters in the bladder and rectum and observers watching them. In our series, only 1348 patients (59.7%) were able to void and some of these did so with abdominal straining. The others were unable to void during the procedure and the voiding data was obtained from the uroflow.

To optimize visibility of the lower urinary tract on fluoroscopy patient positioning must be correct. However, visibility may be poor or absent with very obese patients, or those with anatomic limitations to their positioning. The clinician must also maintain a dialogue with the patient to image crucial events as the patient must relay changes in sensation during filling and may be the first to sense incontinence.

The radiation equipment must be well maintained and undergo regular maintenance and safety inspections. The failure to maintain equipment may lead to inaccurate results. Since fluoroscopy time is short, radiation exposure to the patient is inconsequential; however, the clinician should use radiation protection including aprons and thyroid shields.

Other pitfalls relate to the urodynamic aspects and are similar to those previously outlined by O'Donnell (31). Standardized terminology to communicate results and concepts should

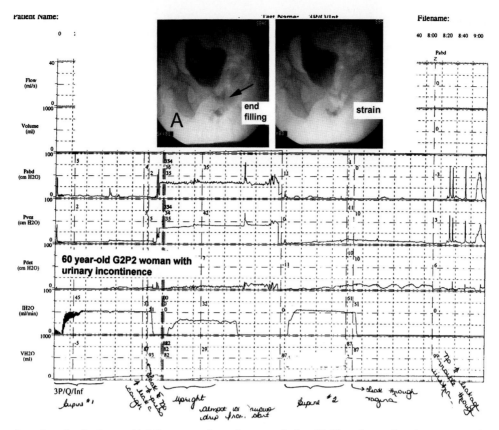

Figure 34.19 Videourodynamic study of a 60-year-old G2P2 woman who underwent an ileal neobladder to her urethra after cystectomy for muscle invasive carcinoma of the bladder. The study was done with a foley catheter blocking the urethra to test compliance (A) which is normal. All of the leakage was demonstrated to exit the fistula at the anastomosis (arrow in A). She underwent a transvaginal fistula repair with a martius labial fat pad flap. *Abbreviatons*: Pabd, abdominal pressure; Pdet, detrusor pressure; Pves, intravesical pressure; IH$_2$O, infused rate of water pumped into the bladder; VH$_2$O, volume of water infused.

always be used (11). The testing procedures and equipment should be compatible with commonly accepted methodologies. The value and limitations of each measurement must be realized that is the VLPP may not be useful in the presence of a large prolapsing cystocele. To confirm reliability within a particular laboratory, it is necessary to have a high test-retest correlation of studies. The validity of a test refers to its ability to measure what it is supposed to measure. The clinician must always be aware of the how it compares to a "gold standard" test, which in urodynamics may be difficult to establish. The urodynamic studies should correlate with other clinical data. The voiding history, physical examination, endoscopic examination, and videourodynamic evaluation should serve to validate one another and strengthen the clinical assessment.

FUTURE DEVELOPMENTS

Videourodynamic techniques have evolved over the years with improvements in technology and refinements in the concepts of lower urinary tract structure, function, treatment. There are exciting developments in other newer imaging technologies. Ultrasound can be used during urodynamic studies but the vaginal probe may alter bladder neck position and perineal probes are undergoing investigation (32). Magnetic resonance imaging has provided significant advances in knowledge about the pelvic floor (33), but it is carried out in the supine position and interventional MR has not yet been adapted to the technique. Near-infrared spectroscopy is a noninvasive technique

that relies on transcutaneous lasers to measure changes in oxyhemoglobin and deoxyhemoglobin concentrations within the detrusor muscle. Early studies have shown differences in oxygenation of the detrusor in obstructed bladders versus nonobstructed bladders (34). Videourodynamic testing when indicated is still as applicable today as when they were first developed more than 50 years ago.

REFERENCES

1. Blaivas JG. Techniques of evaluation. In: Yalla SV, McGuire EJ, Elbadawi A, Blaivas JG, eds. Neurourology and Urodynamics, Principles and Practice. New York: Macmillan, 1988: 166–74.
2. Miller E. The beginnings. Urol Clin North Am 1979; 6: 7–9.
3. Enhoerning G, Miller ER, Hinman F, Jr. Urethral closure studied with cineroentgenography and simultaneous bladder-urethra pressure recording. Surg Gynecol Obstet 1964; 118: 507–16.
4. Webster GD, Guralnick MS. The neurourologic evaluation. In: Walsh PC RA, Vaughan ED, Jr., Wein AJ, eds. Campbell's Urology. Philadelphia: WB Saunders Company, 2002: 900–30.
5. Scarpero HM, Padmanabhan P, Xue X, Nitti VW. Patient perception of videourodynamic testing: a questionnaire based study. J Urol 2005; 173: 555–9.
6. Blaivas JG. Deciding on the right urodynamic equipment. In: Blaivas JG, eds. Atlas of Urodynamics. Baltimore: Williams and Wilkins, 1996: 19–28.
7. Bates CP, Whiteside CG, Turner-Warwick R. Synchronous cine-pressure-flow-cysto-urethrography with special reference to stress and urge incontinence. Br J Urol 1970; 42: 714–23.
8. McGuire EJ, Cespedes RD, Cross CA, O'Connell HE. Videourodynamic studies. Urol Clin North Am 1996; 23: 309–21.
9. Massey A, Abrams P. Urodynamics of the female lower urinary tract. Urol Clin North Am 1985; 12: 231–46.

10. Haylen BT, Ashby D, Sutherst JR, Frazer MI, West CR. Maximum and average urine flow rates in normal male and female populations–the Liverpool nomograms. Br J Urol 1989; 64: 30–8.

11. Abrams P, Cardozo L, Fall M, et al. The standardisation of terminology of lower urinary tract function: report from the Standardisation Sub-committee of the International Continence Society. Neurourol Urodyn 2002; 21: 167–78.

12. Abrams P, Blaivas JG, Stanton SL, Andersen JT. Standardisation of of lower urinary tract function. Neurourol Urodyn 1988; 7: 403–27.

13. Webb RJ, Styles RA, Griffiths CJ, Ramsden PD, Neal DE. Ambulatory monitoring of bladder pressures in patients with low compliance as a result of neurogenic bladder dysfunction. Br J Urol 1989; 64: 150–4.

14. Schafer W, Abrams P, Liao L, et al. Good urodynamic practices: uroflowmetry, filling cystometry, and pressure-flow studies. Neurourol Urodyn 2002; 21: 261–74.

15. Gravina GL, Costa AM, Galatioto GP, et al. Urodynamic obstruction in women with stress urinary incontinence–do nonintubated uroflowmetry and symptoms aid diagnosis? J Urol 2007; 178(3 Pt 1): 959–63; discussion 63–4.

16. Tseng LH, Liang CC, Chang YL, et al. Postvoid residual urine in women with stress incontinence. Neurourol Urodyn 2008; 27: 48–51.

17. Bates P, Bradley WE, Glen E, et al. The standardization of terminology of lower urinary tract function. Eur Urol 1976; 2: 274–6.

18. Awad SA, Flood HD, Acker KL. The significance of prior anti-incontinence surgery in women who present with urinary incontinence. J Urol 1988; 140: 514–7.

19. McGuire EJ. Bladder instability and stress incontinence. Neurourol Urodyn 1988; 7: 563–7.

20. McGuire EJ, Fitzpatrick CC, Wan J, et al. Clinical assessment of urethral sphincter function. J Urol 1993; 150(5 Pt 1): 1452–4.

21. Sinha D, Nallaswamy V, Arunkalaivanan AS. Value of leak point pressure study in women with incontinence. J Urol 2006; 176: 186–8; discussion 8.

22. McGuire EJ, Cespedes RD, O'Connell HE. Leak-point pressures. Urol Clin North Am 1996; 23: 253–62.

23. Blaivas JG. Cystometry. In: Blaivas JG, eds. Atlas of Urodynamics. Baltimore: Williams and Wilkins, 1996: 31–47.

24. McGuire EJ, Woodside JR, Borden TA, Weiss RM. Prognostic value of urodynamic testing in myelodysplastic patients. J Urol 1981; 126: 205–9.

25. Woodside JR, McGuire EJ. Technique for detection of detrusor hypertonia in the presence of urethral sphincteric incompetence. J Urol 1982; 127: 740–3.

26. Farrar D, Warwick RT. Outflow obstruction in the female. Urol Clin North Am 1979; 6: 217–25.

27. Wein A, Barrett DM. Other voiding dysfunctions and related topics. In: Wein A, Barrett DM, eds. Voiding Function and Dysfunction. Chicago: Year Book, 1988: 274–301.

28. Akikwala TV, Fleischman N, Nitti VW. Comparison of diagnostic criteria for female bladder outlet obstruction. J Urol 2006; 176: 2093–7.

29. Fowler C. Electromyography. In: Blaivas JG, eds. Atlas of Urodynamics. Baltimore: Williams and Wilkins, 1996: 60–76.

30. Blaivas JG, Olsson CA. Stress incontinence: classification and surgical approach. J Urol 1988; 139: 727–31.

31. O'Donnell PD. Pitfalls of urodynamic testing. Urol Clin North Am 1991; 18: 257–68.

32. Virtanen HS, Ekholm E, Kiilholma PJ. Evisceration after enterocele repair: a rare complication of vaginal surgery. Int Urogynecol J Pelvic Floor Dysfunct 1996; 7: 344–7.

33. Yang A, Mostwin JL, Rosenshein NB, Zerhouni EA. Pelvic floor descent in women: dynamic evaluation with fast MR imaging and cinematic display. Radiology 1991; 179: 25–33.

34. Stothers L, Guevara R, Macnab A. Classification of male lower urinary tract symptoms using mathematical modelling and a regression tree algorithm of noninvasive near-infrared spectroscopy parameters. Eur Urol 2010; 57: 327–32.

35 Ambulatory Urodynamics

Stefano Salvatore, Vik Khullar, and Linda Cardozo

INTRODUCTION

Laboratory urodynamics is currently the "gold standard" in the objective assessment of urinary symptoms. However, it is necessarily unphysiologic because it measures pressures during retrograde bladder filling using a fast filling rate and during voiding.

In the past, attempts were made to monitor lower urinary tract function on a long-term basis and in an ambulant patient, with the aim of overcoming some of the problems encountered in standard urodynamics.

The first problem is physiological: When monitoring detrusor function using standard urodynamics, fast retrograde bladder filling is employed, which is necessarily provocative. The second is environmental: Incontinence is a benign condition, and reliance is placed on the person's symptoms as evidence of disease; many of these symptoms are related to acts of everyday life, all of which are removed in a laboratory atmosphere. Thirdly, throughout the period of time during which the standard urodynamic tests are being conducted, the individual is the focus of attention and is asked to respond to certain commands. This may lead to cortical suppression of detrusor activity.

The first description of a bladder pressure measurement in an ambulant patient was reported by Mackay (1) using radiotelemetry, followed by many other methods. To allow an individual to be mobile, the system must employ telemetry, long cables, or portable recording units. In the first systems, telemetry was used (2–5). A pressure-sensitive radio pill was inserted into the bladder, allowing intravesical pressure to be monitored without the presence of a foreign body in the urethra. However, the cost, limited range of transmission, and occasional difficulty in retrieval prevented its widespread use.

In standard urodynamics the lines used are fluid filled. A study of natural filling in spinal injury patients (6) demonstrated increased phasic activity. However, in general, fluid-filled lines are not recommended as they are prone to movement artifact and the pressures measured are dependent on the relative position of the pressure transducer to the tip of the fluid-filled line; thus the baseline measurement alters as the woman changes position. Air is not subject to the same movement artifact, and air-filled tubes have been used in ambulatory urodynamics (2). In this system, one end of the tube is filled by a meniscus of urine and the other is covered by a compliant balloon to prevent fluid traveling down the tube and thus producing artifact. In this set-up, the position of the catheter relative to the transducer is unimportant; unfortunately, changes in the temperature can alter pressure measurement.

As time has progressed, tape-recording systems have been used. Initially, these systems had a limited capacity which enabled pressures to be recorded only above a certain pre-set threshold (7). If the patient became symptomatic during the test, but the threshold had not been met, then the pressure was unrecorded, and therefore no substantive diagnosis was provided. Subsequently, Griffiths et al. (8) developed an ambulatory system using micro-tip pressure transducers and a digital solid-state recorder. In this system the information is recorded digitally, transferred, and then reviewed at the end of the test. The trace can then be compressed or expanded without loss of information.

EQUIPMENT

There are three main components to an ambulatory system (Figs. 35.1–35.3): (*i*) the transducers; (*ii*) the recording unit; and (*iii*) the analyzing system.

The transducers are solid state and are mounted on a 5 to 7 Fr bladder and rectal catheter, to measure the pressure impinging on it. Most transducers have the pressure-sensitive membrane a few millimeters beyond the tip of the catheter and, therefore, pressure changes are recorded when the tip touches the side of the bladder. This can be overcome by inserting two catheters, and the intravesical pressure change is deemed significant only if it is recorded on both transducers. The rectal catheter is covered with silicone in order to protect it from deformation (9). There can be problems with drift of the transducers, but this is usually <3 cmH$_2$O within the four-hour test (8).

The recording system must be portable and, ideally, battery powered to allow freedom of movement. Sampling of the pressures should be at 4 Hz and the memory should be digital, allowing the trace to be compressed and expanded. A trace should not be interpreted in isolation: A recording unit should have some means of marking events during the test—the simpler the better, as patients often find multiple buttons confusing and pressing the wrong button can confuse the interpretation. More sophisticated systems, however, are available (10), providing the subject with separate switches on a single remote unit which sends a coded signal to the recorder depending on the button pressed.

As well as marking the event, it is helpful if there is some mechanism of timing, either by having an in-built timer in the unit or by asking the patient to record the time. The recorder should have an option to be connected to an electronic "diaper" (nappy), allowing accurate information about urine loss. In addition, there should be a connector to a gravimetric flowmeter that will calculate pressure–flow curves and check when detrusor overactivity (DO) has occurred.

The pressure traces are downloaded onto a computer, which can then analyze detrusor and urethral function. There is a variety of different formats. The software available today enables the trace to be expanded or compressed, the scales to

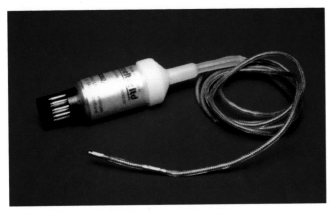

Figure 35.1 Bladder pressure catheter.

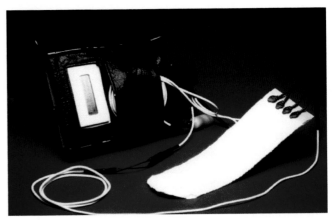

Figure 35.4 Urilos pad connected to the recording unit.

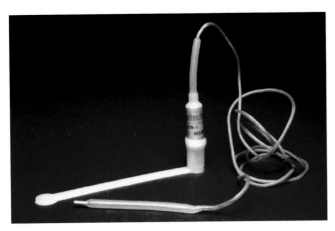

Figure 35.2 Rectal pressure catheter.

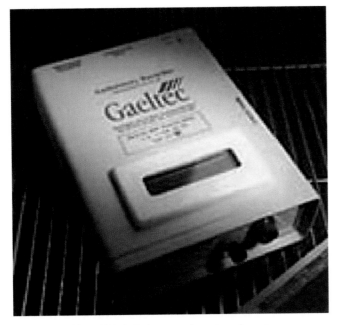

Figure 35.3 Ambulatory urodynamic equipment.

be changed, a pressure–flow study to be analyzed, and a computerized archive of the tests performed to be maintained. It is important to choose the appropriate scale for the pressure and time measurements; the patient's diary and trace should be

reviewed with the patient. This allows further information to be gleaned, which a simple system of pushing buttons might have missed. For some new ambulatory urodynamic equipment the wireless bluetooth techniques allow data to be viewed while recording.

The urine loss itself needs to be evaluated. Using a weighed perineal pad for the length of the test gives some idea of the severity of the incontinence, but gives little information about when the loss occurred. If the timing of the loss can be calculated, then the manometric changes leading to incontinence can be interpreted and may be helpful in determining the cause of urinary leakage. There are three ways of achieving this. The first is the Urilos (Exeter) (Fig. 35.4) electronic diaper, which has already been alluded to. It has elongated, interleaved electrodes embedded in absorbent material. A 50 mV (low voltage) alternating current is passed between the two electrodes; as the urine loss increases, so does this current. Obviously this depends on the electrodes being within the urine, which is definitely not guaranteed, and so the pad has to be preloaded with a known volume of electrolyte solution. This method is suitable only for volumes between 1 and 100 ml and is reproducible within 20%.

The second method is to measure perineal temperature, which is usually 30°C to 40°C. Urine has a higher temperature than that of the body surface, 37°C. When there is leakage of urine there is a transient rise in temperature which then falls rapidly, allowing effective detection of distinct episodes of urine loss. The rate of the temperature increase may correlate well with the quantity of leaked urine. A single temperature detector is ineffective, as the position of the detector in relation to the leaked urine changes; hence, a parallel array of diodes has been used with a separate reference diode. Problems of interpretation can occur if the patient has her legs together when seated, as the perineal temperature may then rise.

The third method relies on a catheter placed within the urethra. Two electrodes are mounted on the catheter and an electrical current is passed between them. If urine is passed, either voluntarily or involuntarily, there is increased conduction and a larger current passes across the electrodes. It is vital that the electrodes are placed correctly. For example, with the electrode in the proximal urethra, a change in the electrical current would indicate the presence of urine. However, this may not have originated from urinary leakage, as this can occur with urethral instability. Conversely, if the electrodes are not in the urethra, then no leakage would be detected. Distal urethral electrical conductance is not used clinically in ambulatory urodynamics, but is mainly a research tool.

STANDARDIZATION OF AMBULATORY URODYNAMIC MONITORING (AUM)

A standardization report (11) on AUM was published by a specific International Continence Society (ICS) committee in 2000. In this document the authors cover different aspects such as indications, technical suggestions, and both clinical and scientific reports for ambulatory urodynamics. In this chapter we will include the most relevant parts of the report for clinical purposes.

Indications for AUM

- Lower urinary tract symptoms which conventional urodynamic investigation fails to reproduce or explain;
- Situations in which conventional urodynamics may be unsuitable;
- Neurogenic lower urinary tract dysfunction;
- Evaluation of therapies for lower urinary tract dysfunction.

Terminology

The terminology applied to observations during AUM should, wherever possible, be consistent with terminology used during conventional urodynamic investigation (12).

Definitions

An ambulatory urodynamic investigation is defined as any functional test of the lower urinary tract predominantly utilizing natural filling of the urinary tract and reproducing the subject's normal activity. The terms introduced by this definition are further explained below.

- *Ambulatory*: This refers to the nature of monitoring rather than the mobility of the subject. Monitoring will usually take place outside a urodynamic laboratory.
- *Natural*: This refers to the natural production of urine rather than an artificial filling medium. Stimulation by forced drinking or pharmacologic manipulation must be stated in the methodology. (The bladder may be pre-filled with an artificial medium but this is not comparable with natural bladder filling. This method of investigation needs further evaluation.)
- *Normal activity*: This refers to the activities of the subject during which symptoms are likely to occur. These may include maneuvers designed specifically to identify the presence of involuntary detrusor or urethral behavior or to provoke incontinence.

Methodology

Signals

The following signals have been recorded by AUM:

- pressure: intravesical, abdominal, urethral, intrapelvic (renal);
- flow rate;
- micturition volume;
- urinary leakage;
- leakage volume;
- urethral electrical conductance;
- perineal integrated surface electromyography (EMG).

Additional information that should be recorded during any AUM investigation as event markers include the following phenomena:

- initiation of voluntary voids;
- cessation of voluntary voids;
- episodes of urgency;
- episodes of discomfort or pain;
- provocative maneuvers;
- time and volume of fluid intake;
- time and volume of urinary leakage;
- time of pad change.

Signal Quality

AUM is more versatile than equivalent conventional urodynamic investigation, but for the same reasons AUM is associated with a greater risk of losing signal quality. Therefore, although all signals should be recorded as outlined in the ICS recommendations on "Good Urodynamic Practices" (13), there are a number of cautions which apply specifically to AUM, as described below.

Intravesical and Abdominal Pressure Measurement
Although it is possible to measure intravesical and abdominal pressures using fluid-filled lines (water or air), the use of catheter-mounted micro-tip transducers allows greater mobility during AUM. In the absence of continuous supervision, stringent checks on signal quality should be incorporated in the measurement protocol. At the start of monitoring, these should include testing of recorded pressure on-line by coughing and abdominal straining in the supine, sitting, and erect positions. The investigator must be convinced that signal quality is adequate before proceeding with the ambulatory phase of the investigation.

Prior to termination of the investigation and at regular intervals during monitoring similar checks of signal quality such as cough tests should be carried out. Such tests will serve as a useful retrospective quality check during the interpretation of traces.

The following considerations must be taken into account when using micro-tip transducers: Transducers should be calibrated prior to every investigation. The "zero point" is atmospheric pressure (there is no fixed reference point). All transducers must be "zeroed" at atmospheric pressure prior to insertion of the catheters.

- Water-filled pressure catheters have a fixed reference point at the upper edge of symphysis pubis whereas catheter-mounted micro-tip pressure transducers have no fixed reference point.
- Micro-tip transducers will record direct contact with solid material (the wall of a viscus or fecal material) as a change in pressure. The use of multiple transducers may eliminate this source of artifact.
- Under some circumstances, the pressure measured at the transducer surface will result in a discrepancy equal to the difference in vertical height between the two transducers. This can result in the estimated detrusor pressure (p_{det}) being <0 (i.e., negative) with, for instance, the patient in the supine position.

Urethral Pressure and Conductance

The recording of urethral pressure is a qualitative measurement with emphasis on changes in pressure rather than absolute values. The use of urethral electrical conductance to identify leakage in association with pressure monitoring facilitates interpretation of urethral pressure traces. Precise positioning and secure fixation are essential to maintain signal quality. The orientation of the transducer should be documented. (The use of multiple pressure transducers facilitates identification of movement artifact but increases catheter stiffness and thereby deformation of the urethra during recording).

Catheter Fixation

As indicated earlier, secure catheter fixation is essential to maintain signal quality. Methods that have been used include adhesive tape, suture fixation, and purpose-designed silicone-fixation devices.

Recording of Urinary Leakage

The method of urine leakage determination should be recorded. It should be stated whether the urinary leakage is recorded as a signal with the pressure measurements, or is dependent on the subject pressing an event marker button or completing a urinary diary.

Instructions to the Patient

Detailed instructions as to recording of symptoms, identification of catheter displacement, and hardware failure should be given to the patient. It is the recommendation of this group that such verbal instructions should be reinforced by written instructions and, in addition to the hardware built into the system, the patient is provided with a simple diary to record events. This facilitates the common primary aim of all urodynamics, i.e., to correlate the test outcome with symptoms.

Analysis

Quality Assessment

The first step in the analysis of an AUM trace is the assessment of the quality of data recorded. The specific points that should be addressed with regard to pressure measurement are:

- Is the trace "active," i.e., fine second to second variation in pressure rather than a fine line?
- Is the baseline static or highly variable?
- Are the cough tests or other activities causing abdominal pressure changes that can be used for signal plausibility check, regularly present?
- Is the subtraction adequate, e.g., minimal change in subtracted p_{det} with coughing?

If the technical quality of the trace is less than perfect, then, although the investigation may yield valuable clinical information, in the context of accurate measurement the pressure recordings must be viewed only as qualitative; further quantitative analysis may well be flawed.

Phase Identification

Depending on the purpose of the investigation, markers must be placed to identify voluntary voids and allow differentiation of such events from involuntary events, which may be associated with changes in recorded pressure. The protocol of the investigation should state specifically the point at which the markers identifying commencement and cessation of a voluntary void are placed. Analysis of the voiding phase follows the same principles and terminology used during conventional pressure–flow investigation.

Events

The use of a patient diary considerably improves the detailed analysis of events occurring during AUM and is strongly recommended. Typical events occurring during the filling phase are detrusor contractions, urethral relaxations, and episodes of urgency and incontinence. (At least for research purposes, it is strongly advised that variables for quantitative interpretation are defined and validated. Validation means to establish data on healthy volunteers and specific patient groups, test–retest reproducibility, interrater validity, and sensitivity to treatment modalities.)

CLINICAL REPORT

The report should be tailored to the urodynamic investigations and can include the following indication(s) and/or urodynamic question(s) (*obligatory*):

- duration of recording;
- filling rate, timing, method and volume of any retrograde filling prior to commencing AUM;
- dose and timing of diuretics if administered;
- volume of fluid drunk during the test;
- number of voids;
- total and range of voided volumes and postmicturition urinary residual;
- episodes of urgency, urinary incontinence, and pain;
- detrusor activity during the filling phase (frequency, time, duration, amplitude, area, form);
- pressure/flow analysis;
- results of provocative maneuvers employed during the test; and
- reasons for termination of recording if prematurely terminated.

COMMENTS

Although the ICS standardization report is accurate and precise, some additional tips are recommended to ensure quality control during ambulatory urodynamics, as follows.

Patient Preparation

- The reasons for the test and all the procedures should be explained in full; patient compliance is essential.
- Urinary tract infection should be excluded before the test.
- All patients should be informed about the duration of the procedure prior to starting it.
- They should be asked to wear loose comfortable separate clothing (e.g., tracksuit).
- Catheters are inserted using an aseptic technique. Both bladder transducers are placed in the bladder in order to exclude artifacts during analysis (Fig. 35.5). The rectal catheter is inserted into the rectum inside a non-lubricated condom to prevent contamination of the silicone coating or vagina.
- Once inserted, the catheters are taped to the inner thigh close to the labia (as close to the urethra as possible) using several pieces of 5 cm micropore tape. The lines are then brought forward, over the abdomen, and arranged to be accessible through the clothing.

Procedure

- The patient is instructed in the use of the diary (Fig. 35.6). This will provide information of activity during the test. It is essential that the woman understands the diary as this is very important in the final analysis. The diary should be checked frequently to ensure compliance.
- The patient should use the timer on the ambulatory box, not her own watch.
- The patient is instructed on how to use the flow-rate machine and the event button, if unable to return to the flowmeter. If this is required, the button is pressed once on entry to a toilet, and once again when void starts. The event button should not be used at any other time. Instructions for the event button should be included on the diary sheet, as are the names and telephone numbers of the test coordinators.
- Contact with the test coordinator should be easy for the patient.
- The patient needs to be checked on-line at least once an hour (or more if deemed necessary); e.g., if the lines have come out, if there is an ambulatory box failure (such as low batteries), if the patient is uncomfortable, or if the test becomes unacceptable.
- At the end of the test period, the patient is asked to carry out a series of activities, with a full bladder (if possible). The use of provocative maneuvers such as 10 coughs, 10 star jumps, hand washing, or heel bouncing, can improve diagnostic yield (14,15). The patient is then asked to void.
- Once the test is complete, the traces are then reviewed by the test coordinator, and the diary is interpreted with the patient present. If possible, another observer should also be present. In our opinion, it is mandatory to interpret the trace and the diary with the patient present at the end of the study. The use of a diary emphasizes the importance of linking urinary symptoms with the investigation; this is as valid for laboratory urodynamics as it is for ambulatory urodynamics. Urinary symptoms are important, as abnormal detrusor activity cannot be diagnosed unless it is associated with symptoms such as urgency

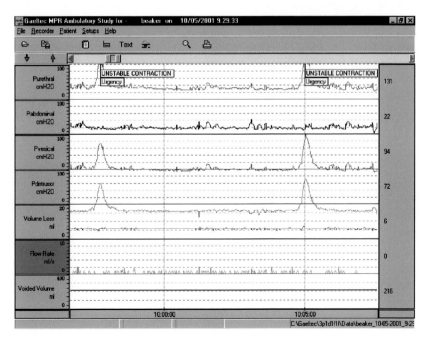

Figure 35.5 Ambulatory urodynamic trace showing abnormal detrusor activity with pressure rise on the detrusor line and on both "intravesical" transducers in the presence of urgency.

AMBULATORY URODYNAMICS DIARY

Use the following codes in the diary below and remember to press the event button and write the time displayed on the side of the recorder.

U = Feeling like you want to/rushing to pass water
P = Passing water   S = Walking up stairs
T = Drinking tea or coffee   D = Drinking any other drink, e.g. orange, water
L = Leaking urine   C = Coughing
W = Walking   R = Sitting

DRINK A CUP OF FLUID EVERY HALF HOUR

TIME	EVENT	TIME	EVENT	TIME	EVENT	TIME	EVENT

Figure 35.6 Ambulatory urodynamic diary.

or urge incontinence. In fact, we found (16) that both the symptom diary and the placement of two transducers in the bladder can decrease, by almost two-thirds, the diagnosis of pathologic detrusor activity on ambulatory urodynamics by minimizing possible artifacts.

• After the test the patient is warned that she may have a stinging sensation in her urethra and bladder for up to 24 hours. For this reason, fluid intake should be maintained and, if symptoms of cystitis are present or the urine becomes offensive, she should seek advice from her doctor. Routine antibiotic prophylaxis is not indicated. In fact, in 91 women who completed a four-hour test, Anders et al. (17) reported an infection rate of 1.1% (1 patient) whereas 17 women reported mild to moderate de novo dysuria without a positive urinary culture. Women who are known to have residuals, reflux, recurrent urinary tract infection, or diabetes should be given antibiotic cover.

CLINICAL STUDIES

Asymptomatic Volunteers

The clinical use of ambulatory urodynamics is limited by the high prevalence (38–69%) of abnormal detrusor contractions

detected with this method in asymptomatic volunteers (5,18–20). These results call ambulatory urodynamics and its validity into question, suggesting that it is oversensitive in the diagnosis of DO (instability). Van Waalwijik van Doorn et al. (19) proposed an equation, the detrusor activity index, to distinguish "abnormal" from "physiologic" detrusor contractions. The mean detrusor activity index is calculated as the sum of the number of uninhibited contractions per hour multiplied by 10, the mean amplitude and the mean duration of these contractions. In a prospective study (21) of 26 asymptomatic women, we showed that the diagnosis of "DO (instability)" is highly dependent on trace interpretation and the technique used to conduct the test. In our population of asymptomatic volunteers, the prevalence of abnormal detrusor contractions varied from 76.9% to 11.5%, according to the definition used of an abnormal event, the use of the diary with the woman present during interpretation, and the placement of two transducers in the bladder. We defined abnormal detrusor contraction as the point at which a simultaneous p_{det} rise on both bladder lines occurred, but only if associated with symptoms (urgency or leakage), in line with the ICS definition of DO.

According to our definition of abnormal detrusor contraction, ambulatory urodynamics findings are normal in almost 90% of asymptomatic women, which is similar to the rate of normal findings in laboratory urodynamic studies. This definition is also applied during our laboratory urodynamic tests, indicating that ambulatory urodynamics does not need new diagnostic standards or methods. Laboratory urodynamics involves the careful observation of urinary symptoms correlated with the cystometric trace. Ambulatory urodynamics does not differ in this respect, and the process becomes even more important in the correct diagnosis of abnormal detrusor contraction.

Variables Recorded on Ambulatory Urodynamics

Voided Volume

Many authors have reported that the volume voided during ambulatory urodynamic studies is less than during laboratory urodynamics (18,22–24). There may be various reasons for this: The irritation of the catheter in an ambulant patient may exacerbate the desire to void.During conventional urodynamics we usually try to reach the maximum functional bladder capacity; presumably, this does not happen in ambulatory urodynamics, with a patient voiding at comfortable bladder fullness. However, Groen et al. (25) compared the voidings from 47 patients at their modal volume (the volume most often voided by the patient as derived from frequency/volume charts) with voidings at maximum cystometric capacity during a routine videourodynamic examination. The authors concluded that the differences between ambulatory and conventional urodynamics could not be explained from possible differences in the voided volume. In fact, they found that although the maximum flow rate depended significantly on the voided volume, the associated p_{det}, urethral resistance, and bladder contraction did not.

Detrusor Pressure

It is not possible to detect low bladder compliance using ambulatory urodynamics (26). Both abnormal detrusor contractions at the maximum p_{det} during the voiding phase are greater in ambulatory urodynamic than in conventional urodynamic studies. Schmidt et al. (27) showed that the p_{det} at maximum flow is dependent on the fluid intake during the test, being higher in a fluid-loaded group.

Flow Rate

The flow rate is higher in ambulatory urodynamic than in laboratory urodynamic studies (28).

Patient Acceptability

AUM evaluation has a longer duration than conventional urodynamics and this could be regarded as a self limiting factor because of reduced patient acceptability. However, a recent study (29) on 40 subjects (33 women and 7 men) from 23 to 72 years of age, comparing AUM to conventional urodynamics showed thatconventional urodynamics brings a significant greater anxiety than AUM (p = 0.045) ; AUM determines a higher degree of boredom (p = 0.013); there was no significant difference in the degree of shame or bother between the two tests; and a total of 74.4% and 84.6% (no significant difference) responded that they were willing to repeat conventional urodynamics and AUM, respectively.

CLINICAL APPLICATIONS

Inconclusive Urodynamics

A proportion of women complaining of urinary symptoms can have an inconclusive laboratory urodynamic evaluation. Vereecken and Van Nuland (24) showed abnormalities on ambulatory urodynamics in 20 of 28 subjects with urinary symptoms but with an inconclusive laboratory urodynamics result.

Patravali showed that AUM can diangose urinary dysfunction in 77% symptomatic women with inconclusive urodynamics (30).

Pannek et al. had onsistent data showing 72% of abnormalities detected on AUM, with treatment modified in 63% of cases, leading to satisfactory results in 42% of patients (31).

Poor Correlation Between Symptoms and Conventional Urodynamics

One hundred patients (32) complaining of urinary symptoms underwent ambulatory urodynamics after having a laboratory urodynamics result that did not correlate with their symptoms or after unsuccessful incontinence surgery. The ambulatory urodynamic studies diagnosed DO twice as often as laboratory urodynamics. The test was described as normal in 32 patients undergoing laboratory urodynamics, but in only five undergoing ambulatory urodynamics. The latter test diagnosed only eight patients as having urethral sphincter incompetence, compared with 13 on laboratory urodynamics.

In another study (14), 52 patients underwent a laboratory urodynamic study, with poor symptom correlation. All of these patients also underwent ambulatory urodynamics, which showed DO in 31 patients with a conventional urodynamic diagnosis of a stable bladder. Of these 31 patients, 11 had DO only after provocative maneuvers, emphasizing the need to carry out this part of the test. This study also showed that incontinence was detected more frequently on ambulatory urodynamics using a Urilos diaper.

Anders et al. (33) compared the diagnosis obtained via ambulatory urodynamics with that obtained by conventional urodynamics in 475 symptomatic women. Ambulatory urodynamics proved to be more sensitive than laboratory urodynamics in the diagnosis of DO, but less sensitive to urodynamic stress incontinence.

Radley et al. (34) compared ambulatory urodynamics and conventional videocystometry findings in 106 women with symptoms of bladder overactivity. DO was detected in 32 and 70 cases on videourodynamics and ambulatory monitoring, respectively (p < 0.001). Stress incontinence was diagnosed in 42 women on videocystometry and in 34 on ambulatory urodynamics (p = 0.629).

Robinson et al. (35), in a blinded prospective study, assessed whether the ultrasound measurement of bladder wall thickness could replace ambulatory urodynamics in a group of 128 women with a conventional urodynamic diagnosis which did not explain their urinary symptoms. The authors concluded that in women with urodynamic stress incontinence ambulatory urodynamics remains the investigation of choice.

Swithinbank et al. (36) analyzed ambulatory urodynamics results in 111 women and 11 men with a conventional urodynamic diagnosis which failed to explain their symptoms. They found that ambulatory urodynamics influenced the management of all but 8.7% patients.

It still has to be demonstrated that changes in patient management after the procedure led to an improvement in outcome, since Gorton and Stanton (37) raised doubts after analyzing 71 ambulatory urodynamic notes of women with inconclusive conventional urodynamics.

Low Compliance

Low bladder compliance does not have a standardized definition and it is characterized by a steep p_{det} rise during the filling phase on laboratory urodynamics. The significance of this is debated: Some feel that this is a passive phenomenon related to the reduced elasticity of the bladder wall, others that increase in pressure is associated with a tonic detrusor contraction. In the former, the pressure rise should not decrease at the end of filling; in the latter, the p_{det} should decay exponentially as the contracting detrusor relaxes.

The predictive value of low bladder compliance for the diagnosis of idiopathic DO, using ambulatory urodynamics as the gold standard investigation for comparison, was retrospectively assessed in 143 patients (38). The comparison of the mean bladder compliance between patients showing no abnormalities or DO on AUM was not statistically significant, being respectively 112 ml/cmH$_2$O and 92 ml/cmH$_2$O. Moreover no set threshold of BC was able to provide sufficient accuracy for the diagnosis of DO.

In a series of patients with neuropathic bladders (26), who developed an increase in p_{det} of more than 25 cmH$_2$O at a filling rate of 100 ml/min during ambulatory urodynamics, there was a much smaller increase in p_{det} on orthograde filling than when these patients underwent cystometry using faster filling rates; however, the frequencies of phasic detrusor instability correlated well with the magnitude of the pressure increase during conventional cystometry. It was also found that the greater number of phasic detrusor contractions during ambulatory monitoring correlated well with the presence of a dilated upper renal tract. However, the diagnosis of low compliance on filling during laboratory urodynamics did not correlate with upper tract dilation.

Preoperative Evaluation

Incontinence surgery is indicated in cases of urodynamic stress incontinence. DO should be excluded prior to surgery, as it is an important cause of operative failure. However, DO can appear after an incontinence operation (such as Burch colposuspension or tension-free vaginal tape-like procedures) and is referred to as de novo. It is still debated whether this could be due to excessive dissection during the operation, or that DO was not diagnosed prior to surgery. Ambulatory urodynamics has been used to predict the appearance of de novo DO after incontinence surgery in two studies (39,40), with conflicting results.

Pressure–Flow Study

Ambulatory urodynamics can be useful to assess the voiding phase in patients who are unable to void during conventional urodynamic studies because of embarrassment or in those who experience suprapubic pain after voiding. The latter can be associated with the post-void uninhibited detrusor contraction, which should be treated as DO; however, these patients may also require cystoscopy and possibly bladder biopsy.

Increased Bladder Sensation

A conventional urodynamic diagnosis of increased bladder sensation may require cystoscopy and biopsies. Where histology is inconclusive it may be appropriate to perform ambulatory urodynamics.

Pharmacologic Treatment Monitoring

Ambulatory urodynamics can be used in the assessment of pharmacologic treatment for overactive bladder. The optimal duration of monitoring in this context appears to be six hours (41). Compared to conventional urodynamics, ambulatory monitoring allows the effects of drugs for the treatment of DO to be assessed and appears to be more sensitive, thus allowing smaller groups of patients to be studied.

Other

Short provocative ambulatory urodynamics was used to assess if women with female ejaculation were more likely to have DO (42). The authors failed to demonstrate any higher risk to have urinary dysfunction in women with female ejaculation.

CONCLUSIONS

Ambulatory urodynamics is a useful tool in the assessment of lower urinary tract disorders, particularly when conventional urodynamics fail to explain the urinary symptoms. Interesting developments of some research applications of ambulatory urodynamics, such as monitoring pharmacologic treatment efficacy, need to be confirmed.

AMBULATORY SYSTEMS
Gaeltec

The Gaeltec NanoLogger™ (Fig. 35.7) has between one and seven input channels and an event marker. There can be up to eight axes on the screen to display the input channels and signals derived from them. Optical isolation allows easy connection to the PC with a serial lead for on-line assessment at any stage of the investigation. The patient simply presses a convenient event marking button in communication with the recorder's built-in clock to keep a reliable and accurate diary. Fast data downloading to the PC allows rapid record processing.

MMS

The Luna (Fig. 35.8) is an easy to use ambulatory urodynamic recorder. Using a bluetooth technique the Luna offers an on-line view of recordings. The Luna weighs <200 g. It has three pressure channels (bladder, urethra, and abdominal), flow, EMG, and automated leak point pressures through conductiv-

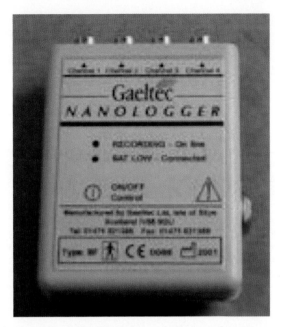

Figure 35.7 The Gaeltec NanoLogger ambulatory urodynamic system.

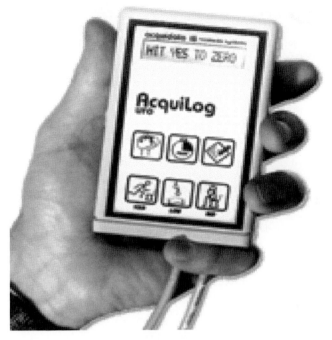

Figure 35.9 The Neomedics Acquilog ambulatory urodynamic system.

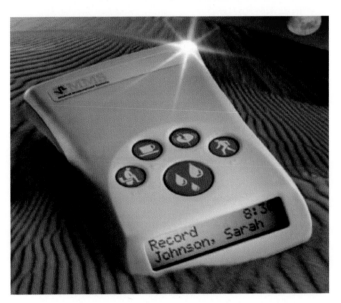

Figure 35.8 The MMS Luna ambulatory urodynamic system.

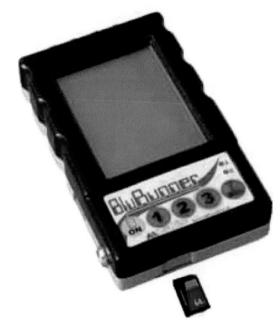

Figure 35.10 The Menfis Blu Runner ambulatory urodynamic system.

ity. More than 24 hours of investigation data can be downloaded. Dedicated Windows® software provides fully automated analysis of all pressure data, in combination with leakage, flow and EMG in a 24 hour study. A complete range of micro-tip catheters is available for use with the Luna, even small sizes such as 3 or 4 Fr for children.

Neomedics
Acquilog (Fig. 35.9) is a multichannel ambulatory urodynamic system that can record for up to 12 or 24 hours. It has two pressures with a third (p_{det}) also displayed when in analysis mode with an optional urine loss detector channel. It employs straightforward patient event commenting and it downloads data into the Acquidata Uromac urodynamics system with a simple,

prompted, step-by-step set-up and download procedure. A range of active microtransducer catheters is available, including miniscule 3 Fr single sensor and 5 Fr dual sensor devices.

Menfis
Blu Runner (Fig. 35.10) is an ambulatory recorder with up to eight channels and a plug-and-play system. It can record pressures, pHmetric, EMG, flow, volume, and conductance signals. It has a large graphic LCD display with a touch-screen type. It is also possible to have a real-time/on-line display of up to four measurement curves.

REFERENCES

1. Mackay RS. Radiotelemetering from within the human body. Institute of Radio Engineers Transactions on Medical Electronics (ME6) 1959; 11: 100–5.

2. Warrell DW, Watson BW, Shelley T. Intravesical pressure measurements in women during movement using a radio-pill and an air-probe. J Obstet Gynaecol Br Commonw 1963; 70: 959–67.

3. Miyagawa I, Nakamura I, Ueda M, et al. Telemetric cystometry. Urol Int 1993; 41: 263–5.

4. Vereecken RL, Puers B, Das J. Continuous telemetric monitoring of bladder function. Urol Res 1983; 11: 15–18.

5. Thuroff JW, Jonas V, Frohneberg D, et al. Telemetric urodynamic investigation in normal males. Urol Int 1980; 35: 427–34.

6. Tsuji I, Kuroda K, Nakajima F. Excretory cystometry in paraplegic patients. J Urol 1960; 83: 839–44.

7. Bhatia NN, Bradley WE, Haldeman S, Johnson BK. Continuous monitoring of bladder and urethral pressure: new technique. Urology 1981; 18: 207–10.

8. Griffiths CJ, Assi MS, Styles RA, et al. Ambulatory monitoring of bladder and detrusor pressure during natural filling. J Urol 1989; 142: 780–4.

9. German K, MacLachlan D, Johnson S, et al. Improvements in the design of equipment used for ambulatory urodynamics. Br J Urol 1994; 74: 377–8.

10. Chu AC. Improved remote event marker for use in ambulatory monitoring. Med Biol Eng Comput 1998; 36: 238–40.

11. Van Waalwijk van Doorn E, Anders K, Khullar V, et al. Standardisation of ambulatory urodynamic monitoring: report of the Standardisation Sub-committee of the International Continence Society for ambulatory urodynamic studies. Neurourol Urodyn 2000; 19: 113–25.

12. Abrams P, Cardozo L, Fall M, et al. The standardisation of terminology of lower urinary tract function: report from the standardisation sub-committee of the international continence society. Neurourol Urodyn 2002; 21: 167–78.

13. Schaefer W, Abrams P, Liao L, et al. Good urodynamic practices: uroflowmetry, filling cystometry, and pressure–flow studies. Neurourol Urodyn 2002; 21: 261–74.

14. Webb RJ, Ramsden PD, Neal DE. Ambulatory monitoring and electronic measurement of urinary leakage in the diagnosis of detrusor instability and incontinence. Br J Urol 1991; 68: 148–52.

15. Athanasiou S, Anders K, Salvatore S, et al. Short term provocative ambulatory urodynamics. Neurourol Urodyn 1996; 4: 276–8.

16. Salvatore S, Khullar V, Anders K, Cardozo LD. Reducing artefacts in ambulatory urodynamics. Br J Urol 1998; 81: 211–14.

17. Anders K, Cardozo L, Ashman O, Khullar V. Morbidity after ambulatory urodynamics. Neurourol Urodyn 2002; 21: 461–3.

18. Robertson AS, Griffiths CJ, Ramsden PD, Neal DE. Bladder function in healthy volunteers: ambulatory monitoring and conventional urodynamic studies. Br J Urol 1994; 73: 242–9.

19. Van Waalwijk Van Doorn ESC, Remmers A, Janknegt RA. Conventional and extramural ambulatory urodynamic testing of the lower urinary tract in female volunteers. J Urol 1992; 47: 1319–26.

20. Heslington K, Hilton P. Ambulatory monitoring and conventional cystometry in asymptomatic female volunteers. Br J Obstet Gynaecol 1996; 103: 434–41.

21. Salvatore S, Khullar V, Cardozo L, et al. Evaluating ambulatory urodynamics: a prospective study in asymptomatic women. Br J Obstet Gynaecol 2001; 108: 107–11.

22. Styles RA, Neal DE, Ramsden PD. Comparison of long-term monitoring and standard cystometry in chronic retention of urine. Br J Urol 1986; 58: 652–6.

23. Yeung CK, Godley ML, Duffy PG, Ransley PG. Natural filling cystometry in infants and children. Br J Urol 1995; 75: 531–7.

24. Vereecken RL, Van Nutland T. Detrusor pressure in ambulatory versus standard urodynamics. Neurourol Urodyn 1998; 17: 129–33.

25. Groen J, van Mastrigt R, Bosch R. Factors causing differences in voiding parameters between conventional and ambulatory urodynamics. Urol Res 2000; 28: 128–31.

26. Webb RJ, Styles RA, Griffiths CJ, et al. Ambulatory monitoring of bladder pressures in patients with low compliance as a result of neurogenic bladder dysfunction. Br J Urol 1989; 64: 150–4.

27. Schmidt F, Jorgensen TM, Djurhuus JC. Twenty-four-hour ambulatory urodynamics in healthy men. Scand J Urol Nephrol Suppl 2004; 215: 75–83.

28. Webb RG, Griffiths CJ, Zacharin KK, Neal DE. Filling and voiding pressures measured by ambulatory monitoring and conventional studies during natural and artificial bladder filling. J Urol 1991; 91: 815–18.

29. Oh SJ, Ku JH, Son H, Jeong JY. A comparative study of patient experiences of conventional fluoroscopic and four-hour ambulatory urodynamic studies. Yonsei Med J 2006; 47: 534–41.

30. Patravali N. Ambulatory urodynamic monitoring: are we wasting our time? J Ostet Gynaecol 2007; 27: 413–15.

31. Pannek J, Pieper P. Clinical usefulness of ambulatory urodynamics in the diagnosis and treatment of lower urinary tract dysfunction. Urol Nephrol 2008; 42: 428–32.

32. Waalwijk Van Doorn ESC, Remmers A, Janknegt RA. Extramural ambulatory urodynamic monitoring during natural filling and normal daily activities: evaluation of 100 patients. J Urol 1992; 146: 124–31.

33. Anders K, Khullar V, Cardozo L, et al. Ambulatory urodynamic monitoring in clinical urogynaecological practice. Neurourol Urodyn 1997; 5: 510–12.

34. Radley SC, Rosario DJ, Chapple CR, Farkas AG. Conventional and ambulatory urodynamic findings in women with symptoms suggestive of bladder overactivity. J Urol 2001; 166: 2253–8.

35. Robinson D, Anders K, Cardozo L, et al. Can ultrasound replace ambulatory urodynamics when investigating women with irritative urinary symptoms? BJOG 2002; 109: 145–8.

36. Swithinbank LV, James M, Shepherd A, Abrams P. Role of ambulatory urodynamic monitoring in clinical urological practice. Neurourol Urodyn 1999; 18: 215–22.

37. Gorton E, Stanton S. Ambulatory urodynamics: do they help clinical management? BJOG 2000; 107: 316–19.

38. Harding C, Dorkin TJ, Thorpe AC. Is low bladder compliance predictive of detrusor overactivity? Neurourol Urodyn 2009; 28: 74–7.

39. Khullar V, Salvatore S, Cardozo L, et al. Ambulatory urodynamics: a predictor of de-novo detrusor instability after colposuspension. Neurourol Urodyn 1994; 13: 443–4.

40. Brown K, Hilton P. The incidence of detrusor instability before and after colposuspension: a study using conventional and ambulatory urodynamic monitoring. BJU Int 1999; 84: 961–5.

41. Rosario DJ, Smith DJ, Radley SC, Chapple CR. Pharmacodynamics of anticholinergic agents measured by ambulatory urodynamic monitoring: a study of methodology. Neurourol Urodyn 1999; 18: 223–33.

42. Cartwright R, Elvy S, Cardozo L. Do women with female ejaculation have detrusor overactivity? J Sex Med 2007; 4: 1655–8.

36 Imaging of the Upper and Lower Urinary Tract (Radiology and Ultrasound)

Andrea Tubaro, Kirsten Kluivers, and Antonio Carbone

INTRODUCTION

This chapter will review indications, techniques, and results of radiological (X ray) and ultrasound (US) imaging of the upper and lower urinary tract (LUT) in women with LUT dysfunction (LUTD). Although some of the techniques may be considered based on their historic importance, a knowledge of radiologic imaging and the information obtained from these images contribute the development of our understanding of pelvic anatomy and function.

The utility of radiographic studies for the diagnosis of stress incontinence and pelvic prolapse—an analysis of the evidence base

The crux of clinical research and ultimately clinical practice concerned with the imaging of urinary incontinence (UI) and pelvic organ prolapse (POP) is to establish if there is a clinical benefit to the measurements that are obtained. Imaging is a method to evaluate anatomy of the individual patient and to diagnose conditions depending on the morphological or functional modifications of individual organs or structures. Imaging can confirm or augment the findings of physical examination, and may provide information that is otherwise unattainable. The identification of the clinical scenarios in which this additional information is beneficial to the management of the patient is the ultimate measure of the utility of the study. Although we may postulate that intraobserver and interobserver variability of physical examination is higher when compared to imaging, this may not necessarily always be true, as well as the assumption that a correlate always exists between the two modalities.

Research into diagnostic accuracy is regulated by the standards for reporting of diagnostic accuracy initiative (1) although the recommendations are rarely adhered to in the (peer-reviewed) literature. To make standardization even more complicated, the Oxford criteria for evidence based medicine (2) does not apply to research in diagnostic accuracy, although they do play a role in the evaluation of clinical benefit. The highest level of evidence according to the Oxford criteria that correlates with the higher grade of recommendation is based on meta-analyses of randomized trials. However, randomization is not a relevant methodology for studies concerning diagnostic accuracy. This significantly limits our ability to develop level 1 evidence and a grade A recommendations for studies dealing with the accuracy of imaging. This is not because the evidence is not robust but because the grading system which has been developed for other areas of clinical research cannot be adequately translated and applied. Clearly, there is no substitute for a properly designed clinical trial.

Analysis of the literature related to the utility of imaging demonstrates that the evaluation of diagnostic accuracy is often

performed properly and the available data include sensitivity and specificity as well as test–retest (intraobserver) and interobserver variability. Of note, a common problem is in the choice of a gold standard that rarely exists in the radiological findings but most commonly is the physical examination. Although this is frequently considered the standard reference, it will ultimately not serve as a comparator, in order to understand whether the new test outperforms the physical examination. As long as imaging is considered an addition to physical examination, the goal may not be to show that there is a high level of agreement between the two, but rather to prove that adding imaging on top of physical examination results is a significant improvement in patient management and treatment outcome. Although it is easy to blame the investigators for a faulty study design, the reality is that designing a study on the clinical benefit of a new imaging technique in patients undergoing diagnostic studies or surgery is a very difficult problem because investigators deal with two different variables—the test under evaluation (e.g., US imaging of the pelvic floor) and the surgical procedure (e.g., surgery for anterior vaginal wall prolapse). In addition, large studies may be needed to evaluate the potential beneficial effects of imaging in certain subgroups of patients. Whenever surgery is involved as the outcome, large multicenter studies are preferable, but when examining the literature in this area, most studies sizes are relatively small and come from single institutions and the variability in patient selection, surgical technique, and outcome assessment must be taken into consideration. Furthermore, a single positive study is rarely compelling enough to change standard practice and confirmatory studies are required. Moving from the identification of the gold standard to defining the best practice is a very long process but it remains the ultimate goal of imaging studies.

Imaging of the pelvic floor in patients with UI and POP is limited by our lack of complete understanding of the physiopathology of these conditions. A classic historical example is the case of patients with stress UI (SUI). Imaging techniques relied for decades on X-ray imaging (e.g., voiding cystograms). This was based upon the assumption that quantification of the bladder neck mobility and the Green classification were of importance (3). Further understanding of the anatomic relationships suggested alternative explanations and demonstrated the limitations of this technique (4–10). Although the images confirmed the observations made during clinical examination, specialists in the field demonstrated a diminished interest in the fluoroscopic imaging of SUI when selecting treatment alternatives, in part due to advances in surgical techniques. When new imaging modalities became available and techniques such as US imaging and MRI were introduced, research in the area of anatomy and anatomic relationships flourished again, since not only the margins of the pelvic floor viscera could be outlined as in X ray, but also images of the organs themselves together with the surrounding structures (muscles and fascias).

In recent years US imaging of the pelvic floor rapidly replaced X-ray imaging because of technological improvements, availability in the office, low cost, lack of radiation hazard, and user friendliness. Research in this area dates back to 1980 when US was first applied in patients with SUI (11). Several papers investigated the relation between X-ray and US imaging (12–19), and the correlation between the two was found to be good (16) while US proved superior, particularly in obese women (19). Although these data are certainly reassuring, they only suggest that US imaging can replace X-ray techniques but they do not establish any additional clinical utility.

In contrast to CT scan and MRI, US imaging is not a "no-touch" technique. Interference between the exploring probe and the target tissue is unavoidable (20,21) although it can certainly be minimized. This is the reason why endo-cavitary imaging (transvaginal or transrectal) has been abandoned in favor of abdominal and perineal techniques. Since, bony structures reflect the beam and affect the US images, but are required as reference points, abdominal imaging has been gradually abandoned in favor of the perineal approach. Two-dimensional (2-D) cineloops or 3-D volumes may be acquired during imaging and can be reviewed offline at a later stage. Similar to CT or MRI techniques, in nowadays 3-D US, images may be obtained through any plane. The depth of the perineal volumes in cranial direction is, however, smaller in US compared with MRI, which may hamper imaging of the central compartment of the pelvic floor in US imaging (20). The availability of high speed computing made real-time or dynamic 3-D US imaging possible, and is currently known as 4-D imaging.

This technique proved particularly interesting in the functional imaging of SUI and POP.

The lack of standardization in US imaging and MRI is impairing research in this area. Of note, there is no consensus as to the ideal patient position (supine or standing) (22), picture orientation in US [caudal part on top (23), bottom, or right side of the picture (24)], reference lines in MRI (25), and degree of bladder filling [empty vs. full (26,27)]. Furthermore, experience has demonstrated how difficult it is to standardize cough and Valsalva maneuvers, which is similarly, a problem in all POP assessment tools (28,29).

In general, the challenge remains that our understanding of the physiopathology of UI and POP is still incomplete and the treatment methods currently applied for correction of the clinical conditions may not be significantly improved, either in selection or performance, by the information obtained by current imaging techniques or the research methods designed to demonstrate their utility.

IMAGING OF THE UPPER URINARY TRACT (UUT)

The rationale for imaging the UUT in female patients with LUTD is twofold: to identify UUT malformations which may be associated with LUTD and to monitor the effect of LUTD on the UUT when necessary. Imaging of the UUT is always indicated in neurogenic UI but in non-neurogenic LUTD the imaging is rarely justified. In extraurethral UI, imaging of the renal moiety, which is sometimes dysplastic or ectopic, is of importance to plan adequate management and surgery. In myelodysplasia, elevated storage pressures in the urinary bladder can cause deterioration of the UUT with hydronephrosis and renal failure, and the kidney morphology and function must be monitored over time (30). Severe POP may results in hydronephrosis because of angulation of the pelvic ureters by the uterine arteries (Fig. 36.1) (31).

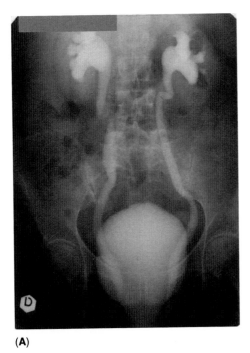
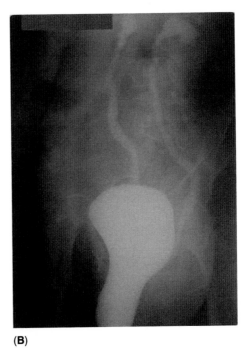

(A)   **(B)**

Figure 36.1 Intravenous pyelography. Bilateral hydronephrosis in a 54-year-old patient with grade IV genital prolapse: (**A**) anteroposterior, (**B**) oblique. *Source:* Courtesy of Professor G. Tomiselli.

With the exception of these three conditions, there is no indication of UUT imaging in the non-neurogenic patient.

Imaging Techniques

Different imaging techniques can be used to picture the UUT—ultrasonography, X rays, CT, MRI, and isotope scanning. In the absence of comparative data on their accuracy and clinical benefit in the management of patients with LUTD, the choice of the technique also depends on availability, expertise, and local policies. In general, the least expensive and hazardous techniques are recommended. Because of the low level of evidence available in the peer-reviewed literature on this subject, recommendations are generally based on expert opinion unless otherwise stated.

Ultrasonography

US is the standard technique for imaging the UUT because of its availability, low cost, and lack of X-ray exposure. Diagnosis of hydronephrosis is straightforward as the collecting system is normally hardly visible on US, imaging is more qualitative (hydronephrosis yes/no) rather then quantitative as there is no relation between the amount of UUT dilatation and the degree of obstruction although there is a relation between the degree of dilatation and cortical damage (32). Doppler analysis of interlobar and arciform arteries has been proposed to diagnose obstruction of the UUT although the technique never gained popularity (33). In the presence of hydronephrosis, additional imaging is usually required to identify the cause and site of the obstruction. US imaging is ideal in the follow-up of patients with LUTD when UUT imaging must be repeated over time.

Intravenous Urography (IVU)

The technique has been the cornerstone of UUT imaging for decades as it provides information on both renal anatomy and function. Indications are limited by the need of normal renal function (creatinine <2.0 ng/dL) and no contraindications for the use of iodinated contrast agents (34). IVU is first line imaging modality for extraurethral incontinence although the renal unit associated with an ectopic ureter is, however, often small, poor functioning, ectopic, and can be sometimes be difficult to image notwithstanding unless delayed films and tomography are used (Fig. 36.2) (35–37). In case the renal moiety cannot be imaged on IVU and CT, MRI or isotope scanning are recommended (38–40). IVU is still recommended in case of ureterovaginal fistula although uro-CT and uro-MR can be also used, and dilatation of the UUT is observed in 84% to 92% of fistula cases (41,42).

CT and MRI

Both techniques have been recommended for the management of patients with a suspected ectopic ureter because of their ability to image small, poor-functioning renal moieties as well as the collecting system (43–46). Both CT and MRI require normal renal function whenever contrast medium is used and, although MR contrast agents were considered safe. They are now to be avoided if they cause adverse effects (47–49).

Isotopes Scanning

Isotope scanning is mainly used to quantify function of the individual renal moieties and to locate ectopic or poorly functioning kidneys. Whenever renal functional impairment is suspected and separate renal function must be quantified, isotope scanning is the technique of choice. Interpretation of isotope scanning is not always straightforward as there are various physiological factors and technical pitfalls that can influence the results. These include the choice of radionucleotide, timing of diuretic injection, state of hydration and diuresis, fullness or back pressure from the bladder, variable renal function, and compliance of the collecting system (50,51). In the suspicion of an ectopic ureter, renal scintigraphy may be successful in imaging hypoplastic kidneys when other techniques have failed (52).

X-RAY IMAGING OF THE LUT

For many years, X-ray imaging of the LUT has been performed in female patients with UI and POP whenever surgery was planned. Quantification of bladder neck mobility and pelvic organ descend was considered of importance for proper patient management, but a more strict evaluation of the available evidence failed to confirm any clinical benefit in the standard patients. X-ray imaging can sometimes help identifying coexisting conditions of the LUT such as bladder diverticula, urethral diverticulum, or comorbidities such as bladder stones, tumors, foreign bodies, etc. (Figs. 36.3–36.6).

X-ray imaging in LUTD mainly consists of voiding cystourethrogram (VCUG) for the quantification of bladder neck mobility (Figs. 36.7 and 36.8) or bladder prolapse (Fig. 36.9); opacification of the vagina and rectum have been proposed to achieve a more complete visualization of the pelvic organs (Figs. 36.10 and 36.11) (53). In the pediatric population, retrograde cystography, and VCUG has been used to diagnose vesicoureteric reflux (54).

In the suspicion of urethral diverticulum, positive pressure urethrography has been shown to be more sensitive than VCUG (55–57) but X-ray imaging has been replaced by US imaging and particularly MRI that is now considered the gold standard for proper delineation of the diverticulum anatomy and the relation with the surrounding structures (58–60).

Quantification of Bladder Neck Mobility

VCUG was pioneered by Mikulicz-Radecki in 1931 (61). The technique was further developed by Stevens and Smith with the introduction of a metallic bead to identify urethra and by Ardran, et al. who proposed the use of cinematographic technique with opacification of the vagina and rectum (62,63). The combined use of imaging and pressure–flow recordings was proposed in the 1960s and 1970s and rapidly gained acceptance in the urological community (64,65). Description of VCUG methodology goes beyond the scope of this chapter but the interested reader can find details about the technique's history and methodology in a nice review by Olesen (57).

A number of different parameters of VCUG have been proposed and assessed for reliability over the years. The posterior urethrovesical (PUV) angle is defined by two lines passing along the posterior urethra and the trigone (8), cut-off values

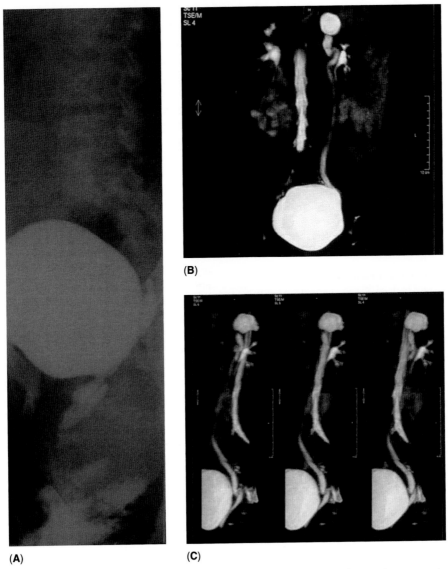

Figure 36.2 Intravenous pyelography in a 16-year-old patient with urinary incontinence. The intravenous pyelogram shows a complete duplex system on the left side. On a lateral projection, the ureter of the upper renal moiety travels below the bladder base, reaching the most distal part of the urethra (**A**); the anatomic condition is confirmed on uro-MR (**B, C**). *Source*: Courtesy of Professor G. Tomiselli.

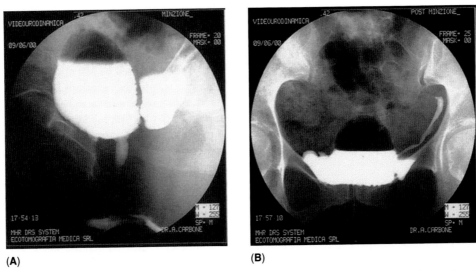

Figure 36.3 Digital fluoroscopy picture obtained during videourodynamics in a 63-year-old female with voiding dysfunction. Dilation of proximal urethra and a bladder diverticulum is evident on a voiding picture (**A**); vesicoureteral reflux is apparent on the post-voiding image (**B**). *Source*: Courtesy of Professor G. Tomiselli.

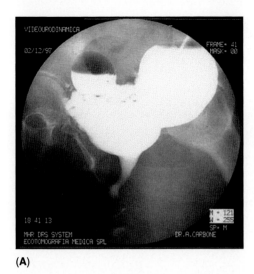 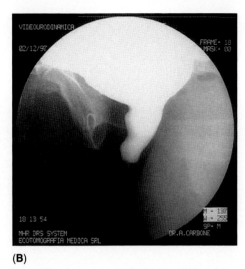

(A)   **(B)**

Figure 36.4 Digital fluoroscopy in a 72-year-old patient with voiding dysfunction. A decompensated bladder is observed during voiding (**A**) and severe dilation of proximal urethra is seen during videourodynamics (**B**). *Source*: Courtesy of Professor G. Tomiselli.

of 115° or more were proposed (Fig. 36.12) (3,9). The degree of urethral inclination is calculated as an angle between the proximal urethral axis and the vertical plane. Unfortunately the angle also varies with pelvic inclination, although, cut-off values of <45° or >45° have been described (3). The angle between a line through the middle of the internal urethral orifice and the urethral knee and a line through the posterior surface of the symphysis and the lowermost part of the obturator foramen closest to the film is defined as the urethropelvic angle (values of 95° are measured in controls and a cut-off value of 70° has been proposed to diagnose bladder descent) (61). The symphysis orifice (SO) distance is measured at rest as the distance on a horizontal line from the symphysis to the internal urethral orifice (normal values are 31 mm and values <20 mm are the cut off points for descent and were used to diagnose anterior bladder suspension defects or bladder base insufficiency) (61,66). In continent women, the urethral axis at rest (UAR) was found to be related to age ($R^2 = 0.28$); patients with UI had a mean UAR value of 25° and a mean UAS (urethral angle during straining) of 43°. Showalter et al. measured UAR and UAS before and after surgery showing that both angles returned close to normal after surgery suggesting a correlation between the correction of the defective bladder support and cure (67). Funneling of the proximal urethra, flatness of the bladder base, and the most dependent portion of the bladder base are important qualitative parameters estimated on straining films (9).

Analysis of the peer-reviewed literature suggest VCUG is not discriminant between continence and incontinence although promising data have also been also published (3,5,10,67,68). Interobserver and intraobserver agreement values of 43% to 79% and 53% to 99%, respectively, have been reported for VCUG parameters (9,69–71).

Overall, specificity and sensitivity values of 44% to 76% and 53% to 100%, respectively, were published (10,72). The type and degree of suspension defects were not related to the degree of SUI (6,69,70), with positive and negative predictive values of 0.70 and 0.52, respectively, on voiding colpocystourethrography (4,66).

Comparison of VCUG and US imaging suggested a good degree of correlation between the two techniques, particularly as regards bladder neck position and mobility, PUV, urethral inclination, SO distance, and rotation angle (6,72–74). Similar values of specificity, sensitivity, and interobserver agreement were also found. The availability and user friendliness of the US technique favor the use of it in most urogynecology practices.

VCUG was also compared to MRI and comparable data for bladder neck position and cystocele descent were found (75,76). Although the difference in the patient position between VCUG (standing) and MRI (lying) is of concern, comparison of standing, and lying colpocystourethrography did not showed any significant difference (76).

Overall, VCUG studies of women with and without UI failed to provide evidence of clinical utility. Several published studies showed significant overlap in the degree of bladder neck mobility and restoration of normal bladder neck mobility following surgery was not necessarily associated with cure of UI. These data, together with the introduction of US imaging and MRI of the pelvic floor, caused the oblivion of VCUG in the management of the standard patient with UI or POP. Although both US imaging and MRI opened a series of new perspective in the imaging of patients with UI, the measurement of bladder neck mobility failed to be of any clinical utility whatever technique was used.

Videourodynamics (VUDN)

The technique is sometimes considered the "gold standard" in the evaluation of LUTD (69). Actually there is no evidence that the combination of retrograde and voiding cystourethrography plus cystometry is superior to the two examinations performed separately; however, VUDN is frequently performed for convenience in the neurogenic population with LUTD (77–80) and in the pediatric population when indicated

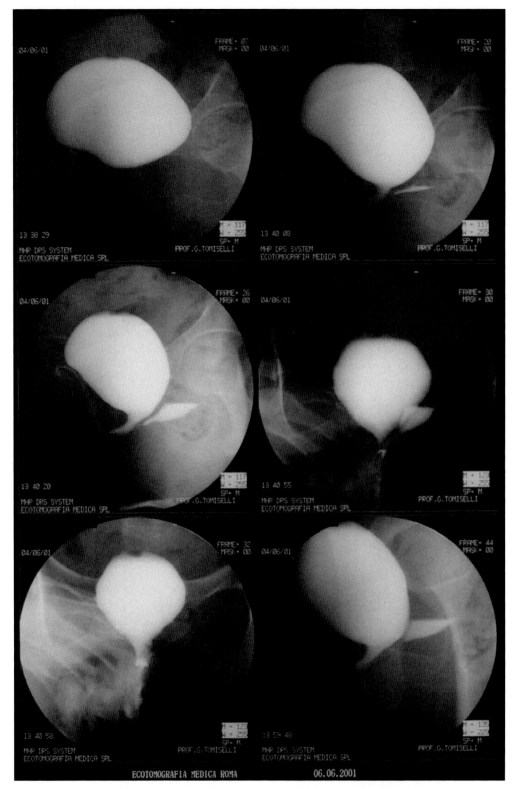

Figure 36.5 Voiding cystourethrogram in a 29-year-old patient with urinary incontinence. During the voiding phase, reflux of contrast medium into an ectopic ureter draining the upper moiety of a complete duplicated left renal system can be seen. In the last phase of the voiding study, the refluxing medium drains into the urethra. *Source*: Courtesy of Professor G. Tomiselli.

(e.g., suspicion of vesico-ureteral reflux) (81,82). The use of VUDN in female patients with UI is not recommended in the standard patients although it may play a role in selected cases. One study compared VCUG with VUDN in women with LUTD and found that in 7.5% out of 200 patients a correct diagnosis could only be made on VUDN (69). Although these data are certainly appealing, the X-ray hazard should also be considered (53,63,83–85).

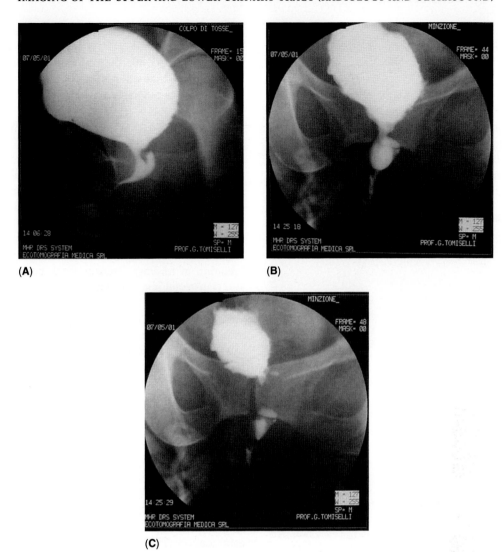

Figure 36.6 Urethral diverticulum of the posterior urethral wall is evident on voiding cystourethrogram in oblique (**A**) and in anteroposterior projections (**B, C**). *Source*: Courtesy of Professor G. Tomiselli.

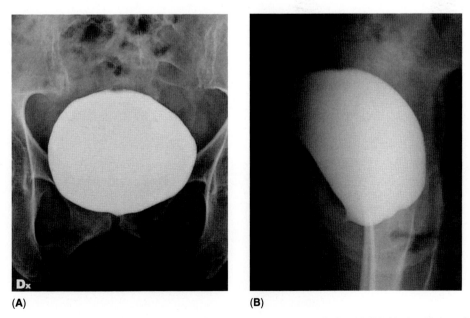

Figure 36.7 Cystourethrography in a 68-year-old patient without urinary incontinence. A symmetrically distended bladder is evident on the anteroposterior image (**A**), with the bladder base above the lower margin of the symphysis pubis; in the true lateral projection (**B**), the anterior and posterior urethrovesical angles are easily observed in the picture taken just before micturition. *Source*: Courtesy of Professor G. Tomiselli.

Conclusions

The use of X-ray imaging in female patients with UI and POP is limited. IVU, CT, and MRI of the UUT maintain a diagnostic role when evaluation of the renal moiety is needed in patients with ectopic ureters and the condition of the UUT needs to be monitored. X-ray imaging of the LUT is not recommended in the standard female patients with UI or POP. Notwithstanding a large body of evidence is available in the peer-reviewed literature concerning diagnostic accuracy, intra- and interobserver variability, and comparison with other

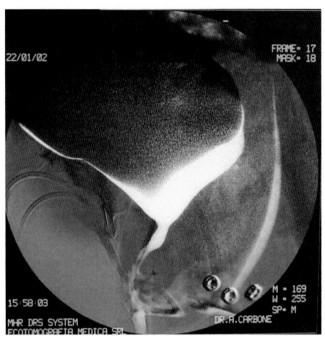

Figure 36.8 Voiding cystourethrogram with digital subtraction. There is normal funneling of the bladder neck with mild downward displacement during micturition. *Source:* Courtesy of Professor G. Tomiselli.

imaging techniques, VCUG cannot be recommended in the evaluation of the standard patient with UI or POP. VCUG is not recommended for the diagnosis or classification of UI. The technique may still have a role in the evaluation of complex patients and in patients with recurrent UI or POP.

ULTRASOUND OF THE LUT IN URINARY INCONTINENCE

In clinical practice, imaging of female urethra is usually performed whenever the presence of a diverticulum is suspected. Although diverticula can easily be shown on US, better anatomical definition is achieved with MRI that is thus considered the "gold standard" technique.

Proper knowledge of the imaging characteristics of the normal female urethra is of importance for adequate interpretation of findings. Transurethral, perineal, transvaginal, and transrectal imaging can be used. The echogenic characteristics of fibrous and muscular structures depend on the angle between the exploring beam and orientation of the muscle fibers. When the female urethra in normal position is imaged from a perineal approach, the US beam is parallel to the structures and the internal sphincter appears hypoechogenic, when the US beam is orthogonal to the structures such as in transvaginal/transrectal imaging, smooth muscle fibers appear hyperechogenic. It is thus difficult to evaluate possible modifications of urethral tissues (e.g., fibrosis) on US since the echogenic pattern of it also depends on how the imaging is performed. Furthermore, the echogenic pattern of female urethra may change during dynamic imaging because of the rotation of the structure on Valsalva and the relative change of incidence between the US beam and the internal sphincter. The external sphincter is known to be hyperechogenic on US (Fig. 36.13) and is more difficult to visualize (86,87). The rationale of assessing the thickness and volume of the female urethra in SUI relies on the hypothesis that

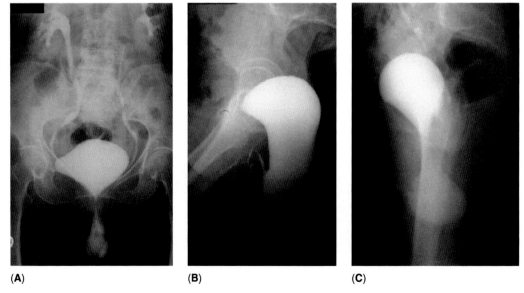

(A)   (B)   (C)

Figure 36.9 Grade IV genital prolapse can be observed in a 63-year-old patient during intravenous pyelography in anteroposterior (**A**) and true lateral projection (**B**); the relationship between pubic bone, bladder trigone, and urethra is best appreciated during voiding cystourethrogram in a true lateral projection (**C**). *Source:* Courtesy of Professor G. Tomiselli.

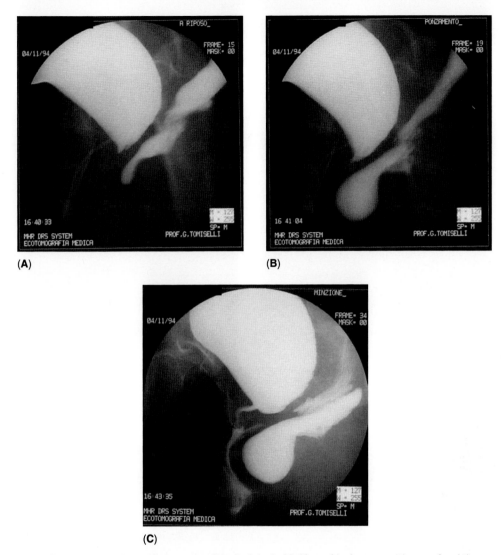

Figure 36.10 Voiding cystourethrogram in a patient with contrast medium both in the bladder and in the rectum. Pictures taken (**A**) at rest, (**B**) during Valsalva, and (**C**) voiding show a gradual distension of the rectocele pouch. *Source:* Courtesy of Professor G. Tomiselli.

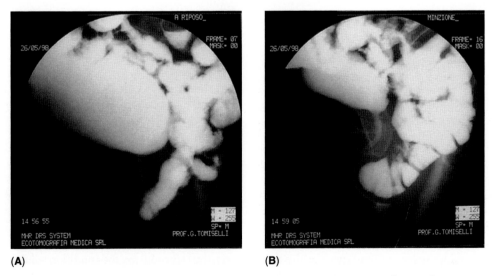

Figure 36.11 Cystourethrography with simultaneous administration of small bowel contrast allows the diagnosis of enterocele in a 61-year-old patient suffering from vaginal vault prolapse. Small bowel protruding down to the perineum level can be observed both at rest (**A**) and during voiding cystourethrogram (**B**), with a significant increase of the enterocele mass when abdominal pressure increases. *Source:* Courtesy of Professor G. Tomiselli.

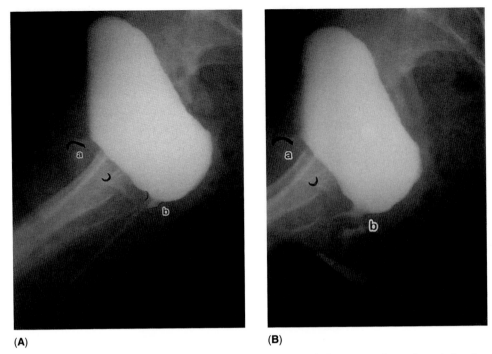

(A)   **(B)**

Figure 36.12 Voiding cystourethrogram: anteroposterior picture with a fully distended bladder (**A**); the acute anterior urethrovesical angle and the obtuse posterior angle are evident on true lateral projection when the bladder neck is filled with contrast medium, at the beginning of the voiding phase (**B**). *Source*: Courtesy of Professor G. Tomiselli.

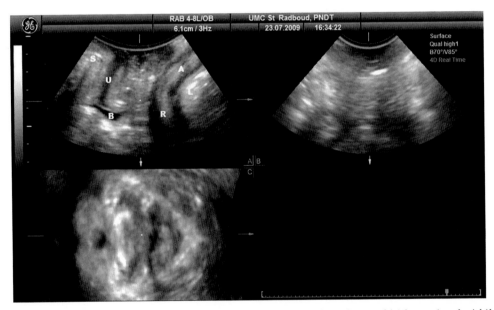

Figure 36.13 Perineal ultrasound imaging in a woman with normal pelvic anatomy. Midsagittal (*left upper*), coronal (*right upper*), and axial (*left lower*) two-dimensional view. *Abbreviation*: S, symphysis pubis; U, urethra; B, bladder; R, rectum; A, anus; L, levator ani muscle.

these measurements and the strength are related, so that measurement of sphincter volume could be a proxy for the parameters of the urethral pressure profile (UPP). Measurement of urethral sphincter proved to be reproducible (87–89), but urethral volumes as assessed with a formula using 2-D measurements and 3-D volume measurements differed significantly (89). Measurement of striated sphincter volume seemed of importance as this was found to be related to symptoms and signs of SUI (87,88) and with UPP (90–93). Urethral sphincter volume was associated with the outcome of surgery for SUI (94).

Rightly or wrongly, pelvic floor imaging in SUI patients aims mainly at the quantification of bladder neck mobility. The bladder outlet is easily visible on US, independently from the degree of filling. The position of bladder neck with respect to the lower margin of the pubic bones is measured at rest and during provocative maneuvers (coughing, Valsalva maneuver), thus reproducing the conditions under which SUI occurs in a particular patient. Bladder neck displacement can also be measured during squeezing (95). During Valsalva, bladder neck, and urethra are considered to rotate posteriorly and inferiorly (caudally and dorsally), and the displacement can be measured in different ways (96–100) with reasonable clinical reproducibility (101,102). The large variability of urethral mobility in continent nulliparous women (1–40 mm) (103–106) made the provision of normative data impossible. Parous women are known to have a larger degree of bladder neck mobility than nulliparous (93,95,107–109) and hypermobility is considered to be associated with SUI (24,107). The sensitivity and specificity of US imaging of the bladder neck mobility for the diagnosis of SUI varies between 92% and 96% (110) and 83% and 68% (111), respectively. Analysis of urethrovesical movement patterns on dynamic perineal US imaging in continent and incontinent women did not result in any characteristic movement pattern being associated with SUI (112). Notwithstanding a huge research effort, US imaging of the bladder neck failed to provide a significant advantage in the management of patients with SUI (113,114). Comparison of interobserver variability of different methods to quantify urethral mobility, such as Q-tip test, Sensor-Q™ test, and US, showed a lower interobserver reliability for the US imaging technique (115).

Post Void Residual (PVR) Urine

Measuring PVR in patients with UI and POP is considered part of the safety assessment before and after surgery. PVR is not uncommon in women with LUTD and is considered to be associated with an increased risk of urinary tract infection. The condition may develop de novo following surgery for SUI and POP. Since US imaging was first applied in the evaluation of PVR, it self-imposed as the gold standard against catheterization (116–119). To correct for deviations of the bladder shape from a sphere, various formulas have been proposed with different correction factors. In a study comparing 12 formulas, the formula "$\pi \times$ height $\times$ width $\times$ depth in centimeters/6" showed the best agreement between US volume and catheterized volume (120). In daily clinical practice, the residual volume is probably best approximated by height $\times$ width $\times$ depth in centimeters $\times$ 0.5. Automated US systems are widely used as they have been shown to be accurate and usable by nursing staff (121). Data from asymptomatic peri- and postmenopausal women suggest a median PVR of 19 ml with 95% of subjects having a PVR <100 ml (117). In another study, women with LUT symptoms showed an average PVR < 30 ml in 81% of cases, larger volumes were associated with increasing age, higher grades of POP, and increased prevalence of recurrent urinary tract infections (122).

Bladder Wall Thickness (BWT) Measurement for the Diagnosis of Detrusor Overactivity (DO)

In 1994, Khullar et al. showed a significant difference in the BWT of female patients with DO and controls (6.7 ± 0.6 mm vs. 3.5 ± 0.6 mm, respectively). In 1996, US evaluation of BWT was proposed as a diagnostic tool to identify patients with DO, since 94% of women with a urodynamics diagnosis of DO had a BWT > 5 mm. Confirmatory data were published in 2002 and 2003. The lack of standardization in the US measurement of BWT hampered a more widespread adoption in daily practice.

Promising results on automated measurement of BWT were published and confirmatory data are eagerly awaited (123,124). Although several papers confirmed the diagnostic value of BWT measurement for the diagnosis of DO, a retrospective analysis of a patient cohort undergoing perineal US for pelvic floor evaluation showed only a low diagnostic accuracy of BWT measurement (125). New automated systems for the measurement of BWT and US estimated bladder weight are currently under evaluation and may translate clinical research into our daily practice.

Imaging of Pelvic Floor Muscles

Different groups have investigated pelvic floor biomechanics (126–131) and much progress has been made in recent years. Computer models have shown that the pelvic floor muscles need to stretch 3.3 times their normal muscle length (131). Avulsion traumas of the lavatory ani muscle from the pubic bone have shown to be associated with POP in the anterior and central compartment (132,133). From a clinical standpoint, however, research on imaging still needs to provide an answer to the hypothesis that information on pelvic muscles morphology can predict the outcome of physical and surgical intervention for UI and POP.

Evaluation of the pelvic floor function may be considered as an integral part of the physical examination in patients with UI or POP, and US is increasingly used for the purpose. US imaging of pelvic floor muscle during exercise have been used as a biofeedback for the patient undergoing pelvic floor rehabilitation (134,135). The importance of good pelvic floor function is proven by the significant therapeutic effect of pelvic floor rehabilitation in UI. Significant change in imaging parameters were found following exercise, including bladder neck resting position (136), and pelvic floor muscle thickness (137). Parameters like the cranial lift of the urethra in relation to the pubic bones during squeezing, the dimension of the genital hiatus, and the posterior ano-rectal angle were measured on US and found to be comparable with data obtained with palpation and perineometry (27,138–141).

Measurements of pelvic muscle thickness and volume may be performed with 3D US (Fig. 36.14) and MRI (22,142–145), but only low test–retest and interobserver variability have been observed (22,146,147). Normative data in healthy controls and athletes have been published (103,137,148). As one could expect, pelvic floor muscles were found to be thinner in women with POP (24,149–151) or UI (149,152) and their genital hiatus was larger (153). Women who undergo regular exercise had thicker muscles compared to controls (148) and Chinese women had thinner muscles than Caucasians (145).

Pelvic floor function depends on the integrity of its different muscles (Fig. 36.15). The levator ani, or in more detail the sling of the puborectal muscle, may suffer avulsion from the pubic bones in vaginally parous women, and the risk of trauma increases with maternal age at first delivery (154). Levator trauma has been observed at the time of labor but no effective therapeutic measures have been identified (155,156). Muscle detachment is best visualized when the muscle contracts as this maneuver increases the gap with the pubic bone. On an

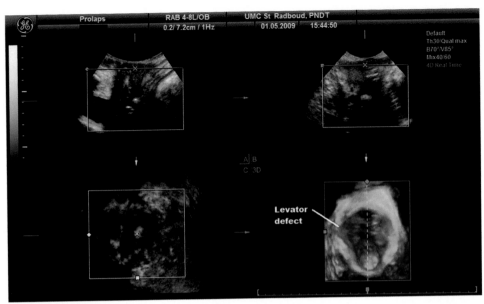

Figure 36.14 Perineal midsagittal (*left upper*), coronal (*right upper*), and axial (*left lower*) two-dimensional view and three-dimensional rendered image (*right lower*). The rendered image suggests a right-sided levator defect, which needs to be confirmed in the tomographic ultrasound imaging.

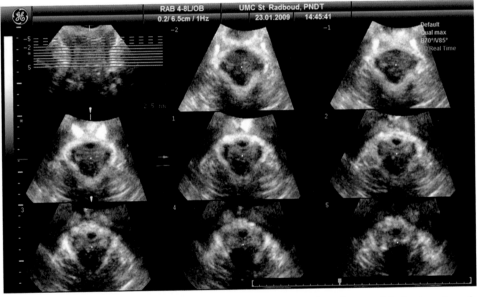

Figure 36.15 Tomographic ultrasound imaging in oblique axial plane. Normal attachments of the levator ani muscle.

axial plane, the loss of the characteristics H shape of the vagina is an indirect sign of levator ani detachment (113,157) and is considered to correspond to what previously described as paravaginal defects (158–161). Methods for quantification of muscle defects on MRI (162) and US imaging (144) have been proposed.

Levator ani detachment (Fig. 36.16) observed on US is associated with a two to sixfold increase in the risk of POP (155) in the anterior and central compartments (132,163). Avulsion of the muscle did not seem to be associated with an increased risk of SUI (164). Muscle detachment from the pubic bone is associated with decreased muscle strength at physical examination (158). The correlation between detection of avulsion on 3-D US imaging and palpation was however only poor (165) mainly due to high interobserver variability in the physical examina-

tion of muscle defects (166). Measurement of the genital hiatus on US (Fig. 36.17) is a reproducible measurement (22,157) and data at rest correlate well with MRI data, although a lower degree of correlation was found during Valsalva (143). Values of >30, >35, and >40 cm^2 were described as mild, moderate, and severe ballooning of the genital hiatus (167). In nulliparous women, areas of 6 to 36 cm^2 have been measured (148,153). Vaginal delivery was associated with an enlargement of the levator hiatus (168). Hiatal dimensions at Valsalva were furthermore correlated with the severity of POP (130,144,150).

On MRI of the dimensions of the bony pelvis at the level of the muscular pelvic support, no differences in these dimensions could be found between women with and without POP (162).

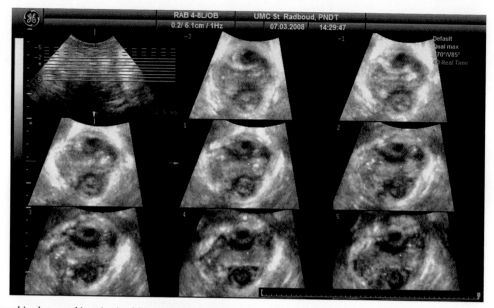

Figure 36.16 Tomographic ultrasound imaging in oblique axial plane. Right-sided avulsion of the levator ani muscle from the symphysis pubis (levator defect).

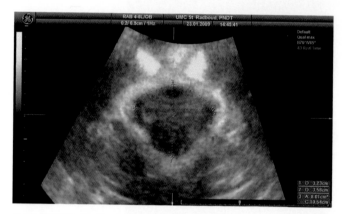

Figure 36.17 Perineal two-dimensional image in oblique axial plane. Measurement of hiatal dimensions.

US imaging and MRI are both appropriate methods in the investigation of the integrity of sphincter ani muscle. On US, the internal anal spincter can easily be visualized, whereas in case of the external sphincter more expertise may be needed (169). A recent study has shown that thickening of the internal sphincter occurred with increasing age, whereas only thinning of the external sphincter correlated with fecal incontinence but not with aging (170).

Imaging of POP

There is a large natural variability in the degree of pelvic organ descent for all three compartments in nulliparous and parous women. After delivery, an increase of pelvic organ mobility was found in all compartments (171). A correlation was also found between increase of organ mobility, length of the second stage of labor, and delivery mode. Operative vaginal delivery was associated with the highest rate of increase in pelvic organ mobility. Generally speaking, the effect of vaginal delivery on pelvic organ descent is more evident in the anterior and central compartments than in the posterior one (172,173). The first delivery has a larger impact on bladder neck descent

than the subsequent ones (90). Interestingly, pelvic organ mobility is not merely a negative factor as US imaging performed during pregnancy showed that a larger bladder neck mobility and a larger and more distensible genital hiatus were associated with natural vaginal delivery (173,174). Unfortunately, a large bladder neck descent is also associated with a higher risk of UI (28).

The sensation or visualization of a bulge in the vagina has shown to be the only symptom that correlated with the degree of POP (175). This finding was irrespective of the method used for the quantification of the degree of POP: POP-quantification (POP-Q), dynamic MRI, or US imaging (176). There is only one study available where POPQ predicted prolapse symptoms better than US (177).

In MRI, various reference lines for quantification of POP have been studied, and the pubococcygeal line showed minor superiority (25,178). For the sake of standardization, the use of this line is advocated. In US, the lack of a reference line through two bony points is an obvious limitation. A horizontal line passing through the lower margin of the symphysis pubis has been used (179), whereas a line through the anal canal is used as a reference point to quantify the severity of rectocele (Fig. 36.18) (177). A cut-off value of 15 mm for descent below the line through the symphysis, and of 20 mm for the depth of a rectocele, has been proposed as a threshold for symptomatic prolapse (180).

Good reproducibility and correlation has been shown for the anterior compartment as assessed on MRI and US imaging (20,179,181) and physical examination. The assessments may thus be interchangeable and the additional value of imaging techniques seems limited in this compartment.

Imaging of the posterior compartment has also been explored in several studies (180,182–189). Poor, moderate, and good interobserver variability in US imaging and MRI has been described (101,178,185,190). [Comparison of X-ray imaging and US showed similar rates of detection for enteroceles (71%) (189)]. Although US and clinical staging or

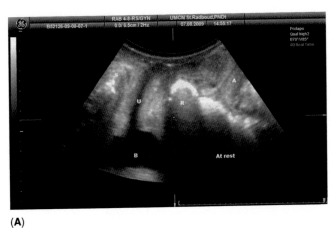
(A)

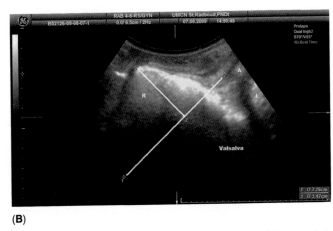
(B)

Figure 36.18 Perineal midsagittal two-dimensional view (**A**) at rest and (**B**) on Valsalva in a woman with rectocele. Measurement of the depth of the rectocele is performed perpendicular to a straight line through the anterior border of the anal sphincter complex (3.47 cm). *Abbreviations*: S, symphysis pubis; U, urethra; B, bladder; R, rectum; A, anus; L, levator ani muscle.

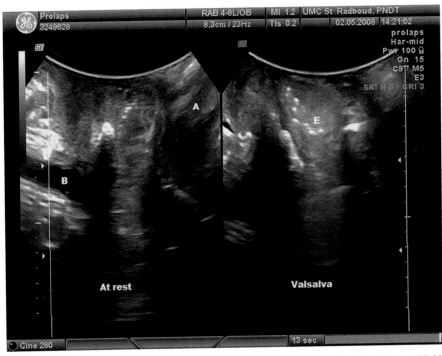

Figure 36.19 Perineal midsagittal two-dimensional view at rest and on Valsalva in a woman with enterocele. *Abbreviations*: B, bladder; E, enterocele; A, anus.

intraoperative findings correlated well (24,182,186), one-third of patients with clinical enterocele (Fig. 36.19) were negative on US. Furthermore, no clinical benefit has been identified from US imaging of enteroceles. The posterior anorectal angle can be measured on US with a good degree of correlation with defecography (180,189,191). The clinical meaning of perineal descent and the best assessment method has not been fully unraveled. In four studies, which have assessed the correlation between POP symptoms and perineal descent on US imaging, MRI, and defecography, a statistically significant correlation was observed in all studies (175,176,189,192).

Although imaging of POP is captivating, the question whether imaging is superior to clinical examination remains open.

US Imaging and Surgery for UI and POP

The role of US imaging during and after incontinence surgery has been investigated. Researchers tried to standardize the amount of bladder neck suspension during the Burch procedure and to correlate the relative position of urethral slings and urethra with the outcome of surgery. Actually no definitive conclusions can be drawn on the relation of sling position, resolution of UI, or postoperative complications (173,193–201). In some studies, tension-free vaginal tapes slings were found to be positioned more cranially compared to transobturator tapes and caused more often urethral kinking during straining, nevertheless, comparable cure rates were achieved (202,203). US imaging is clearly superior as compared to other imaging techniques regarding the visualization of polypropylene mesh materials (Fig. 36.20) as used in POP

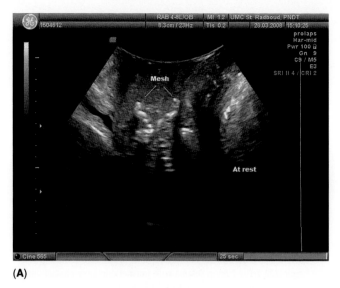

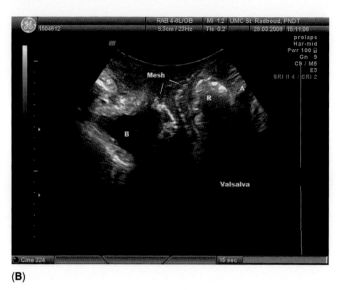

(A)   (B)

Figure 36.20 Perineal midsagittal two-dimensional view (**A**) at rest and (**B**) on Valsalva in a woman with polypropylene mesh (prolift anterior and posterior). *Abbreviations*: S, symphysis pubis; B, bladder; R, rectum; A, anus.

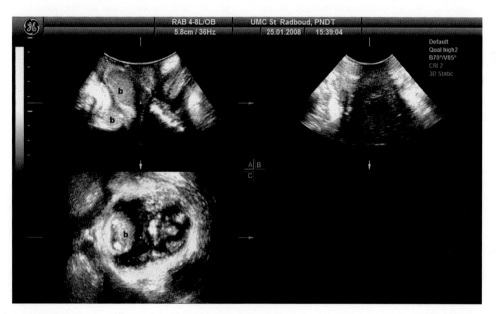

Figure 36.21 Perineal ultrasound imaging in a woman following periuretral bulking agents for stress urinary incontinence. Midsagittal (*left upper*), coronal (*right upper*), and axial (*left lower*) two-dimensional view. *Abbreviation*: b, periuretral bulking agent.

and UI surgery. Various studies have recently explored the causes for POP relapse but no conclusive data have been obtained yet (204–206).

US imaging of bulking agents injected for SUI (Fig. 36.21) showed a good correlation between the height and volumes of the injected collagen bulges and clinical outcome, with a collagen volume of 2.8 ml considered to be ideal (207,208).

CONCLUSIONS
Research into US imaging of the pelvic floor in UI and POP is vibrant and quality of the published data increased significantly over the last decade. Imaging has already proved to be comparable to physical examination and sometimes superior. Research in this area proved to be inventive, innovative, and prolific thanks to a widespread use of US systems in urological and

urogynecological offices. The evidence currently available should be carefully scrutinized to identify areas of consensus and areas that still need further verification and confirmation. The lack of proven clinical utility should not reduce our research effort and imaging is a powerful approach to improve our knowledge on the physiopathology of continence and POP. A new paradigm for proper evaluation of the level of evidence and grade of recommendations in this area is eagerly awaited.

REFERENCES
1. Bossuyt PM, Reitsma JB, Bruns DE, et al. The STARD statement for reporting studies of diagnostic accuracy: explanation and elaboration. Clin Chem 2003; 49: 7–18.
2. Medicine CFEB. 2009 [updated 2009 March 2009; cited 2009 15/08/2009]. [Available from: http://www.cebm.net/index.aspx?o=1025].

3. Green TH Jr. Development of a plan for the diagnosis and treatment of urinary stress incontinence. Am J Obstet Gynecol 1962; 83: 632–48.

4. Stage P, Fischer-Rasmussen W, Hansen RI. The value of colpo-cysto-urethrography in female stress- and urge incontinence and following operation. Acta Obstet Gynecol Scand 1986; 65: 401–4.

5. Pelsang RE, Bonney WW. Voiding cystourethrography in female stress incontinence. AJR Am J Roentgenol 1996; 166: 561–5.

6. Mouritsen L, Strandberg C, Jensen AR, et al. Inter- and intra-observer variation of colpo-cysto-urethrography diagnoses. Acta Obstet Gynecol Scand 1993; 72: 200–4.

7. Klarskov P, Vedel Jepsen P, Dorph S. Reliability of voiding colpo-cysto-urethrography in female urinary stress incontinence before and after treatment. Acta Radiol 1988; 29: 685–8.

8. Fantl JA, Hurt WG, Beachley MC, et al. Bead-chain cystourethrogram: an evaluation. Obstet Gynecol 1981; 58: 237–40.

9. Drutz HP, Shapiro BJ, Mandel F. Do static cystourethrograms have a role in the investigation of female incontinence? Am J Obstet Gynecol 1978; 130: 516–20.

10. Bergman A, McKenzie C, Ballard CA, Richmond J. Role of cystourethrography in the preoperative evaluation of stress urinary incontinence in women. J Reprod Med 1988; 33: 372–6.

11. White RD, McQuown D, McCarthy TA, Ostergard DR. Real-time ultrasonography in the evaluation of urinary stress incontinence. Am J Obstet Gynecol 1980; 138: 235–7.

12. Bernaschek G, Kratochwil A. Sonographic method for the measurement of the posterior urethrovesical angle. Gynakol Rundsch 1980; 20(Suppl 2): 208–11.

13. Koelbl H, Bernaschek G. A new method for sonographic urethrocystography and simultaneous pressure-flow measurements. Obstet Gynecol 1989; 74(3 Pt 1): 417–22.

14. Bergman A, Koonings P, Ballard CA, Platt LD. Ultrasonic prediction of stress urinary incontinence development in surgery for severe pelvic relaxation. Gynecol Obstet Invest 1988; 26: 66–72.

15. Kohorn EI, Scioscia AL, Jeanty P, Hobbins JC. Ultrasound cystourethrography by perineal scanning for the assessment of female stress urinary incontinence. Obstet Gynecol 1986; 68: 269–72.

16. Mouritsen L, Strandberg C. Vaginal ultrasonography versus colpo-cysto-urethrography in the evaluation of female urinary incontinence. Acta Obstet Gynecol Scand 1994; 73: 338–42.

17. Schaer GN, Koechli OR, Schuessler B, Haller U. Perineal ultrasound for evaluating the bladder neck in urinary stress incontinence. Obstet Gynecol 1995; 85: 220–4.

18. Troeger C, Gugger M, Holzgreve W, Wight E. Correlation of perineal ultrasound and lateral chain urethrocystography in the anatomical evaluation of the bladder neck. Int Urogynecol J Pelvic Floor Dysfunct 2003; 14: 380–4.

19. Shah W, Honeck P, Kwon ST, et al. The role of perineal ultrasound compared to lateral cysturethrogram in urogynecological evaluations. Aktuelle Urol 2007; 38: 144–7.

20. Broekhuis SR, Kluivers KB, Hendriks JC, et al. POP-Q, dynamic MR imaging, and perineal ultrasonography: do they agree in the quantification of female pelvic organ prolapse? Int Urogynecol J Pelvic Floor Dysfunct 2009; 20: 541–9.

21. Wise BG, Burton G, Cutner A, Cardozo LD. Effect of vaginal ultrasound probe on lower urinary tract function. Br J Urol 1992; 70: 12–16.

22. Braekken IH, Majida M, Ellstrom-Engh M, et al. Test-retest and intra-observer repeatability of two-, three- and four-dimensional perineal ultrasound of pelvic floor muscle anatomy and function. Int Urogynecol J Pelvic Floor Dysfunct 2008; 19: 227–35.

23. Tunn R, Schaer G, Peschers U, et al. Updated recommendations on ultrasonography in urogynecology. Int Urogynecol J Pelvic Floor Dysfunct 2005; 16: 236–41.

24. Dietz HP. Ultrasound imaging of the pelvic floor. Part I: two-dimensional aspects. Ultrasound Obstet Gynecol 2004; 23: 80–92.

25. Broekhuis SR, Futterer JJ, Barentsz JO, Vierhout ME, Kluivers KB. A systematic review of clinical studies on dynamic magnetic resonance imaging of pelvic organ prolapse: the use of reference lines and anatomical landmarks. Int Urogynecol J Pelvic Floor Dysfunct 2009; 20: 721–9.

26. Martan A, Drbohlav P, Masata M, Halaska M, Voigt R. Changes in the position of the urethra and bladder neck during pregnancy and after delivery. Ceska Gynekol 1996; 61: 35–9.

27. Dietz HP, Wilson PD. The influence of bladder volume on the position and mobility of the urethrovesical junction. Int Urogynecol J Pelvic Floor Dysfunct 1999; 10: 3–6.

28. King JK, Freeman RM. Is antenatal bladder neck mobility a risk factor for postpartum stress incontinence? Br J Obstet Gynaecol 1998; 105: 1300–7.

29. Howard D, Miller JM, Delancey JO, Ashton-Miller JA. Differential effects of cough, valsalva, and continence status on vesical neck movement. Obstet Gynecol 2000; 95: 535–40.

30. McGuire EJ, Woodside JR, Borden TA, Weiss RM. Prognostic value of urodynamic testing in myelodysplastic patients. J Urol 1981; 126: 205–9.

31. Kontogeorgos L, Vassilopoulos P, Tentes A. Bilateral severe hydroureter-onephrosis due to uterine prolapse. Br J Urol 1985; 57: 360–1.

32. Konda R, Sakai K, Ota S, et al. Ultrasound grade of hydronephrosis and severity of renal cortical damage on 99m technetium dimercaptosuccinic acid renal scan in infants with unilateral hydronephrosis during followup and after pyeloplasty. J Urol 2002; 167: 2159–63.

33. Platt JF, Rubin JM, Ellis JH. Distinction between obstructive and nonobstructive pyelocaliectasis with duplex Doppler sonography. AJR Am J Roentgenol 1989; 153: 997–1000.

34. Toprak O. Conflicting and new risk factors for contrast induced nephropathy. J Urol 2007; 178: 2277–83.

35. Braverman RM, Lebowitz RL. Occult ectopic ureter in girls with urinary incontinence: diagnosis by using CT. AJR Am J Roentgenol 1991; 156: 365–6.

36. Utsunomiya M, Itoh H, Yoshioka T, Okuyama A, Itatani H. Renal dysplasia with a single vaginal ectopic ureter: the role of computerized tomography. J Urol 1984; 132: 98–100.

37. Prewitt LH Jr, Lebowitz RL. The single ectopic ureter. AJR Am J Roentgenol 1976; 127: 941–8.

38. Borer JG, Bauer SB, Peters CA, et al. A single-system ectopic ureter draining an ectopic dysplastic kidney: delayed diagnosis in the young female with continuous urinary incontinence. Br J Urol 1998; 81: 474–8.

39. Bozorgi F, Connolly LP, Bauer SB, et al. Hypoplastic dysplastic kidney with a vaginal ectopic ureter identified by technetium-99m-DMSA scintigraphy. J Nucl Med 1998; 39: 113–15.

40. Carrico C, Lebowitz RL. Incontinence due to an infrasphincteric ectopic ureter: why the delay in diagnosis and what the radiologist can do about it. Pediatr Radiol 1998; 28: 942–9.

41. Mandal AK, Sharma SK, Vaidyanathan S, Goswami AK. Ureterovaginal fistula: summary of 18 years' experience. Br J Urol 1990; 65: 453–6.

42. Murphy DM, Grace PA, O'Flynn JD. Ureterovaginal fistula: a report of 12 cases and review of the literature. J Urol 1982; 128: 924–5.

43. Pantuck AJ, Barone JG, Rosenfeld DL, Fleisher MH. Occult bilateral ectopic vaginal ureters causing urinary incontinence: diagnosis by computed tomography. Abdom Imaging 1996; 21: 78–80.

44. Leyendecker JR, Barnes CE, Zagoria RJ. MR urography: techniques and clinical applications. Radiographics 2008; 28: 23–46; discussion 46–7.

45. Avni EF, Matos C, Rypens F, Schulman CC. Ectopic vaginal insertion of an upper pole ureter: demonstration by special sequences of magnetic resonance imaging. J Urol 1997; 158: 1931–2.

46. Kaneko K, Ohtsuka Y, Suzuki Y, et al. Masked ureteral duplication with ectopic ureter detected by magnetic resonance imaging. Acta Paediatr Jpn 1996; 38: 291–3.

47. Grobner T. Gadolinium—a specific trigger for the development of nephrogenic fibrosing dermopathy and nephrogenic systemic fibrosis? Nephrol Dial Transplant 2006; 21: 1104–8.

48. Marckmann P, Skov L, Rossen K, et al. Nephrogenic systemic fibrosis: suspected causative role of gadodiamide used for contrast-enhanced magnetic resonance imaging. J Am Soc Nephrol 2006; 17: 2359–62.

49. Perazella MA. Gadolinium-contrast toxicity in patients with kidney disease: nephrotoxicity and nephrogenic systemic fibrosis. Curr Drug Saf 2008; 3: 67–75.

50. Conway JJ. "Well-tempered" diuresis renography: its historical development, physiological and technical pitfalls, and standardized technique protocol. Semin Nucl Med 1992; 22: 74–84.

51. O'Reilly PH. Diuresis renography. Recent advances and recommended protocols. Br J Urol 1992; 69: 113–20.

52. Pattaras JG, Rushton HG, Majd M. The role of 99 m technetium dimercapto-succinic acid renal scans in the evaluation of occult ectopic ureters in girls with paradoxical incontinence. J Urol 1999; 162(3 Pt 1): 821–5.

53. Olesen KP, Walter S. Colpo-cysto-urethrography: a radiological method combined with pressure-flow measurements. Dan Med Bull 1977; 24: 96–101.

54. Bellinger MF. The management of vesicoureteric reflux. Urol Clin North Am 1985; 12: 23–9.

55. Jacoby K, Rowbotham RK. Double balloon positive pressure urethrography is a more sensitive test than voiding cystourethrography for diagnosing urethral diverticulum in women. J Urol 1999; 162: 2066–9.

56. Romanzi LJ, Groutz A, Blaivas JG. Urethral diverticulum in women: diverse presentations resulting in diagnostic delay and mismanagement. J Urol 2000; 164: 428–33.

57. Olesen KP. Descent of the female urinary bladder. A radiological classification based on colpo-cysto-urethrography. Dan Med Bull 1983; 30: 66–84.

58. Neitlich JD, Foster HE Jr, Glickman MG, Smith RC. Detection of urethral diverticula in women: comparison of a high resolution fast spin echo technique with double balloon urethrography. J Urol 1998; 159: 408–10.

59. Foster RT, Amundsen CL, Webster GD. The utility of magnetic resonance imaging for diagnosis and surgical planning before transvaginal periurethral diverticulectomy in women. Int Urogynecol J Pelvic Floor Dysfunct 2007; 18: 315–19.

60. Rovner ES. Urethral diverticula: a review and an update. Neurourol Urodyn 2007; 26: 972–7.

61. V. Mikulicz-Radecki F. Röntgenologische studien zur ätiologie der urethralen inkontinenz. Zbl Gynäk 1931; 55: 795–810.

62. Stevens WE, Smith SP. Roentgenological examination of the female urethra. J Urol 1937; 37: 194–2001.

63. Ardran GM, Simmons CA, Stewart JH. The closure of the female urethra. J Obstet Gynaecol Br Emp 1956; 63: 26–35.

64. Enhoerning G, Miller ER, Hinman F Jr. Urethral closure studied with cineroentgenography and simultaneous bladder-urethra pressure recording. Surg Gynecol Obstet 1964; 118: 507–16.

65. Bates CP, Whiteside CG, Turner-Warwick R. Synchronous cine-pressure-flow-cysto-urethrography with special reference to stress and urge incontinence. Br J Urol 1970; 42: 714–23.

66. Gjorup T. Reliability of diagnostic tests. Acta Obstet Gynecol Scand Suppl 1997; 166: 9–14.

67. Showalter PR, Zimmern PE, Roehrborn CG, Lemack GE. Standing cystourethrogram: an outcome measure after anti-incontinence procedures and cystocele repair in women. Urology 2001; 58: 33–7.

68. Kitzmiller JL, Manzer GA, Nebel WA, Lucas WE. Chain cystourethrogram and stress incontinence. Obstet Gynecol 1972; 39: 333–40.

69. Barnick CG, Cardozo LD, Benness C. Use of routine videocystourethrography in the evaluation of female lower urinary tract dysfunction. Neurourol Urodyn 1989; 8: 447–9.

70. Fischer-Rasmussen W, Hansen RI, Stage P. Predictive values of diagnostic tests in the evaluation of female urinary stress incontinence. Acta Obstet Gynecol Scand 1986; 65: 291–4.

71. Gordon D, Pearce M, Norton P, Stanton SL. Comparison of ultrasound and lateral chain urethrocystography in the determination of bladder neck descent. Am J Obstet Gynecol 1989; 160: 182–5.

72. v. Christ F, Meyer-Delpho W. Röntgendiagnostik bei der weiblichen harninkontinenz. Fortschr Röntgenstr 1981; 134: 551–6.

73. Kolbl H, Bernaschek G, Wolf G. A comparative study of perineal ultrasound scanning and urethrocystography in patients with genuine stress incontinence. Arch Gynecol Obstet 1988; 244: 39–45.

74. Dietz HP, Wilson PD. Anatomical assessment of the bladder outlet and proximal urethra using ultrasound and videocystourethrography. Int Urogynecol J Pelvic Floor Dysfunct 1998; 9: 365–9.

75. Gufler H, DeGregorio G, Allmann KH, Kundt G, Dohnicht S. Comparison of cystourethrography and dynamic MRI in bladder neck descent. J Comput Assist Tomogr 2000; 24: 382–8.

76. Gufler H, Ohde A, Grau G, Grossmann A. Colpocystoproctography in the upright and supine positions correlated with dynamic MRI of the pelvic floor. Eur J Radiol 2004; 51: 41–7.

77. Sakakibara R, Hattori T, Uchiyama T, Yamanishi T. Videourodynamic and sphincter motor unit potential analyses in Parkinson's disease and multiple system atrophy. J Neurol Neurosurg Psychiatry 2001; 71: 600–6.

78. Hinman F. Urinary tract damage in children who wet. Pediatrics 1974; 54: 143–50.

79. Allen TD. The non-neurogenic neurogenic bladder. J Urol 1977; 117: 232–8.

80. Williams DI, Hirst G, Doyle D. The occult neuropathic bladder. J Pediatr Surg 1974; 9: 35–41.

81. Podesta ML, Castera R, Ruarte AC. Videourodynamic findings in young infants with severe primary reflux. J Urol 2004; 171(2 Pt 1): 829–33; discussion 833.

82. Soygur T, Arikan N, Tokatli Z, Karaboga R. The role of video-urodynamic studies in managing non-neurogenic voiding dysfunction in children. BJU Int 2004; 93: 841–3.

83. Pick EJ, Davis R, Stacey AJ. Radiation dose in cinecystourethrography of the female. Br J Radiol 1960; 33: 451–4.

84. Westby M, Ulmsten U, Asmussen M. Dynamic urethrocystography in women. Urol Int 1983; 38: 329–36.

85. Rud T, Ulmsten U, Westby M. Initiation of micturition: a study of combined urethrocystometry and urethrocystography in healthy and stress incontinent females. Scand J Urol Nephrol 1979; 13: 259–64.

86. Kondo Y, Homma Y, Takahashi S, Kitamura T, Kawabe K. Transvaginal ultrasound of urethral sphincter at the mid urethra in continent and incontinent women. J Urol 2001; 165: 149–52.

87. Umek WH, Obermair A, Stutterecker D, et al. Three-dimensional ultrasound of the female urethra: comparing transvaginal and transrectal scanning. Ultrasound Obstet Gynecol 2001; 17: 425–30.

88. Athanasiou S, Khullar V, Boos K, Salvatore S, Cardozo L. Imaging the urethral sphincter with three-dimensional ultrasound. Obstet Gynecol 1999; 94: 295–301.

89. Toozs-Hobson P, Khullar V, Cardozo L. Three-dimensional ultrasound: a novel technique for investigating the urethral sphincter in the third trimester of pregnancy. Ultrasound Obstet Gynecol 2001; 17: 421–4.

90. Khullar V, Salvatore S, Cardozo L. Three dimensional ultrasound of the urethra and urethral pressure profiles. Int Urogynecol J 1994; 5: 319.

91. Robinson D, Toozs-Hobson P, Cardozo L, Digesu A. Correlating structure and function: three-dimensional ultrasound of the urethral sphincter. Ultrasound Obstet Gynecol 2004; 23: 272–6.

92. Wiseman OJ, Swinn MJ, Brady CM, Fowler CJ. Maximum urethral closure pressure and sphincter volume in women with urinary retention. J Urol 2002; 167: 1348–51; discussion 1351–2.

93. Dietz HP, Clarke B. The urethral pressure profile and ultrasound imaging of the lower urinary tract. Int Urogynecol J Pelvic Floor Dysfunct 2001; 12: 38–41.

94. Digesu GA, Robinson D, Cardozo L, Khullar V. Three-dimensional ultrasound of the urethral sphincter predicts continence surgery outcome. Neurourol Urodyn 2009; 28: 90–4.

95. Hol M, van Bolhuis C, Vierhout ME. Vaginal ultrasound studies of bladder neck mobility. Br J Obstet Gynaecol 1995; 102: 47–53.

96. Shek KL, Dietz HP. The urethral motion profile: a novel method to evaluate urethral support and mobility. Aust N Z J Obstet Gynaecol 2008; 48: 337–42.

97. Dietz HP, Eldridge A, Grace M, Clarke B. Pelvic organ descent in young nulligravid women. Am J Obstet Gynecol 2004; 191: 95–9.

98. Martan A, Masata J, Halaska M, Voigt R. Ultrasound imaging of the lower urinary system in women after Burch colposuspension. Ultrasound Obstet Gynecol 2001; 17: 58–64.

99. Alper T, Cetinkaya M, Okutgen S, Kokcu A, Malatyalioglu E. Evaluation of urethrovesical angle by ultrasound in women with and without urinary stress incontinence. Int Urogynecol J Pelvic Floor Dysfunct 2001; 12: 308–11.

100. Voigt R, Halaska M, Michels W, et al. Examiantion of the urethrovesical junction using perineal sonography compared to urethrocystography using a bead chain. Int J Urogynecol 1994; 5: 212–14.

101. Gottlieb D, Dvir Z, Golomb J, Beer-Gabel M. Reproducibility of ultrasonic measurements of pelvic floor structures in women suffering from urinary incontinence. Int Urogynecol J Pelvic Floor Dysfunct 2009; 20: 309–12.

102. Dietz HP, Eldridge A, Grace M, Clarke B. Test-retest reliability of the ultrasound assessment of bladder neck mobility. Int J Urogynecol 2003; 14(Suppl 1): S57–8.

103. Dietz HP, Steensma AB, Vancaillie TG. Levator function in nulliparous women. Int Urogynecol J Pelvic Floor Dysfunct 2003; 14: 24–6; discussion 26.

104. Peschers UM, Fanger G, Schaer GN, et al. Bladder neck mobility in continent nulliparous women. BJOG 2001; 108: 320–4.

105. Brandt FT, Albuquerque CD, Lorenzato FR, Amaral FJ. Perineal assessment of urethrovesical junction mobility in young continent females. Int Urogynecol J Pelvic Floor Dysfunct 2000; 11: 18–22.

106. Di Pietto L, Scaffa C, Torella M, et al. Perineal ultrasound in the study of urethral mobility: proposal of a normal physiological range. Int Urogynecol J Pelvic Floor Dysfunct 2008; 19: 1405–9.

107. Tunn R, Petri E. Introital and transvaginal ultrasound as the main tool in the assessment of urogenital and pelvic floor dysfunction: an imaging panel and practical approach. Ultrasound Obstet Gynecol 2003; 22: 205–13.

108. Quinn MJ, Beynon J, Mortensen NJ, Smith PJ. Transvaginal endosonography: a new method to study the anatomy of the lower urinary tract in urinary stress incontinence. Br J Urol 1988; 62: 414–18.

109. Petri E, Koelbl H, Schaer G. What is the place of ultrasound in urogynecology? A written panel. Int Urogynecol J Pelvic Floor Dysfunct 1999; 10: 262–73.

110. Chen GD, Su TH, Lin LY. Applicability of perineal sonography in anatomical evaluation of bladder neck in women with and without genuine stress incontinence. J Clin Ultrasound 1997; 25: 189–94.

111. Pregazzi R, Sartore A, Bortoli P, et al. Perineal ultrasound evaluation of urethral angle and bladder neck mobility in women with stress urinary incontinence. BJOG 2002; 109: 821–7.

112. Lewicky-Gaupp C, Blaivas J, Clark A, et al. "The cough game": are there characteristic urethrovesical movement patterns associated with stress incontinence? Int Urogynecol J Pelvic Floor Dysfunct 2009; 20: 171–5.

113. Enzelsberger H, Kurz C, Adler A, Schatten C. Effectiveness of Burch colposuspension in females with recurrent stress incontinence—a urodynamic and ultrasound study. Geburtshilfe Frauenheilkd 1991; 51: 915–19.

114. Richmond DH, Sutherst JR. Burch colposuspension or sling for stress incontinence? A prospective study using transrectal ultrasound. Br J Urol 1989; 64: 600–3.

115. Salvatore S, Serati M, Uccella S, et al. Inter-observer reliability of three different methods of measuring urethrovesical mobility. Int Urogynecol J Pelvic Floor Dysfunct 2008; 19: 1513–17.

116. Nwosu CR, Khan KS, Chien PF, Honest MR. Is real-time ultrasonic bladder volume estimation reliable and valid? A systematic overview. Scand J Urol Nephrol 1998; 32: 325–30.

117. Gehrich A, Stany MP, Fischer JR, Buller J, Zahn CM. Establishing a mean postvoid residual volume in asymptomatic perimenopausal and postmenopausal women. Obstet Gynecol 2007; 110: 827–32.

118. Choe JH, Lee JY, Lee KS. Accuracy and precision of a new portable ultrasound scanner, the BME-150A, in residual urine volume measurement: a comparison with the BladderScan BVI 3000. Int Urogynecol J Pelvic Floor Dysfunct 2007; 18: 641–4.

119. Teng CH, Huang YH, Kuo BJ, Bih LI. Application of portable ultrasound scanners in the measurement of post-void residual urine. J Nurs Res 2005; 13: 216–24.

120. Yip SK, Sahota D, Chang AM. Determining the reliability of ultrasound measurements and the validity of the formulae for ultrasound estimation of postvoid residual bladder volume in postpartum women. Neurourol Urodyn 2003; 22: 255–60.

121. Resnick B. A bladder scan trial in geriatric rehabilitation. Rehabil Nurs 1995; 20: 194–6, 203.

122. Haylen BT, Lee J, Logan V, et al. Immediate postvoid residual volumes in women with symptoms of pelvic floor dysfunction. Obstet Gynecol 2008; 111: 1305–12.

123. Oelke M, Mamoulakis C, Ubbink DT, de la Rosette JJ, Wijkstra H. Manual versus automatic bladder wall thickness measurements: a method comparison study. World J Urol 2009; 27: 747–53.

124. Chalana V, Dudycha S, Yuk JT, McMorrow G. Automatic measurement of ultrasound-estimated bladder weight (UEBW) from three-dimensional ultrasound. Rev Urol 2005; 7(Suppl 6): S22–8.

125. Lekskulchai O, Dietz HP. Detrusor wall thickness as a test for detrusor overactivity in women. Ultrasound Obstet Gynecol 2008; 32: 535–9.

126. Wijma J, Potters AE, de Wolf BT, Tinga DJ, Aarnoudse JG. Anatomical and functional changes in the lower urinary tract following spontaneous vaginal delivery. BJOG 2003; 110: 658–63.

127. Wijma J, Weis Potters AE, van der Mark TW, Tinga DJ, Aarnoudse JG. Displacement and recovery of the vesical neck position during pregnancy and after childbirth. Neurourol Urodyn 2007; 26: 372–6.

128. Constantinou CE, Omata S. Direction sensitive sensor probe for the evaluation of voluntary and reflex pelvic floor contractions. Neurourol Urodyn 2007; 26: 386–91.

129. Jung SA, Pretorius DH, Padda BS, et al. Vaginal high-pressure zone assessed by dynamic 3-dimensional ultrasound images of the pelvic floor. Am J Obstet Gynecol 2007; 197: 52 e1–7.

130. Thyer I, Shek C, Dietz HP. New imaging method for assessing pelvic floor biomechanics. Ultrasound Obstet Gynecol 2008; 31: 201–5.

131. Ashton-Miller JA, Delancey JO. On the biomechanics of vaginal birth and common sequelae. Annu Rev Biomed Eng 2009; 11: 163–76.

132. Dietz HP, Simpson JM. Levator trauma is associated with pelvic organ prolapse. BJOG 2008; 115: 979–84.

133. Chen L, Ashton-Miller JA, Hsu Y, DeLancey JO. Interaction among apical support, levator ani impairment, and anterior vaginal wall prolapse. Obstet Gynecol 2006; 108: 324–32.

134. Dietz HP, Wilson PD, Clarke B. The use of perineal ultrasound to quantify levator activity and teach pelvic floor muscle exercises. Int Urogynecol J Pelvic Floor Dysfunct 2001; 12: 166–8; discussion 168–9.

135. Whittaker JL, Thompson JA, Teyhen DS, Hodges P. Rehabilitative ultrasound imaging of pelvic floor muscle function. J Orthop Sports Phys Ther 2007; 37: 487–98.

136. Balmforth JR, Mantle J, Bidmead J, Cardozo L. A prospective observational trial of pelvic floor muscle training for female stress urinary incontinence. BJU Int 2006; 98: 811–17.

137. Bernstein IT. The pelvic floor muscles: muscle thickness in healthy and urinary-incontinent women measured by perineal ultrasonography with reference to the effect of pelvic floor training. Estrogen receptor studies. Neurourol Urodyn 1997; 16: 237–75.

138. Dietz HP, Jarvis SK, Vancaillie TG. The assessment of levator muscle strength: a validation of three ultrasound techniques. Int Urogynecol J Pelvic Floor Dysfunct 2002; 13: 156–9; discussion 159.

139. Thompson JA, O'Sullivan PB, Briffa NK, Neumann P. Comparison of transperineal and transabdominal ultrasound in the assessment of voluntary pelvic floor muscle contractions and functional manoeuvres in continent and incontinent women. Int Urogynecol J Pelvic Floor Dysfunct 2007; 18: 779–86.

140. Peschers UM, Gingelmaier A, Jundt K, Leib B, Dimpfl T. Evaluation of pelvic floor muscle strength using four different techniques. Int Urogynecol J Pelvic Floor Dysfunct 2001; 12: 27–30.

141. Yang SH, Huang WC, Yang SY, Yang E, Yang JM. Validation of new ultrasound parameters for quantifying pelvic floor muscle contraction. Ultrasound Obstet Gynecol 2009; 33: 465–71.

142. Weinstein MM, Jung SA, Pretorius DH, et al. The reliability of puborectalis muscle measurements with 3-dimensional ultrasound imaging. Am J Obstet Gynecol 2007; 197: 68 e1–6.

143. Kruger JA, Heap SW, Murphy BA, Dietz HP. Pelvic floor function in nulliparous women using three-dimensional ultrasound and magnetic resonance imaging. Obstet Gynecol 2008; 111: 631–8.

144. Dietz HP. Quantification of major morphological abnormalities of the levator ani. Ultrasound Obstet Gynecol 2007; 29: 329–34.

145. Yang JM, Yang SH, Huang WC. Biometry of the puboviseral muscle and levator hiatus in nulliparous Chinese women. Ultrasound Obstet Gynecol 2006; 28: 710–16.

146. Majida M, Braekken IH, Umek W, et al. Interobserver repeatability of three- and four-dimensional transperineal ultrasound assessment of pelvic floor muscle anatomy and function. Ultrasound Obstet Gynecol 2009; 33: 567–73.

147. Lockhart ME, Fielding JR, Richter HE, et al. Reproducibility of dynamic MR imaging pelvic measurements: a multi-institutional study. Radiology 2008; 249: 534–40.

148. Kruger JA, Dietz HP, Murphy BA. Pelvic floor function in elite nulliparous athletes. Ultrasound Obstet Gynecol 2007; 30: 81–5.

149. Hoyte L, Jakab M, Warfield SK, et al. Levator ani thickness variations in symptomatic and asymptomatic women using magnetic resonance-based 3-dimensional color mapping. Am J Obstet Gynecol 2004; 191: 856–61.

150. Athanasiou S, Chaliha C, Toozs-Hobson P, et al. Direct imaging of the pelvic floor muscles using two-dimensional ultrasound: a comparison of women with urogenital prolapse versus controls. BJOG 2007; 114: 882–8.

151. Dietz HP. Ultrasound imaging of the pelvic floor. Part II: three-dimensional or volume imaging. Ultrasound Obstet Gynecol 2004; 23: 615–25.

152. Morkved S, Salvesen KA, Bo K, Eik-Nes S. Pelvic floor muscle strength and thickness in continent and incontinent nulliparous pregnant women. Int Urogynecol J Pelvic Floor Dysfunct 2004; 15: 384–9; discussion 390.

153. Dietz HP, Shek C, Clarke B. Biometry of the puboviseral muscle and levator hiatus by three-dimensional pelvic floor ultrasound. Ultrasound Obstet Gynecol 2005; 25: 580–5.

154. Dietz HP, Simpson JM. Does delayed child-bearing increase the risk of levator injury in labour? Aust N Z J Obstet Gynaecol 2007; 47: 491–5.

155. Dietz HP. Why pelvic floor surgeons should utilize ultrasound imaging. Ultrasound Obstet Gynecol 2006; 28: 629–34.

156. Dietz HP. Levator trauma in labor: a challenge for obstetricians, surgeons and sonologists. Ultrasound Obstet Gynecol 2007; 29: 368–71.

157. Dietz HP, Lanzarone V. Levator trauma after vaginal delivery. Obstet Gynecol 2005; 106: 707–12.

158. Dietz HP, Shek C. Levator avulsion and grading of pelvic floor muscle strength. Int Urogynecol J Pelvic Floor Dysfunct 2008; 19: 633–6.

159. Dietz HP, Pang S, Korda A, Benness C. Paravaginal defects: a comparison of clinical examination and 2D/3D ultrasound imaging. Aust N Z J Obstet Gynaecol 2005; 45: 187–90.

160. Wisser J, Schar G, Kurmanavicius J, Huch R, Huch A. Use of 3D ultrasound as a new approach to assess obstetrical trauma to the pelvic floor. Ultraschall Med 1999; 20: 15–18.

161. Dietz HP, Steensma AB, Hastings R. Three-dimensional ultrasound imaging of the pelvic floor: the effect of parturition on paravaginal support structures. Ultrasound Obstet Gynecol 2003; 21: 589–95.

162. Morgan DM, Umek W, Stein T, et al. Interrater reliability of assessing levator ani muscle defects with magnetic resonance images. Int Urogynecol J Pelvic Floor Dysfunct 2007; 18: 773–8.

163. Dietz HP, Steensma AB. The prevalence of major abnormalities of the levator ani in urogynaecological patients. BJOG 2006; 113: 225–30.

164. Dietz HP, Kirby A, Shek KL, Bedwell PJ. Does avulsion of the puborectalis muscle affect bladder function? Int Urogynecol J Pelvic Floor Dysfunct 2009; 20: 967–72.

165. Dietz HP, Hyland G, Hay-Smith J. The assessment of levator trauma: a comparison between palpation and 4D pelvic floor ultrasound. Neurourol Urodyn 2006; 25: 424–7.

166. Dietz HP, Shek C. Validity and reproducibility of the digital detection of levator trauma. Int Urogynecol J Pelvic Floor Dysfunct 2008; 19: 1097–101.

167. Dietz HP, Hoyte LP, Steensma AB. Atlas of Pelvic Floor Ultrasound, 1st edn. London: Springer-Verlag, 2008.

168. Shek KL, Dietz HP. The effect of childbirth on hiatal dimensions. Obstet Gynecol 2009; 113: 1272–8.

169. Williams AB, Bartram CI, Halligan S, et al. Endosonographic anatomy of the normal anal canal compared with endocoil magnetic resonance imaging. Dis Colon Rectum 2002; 45: 176–83.

170. Lewicky-Gaupp C, Hamilton Q, Ashton-Miller J, et al. Anal sphincter structure and function relationships in aging and fecal incontinence. Am J Obstet Gynecol 2009; 200: 559 e1–5.

171. Dietz HP. Prolapse worsens with age, doesn't it? Aust N Z J Obstet Gynaecol 2008; 48: 587–91.

172. Dietz HP, Bennett MJ. The effect of childbirth on pelvic organ mobility. Obstet Gynecol 2003; 102: 223–8.

173. Toozs-Hobson P, Balmforth J, Cardozo L, Khullar V, Athanasiou S. The effect of mode of delivery on pelvic floor functional anatomy. Int Urogynecol J Pelvic Floor Dysfunct 2008; 19: 407–16.

174. Dietz HP, Lanzarone V, Simpson JM. Predicting operative delivery. Ultrasound Obstet Gynecol 2006; 27: 409–15.

175. Blain G, Dietz HP. Symptoms of female pelvic organ prolapse: correlation with organ descent in women with single compartment prolapse. Aust N Z J Obstet Gynaecol 2008; 48: 317–21.

176. Broekhuis SR, Futterer JJ, Hendriks JC, et al. Symptoms of pelvic floor dysfunction are poorly correlated with findings on clinical examination and dynamic MR imaging of the pelvic floor. Int Urogynecol J Pelvic Floor Dysfunct 2009; 20: 1169–74.

177. Kluivers KB, Hendriks JC, Shek C, Dietz HP. Pelvic organ prolapse symptoms in relation to POPQ, ordinal stages and ultrasound prolapse assessment. Int Urogynecol J Pelvic Floor Dysfunct 2008; 19: 1299–302.

178. Broekhuis SR, Kluivers KB, Hendriks JC, et al. Dynamic magnetic resonance imaging: reliability of anatomical landmarks and reference lines used to assess pelvic organ prolapse. Int Urogynecol J Pelvic Floor Dysfunct 2009; 20: 141–8.

179. Dietz HP, Haylen BT, Broome J. Ultrasound in the quantification of female pelvic organ prolapse. Ultrasound Obstet Gynecol 2001; 18: 511–14.

180. Beer-Gabel M, Teshler M, Schechtman E, Zbar AP. Dynamic transperineal ultrasound vs. defecography in patients with evacuatory difficulty: a pilot study. Int J Colorectal Dis 2004; 19: 60–7.

181. Dietz HP, Eldridge A, Grace M, Clarke B. Does pregnancy affect pelvic organ mobility? Aust N Z J Obstet Gynaecol 2004; 44: 517–20.

182. Vierhout ME, van der Plas-de Koning YW. Diagnosis of posterior enterocele: comparison of rectal ultrasonography with intraoperative diagnosis. J Ultrasound Med 2002; 21: 383–7; quiz 9.

183. Karaus M, Neuhaus P, Wiedenmann TB. Diagnosis of enteroceles by dynamic anorectal endosonography. Dis Colon Rectum 2000; 43: 1683–8.

184. Grasso RF, Piciucchi S, Quattrocchi CC, et al. Posterior pelvic floor disorders: a prospective comparison using introital ultrasound and colpocystodefecography. Ultrasound Obstet Gynecol 2007; 30: 86–94.

185. Dietz HP, Steensma AB. Posterior compartment prolapse on two-dimensional and three-dimensional pelvic floor ultrasound: the distinction between true rectocele, perineal hypermobility and enterocele. Ultrasound Obstet Gynecol 2005; 26: 73–7.

186. Dietz HP, Korda A. Which bowel symptoms are most strongly associated with a true rectocele? Aust N Z J Obstet Gynaecol 2005; 45: 505–8.

187. Dietz HP, Clarke B. Prevalence of rectocele in young nulliparous women. Aust N Z J Obstet Gynaecol 2005; 45: 391–4.

188. Brusciano L, Limongelli P, Pescatori M, et al. Ultrasonographic patterns in patients with obstructed defaecation. Int J Colorectal Dis 2007; 22: 969–77.

189. Beer-Gabel M, Assoulin Y, Amitai M, Bardan E. A comparison of dynamic transperineal ultrasound (DTP-US) with dynamic evacuation proctography (DEP) in the diagnosis of cul de sac hernia (enterocele) in patients with evacuatory dysfunction. Int J Colorectal Dis 2008; 23: 513–19.

190. Steensma AB, Oom DM, Burger CW, Rudolph Schouten W. Assessment of posterior compartment prolapse; a comparison of evacuation proctography and 3D transperineal ultrasound. Colorectal Dis 2009; doi: 10.1111/j.1463-1318.2009.01936.x.

191. Barthet M, Portier F, Heyries L, et al. Dynamic anal endosonography may challenge defecography for assessing dynamic anorectal disorders: results of a prospective pilot study. Endoscopy 2000; 32: 300–5.

192. Dietz HP, Lekskulchai O. Ultrasound assessment of pelvic organ prolapse: the relationship between prolapse severity and symptoms. Ultrasound Obstet Gynecol 2007; 29: 688–91.

193. Yalcin OT, Hassa H, Tanir M. A new ultrasonographic method for evaluation of the results of anti-incontinence operations. Acta Obstet Gynecol Scand 2002; 81: 151–6.

194. Lo TS, Horng SG, Liang CC, Lee SJ, Soong YK. Ultrasound assessment of mid-urethra tape at three-year follow-up after tension-free vaginal tape procedure. Urology 2004; 63: 671–5.

195. Lo TS, Wang AC, Horng SG, Liang CC, Soong YK. Ultrasonographic and urodynamic evaluation after tension free vagina tape procedure (TVT). Acta Obstet Gynecol Scand 2001; 80: 65–70.

196. Virtanen HS, Kiilholma P. Urogynecologic ultrasound is a useful aid in the assessment of female stress urinary incontinence—a prospective study with TVT procedure. Int Urogynecol J Pelvic Floor Dysfunct 2002; 13: 218–22; discussion 23.

197. Ng CC, Lee LC, Han WH. Use of three-dimensional ultrasound scan to assess the clinical importance of midurethral placement of the tension-free vaginal tape (TVT) for treatment of incontinence. Int Urogynecol J Pelvic Floor Dysfunct 2005; 16: 220–5.

198. Chene G, Cotte B, Tardieu AS, Savary D, Mansoor A. Clinical and ultrasonographic correlations following three surgical anti-incontinence procedures (TOT, TVT and TVT-O). Int Urogynecol J Pelvic Floor Dysfunct 2008; 19: 1125–31.

199. Martan A, Svabik K, Masata J, et al. The solution of stress urinary incontinence in women by the TVT-S surgical method—correlation between the curative effect of this method and changes in ultrasound findings. Ceska Gynekol 2008; 73: 271–7.

200. Yang JM, Yang SH, Huang WC. Dynamic interaction involved in the tension-free vaginal tape obturator procedure. J Urol 2008; 180: 2081–7.

201. Yang JM, Yang SH, Huang WC. Correlation of morphological alterations and functional impairment of the tension-free vaginal tape obturator procedure. J Urol 2009; 181: 211–18.

202. Reich A, Wiesner K, Kohorst F, Kreienberg R, Flock F. Comparison of transobturator vaginal tape and retropubic tension-free vaginal tape: clinical outcome and sonographic results of a case-control study. Gynecol Obstet Invest 2009; 68: 137–44.

203. Long CY, Hsu CS, Liu CM, et al. Clinical and ultrasonographic comparison of tension-free vaginal tape and transobturator tape procedure for the treatment of stress urinary incontinence. J Minim Invasive Gynecol 2008; 15: 425–30.

204. Shek C, Dietz HP. Transobturator mesh anchoring for the repair of large or recurrent cystocele. Neurourol Urodyn 2006; 25: 554.

205. Shek KL, Dietz HP, Rane A, Balakrishnan S. Transobturator mesh for cystocele repair: a short- to medium-term follow-up using 3D/4D ultrasound. Ultrasound Obstet Gynecol 2008; 32: 82–6.

206. Shek KL, Rane A, Goh J, Dietz HP. Stress urinary incontinence after transobturator mesh for cystocele repair. Int Urogynecol J Pelvic Floor Dysfunct 2009; 20: 421–5.

207. Poon CI, Zimmern PE. Role of three-dimensional ultrasound in assessment of women undergoing urethral bulking agent therapy. Curr Opin Obstet Gynecol 2004; 16: 411–17.

208. Defreitas GA, Wilson TS, Zimmern PE, Forte TB. Three-dimensional ultrasonography: an objective outcome tool to assess collagen distribution in women with stress urinary incontinence. Urology 2003; 62: 232–6.

37 Magnetic Resonance Imaging and the Female Pelvic Floor
Lennox Hoyte

INTRODUCTION

Female pelvic floor dysfunction (PFD) includes pelvic organ prolapse (POP), and urinary and fecal incontinence. Appropriate therapy for PFD depends on a proper diagnosis, which requires an understanding of the female pelvic anatomy, relative to continence and pelvic support. Cadaveric dissections have been used to aid understanding of the pelvic anatomy but these have been limited by artifacts of fixation and other changes which occur when living tissues become non-viable.

An understanding of the anatomic relationships in living symptomatic and asymptomatic (ASY) women is possible with detailed, high resolution imaging. Magnetic resonance imaging (MRI) has evolved as a useful tool for evaluating the living anatomy in the female pelvis, both in the upright and supine positions, and under differing physiologic conditions, such as rest, squeeze, and strain. With MRI, high resolution images with a wide field of view are made possible in multiple planes. The results from such imaging studies have shed new light on our understanding of the behavior of the ASY and symptomatic female pelvic floor, and may yet pave the way to help triage those with PFD for appropriate therapy, and possibly aid in predicting which women may be at risk for PFD. At present, however, there is no currently agreed-upon role for MRI in the diagnostic evaluation of female PFD.

With the above reality in mind, the aims of this chapter are:

- to review the development of MRI as a tool for understanding female pelvic floor anatomy;
- to show the range and variability of the female pelvic anatomy;
- to show how pelvic anatomic changes may relate to various forms of PFD;
- to study the possible effects of childbirth on the pelvic floor;
- to introduce MR-based methods for advanced study of the female pelvic floor—e.g., MR-based three-dimensional (3D) reconstruction and computer-based pelvic floor simulation models (which may be used to gain a better understanding of the parameters of childbirth-related female pelvic floor injury);
- to describe the basic MRI techniques, their interpretation, and pitfalls in application;
- to briefly present current public domain tools for visualization, analysis, and management of the MR images.

MRI FOR UNDERSTANDING FEMALE PELVIC FLOOR ANATOMY

MRI has been used to assess the normal anatomy of the female pelvic floor, as well as to study the anatomic determinants of pelvic organ dysfunction. When Strohbehn et al. compared MRI findings with anatomy at dissection in two cadavers (1) (Fig. 37.1), they found that sagittal and axial MRI demonstrated the levator ani muscle from its fascial origination at the pubic bone, along its course passing alongside the urethra, distal vagina, and posterior to the rectum, noting its insertion between the internal and external anal sphincters (Fig. 37.2). Furthermore, MRI showed the iliococcygeus muscle attachment to the arcus tendineus laterally, as well as the relative thickness of the medial aspect of the levators when compared to the thinner, more lateral aspect. Their work demonstrated that MRI findings reflected actual anatomy; however, they did have the benefit of long MRI scan times which increased resolution without introducing the motion artifact that would limit scan times in living subjects.

Basic Female Pelvic MR Anatomy

MR images are routinely obtained in the axial, coronal, and sagittal planes. By convention, coronal slices are presented with the subject facing the observer, axial images are presented with the subject's feet closest to the observer, and sagittal images are presented with the subject facing to the left of the observer. Examples of these three slice orientations are illustrated in Figure 37.3. Axial slices are obtained for best visualization of the puborectalis, the urethra, and the distal vagina; coronal slices best demonstrate the iliococcygeus portion of levator ani and also the external anal sphincter; midsagittal images are usually obtained in order to evaluate descent of the pelvic floor structures with straining versus rest or squeeze maneuvers. Oblique slices may also be collected, depending on the specific question to be answered.

Typical MRI findings in the ASY nullipara include a urethra and bladder neck that are close to the symphysis, puborectalis muscle arms which come into close proximity with the superior pubic rami, and a downwardly convex distal vagina with upwardly curving edges bilaterally. The general shape of the puborectalis muscle is that of a "V". These findings are shown in Figure 37.4.

Findings in the ASY vaginal multipara are much more variable. They can range from closely resembling the nullipara, all the way to having a lower urethra and bladder neck, loss of puborectalis approximation to the superior rami, loss of the downward concavity of the distal vagina, and a "bowing" of the puborectalis muscle, causing it to resemble a "U" instead of the nulliparous "V." The range of multiparous variation is shown in Figure 37.5.

Findings in symptomatic women are also quite variable, as can be seen from the following discussion.

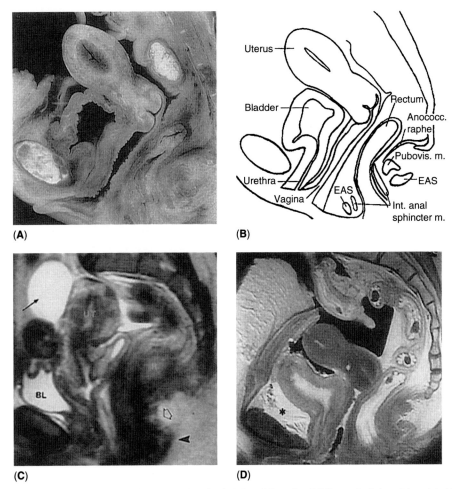

Figure 37.1 Comparison of cadaveric anatomy from magnetic resonance imaging (MRI) and dissection. Midline sagittal view of the pelvis. (**A**) Cross-sectional anatomy. (**B**) Corresponding diagram. EAS, external anal sphincter muscle. (**C**) Fast spin-echo T2-weighted 1.5-tesla MRI of a 26-year-old living patient (repetition time 3600 msec, echo delay time 85 msec, field of view 24 cm, scan time 11:44 min). Incidental ovarian cyst (black arrow) is seen anterior to the uterus. BL, bladder; UT, uterus; R, rectum. (**D**) T2-weighted MRI of cadaver specimen at the same level. (*Note: The asterisk posterior to the symphysis on the cadaver MRI represents fixation artifact from a fluid collection in the space of Retzius in this and subsequent figures.) The fibers of the pubovisceralis muscle (puborectalis) that decussate behind the rectum are seen in relationship to the internal and external anal sphincter muscles. The image clarity is less in the patient MRI compared with the cadaver MRI because of motion artifact and shorter scan time, but the external anal sphincter muscle (arrowhead) and the pubovisceralis muscle (open arrow) are seen. *Source*: From Ref. 1.

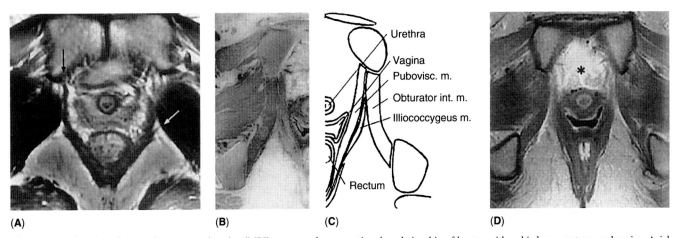

Figure 37.2 Cadaveric and magnetic resonance imaging (MRI) anatomy, demonstrating the relationship of levator with pubic bone, rectum, and vagina. Axial views of the pelvis near the level of the symphysis pubis. (**A**) Proton density MRI of 28-year-old living patient, using a pelvic phased-array coil (repetition time 3800 msec, echo delay time 18 msec, field of view 20 cm, scan time 8:59 min). Note a small group of distinct fibers of the left iliococcygeus muscle (white arrow) originating laterally at the oburator internus muscle, and fibers from the pubovisceralis muscccle (black arrow) originating at the symphysis pubis. (**B**) Cross-sectional anatomy of the right hemipelvis. (**C**) Corresponding diagram of the left hemipelvis. (**D**) T2-weighted MRI at the same level. This plane demonstrates the relationship of the modline viscera to the pubovisceralis muscle. The patient MRI also demonstrates the difference in origin of the pubovisceralis muscle and the iliococcygeus muscle. *Source*: From Ref. 1.

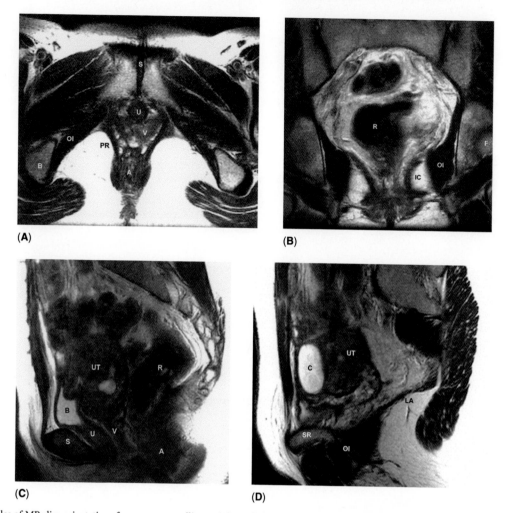

Figure 37.3 Examples of MR slice orientations from a young nullipara. (**A**) Axial slice at the level of the bladder neck (B, bones). (**B**) Coronal slice at the level of the distal rectum: note the left to right asymmetry of the slice; the femoral head (F) is seen on the left, but not on the right. (**C**) Sagittal slice: Midsagittal view (B, bladder). (**D**) Left parasagittal slice: note the left simple ovarian cyst (C) anterior to the uterus. Levator ani (LA) is seen running posterior to anterior. The superior pubic ramus (SR) is seen as well as the obturator internus (OI). *Abbreviations*: A, anus; IC, iliococcygeus; MR, magnetic resonance; PR, puborectalis; R, rectum; S, symphysis; U, urethra; UT, uterus; V, vagina.

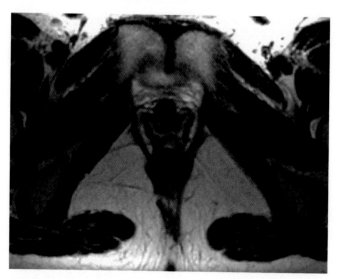

Figure 37.4 Typical magnetic resonance imaging findings in the nullipara include a urethra and bladder neck which are close to the symphysis, puborectalis muscle arms which come into close proximity with the superior pubic rami, and a downwardly convex distal vagina with upwardly curving edges bilaterally. The general shape of the puborectalis muscle is that of a "V".

Symptomatic Pelvic MRI Findings

Huddleston et al. (2) demonstrated MRI findings of three alterations in vaginal shape that were associated with clinical POP, showing a relationship between pathologic MR and clinical findings (Fig. 37.6). Kirshner-Hermanns et al. reported increased T1 signal intensity as evidence of muscle atrophy in 66% of their subjects with stress incontinence (3), suggesting a relationship between levator weakness and stress urinary incontinence (SUI). Their conclusions were supported by Fielding et al. (4) who found a trend towards levator muscle laxity and thinning in women with SUI. However, it is possible that their results were a reflection of the wide normal range of levator variation. This idea was demonstrated by Tunn et al. who used pelvic MRI to show two- to three-fold differences in distance, area, and volume of pelvic floor structures among a group of 20 ASY nulliparas (5).

Klutke et al. studied bladder neck MRI findings taken in the supine position in normals compared to those with a urodynamic diagnosis of stress incontinence (6). They found that, when compared to patients with stress incontinence, normal subjects were characterized by MR findings of a

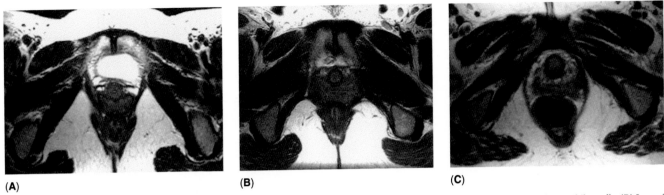

Figure 37.5 Magnetic resonance imaging Findings in the vaginal multipara. (**A**) A V-shaped puborectalis, with loss of upward vaginal curve bilaterally. (**B**) Loss of puborectalis approximation to the pubic rami, with flattened vagina. (**C**) Bilateral bowing of the puborectalis, and sagging of the vagina on the left.

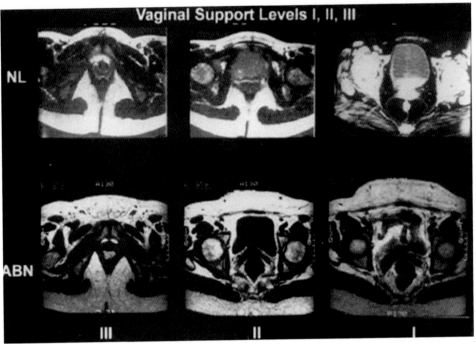

Figure 37.6 Alterations in vaginal shape associated with pelvic organ prolapse. Upper panel: magnetic resonance imaging (MRI) of normal support. Lower panel: MRI of abnormal support, both at DeLancey's levels I, II, and III. *Abbreviations*: NL, normal; ABN, abnormal. *Source*: From Ref. 2.

bladder neck positioned close to the symphysis, a vaginal lumen with a widened "H" shape, and nearly horizontal "urethropelvic" ligaments. It should be noted that they considered the urethropelvic ligaments to attach the lateral aspect of the urethra to the medial aspect of the levator sling (Fig. 37.7). This point was also emphasized by Tunn et al. who identified these lateral attachments on MR scans in 20 continent nulliparas (7).

Looking retrospectively at women with PFD, Handa et al. compared pelvic MRI findings of the bony pelvis in 59 women with PFD with 39 controls (8). They found that women with PFD tended to have a wider transverse inlet, intertuberous and interspinous diameter, a longer sacrum with a deeper curve, and a narrower anteroposterior outlet, when compared to those without PFD. Their findings were independent of race. These results echoed the findings of Sze et al. who previously used CT pelvimetry to correlate the

bony pelvic shape with the risk of female PFD. They found wider transverse pelvic inlet diameters in 34 multiparous white women with prolapse, compared to 34 matched controls with normal pelvic support (9). These findings also suggest a relationship between the wide, deep bony pelvis and the presence of PFD among parous women.

In seeking a better understanding of the specific anatomic defects that might correlate to female PFD, our group evaluated the morphology, volume, and integrity of the levator ani and the bladder neck, using reconstructed 3D MR-based models in living women. Fielding and colleagues demonstrated the feasibility of the 3D technique and yielded early estimates of the normal range of levator volume in a group of 10 ASY women aged 22 to 33 years (10). Our subsequent study used MR-based 3D reconstruction techniques to evaluate a group of 30 women, divided into three groups (11): 10 were ASY, 10 had urodynamic stress incontinence (USI), and 10 had symptomatic

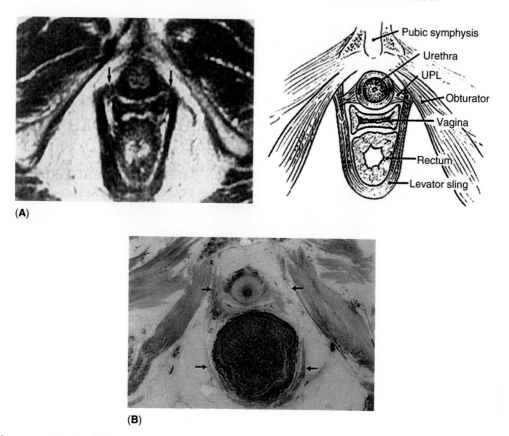

Figure 37.7 Magnetic resonance imaging findings in asymptomatics and those with stress incontinence. (**A**) Axial magnetic resonance image at level of bladder neck in well-supported continent woman shows urethropelvic ligaments (UPL, arrows) supporting the bladder neck. (**B**) Corresponding step-section at the same level shows urethropelvic ligaments attaching to levator (arrows) at level of arcus tendineus. *Source*: From Ref. 6.

POP. The data showed significant differences in levator volume, integrity, and shape across the range of ASY to USI to POP, suggestive of a continuum of disease. In that study, we identified a marker for anterior puborectalis attachment disruption—the levator–symphysis gap (LSG)—which is measured as the distance from the inferior symphysis to the nearest occurrence of the puborectalis muscle on each side. Shorter distances suggest closer approximation of levator to pubis, and longer distances suggest disruption of the puborectalis attachment. Our findings of LSG indicated greater disruption in POP and USI subjects, compared to ASYs. As will be discussed in the next section, DeLancey's group showed that these levator disruptions appear to occur only in parous women.

MRI has also been used to study the anatomy of the urethra. Aronson's group looked at MRI anatomy of the female urethra using an endoanal coil, placed vaginally (12). They compared MR images from four continent nulliparas with four incontinent women. They found that they were able to effectively image the periurethral and paravaginal connective tissues, and found that the MR images correlated well with each subject's assessed clinical defects. They measured the volume of the space of Retzius, and observed that the volume was twice as high in the incontinent versus the continent, but this was not statistically significant. DeLancey's group looked at the position of the striated urethral sphincter in a cohort of 78, young, healthy nulliparas using MRI (13). They observed the urethra to start between 0.5 and 2.5 cm distal to the bladder base, extending to

the perineal membrane, which was located 2 to 3 cm distal to the bladder base. Examples of urethral MR images are given in Figure 37.8. These two studies demonstrated the ability of MRI to identify the urethral and periurethral structures.

CHILDBIRTH-RELATED CHANGES AS SEEN ON MRI
Childbirth-related damage to the levator muscle, as well as to nerves and connective tissues in the pelvis, is believed to be a major contributor to female PFD (14–18). Notably, approximately three-quarters of the over four million annual US births are delivered vaginally (19,20). There is epidemiologic evidence of a relationship between childbirth and PFD (21,22). However, not all women who undergo vaginal childbirth develop PFD (23). Furthermore, not all nulliparous women are free of PFD (24). This apparently variable response of the pelvic floor to childbirth has prompted investigators to use MRI to look more closely at the possible effects of birth on the pelvic floor.

When DeLancey examined MRI scans of 80 nulliparas, he found intact puborectalis muscle arms in 100%. Among 160 primiparas, however, 20% demonstrated disruptions in one or both puborectalis arms. These findings suggested that childbirth may have caused injury to the puborectalis attachment at the superior pubic ramus. Of the primiparas with these disruptions, 71% were found to have SUI (17). This suggests that SUI is correlated with puborectalis disruptions, probably caused by vaginal childbirth. Furthermore, Miller compared maximum urethral closure pressures (MUCPs) in 17 women

Bladder base	Bladder neck	SUS	CU / UVS	PM

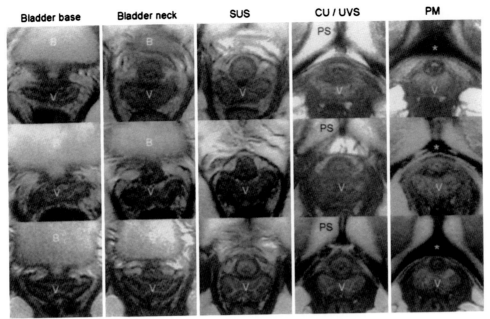

Figure 37.8 The female striated urethra as seen on magnetic resonance imaging. Variations of normal urethral anatomy. Each column shows three examples of typical urethral anatomy, each from a different woman. Rows do not represent individual urethrae. *Abbreviations*: B, bladder; CU/CVS, region of the compressor urethrae and urethrovaginal sphincter muscles; PM, region of the perineal membrane; PS, pubic symphysis; SUS, region of the striated muscle sphincter; V, vagina. *Arcuate pubic ligament below the symphysis pubis. *Source*: From Ref. 13.

with MRI-proven puborectalis disruptions to MUCPs in 28 women without such disruptions. Those women with disruptions in the puborectalis muscles were seen to generate lower MUCPs with voluntary pelvic muscle contractions when compared to those without the disruptions (25). Taken together, these findings would suggest that vaginal childbirth may weaken the urethral closure mechanism, thereby disposing the patient to urinary incontinence.

Our group looked at the impact of childbirth on the levator ani and bladder neck in 10 nulliparas and 9 parous women, all of whom were ASY with respect to PFD (26). We found that the nulliparas had a narrower levator hiatus, a higher bladder neck, and closer approximation of the puborectalis to the superior rami when compared to the parous women. In addition, all of the nulliparas had a V-shaped puborectalis (Fig. 37.4), but 33% of the parous women had U-shaped puborectalis muscles (Fig. 37.5b). Despite the study limitations, these results point to demonstrable anatomic changes in key pelvic floor structures, associated with childbirth.

RACE AND PELVIC MRI FINDINGS
Previous investigators have reported striking differences in the prevalence and incidence of PFD among different races (27–33). There is, however, no consensus in the medical literature on exactly how race affects the development of PFD.

Anecdotally, urinary incontinence and POP may occur less often in women of African descent, when compared to Caucasians (27,34,35). Work by Handa et al. (8) and Sze et al. (9) suggested that bony pelvic shape, rather than race, may be a factor in the development of PFD among parous women. Our group attempted to ascertain if there were bony and soft tissue differences in pelvic geometry between well-characterized, ASY nulliparous Caucasian and African–American women. In

this prospective observational cohort study, we examined MRI data from two groups of nulliparous women: 12 African–American and 10 Caucasian–American (36). All were premenopausal, and had stage zero or one pelvic support as defined by the POPQ system (37) by examination in the supine straining position. To be eligible for inclusion, each subject had to deny pelvic floor symptoms of chronic pain, urinary incontinence, prolapse, or defecatory dysfunction.

Our study data showed statistically significant increased levator ani muscle volume among African–American nulliparas when compared to age-matched Caucasian nulliparas. In addition, the arms of the puborectalis muscle were carried closer to the superior pubic rami bilaterally, suggestive of closer, more extensive attachments between muscle and bone. The bladder neck is held higher and closer to the symphysis in the African–Americans than in the Caucasians, and the pubic arch is slightly wider among the African–Americans. All levators were V-shaped. Taken collectively, these differences suggest a levator ani complex in African–American subjects that is bulkier and more intimately associated with its bony attachments.

Downing, using advanced color thickness mapping techniques applied to MRIs from these subjects, demonstrated significantly thicker levator ani muscles in the African–American compared to the Caucasian nulliparas (38). Notably, obturator internus muscle thickness was similar in the two groups, suggesting that levator muscle bulk was singularly increased in African–American nulliparas.

DeLancey's group also looked at racial differences in the female continence mechanism using MRI and other techniques (39). Their study groups consisted of 18 African-American women and 17 Caucasian women, all young, ASY nulliparas. Their data showed that the African–American women had

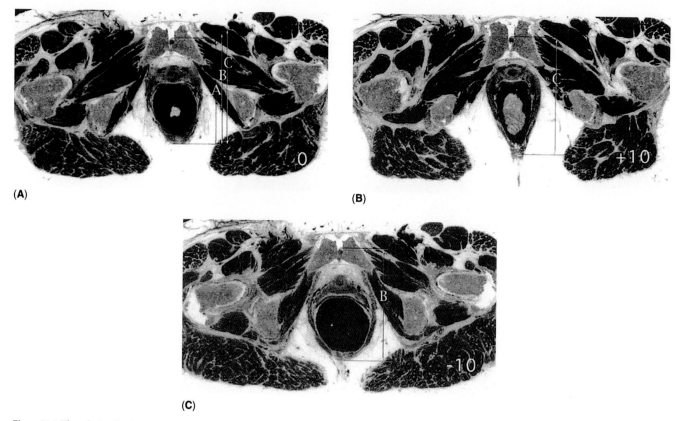

Figure 37.9 The relationship between slice acquisition angle and linear measurement. (**A**) The reference (0°) axial image is presented and marked to show the parameter levator hiatus. For reference (line A) and resliced (lines B, C) axes. (**B**) Resliced images at +10°, with levator hiatus measurements marked. (**C**) Resliced images at −10°, with levator hiatus measurements marked. *Source:* From Ref. 42.

a higher urethral volume and demonstrated higher resting and squeezing MUCPs, when compared to the Caucasians in the study.

It is possible that increased levator bulk allows for better tonic support of the vagina, thus reducing the risk of prolapse. Similarly, increased urethral bulk might lead to increased baseline closure pressure, thus decreasing the risk of incontinence, even after childbirth related injury. These factors may account the apparent differences in prolapse and urinary incontinence rates in African–American women compared to Caucasions. However, definitive answers must await more rigorous, well designed, prospective studies.

PITFALLS IN MR-BASED ANALYSIS

MR analysis affords excellent visualization of soft tissue relationships in the female pelvis. However, it is possible to encounter pitfalls in the interpretation of MRI studies. The attentive observer will be alert to these, and will have methods available to account for the artifacts which can occur in the acquisition of MR data. Two important pitfalls in MR-based analysis relate to the slice acquisition angle and the chemical shift artifact.

Slice Acquisition Angle

MR images are acquired in multiple parallel "slices," oriented in some way with respect to the subject being scanned. This "angle of orientation," or "slice angle," can introduce errors in linear and angular measurements made on the acquired images. These "slice angle errors" are unrelated to the actual anatomy being studied.

Using data from the visible human project (40,41), and specialized image reslicing tools (42), our group demonstrated that identical linear measurements made on two-dimensional (2D) source images can vary based solely upon the slice acquisition angle. From our simple experiments, we demonstrated measurement variations of up to 15% for slice angle variations as low as 20°. Furthermore, for similar appearing axial slices rotated slightly with respect to each other, identical measurements varied by up to 16% (43). These findings are illustrated in Figure 37.9.

These findings suggest that in order to evaluate linear measurements on 2D images accurately, a consistent method for standardizing the slice acquisition angle must be adopted. This could be accomplished in a number of ways:

The MR slice acquisition angle could be rigorously standardized with respect to a known landmark (e.g., ischial tuberosities, femoral heads). This would result in consistent slice angles across multiple scans, but would require agreement between centers regarding the standardization protocol. Examples of properly and poorly aligned axial slices are given in Figure 37.10a and 37.10b, respectively.

Another method would involve reorienting (mathematically transforming) the MRI data into standardized planes after it has been acquired. This approach has the advantage of eliminating the need for exact slice alignment prior to scanning; however, it is likely that the reorienting would result in a

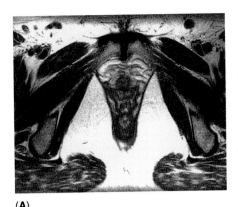 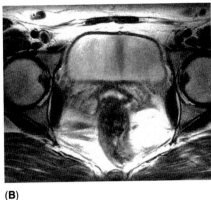 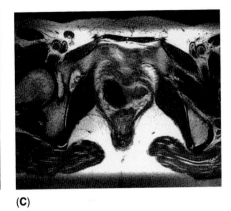

(A) **(B)** **(C)**

Figure 37.10 Variations in slice angle alignment. (**A**) Well-aligned axial slice: note structural symmetry to the left and right of the symphysis at the bladder neck. (**B**) Another slice taken from the femoral heads: note symmetry about the midline. (**C**) A misaligned MR slice: note the femoral head is seen on the right, but not on the left. This MR series was misaligned by about 12°. Such misalignments can account for discrepancies in linear measurements made on MR images.

degradation of the image quality, which might be unacceptable in some cases.

Additionally, optimal slice angle standardization would depend upon the measurement goals. For evaluating puborectalis integrity, levator hiatus width and height, a plane parallel to the puborectalis sling is optimal. An example of such a plane is shown in Figure 37.5, defined by the line running from the inferior-most point of the symphysis to the external sphincter. A sound definition of a plane that could become an accepted standard will require further assessment.

To evaluate the bladder neck descent, levator plate angle, and posterior urethrovesical angle, the well-known midsagittal plane is appropriate. However, it is important that this plane be rigorously specified in order to avoid measurement artifacts. To date, we have not been successful in using the coronal plane for making measurements.

The slice angle artifact can also be overcome by converting the 2D stack into a 3D image, which can then be directly measured. This option is discussed in the next section.

Chemical Shift Artifact

The second important potential MR pitfall is the so-called "chemical shift" artifact. This effect can result in changes to the width of anatomic structures, depending on certain MRI scan parameters. For example, a structure on the right side of an axial slice (e.g., puborectalis) can appear to be thinner or thicker than its contralateral counterpart. For this reason, left to right thickness comparisons should not be attempted on axial or coronal scans. Furthermore, if data from multiple MR datasets are to be compared, all of the MRI scanning parameters should be established and consistent across all of the acquisitions.

In order to avoid these and other potential pitfalls, it will be important to consult a trained radiologic expert, in order to define and standardize appropriate MRI scanning protocols, well before beginning any investigation involving multiple MRI datasets.

MR IMAGING PROTOCOLS

While many protocols for MR image acquisition exist, we have had good success with the particular sequence publicized by Fielding (10,11) and summarized here. Prior to imaging, the patient is asked to void so that a distended bladder will not distort the adjacent anatomy. A pelvic or torso multicoil array is wrapped

around the lower aspect of the pelvis, low enough to capture data from prolapsing structures. In the absence of a multicoil array, the body coil can be used. A standard axial fast spin echo sequence with the following imaging parameters is typically employed: TR = 4200 ms, TE(eff) = 108 ms, 128 phase encoding steps, 24 cm field of view, 3 mm slice thickness, no gap. This sequence obtains high-resolution axial images of the puborectalis, vagina, urethra, anus, and rectum, along with pubocervical fascia and fascial condensations supporting the urethra. The axial scan should encompass points 5 to 10 mm inferior to the ischial tuberosities, up to points 10 mm superior to the femoral heads. This scan should also include all pelvic anatomy medial to the femoral necks. To obtain rest and strain images, a midline slice 10 mm thick should include the symphysis, bladder neck, vagina, rectum, and coccyx. If all the relevant structures cannot be imaged on a single slice, two contiguous locations may be specified. The patient is then asked to valsalva at maximum effort. Using a fast, T2-weighted imaging technique, sagittal midline images are then obtained at rest and at maximal strain. Typical imaging parameters are: TR = 10,000 ms, TE1/TE2 = 90 ms, ETL = 8, one acquisition, 10 mm section thickness, 256 phase encoding steps, 24 to 30 cm field of view. Using these parameters, each image is obtained in less than three seconds. The strain images can be repeated with additional verbal coaching if necessary. If a perineal hernia or ballooning of the puborectalis is suspected, this same series of images should be repeated in the coronal plane. T1-weighted and contrast-enhanced images are usually not required.

ADVANCED MR-BASED TECHNIQUES
Magnetic Resonance Defecography

Functional pelvic floor symptoms include defecatory dysfunction (outlet constipation), fecal incontinence, and pelvic pain. These problems can be caused by defects in the posterior vaginal wall (e.g., rectocele), compression of the rectosigmoid by the descending uterus or vaginal walls during straining, nonrelaxing pelvic floor muscles, rectal prolapse, intussusception, or combinations of these. MR defecography is a useful technique for evaluating complaints of disordered defecation, fecal incontinence, and pain with defecation (44) For the MR defecography study, rectal and vaginally placed contrast gel is inserted, and the patient is asked to rest, squeeze, strain, and defecate during high speed MR scanning. This study is best performed in an upright MR scanner, but can also be done with the patient supine, and wearing a large adult diaper. The MR defecography study can highlight rectovaginal interface defects, rectal intussusception, perineal defects, and obstructions due to a compressive, hypermobile vaginal wall, or descending uterus. We have found the results useful in pinpointing these correctable anatomic defects in women with outlet constipation. In our experience, these patients respond well to either sacrocolpopexy, rectopexy, site specific posterior wall repair, or ocassionally myofascial release pelvic floor physical therapy, depending on the specific findings on the MR defecography study.

D Female Pelvic Floor Reconstruction

As noted earlier, MR data are acquired and presented as "stacks" of 2D images. While these stacks contain all of the information required to analyze the study, many surgeons prefer to think of pelvic anatomy in three dimensions. For this reason, Fielding and colleagues (45) built MR-based 3D reconstructions of the female pelvic floor structures, as follows.

Acquired MRI data were electronically transferred to a Sun UltraSparc-30 graphics computer workstation. The axial image data were segmented into anatomically significant components, including bladder, urethra, vagina, levator ani, symphysis, and coccyx, and then labeled using a combination of semi-automated

and manual editing using the 3DSlicer, a computer tool developed by our group (43). A gynecologist experienced in pelvic radiologic anatomy performed the manual segmentation, which required approximately two hours per subject. 3D surface models were generated using a pipeline consisting of dividing cubes, triangle reduction, triangle smoothing, and a surface-rendering method (47–49). The computer processing time for 3D model generation was <10 minutes per subject. The resulting reconstructions permitted outstanding 3D visualization of the intimate anatomic relationships in the living female pelvis for the first time. Examples of the 3D reconstructions are given in Figure 37.11a (dorsal lithotomy view) and 37.11b (left sagittal view). The reconstructed 3D models also permitted linear, angular, and volumetric measurements to be made, allowing parametric comparison between groups of MR datasets (10,11,50).

The 3D reconstructions have also proven useful in planning surgical interventions for gynecologic (51,52) and obstetric (53) applications. Public domain tutorials (including videos) of MR-based female pelvic reconstruction may be found at http://splweb.bwh.harvard.edu:8000/pages/ppl/lennox/tutorial/img0.html.

Cornella et al. (54) also used the 3DSlicer to reconstruct 3D models of the external anal sphincter in 10 healthy nulliparous women who also underwent anal manometry. They were able to visualize the external sphincter as a funnel-shaped structure,

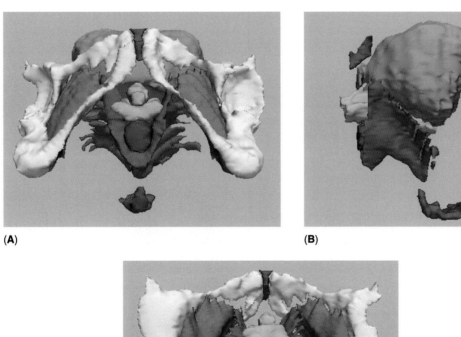

(A)   (B)

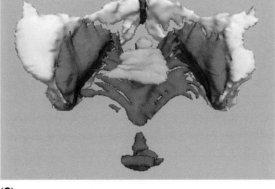

(C)

Figure 37.11 Representative 3D reconstructions from a young nullipara. (**A**) Viewed in the dorsal lithotomy position. (**B**) Left sagittal view, with bones and obturator removed. (**C**) Posterior view, with bladder removed. Color legend: Pubic bones, white; Obturator internus, rose; Urethra and bladder, yellow; Vagina, pink; Levator, brown; Symphysis and coccyx, gray.

with the internal sphincter appearing more cylindrical. Both sphincters appeared somewhat elongated in the anteroposterior dimension. They also found that the volume of the internal anal sphincter was correlated with the length of the high-pressure zone at squeeze. This group also noted very high interrater reliability of the sphincter volume measurements, with a 95% confidence interval of 94% to 98% for external and internal sphincter volume assessment.

In these and other applications, the 3D reconstructions permitted improved visualization of the pelvic floor structures, leading to a better appreciation of the pelvic anatomy. It also afforded straightforward evaluation of the volumes and complex linear measurements on the reconstructured structures when compared to the 2D MR source images.

Color Thickness Mapping

MR-based segmentations have also been used to generate color maps of the levator ani, with the color varying according to the muscle thickness at each point. This color thickness mapping technique consists of a computer algorithm which was first used by Fielding et al. to detect bladder tumors, based on wall thickness variations (55). When this technique was adapted to study the levator ani muscles (56), it demonstrated thinning of the puborectalis muscle in female stress incontinent and prolapse subjects when compared to ASYs. The technique can be used to evaluate

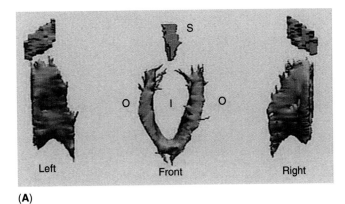

(A)

(B)

Figure 37.12 An example of an magnetic resonance imaging (MRI)-based color-mapped levator. (**A**) A reconstructed levator is shown in brown, with the symphysis (S). Views of the front, left, and right sides are shown. In the front view, the inner layer faces the label I, and the outer layer faces the label O. (**B**) Three views of a color-mapped levator are shown. The color bar on the left shows the thickness (in millimeters) corresponding to the colors seen. *Source:* From Ref. 54.

thickness variations among large groups of levator muscles. An example of a color-mapped levator is illustrated in Figure 37.12.

Pelvic Floor Childbirth Simulation

MRI has also been used to generate pelvic floor models for childbirth simulation. DeLancey's group used MR-based information from a 32-year-old nulliparous woman in order to build a simulation model of the bony pelvis and levator ani, through which they simulated passage of a fetal head as in vaginal

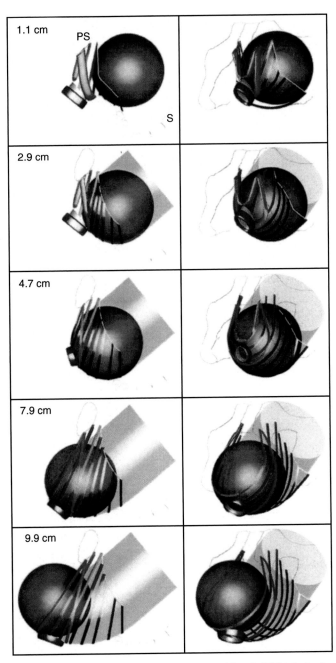

Figure 37.13 An magnetic resonance imaging (MRI)-based childbirth simulation at the point of cranial delivery. Simulated effect of fetal head descent on the levator ani muscles in the second stage of labor. At top left, a left lateral view shows the fetal head (blue) located posteriorly and inferioly to the public symphysis (PS) in front of the sacrum (S). The sequence of five images at left show the fetal head as it descends 1.1, 2.9, 4.7, 7.9, and 9.9 cm below the ischial spines as the head passes along the curve of carus (indicated by the transparent, light blue, curved tube). The sequence of five images at right are front-left, three-quarter views corresponding to those shown at left. *Source:* From Ref. 55.

performed in an upright MR scanner, but can also be done with the patient supine, and wearing a large adult diaper. The MR defecography study can highlight rectovaginal interface defects, rectal intussusception, perineal defects, and obstructions due to a compressive, hypermobile vaginal wall, or descending uterus. We have found the results useful in pinpointing these correctable anatomic defects in women with outlet constipation. In our experience, these patients respond well to either sacrocolpopexy, rectopexy, site specific posterior wall repair, or ocassionally myofascial release pelvic floor physical therapy, depending on the specific findings on the MR defecography study.

D Female Pelvic Floor Reconstruction

As noted earlier, MR data are acquired and presented as "stacks" of 2D images. While these stacks contain all of the information required to analyze the study, many surgeons prefer to think of pelvic anatomy in three dimensions. For this reason, Fielding and colleagues (45) built MR-based 3D reconstructions of the female pelvic floor structures, as follows.

Acquired MRI data were electronically transferred to a Sun UltraSparc-30 graphics computer workstation. The axial image data were segmented into anatomically significant components, including bladder, urethra, vagina, levator ani, symphysis, and coccyx, and then labeled using a combination of semi-automated

and manual editing using the 3DSlicer, a computer tool developed by our group (43). A gynecologist experienced in pelvic radiologic anatomy performed the manual segmentation, which required approximately two hours per subject. 3D surface models were generated using a pipeline consisting of dividing cubes, triangle reduction, triangle smoothing, and a surface-rendering method (47–49). The computer processing time for 3D model generation was <10 minutes per subject. The resulting reconstructions permitted outstanding 3D visualization of the intimate anatomic relationships in the living female pelvis for the first time. Examples of the 3D reconstructions are given in Figure 37.11a (dorsal lithotomy view) and 37.11b (left sagittal view). The reconstructed 3D models also permitted linear, angular, and volumetric measurements to be made, allowing parametric comparison between groups of MR datasets (10,11,50).

The 3D reconstructions have also proven useful in planning surgical interventions for gynecologic (51,52) and obstetric (53) applications. Public domain tutorials (including videos) of MR-based female pelvic reconstruction may be found at http://splweb. bwh.harvard.edu:8000/pages/ppl/lennox/tutorial/img0.html.

Cornella et al. (54) also used the 3DSlicer to reconstruct 3D models of the external anal sphincter in 10 healthy nulliparous women who also underwent anal manometry. They were able to visualize the external sphincter as a funnel-shaped structure,

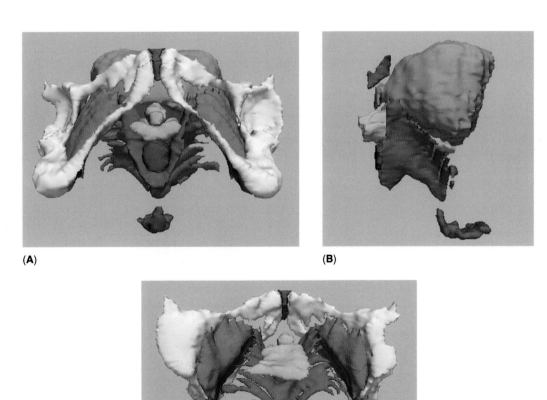

(A)

(B)

(C)

Figure 37.11 Representative 3D reconstructions from a young nullipara. (**A**) Viewed in the dorsal lithotomy position. (**B**) Left sagittal view, with bones and obturator removed. (**C**) Posterior view, with bladder removed. Color legend: Pubic bones, white; Obturator internus, rose; Urethra and bladder, yellow; Vagina, pink; Levator, brown; Symphysis and coccyx, gray.

with the internal sphincter appearing more cylindrical. Both sphincters appeared somewhat elongated in the anteroposterior dimension. They also found that the volume of the internal anal sphincter was correlated with the length of the high-pressure zone at squeeze. This group also noted very high interrater reliability of the sphincter volume measurements, with a 95% confidence interval of 94% to 98% for external and internal sphincter volume assessment.

In these and other applications, the 3D reconstructions permitted improved visualization of the pelvic floor structures, leading to a better appreciation of the pelvic anatomy. It also afforded straightforward evaluation of the volumes and complex linear measurements on the reconstructured structures when compared to the 2D MR source images.

Color Thickness Mapping

MR-based segmentations have also been used to generate color maps of the levator ani, with the color varying according to the muscle thickness at each point. This color thickness mapping technique consists of a computer algorithm which was first used by Fielding et al. to detect bladder tumors, based on wall thickness variations (55). When this technique was adapted to study the levator ani muscles (56), it demonstrated thinning of the puborectalis muscle in female stress incontinent and prolapse subjects when compared to ASYs. The technique can be used to evaluate

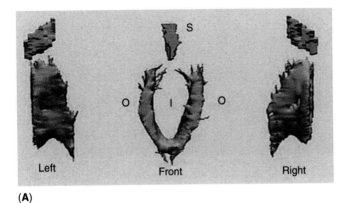

Figure 37.12 An example of an magnetic resonance imaging (MRI)-based color-mapped levator. (**A**) A reconstructed levator is shown in brown, with the symphysis (S). Views of the front, left, and right sides are shown. In the front view, the inner layer faces the label I, and the outer layer faces the label O. (**B**) Three views of a color-mapped levator are shown. The color bar on the left shows the thickness (in millimeters) corresponding to the colors seen. *Source:* From Ref. 54.

thickness variations among large groups of levator muscles. An example of a color-mapped levator is illustrated in Figure 37.12.

Pelvic Floor Childbirth Simulation

MRI has also been used to generate pelvic floor models for childbirth simulation. DeLancey's group used MR-based information from a 32-year-old nulliparous woman in order to build a simulation model of the bony pelvis and levator ani, through which they simulated passage of a fetal head as in vaginal

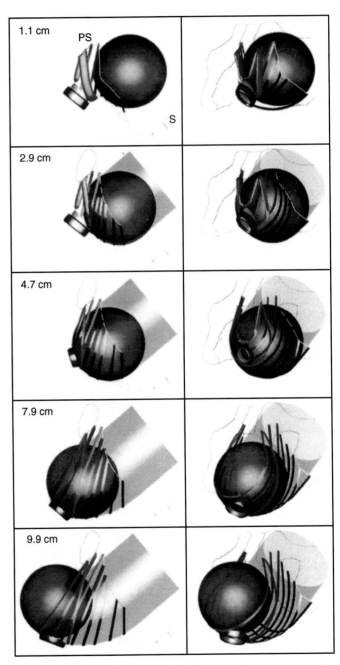

Figure 37.13 An magnetic resonance imaging (MRI)-based childbirth simulation at the point of cranial delivery. Simulated effect of fetal head descent on the levator ani muscles in the second stage of labor. At top left, a left lateral view shows the fetal head (blue) located posteriorly and inferioly to the public symphysis (PS) in front of the sacrum (S). The sequence of five images at left show the fetal head as it descends 1.1, 2.9, 4.7, 7.9, and 9.9 cm below the ischial spines as the head passes along the curve of carus (indicated by the transparent, light blue, curved tube). The sequence of five images at right are front-left, three-quarter views corresponding to those shown at left. *Source:* From Ref. 55.

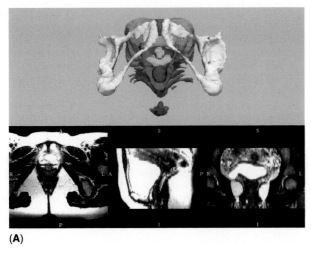 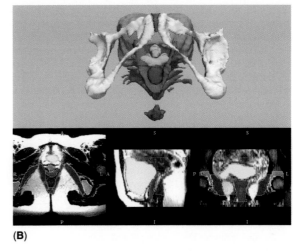

(A) (B)

Figure 37.14 Interactive windows from the 3DSlicer (www.slicer.org). (**A**) The 3D window (*top*), and the axial, sagittal, and coronal 2D windows (*bottom*). (**B**) The 2D windows (*bottom*), with selected anatomic structures outlined.

childbirth (57). Their results showed stretching of all portions of the levator muscle, with maximum stretch of 300% occurring in a band of the muscle corresponding to the pubococcygeus portion. This was the same portion of levator found on other studies to be intact in nulliparas, but disrupted in 20% of their primiparous subjects. An example of the childbirth simulation at the point of cranial delivery is illustrated in Figure 37.13. Our work demonstrated similar results (58), and further showed that maximal levator stretch increases with the stiffness of the levator ani attachments to the pelvic sidewall. This finding implies that the stiffer collagen attachments in the nulliparous pelvic floor may lead to more stretching during vaginal childbirth, compared to birth via the same pelvis on a subsequent delivery when the collagen attachments are less stiff. This may explain Rortveit's observation that the first vaginal birth seems to confer the highest risk of pelvic floor damage (as registered by SUI), compared to subsequent deliveries (59). Ongoing work in this area will likely yield improved insights into the mechanisms of childbirth-related pelvic floor injury.

Tools for Processing and Evaluating MRI Data

The analysis of MRI and other imaging data was previously limited by the need to use expensive, specialized hardware to view the acquired MR images. With the advent of ever more powerful personal computers, software tools for viewing MR images on personal computers have become available. With inexpensive, standardized storage afforded by z disks, and portable memory disks, the MR data can be moved easily from the MR scanner to most personal computers for viewing and analysis.

For research purposes, our group has developed and evolved a comprehensive, public domain, PC-based software tool (3DSlicer) to support all aspects of MR and CT image analysis (46). The 3DSlicer can be used for visualization, measurement, segmentation, 3D reconstruction, animation, and recording of images based on MR or CT data. It is available for download at no charge at www.slicer.org for Windows™, Macintosh™, and other computing platforms. The 3DSlicer is user friendly, and reads many commercial MR image data formats from standard media (e.g., DVD and CD-ROM). Examples of 3DSlicer interactive windows are shown in Figure 37.14. This tool has proven instrumental in permitting analysis of large groups of MR datasets.

CONCLUSION

MRI affords a closer view into the anatomy and interactions of the female pelvic structures in living women. Advanced processing techniques have further improved visualization and enabled simulation models to be built and tested. This work will continue to be built upon. Most of the work in pelvic MRI to date has been performed with MR images acquired in the supine position. Images may also be acquired with the subject in the sitting position, at some cost in image resolution. Such upright imaging may better capture the effects of gravity. In addition, more powerful MR scanners are becoming available, and will undoubtedly offer higher resolution images, with wide fields of view, and perhaps better views of the pelvic connective tissues, to further elucidate their role in supporting the pelvic viscera.

REFERENCES

1. Strohbehn K, Ellis J, Strohbehn JA, DeLancey JOL. Magnetic resonance imaging of the levator ani with anatomic correlation. Obstet Gynecol 1996; 87: 277–85.
2. Huddleston HT, Dunnihoo DT, Huddleston PM III, Meyers PC. Magnetic resonance imaging of defects in DeLancey's support levels I, II, and III. Am J Obstet Gynecol 1995; 172: 1778–84.
3. Kirshner-Hermanns R, Wein B, Niehaus S, Schaeffer W, Jakse G. The contribution of magnetic resonance imaging of the pelvic floor to the understanding of urinary incontinence. Br J Urol 1993; 72: 715–18.
4. Fielding JR, Griffiths DJ, Versi E, et al. MR imaging of pelvic floor continence mechanisms in the supine and upright positions. Am J Radiol 1998; 171: 1607–10.
5. Tunn R, DeLancey JOL, Howard D, Ashton-Miller J, Quint LE. Anatomic variations in the levator ani muscle, endopelvic fascia, and urethra in nulliparas evaluated by magnetic resonance imaging. Am J Obstet Gynecol 2003; 188: 116–21.
6. Klutke C, Golomb J, Barbaric Z, Raz S. The anatomy of stress incontinence: magnetic resonance imaging of the female bladder neck and urethra. J Urol 1990; 143: 563–6.
7. Tunn R, DeLancey JOL, Quint LE. Visibility of pelvic organ support system structures in magnetic resonance images without an endovaginal coil. Am J Obstet Gynecol 2001; 184: 1156–63.
8. Handa VL, Pannu HK, Siddique S, et al. Architectural differences in the bony pelvis of women with and without pelvic floor disorders. Obstet Gynecol 2003; 102: 1283–90.

375

9. Sze EHM, Kohli N, Miklos JR, Roat T, Karram MM. Computed tomography comparison of bony pelvis dimensions between women with and without genital prolapse. Obstet Gynecol 1999; 93: 229–32.

10. Fielding JR, Dumanli H, Schreyer A, et al. MR-based three dimensional modeling of the normal pelvic floor in women: quantification of muscle mass. Am J Radiol 2000; 174: 657–60.

11. Hoyte L, Schierlitz L, Zou K, Flesh G, Fielding JR. Two and 3 dimensional MRI comparison of levator ani structure, volume and integrity in women with stress incontinence and prolapse. Am J Obstet Gynecol 2001; 185: 11–19.

12. Aronson MP, Bates SM, Jacoby AF, Chelmow D, Sant GR. Periurethral and paravaginal anatomy: an endovaginal magnetic resonance imaging study. Am J Obstet Gynecol 1995; 173: 1702–8; discussion 1708–10.

13. Umek WH, Kearney R, Morgan DM, Ashton-Miller JA, DeLancey JO. The axial location of structural regions in the urethra: a magnetic resonance study in nulliparous women. Obstet Gynecol 2003; 102: 1039–45.

14. Gregory WT, Lou J, Stuyvesant A, Clark AL. Quantitative electromyography of the anal sphincter after uncomplicated vaginal delivery. Obstet Gynecol 2004; 104: 327–35.

15. Snooks SJ, Swash M, Mathers SE, Henry MM. Effect of vaginal delivery on the pelvic floor: a 5-year follow-up. Br J Surg 1990; 77: 1358–60.

16. Dietz HP, Bennett MJ. The effect of childbirth on pelvic organ mobility. Obstet Gynecol 2003; 102: 223–8.

17. DeLancey JOL, Kearney R, Chou Q, Speights S, Binno S. The appearance of levator ani muscle abnormalities in magnetic resonance images after vaginal delivery. Obstet Gynecol 2003; 101: 46–53.

18. Allen RE, Hosker GL, Smith ARB, Warrel DW. Pelvic floor damage and childbirth: a neurophysiological study. Br J Obstet Gynaecol 1990; 97: 770–9.

19. Menacker F, Curtin SC. Trends in cesarean birth and vaginal birth after previous cesarean. Natl Vital Stat Rep 2001; 49: 1–16.

20. Martin JA, Park MM, Sutton PD. Births: preliminary data for 2001. Natl Vital Stat Rep 2002; 50: 1–20.

21. Hendrix SL, Clark AM, Nygaard I, et al. Pelvic organ prolapse in the women's health initiative: gravity and gravidity. Am J Obstet Gynecol 2002; 186: 1160–6.

22. Madoff RD, Williams JG, Caushaj PF. Fecal incontinence. N Engl J Med 1992; 326: 1002–7.

23. Rortveit G, Daltveit AK, Hannestad YS, Hunskaar S. Urinary incontinence after vaginal delivery or cesarean section. N Engl J Med 2003; 348: 900–7.

24. Buchsbaum GM, Chin M, Glantz C, Guzick D. Prevalence of urinary incontinence and associated risk factors in a cohort of nuns. Obstet Gynecol 2002; 100: 226–9.

25. Miller JM, Umek WH, DeLancey JO, Ashton-Miller JA. Can women without visible pubococcygeal muscle in MR images still increase urethral closure pressures? Am J Obstet Gynecol 2004; 191: 171–5.

26. Hoyte L, Jakab M, Shott S, Brubaker L. Does your bony pelvic shape determine your soft tissue destiny? Results from a 3D MRI study. International Continence Society Meeting August 2004; Paris, France.

27. Bump RC. Racial comparisons and contrasts in urinary incontinence and pelvic organ prolapse. Obstet Gynecol 1993; 81: 421–5.

28. Duong TH, Korn AP. A comparison of urinary incontinence among African–American, Asian, Hispanic, and white women. Am J Obstet Gynecol 2001; 184: 1083–6.

29. Grodstein F, Fretts R, Lifford K, Resnick N, Curhan G. Association of age, race, and obstetric history with urinary symptoms among women in the nurses' health study. Am J Obstet Gynecol 2003; 189: 428–34.

30. Hendrix SL, Clark A, Nygaard I, et al. Pelvic organ prolapse in the women's health initiative: gravity and gravidity. Am J Obstet Gynecol 2002; 186: 1160–6.

31. Klingele CJ, Carley ME, Hill RF. Patient characteristics that are associated with urodynamically diagnosed detrusor instability and genuine stress incontinence. Am J Obstet Gynecol 2002; 186: 866–8.

32. Knobel J. Stress incontinence in the black female. S Afr Med J 1975; 49: 430–2.

33. Vandongen L. The anatomy of genital prolapse. S Afr Med J 1981; 60: 657–9.

34. Sampselle CM, Harlow SD, Skurnick J, Brubaker L, Bondarenko I. Urinary incontinence predictors and life impact in ethnically diverse perimenopausal women. Obstet Gynecol 2002; 100: 1230–8.

35. Howard D, DeLancey JOL, Tunn R, Ashton-Miller JA. Racial differences in the structure and function of the stress urinary continence mechanism. Obstet Gynecol 2000; 95: 713–17.

36. Hoyte L, Thomas J, Foster RT, et al. Racial differences in pelvic geometry among asymptomatic nulliparas as seen on three-dimensional MR images. Am J Obstet Gynecol 2005; 2005 Annual Meeting, Society of Gynecologic Surgeons.

37. Bump RC, Mattiasson ABK, Brubaker LP, et al. The standardization of terminology of female pelvic organ prolapse and pelvic floor dysfunction. Am J Obstet Gynecol 1996; 175: 10–17.

38. Downing KT, Hoyte LP, Warfield SK, Weidner AC. Racial differences in pelvic floor muscle thickness in asymptomatic nulliparas as seen on magnetic resonance imaging-based three-dimensional color thickness mapping. Am J Obstet Gynecol. 2007; 197: 625.

39. Howard D, DeLancey JO, Tunn R, Ashton-Miller JA. Racial differences in the structure and function of the stress urinary continence mechanism. Obstet Gynecol 2000; 95: 713–17.

40. Hersch RD, Gennart B, Figueiredo O, et al. The visible human slice web server: a first assessment. In: Proceedings IS&T/SPIE Conference on Internet Imaging. CA: San Jose, 2000 (vol 3964).

41. Spitzer V, Whitlock DG. The visible human dataset: the anatomical platform for human simulation. Anat Rec (New Anatomist) 1998; 253: 49–57.

42. Messerli V, Figueiredo O, Gennart B, Hersch RD. Parallelizing I/O intensive image access and processing applications. IEEE Concurrency 1999; 7: 28–37.

43. Hoyte L, Ratiu P. Linear measurements in 2-dimensional pelvic floor imaging: the impact of slice tilt angles on measurement reproducibility. Am J Obstet Gynecol 2001; 185: 537–44.

44. Mortele KJ, Fairhursta J. Dynamic MR defecography of the posterior compartment: indications, techniques and MRI features. Eur J Radiol 2007; 61: 462–72.

45. Fielding J, Ratiu P, Hoyte L, et al. Three-dimensional MR-based imaging of the female pelvic floor in vivo. Annual meeting, Radiologic Society of North America, Chicago, 1997.

46. Gering DT, Nabavi A, Kikinis R, et al. An integrated visualization system for surgical planning and guidance using image fusion and interventional imaging. Second International Conference on Medical Image Computing and Computer-assisted Interventions (MICCAI). Cambridge, U.K, 1999.

47. Lorensen W, Cline H. Marching cubes: a high resolution 3D surface construction algorithm. Comput Graph 1987; 21: 163–89.

48. Schroeder WZJ, Lorenson W. Decimation of triangle meshes. Comput Graph 1992; 26: 65–70.

49. Taubin G. Curve and surface smoothing without shrinkage. IBM Research Report 1994; RC-19536.

50. Singh K, Jakab M, Reid WM, Berger LA, Hoyte L. Three-dimensional magnetic resonance imaging assessment of levator ani morphologic features in different grades of prolapse. Am J Obstet Gynecol 2003; 188: 910–15.

51. Hoyte L, Lu K, Muto M, et al. Magnetic resonance imaging based three dimensional modeling of a complex vulvar tumor as a component of presurgical planning. J Women's Imaging 2000; 2: 138–40.

52. Hundley AF, Fielding JR, Hoyte L. Double cervix and vagina with septate uterus: an uncommon mullerian. Obstet Gynecol 2001; 98: 982–5.

53. Norwitz ER, Hoyte LPJ, Jenkins K, et al. Conjoined twins with twin reversed arterial perfusion sequence: a novel technique for antenatal surgical planning. N Engl J Med 2000; 343: 399–402.

54. Cornella JL, Hibner M, Fenner DE, et al. Three-dimensional reconstruction of magnetic resonance images of the anal sphincter and correlation between sphincter volume and pressure. Am J Obstet Gynecol 2003; 189: 130–5.

55. Fielding JR, Hoyte L, Okon S, et al. Tumor detection by virtual cystoscopy with color mapping of bladder wall thickness. J Urol 2002; 167: 559–62.

56. Hoyte L, Jakab M, Warfield SK, et al. Levator ani thickness variations in symptomatic and asymptomatic women using magnetic resonance-based 3-dimensional color mapping. Am J Obstet Gynecol 2004; 191: 856–61.

57. Lien K-C, Mooney B, DeLancey JOL, Ashton-Miller JA. Levator ani muscle stretch induced by simulated vaginal birth. Obstet Gynecol 2004; 103: 31–40.

58. Hoyte L, Damaser MS, Warfield SK, et al. Quantity and distribution of levator ani stretch during simulated vaginal childbirth. Am J Obstet Gynecol 2008; 199: 198 e1–5.

59. Rortveit G, Daltveit AK, Hannestad YS, Hunskaar S. Urinary incontinence after vaginal delivery or cesarean section. N Engl J Med 2003; 348: 900–7.

38 Endoscopy

Lesley Carr and Geoffrey W Cundiff

EVALUATION OF URINARY INCONTINENCE

Urinary incontinence is a non-specific symptom resulting from a variety of different conditions, and the differential diagnosis of urinary incontinence in women is broad, including urodynamic stress incontinence (USI), overactive bladder disorders, overflow incontinence, urinary tract fistulae, and urethral diverticula. Distinguishing these different etiologies is imperative as each condition warrants a different therapeutic approach.

Prior to the advent of sophisticated diagnostic modalities, most physicians depended on historical information related to inciting events and associated symptoms combined with physical findings to determine the etiology of incontinence. During the 1980s and 1990s a body of literature was published addressing the inaccuracy of historical and physical findings (1–3). Although physiologic subtypes of urinary incontinence demonstrate significant population differences in the distribution of symptoms, the considerable overlap in symptoms limits the predictive value in the individual patient. Attempts to improve this sensitivity by using pure symptoms or symptom complexes have proven equally inaccurate (4). Consequently, while historical and physical examination findings are valuable to correlate findings with patient complaints, more sophisticated diagnostic modalities are useful in evaluating complicated lower urinary tract symptoms.

More recently, the development of the minimally invasive mid-urethral sling techniques for surgically managing stress incontinence, have improved safety and shortened hospital stays, while maintaining the efficacy of traditional open incontinence surgery (5). Management of mixed symptoms of urinary incontinence with behavioral therapies and pharmacotherapy is generally quite successful leading some to recommend that cystoscopy and urodynamics should be reserved for patients that fail behavioral and initial pharmacotherapy or when other complicating conditions are identified (6). Should this pragmatic approach apply only to nonsurgical therapy? In a recent retrospective cohort study, mixed urinary incontinence symptoms, and previous incontinence surgery were associated with failure of a mid-urethral sling, while universal preoperative urodynamics failed to predict failure (7). Consequently, many surgeons are reserving urodynamics and cystoscopic evaluation for patients who have failed treatment or have known risk factors for failure.

More than 40 years ago, dynamic urethroscopy was proposed as an alternative to overcome the inaccuracy of symptomatology as the sole basis for diagnosing urinary incontinence (8). The subsequent refinement of urodynamic evaluation demonstrated its superiority for defining subtleties of pathophysiology causing urinary incontinence. In comparing urodynamics directly to cystourethroscopy, several authors concluded that it is a more sensitive method of diagnosing USI and detrusor overactivity (DO) (9,10). While these comparisons illustrate the superiority of urodynamics in evaluating abnormalities of lower urinary tract physiology, they fail to recognize the unique anatomic information provided by cystourethroscopy. When combined with urodynamics, cystourethroscopy contributes an anatomic assessment of the urethra and bladder, enabling the diagnosis of benign and malignant mucosal lesions that would remain undiagnosed by urodynamics alone. The value of cystourethroscopy as an adjunct to urodynamics was demonstrated in a study of women undergoing combined urodynamics and cystourethroscopy in which cystourethroscopy was considered important to 19% of the final diagnoses (11). Specifically, it provided new information in patients with anatomic abnormalities including intravesical lesions, intravesical foreign bodies, and urethral diverticulum. While not present in this series, urogenital fistula should be included in this category of anatomic lesions amenable to diagnosis by endoscopy.

INDICATIONS

The modern era of cost containment in medicine challenges physicians to determine a cost-effective approach to diagnosis that does not compromise the accuracy of the evaluation. In this context, it is important to define those women presenting with urinary incontinence who will benefit from diagnostic testing including urodynamics and cystourethroscopy. There are several clear indications for the anatomic assessment provided by that will be addressed individually.

Suspected Anatomic Lesions

Anatomic abnormalities, such as urogenital fistulae and urethral diverticula, might be suspected based on history or urodynamics but require an anatomic assessment for confirmation. For example, a diverticulum can be suspected based on a history of recurrent urinary tract infections, post-void dribbling, or pelvic pain. In such a patient, a biphasic urethral pressure profile is supportive of the diagnosis of a urethral diverticulum; however, Leach and Bavendam found that only 72% of patients with a urethral diverticulum demonstrated a biphasic pattern (12). This contrasts with the reported diagnostic accuracy for cystourethroscopy of 84% to 90% (13,14). Beyond diagnosis, cystourethroscopy also provides important information about the size and location of the ostia, as well as the presence of multiple diverticula. The ability of cystourethroscopy to define the location, size, and surrounding anatomic relationships also pertains for urogenital fistulae, and both Massee et al. (15) and Symmonds (16) consider it the simplest method of evaluating urinary tract fistulae.

Recurrent Incontinence

Women with recurrent urinary incontinence following a prior therapeutic intervention are a complex group of patients that may suffer from preoperative misdiagnosis, failed intervention, or a complication of the intervention. The fallibility of symptoms in determining the etiology of incontinence is high in this group of patients, and they all deserve a thorough evaluation, including multichannel urodynamics as well as the anatomic assessment provided by cystourethroscopy.

When recurrent incontinence is associated with a urodynamic diagnosis of DO, the differential diagnosis includes new onset DO, persistent but previously undiagnosed DO, DO related to obstruction, and mucosal irritation leading to DO. Mucosal irritation may be due to foreign bodies, such as urolithiasis or an intravesical suture, which are easily diagnosed at cystourethroscopy (17). Outflow obstruction due to overzealous elevation of the urethrovesical junction (UVJ) at the time of surgery has also been shown to be a cause of DO in recurrent incontinence (18). Cystourethroscopy is useful in these patients to achieve a visual evaluation of UVJ elevation and eliminate other possible etiologies in the differential diagnosis.

Recurrent USI after continence surgery may result from persistent urethral hypermobility or poor coaptation. Persistent urethral hypermobility occurs from inadequate elevation of the UVJ or failed UVJ stabilization secondary to sling or suture failure, poor tissue quality, or excessive stress on the repair (19). Poor coaptation, whether due to a damaged sphincter muscle, poor compressibility due to urethral fibrosis, or a lack of compressibility by surrounding organs, results in intrinsic sphincteric deficiency (ISD). This is another group of women that may also benefit from an anatomic assessment such as that provided by cystourethroscopy.

Intrinsic Sphincteric Deficiency

The Agency for Health Care Policy and Research coined the term "intrinsic sphincteric deficiency," defining it as a condition in which "the urethral sphincter is unable to coapt and generate enough resistance to retain urine in the bladder" (20). ISD is generally contrasted with the more common form of USI caused by bladder neck hypermobility, although most women with USI have varying degrees of both. Unfortunately, clinical criteria for ISD have not been standardized. In the absence of validated standard criteria for diagnosing ISD, an approach that combines historical risk factors with measures of incontinence severity, urodynamic evidence of poor urethral resistance, and an anatomic evaluation of urethral coaptation appears to be warranted. Cystourethroscopy is perhaps the simplest approach to the anatomic evaluation of the UVJ.

Fluoroscopic evaluation during video urodynamics is an alternative method to achieve the anatomic evaluation provided by cystourethroscopy. Transrectal and perineal ultrasound have been used to evaluate women with urinary incontinence, and while most investigators have utilized ultrasound to assess UVJ mobility (21–23), others have advocated it as a means of differentiating between USI and ISD (24). This might be an alternative to urethroscopy for evaluating the UVJ but does not provide the mucosal evaluation of the lower urinary tract achieved with cystourethroscopy. The same is true of fluoroscopy, although some authors feel that it is superior to cystourethroscopy for diagnosing ISD. Moreover, while videourodynamics can provide an equivalent anatomic evaluation of the UVJ, the cost for providing such a service is considerably higher than the cost of basic cystourethroscopy.

Universal Evaluation

There is general agreement that cystoscopy is indicated for patients complaining of irritative symptoms, persistent incontinence or voiding dysfunction following incontinence surgery. There is less agreement about the role of cystoscopy in the baseline evaluation of all women with urinary incontinence and there are relatively few analyses to define its role in this capacity. One series suggests that at the time of cystourethroscopy, up to 5% of patients presenting with urinary incontinence may have unsuspected neoplastic lesions, including bladder malignancies and potentially premalignant lesions such as cystitis glandularis (11). The annual age-adjusted incidence rate per 100,000 for bladder cancer in women is reported as 6.2. It rises with increasing age, approaching 20 for age 55 years, and there are also regional variations (25,26). Whether women presenting with urinary incontinence have a higher incidence of bladder cancer is poorly studies. Ideally, historical factors should distinguish those patients that merit cystourethroscopy based on risks for neoplastic lesions; however, in this relatively small series, age over 60, symptoms of urgency, pain, and hematuria were not predictive of these mucosal lesions. Individual clinicians should determine the benefits of cystourethroscopy in the evaluation for women presenting with urinary incontinence, although most utilize it based on indications rather than universally.

Intraoperative Evaluation of the Lower Urinary Tract

While some authors began advocating universal cystoscopy for reconstructive surgery in the mid 1990s, it was not until the advent of the tension free vaginal tape that this concept was widely embraced (27,28). Cystotomy is clearly a risk during placement of a retropubic mid-urethral sling, but is not a serious morbidity provided it is detected and corrected. The subsequent introduction of the transobturator mid-urethral slings promised a safer technique with respect to bladder Injury. One recent study comparing the rate of bladder injury between the two techniques found an overall cystotomy rate of 3.7% for retropubic mid-urethral slings compared to 0.3% for the transobturator approach (29). Some have suggested that cystoscopy is no longer necessary when using the transobturator approach, although other warn that urethral injury is sufficiently common with this technique to continue universal cystoscopy during all mid-urethral slings (30).

INSTRUMENTATION

Rigid Cystoscopy

There are three components to the rigid cystoscope: the telescope, the sheath, and the bridge (Fig. 38.1). Each component performs a different function and is available with various options to facilitate its role under different circumstances.

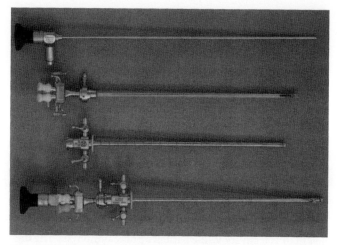

Figure 38.1 Components of a rigid cystoscope (from *top* to *bottom*): telescope, diagnostic (17 Fr) sheath, bridge, and assembled cystoscope.

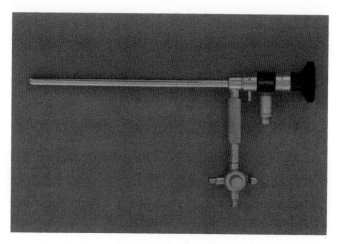

Figure 38.2 Urethroscope.

Telescopes

The telescope transmits light to the bladder cavity as well as an image to the viewer. Today, virtually all-rigid telescopes use a rod lens system. Telescopes designed for cystoscopy are available with several viewing angles, including 0° (straight), 30° (forward-oblique), 70° (lateral), and 120° (retroview). The angled telescopes have a field marker that helps maintain orientation. It is visible as a blackened notch at the outside of the visual field and opposite the angle of deflection.

The different angles facilitate the inspection of the entire bladder wall. Although the 0° lens is essential to adequate urethroscopy, it is insufficient for cystoscopy. The 30° lens provides the best view of the bladder base and posterior wall, while the 70° lens permits inspection of the anterolateral walls. The retroview of the 120° lens is not usually necessary for cystoscopy of the female bladder but can be useful for evaluating the urethral opening into the bladder. For many applications, a single telescope is preferable. In diagnostic cystoscopy, the 30° telescope is usually sufficient, although a 70° telescope may be required in the presence of fixation of the UVJ. For operative cystoscopy, the 70° telescope is preferable.

Sheaths

The cystoscope sheath provides a vehicle for introducing the telescope and distending media into the vesicle cavity. Sheaths are available in various calibers, ranging from 17 to 28 Fr. When placed within the sheath, the telescope, which is 15 Fr, only partially fills the lumen, leaving an irrigation-working channel. The smallest diameter sheath is useful for diagnostic procedures; those of larger caliber provide space for the placement of instruments into the irrigation-working channel. The proximal end of the sheath has two irrigating ports: one for introduction of the distending media and another for its exit. The distal end of the cystoscope sheath is fenestrated to permit use of instrumentation in the angled field of view. It is also beveled, opposite the fenestration, to increase the comfort of introduction of the cystoscope into the urethra. Bevels increase with the diameter of the cystoscope and larger diameter sheaths may require an obturator for placement.

Bridges

The bridge serves as a connector between the telescope and sheath, and forms a watertight seal with both. It may also have one or two ports for introduction of instruments into the irrigation-working channel. The Albarran bridge is a variation of the bridge that has a deflector mechanism at the end of an inner sheath. When placed within the cystoscope sheath, the deflector mechanism is located at the distal end of the inner sheath within the fenestra of the outer sheath. In this location, elevation of the deflector mechanism assists the manipulation of instruments within the field of view.

Urethroscopes Vs. Cystoscopes

The architectural differences between the urethra and bladder place unique demands on the endoscopes used to evaluate these two structures. The narrow caliber, straight lumen of the urethra is not adequately assessed by the angled cystoscope. The rigid urethroscope is a modification of the cystoscope designed exclusively for evaluation of the female urethra (Fig. 38.2). The urethroscope uses a telescope that is shorter and has a 0° viewing angle that provides a circumferential view of the urethral lumen as the mucosa in front of the urethroscope is distended by the distension media. The 0° lens is essential for adequate urethroscopy.

The urethroscope sheath is designed to maximize distension of the urethral lumen. The proximal end of the sheath has a single irrigating port and the telescope only partially fills the sheath, leaving space for the irrigant to flow around it. Sheaths are available in 15 and 24 Fr calibers. The larger diameter sheath is useful, if tolerated, as it provides the best view of the urethral lumen by providing more rapid fluid flow for maximal distension. As the rigid urethroscope is primarily a diagnostic instrument, it does not have a bridge. Just as the cystoscope is inadequate for evaluation of the urethra, the urethroscope is inadequate for a complete assessment of the bladder.

There are other urethroscopes with lenses angled up to 30° from the horizontal, thus permitting a more panoramic view of the urethra.

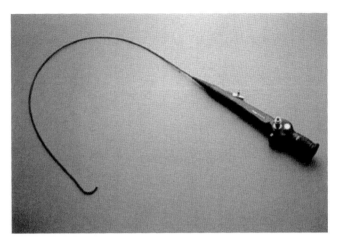

Figure 38.3 Flexible cystourethroscope.

Flexible Endoscopes

Unlike the rigid cystoscope, the flexible cystoscope combines the optical systems and irrigation-working channel in a single unit. The optical system consists of a single image-bearing fiber optic bundle and two light-bearing fiber optic bundles. The fibers of these bundles are coated parallel coherent optical fibers that transmit light even when bent. This permits incorporation of a distal tip-deflecting mechanism that will deflect the tip 290° in a single plane. A lever at the eyepiece controls the deflection. The optical fibers are fitted to a lens system that magnifies and focuses the image. A focusing knob is located just distal to the eyepiece. The irrigation-working port enters the instrument at the eyepiece opposite the deflecting mechanism. The coated tip is 15 to 18 Fr in diameter and 6 to 7 cm in length, with the working unit comprising half the length (Fig. 38.3).

Because of the individual coating of the fibers, there is a small space between each fiber in the image guide. Consequently, the image appears somewhat granular, although newly designed video flexible telescopes in which a video-camera is incorporated into the eyepiece have managed to eliminate the granular appearance entirely. The delicate 5 to 10 μm diameter of the fibers makes them susceptible to damage that will further compromise the image or light transmission. Gentle handling is, therefore, essential not only to good visualization but also to the longevity of the instrument. The flow rate of the irrigation-working channel is approximately one-quarter that of a similar size rigid cystoscope and is further curtailed by passage of instruments down this channel. Some tip deflection is also lost with use of the instrument channel.

In spite of these restrictions, several studies have compared rigid to flexible cystoscopy and found no compromise of diagnostic capabilities (31,32). Many urologists prefer the flexible cystoscope because of improved patient comfort, although the improvement in patient comfort primarily applies to male patients. The absence of a prostate and the short length of the female urethra make rigid cystoscopy well tolerated by women (33). This may offset any perceived advantage of flexible cystoscopy in female patients.

ENDOSCOPIC TECHNIQUES

Since a complete endoscopic evaluation for urinary incontinence demands evaluation of both the bladder and the urethra, diagnostic urethroscopy and cystoscopy are usually combined. Diagnostic cystourethroscopy in women is well tolerated as an office procedure without anesthesia. Urethroscopy usually precedes the cystoscopic examination to prevent sheath-associated trauma from compromising the urethroscopic evaluation. Both rigid and flexible endoscopes will provide adequate visualization of the lower urinary tract, but only rigid endoscopy is described. The approach using a flexible cystoscope is similar to the technique described for rigid cystoscopy.

Dynamic Urethroscopy

Sterile water and saline at room temperature are the most commonly used distending media. Instillation is by gravity through a standard intravenous infusion set with the bag at a height of 100 cm above the patient's pubic symphysis. The urethroscope has a 0° viewing angle (straight), ideal for viewing the urethral lumen directly in front of the urethroscope. The urethral meatus is cleansed with a disinfectant and, with the distension medium flowing; the urethroscope is introduced into the urethral meatus. The center of the urethral lumen is maintained in the center of the operator's visual field and the urethral lumen, distended by the infusing medium, is followed to the UVJ. The urethral mucosa is examined for redness, pallor, exudate, and polyps as the urethroscope is advanced.

Dynamic urethroscopy, as originally described by Robertson (34), provides a subjective evaluation of urethral function. With a bladder volume of at least 300 ml, the urethroscope is withdrawn until the UVJ closes one-third of the way, and the response of the UVJ to "hold your urine" and "squeeze your rectum" commands, as well as Valsalva maneuver and cough, is observed. The UVJ should close with all of these commands. The urethroscope is then withdrawn while a finger in the vagina obstructs the urethral lumen proximal to the urethroscope. This maximizes distension of the urethral lumen, providing the best possible view of the urethral mucosa. Gentle massage of the urethra against the scope milks exudate from glands and diverticular openings, which helps to localize the ostia.

Diagnostic Cystoscopy

Cystoscopy is performed using a 30° or 70° angled telescope in a 17 Fr sheath. Topical anesthetics should be avoided during urethroscopy since they can affect the color of the urethral mucosa. Following urethroscopy, however, 1% lidocaine jelly may be used as a lubricant and topical anesthetic. The cystoscope is placed into the urethral meatus with the blunt beak of the sheath directed posteriorly and advanced to the bladder under direct visualization. An obturator is not usually necessary since downward pressure on the posterior urethral lumen with the blunt bleak of a 17 Fr sheath fully opens the urethral lumen and is well tolerated by the majority of women. The infusion of water is maintained at a slow rate until a volume of 300 to 400 ml is reached or until the patient reports fullness. At this volume, the flow may be stopped unless it is required to improve the endoscopic view, in which case a small volume can be removed for patient comfort. Orientation is easily established by identifying an air bubble at the anterior dome of the bladder. This serves as a landmark during the remainder of the examination of the bladder mucosa. Beginning at the superior dome to the UVJ, the survey progresses in 12 sweeps, mimicking the points of a clock. Orientation is maintained by placing the field marker directly opposite that portion of the bladder to be inspected. Visualization of the bladder base can be difficult in patients with a large cystocele although reduction of the prolapse with a finger in the vagina easily circumvents this problem. The mucosa is examined for color, vascularity, trabeculation, and abnormal lesions such as plaques or masses.

"Flat Tire" Test

Endoscopic evaluation for urinary vaginal fistulae requires several modifications from the usual diagnostic technique. The "flat tire" technique permits differentiation of a vesicovaginal from an ureterovaginal fistula, while also identifying the vaginal fistula opening. Prior to cystoscopy, the vaginal vault is filled with 10% dextrose solution, and CO_2 gas is used in place of sterile water as a distending medium through the cystoscope. The CO_2 distends the bladder and, if a vesicovaginal fistula is present, CO_2 bubbles into the water-filled vaginal vault, identifying the fisutla opening. Simultaneous administration of intravenous indigo carmine will identify an ureterovaginal fistula, as the dye seeps into the hypertonic fluid in the vagina. A vesicovaginal fistula following hysterectomy is most commonly identified in the supratrigonal area of the bladder.

ENDOSCOPIC FINDINGS
Normal Endoscopic Findings

Normally, the urethral mucosa is pink and smooth with a posterior longitudinal ridge, called the urethral crest (Fig. 38.4). The UVJ is typically round or an inverted horseshoe shape and is completely coapted until the lumen is opened by the irrigant. The UVJ normally closes briskly and has minimal mobility on Valsalva maneuver.

In its normal state, the bladder mucosa has a smooth surface with a pale pink to glistening white hue. The translucent mucosa affords easy visualization of the branched submucosal vasculature. As the mucosa of the dome gives way to the trigone, it thickens and develops a granular texture. The trigone is triangular in shape, with the inferior apex directed toward the UVJ and the ureteral orifices forming the superior apices. As the cystoscope is advanced past the UVJ, the trigone is apparent at the bottom of the field. The interureteric ridge is a visible elevation that forms the superior boundary of the trigone, running between the ureteral orifices. The intramural portion of the ureters can often be seen as they course from the lateral aspect of the bladder towards the trigone and ureteral orifices. Although there is marked variation in the ureteral orifices, they are generally circular or slit-like openings at the apex of a small mound (Fig. 38.5). With efflux of urine, the slit opens and the mound retracts in the direction of the intramural ureter.

When distended, the bladder is roughly spherical in shape, but numerous folds of mucosa are evident in the empty or partially filled bladder. The uterus and cervix can usually be seen indenting the posterior wall of the bladder, which creates posterolateral pouches where the bladder drapes over the

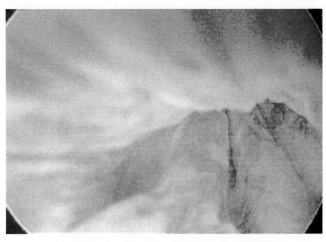

Figure 38.4 Urethral lumen showing urethral crest and normal coaptation.

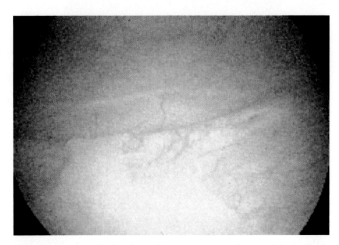

Figure 38.5 Left urethral orifice with squamous metaplasia overlying trigone. The interureteric ridge is also visible.

uterus into the paravaginal spaces. At times, visualization of the anterior bladder dome requires manual pressure on the lower abdomen.

Urethral Findings

While congenital urethral anomalies are quite uncommon, urethral duplication has been reported, and typically the most anterior lumen drains the true bladder (Fig. 38.6). Due to the blind ending and the possibility of urine deposition and entrapment in the false urethra, resection of the duplicate urethra may be required.

Polyps and Fronds

Fibroepithelial polyps of the bladder and ureter (which can extend into the bladder) have also been identified and usually appear as smooth lesions, commonly on a long stalk. Diagnosis is made by endoscopic resection. Bladder neck and/or urethral pseudopolyps appear as pink frondular lesions within the urethra proper or extending into the bladder. They are nonmalignant lesions that do not require histological confirmation, and have been associated with irritative symptoms. It has not been clearly demonstrated that fulguration is associated with long-lasting symptom resolution.

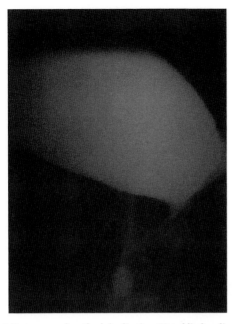

Figure 38.6 Cystogram of urethral duplication. Note blind ending posterior urethral lumen. *Source*: Courtesy of Dr. P. Zimmern, University of Texas Southwestern Medical Center, Dallas, Texas.

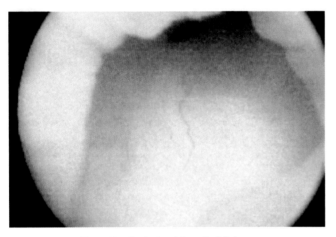

Figure 38.7 Intrinsic sphincteric deficiency.

Urodynamic Stress Incontinence

The urethral hypermobility typical of USI causes the UVJ to open and descend in response to cough and Valsalva maneuver, and the patient may not be able to close the UVJ to the "hold" and "squeeze" commands. Urethroscopic findings typical of the patient with ISD include a rigid, immobile urethra with poor coaptation (Fig. 38.7). In severe cases, the UVJ is unresponsive to commands and the lumen is visualized in its entirety from meatus to UVJ. DO should be suspected if there is uncontrollable urethral opening during filling.

Diverticula

Urethral diverticula occur in 1% to 3% of women, and are located along the posterolateral wall of the urethra as single or multiple outpouchings. Over half of the diverticular openings are at the mid-urethra, with a number more proximal, and some more distal (Fig. 38.8). The urethroscopic diagnosis is

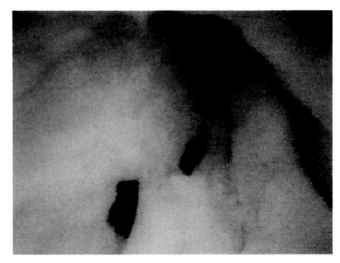

Figure 38.8 Urethral diverticula.

most accurate when the bladder is filled, and a finger in the vagina occludes the bladder neck or proximal urethra. A steady flow of fluid into the urethra is maintained as the scope is withdrawn and the urethra massaged by the finger pressing upward from below.

ABNORMAL BLADDER FINDINGS
Non-malignant Bladder Lesions
One of the more common findings on initial cystoscopic evaluation is squamous metaplasia, seen as a whitish, cobble stoning appearance of the trigone found exclusively in women. A benign lesion that may represent ectopic vaginal epithelium, it does not require bladder biopsy. Cystitis cystica and cystitis glandularis are histological diagnoses of bladder lesions that typically appear as reddened, inflamed areas, often indistinguishable from carcinoma in situ, and are associated with recurrent and chronic infections. They appear to result from Brunn's nests (subepithelial islands of transitional cells that form cystic lesions). Though both are benign lesions, adenocarcinoma of the bladder occurring in conjunction with cystitis glandularis has been reported (35). Eosinophilic cystitis may appear as a red–brown patch cystoscopically, and the diagnosis can only be made by histological evaluation. Steroid treatment has been employed in patients with this form of cystitis. Malakoplakia of the bladder results from some form of chronic irritation, often as a result of recurrent infection. The cystoscopic appearance is non-diagnostic, often appearing as yellow or brown flat plaques, although the pathologic finding of Michaelis–Gutmann bodies (partially digested cell wall fragments) is confirmatory. Long-term antibiotic treatment may be required in symptomatic patients.

Bladder trabeculations have been most commonly described in association with bladder outlet obstruction (Fig. 38.9), though this is a non-specific finding. Grades of trabeculation have been proposed, though none is universally accepted. In general, more severe trabeculation has been associated with detrusor compromise. Histological analysis of trabeculations has demonstrated a mixture of smooth muscle bundles with an abundance of interfascicular collagen deposition.

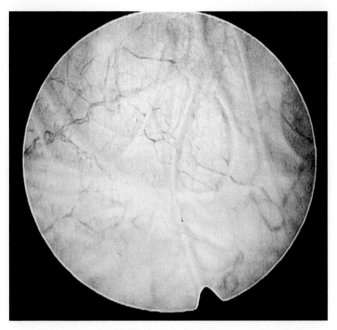

Figure 38.9 Bladder trabeculations.

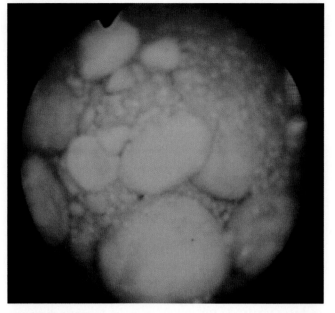

Figure 38.11 Bladder stones in setting of poorly draining bladder secondary to severe anterior vaginal wall prolapse.

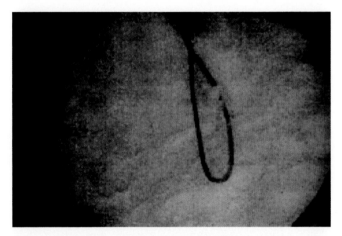

Figure 38.10 Intravesical suture with adherent calculi.

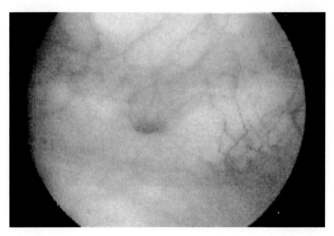

Figure 38.12 Supratrigonal fistula.

Diverticula are urothelial-lined pockets without smooth muscle backing that can either be congenital (i.e., Hutch diverticula located adjacent to a ureteral orifice) or acquired (commonly in the setting of outlet obstruction). They may have either a large or a narrow neck, and if poorly draining can be a source of recurrent infection. As noted above, each must be carefully examined at the time of cystoscopy to evaluate for mucosal tumors.

Foreign Bodies

Intravesical foreign bodies may present with hematuria or as urge incontinence due to mucosal irritation. Bladder calculi may result from urinary stasis or the presence of a foreign body, or an inflammatory exudate may coalesce and serve as a nidus for stone formation (Figs. 38.10, 38.11). Stones have an extremely variable cystoscopic appearance in terms of color, size, and shape, but generally have an irregular surface. Foreign bodies and stones are usually accompanied by varying degrees

of general or localized inflammatory reaction. Cystourethroscopy can provide valuable information in making these diagnoses.

Fistulae

Diagnosis is made in three steps after a fistula is suspected. Step one is to confirm that watery drainage is urine; Pyridium may be used for this purpose. The next step is to exclude urinary incontinence occurring from the urethra by filling the bladder and observing for loss from the urethra or vagina. Finally, the source of the fistula needs to be determined. This commences with a thorough speculum inspection, which may reveal a fistula site to the vagina. The double-contrast test is also useful, although cystoscopy and the flat tire test are the best ways to visualize the fistula site in the bladder. A post hysterectomy vesicovaginal fistula on the bladder side appears above the trigone medial to the ureters (Fig. 38.12); at vaginoscopy it is at the vaginal vault. Cystoscopy may show edema and congestion, or even mucosal papillomatous hyperplasia in enterovesical fistulae. Sometimes a ureteral catheter can be passed into a visible fistula opening to outline its path.

Enterovesical fistulae are not uncommon, particularly among patients with a history of diverticulitis (colovesical fistulae). Often noted as a "herald" patch on diagnostic cystoscopy (reddened appearance typically at the dome or on the left lateral wall), the diagnosis can be confirmed by cystography or pelvic computed tomography scanning. Occasionally, oral administration of charcoal will help confirm the diagnosis (apparent in urinary sediment) when radiologic studies are equivocal.

Bladder Pain Syndrome (BPS)/Painful Bladder Syndrome (PBS)/Interstitial Cystitis (IC)

The triad of bladder pain, urinary frequency, and urgency defines the BPS/PBS/IC syndrome. BPS/PBS/IC is a distinct condition and it is likely that the urgency experienced by these patients differs from that experienced by those with overactive bladder (36). While BPS/PBS/IC remains largely a diagnosis made by symptom assessment, the inclusion of typical cystoscopic findings in the original National Institute of Arthritis, Diabetes, Digestive and Kidney Disease criteria (37) highlights the historical role of cystoscopy in the evaluation of patients with BPS/PBS/IC. More recent studies have downplayed the importance of cystoscopy for making the diagnosis (38).

Office cystoscopy in patients with BPS/PBS/IC will typically reveal a small capacity bladder (<200 cc) that is readily inflamed with the slightest provocation. Petechial hemorrhages at sites of mucosal glomerulations are common with slight distension (Fig. 38.13); discrete areas of mucosal breaks can also be seen with more aggressive distension. Therapeutic hydrodistension under anesthesia will usually lead to significant petechial hemorrhaging, which is common in patients with BPS/PBS/IC, though certainly non-diagnostic, as patients with altered compliance (e.g., secondary to radiation cystitis) may have a similar response to distension. Hunner's ulcers, which appear as discrete areas of ulcerated mucosa, are thought to be characteristic (and perhaps diagnostic) of BPS/PBS/IC. Overall, there are few data to suggest that the presence of petechial hemorrhaging is specific for BPS/PBS/IC, and although Hunner's ulcers are certainly uncommon in other conditions, they may be present in only 5% to 20% of patients with BPS/PBS/IC (39,40). A recent study evaluating the role of cystoscopy in diagnosing BPS/PBS/IC concluded the standard clinical evaluation cannot reliably distinguish patients with and without Hunner's ulcers (41).

Malignant Bladder Lesions

Transitional cell carcinoma (TCC) of the bladder typically has a papillary appearance (Fig. 38.14) and may be multifocal. Patients found to have a bladder mass should undergo careful cystoscopy with both 30° and 70° lenses or a flexible cystoscope to evaluate the complete mucosal surface, including the bladder neck circumferentially. With a flexible cystoscope, this is best achieved by advancing the cystoscope and retroflexing the scope on itself to view the bladder neck. If diverticula are noted in the bladder, each diverticulum must be carefully

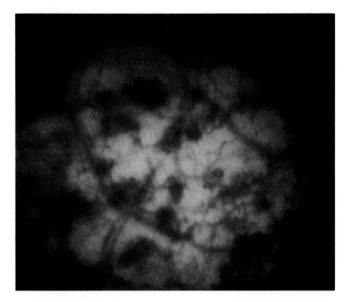

Figure 38.13 Glomerulations secondary to minimal hydrodistension in presumed case of interstitial cystitis. *Source*: Courtesy of Dr. P. Zimmern, University of Texas Southwestern Medical Center, Dallas, Texas.

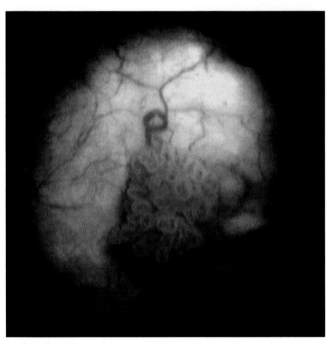

Figure 38.14 Papillary transitional cell carcinoma. *Source*: Courtesy of Dr. A. Sagalowsky, University of Texas Southwestern Medical Center, Dallas, Texas.

inspected to rule out the presence of TCC, which can be difficult to detect in these poorly draining areas. Other TCC lesions may have a more sessile appearance (Fig. 38.15). Generally, this type of appearance portends a more aggressive, potentially invasive tumor. Carcinoma in situ typically has a flat, red, velvety appearance that may be multifocal (Fig. 38.16). Other malignant bladder lesions include squamous cell tumors, sometimes associated with chronic infections or chronic indwelling catheters (42), and metastatic lesions. Melanoma (Fig. 38.17), breast adenocarcinoma, as well as several other

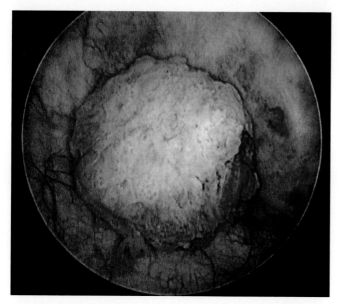

Figure 38.15 Sessile transitional cell carcinoma. *Source*: Courtesy of Dr. Y. Lotan, University of Texas Southwestern Medical Center, Dallas, Texas.

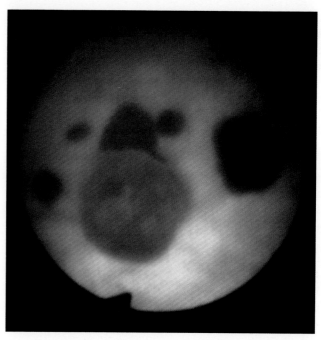

Figure 38.17 Metastatic melanoma to the bladder. *Source*: Courtesy of Dr. Y. Lotan, University of Texas Southwestern Medical Center, Dallas, Texas.

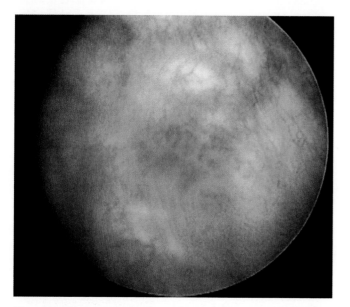

Figure 38.16 Carcinoma in situ. *Source*: Courtesy of Dr. Y. Lotan, University of Texas Southwestern Medical Center, Dallas, Texas.

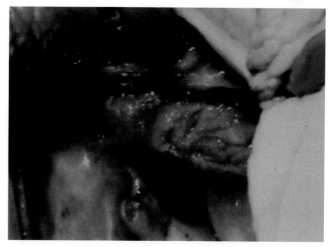

Figure 38.18 Urethral duplication. Note ectopic urethral orifice. *Source*: Courtesy of Dr. P. Zimmern, University of Texas Southwestern Medical Center, Dallas, Texas.

tumors, have been noted to metastasize to the bladder, often resulting in repeated bouts of gross hematuria. Locally advanced malignancies, typically of the colon, can also directly invade the bladder wall and eventually disrupt the bladder mucosa, resulting in an abnormal cystoscopic appearance and hematuria.

Bladder lesions of uncertain etiology on initial evaluation must be investigated under anesthesia, as often cold cup biopsies and fulguration will be required to determine their malignant potential. Although both urinary cytologies and other urinary markers are helpful in determining if malignant cells are present in bladder washings, none at this point is sensitive enough to preclude the need for tissue diagnosis, particularly when the lesion is not a typical papillary mass. Bladder masses

of likely malignant nature require complete transurethral endoscopic removal, and may require adjuvant intravesical chemotherapy or further surgical endeavors, depending on the depth of invasion and grade of tumor present.

Ureteral and Urethral Anomalies

Ureteral anomalies are not uncommonly found in patients undergoing diagnostic cystoscopy. Duplicated systems can occur bilaterally or unilaterally, with two orifices from the same renal unit typically being adjacent to one another. The medial and caudal-most of the ureteral orifices normally serve the upper pole system. Vesicoureteral reflux is often present in the ureter serving the lower pole system (a finding confirmed on cystography). In women, ectopic ureters may also be found to drain into the urethra and vaginal vestibule, though most of these abnormalities will be found in childhood secondary to ongoing incontinence.

Asymptomatic, single system ureteroceles are also not uncommon in adults, with the typical appearance being a thin layer of urothelium covering a bulging orifice in a normal location. Often, a pinpoint opening is noted on the membrane, and, due to urinary stasis, ureteral stone formation can occur proximal to this opening, particularly in children. Upper tract imaging may be required to evaluate the collecting system in these instances. Occasionally, ureteroceles will be ectopic in location, at times presenting as far distally as the mid and distal urethra.

In contrast, urethral anomalies are quite uncommon. Urethral duplication has been reported, and typically the most anterior lumen drains the true bladder (Figs. 38.6, 38.18). Due to the blind ending and the possibility of urine deposition and entrapment in the false urethra, resection of the duplicate urethra may be required.

CONCLUSION

Endoscopy of the lower urinary tract is an invaluable tool to the physician treating women for urinary incontinence. While it is not the best method for diagnosing USI and DO, it does provide unique anatomic information with a simple, minimally invasive approach. Endoscopy is a useful adjunct to multichannel urodynamics in women with possible ISD, urethral diverticula, urogenital fistulae, foreign bodies or urothelial lesions and should be considered in women with complex lower urinary symptoms. It should also be used intraoperatively following surgery for urinary incontinence to insure the integrity of the lower urinary tract.

REFERENCES

1. Largo-Janssen ALM, Debruyne FMJ, Van Weel C. Value of the patient's case history in diagnosing urinary incontinence in general practice. Br J Urol 1991; 67: 569–72.
2. Sand PK, Hill RC, Ostergard DR. Incontinence history as a predictor of detrusor stability. Obstet Gynecol 1988; 71: 257–9.
3. Korda A, Krieger M, Hunter P, Parkin G. The value of clinical symptoms in the diagnosis of urinary incontinence in the female. Aust N Z Obstet Gynaecol 1987; 27: 149–51.
4. Cundiff GW, Harris RL, Coates KW, Bump RC. Clinical predictors of urinary incontinence in women. Am J Obstet Gynecol 1997; 177: 262–7.
5. Balmforth J, Cardozo LD. Trends toward less invasive treatment of female stress urinary incontinence. Urology 2003; 62(4 Suppl 1): 52–60.
6. Carr LK. Overactive bladder. Can J Urol 2008; 15(Suppl 1):32–6; discussion 36.
7. Houwert RM, Venema PL, Aquarius AE, et al. Predictive value of urodynamics on outcome after midurethral sling surgery for female stress urinary incontinence. Am J Obstet Gynecol 2009; 200: 649.e1–12. [Epub 2009 Apr].
8. Robertson JR. Air cystoscopy. Obstet Gynecol 1968; 32: 328–30.
9. Sand PK, Hill RC, Ostergard DR. Supine urethroscopic and standing cystometry as screening methods for detection of detrusor instability. Obstet Gynecol 1987; 70: 57–60.
10. Scotti RJ, Ostergard DR, Guillaume AA, Kohatsu KE. Predictive value of urethroscopy as compared to urodynamics in the diagnosis of genuine stress incontinence. J Repro Med 1990; 35: 772–6.
11. Cundiff GW, Bent AE. The contribution of cystourethroscopy to a combined urodynamic and urethrocystoscopic evaluation of urinary incontinence in women. Int J Urogynecol 1996; 7: 307–11.
12. Leach GE, Bavendam TG. Female urethral diverticula. Urology 1987; 30: 407–15.
13. Robertson JR. Urethral diverticula. In: Ostergard DR, Bent AE, eds. Urogynecology and Urodynamics: Theory and Practice, 3rd edn. Baltimore: Williams and Wilkins, 1991; 283–91.
14. Drutz HP. Urethral diverticula. Obstet Gynecol Clin North Am 1989; 16: 923–9.
15. Massee JS, Welch JS, Pratt JH, Symmonds RE. Management of urinary–vaginal fistula. JAMA 1964; 190: 124–8.
16. Symmonds RE. Incontinence: vesical and urethral fistulas. Clin Obstet Gynecol 1984; 27: 499–514.
17. Quiroz LH, Cundiff GW. Transurethral resection of tension-free vaginal tape under tactile traction. Int Urogynecol J Pelvic Floor Dysfunct 2009; 20: 873–5. [Epub 2008 Nov].
18. Bump RC, Hurt WG, Theofrastous JP, et al. Continence program for women research group. Randomized prospective comparison of needle colposuspension versus endopelvic fascia plication for potential stress incontinence prophylaxis in women undergoing vaginal reconstruction for stage II or IV pelvic organ prolapse. Am J Obstet Gynecol 1996; 175: 326–35.
19. Bruskewitz R, Nielsen K, Graversen P, et al. Bladder neck suspension material investigated in a rabbit model. J Urol 1989; 142: 1361–3.
20. Urinary Incontinence Guideline Panel. Urinary incontinence in adults: clinical practical guidelines. AHCPR Pub. No. 92-0038. Rockville, MD: Agency for Health Care Policy and Research, Public Health Service, U.S. Department of Health and Human Services, 1992.
21. Bergman A, McKenzie CJ, Richmond J, Ballard CA, Platt LD. Transrectal ultrasound versus cystography in the evaluation of anatomical stress urinary incontinence. Br J Urol 1988; 62: 228–34.
22. Chang HC, Chang SC, Kuo HC, Tsai TC. Transrectal sonographic cystourethrography: studies in stress urinary incontinence. Urology 1990; 36: 488–92.
23. Gordon D, Pearce M, Norton P, Stanton S. Comparison of ultrasound and lateral chain urethrocystography in the determination of bladder neck descent. Am J Obstet Gynecol 1989; 160: 182–5.
24. Weil EHK, van Waalaijk van Doorn ESC, et al. Transvaginal ultrasonography: a study with healthy volunteers and women with genuine stress incontinence. Eur Urol 1993; 24: 226–30.
25. Young JL Jr, Percy CL, Asire AJ, eds. Surveillance, epidemiology, end results: incidence and mortality data, 1973–77. Natl Cancer Inst Monogr 1981; 57: 1–1082.
26. Anton-Culver H, Lee-Feldstein A, Taylor TH. Occupation and bladder cancer risk. Am J Epidemiol 1992; 136: 89–94.
27. Harris RL, Cundiff GW, Theofrastous JT, et al. The value of intraoperative cystoscopy in urogynecologic and reconstructive pelvic surgery. Am J Obstet Gynecol 177: 1367–9.
28. Ulmsten U. An introduction to tension-free vaginal tape (TVT)—a new surgical procedure for treatment of female urinary incontinence. Int Urogynecol J Pelvic Floor Dysfunct 2001; 12(Suppl 2): S3–4.
29. Stav K, Dwyer PL, Rosamilia A, et al. Risk factors for trocar injury to the bladder during mid urethral sling procedures. J Urol 2009; 182: 174–9. [Epub 2009 May 17].
30. Morton HC, Hilton P. Urethral injury associated with minimlly invasive mid-urethral sling procedures for the treatment of stress uriarny incontincne: a case series ans systematic literature review. BJOG 2009; 116: 1120–6. [Epub 2009 May 11].
31. Figueroa TE, Thomas R, Moon TD. Taking the pain out of cystoscopy: a comparison of rigid with flexible instruments. J La State Med Soc 1987; 139: 26–8.
32. Clayman RV, Reddy P, Lange PH. Flexible fiberoptic and rigid-rod lens endoscopy of the lower urinary tract: a prospective controlled comparison. J Urol 1984; 131: 715–16.
33. Ellerkman RM, Dunn JS, McBride AW, et al. A comparison of anticipated pain before and pain rating after the procedure in patients who undergo cystourethroscopy. Am J Obstet Gynecol 2003; 189: 66–9.

34. Robertson JR. Endoscopic examination of the urethra and bladder. Clin Obstet Gynecol 1983; 26: 347–8.

35. Sozen S, Gurocak S, Uzum N, Biri H, Memis L, Bozkirli I. The importance of re-evaluation in patients with cystitis glandularis associated with pelvic lipomatosis: a case report. Urol Oncol 2004; 22: 428–30.

36. HannoPM, Chapple CR, Cardozo LD. Bladder pain syndrome/interstitial cystitis: a sense of urgency. World J Urol 2009. [Epub ahead of print].

37. Gillenwater JY, Wein AJ. Summary of the National Institute of Arthritis, Diabetes, Digestive and Kidney Diseases Workshop on Interstitial Cystitis. J Urol 1988; 140: 203–6.

38. Seth A, Teichman JM. What's new in the diagnosis and management of painful bladder syndrome/interstitial cystitis? Curr Urol Rep 2008; 9: 349–57.

39. Sant GR. Interstitial cystitis. Monograms in Urology 1991; 12: 37–63.

40. Koziol JA. Epidemiology of interstitial cystitis. Urol Clin North Am 1994; 21: 7–20.

41. Braunstien R, Shapiro E, Kaye J, Moldwin R. The role of cystoscopy In the diagnosis of Hunner's ulcer disease. J Urol 2008; 180: 1383–6. [Epub 2008 Aug 15].

42. Delnay KM, Stonehill WH, Goldman H, Jukkola AF, Dmochowski RR. Bladder histological changes associated with chronic indwelling urinary catheter. J Urol 1999; 161: 1106–9.

39 The Role of the Continence Nurse
Angie Rantell

INTRODUCTION

The role of the continence nurse (CN) is multifaceted and ever expanding. It has developed rapidly in the United Kingdom since the 1980s and now most health authorities (Trusts) offer a continence service that is run by specialist nurses.

These specialists provide a comprehensive assessment of all patients with continence needs and if applicable will implement conservative and pharmacological management plans. CNs have a role in education and health promotion for patients and other health care professionals (HCPs). They also act as counsellors when dealing with the negative psychosexual, emotional, and social impact that incontinence can have on individual's quality of life. Generally, CNs are the first HCP that patients are referred to following disclosure of an incontinence problem, this places them in a prime position to undertake further research into the field especially with regards to etiology, epidemiology, quality of life improvements, and assessment of successful management.

Continence care is considered to be the total care package tailored to meet individual needs of patients with bladder and bowel problems. This chapter will further discuss the varied roles that CNs perform to be able to provide a continence care package for all patients.

THE RANGE OF NURSING ROLES WITHIN CONTINENCE CARE

When continence services were first introduced they would often provide care for all patient groups. However, now with the expanding needs of these services, specialized areas have emerged. Box 39.1 shows the different nursing specialities within continence care. These sub-specialities are essential to offer expert care to all patients in primary, secondary, and tertiary care.

There is also a distinct range of nursing roles within the field including nurse consultants, clinical nurse specialists, continence advisors, staff nurses, and health support workers. Some may work alone or as part of a larger multi-disciplinary team.

Austin (1) undertook a postal survey of continence advisors working in one health region to assess the differences in their roles, in total 41 responded. All of them had clinical contact with patients. Fifty percent had been involved in research relating to their specialty. A high proportion of respondents were involved in the education of nurses, medical staff, and other HCPs. Most were involved in producing standards, protocols, and guidelines and all had an organizational-wide remit in an advisory role. Many were responsible for auditing the practice of others and 65% managed other staff in their team. Ninety percent were responsible for providing advice or approval regarding purchasing and supply of specialist products and half of them held their own budget. This paper demonstrates

the many different roles which a CN must perform to provide a full service.

ASSESSMENT

Incontinence is a symptom of an underlying disorder. A complete continence assessment will help to identify possible causes by building a complete picture of bladder and bowel dysfunction. A thorough initial assessment is important to determine incontinence type and rule out infections or other causes (2). According to Lloyd and Craig (3), the procedure of taking a patient history allows the patient to present their account of the problems and provides essential information to the practitioner. There are many different models of assessment that can be utilized for this, however, many units will have developed their own pro-forma to standardize assessment in their specialist area. These may not only be used for specialist assessment but can also be used to standardize continence assessment for general nurses and help to ensure appropriate referral for patients with continence issues. Figure 39.1 demonstrates a continence assessment proforma that is designed for general nurses to help identify and assess hospital in-patients with bladder or bowel dysfunction.

Nolan and Caldock (4) stated that any framework for assessment should be:

- Flexible and able to be adapted to a variety of circumstances
- Appropriate to the audience it is intended for
- Capable of balancing and incorporating the views of a number of carers, users, and agencies
- Able to provide a mechanism for bringing different views together, while recognizing the diversity and variation within individual circumstances.

The quality of assessment will be greatly enhanced by the participation of the patient and carers to the assessment process ensuring that the patient's wishes are foremost and, wherever possible, her own words are used to reflect her needs (5).

Box 39.1 List of the Variety of Nursing Roles Involved in Continence Care

General continence nurse specialist
Urogynecology nurse specialist
Urology nurse specialists
Colorectal nurse specialist
Stoma nurse specialists
Pediatric continence specialist
Geriatric continence specialist
Neurology nurse specialist, e.g., stroke, multiple sclerosis, Parkinson's disease

---

King's College Hospital **NHS**

NHS Trust

CONTINENCE ASSESSMENT FORM

CLIENT'S NAME:	
NAME OF ASSESSOR:	

WARD:	ASSESSMENT DATE:
ADDRESS:	DESIGNATION:
TEL NO:	

DATE OF BIRTH:	AGE:

N.O.K/CARER:	
GP NAME:	
ADDRESS:	
CONSULTANTS:	

1. MEDICAL/SURGICAL HISTORY

OBSTETRIC HISTORY – PARITY ☐

2. MEDICATION

3. HISTORY OF INCONTINENCE

Onset: 0–12 Mths ☐   1–3 Yrs ☐   Over 3 Yrs ☐   Over 10 Years ☐

4. FAMILY HISTORY OF INCONTINENCE?

Figure 39.1 Continence assessment form. *Abbreviations*: GP, general practitioner; Physio, physiotherapist; OT, occupational therapist; D/N, district (community) nurse.

SYMPTOMS IDENTIFIED (PLEASE CIRCLE)	MANAGEMENT REQUIRED
FREQUENCY　　URGENCY　　LEAKS WITH URGENCY　　NOCTURIA	**URGE** INCONTINENCE
LEAKING ON COUGHING, SNEEZING, PHYSICAL ACTIVITY	**STRESS** INCONTINENCE
POOR STREAM　　HESITANCY　　STRAINING　　HISTORY OF UTI	VOIDING DIFFICULTIES **/ OVERFLOW** INCONTINENCE
LEAKAGE ASSOCIATED WITH FUNCTIONAL / COGNITIVE / MENTAL IMPAIRMENT.	**PASSIVE** / FUNCTIONAL INCONTINENCE

5. SEXUAL DIFFICULTIES *(RELATED TO INCONTINENCE)*

6. BOWELS

NO PROBLEM ☐　　CONSTIPATION ☐　　DIARRHOEA ☐　　FAECAL INCONTINENCE ☐

IMPACTION

NORMAL FOR CLIENT

7. FLUID INTAKE

SUFFICIENT (AT LEAST 8 CUPS) ☐　　INSUFFICIENT ☐　　IN EXTREME ☐

8. MOBILITY

NO PROBLEM ☐　　PROBLEM ☐

PLEASE SPECIFY

9. DEXTERITY

NO PROBLEM ☐　　PROBLEM ☐　　DIFFICULTY WITH CLOTHING, ETC. ☐

PLEASE SPECIFY

10. ATTITUDE TO INCONTINENCE

CARER　　POSITIVE ☐　APATHY ☐　DISTRESS ☐　ACCEPTANCE ☐　DENIAL ☐

CLIENT　　POSITIVE ☐　APATHY ☐　DISTRESS ☐　ACCEPTANCE ☐　DENIAL ☐

11. MENTAL STATE OF CLIENT

ALERT ☐　　ANXIOUS ☐　　CONFUSED ☐　　DEPRESSED ☐

DEMENTIA ☐　　LEARNING DIFFICULTY ☐

OTHER

Figure 39.1 (Continued)

12. SOCIAL NETWORK

LIVES ALONE ☐   CARER ☐   COMMUNITY NURSE ☐

OTHER

13. TOILET FACILITIES

EASILY ACCESSIBLE ☐   ADAPTED TOILET ☐   COMMODE ☐

INSIDE TOILET ☐   OUTSIDE TOILET ☐

PLEASE SPECIFY

14. PHYSICAL EXAMINATION BY NURSE, IF APPROPRIATE

GENITALIA/VAGINAL ☐   RECTAL EXAMINATION

RASH/EXCORIATION ☐   BLEEDING ☐

LOADED RECTUM ☐

15. INVESTIGATIONS UNDERTAKEN

URINE TEST (LABSTIX) ☐   MSU ☐   CSU ☐

RESULT _____

DATE _____

RESIDUAL URINE MLS _____

BASELINE CHART ☐   BLADDER SCAN ☐

16. PATIENT INFORMATION

SERVICE LEAFLET(S) ☐   SPECIFY: _____

TREATMENT LEAFLET(S) ☐   SPECIFY: _____

PRODUCT INFORMATION ☐   SPECIFY: _____

17 INCONTINENCE AIDS & EQUIPMENT

PRODUCTS USED AT PRESENT – PRIVATE PURCHASE?   YES ☐   NO ☐

STATE PRODUCT USED AT TIME OF ASSESSMENT _____

IF PRODUCT REQUIRED STATE PRODUCT GIVEN ON THE WARD _____ _____

18. ANY OTHER INFORMATION

19. SUMMARY

Figure 39.1 (Continued)

OTHER – *PLEASE SPECIFY* _____

TYPE	SYMPTOMS	TREATMENT	ACTIONS
STRESS Incontinence	• Leakage of urine upon physical exertion, e.g. cough, laugh, sneeze, or strain in any way.	• Pelvic floor exercises • Dietary a dvice • Surgical intervention	• Give out patient information sheet. • Inform medical staff Date ____ Sign ____
URGE Incontinence	• Urgency - urge incontinence • Frequency - nocturnal enuresis	• Bladder re training • Drug therapy – anticholinergics (slows the bladders activity down).	• Give out patient information sheet. • Refer to link nurse. Date ____ Sign ____
OVERFLOW Incontinence	• Bladder does not empty properly • Possesses residual urine • Frequent urinary tract infection • Hesitancy, straining, dribbling • Poor flow	• Bowel management • Instruction in voiding technique • Intermittent catheterisation • Indwelling catheter	• Give out patient information sheet. • Refer to medical staff • Refer to link nurse Date ____ Sign ____
PASSIVE Incontinence	• Incontinent without warning or no apparent reason. • Reduced awareness • Mental impairment • Confusion • Dementia • Nocturnal Enuresis – Bed wetting	• Bladder training • Toileting programme combined with reality orientation • Behaviour modification	• Give out patient information sheet. • Commence toileting chart. • Refer to link nurse. Date ____ Sign ____

20. REASON FOR REFERRAL

WHEN REFERRING TO THE CONTINENCE ADVISOR, PLEASE LIASE WITH YOUR WARD CONTINENCE LINK NURSE, FIRST

21. DISCHARGE PLAN

GP ☐　　　　　DIETICIAN ☐

　　　　　　　　　　　　　　　　　D/N ☐

PHYSIO ☐　　　CONTINENCE NURSE ☐

OT ☐　　　　　MEDICAL STAFF ☐

Figure 39.1 (Continued)

Box 39.2 Key Components of a Continence Assessment

- Review of symptoms and their effect on quality of life
- Assessment of the patient's desire for treatment and possible alternative management
- Examination of the patient's abdomen for palpable mass or retention of urine
- Examination of the perineum to identify prolapse, excoriation, and assess pelvic floor contraction
- Rectal examination to exclude fecal impaction
- Urinalysis to exclude urinary tract infection
- Assessment of manual dexterity
- Assessment of the patient's environment—access to the toilet
- Use of a bladder diary/frequency-volume chart/bladder scan.
- Identification of conditions that may exacerbate the patient's incontinence—medication, chronic cough, and drinking habits

Source: From Ref. 6.

Box 39.3 Environmental Considerations for the Assessment

The environment that the assessment takes place in should be:
Accessible
Maintains privacy and dignity
Hand washing facilities
Male/female toilets
Clean
Warm
Good lighting
Appropriately equipped
Free from distraction
Safe for the patient and the nurse
Sensitive to religious and cultural needs

Source: From Ref. 8.

For this to be put into practice, the CN needs to have excellent inter-personal skills to build a trusting and open relationship with the patients and carers, encouraging them to voice their feelings and views about their problems.

There are many components that are needed to perform a full continence assessment and these will differ depending on local/national policies, the CN's level of experience/expertise, and the specialization within the field. It will also depend on the wishes of the patients and their desire for treatment or management. In 2000, the Department of Health published a paper on good practice in continence services. This suggested key components that should be performed during a routine continence assessment. These are listed in Box 39.2.

SPECIALIST INVESTIGATION

CNs need a full understanding of different investigations that can be performed to assess and diagnose the causes of a patient's incontinence. They will not only be responsible for referring patients for further testing but also for performing investigations on their patients This may be simple procedures such as urinalysis or more complex studies such as uroflowmetry, bladder scanning, subtracted cystometry, video cystourethrography (VCU), ambulatory urodynamics, ano-rectal physiology and manometry, and barium meals/enemas. To be able to perform these investigations CNs may need specialist training in the procedures and may also need to gain further qualifications, e.g., good urodynamic practice. For CNs performing VCUs and barium studies, they may also have to be assessed and work within regulations for ionizing radiation (IR medical exposure) which can involved a theoretical exam and clinical assessment. This should be addressed in line with local policies.

There are many different levels to which CNs will perform investigations depending on their level of expertise and training. Some may be technically experienced but unable to interpret the results of the tests in relation to the patient's symptoms; however, the more experienced nurses will be able to assess, analyze, and interpret the results of any investigation that they perform.

Part of these investigations may involve internal examinations (vaginal and rectal). Prior to performing these examinations it is essential to consider what information you will be achieving, whether it is a screening or diagnostic procedure and whether it is necessary at the time (7). Informed consent should be gained verbally from all patients prior to investigation and in some cases, written consent may also be necessary. Consideration should also be taken to ensure that the environment in which the assessment or investigation takes place is appropriate to meet the needs of the patient and the requirements of the investigation. Box 39.3 lists some of these environmental considerations.

DECISION MAKING

Hamilton and Martin (9) state that "Information acquisition is not the end point for practitioners. Having the information is one thing but deciding on the implications of it and on what to do with the information is the essence of professionalism in nursing." Specialist practice is the exercising of higher levels of judgement, discretion, and decision making in clinical care (10).

Management of incontinence should take into consideration patients' individual needs and preferences, and patients should have the opportunity to make informed choices about their care and treatment (11). It has been shown that patient empowerment is the most dynamic, effective, and efficient approach to care (12). This places choices and decisions into the hands of those with incontinence.

Working as autonomic practitioners CNs play a large role in decision making. This includes the analysis and interpretation of investigations along with clinical observations and the information gained from taking a patients history to make a clinical diagnosis and appropriate management plan. Once a diagnosis has been made, CNs have a responsibility to fully inform patients and carers what type of incontinence they have and the treatment options available. With this knowledge a management plan can be set based on the CN's recommendations and patients choice and in line with local policies.

Kurtz et al. (13) developed the Calgary Cambridge Observation guide model of consultation. It facilitates continued

Box 39.4 The Five Stages of the Calgary Cambridge Observation guide

1. Explanation and planning—giving patients information, checking that it is correct and that you both agree that the history has been taken
2. Aiding accurate recall and understanding—making information easier for the patient using reflection
3. Achieving a shared understanding—incorporating the patients perspective to encourage an interaction rather that a one way transmission
4. Planning through shared decision making—working with patients to assist understanding and involving patients in the decision making process
5. Closing the consultation—explaining, checking, and offering a plan acceptable to the patients needs and expectations

Source: From Ref. 13.

learning and refining of consultation skills for nurses through five stages as described in Box 39.4.

Along with diagnosing and outlining and implementing management strategies, CNs must also be able to make clinical decisions as to when patients needs to be referred on for further investigation or more specialist care. This may be to a specialist within the field—a urogynecologist/urologist or colorectal team for surgery or to a different specialty following abnormal findings during assessment or exacerbation of a pre-existing co-morbidity that may be impacting upon their incontinence, e.g., heart failure or diabetes.

CONSERVATIVE MANAGEMENT

The most recently published guidelines on urinary incontinence from the Fourth International Consultation on Incontinence (2008) and National Institute for Health and Clinical Excellence (11) recommend initial lifestyle interventions followed by conservative management, which is usually pelvic floor physiotherapy for stress urinary incontinence and behavioral therapy, such as bladder re-training. CNs play a major role in the implementation of these conservative management strategies through patient education and health promotion. This is further discussed later in the chapter.

PHARMACOLOGICAL MANAGEMENT

Many CNs are not only working as advanced but autonomic practitioners and this has been helped with the advances in nurse prescribing. Whether CNs are working as an independent or supplementary prescriber or within the bounds of Patient Group Directives it has meant that patients can also access pharmacological treatment if appropriate for their type of incontinence through the nurse led service. Long-term monitoring and adjustments of these medications can also be performed through the nurse led service thus reducing waiting lists for medical teams within the specialty. Additionally, some general practitioners may not have an in depth knowledge of the different medications available, their modes of action, and how to monitor progress.

PADS, CATHETERS, AND ANTI-INCONTINENCE DEVICES

Management of incontinence with the use of pads, catheter, or nonsurgical devices is appropriate for some patients. CNs are responsible for assessing the need for these and providing the necessary education for patients using them as a coping strategy either in the short term while awaiting further treatment or surgery or long term for people with intractable incontinence. Some CNs who hold a budget may also have a role in the negotiation of contracts and provision of these products in line with local policy and needs assessment.

MINOR SURGERY

One of the expanding roles of all specialist nurses has been in the training to perform minor surgery. For CNs this has included performing procedures such as flexible cystoscopies and insertion of supra-pubic catheters, colonoscopies under local anesthetics or mild sedation. To perform this role CNs must have an advanced level of understanding of anatomy and physiology and be experienced and proficient clinical decision makers. A formal assessment pathway to ensure competency must be performed by an appropriate medical professional to ensure safe practice in line with regulatory bodies and individual trust protocols. With the invention of more surgical devices for incontinence that can be inserted under local anesthetic this role may soon expand further.

COUNSELLING SKILLS

People with incontinence often adopt coping behaviors to manage or reduce their symptoms, e.g., toilet mapping or dietary and fluid restrictions. Coping strategies and symptoms of incontinence can have a profound effect on health-related quality of life, negatively impacting on even simple daily activities. People with incontinence may be reluctant to travel, visit friends and family, or pursue leisure activities for fear of embarrassment (14). The psychological burden of incontinence can be severe, leading to depression and low self-esteem. Furthermore, some coping strategies are not only inconvenient but can also have serious medical sequelae (15).

Despite the debilitating effects of overactive bladder, almost half of symptomatic people do not seek healthcare advice, often because of shame and embarrassment (16).

Barriers to treatment seeking can include:

- Embarrassment
- Lack of knowledge about the condition and management
- Belief that incontinence is a normal part of aging and not a medical condition
- Availability of products to contain incontinence
- Fear of physical examinations, invasive testing, and surgery
- Low expectations regarding treatment

To overcome these barriers CNs need to aim to improve patient education to allay fears and misconceptions, and promote awareness of symptoms and treatments.

HEALTH PROMOTION

CNs are often in the prime position to provide information to patients and relatives/carers on health promotion. This may be in the form of diet and lifestyle advice, weight loss, or smoking cessation, and information on what are considered to be normal bladder and bowel habits.

Continence is now becoming a more public subject. In the past it has been counted a taboo that should not be discussed in public, however, with large numbers of women experiencing continence problems it is the ideal time to improve awareness and knowledge. This has been achieved in many ways. In the United Kingdom every year there is a "National Continence Week" where many HCPs working within the field will actively promote the specialty and services offered and address any myths associated with the subject.

In modern times the increase in women seeking information and help from the internet provides HCPs and charitable foundations with the opportunity to provide accurate health promotion information to a wider audience.

Many of the charities associated with this field (e.g., The Bladder and Bowel Foundation and the Overactive Bladder and Interstitial Cystitis Group) also provide user support groups where women with similar problems can share their experiences and help each other through the difficulties associated with the diagnosis and management of chronic conditions.

EDUCATION

Education forms a large part of the CN's role. They do not only educate patients but also carers, relatives, colleagues, and other HCPs. Patient education can often be the most difficult. Not only does it have to be tailored to individual patient need taking into account their degree of understanding, cultural sensitivities, and the level of knowledge that they need or wish to have. However, there is a growing trend toward "The Expert Patient" (17) where, in all probability, the patient with a chronic condition will actually know at least the same if not more on disease management than the HCP giving the care.

CNs are considered to have an in-depth knowledge and experience in the field and therefore act as clinical advisors and educators to other HCP to raise awareness of continence issues in different medical settings. Box 39.5 sets out the responsibilities of the CNs with regard to education as suggested by the Royal College of Nursing (18).

MAXIMIZING COMPLIANCE

Compliance is a medical term that is used to indicate a patient's correct following of medical advice. It applies to medication, the use of surgical appliances, or attending courses of therapy. It is also known as adherence, persistence, or concordance. There are several reasons as to why we should promote compliance to therapy as shown in Box 39.6.

Poor adherence to medication represents a major challenge in the management of urinary incontinence (19). There are many factors that can influence compliance with therapy and these are demonstrated in Box 39.7. Before starting therapy it is important to ensure that patients are counselled regarding the role of therapy, medication, or surgery. This should include

---

Box 39.5 The Educational Responsibilities of Nurses Specializing in Continence Care

- Be involved with other members of the team in the assessment, planning, delivery, and evaluation of initial education to patients, their families, and carer about incontinence
- Be involved in providing continuing education for all patients with incontinence and planning educational programmes for the area, the nurse specialist should also be involved with the team in setting, reviewing, and monitoring standards of continence care in the health district
- Participate in the planning and delivery of education about continence care for both nursing colleagues and those working in other disciplines. This may take place in the college of nursing, university, hospital, or community
- Act as a source of expert advice for all who cope with incontinence—including patients, other nurses, health care staff, and agencies that work with people with incontinence, e.g., local voluntary organizations

---

Box 39.6 Why Promote Compliance to Therapy?

- Reduce therapeutic failure
- Reduce wastage of resources
- Cost
- Improve patient satisfaction
- Increase efficacy of service provided

Box 39.7 Reasons for Nonadherence to Treatment

- Forgetfulness
- Purpose of treatment not clear
- Perceived lack of effect
- Side effects
- Instructions for administration not clear
- Complicated regimen
- Physical difficulty in complying
- Experiences since diagnosis
- Lack of time/money
- Health care provision

---

information on the side effects, the estimated length of treatment, other therapies available, how medication will improve their symptoms and how long it may take to be able to notice these differences, postoperative recovery, and risks and benefits of each intervention. This may help the patient to make an informed decision about her treatment and improve compliance with treatment. Often patients can become disillusioned with the expected outcome of treatment and this directly affects motivation and concordance which are paramount to the success of certain treatments. Regular assessment, good communication, and patient education are key skills for CNs to ensure that patients are making informed choices about their care and management. This is set out in The Code (20), which advises nurses to act as an advocate for those in their care, helping them to access relevant health and social care, information, and support. This will not only aid in maximizing compliance but in overall patient satisfaction through their continence care package.

MANAGEMENT

As well as the clinical responsibilities of CNs many staff in these posts will also have a management role within their trust. They may be leading or actively involved in the commissioning of integrated continence services and participating in regular policy reviews on nursing issues in their service (RCN). For new services, the CNs may be drafting policies in line with evidence based practice and setting out the aims and needs of their service by developing a service model.

In primary care CNs may hold a budget to provide containment products for their patients and in secondary care may be responsible for the standardization of products across the trust. In these roles the CNs act as buyers to negotiate the best contracts as well as accountants managing budgets and trying to make cost improvements in line with set targets. They will also have to design policies to outline those patients who are entitled to such services and how needs are assessed and standardized.

As part of a standard management role the CNs will also need to be proficient in tasks such as risk assessment, quality assurance as well as having strong leadership skills, and expertise in effective staff management.

CNs also have a role in the auditing of current services to ensure that they are working in line with the current evidence base and also of identifying and assessing the needs of the service and how these can be developed.

COORDINATION OF CARE

Some patients seen in continence clinics may require input from other services. As CNs have often performed the initial assessment it is their role to make direct referrals to these other teams and they often play a pivotal role in the coordination of care between these specialties to ensure that care is integrated and continuous. Box 39.8 lists some of the other services that continence patients may need referral too.

RESEARCH AND AUDIT

As a consequence of the advanced nursing practice within continence care, more CNs are participating in further

education by completing degree, masters, and even doctorate programs. As part of these courses they are undertaking innovative and original research into the field that previously had only been completed by the doctors. CNs are often best placed to recruit patients into clinical trials as they have more direct patient contact and are the first HCP that patients will meet along their pathway. With this in mind CNs are in an ideal place to actively promote research and can collect a multitude of data with regards to initial presentation of symptoms, epidemiology, etiology, success of conservative and pharmaceutical management, etc.

For those who do not wish to undertake formal research clinical audits can also be used to inform practice. For CNs with management duties service audits may also be completed to assess how services are running, ensure that patient needs are being met and as a scoping exercise when looking to further develop services.

COMMUNICATION

Communication is very important in the health care setting. Smith (21) said that the ability to communicate effectively with patients, relatives, and other staff is essential if nurses are to build trusting relationships in which patients feel that they are accepted and understood. According to Payton (22) communication has two functions in health care. Firstly, it is essential to establish and maintain effective inter-professional relationships with the patients, relatives, HCPs, and any other persons whom we come into contact with. The second function is the successful achievement of professional tasks, such as patient care, education, research, administration, supervision, and consultation. Wojinicki-Johansson (23) suggests that certain behaviors and devices have been found to facilitate and improve communication between nurses and patients, these include the use of body language, eye contact, and touch. Nurses can facilitate successful and therapeutic patient contact through questioning, listening, summarizing, reflecting, paraphrasing, set induction, and closure (9). CNs use these skills every day to assess, reassure, reduce anxiety, educate staff and patients, plan care, encourage critical thinking, liase with other HCPs, and promote continence care.

MAINTAINING PRIVACY AND DIGNITY

In the field of continence, ensuring complete privacy and dignity can be difficult. Although basic environmental issues are often met in order for CNs to assess incontinence we need to understand and know many personal pieces of information about the patient and often perform internal examinations. Some patients may find this information difficult to disclose to a nurse that they have never met before. It can therefore be difficult for CNs to strike a balance between protecting privacy and dignity and maintaining modesty whilst assessing, diagnosing and managing incontinence. To compensate for this every effort should be made to ensure all other areas of privacy and dignity are maintained, e.g., appropriate clinical area for review, appropriate use of chaperones during examination, confidentiality, etc.

Box 39.8 Examples of Additional Services Needed by Continence Patients

Urogynecologists
Gynecologists
Urologists
Colorectal surgeons
Gastroenterologists
Geriatricians
Psychologists
Social workers
Physiotherapists
Occupational therapists
Pharmacists
General practitioners

CONCLUSIONS

The role of the CN does not just involve clinical care of the incontinence patient. They aim to provide holistic care for patients and to act as educators and advisors to all other HCP who encounter continence issues in their practice. As the scope of nursing practice continues to expand, CNs will further develop to meet these demands and the level of nursing expertise with increase, not only with regard to the clinical aspects of care but also in service development to ensure integrated services and optimal continence care packages for patients.

REFERENCES

1. Austin L. A survey of continence nurse advisors working in one health region. J Commun Nursing 2003; 17: 7.
2. White C. Improving continence management for women. Nurs Times 2007; 103: 14–15, 49.
3. Lloyd H, Craig S. A guide to taking a patient's history. Nurs Stand 2007; 22: 13, 42–8.
4. Nolan M, Caldock K. Assessment: identifying the barriers to good practice. Health Soc Care Commun 1996; 4: 77–85.
5. Royal College of Nursing. Nursing Assessment and Older People—A RCN Toolkit. London: RCN, 2004.
6. Department of Health. Good Practice in Continence Services. London: DH, 2000.
7. Royal College of Obstetricians and Gynaecologists. Gynaecological Examinations: Guidelines for Specialist Practice. London: RCOG, 2002.
8. Crouch A, Meurier C. Vital Notes for Nurses: Health Assessment. Oxford: Blackwell Publishing, 2005.
9. Hamilton S, Martin D. A framework for effective communication skills. Nurs Times 2007; 103: 30–1, 48.
10. Hudson L. Best practice in care planning and documentation. In: Addison R, ed. Nurse Led Continence Clinics. Peterborough: Coloplast, 2005.
11. National Institute for Health and Clinical Excellence. Urinary Incontinence: The Management of Urinary Incontinence in Women. Clinical Guideline 40. Implementation Advice. October. London: NICE, 2006.
12. Addison R. Fluid intake: how coffee and caffeine affect continence. Nurs Times 2000; 96: 7–8.
13. Kurtz S, Silverman J, Benson J, Draper J. Marrying the content and process in clinical method teaching: enhancing the Calgary-Cambridge guides. Acad Med 2003; 78: 802–9.
14. Irwin DE, Milsom I, Kopp Z, Abrams P, Cardozo L. Impact of overactive bladder symptoms on employment, social interactions and emotional well-being in six European countries. BJU Int 2006; 97: 96–100.
15. Miller J, Hoffman E. Causes and consequences of overactive bladder. J Womens Health (Larchmt) 2006; 15: 251–60.
16. Shaw C. Barriers to help seeking in people with urinary symptoms. Fam Pract 2001; 18: 48–52.
17. Department of Health. The Expert Patient: A New Approach to Chronic Disease Management for the 21st Century. London: DOH, 2001.
18. Royal College of Nursing. Improving Continence Care for Patients—The Role of the Nurse. London: RCN, 2006.
19. Basra R, Wagg A, Chapple C, et al. A review of adherence to drug therapy in patients with overactive bladder. BJU Int 2008. [Available from: http://www.ncbi.nlm.nih.gov/pubmed/18616691?ordinalpos=1&itool=EntrezSystem2.PEntrez.Pubmed.Pubmed_ResultsPanel.Pubmed_RVDocSum].
20. Nursing and Midwifery Council. The Code. London: NMC, 2008.
21. Smith C. Learning about yourself can help patient care: using self-awareness to improve practice. Prof Nurse 1995; 10: 6, 390–2.
22. Payton OD. Psychosocial Aspects of Clinical Practice. New York: Churchill Livingstone, 1986.
23. Wojinicki-Johansson G. Communication between nurse and patients during ventilator treatment: patient reports and RN evaluations. Intensive Crit Care Nurs 2001; 17: 29–39.

40 Behavioral Therapies and Management of Urinary Incontinence in Women

Kathryn L Burgio

INTRODUCTION

Behavioral therapies are a group of interventions that improve bladder control by teaching patients skills for preventing urine loss or changing their daily habits. In clinical practice, behavioral interventions are usually comprised of multiple components, tailored to the individual needs of the patient, the characteristics of her symptoms, and her life circumstances. Behavioral treatment programs generally take one of two approaches. One approach focuses on improving bladder function through voiding schedules, such as with bladder training. Another basic approach targets the bladder *outlet*, such as with pelvic floor muscle training and exercise. Among the techniques included in behavioral treatment programs are: self-monitoring with a bladder diary, pelvic floor muscle training techniques (including biofeedback or digital teaching), pelvic floor muscle exercise regimens, active use of pelvic floor muscles for urethral occlusion, urge control and suppression strategies, urge avoidance strategies, scheduled voiding (including bladder training), delayed voiding, fluid management, dietary changes to avoid bladder irritants (including caffeine), weight loss, and other life style changes.

Although they are not curative in most patients, behavioral interventions are widely used because their efficacy is well established. They are safe and without the risks and side effects associated with some other therapies. However, they do depend on the active participation of a motivated patient and usually require some time and persistence to reach optimum benefit. Behavioral treatments have been recognized as effective by the 1988 Consensus Conference on Urinary Incontinence in Adults (1), the Guideline for Urinary Incontinence in Adults developed by the Agency for Health Care Policy and Research (2), and the International Consultation on Incontinence (3).

VOIDING HABITS AND BLADDER TRAINING
Decreasing Voiding Frequency: Bladder Training

It has long been thought that habitual frequent urination can over time contribute to reduced bladder capacity and lead to detrusor overactivity, which in turn causes urgency and urge incontinence. Bladder training is a behavioral intervention that was developed to break the cycle of urgency and frequency using consistent, incremental voiding schedules. When it was first introduced, it was known as bladder drill. Bladder drill was an intensive intervention, often conducted in an inpatient setting, in which women were placed on a strict expanded voiding schedule for 7 to 10 days to establish a normal voiding interval (4,5). Urgency and anxiety about possible urine loss were sometimes managed with Valium. Bladder training is a sequel to this procedure that increases the voiding interval more gradually, over a longer period of time, and is conducted in the outpatient setting (6–15).

Patients are given instructions to void at predetermined intervals, and over a period of several weeks, the voiding interval is gradually increased. To follow this regimen, patients must resist the sensation of urgency and postpone urination. This is believed to increase bladder capacity and decrease overactivity, resulting in improved bladder control. Bladder training programs have differed widely in terms of the instructional approach, intensity of clinical supervision, scheduling parameters, strategies for controlling urgency, frequency of schedule adjustments, criteria for increasing the voiding interval, length of treatment, and use of adjunctive treatments. At present there is no evidence for determining which parameters are most effective. However, the International Consultation on Incontinence recommends that clinicians should provide the most intensive bladder training supervision that is possible within service constraints. Guidelines for conducting bladder training appear in Table 40.1.

Several clinical series studies and two randomized trials have demonstrated efficacy of outpatient bladder training or a mixture of inpatient and outpatient intervention (6–15). The most definitive study of outpatient bladder training is a randomized clinical trial that demonstrated a mean 57% reduction in frequency of incontinence in older women (13). In this trial, bladder training not only reduced incontinence associated with detrusor overactivity, but also incontinence associated with sphincter insufficiency, possibly because patients acquired a greater awareness of bladder function or that the exercise of postponing urination increased the use of pelvic floor muscles.

Increasing Voiding Frequency

It is quite common for health care providers to advise patients with incontinence to simply increase their frequency of urination as a way to avoid a full bladder and its increased risk of incontinence. While increased frequency of urination can have an immediate benefit in terms of avoiding incontinent episodes, the long-term result is most likely counterproductive, because the patient can lose the ability to accommodate larger volumes and tolerate bladder fullness. In addition, it feeds the cycle of urgency and frequency thought to perpetuate overactive bladder and exacerbate urge incontinence in the long run.

Increasing the frequency of voiding is generally reserved for patients who clearly void infrequently (<5 times per day) or for patients with cognitive impairment who are unable to inhibit bladder contraction and unable to learn new skills for bladder control. Although we often describe voiding in terms of schedules, most patients have irregular daily voiding patterns. For many patients it is possible to identify times in their day when they are at increased risk of incontinence, for example, two hours after morning coffee or during exercise, and they can plan strategic voids before those times.

Table 40.1 Guidelines for Bladder Training

1. Review voiding diary with the patient, noting the various voiding intervals
2. Identify with the patient the longest voiding interval that is comfortable for her
3. Patient Instructions: Empty your bladder…
   - First thing in morning
   - Every time your voiding interval passes during the day
   - Just before bed
4. Teach coping strategies for occurrence of urge
   - Self-statements (affirmations)
   - Distraction to another task
   - Relaxation
   - Urge suppression strategy (using pelvic floor muscle contraction)
5. Gradually increase interval
   - When patient is comfortable for at least 3 days
   - By 30-minute intervals or clinical judgment based on patient confidence

BEHAVIORAL TRAINING AND PELVIC FLOOR MUSCLE TRAINING

Pelvic floor muscle training and exercise were first described by Margaret Morris in 1936 (16). In her paper she described tensing and relaxing of the pelvic floor muscles as an approach to the prevention and treatment of urinary and fecal incontinence. Pelvic floor muscle training was first popularized in the 1950s by Arnold Kegel, a gynecologist who proposed that women with stress incontinence lacked awareness and coordination of their muscles (17). He also demonstrated that women could improve their stress incontinence through pelvic floor muscle training and exercise to improve strength and coordination (17,18). Over the ensuing decades, this intervention has evolved both as a behavior therapy and as a physical therapy, combining principles from both fields into a widely accepted conservative treatment for stress and urge incontinence. The literature on pelvic floor muscle training and exercise has demonstrated that it is effective for reducing stress, urge, and mixed incontinence in most outpatients who cooperate with training (19–31). Pelvic floor muscle training and exercise is now a cornerstone of behavioral treatment for both stress and urge urinary incontinence.

Teaching Pelvic Floor Muscle Control

The goal of behavioral treatment for stress incontinence is to teach patients how to improve urethral closure and bladder neck support by voluntarily contracting pelvic floor muscles during whatever physical activities precipitate urine leakage. The first step in training is to properly identify the pelvic floor muscles and to contract and relax them selectively (without increasing intra-abdominal pressure on the bladder or pelvic floor). It is an essential and often overlooked step to confirm that patients have identified the correct muscles. Failure to find the pelvic floor muscles or to exercise them correctly is an important source of failure with this treatment modality. While it is easy for the clinician to give patients a pamphlet or brief verbal instructions to "lift the pelvic floor" or to interrupt the urinary stream during voiding, this approach does not ensure that she knows which muscles to use before she is sent

home to do daily exercises. Verification of proper muscle contraction can be accomplished by palpating the vagina during pelvic examination and giving her verbal feedback. Pelvic floor muscle control can also be taught using biofeedback or electrical stimulation.

Biofeedback is a teaching technique that helps patients learn control by giving them instantaneous, accurate feedback of their pelvic floor muscle activity. In his original work, Kegel used a biofeedback device he designed and named the perineometer (17). It consisted of a pneumatic chamber (which was placed in the vagina) and a hand-held pressure gauge, which visually displayed the pressure generated by circumvaginal muscle contraction. This device provided immediate visual feedback of pelvic floor muscle contraction to the woman learning to identify her muscles and monitor her practice.

Most biofeedback instruments in current use are computerized and display feedback visually on a computer monitor. Pelvic floor muscle activity can be measured by manometry or electromyography, using vaginal or anal probes or surface electrodes. Signals are augmented through the computer, and immediate feedback is provided on a monitor for visual feedback or via speakers for auditory feedback. When patients observe the results of their attempts to control bladder pressure and pelvic floor muscle activity, learning occurs by means of operant conditioning (trial and error learning). Biofeedback-assisted behavioral training has been tested in several studies, producing mean reductions of incontinence ranging from 60% to 85% (19,20,23,30–35).

A common problem encountered in learning to control the pelvic floor muscles is that patients tend to recruit other muscles, such as the rectus abdominis muscles or gluteal muscles, when they contract the pelvic floor muscles. Contracting certain abdominal muscles can be counterproductive, when it increases pressure on the bladder or pelvic floor, and therefore tends to push urine out rather than holding it in. Thus, it is important to observe for this bearing down valsalva response and to help patients to exercise pelvic floor muscles selectively while relaxing these abdominal muscles.

Daily Pelvic Floor Muscle Exercise

Once patients learn to properly contract and relax the pelvic floor muscles selectively, a regimen of daily practice and exercise is prescribed. The purpose of daily practice is twofold: to increase muscle strength and to enhance motor skills through practice. It has also been suggested that intensive strength training may increase resting tone and structural support of the pelvis by elevating the levator plate and enhancing the hypertrophy and stiffness of its connective tissues (36).

Exercise regimens vary considerably in frequency and intensity, and the optimal exercise regimen has yet to be determined. However good results are generally achieved using 45 to 50 exercises per day (19,31). To avoid muscle fatigue, it is usually recommended that patients space the exercises across the day, typically in two to three sessions per day. Patients may practice the exercises in the lying position at first, but it is important to progress them to sitting or standing positions as well, so that they become comfortable and skilled using their muscles to avoid incontinence in any position.

Table 40.2 Instructions for Daily Pelvic Floor Muscle Practice

- Do 45 pelvic floor muscle exercises EVERY day:
  15 at a time, 3 times per day.
    - Do _____ lying down
    - Do _____ sitting
    - Do _____ standing
- For each exercise, squeeze your pelvic floor muscles as quickly and as hard as you can.
- Hold the squeeze for: _____ seconds
- Relax completely after each squeeze for: _____ seconds
- Remember to relax all the muscles in your abdomen when you do these exercises and continue to breathe normally.

To improve muscle strength, contractions should be sustained for 2 to 10 seconds (37,38), depending on the patient's initial ability. Exercise regimens should be individualized so that patients begin with a comfortable duration and gradually progress to 10 seconds (38). Each exercise consists of muscle contraction followed by a period of relaxation using a 1:1 or 1:2 ratio (38). This allows the muscles to recover between contractions. A template for individualized instructions for daily pelvic floor muscle exercise appears in Table 40.2.

One of the challenges of pelvic floor muscle training and exercise is motivating patients to adhere to the regimen and to sustain their efforts over time. It can be helpful to educate them that sustained improvement depends upon their continued exercise. Among the barriers to daily exercise are difficulty remembering to do the exercises and difficulty finding time. To assist patients to remember their exercises, a variety of cues can be considered, including alarms or notes in prominent places in the home or car. Another approach is to teach them to integrate their pelvic floor muscle contractions into several daily activities. Once they are proficient, they no longer need to set time asides to concentrate on their exercises. Rather they can do a few exercises during certain daily activities, such as taking a shower or sitting at a traffic light. Not only does this not add time to their busy schedules, but the activities eventually become cues, reminding them to exercise. This can improve adherence during active treatment, and supports continued exercise during the maintenance phase when motivation tends to subside.

Using Muscles to Prevent Stress Incontinence

Although exercise alone has been known to improve urethral pressure and structural support and reduce incontinence (39), the best results seem to be achieved when patients contract their muscles consciously before and during coughing, sneezing, or any other activities that precipitate urine loss (27,36). Initially, this new skill requires a conscious effort, but with consistent practice, patients can develop the habit of automatically contracting their muscles to occlude the urethra in situations of physical exertion. This skill has been referred to varyingly as the "stress strategy" (30), "counterbracing," "the Knack" (40), and "the perineal blockage before stress technique" (41).

Even when their muscles are weak, some women will benefit from simply learning how to control their pelvic floor muscles and use them to prevent urine loss. In one trial, women were taught to voluntarily contract pelvic floor muscles before or during a cough and demonstrated reduction in leakage after only one week of training (40). Pelvic floor muscle precontraction has been recommended, not only during coughing, but during any daily activity that results in increased intra-abdominal pressure (42). The strength that is needed to occlude the urethra and prevent urine leakage is not known, and some women will still need a more comprehensive program of pelvic floor muscle rehabilitation to increase strength in addition to learning this skill.

BEHAVIORAL TRAINING FOR URGE INCONTINENCE

Historically, pelvic floor muscle training and exercise was used almost exclusively for the treatment of stress incontinence. It is now established as a component in the treatment of urge incontinence as well. Initially, it was observed that detrusor contraction could be inhibited by pelvic floor muscle contraction that was induced by electrical stimulation (43–45). Then, in the 1980s, it was shown that voluntary pelvic floor muscle contraction can be used not only to occlude the urethra, but also to inhibit detrusor contraction (19,31,46).

Using Muscles to Prevent Urge Incontinence: Urge Suppression Strategies

Most patients with urge incontinence feel compelled to rush to the toilet to void. This behavior can make incontinence more likely, because it increases intra-abdominal pressure on the bladder, increases the feeling of fullness, and when the patient reaches the vicinity of the toilet, she is exposed to visual cues that can trigger incontinence. Behavioral training teaches patients a new way to respond to the sensation of urge. The urge suppression strategy encourages patients to pause, sit down if possible, relax the entire body, and contract pelvic floor muscles repeatedly to diminish urgency, inhibit detrusor contraction, and prevent urine loss. After the urge sensation subsides, they are to proceed to the toilet at a normal pace (47). A handout for teaching patients about the urge suppression strategy appears in Figure 40.1.

Detrusor inhibition can be taught and documented in the clinic (Fig. 40.2). Then patients are encouraged to practice this urge suppression technique to manage urge and prevent incontinence episodes in their daily lives.

Behavioral training for urge incontinence has been tested in several clinical series utilizing pre-post designs. Mean reductions of incontinence range from 76% to 86% (19,33,35,46). In randomized controlled trials using intention-to-treat models, mean reductions of incontinence range from 60% to 80% (31,32).

This urge suppression strategy can be combined with bladder training as one of several coping techniques that can help patients make it to their next scheduled void. It can also be combined with a delayed voiding approach, in which patients are encouraged to wait a specified period of time after they have suppressed the urge. Beginning with short delays (five-minute) and increasing them incrementally, it is possible to expand the voiding interval and bladder capacity.

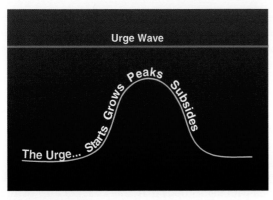

When the urge strikes…

- Stop and stay still. Do NOT rush to the toilet
- Sit down if you can.
- Squeeze your pelvic floor muscles quickly 3 to 5 times and repeat as needed.
- Relax the rest of your body. Take a deep breath.
- Concentrate on suppressing the urge.
- Wait until the urge calms down.
- Walk to the bathroom at a normal pace.
- If the urge returns on the way to the bathroom, stop and repeat.

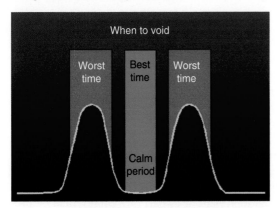

Figure 40.1 Urge suppression strategy.

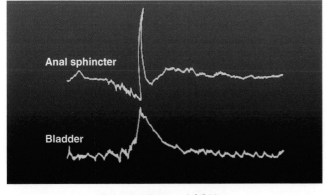

Figure 40.2 Detrusor inhibition.

THE BLADDER DIARY

The bladder or voiding diary is a widely used tool in the evaluation and monitoring of incontinence in women. It provides information on the timing of symptoms and events that helps the clinician to understand the type, severity, and circumstances

of urine loss and plan appropriate components of behavioral intervention. The diary is less recognized for its value in the treatment phase when it can be reviewed periodically to track the efficacy of various treatment components and guide the intervention. In research, it provides a validated measure of the frequency of voids and incontinence episodes and has also been used to measure the number and severity of urgency episodes.

In addition to its value for the clinician, completing a daily diary can have direct benefit to the patient. Its self-monitoring effect enhances the patient's awareness of voiding habits and patterns of incontinence. It encourages patients' recognition of how their incontinence is related to their activities, e.g., their physical activities or drinking patterns. In particular, understanding clearly the immediate precipitants of urine leakage optimizes the patient's vigilance and readiness to implement the continence skills learned through behavioral treatment.

At a minimum, the patient should record the time of each incontinent episode and the circumstances or reasons for the leakage (47). In behavioral treatment, the circumstances of each incontinent episode noted in the diary can be reviewed with the patient and used to develop instructions that are specific to that patient's situation. Through the process of reviewing the bladder diary, patients can identify certain times when they are more likely to have incontinence and activities that seem to trigger incontinence. Most commonly, patients can be made more aware of the antecedents of stress incontinence (e.g., coughing, sneezing) and develop the habit of contracting their pelvic floor muscles in preparation for these situations.

In addition to documenting incontinence, it is also very useful to have the patient record the times she urinates, both during the day and at night. These recordings can be used to identify patients who urinate too frequently and to establish appropriate voiding intervals for interventions like bladder training and delayed voiding.

Many clinicians are skeptical of the bladder diary, partly because of reports that patients have not completed them in real time, but rather just before the visit in the waiting room. Despite these anecdotes, we have observed that most patients are capable of using the diary correctly if they are educated about its purpose and how it will be used. Sending a blank diary to patients along with other routine forms in preparation for their first visit may not accomplish this. To improve the chances of obtaining a useful diary, it is best look at the diary with the patient in person, review its parts, and explain how and when to fill it out. Patients should be encouraged to carry the diary with them at all times and to make entries as soon as it is feasible. Some patients prefer that the diary be small enough to fit in a purse. Alternatively, they can be given explicit permission to fold it. Further, it seems to be helpful to tell patients that it is okay to get it dirty or spill on it, that we expect to see coffee stains and ragged edges.

Equally important is how the diary is handled when the patient returns it to the clinician. If we merely collect the diary and put it in the chart, we can devalue this carefully collected information in the patient's eyes. If she does not believe that her diary entries will be used to understand her condition and

401

inform decisions about her treatment, she is not likely to put effort into daily recording in the future. If the clinician takes an interest in her diary entries by reviewing each day's events, we communicate that the information is useful in guiding her treatment, and this encourages continued accurate recordings.

LIFE STYLE CHANGES

Life style changes are generally used as adjuncts to a primary behavioral intervention in selected cases. Life style changes include fluid management, caffeine reduction, weight loss, avoiding bladder irritants, and bowel management.

Fluid Management

Fluid management is a common practice used to make it easier for patients to control their bladders. Recommendations include alterations in the volume or type of fluids that patients consume. Many patients with incontinence restrict fluid intake as a self-management technique to help avoid incontinence by avoiding bladder fullness. In some cases, particularly among older women, this results in an inadequate intake of fluid and places them at risk of dehydration. It is important to recognize these cases and encourage patients, for their overall health and well-being, to consume an adequate amount of fluid, such as the often recommended six to eight glasses of fluid each day.

In patients who consume an abnormally high volume of liquids, fluid restriction is often appropriate. Some patients maximize their fluid intake deliberately in the belief that they need to "flush" their kidneys, to avoid dehydration, or an effort to lose weight. It is not uncommon to see women carry a water bottle throughout the day taking frequent drinks for health reasons. In these cases, reducing excess fluids can relieve problems with sudden bladder fullness and urgency. Avoiding fluids in the evening hours is also helpful for reducing nocturia.

Caffeine Reduction

Caffeinated beverages in particular can exacerbate incontinence, because in addition to its diuretic effect, caffeine is a bladder irritant for many people. Research has demonstrated that caffeine increases detrusor pressure (48) and that it is a risk factor for detrusor instability (49,50). Evidence also exists that reducing caffeine intake helps to reduce episodes of incontinence (51–53).

Although it is very difficult for most coffee drinkers to completely eliminate it from their diet, provided with the knowledge that caffeine may be aggravating their incontinence, many will be willing to reduce caffeine intake. This can be done gradually by mixing decaffeinated beverages with caffeinated beverages in increasing increments. For example, coffees can be mixed to consist of one-fourth decaffeinated coffee in week 1, one-half in week 2, three-quarters in week three, and full decaffeinated coffee in week 4.

Avoiding Bladder Irritants

Many clinicians recommend, even as a first-line approach, restricting certain foods and beverages that are believed to irritate the bladder, including sugar substitutes, citrus fruits, spicy foods, and tomato products. Although there is little scientific evidence on dietary factors, there are many cases in which these substances appear to be aggravating incontinence, and reducing or eliminating them has provided clinical improvement. A diary of food and beverage intake can sometimes be useful in identifying which substances are irritants for individual patients. Rather than recommending that all patients restrict their intake of these substances, a diary or trial restriction can help to identify which patients are sensitive and may chose to reduce their intake.

Weight Loss

Obesity is an established risk factor for urinary incontinence. Women with higher body mass index are not only more likely to develop incontinence, but they also tend to have more severe incontinence than women with lower body mass index. Research on the relationship between body mass index and incontinence reports that each five-unit increase in body mass index increases the risk of daily incontinence by approximately 60% (54,55).

Intervention studies of morbidly obese women report significant improvement in symptoms of incontinence with weight loss of 45 to 50 kg following bariatric surgery (56–58). Similarly, significant improvements in continence status have been demonstrated with as little as 5% weight reduction in more traditional weight loss programs (59). A recent randomized controlled trial (the PRIDE study) compared an intensive six-month weight-loss program of diet, exercise, and behavior modification to a structured education control program in overweight and obese women with incontinence (60). The weight-loss program, which resulted in a mean weight loss of 8%, showed significantly greater reductions in number of incontinence episodes (47% vs. 28%).

Because moderate weigh loss is an achievable goal for many women, it is rational to recommend weight loss as a first-line treatment or as part of a comprehensive program to treat incontinence in overweight and obese women.

Bowel Management

Fecal impaction and constipation have been cited as factors contributing to urinary incontinence in women, particularly in nursing home populations (61). In severe cases, fecal impaction can be an irritating factor in overactive bladder or obstruct normal voiding, causing incomplete bladder emptying and overflow incontinence. Disimpaction relieves symptoms for some patients, but it can recur in the absence of a bowel management program. Bowel management may consist of recommendations for a normal fluid intake and dietary fiber (or supplements) to maintain normal stool consistency and regular bowel movements. When hydration and fiber are not enough, enemas may be used to stimulate a regular daily bowel movement, preferably after a regular meal such as breakfast to take advantage of postprandial motility.

ENCOURAGING PATIENT PARTICIPATION

The success of behavioral treatments depends on the active participation of a motivated patient, and this reliance on patient behavior change represents the major limitation of this treatment approach. Like any new habit or skill, changing daily bladder habits and learning new skills requires some effort and persistence over time. It can be challenging to remember to use muscles strategically in daily life, as well as to maintain a regular exercise regimen for strength and skill. Unlike with some therapies, progress with behavioral treatment is often gradual. This gradual change makes it difficult for patients to appreciate even steady improvement over time and represents the primary challenge for behavioral treatment—how to sustain the patient's motivation for a long enough time that she will experience noticeable change in her bladder control. A key ingredient in addressing this problem is to maintain contact with the patient during this period of time when her benefit is not yet appreciable. Rather than leaving the patient on her own, it is essential that clinicians support the patient's efforts to persist by scheduling follow-up appointments to review and reinforce her progress, encourage persistence, and make any needed adjustments to her daily regimen.

In addition, when initiating behavioral treatment, it is important to make it clear to the patient that her improvement, as with any new skill, will likely be gradual, and that it will depend on her consistent practice. The patient who expects this course of treatment will be better prepared to persist over time until results can be achieved.

REFERENCES

1. NIH Consensus Conference. Urinary incontinence in adults. JAMA 1989; 261: 2685–96.
2. Fantl JA, Newman DK, Colling J, et al. Urinary Incontinence in Adults: Acute and Chronic Management. Clinical Practice Guideline, No. 2 1996 Update. Rockville, MD: U.S. Department of Health and Human Services. Public Health Service, Agency for Health Care Policy and Research. AHCPR Publication No.96-0682, 1996.
3. Hay Smith J, Berghmans B, Burgio K, et al. Adult Conservative Management. In: Abrams P, Cardozo L, Khoury S, Wein A, eds. Incontinence, 4th edn. International Consultation on Incontinence. Paris: Health Publication Ltd., 2009.
4. Frewen WK. Role of bladder training in the treatment of the unstable bladder in the female. Urol Clin North Am 1979; 6: 273–7.
5. Frewen WK. A reassessment of bladder training in detrusor dysfunction in the female. Br J Urol 1982; 54: 372–3.
6. Elder DD, Stephenson TP. An assessment of the Frewen regime in the treatment of detrusor dysfunction in females. Br J Urol 1980; 52: 467–71.
7. Jarvis GJ, Millar DR. Controlled trial of bladder drill for detrusor instability. Br Med J 1980; 281: 1322–3.
8. Jarvis GJ. A controlled trial of bladder drill and drug therapy in the management of detrusor instability. J Urol 1981; 53: 565–6.
9. Jarvis GJ. The management of urinary incontinence due to primary vesical sensory urgency by bladder drill. Br J Urol 1982; 54: 374–6.
10. Pengelly AW, Booth CM. A prospective trial of bladder training as treatment for detrusor instability. Br J Urol 1980; 52: 463–6.
11. Svigos JM, Matthews CD. Assessment and treatment of female urinary incontinence by cystometrogram and bladder retraining programs. Obstet Gynecol 1977; 50: 9–12.
12. Jeffcoate TNA, Francis WJ. Urgency incontinence in the female. Am J Obstet Gynecol 1966; 94: 604–18.
13. Fantl JA, Wyman JF, McClish DK, et al. Efficacy of bladder training in older women with urinary incontinence. JAMA 1991; 265: 609–13.
14. Colombo M, Zanetta G, Scalambrino S, Milani R. Oxybutynin and bladder training in the management of female urinary urge incontinence: a randomized study. Int Urogynecol J 1995; 6: 63–7.
15. Lagro-Janssen AL, Debruyne FM, Smits AJ, van Weel C. The effects of treatment of urinary incontinence in general practice. Fam Pract 1992; 9: 284–9.
16. Morris M. Maternity and Post-operative Exercises. London: William Heinemann, 1936.
17. Kegel AH. Progressive resistance exercise in the functional restoration of the perineal muscles. Am J Obstet Gynecol 1948; 56: 238–48.
18. Kegel AH. Stress incontinence of urine in women: physiologic treatment. J Int Coll Surg 1956; 25: 487–99.
19. Burgio KL, Whitehead WE, Engel BT. Urinary incontinence in the elderly: bladder-sphincter biofeedback and toileting skills training. Ann Intern Med 1985; 104: 507–15.
20. Burns PA, Pranikoff K, Nochajski TH, et al. A comparison of effectiveness of biofeedback and pelvic muscle exercise treatment of stress incontinence in older community-dwelling women. J Gerontol 1993; 48: 167–74.
21. Wells TJ, Brink CA, Diokno AD, Wolfe R, Gillis GL. Pelvic muscle exercise for stress urinary incontinence in elderly women. J Am Geriatr Soc 1991; 39: 785–91.
22. Dougherty M, Bishop K, Mooney R, Gimotty P, Williams B. Graded pelvic muscle exercise. Effect on stress urinary incontinence. J Reprod Med 1993; 39: 684–91.
23. Berghmans LCM, Frederiks CMA, de Bie RA. Efficacy of biofeedback when included with pelvic floor muscle exercise treatment for genuine stress incontinence. Neurourol Urodyn 1996; 15: 37–52.
24. Nygaard IE, Kreder KJ, Lepic MM, Fountain KA, Rhomberg AT. Efficacy of pelvic floor muscle exercises in women with stress, urge, and mixed urinary incontinence. Am J Obstet Gynecol 1996; 174: 120–5.
25. Bo K, Talseth T. Single blind randomized controlled trial of pelvic floor exercises, electrical stimulation, vaginal cones, and no treatment in management of genuine stress incontinence in women. BMJ 1999; 318: 487–93.
26. Wilson PD, Herbison GP. A randomized controlled trial of pelvic floor muscle exercises to treat postnatal urinary incontinence. Int Urogynecol J 1998; 9: 257–64.
27. Wilson PD, Herbison GP, Glazener CMA, et al. Postnatal incontinence: a multicenter, randomized controlled trial of conservative treatment. Neurourol Urodyn 1997; 16: 349–50.
28. Glazener CM, Herbison GP, Wilson PD, et al. Conservative management of persistent postnatal urinary and faecal incontinence: a randomized controlled trial. BMJ 2001; 323: 1–5.
29. Morkved S, Bo K. Effect of postpartum pelvic floor muscle training in prevention and treatment of urinary incontinence: a one-year follow-up. Br J Obstet Gynaecol 2000; 107: 1022–8.
30. Goode PS, Burgio KL, Locher JL, et al. Effect of behavioral training with or without pelvic floor electrical stimulation on stress incontinence in women: a randomized controlled trial. JAMA 2003; 290: 345–52.
31. Burgio KL, Locher JL, Goode PS, et al. Behavioral versus drug treatment for urge incontinence in older women: a randomized clinical trial. JAMA 1998; 23: 1995–2000.
32. Burgio KL, Goode PS, Locher JL, et al. Behavioral training with and without biofeedback in the treatment of urge incontinence in older women: a randomized controlled trial. JAMA 2002; 288: 2293–9.
33. Baigis-Smith J, Smith DAJ, Rose M, Newman DK. Managing urinary incontinence in community-residing elderly persons. Gerontologist 1989; 229: 33.
34. Burgio KL, Robinson JC, Engel BT. The role of biofeedback in Kegel exercise training for stress urinary incontinence. Am J Obstet Gynecol 1986; 157: 58–64.
35. McDowell BJ, Burgio KL, Dombrowski M, Locher JL, Rodriguez E. Interdisciplinary approach to the assessment and behavioral treatment of urinary incontinence in geriatric outpatients. J Am Geriatr Soc 1992; 40: 370–4.
36. Bø K. Pelvic floor muscle training is effective in treatment of female stress urinary incontinence, but how does it work? Int Urogynecol J Pelvic Floor Dysfunct 2004; 15: 76–84.
37. American College of Sport's Medicine. ACSM's Guidelines for Exercise Testing and Prescription, 2nd edn. Philadelphia: Lea & Febiger, 1993.
38. Kisner C, Colby LA. Therapeutic Exercise. Foundations and Techniques, 4th edn. Philadelphia: F.A. Davis, 2003.
39. Bo K. Pelvic floor muscle exercise for the treatment of stress urinary incontinence: an exercise physiology perspective. Int Urogynecol J 1995; 6: 282–91.
40. Miller JM, Ashton-Miller JA, DeLancey J. A pelvic muscle pre-contraction can reduce cough-related urine loss in selected women with mild SUI. J Am Geriatr Soc 1998; 46: 870–4.

41. Bourcier AP, Juras JC, Jacquetin B. Urinary incontinence in physically active and sportswomen. In: Appell RA, Bourcier AP, La Torre F, eds. Pelvic Floor Dysfunction: Investigations and Conservative Treatment. Rome: C.E.S.I., 1999: 9–17.

42. Carrière B. The pelvic floor. Stuttgard: Georg Thieme Verlag, 2006.

43. Godec C, Cass AS, Ayala GF. Bladder inhibition with functional electrical stimulation. Urology 1975; 6: 663–6.

44. Morrison JFB. The excitability of the micturition reflex. Scand J Urol Nephrol 1995; 29(Suppl 175): 21–5.

45. de Groat WC, Fraser MO, Yoshiyama M, et al. Neural control of the urethra. Scand J Urol Nephrol 2001; (Suppl 207): 35–43.

46. Burton JR, Pearce KL, Burgio KL, Engel BT, Whitehead WE. Behavioral training for urinary incontinence in elderly ambulatory patients. J Am Geriatr Soc 1988; 36: 693–8.

47. Burgio KL, Pearce KL, Lucco AJ. Staying Dry: A Practical Guide to Bladder Control. Baltimore: Johns Hopkins University Press, 1989.

48. Creighton SM, Stanton SL. Caffeine: does it affect your bladder? Br J Urol 1990; 66: 613–14.

49. Arya LA, Myers DL, Jackson ND. Dietary caffeine intake and the risk for detrusor instability: a case-control study. Obstet Gynecol 2000; 96: 85–9.

50. Holroyd-Leduc JM, Straus SE. Management of urinary incontinence in women: scientific review. JAMA 2004; 291: 986–95.

51. Tomlinson BU, Dougherty MC, Pendergast JF, et al. Dietary caffeine, fluid intake and urinary incontinence in older rural women. Int Urogynecol J Pelvic Floor Dysfunct 1999; 10: 22–8.

52. Bryant CM, Dowell CJ, Fairbrother G. Caffeine reduction education to improve urinary symptoms. Br J Nurs 2002; 11: 560–5.

53. Gray M. Caffeine and urinary continence. J Wound Ostomy Continence Nurs 2001; 28: 66–9.

54. Brown J, Seeley D, Feng J, et al: Urinary incontinence in older women: who is at risk? Study of Osteoporotic Fractures Research Group. Obstet Gynecol 1996; 87: 715.

55. Brown J, Grady D, Ouslander J, et al. Prevalence of urinary incontinence and associated risk factors in postmenopausal women. Heart & Estrogen/Progestin Replacement Study (HERS) Research Group. Obstet Gynecol 1999; 94: 66.

56. Bump R, Sugerman H, Fantl J, et al: Obesity and lower urinary tract function in women: effect of surgically induced weight loss. Am J Obstet Gynecol 1992; 166: 392.

57. Deitel M, Stone E, Kassam HA, et al. Gynecologic-obstetric changes after loss of massive excess weight following bariatric surgery. J Am Coll Nutr 1988; 7: 147.

58. Burgio KL, Richter HE, Clements RH, Redden DT, Goode PS. Changes in urinary and fecal incontinence symptoms with weight loss surgery in morbidly obese women. Obstet Gynecol 2007; 110: 1034–40.

59. Subak LL, Johnson C, Whitcomb E, et al. Does weight loss improve incontinence in moderately obese women? Int Urogynecol J Pelvic Floor Dysfunct 2002; 13: 40.

60. Subak LL, Wing R, West DS, et al., for the Program to Reduce Incontinence by Diet and Exercise (PRIDE). Weight loss to treat urinary incontinence in overweight and obese women. N Engl J Med 2009; 360: 481–90.

61. Ouslander JG, Schnelle JF. Incontinence in the nursing home. Ann Intern Med 1995; 122: 438–49.

41 Physiotherapy for Urinary Incontinence
Bary Berghmans

SUMMARY

This chapter will focus on physiotherapeutic management for the diagnosis, analysis, evaluation, and treatment of female urinary incontinence, with more specific stress (urinary) incontinence, (urinary) incontinence due to detrusor overactivity, and mixed (urinary) incontinence. For these health problems pelvic physiotherapy is often considered as first line treatment. Most patients can be treated to a satisfactory level. In several countries clinical practice guidelines have been published. The physiotherapeutic processes, algorithms, and flowcharts, described in this chapter, are based on these guidelines. For the time being, little is known about the implementation of these guidelines and their use in daily pelvic floor rehabilitation.

In stress urinary incontinence (SUI), to improve the extrinsic closing mechanism of the urethra, physiotherapy is especially aimed on strength improvement and coordination of the peri-urethral and pelvic floor muscles (PFMs). Treatment modalities are patient information and education, PFM training (PFMT), with or without biofeedback, electrical and magnetic stimulation, and vaginal cones. In particular, PFMT is effective.

For detrusor overactivity physiotherapy is aimed at the reduction or elimination of involuntary detrusor muscle contractions through reflex inhibition. Treatment modalities are patient information and education, toilet training, bladder (re-)training, or behavioral therapy, PFMT with or without biofeedback, electrical stimulation, and magnetic stimulation. Especially, electrical therapy appears to be an effective treatment modality.

Conclusion: pelvic physiotherapy is in many cases of urinary incontinence an effective treatment option.

INTRODUCTION

World wide, urinary incontinence is a common and distressing health problem with often high social consequences. In western countries approximately 5% of the population suffer from incontinence (1). Increasing prevalence of 20% to 30% during young adult life to 30% to 40% around the menopause to 30% to 50% in the elderly have been reported by some authors (2,3). Others report a prevalence of any urinary incontinence of 22% (4) to 29% (5) in older women, severe urinary incontinence in 7% (5). Among nursing home residents this percentage increases over 50% (6). Incontinence is predominantly a problem among women: 9% of them suffer from incontinence compared to "only" 1.6% of all men (7). Usually, male incontinence is seen only in elderly men (8).

The yearly incidence of urinary incontinence varies between 1% and 11%, the yearly remission between 6% and 11% (2).

Mainly due to shame, taboo, and unawareness of treatment possibilities, only a minority of people suffering from incontinence seeks professional help (9). In daily general practice patients usually go for help when the loss of urine leads to mental, physical, or social problems or discomfort for the patient or his/her social environment. Because of more and better patient information, in the Netherlands now about half of the women suffering from urinary incontinence consult a medical doctor (10).

Several forms of urinary incontinence such as stress incontinence, mixed incontinence, and incontinence due to detrusor overactivity can be differentiated (11). Symptoms of the latter are urgency, frequent micturition, nocturia, and/or urgency incontinence (11).

In women the most prevalent form is stress incontinence, being responsible for 49% of all cases (5). Next to stress incontinence, detrusor overactivity is the second most prevalent cause of incontinence (21%) (5). Combinations of the aforementioned symptoms of stress and urgency incontinence are considered to reflect mixed incontinence (12). Its prevalence is 29% (5).

A patient suffering from stress incontinence usually has a normal voiding frequency (≤8 times in 24 hours) and bladder volume, has mean micturitions between 200 and 400 cc/void, but with neither urgency nor nycturition. The patient complaints of losing small amounts of urine during exertion.

A patient with urgency incontinence usually loses more urine (up to the complete content of the bladder) than a patient with stress incontinence. On the other hand the patient may loose less than 150 ml urine during micturition, suggesting a reduced functional capacity of the bladder.

Incontinence has several treatment options such as physiotherapy, drug treatment, and surgical procedures. Most patients can be treated to a satisfactory level (13). In several countries guidelines have been published recently (13–20). For the time being, little is known about the implementation of these guidelines and their use in daily practice (13).

For patients with incontinence physiotherapy is often considered as first-line treatment, due to its non-invasive character, the results in terms of symptom relief, the possibility of combining physiotherapy with other treatments, the low risk of side effects, and the moderate to low costs. Important restrictions are that the success depends on the motivation and perseverance of both the patient and the physiotherapist and the time needed for therapy (16).

In this chapter we review and discuss the diagnosis, analysis, evaluation, and therapeutic possibilities of physiotherapy for stress incontinence, urgency incontinence, and mixed incontinence.

MEDICAL DIAGNOSIS

For women with urinary incontinence the International Consultation of Incontinence (ICI) distinguishes between initial management and, in case of failure, specialized management (21,22). For initial management the ICI (2005) recommends a simple clinical assessment leading to a *presumed* medical diagnosis. First-line health care providers such as general practitioners (GPs) should use simple diagnostic tools like structured history taking, micturition or voiding diaries (to assess drinking habits, voiding pattern, type, pattern and volume of urine loss, impact) filled in by the patient, and physical examination (6,23–25). Recently, to help the GP to improve his accuracy of medical diagnosis, short questionnaires for the triage of women with urinary incontinence to quickly differentiate between stress, urgency and mixed incontinence are developed and methodologically tested (26). An example of such a questionnaire is the two-items stress/urgency incontinence questionnaire, (S/UIQ) (26).

S/UIQ and Classification System
S/UIQ

1. How many times in the last seven days have you had an accidental leakage of urine onto your clothing, underwear, or pad during an activity such as coughing, sneezing, laughing, running, exercising, or lifting?
2. How many times in the last seven days have you had an accidental leakage of urine onto your clothing, underwear, or pad with such a sudden strong need to urinate (US)/pass water (UK) that you could not reach the toilet in time?

Incontinence Symptom Classification System with S/UIQ

- SUI ≥ 4; UUI = 0 Pure stress urinary incontinence
- SUI > 0; SUI > UUI; UUI > 0 Stress predominant mixed urinary incontinence
- SUI > 0; SUI = UUI Balanced mixed urinary incontinence
- SUI > 0; UUI > 0; UUI > SUI Urge predominant mixed urinary incontinence
- UUI ≥ 4; SUI = 0 Pure urge urinary incontinence

where SUI is stress urinary incontinence episodes per week and UUI is urge urinary incontinence episodes per week.

For the GP, who is in many countries throughout the world the first physician whom the patient refers to for consultation, with these simple tools still it is very difficult to find the exact cause of urinary incontinence. Specialists, like the urologist or the gynecologist, may fall back on specific diagnostic tests such as urodynamic evaluation. Usually, GPs have no access to such tests and therefore GPs must rely on their history taking, physical examination, and questionnaires like the SUIQ. For GPs urodynamic tests are—by and large—only needed if there is doubt about the type of incontinence and, consequently, about the necessity and choice of treatment. This statement is supported by reports concluding that under optimal conditions (after GP training) the sensitivity and specificity of the GPs history taking and physical examination to detect urodynamic stress incontinence is 78% and 84%, with a positive predictive value of 87% (24). Using simple diagnostic tools as the SUIQ these percentages even can be enhanced (22). A recent

meta-analysis of primary care diagnostical methods of urinary incontinence (initial management) showed a sensitivity of 0.92 (95% C.I.: 0.91–0.93) and a specificity of 0.56 (0.53–0.60) to correctly identify women with urodynamic stress incontinence (27). A clinical history for the diagnosis of detrusor overactivity (DO) was found to be 0.61 (0.57–0.65) sensitive and 0.87 (0.85–0.89) specific (27).

Unfortunately, in daily practice with busy GPs such optimal conditions can usually not be met over a prolonged period of time. Moreover, the symptoms of incontinence may be vague and less clear-cut as written in hand books. Altogether, this may impair the reliability of history taking and physical examination (13).

In case of a referral to a pelvic physiotherapist, it is very important to have a medical diagnosis that is as accurate as possible to determine the impact of the complaints of the patient and to estimate the success or failure aspects of pelvic floor physiotherapy (28). However, in the initial management of urinary incontinence in women, in many cases the *presumed* medical diagnosis lacks accuracy, confronting the physiotherapists with heterogeneity or complexity of indications and unclear grade of severity that might result in a minor degree of success or even failure.

Probably because of its impredictable prognosis, urgency incontinence due to detrusor overactivity has a greater impact on quality of life than stress incontinence (29). Younger people in particular experience detrusor overactivity as very intrusive (30). After a child-birth stress incontinence sometimes goes together with a total denervation of the PFMs or with great damage to surrounding connective and structure tissue. In such cases physiotherapy has normally little or no effect. Also, in patients with detrusor overactivity as a result of an infection or a spinal cord lesion the effect of physiotherapy is not likely (31). Incontinence can also develop as a result of a neurologic problem, a trauma, or a birth dysfunction. For a great deal the pathophysiological character of the health problem(s) determine(s) prognosis and result of treatment (32).

Whether or not there is a causal relationship between (grade of) pelvic organ prolapse (POP) and (stress) urinary incontinence has yet to be determined. Some authors consider that POP and SUI share similar pathophysiologies and might be etiologically connected (33). DeLancey et al. showed in a study of 151 women with prolapse and 135 controls with normal support determined by POP quantification examination, that women with prolapse have reduced PFM strength and generated less vaginal closure force during pelvic muscle contraction than controls, potentially leading to urinary incontinence (34).

Hagen et al. reported that in the United Kingdom physicians referred a number of women with a presumed diagnosis of both POP and urinary incontinence to the pelvic physiotherapist and that—although there are no guidelines for the treatment of POP available so far and although it is up to now unclear whether or not and to what extent pelvic physiotherapy is effective in women with POP—92% of the physiotherapists assessed and treated the combination of these two pelvic floor dysfunctions (35).

Also other etiological and prognostic factors such as age, hysterectomy, estrogen depletion during the menopause, chronic diseases such as diabetes mellitus, immobility, adipositas, number, duration, and mode of delivery play a role in incontinence (36).

If and to what extent there is an association or causal relationship between these factors and the incidence of incontinence is by far not clear yet (37).

Still, identification of relevant etiological and prognostic factors that might hinder—locally and/or in general—recovery and compensation and whether or not these factors can be influenced by physiotherapy is important, because these might have consequences for the strategy, routing, and outcome of treatment.

So, following relevant guidelines recommendations, the referral to a pelvic physiotherapist should contain the following data (38):

- Date of referral and personal data patient
- An as accurate as possible medical diagnosis
- Severity of urine loss and patient's experience and impact of the complaints of the patient
- Diagnostic findings: capacity to contract, either voluntarily or unvoluntarily, and relax the PFMs and indication of (level of) PFM strength
- Presence of and grade of prolapse and/or other relevant urogynecological health problems
- Data of the voiding diary
- Requested intervention and, if applicable, former interventions
- Potential (causal) (risk) factors and prognostic factors (e.g., rupture after vaginal delivery, a neurological damage of the pudendal nerve, diabetes mellitus, earlier urogynecological surgery)
- Use of medication (related to incontinence interfering with treatment)

PHYSIOTHERAPEUTIC DIAGNOSTIC PHASE

Based on the medical diagnosis of the referring physician the physiotherapist starts his physiotherapeutic diagnostic process. The aim is to assess, analyze, and evaluate the often unclear (16) nature and severity of the urinary incontinence problem and to determine if and to what extent a physiotherapeutical intervention can be effective. What is the nature of the underlying pathology, are there any local or general obstructing factors for recovery and improvement, and to what extent can these factors be influenced by physiotherapy?

Using the International Classification of Functions (37) (Table 41.1), the physiotherapist tries to influence the *consequences* of the health problem on three different levels: organ level (impairment level, e.g., urine loss while coughing), persons level (disability level, e.g., sanitation), and social-societal level (restriction of participation, e.g., social isolation).

Systematic history taking aims to establish and record:

- the severity of the health problem by noting impairment(s), disability(ies), and restrictions in participation;

Table 41.1 Definitions of the ICF-Terms Impairment, Disability, and Handicaps

Impairment	Loss or abnormality of psychological, physiological, or anatomical structure or function at organ level. With respect to the classification of disorders in the storage and voiding of urine and feces, this means the impairment of stress incontinence or detrusor overactivity.
Disability	Restriction or loss of ability of a person to perform functions/activities in a normal manner. With respect to the classification of disabilities of voiding and stool, this means the disability of involuntary loss of urine.
Restriction in participation	Disadvantage due to impairment or disability that limits or prevents fulfillment of a normal role (depends on age, sex, sociocultural factors) for the person.

Abbreviations: ICF, International Classification of Functions.
Source: From Ref. 37.

- the likely nature of the underlying pathology by noting causal factors [e.g., in stress incontinence trauma during vaginal delivery(ies)];
- local factors, which may prevent the recovery and improvement (e.g., prolaps uteri);
- general or systematic factors, which may prevent recovery and improvement (e.g., diabetes mellitus); and
- personal factors (e.g., what efforts does the patient make to alleviate stress or urgency incontinence).

A physical examination of the patient is important in order to verify and support the patient-profile gained from the patient's history. To conduct the physical examination, a number of diagnostic tests are available to the physiotherapist. The severity of the stress, urgency or mixed incontinence depends not only on the condition of the pelvic floor and the bladder, but also on the posture, respiration, movement, as well as the general physical and psychological condition (39,40). Information on the severity of stress, urgency, or mixed incontinence can also be obtained by studying the voiding diaries mentioned above with relevant data about incontinence. Also, subjective self-report, quality-of-life questionnaires and/or symptom questionnaires, such as the PRAFAB-score (which combines the most important objective and subjective elements of the degree of urinary incontinence) are helpful (41); **p**rotection (use of pads), **a**mount of urine loss, **f**requency of the complaint, **a**djustment in behavior due to the complaint, and **b**ody image as result of the urine loss are the five elements of the PRAFAB-score. With such questionnaires it is possible to illustrate the degree of incontinence in a reproducible manner (41). Especially in patients with stress incontinence a pad test can be useful to test the extent and severity of the involuntary loss of urine (42).

The objective of physical examination is to understand:

- the functionality of the pelvic floor in rest and during activities in terms of coordination, tonus, endurance, and strength;

407

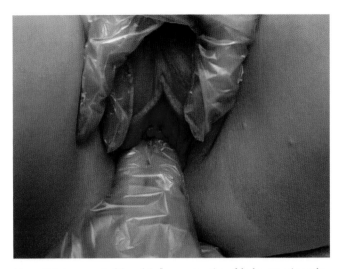

Figure 41.1 Assessment of the pelvic floor, contraction of the levator ani muscles.

- the possibility and degree of contraction (with or without awareness) and relaxation of the PFMs; and
- the influence of other parts of the body on the function of the pelvic floor, by inspection at rest and while moving.

For quantification of strength of contraction, level of relaxation, coordination, endurance, and exhaustibility manual assessment of the function of the PFMs is the most commonly performed technique by physiotherapists. It is done either by digital intra-vaginal (Fig. 41.1) or intra-anal palpation with the patient in supine position (38). To test maximal strength the patient is instructed to contract the PFMs as hard as possible. Endurance is tested by asking the patient to sustain a contraction, exhaustibility to repeat as many contractions as possible. Digital palpation is also used to determine PFM tone, tone differences, and differences between left and right side of the pelvic floor.

With PFM palpation vaginal squeeze pressure and inward/upward lift of the PFMs can be registered. For assessment of contraction of the levator ani muscles the pelvic physiotherapist inserts his fingers from below inside the vagina until he feels the levator ani muscles. The patient is instructed to contract the PFMs ("withhold a flatus, contract the anus inwards, stop the urine"). A correct contraction is a simultaneous squeezing around the physiotherapist's index or index and middle finger and inward/upward movement or elevation of the levator ani muscles. To quantify the strength of the contraction often the modified Oxford grading scale is used.

The Modified Oxford scale (43)

- 0 = no contraction
- 1 = flicker
- 2 = weak
- 3 = moderate contraction (PF lift is checked)
- 4 = good contraction (PF lift is checked)

PFMs relaxation should be tested after a contraction. Therefore the investigator should always start with a contraction and then ask for relaxation.

The strength of the PFMs can also be measured by a vaginal squeeze pressure device connected to a manometer (pressure manometry, perineometer) (44) or pelvic floor dynamometer (a kind of strain gage device for the pelvic floor to measure precisely forces produced during a PFM contraction independently of the evaluator's judgement) (45). These methods are complicated to perform, demanding clinical experience and skills to produce high methodologically quality results or are not yet clinically available (46).

More recently, an increasing number of pelvic physiotherapists assess the pelvic floor function also with perineal ultrasound. Dynamic evaluation of pelvic floor function includes position and elevation or descent of the bladder neck. Also the puborectalis muscle at rest as well as pelvic floor pre-contraction, voluntary pelvic floor maximal and submaximal contractions, hold during respiration and sneezing or coughing, stabilization of the urethra, hold of bladder neck position during coughing or abdominal maneuvers can be evaluated. However, although pelvic floor imaging using ultrasound becomes more and more popular, diagnostic ultrasound is reported to be well known for its operator-dependent nature and should only be used after appropriate and effective education (47).

Overviewing the different measurement methods a limitation is that all clinic based measurements of PFM function are performed in the supine position or other standard positions. One should keep in mind that this might not reflect functional or automatic activity of the pelvic floor during daily life activities as a response to increased abdominal pressure (46).

After the history taking, physical examination, and functional tests, analysis and evaluation of the results of physiotherapeutic diagnostic phase and relevant medical data will complete this process. The diagnosis of the referrer can be stated and the indication for physiotherapy ascertained. Therefore, answering the following questions is necessary:

- Is referral diagnosis likely?
- Are there any urinary incontinence related health problems?
- What is the nature of the stress incontinence, urgency incontinence, or mixed incontinence?
- What is the severity and the extent of the health problem?
- Is there a dysfunction of the pelvic floor?
- What caused this dysfunction?
- Are there any local factors which may prevent recovery or improvement and can physiotherapeutic intervention have an influence on these factors?
- Are there any general factors which may prevent recovery or improvement?
- Is physiotherapy indicated?

A given severity of the health problem at referral has impact on the prognosis and the evaluation of the likely effect of the physiotherapeutic intervention.

It is important to take into account also other prognostic and patient variables, such as age, obesity, and vaginal childbirth, which will have their impact on the process of intervention. In Table 41.2 a flowchart for the referral and physiotherapeutic diagnostic process is given.

Table 41.2 Flowchart of Referral and Physiotherapeutic Process

Referral for physiotherapy intervention

Specialist:

Medical diagnosis (urodynamics)
Referral diagnosis
Referral data

General practitioner:

Medical diagnosis (?) (NO urodynamics)
Referral diagnosis
Referral data

Physiotherapy
Patient education and information on
  Anatomy, physiology:
    • pelvic floor, bladder
    • toilet behavior/-regimen
Process of diagnosis
  History taking
  Physical examination:
    • General examination
    • Local examination
  Relevant data from:
  Subjective self-report:
    • Questionnaires (e.g., PRAFAB)
    • Diaries (e.g., voiding diary)
  Functional tests (e.g., padtest)
  Observation
  Palpation:
    • Vaginal/anal
  Physiotherapist's diagnosis
  Inventory of health problem USI:
    • Nature
    • Severity
    • Obstructing factors
  Conclusion: Indication for physiotherapy →
  continue with treatment plan
  No indication for physiotherapy →
  back to referring physician
Formulation of treatment plan
    • Treatment objectives
    • Treatment strategy
    • Treatment procedures
    • Expected outcome
    • Prognosis of treatment duration
  In terms of total time and number
  of treatment sessions

Abbreviations: PRAFAB, protection (use of pads), amount of urine loss, frequency of the complaint, adjustment in behavior due to the complaint, and body image as result of the urine loss; USI, urodynamic stress incontinence.

INTERVENTION PHASE

As a general rule, the least invasive and the least troublesome treatment procedure should be considered as a first choice. After analysis and evaluation, the physiotherapist formulates his treatment plan. He estimates whether full recovery can be achieved or only compensation of the complaints is possible. Also, he determines his strategy, procedure, methods of treatment to reach the goal, and whether or not he has the skills and capability to do the job.

Approach and treatment modalities will be different for patients with stress incontinence, detrusor overactivity, or mixed incontinence, but all these low-risk interventions involve educating the patient and providing positive reinforcement for effort and progress (17).

Patient education embraces all relevant concepts (e.g., what is the function of the bladder) and information for the patient. Comprehension on the part of the patient will promote the motivation to start on other stages of treatment. The interplay between patient and physiotherapist is very important in this process. Before starting the specific therapy modalities of the pelvic floor, it is important to know and appreciate the position and the function of the pelvic floor and how to contract and relax the PFMs. To achieve satisfactory results from intervention (in the long term), information and supervision by the physiotherapist throughout the intervention phase are essential, especially concerning the adequate use of the PFMs and behavior of micturition.

Stress Incontinence

Physiotherapeutic treatment modalities for SUI are PFMT with or without biofeedback, electrical stimulation, magnetic stimulation, and/or vaginal cones.

The biological rationale for PFMT in the management of stress incontinence is that a strong and fast PFMs contraction will clamp the urethra, increasing the urethral pressure, to prevent leakage during an abrupt increase in intra-abdominal pressure (48). If the PFMs are normally innervated and sufficiently attached to the endopelvic fascia, and if by contracting her pelvic muscles before and during a cough a woman is able to decrease that leakage (49), then simply learning when and how to use her pelvic muscles may be an effective therapy. In such cases the subject needs to train to use this skill during those activities that transiently increase abdominal pressure (50). DeLancey has also suggested that an effective PFMs contraction may press the urethra against the pubic symphysis, creating a mechanical pressure rise (30). PFMs contraction also supports the pelvic organs (30). Timing might also be important; Bø has suggested that a well-timed, fast, and strong PFMs contraction may prevent urethral descent during intra-abdominal pressure rise (50,51). So, PFMs training is especially focused on strength improvement and coordination of the peri-urethral and the PFMs.

Appropriate treatment with PFMT should always include an assessment of PFM contraction and relaxation, because the effect of PFMT is dependent on whether the contractions and relaxations are performed correctly (52).

Repeated correct contractions of the pelvic floor, strengthening the PFMs in a regular, intensive and long-lasting training program, are essential for an effective improvement through PFMT (52–54).

Extrapolation of exercise prescription guidelines suggests that PFMT should include short and long duration exercises, based on diagnostic findings, as both type I and type II muscle fibers need to be exercised with overload strategies. The frequency and the number of repetitions of exercises should be selected following assessment of the PFMs. Daily regimes of increasing repetitions to the point of fatigue seem to be recommended [8–12 *maximal* PFMs contractions, 1–3 seconds to 6–8 seconds hold/relax, 3 extra quick peak contractions super imposed on the maximal contraction, 3 times a day for at least 6 months (54)]. A process of patient awareness of isolated contractions to fully automatic controlled function of the pelvic floor during multiple complex tasks is required (16).

It is very important to select relevant, tailored to the individual patient starting positions while training and functional activities must be incorporated into the training program as soon as possible (36). An individually tailored home exercises program manageable in daily live activity is essential (52).

Because the total urethral closing mechanism also depends on a competent intrinsic urethral sphincter [in case of incompetence this is intrinsic sphincter deficiency (ISD)] there is no guarantee that improvement of absolute power and endurance of the pelvic floor, the extrinsic part of the total urethral closing mechanism, will fully restore continence (50) (Fig. 41.2).

Meanwhile, there is sufficient evidence that PFMT is effective in the reduction of involuntary loss of urine in patients with stress incontinence, also for the long term (55–58).

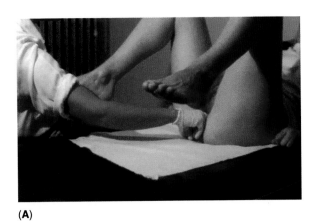

(A)

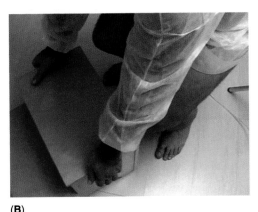

(B)

Figure 41.2 Pelvic floor muscle training for SUI (and MUI with predominant stress factor).

- Explain correct PFM contraction
- Practice before checking ability to contract
- First intensive guidance in office to perform conscious and selective PFM contractions
- Prepare for PFMT at home.
- Set up individual home training program
- Follow-up with weekly or more often supervised training

The first part of PFMT can involve digital palpation to support and control PFM contractions during coughing, lift of one or two legs as can be seen in (**A**), followed by more functional exercises such as lifting weights (**B**), sitting down, or standing up. Note: Images of the model authorized for publication by the IRPP representative Dabbadie L. *Abbreviations:* PFM, pelvic floor muscle; PFMT, PFM training; SUI, stress urinary incontinence

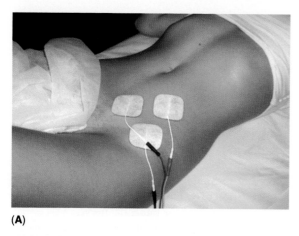

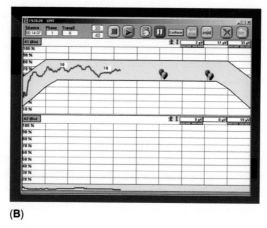

(A)   **(B)**

Figure 41.3 EMG biofeedback. EMG biofeedback, here registered by surface electrodes (**A**), can be used to visualize on screen (**B**) selective pelvic floor muscle activity (blue line) together with control of any synergistic abdominal muscle activity (red line) (1). *Abbreviations*: EMG, electromyography signals. *Source*: VIVALTIS, France.

In general, intensive training showed better results than a low intensity program (36,59,60).

Twenty-five percent of the females are still dry after five years, while two-thirds of them indicate by follow-up that they are very satisfied with their present state and that they wish no further treatment (58).

Biofeedback is the technique whereby information regarding "hidden" physiological processes, in this case PFMs contractions and relaxations, is displayed in a form understandable to the patient, to permit self-regulation of these events (36). This technique can be applied either by the use of electromyography signals (EMG), manometry, a combination of both, or ultrasound. Biofeedback is not a treatment on its own. It is an adjunct to PFMT.

Biofeedback is based on operant conditioning and a cognitive learning process. An incontinence patient can be taught, with the aid of biofeedback, to be selective in the use of the PFMs. Through registration by means of surface electrodes (Fig. 41.3) or an intravaginal or intrarectal electrode the patient can see on a monitor if and to what extent contraction or relaxation of the PFMs is possible and adequate (Fig. 41.3).

Usually, at the onset of therapy with biofeedback, first the motor unit activity (EMG) or the intravaginal/anal pressure of the PFMs (manometry) at rest, during a maximal PFMs contraction (P_{max}), and relaxation after P_{max} are measured.

In a randomized clinical trial (RCT) comparing a group using PFMT with biofeedback and a group without biofeedback Berghmans et al. demonstrated quicker progress in the first group. At the long run, for the treatment of stress incontinence, biofeedback in combination with PFMT seems equally effective as only PFMT (42). Nevertheless, in patients with urinary incontinence who have insufficient or no awareness of the PFMs and therefore are not able to voluntary contract or relax their PFMs or have very poor quality (intensity) of contraction at initial assessment, biofeedback is suggested to be an important strategy to quicken up and restore this awareness (36,42,51,61). However, further large, high quality RCTs in order to proof this hypothesis are required (36,42,51).

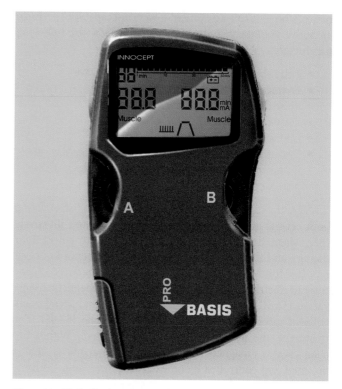

Figure 41.4 Biofeedback equipment for urinary incontinence. *Source*: From INNOCEPT, Biobedded Medizintechnik GmbH, Am Wiesenbusch 1, D-45966 Gladbeck, Germany.

Electrical stimulation is provided by clinic based mains powered machines (i.e., those that need to be plugged into a wall socket) or portable battery powered stimulators (Fig. 41.4).

Although relevant studies poorly report the biological rationale underpinning the application of electrical stimulation for the treatment of SUI (36), the aim of electrical stimulation here appears to be to improve the function of the PFMs, while for patients with urgency incontinence the objective seems to be to inhibit detrusor overactivity.

For stress incontinence electrical stimulation is focused on the restoration of the reflex activity through stimulation of the

411

fibers of the pudendal nerve with the purpose to create a contraction of the PFMs (62). Electrical stimulation is suggested to lead to a motor response by patients for whom a voluntary contraction is not possible as a result of an insufficient pelvic floor, on the condition that the nerve is (partly) intact (63).

Although electrical stimulation appeared to be better than placebo; yet, its effect in stress incontinence is insufficiently demonstrated as a result of inconsistency in protocols (64).

There are many differences in clinical application that have not yet been investigated. For example, some clinicians suggest that "active" electrical stimulation (i.e., the patient voluntarily contracts the PFMs during stimulation) is better than "passive" electrical stimulation but the effect of these two approaches has not yet been evaluated (64). Equally it may be that some populations or subgroups of patients benefit from electrical stimulation more than others.

Although to date there is still insufficient evidence, in clinical practice we suggest to use in patients with stress incontinence, who—during assessment—were not capable to perform an active voluntary contraction of the PFMs, the following parameters as a starting point:

- Pulse shape: bipolar rectangular square wave
- Frequency: 50 Hz
- Pulse duration: 200 mseconds
- Duty circle: ratio 1:2
- Intensity of current: maximal tolerance
- Two times/week office-bound, two times/day at home, until voluntary contraction by the patient him- or herself is possible and adequate.

Magnetic stimulation has been developed for stimulating both central and peripheral nervous systems non-invasively (65). Magnetic stimulation has been applied to pelvic floor therapy and the treatment of urinary incontinence has been reported for the first time in 1999 by Galloway et al. (66). Contrary to electrical stimulation, extracorporeal magnetic innervation (ExMI) aims to stimulate the PFMs and sacral roots without insertion of an anal or vaginal probe (67,68). For treatment, the patient is positioned in a chair. Within the chair's seat is a magnetic field generator (therapy head) that is powered and controlled by an external power unit. Conventional stimulators deliver, at frequencies of 10 to 50 Hz, repetitive pulses of current between <100 μsec (67) and 275 μsec (66) in duration. Size and strength of the magnetic field is determined by adjusting this amplitude by the physiotherapist (66). A concentrated steep gradient magnetic field is directed vertically through the seat of the chair. When seated, the patient's perineum is centered in the middle of the seat, which places the PFMs and sphincters directly on the primary axis of the pulsing magnetic field. Because of this all tissues of the perineum can be penetrated by the magnetic field. Galloway indicated that no electricity, but only magnetic flux enters the patient's body from the device. Goldberg indicated that, in contrast to electrical current, the conduction of magnetic energy is unaffected by tissue impedance, creating a major advantage in its clinical application compared to electrical stimulation. In that way structures, such as sacral roots or pudendal nerves, might therefore be magnetically stimulated

without patient's discomfort or inconvenience of probe insertion for electrical stimulation.

Therefore, advantages of ExMI seems to be that it is performed through full clothing, entailing no probes, skin preparation, or physical or electrical contact with the skin surface. On the other hand, the need for repeated office-based treatment sessions represents an inherent disadvantage. In contrast to electrical stimulation units, this kind of technology lacks portability, and, because both the depth and width of magnetic field penetration is proportional to coil diameter, the present technology according to Goldberg is best suited for stimulation of a field, rather than a narrowly focused target as the sacral roots or the pudendal nerve.

Magnetic stimulation of the sacral nerve roots and pelvic floor is suggested to be effective for SUI (67,68), although the mechanism of action on the continence mechanism is not fully understood (68). Some authors suggested that in SUI it stimulates pelvic floor musculature causing external sphincter contraction (69), acting as a kind of a passive PFM exercise (70), and increase of maximal urethral closing pressure (71). Stimulation of sympathetic fibers maintaining smooth muscle tone within the intrinsic urethral sphincter seems to be involved in this mechanism of action (72,73). Previous studies suggested a stimulation frequency of 50 Hz to be the most effective for urethral closure (66).

Up to now, there is only limited evidence of the effect of magnetic stimulation treatment in women with SUI. There was considerable variation in diagnostic groups, the regimen, protocols, intensity, and duration of treatment. Sample sizes were small, outcomes were contradictory. Only short term results were available. At the moment there is not enough evidence for the efficacy of magnetic stimulation in women with SUI.

In women with stress incontinence, sometimes weighted vaginal cones in combination with PFMT are used (56,74). All cones are identical in size, but have increasing weight. The idea is that the stronger the PFMs grow, the higher the weight of a cone must be to stimulate the PFMs to hold the cone inside the vagina. A review by Herbison et al. (75) provided some evidence that weighted vaginal cones are better than no active treatment but on the other hand add no benefit to a PFMs training program (36). Vaginal cones may add benefit to a training protocol if subjects are asked to contract around the cone and simultaneously try to pull it out in lying or standing position while performing their PFM exercises in the way described above (76).

Because of the lack of evidence about their efficacy, widespread use is not recommended (74).

Guidelines for SUI

In the Royal Dutch Association of Physiotherapy (KNGF) guidelines for stress incontinence, the following problem areas are differentiated (16,38):

- Stress incontinence with a dysfunction of the pelvic floor
  o with awareness of the pelvic floor
  o without awareness of the pelvic floor
  o the function of the pelvic floor is compromised by dysfunctions in the respiratory or the locomotive tract

- Stress incontinence without a dysfunction of the pelvic floor
- Stress incontinence (with or without a dysfunction of the pelvic floor) in combination with general factors that inhibit or delay improvement or recovery

Stress Incontinence with a Dysfunction of the Pelvic Floor
The primary aim of treatment is to obtain a good awareness of the PFMs. During the treatment the following techniques are used: digital palpation either by the patient herself or by the physiotherapist, electrical stimulation, and/or biofeedback in combination with PFMs training. If the patient is aware of contraction and relaxation of the PFMs, the therapy continues with the use of PFMT only. If a pelvic floor dysfunction coexists with dysfunctions of the respiration or the locomotive tract or with inadequate toilet behavior, these issues need to be addressed additionally. The ultimate aim of the treatment is a complete restoration of the functionality of the pelvic floor.

Stress Incontinence Without a Dysfunction of the Pelvic Floor
Without a dysfunction of the pelvic floor, an ISD is likely. Here, pelvic floor training can only realize compensation at the most. A complete cure is merely impossible.

Stress Incontinence in Combination with General Factors That Inhibit or Delay Improvement or Recovery
In this case, physiotherapy will aim at the reduction of these negative general factors. Avoiding specific situations by the patient, impaired social participation and feelings of shame related to involuntary urine loss can be reduced by the physiotherapist using relevant information, education, counselling, and care.

In Table 41.3 an algorithm of the process of therapy for stress incontinence in women is given.

Detrusor Overactivity
In this condition, the patient has no or insufficient control over involuntary detrusor contractions, which can result in involuntary urine loss (77). Physiotherapy for detrusor overactivity consists of patient information and education, toilet training, bladder (re-)training or behavioral therapy, PFMT with or without biofeedback, electrical stimulation, and magnetic stimulation. All physiotherapeutic modalities can be used alone or in combination with each other or in combination with medication.

Patient information and education is provided about the lower urinary tract function, the function of the pelvic floor, and the way to contract and relax the pelvic floor.

The goal of toilet training is to change inadequate toilet behavior and regimens, i.e., aiming at the aspects of the micturition process itself.

Bladder (re-)training (BlT) aims to restore normal bladder function using patient education together with a scheduled voiding regimen in order to increase the time interval between two consecutive voidings (78). It consists of four components. The first is an educational program that addresses lower urinary tract function. The next component involves training to inhibit the sensation of urgency and to postpone voiding. The third is to urinate according to a timetable in patients with an interval less

Table 41.3 Algorithm of Process of Therapy for Stress Incontinence in Women

Process of therapy
Therapeutic training/management for distinguished problem areas
- USI + dysfunction pelvic floor + NO awareness of pelvic floor:
  ° Digital palpation by patient and/or physiotherapist
  ° Electrostimulation (intravaginal/extravaginal) + PFMT
  ° Biofeedback + PFMT
  Objective: restoration of awareness of the pelvic floor
  ° If awareness restored → see below
  ° Unsatisfactory results → back to referring physician
- USI + dysfunction pelvic floor + awareness of the pelvic floor:
  ° PFMT +home exercises; isolated contractions of the pelvic floor → with awareness of pelvic floor, single tasks → double tasks→ multiple tasks→ automatic controlled tasks; optional: vaginal cones
  Objective: total recovery (of the functionality of the pelvic floor)
  ° Unsatisfactory results → back to referring physician
- USI + dysfunction pelvic floor + function pelvic floor mal-influenced by disorders tractus respiratorius, other parts tractus motorius, toilet regimen, toilet behavior
  ° PFMT + home exercises
  ° Exercises to achieve adequate respiration, postural exercises, relaxation exercises, lift-instruction
  Objective: reduction or elimination mal-influence disorders, improvement functionality pelvic floor
  ° Unsatisfactory results → back to referring physician
- USI + NO dysfunction of the pelvic floor
  ° PFMT + home exercises; optional: vaginal cones
  Objective: compensation. Expectation: total recovery is not likely
  ° Unsatisfactory results → back to referring physician
- USI + general obstructing factors
  Objective: maximal possible reduction of these negative factors
  ° Unsatisfactory results → back to referring physician
Evaluation
Treatment results, (changes in) patient's health status, course of action physiotherapist
Concluding treatment period and reporting to referring physician

Abbreviations: PFMT, pelvic floor muscle training; USI, urodynamic stress incontinence.

than two hours between two consecutive micturitions in order to reach an interval of at least three hours between two consecutive voidings and to reach larger voided volumes. As a fourth step, reinforcement of patient motivation by the physiotherapist;

Especially in those patients whose functional capacity of the bladder is too small, a bladder (re-)training program can provide normalization of bladder capacity.

So far, the exact working mechanism of BlT remains unclear (79). Improvement of cortical inhibition over involuntary detrusor contractions (80), central modulation of afferent sensory impulses or cortical facilitation over urethral closure during bladder filling (81), and behavioral changes leading to an increase of "reserve capacity" of the lower urinary tract system (82) have been reported.

The efficacy of bladder training in women with detrusor overactivity varies from 12% to 90% (36). From the few trials available the ICI concluded that there is scant Level 1 evidence that BlT may be an effective treatment for women with UUI and MUI (Level of Evidence: 1). If there is no reduction in incontinent episodes after three weeks of bladder training, the ICI recommends re-evaluation and the consideration of other treatment options (36).

Specific PFMT *probably* facilitates and restores the detrusor inhibition reflex (DIR) by selective contraction of the PFMs. PFMT consists of PFME and general or specific relaxation exercises. Different from the mechanism in stress incontinence, in patients with detrusor overactivity selective contractions of the PFMs during the therapy are focused on the inhibition of involuntary detrusor contractions (reflex inhibition) (83).

In many patients with a detrusor overactivity there is a concurrent high PFMs tone (84). The level of activation is so high that selective contraction of the PFMs in order to achieve reciproqual inhibition of the bladder is very difficult or not possible (85). Teaching selective contraction and relaxation of the PFMs is then an important first step. Once this is achieved, selective contraction of the PFMs focuses on facilitation of the DIR. After testing a patient's ability to hold contractions for at least 20 seconds by digital palpation by the physiotherapist, patients are instructed to do so, followed by a relaxation period of 10 seconds. A more functional training (pelvic floor exercises during daily living activities) completes the exercise program.

Also combinations of bladder (re-)training and PFMT are used in patients with detrusor overactivity. In the study of Berghmans et al. this kind of program was called Lower Urinary Tract Exercises (LUTE) (63).

Like in patients with stress incontinence, in patients with detrusor overactivity with insufficient or no awareness of the pelvic floor, biofeedback can be used to learn to control muscle function such as reduction of an increased muscle activity or a better timing and coordination of contraction or relaxation (42).

Wyman et al. suggested that a combination of biofeedback, PFMT, and bladder training was more effective immediately after the therapy than separate application of each treatment modality (82).

In patients with detrusor overactivity electrical stimulation theoretically stimulates the detrusor inhibition reflex (DIR) and pacifies the micturition reflex, resulting in a decrease of overactive bladder dysfunction (62).

Electrical stimulation aims through selective stimulation of afferent and efferent nerve fibers in the pelvic floor, resulting in contraction of the para- and periurethral musculature, either direct or via spinal reflexes, to inhibit involuntary detrusor contractions (63).

Although sometimes external electrodes have been used, mostly electrical stimulation is applied vaginally or anally through plug mounted electrodes (25,36). A patient is instructed to use the maximal tolerable level during stimulation. In relevant studies the following treatment characteristics were used: frequency modulation of 0.1 second trains of rectangular biphasic 200 μsec (63,86) or 400 μsec (87) long pulses which varied stochastically between 4 and 10 Hz (63) or with a fixed frequency of 10 Hz (86,87). Acute electrical stimulation can be applied (mostly one to two times a week during 20 minutes) or chronic electrical stimulation (daily at home, e.g., every 6 hours 20 minutes).

Besides office-based electrical stimulation, portable electrical stimulation devices for self care by patients themselves at home have been developed (63) (Fig. 41.5).

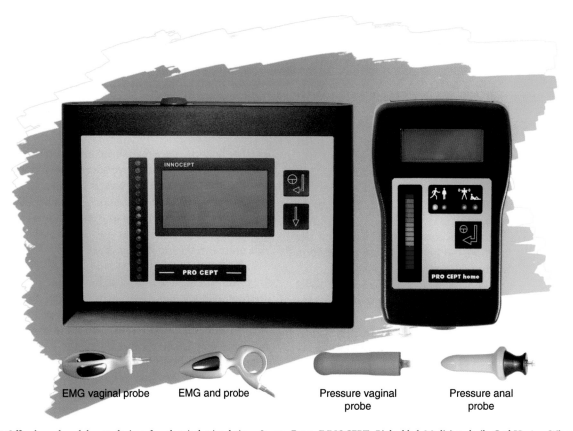

Figure 41.5 Office-bound and home devices for electrical stimulation. *Source*: From INNOCEPT, Biobedded Medizintechnik GmbH, Am Wiesenbusch 1, D-45966 Gladbeck, Germany.

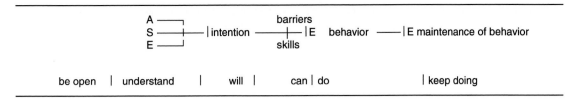

Figure 41.6 Parallels between the ASE-model and the Steps-model. *Source*: From Ref. 88.

Magnetic stimulation of the sacral nerve roots and pelvic floor is suggested to be an effective treatment modality also for urgency urinary incontinence (67,68). The mechanism of action to improve or restore urgency urinary incontinence is still not fully clear (68). Using low frequency stimulation (e.g., 10 Hz) (71), in urgency urinary incontinence magnetic stimulation might suppress detrusor overactivity through at least two autonomic effects: activation of pudendal nerve afferents blocking parasympathetic detrusor motor fibers at the spinal reflex arc, activation of inhibitory hypogatric sympathetic neurons, or a combination of both mechanisms (73). Modulation of pudendal nerve afferent branches stimulating an inhibitory spinal reflex at the S3 nerve root, are also suggested to play a role in this mechanism of action (73).

Only sparse evidence of the effect of magnetic stimulation versus no treatment, placebo or control treatment in women with urgency urinary incontinence is available. So far, only short term results were reported. At the moment there is not enough evidence for the efficacy of magnetic stimulation in women with urgency urinary incontinence.

Overviewing the evidence for the different treatment modalities for detrusor overactivity the following conclusions can be made: The efficacy of bladder training in women with detrusor overactivity is still pending and varies from 12% to 90% (36). Despite a positive trend in several studies (63,87) with reported success percentages around 45% to 50%, today there is still insufficient evidence for the efficacy of PFMT programs with or without biofeedback in patients with detrusor overactivity (25,36,63). Recent studies show that acute and chronic electrical stimulation, office- and home-based, are effective in 70% of all cases (63,86,87). This treatment modality may be the treatment of first choice in patients with detrusor overactivity (36,63,86,87).

Mixed Incontinence

The physiotherapeutic diagnostic and therapeutic process focuses on the predominant factors of the mixed urinary incontinence. If the symptoms of urgency/frequency appear to be dominant, mostly the aim will be to reduce and improve these factors. In case the physiotherapist starts with the stress component this can provide a negative influence on the urgency component, maybe introducing more severe urgency/frequency. Reduction or improvement of the latter symptoms will provide a solid base for the following treatment of the stress component. The choices of therapy modalities depend on the nature, extent, and severity of the health problem, and are based on the analysis and evaluation of the physiotherapeutic diagnostic process.

PATIENT EDUCATION IN PHYSIOTHERAPY PRACTICE

In order to achieve a permanent positive result from physiotherapy, patients have to incorporate the newly acquired abilities into daily life. The physiotherapist is the most important mentor in this behavioral modification. Patient education is a very important aspect of this kind of care and a professional attitude towards providing patient education is required. Van der Burgt and Verhulst developed a model for allied health professions as an instrumental tool for patient education (88). This model is a combination of the ASE-model and the so-called Steps-model of Hoenen et al., developed for individual patient education (89). In the ASE-model the premise is that the interplay between attitude, social influence, and own efficacy determines the willingness to modify behavior (Fig. 41.6).

In the model of Van der Burgt and Verhulst, a number of stages are distinguished, such as thinking, feeling, and doing. In patients with urinary incontinence this model can be transformed into an exchange of information and explanation (*thinking*), in awareness and feeling of the pelvic floor, posture and movement (*feeling*), and in training of the pelvic floor and promotion of short and long term compliance (*doing*). The standardized patient education model of Van der Burgt and Verhulst can be seen as an example of how to facilitate best practice and thus can provide physiotherapists with a framework upon which to base patient education in urinary incontinence.

CONCLUSION

Pelvic physiotherapy often appears to be effective in the treatment of incontinence. For this reason, physiotherapy is a valuable treatment option in the management of patients with urinary incontinence.

REFERENCES

1. Rekers H, Drogendijk AC, Valkenburg H, et al. Urinary incontinence in women from 35 to 79 years of age: prevalence and consequences. Eur J Obstet Gynecol Reprod Biol 1992; 43: 229–34.
2. Hunskaar S, Burgio K, Diokno AC, et al. Epidemiology and natural history of urinary incontinence in women. Urology 2003; 62(Suppl 4A): 16–23.
3. Hannestad YS, Rortveit G, Sandvik H, Hunskaar S. A community-based epidemiological survey of female urinary incontinence: The Norwegian EPINCONT Study. J Clin Epidemiol 2000; 53: 1150–7.
4. Maggi S, Minicuci N, Langlois J, et al. Prevalence rate of urinary incontinence in community-dwelling elderly women, the Veneto Study. J Gerontol A Biol Sci Med Sci 2001; 56A: M14.
5. Hunskar S, Burgio K, Diokno AC, et al. Epidemiology. In: Abrams P, Cardozo L, Khoury S, Wein A, eds. Incontinence. Plymouth, UK: Health Publication Ltd., 2002: 177.
6. Valk M. Urinary incontinence in psychogeriatric nursing home patients. Prevalence and determinants (Dissertation). Utrecht: Universiteit Utrecht, 1999.

7. Newman DK. How much society pays for urinary incontinence. Ostomy Wound Manage 1997; 43: 18–25.

8. Schulman C, Claes H, Matthijs J. Urinary incontinencein Belgium: a population-based epidemiological survey. Eur Urol 1997; 32: 315–20.

9. Lagro-Janssen TL, Smits AJ, van Weel C. Women with urinary incontinence: self perceived worries and general practitioners' of knowledge of the problem. Br J Gen Pract 1990; 40: 331–4.

10. Teunissen D, van Weel C, Lagro-Janssen T. Urinary incontinence in older people living in the community: examining help-seeking behaviour. Br J Gen Pract 2005; 55: 776–82.

11. Abrams P, Cardozo L, Fall M, et al. The standardization of terminology of lower urinary tract function. Neurourol Urodyn 2002; 21: 167–78.

12. ICS Pelvic Floor Clinical Assessment Group. Terminology of pelvic floor function and dysfunction. ICS report 2001.

13. Gezondheidsraad: Urine-incontinentie. Den Haag: Gezondheidsraad, 2001; publicatie nr 2001/12.

14. Lagro-Janssen ALM, Breedvelt Boer HP, van Dongen JJA, et al. NHG-standaard Incontinentie voor urine. Huisarts Wet 1995; 38: 71–80.

15. Klomp MLF, Gercama AJ, de Jong-Wubben JGM, et al. NHG-standaard Bemoeilijkte mictie bij oudere mannen (eerste herziening). Huisarts Wet 1997; 40: 114–24.

16. Berghmans LCM, Bernards ATM, Bluyssen AMW, et al. KNGF-richtlijn Stress urine-incontinentie. Ned Tijdschr Fysiother 1998; 108(Suppl): 1–35.

17. Fantl JA, Newman DK, Colling J, et al. Urinary Incontinence in Adults: Acute and Chronic Management. Clinical Practice Guideline No.2, 1996 Update. AHCPR publication 96-0682. Rockville MD: US Dept of Health and Human Services, Public Health Service, Agency for Health Care Policy and Research, 1996.

18. Scottisch Intercollegial Guideline Network (SIGN). Management of Urinary Incontinence in Primary Care. A National Clinical Guideline, 2004.

19. Robert M, Ross S. SOGC clinical Practice Guideline, Conservative Management of Urinary Incontinence. J Obstet Gynaecol Can 2006; 28: 1113–18.

20. National Collaborating Centre for Women's and Children's Health. Urinary Incontinence: The Management of Urinary Incontinence in Women. London: RCOG Press, 2006.

21. Viktrup L, Summers KH, Dennett SL. Clinical practice guidelines for the initial management of urinary incontinence in women: a European-focused review. BJU Int 2004; 94(Suppl 1): 14–22.

22. Abrams P, Cardozo L, Khoury S, Wein A, eds. Incontinence, 3rd edn. Paris, France: Health Publication Ltd., 2005.

23. Abrams P. Assessment and treatment of urinary incontinence. Lancet 2000; 355: 2153–8.

24. Lagro-Janssen ALM, Debruyne FMJ, Smits AJA, van Weel C. The effects of treatment of urinary incontinence in general practice. Fam Pract 1992; 9: 284–9.

25. Berghmans LCM, Hendriks HJM, De Bie RA, et al. Conservative treatment of urge urinary incontinence in woman, a systematic review of randomized clinical trials. BJU Int 2000; 85: 254–63.

26. Bent AE, Gousse AE, Hendrix SL, et al. Validation of a two-item quantitative questionnaire for the triage of women with urinary incontinence. Obstet Gynecol 2005; 106: 767–73.

27. Martin JL,Williams KS, Sutton AJ, Abrams KR, Assassa RP. Systematic review and meta-analysis of methods of diagnostic assessment for urinary incontinence. Neurourol Urodyn 2006; 25: 674–83.

28. DeLancey JOL. Genuine stress incontinence: Where are we now, where should we go? Am J Obstet Gynecol 1996; 175: 311–19.

29. Grimby A, Milson I, Molander U, Wiklund I, Ekelund P. The influence of urinary incontinence on the QOL of elderly women. Age Ageing 1993; 22: 82–9.

30. DeLancey JOL. Structural aspects of urethrovesical function in the female. Neurourol Urodyn 1988; 7: 509–19.

31. Van Kampen M, De Weerdt W, Van Poppel H, Baert L. Urinary incontinence following transurethral, transvesical and radical prostatectomy. Acta Urol Belg 1997; 65: 1–7.

32. Van Kampen M, De Weerdt W, Van Poppel H, et al. Prediction of urinary continence following radical prostatectomy. Urol Int 1998; 60: 80–4.

33. Bump RC, Norton PA. Epidemiology and natural history of pelvic floor dysfunction. Obstet Gynecol Clin North Am 1998; 25: 723–46.

34. DeLancey JO, Morgan DM, Fenner DE, et al. Comparison of levator ani muscle defects and function in women with and without pelvic organ prolapse. Obstet Gynecol 2007; 109(2 Pt 1): 295–302.

35. Hagen S, Stark D, Cattermole D. United Kingdom-wide survey of physiotherapy practice in the treatment of pelvic organ prolapse. Physiotherapy 2004; 90: 19–26.

36. Wilson PD, Hay-Smith J, Berghmans L. Adult conservative management. In: Abrams P, Cardozo L, Khoury S, Wein A, eds. Incontinence. Paris, France: Health Publication Ltd., 2005: 857–964.

37. WHO publication. International Classification of Functioning, Disability and Health: ICF. Geneva: WHO, 2001.

38. Berghmans LCM, Bernards ATM, Hendriks HJM, et al. Update of Royal Dutch Association of Physiotherapy—Guidelines: Stress Urinary Incontinence. In press.

39. Wells TJ, Brink CA, Diokno AC, Wolfe R, Gillis GL. Pelvic muscle exercise for stress urinary incontinence in elderly women. J Am Geriatr Soc 1991; 39: 785–91.

40. Tapp AJS, Hills B, Cardozo LD. Randomized study comparing pelvic floor physiotherapy with the Burch colposuspension. Neurourol Urodyn 1989; 8: 356–7.

41. Hendriks EJM, Bernards ATM, Berghmans LCM, de Bie RA. The psychometric properties of the PRAFAB questionnaire: a brief assessment questionnaire to evaluate severity of urinary incontinence in women. Neurourol Urodyn 2007; 26: 998–1007.

42. Berghmans LCM, Frederiks CMA, De Bie RA, et al. Efficacy of biofeedback, when included with pelvic floor muscle exercise treatment, for genuine stress incontinence. Neurourol and Urodyn 1996; 15: 37–52.

43. Laycock J. Clinical evaluation of the pelvic floor. In: Schüssler B, Laycock J, Norton PA, Stanton SL, eds. Pelvic floor re-education. London: Springer-Verlag, 2003: 42–8.

44. Bø K. Pressure measurements during pelvic floor muscle contractions: the effect of different positions of the vaginal measuring device. Neurourol Urodyn 1992; 11: 107–13.

45. Dumoulin C, Bourbonnais D, Lemieux MC. Development of a dynamometer for measuring the isometric force of the pelvic floor musculature. Neurourol Urodyn 2003; 23: 134–42.

46. Bø K, Sherburn M. Evaluation of female pelvic-floor muscle function and strength. Phys Ther 2005; 85: 269–82.

47. Dietz H. Ultrasound in the assessment of pelvic floor muscle and pelvic organ descent. In: Bø K, Berghmans B, Mørkved S, Van Kampen M, eds. Evidence-Based Physical Therapy for the Pelvic Floor: Bridging Science and Clinical Practice. London: Churchill Livingstone Elsevier, 2007: 81–93.

48. Howard D, Miller J, DeLancey J, et al. Differential effects of cough, valsalva, and continence status on vesical neck movement. Obstet Gynecol 2000; 95: 535–40.

49. Miller JM, Ashton-Miller JA, DeLancey J. A pelvic muscle precontraction can reduce cough-related urine loss in selected women with mild SUI. J Am Geriatr Soc 1998; 46: 870–4.

50. Ashton-Miller JA, DeLancey JOL. Functional anatomy of the female pelvic floor. In: Bø K, Berghmans B, Mørkved S, Van Kampen M, eds. Evidence-Based Physical Therapy for the Pelvic Floor: Bridging Science and Clinical Practice. London: Churchill Livingstone Elsevier, 2007: 19–35.

51. Bø K. Pelvic floor muscle exercise for the treatment of stress urinary incontinence: an exercise physiology perspective. Int Urogynecol J Pelvic Floor Dysfunct 1995; 6: 282–91.

52. Bø K. Physiotherapy to treat genuine stress incontinence. Int Cont Surv 1996; 6: 2–8.

53. DiNubile NA. Strenght training. Clin Sports Med 1991; 10: 33–62.

54. Bø K, Hage RH, Kvarstein B, Jorgensen J, Larsen S. Plevic floor muscle exercise for the treatment of female stress urinary incontinence. III Effects of two different degrees of pelvic floor muscle exercises. Neurourol Urodyn 1990; 9: 489–502.

55. Berghmans LCM, Hendriks HJM, Bø K, et al. Conservative treatment of stress urinary incontinence in women: a systematic review of randomized clinical trials. Br J Urol 1998; 82: 181–91.

56. Hay-Smith EJC, Bø K, Berghmans LCM, et al. Pelvic floor muscle training for urinary incontinence in women. Cochrane Database Syst Rev 2001; (4): CD001407.

57. Bø K, Kvarstein B, Nygaard I. Lower urinary tract symptoms and pelvic floor muscle exercise adherence after 15 years. Obstet Gynecol 2005; 105(5 Pt 1): 999–1005.

58. Cammu H, Van Nijlen M, Amy J. A ten-year follow-up after Kegel pelvic floor muscle exercises for genuine stress incontinence. Br J Urol 2000; 85: 655–8.

59. Glavind K, Nohr S, Walter S. Biofeedback and physiotherapy versus physiotherapy alone in the treatment of genuine stress incontinence. Int Urogynecol J Pelvic Floor Dysfunct 1996; 7: 339–43.

60. Goode P, Burgio KL, Locher JL, et al. Effect of behavioral training with or without pelvic floor electrical stimulation on stress incontinence in women. A randomized clinical trial. JAMA 2003; 290: 345–52.

61. Wall LL, Davidson TG. The role of muscular re-education by physical therapy in the treatment of GSI. Obstet Gynecol Surv 1992; 47: 322–31.

62. Eriksen BC. Electrostimulation of the pelvic floor in female urinary incontinence (Thesis). Norway: University of Trondheim, 1989.

63. Berghmans LCM, Van Waalwijk van Doorn ESC, Nieman FHM, et al. Efficacy of physical therapeutic modalities in women with proven bladder overactivity. Eur Urol 2002; 41: 581–8.

64. Berghmans B. Physical therapies—electrical stimulation. In: Abrams P, Cardozo L, Khoury S, Wein A, eds. Incontinence, Vol. 2, Management. Paris, France: Health Publication Ltd., 2005: 889–900.

65. Barker AT, Freeston IL, Jalinous R, et al. Magnetic stimulation of the human brain and peripheral nerve system: an introduction and the results of an initial clinical evaluation. Neurosurgery 1997; 20: 100.

66. Galloway NT, El-Galley RE, Sand PK, et al. Extracorporeal magnetic innervation therapy for stress urinary incontinence. Urology 1999; 53: 1108.

67. Goldberg RP, Sand PK. Electromagnetic pelvic floor stimulation: applications for the gynecologist. Obstet Gynecol Surv 2000; 55: 715.

68. Quek P. A critical review on magnetic stimulation: what is its role in the management of pelvic floor disorders? Curr Opin Urol 2005; 15: 231–5.

69. Craggs MD, Sheriff MK, Shah PJ. Response to multi-pulse magnetic stimulation of spinal nerve roots mapped over the sacrum in man. J Physiol 1995; 483: 127.

70. Kralj B. Conservative treatment of female stress urinary incontinence with functional electrical stimulation. Eur J Obstet Gynecol Reprod Biol 1999; 85: 53.

71. But I. Conservative treatment of female urinary incontinence with functional magnetic stimulation. Urology 2003; 61: 558.

72. Yokoyama T, Nishiguchi J, Watanabe T, et al. Comparative study of effects of extracorporeal magnetic innervation versus electrical stimulation for urinary incontinence after radical prostatectomy. Urology 2004; 63: 264.

73. Lindström S, Fall M, Carlsson CA, et al. The neurophysiological basis of bladder inhibition in response to intravaginal electrical stimulation. J Urol 1983; 129: 405.

74. Bø K. Vaginal weight cones. Theoretical framework, effect on pelvic floor muscle strength and female stress urinary incontinence. Acta Obstet Gynecol Scand 1995; 74: 87.

75. Herbison P, Plevnik S, Mantle J. Weighted vaginal cones for urinary incontinence. Cochrane Database Syst Rev 2002; (1): CD002114.

76. Arvonen T, Fianu-Jonasson A, Tyni-Lenne R. Effectiveness of two conservative modes of physiotherapy in women with urinary stress incontinence. Neurourol Urodyn 2001; 20: 591–9.

77. Van Waalwijk van Doorn ESC, Ambergen AW. Diagnostic assessment of the overactive bladder during the filling phase: the detrusor activity index. Br J Urol 1999; 83(Suppl 2): 16–21.

78. Wyman JF, Fantl JA. Bladder training in ambulatory care management of urinary incontinence. Urol Nurs 1991; 11: 11–17.

79. Fantl JA. Behavioral intervention for community-dwelling individuals with urinary incontinence. Urology 1998; 51(Suppl 2A): 30–4.

80. Fantl JA, Hurt WG, Dunn LJ. Detrusor instability syndrome: the use of bladder retraining drills with and without anticholinergics. Am J Obstet Gynecol 1981; 140: 885–90.

81. Fantl JA, Wyman JF, McClish DK, et al. Efficacy of bladder training in older women with urinary incontinence. JAMA 1991; 265: 609–13.

82. Wyman JF, Fantl JA, McClish DK, et al. Comparative efficacy of behavioural interventions in the management of female urinary incontinence. Continence program for women Research Group. Am J Obstet Gynecol 1998; 179: 999–1007.

83. Bø K, Berghmans LCM. Nonpharmacologic treatments for overactive bladder—Pelvic floor exercises. Urology 2000; 55(Suppl 5a): 7–11.

84. Houston KA. Incontinence and the older woman. Clin Geriatr Med 1993; 9: 157–71.

85. Messelink EJ. The overactive bladder and the role of the pelvic floor muscles. Br J Urol 1999; 83(Suppl 2); 31–5.

86. Yamanishi T, Yasuda K, Sakakibara R, Hattori T, Suda S. Randomized, double blind study of electrical stimulation for urinary incontinence due to detrusor overactivity. Urology 2000; 55: 353–7.

87. Wang AC, Wang YY, Chen MC. Single-blind, randomized trial of pelvic floor muscle training, biofeedback-assisted pelvic floor muscle training, and electric stimulation in the management of overactive bladder. Urology 2004; 63: 61–6.

88. Van der Burgt M, Verhulst F. Gedragsmodellen. In: van der Burgt M, Verhulst F, eds. Doen en blijven doen. Houten: Bohn Stafleu Van Loghum, 1996: 31.

89. Hoenen JA, Tielen LM, Willink AE. Patiëntenvoorlichting stap voor stap: suggesties voor de huisarts voor de aanpak van patiëntenvoorlichting in het consult. Uitgeverij voor de gezondheidsbevordering, Stichting O&O, 1988.

42 Drug Treatment of Voiding Dysfunction in Women
Ariana L Smith and Alan J Wein

INTRODUCTION

The lower urinary tract (LUT) has two basic functions: storage of urine and emptying of urine. These functions are achieved in two discrete phases of micturition (1).

Phase one involves filling and storage of urine in the bladder and is accomplished through:

1. accommodation of increasing volumes of urine at low intravesical pressure,
2. appropriate sensation of bladder filling without allodynia,
3. a bladder outlet that *is closed at rest* remains closed despite increases in intra-abdominal pressure, and
4. the absence of involuntary detrusor contractions (IVCs) secondary to neurogenic or non-neurogenic detrusor overactivity (DO).

Phase two involves voiding and emptying of the bladder and is accomplished through:

1. coordinated contraction of the bladder smooth muscle with adequate magnitude and duration,
2. concomitant lowering of resistance at the level of the smooth and striated urethral sphincter, and
3. the absence of anatomic obstruction.

Voiding dysfunction is a broad term that results from disruption of any one of the factors listed above; essentially a failure store, a failure to empty, *or any combination of these factors*. Likewise, all treatments of voiding dysfunction can be classified under the categories of facilitating urinary storage or facilitating urinary emptying. These actions are achieved pharmacologically primarily by acting selectively or non-selectively on bladder smooth muscle or bladder outlet smooth or striated muscle. As a result of advances in the fields of neuropharmacology and neurophysiology of the LUT, effective pharmacologic therapy now exists for the management of many categories of voiding dysfunction. In fact, in some categories so many drug therapies are available for use with varying quality and quantity of research performed on them, the International Consultation on Incontinence has assessed and made recommendations on many of the available agents (Tables 42.1 and 42.2). The clinical drug recommendations are based on evaluations made using a modification of the Oxford system (Table 42.3).

CLINICAL UROPHARMACOLOGY OF THE LUT

LUT uropharmacology addresses the innervations and receptor contents of the bladder, urethra, and pelvic floor. The targets of pharmacologic intervention include not only these structures, but also the peripheral nerves and ganglia that supply these tissues and the central nervous system (CNS), including the spinal cord and supraspinal areas. Specifically, pharmacologic targets include nerve terminals which alter the release of neurotransmitters, receptor subtypes, cellular second messenger systems, and ion channels. The autonomic nervous system assumes primary control over the two functions of the LUT, however, due to its lack of specificity and ubiquitous nature of its receptors there are no pharmacologic agents that are purely selective for the LUT. Consequently, side effects of treatment are common and are the result of collateral effects on organ systems that share some of the same neurophysiologic or pharmacologic characteristics as the bladder and urethra.

Our approach to pharmacologic management is to start with the simplest and least perilous form of treatment first. After appropriate dose escalation, other, potentially more toxic, therapeutic options can be offered. Alternatively, a combination of agents or drugs can be used, ideally with synergistic mechanisms of action and non-synergistic side effects. In our experience, although great improvement can occur with rational pharmacologic therapy, a perfect result, i.e., the restoration to normal function, is seldom achieved.

FACILITATION OF URINE STORAGE

Failure of the LUT to adequately fill and store urine may be secondary to pathology in the bladder, the outlet, or both (2). The most common etiology in women is DO which manifests symptomatically as overactive bladder (OAB), a syndrome of urgency, with or without urge urinary incontinence (UUI), which may be associated with frequency and nocturia (3). DO includes IVCs of the bladder, discrete or phasic, and decreased compliance. IVCs are commonly associated with neurologic disease, inflammatory processes of the bladder, bladder outlet obstruction (BOO), aging, can be stress induced, or may be idiopathic. Decreased compliance is usually the sequelae of neurologic disease but may also result from any process that destroys the elastic or viscoelastic properties of the bladder wall. Treatment for these conditions is aimed at decreasing bladder activity or increasing bladder capacity.

Heightened or altered sensation of the bladder may manifest as urgency with or without DO or as painful bladder syndrome. This may result from inflammatory, infectious, neurologic, or psychological factors, or it may be idiopathic. Therapy is aimed at increasing bladder capacity or decreasing sensory (afferent) input. The various therapeutic options for painful bladder syndrome will be dealt with in a separate chapter.

Decreased outlet resistance may manifest from damage to the smooth or striated sphincter secondary to surgical, obstetric or other mechanical trauma, or degeneration of innervation with loss of neuronal mass secondary to neurologic disease, aging, or trauma (4). In addition, in women it may

Table 42.1 Drugs used in the Treatment of OAB/DO. Assessments According to the Modified Oxford System

	Level of evidence	Grade of recommendation
Antimuscarinic drugs		
Tolterodine	1	A
Trospium	1	A
Solifenacin	1	A
Darifenacin	1	A
Propantheline	2	B
Atropine, hyoscyamine	3	C
Drugs acting on membrane channels		
Calcium antagonists	2	D
K-Channel openers	2	D
Drugs with mixed actions		
Oxybutynin	1	A
Propiverine	1	A
Dicyclomine	3	C
Flavoxate	2	D
Antidepressants		
Imipramine	3	C
Duloxetine	2	C
α-AR antagonists		
Alfuzosin	3	C
Doxazosin	3	C
Prazosin	3	C
Terazosin	3	C
Tamsulosin	3	C
β-AR antagonists		
Terbutaline (β_2)	3	C
Salbutamol (β_2)	3	C
YM-178 (β_3)	2	B
PDE-5 inhibitors[a]		
(Sildenafil, Taladafil, Vardenafil)	2	B
COX-inhibitors		
Indomethacin	2	C
Flurbiprofen	2	C
Toxins		
Botulinum toxin (neurogenic)[d]	2	A
Botulinum toxin (idiopathic)[d]	3	B
Capsaicin (neurogenic)[c]	2	C
Resiniferatoxin (neurogenic)[c]	2	C
Other drugs		
Baclofen[b]	3	C
Hormones		
Estrogen	2	C
Desmopressin[e]	1	A

[a]Male LUTS/OAB; [b]intrathecal; [c]intravesical; [d]bladder wall; [e]nocturia (nocturnal polyuria), caution hyponatremia especially in the elderly.
Abbreviations: AR, adrenoceptor; COX, cyclo-oxygenase; DO, detrusor overactivity; LUTS, lower urinary tract symptoms; OAB, overactive bladder; PDE, phosphodiesterase.
Source: Adapted from Ref. 12.

Table 42.2 Drugs used in the Treatment of Stress Urinary Incontinence. Assessments According to the Modified Oxford System

Drug	Level of evidence	Grade of recommendation
Duloxetine	1	A
Imipramine	3	D
Clenbuterol	3	C
Midodrine	2	C
Ephedrine	3	D
Phenylpropanolamine	3	D
Estrogen	2	D

Source: Adapted from Ref. 12.

Table 42.3 International Consultation on Incontinence Assessments 2008: Modified Oxford Guidelines

Levels of evidence
Level 1: Systematic reviews, meta-analyses, good quality RCTs
Level 2: RCTs, good quality prospective cohort studies
Level 3: Case-control studies, case series
Level 4: Expert opinion
Grades of recommendation
Grade A: Based on level 1 evidence (highly recommended)
Grade B: Consistent level 2 or 3 evidence (recommended)
Grade C: Level 4 studies or "majority evidence" (optional)
Grade D: Evidence inconsistent/inconclusive (no recommendation possible) or the evidence indicates that the drug should not be recommended

Abbreviation: RCTs, randomized controlled trials.
Source: Adapted from Ref. 12.

result from decreased pelvic floor support of the bladder outlet. Clinically, this manifests as effort related or stress urinary incontinence (SUI) or, when severe, as complete gravitational incontinence. Treatment is aimed at increasing outlet resistance.

Disruption in the filling and storing function of the bladder can, in theory, be improved by agents that decrease detrusor activity, increase bladder capacity, decrease sensory input, or increase outlet resistance (2).

Decreasing Bladder Contractility
Antimuscarinic Agents
Physiologic bladder contractions are thought to be primarily triggered by acetylcholine (ACh) induced stimulation of post-ganglionic parasympathetic muscarinic cholinergic receptor sites on bladder smooth muscle (1,5). Atropine and other antagonists of ACh which bind these receptor sites will depress normal bladder contractions and IVCs of any cause (5,6). In addition, these agents increase the volume to first IVC and the total bladder capacity, and decrease the amplitude of the contraction (7).

The commonly held belief regarding antimuscarinic drugs is that they bind receptors on the detrusor that are stimulated by ACh, thereby decreasing the ability of the bladder to contract.

419

However, during bladder filling and storage, there is no sacral parasympathetic outflow (8), which raises the question: "Why do antimuscarinics affect the filling/storage phase of the micturition cycle, increasing, in patients with OAB and without DO, bladder capacity, and decreasing urgency?" Muscarinic receptors are also present in bladder urothelium and suburothelium (9) and there is a basal ACh release in human detrusor muscle which may be produced, at least partly, by the urothelium and suburothelium (10). This suggests that detrusor tone may be affected by ongoing ACh mediated stimulation. There is now good direct experimental evidence that the antimuscarinics decrease activity in both C and A-delta afferent nerve fibers from the bladder during filling/storage (11,12).

ACh acts on two classes of receptors, nicotinic and muscarinic. Signal transduction between parasympathetic nerves and smooth muscle of the detrusor involves muscarinic receptors (13). At least five different muscarinic receptor subtypes exist which are designated M_1 to M_5. Although it appears that the majority of the muscarinic receptors in human smooth muscle are of the M_2 subtype, in vitro data indicate that most smooth muscle contraction, including that of the bladder, is mediated by the M_3 receptor subtype. The muscarinic receptors are found not only on smooth muscle cells of the bladder, but also on urothelial cells, suburothelial nerves, and on suburothelial structures such as interstitial cells with a M_2 and M_3 preponderance (9). Based on work in animals, the M_2 receptors have been implicated in the contraction of diseased bladders (denervated, hypertrophied rat bladders) (11).

Antimuscarinics can be divided into tertiary and quaternary amines which differ in molecular size, molecular charge, and lipophilicity (13). Small molecular size with little charge and greater lipophilicity increase the passage through the blood brain barrier with the theoretical potential of greater CNS side effects. Tertiary compounds have higher lipophilicity and less molecular charge than quaternary agents. Quaternary compounds have greater molecular charge and less lipophilicity resulting in limited passage into the CNS and a low incidence of CNS side effects (14).

A recent meta-analysis on antimuscarinic agents found that these agents are more effective than placebo in improving continent days, mean voided volume, urgency episodes, and micturition frequency (15). The vast majority of agents studied provided improvement in health related quality of life (HRQL). Across large patient samples, all of the currently available antimuscarinics appear to have comparable efficacy but do show some measurable differences in tolerability (16). Since the profiles of each drug and the dosing schedules differ, these things along with medical co-morbidities and concomitant medications should be considered when individualizing treatment for patients.

The currently available antimuscarinic drugs lack selectivity for the bladder and as a result produce side effects on other organ systems (Fig. 42.1). The most common adverse effects include dry mouth, blurred vision, pruritis, tachycardia, somnolence, impaired cognition, and headache. Constipation is reported as the most burdensome side effect (15). This class of drug is contraindicated in patients with urinary retention, gastric retention, and other severe decreased gastrointestinal motility conditions, and uncontrolled narrow-angle glaucoma. The concomitant use with other anticholinergic agents may

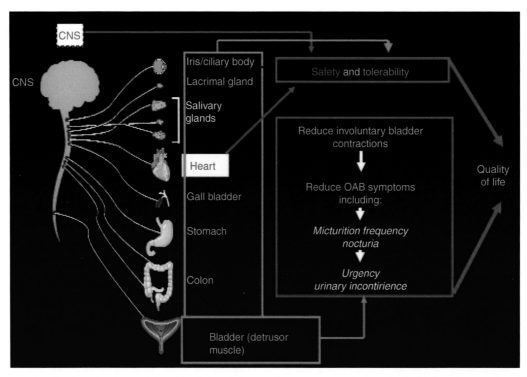

Figure 42.1 Important sites of action of antimuscarinics. *Abbreviations:* CNS, central nervous system; OAB, overactive bladder. *Source:* Adapted from Ref. 12.

increase the frequency and/or severity of these effects. Specific patient populations including those with renal or liver impairment and those with genetic heterogeneity in drug-metabolizing enzymes may experience increased side effects due to altered pharmacokinetic behavior of a given drug (16). Many of these drugs should not be used with potent cytochrome p450 (CYP) 3A4 inhibitors including ritonavir, ketoconazole, itraconazole, verapamil, and cyclosporine (17–20).

It is estimated that about one-third of all OAB patients have at least one risk factor for altered drug metabolism (16). While relative muscarinic receptor selectivity exists for some agents, there is no uroselective option that avoids unpleasant systemic side effects. As a result, patient compliance is extremely low and the search for uroselectivity continues. Intravesical administration in the absence of systemic absorption would greatly diminish the antimuscarinic side effects; however, this is practical only in patients who perform clean intermittent catheterization (CIC).

Antimuscarinic agents are considered first-line pharmacotherapy for OAB (21). Specific antimuscarinic drugs are listed below with available data on efficacy and comparative efficacy with other drugs in class.

Atropine

Atropine, along with hyoscyamine and scopolamine, are active belladonna alkaloids, derived from the toxic belladonna plant with anticholinergic properties (12). Atropine has significant systemic side effects including ventricular fibrillation, tachycardia, dizziness, nausea, blurred vision, loss of balance, dilated pupils, photophobia, extreme confusion, and dissociative hallucinations which limit its oral use for the treatment of OAB. Intravesical atropine at a dose of 6 mg four times per day was shown to be as effective as intravesical oxybutynin (OXY) for increasing bladder capacity with minimal systemic side effects in patients with multiple sclerosis in a double blind, randomized placebo controlled trial (RCT) with cross over design (22). Its mention in this chapter is more of a historic one.

Darifenacin

Darifenacin is a tertiary amine with moderate lipophilicity and is a relatively selective M_3 receptor antagonist. At least theoretically, darifenacin's advantage is the ability to relatively selectively block the M_3 receptor which although less prevalent than the M_2 receptor, appears to be more important in bladder contraction. This selectivity is expected to increase efficacy in patients with OAB while reducing the adverse events related to the blockade of other muscarinic subtypes (23). Darifenacin has been developed as a controlled release formulation to allow daily dosing and is available at 7.5 and 15 mg/day. Several RCTs have documented the clinical effectiveness of the drug. Haab et al. performed a multicenter, double blind RCT comparing darifenacin 3.75 mg, 7.5 mg, 15 mg, and placebo once daily for 12 weeks (24). The study enrolled 561 patients (85% female) age 19 to 88 years with OAB symptoms for at least six months, and included patients with prior exposure to antimuscarinic therapy. The 7.5 and 15 mg doses of darifenacin had rapid onset of effect with significant improvement in symptoms over placebo at two-week follow up. The clinical parameters in

which the treatment arm was significantly better than placebo included: micturition frequency, bladder capacity, frequency of urgency, severity of urgency, and number of incontinence episodes. No significant change in nocturia was seen. The most common side effects were mild to moderate dry mouth and constipation. The CNS and cardiac safety profiles were similar to placebo. Discontinuation was rare.

A review of the pooled data from three phase III, multicenter, double blind RCTs was performed by Chapple et al. in 2005 (25). A total of 1059 patients (85% female) with urgency, UUI, and frequency were treated with darifenacin 7.5 mg, 15 mg, or placebo daily for 12 weeks. Significant dose related improvements in number of incontinence episodes per week were seen: 8.8 less episodes per week with the 7.5 mg dose and 10.6 less episodes per week with the 15 mg dose. Improvements in micturition frequency, bladder capacity, and severity of urgency were also seen. The most common side effects were dry mouth and constipation resulting, in few discontinuations.

The ability to postpone urination is one of the most noticeable clinical effects of antimuscarinic therapy. Often measured as "warning time," which is defined as the time from first sensation of urgency to the time of voluntary micturition or incontinence, the ability to postpone a few extra minutes can be the difference between wet and dry. Cardozo and Dixon performed a multicenter, double-blind RCT looking at the effects of darifenacin on warning time (26). Overall, 47% of the darifenacin group compared to 20% of the placebo group achieved a >30% increase in mean warning time. The patients in this study received a 30mg dose of darifenacin which is higher than the clinically recommended dose. These results have not been replicated using the 15 mg dose.

The effects of darifenacin on cognitive function in elderly volunteers was tested in a randomized, double blind, three-period crossover study with 129 patients 65 years of age or older (27). After two weeks of treatment no effect on cognitive function compared with baseline was found. The authors hypothesized that this was related to its M3 receptor selectivity.

Fesoterodine

Fesoterodine is a newer antimuscarinic drug that is metabolized rapidly and extensively to 5-hydroxymethyl tolterodine (5-HMT), the same active metabolite of tolterodine (TOLT) (28). Fesoterodine relies on nonspecific esterases that produce a rapid and complete conversion to 5-HMT with little pharmacokinetic variability. 5-HMT is further metabolized in the liver, but a modest percentage of 5-HMT undergoes renal excretion without additional metabolism, raising the possibility that 5-HMT could also work from the luminal side of the bladder (29). Whether this contributes to clinical efficacy in humans remains unknown at this time. Like TOLT, this compound is a non-subtype selective muscarinic receptor antagonist (30).

Fesoterodine is indicated for the treatment of DO at doses of 4 and 8 mg daily. In a multicenter, double-blind, double-dummy RCT with TOLT extended release (ER), 1132 patients were enrolled and received treatment (28). The trial showed that both the 4 mg and 8 mg doses of fesoterodine were effective in improving symptoms of OAB with the 8 mg dose have greater effect at the expense of a higher rate of dry mouth. Only one subject from the fesoterodine 8 mg group and one subject from the TOLT ER 4 mg group withdrew from the study due to dry mouth. The dose response relationship was confirmed in another study that pooled data from two phase III RCTs (31). Fesoterodine 8 mg performed better than the 4 mg dose in improving urgency and UUI as recorded by three-day bladder diary, offering the possibility of dose titration. A study on the effect of fesoterodine on HRQL in patients with OAB confirmed improvement for both the 4 and 8 mg dose of the drug (32).

Hyoscyamine
Hyoscyamine is a pharmacologically active antimuscarinic component of atropine that is reported to have similar actions and side effects (12). Few clinical studies are available to evaluate efficacy in the treatment of DO (33). A sublingual formulation of hyoscyamine sulfate is available.

Propantheline Bromide
The classic oral agent for antimuscarinic effects on the LUT was propantheline bromide, a nonselective quaternary ammonium compound that is poorly absorbed after oral administration (12). It has a short plasma half-life of <2 hours and varying biologic availability requiring individual titration. It is initially prescribed at 15 to 30 mg four times daily but larger doses are often required (34). Despite having antimuscarinic binding potential quite similar to atropine there is a lack of convincing data on the effectiveness for the treatment of OAB/DO. Contradictory studies are available that show complete response in 25/26 patients (35) and no difference from placebo in 154 and 23 patients respectively (36,37). By today's standards, the effect of propantheline on DO has not been well documented in RCTs; however, with its long history of use, it can be considered effective and may, in individually titrated doses, be clinically useful.

Scopolamine
Scopolamine, a belladonna alkaloid, has greater penetration through the blood-brain barrier than atropine and as a result produces more prominent central depressive effects even at low doses (12). Transdermal scopolamine has been used for treating DO at a continuous dose of 0.5 mg for three days (38). A double blind RCT was performed in 20 patients with DO. After 14 days, patients in the treatment group showed significant improvements in frequency, nocturia, urgency, and UUI over the placebo group. Side effects included dizziness, ataxia, blurred vision, dry mouth, and skin irritation at patch site. No patients discontinued use during the study period (33).

Solifenacin
Solifenacin is a tertiary amine with modest selectivity for the M3 receptor over the M2 and marginal selectivity over the M1 receptors (13,39). Solifenacin is metabolized in the liver utilizing the cytochrome P450 enzyme system (CYP3A4), but a modest percentage undergoes renal excretion without additional metabolism, raising the possibility that solifenacin could also work from the luminal side of the bladder. Whether this contributes to clinical efficacy in humans remains unknown at this time.

Solifenacin is a once a day antimuscarinic that is being marketed at the 5 mg and 10 mg doses. There have been several large trials examining the effects of solifenacin. A large phase II multinational RCT was performed comparing solifenacin 2.5, 5, 10, and 20 mg daily to TOLT immediate release (IR) 2 mg twice daily and placebo (40). A total of 225 patients with urodynamically confirmed DO were enrolled, treated for four weeks, and followed for two additional weeks. There was a significant decrease in micturition frequency, incontinence episodes, and urgency episodes, and an increase in volume voided in the 5, 10, and 20 mg solifenacin groups compared to placebo. The mean effects with TOLT were generally smaller than with solifenacin. The 5 and 10 mg doses of solifenacin had a lower dry mouth rate than TOLT. Discontinuation rates were highest for solifenacin 20 mg.

Cardozo and colleagues performed a multinational RCT comparing solifenacin 5 and 10 mg daily to placebo in 857 patients (41). Both doses significantly improved micturition frequency, urgency, volume voided, and incontinence episodes compared to placebo as determined by three-day micturition diaries. Of patients who reported any incontinence at baseline, 50% achieved continence after treatment with solifenacin compared with 27.9% after placebo. Dry mouth was reported in 7.7% of patients taking solifenacin 5 mg, 23.1% in solifenacin 10 mg, and 2.3% in the placebo arm. Only a small percentage of patients (2–4%) did not complete the study due to adverse events and this was comparable in all groups.

The STAR (Solifenacin and Tolterodine as an Active comparator in a Randomized) trial was a prospective double blind, parallel group 12 week study comparing solifenacin 5 and 10 mg once daily to TOLT ER 4 mg once daily (42). After four weeks of treatment, patients were given the option to increase medication dosage. However, only those on solifenacin actually received the dose increase. The results showed non-inferiority of solifenacin's flexible dosing regimen compared to TOLT ER for voiding frequency. Solifenacin showed increased efficacy in decreasing urgency episodes, incontinence, and pad usage compared with TOLT ER. Additionally, more solifenacin patients achieved dryness, as documented by three-day voiding diary, by the end of the study (59% vs. 49%). However, these symptomatic improvements were accompanied by an increase in adverse events with dry mouth and constipation occurring in 30% and 6.4% of the solifenacin group, respectively, versus 23% and 2.5% in the TOLT group. The discontinuation rate was comparably low in both groups.

Efficacy in the mixed urinary incontinence group (43), and the elderly has been shown (44), as has an improvement in HRQL (45).

Tolterodine
TOLT is a tertiary amine with a major active metabolite, 5-HMT, which significantly contributes to the therapeutic effect of the drug (46). Both TOLT and its metabolite have plasma half-lives of two to three hours, but their effects on the bladder seem to be more long lasting. Whether this could be the result of urinary excretion of the drug with direct bladder mucosal effects remains unknown. TOLT does not have muscarinic subtype selectivity but there is evidence in some experimental models that it has functional selectivity for the bladder over the salivary glands (47). This has been shown in the guinea

pig where the binding affinity of TOLT and OXY to muscarinic receptors in the bladder were very similar, but the affinity of TOLT for muscarinic receptors in the parotid gland was eight times lower than that of OXY (48). TOLT is available in two formulations: an IR form prescribed as 2 mg twice daily, and an ER form prescribed as 2 or 4 mg once daily. There appears to be advantages in both efficacy and tolerability with the ER form (49). There appears to be a very low incidence of cognitive side effects with TOLT which is likely due to the low lipophilicity of the drug and its metabolite, minimizing penetration into the CNS (50). A notable subset of patients, up to 10% of whites and up to 19% of blacks, lack the specific CYP enzyme, 2D6, that metabolizes TOLT to 5-HMT (51). In these patients a higher side effect profile, specifically including sleep disturbance, is seen (52). Drugs that do not require CYP2D6 metabolism have the potential for less pharmacokinetic variability.

The efficacy of TOLT has been documented by several double-blind RCT on patients with DO. The OBJECT (Overactive Bladder: Judging Effective Control and Treatment) trial compared TOLT IR 2 mg twice daily to OXY ER 10 mg daily (53). This was a double-blind, parallel group RCT which included 378 patients with OAB treated for 12 weeks. The study showed OXY ER to be significantly more effective than TOLT in reducing UUI episodes, total incontinence, and micturition frequency. The most common adverse event, dry mouth, was reported in 28% of those taking OXY ER and 33% of those taking TOLT IR. Rates of other adverse events including CNS effects were generally low and comparable between the groups.

The OPERA (Overactive Bladder: Performance of Extended Release Agents) trial compared TOLT ER 4 mg daily to OXY ER 10 mg daily in 790 women with OAB symptoms (54). This was a double-blind RCT with duration of 12 weeks. Improvements in UUI episodes were similar between the two groups but cure of UUI was greater in the OXY ER group (23.0% vs. 16.8%). OXY ER was also more effective in reducing micturition frequency at the price of increased rates of dry mouth. Adverse events were mild and occurred at low rates, with both groups having similar rates of discontinuation of treatment.

The ACET (Antimuscarinic Clinical Effectiveness Trial) was an open label study of 1289 patients with OAB comparing TOLT ER 2 or 4 mg daily to OXY 5 or 10 mg daily (55). After eight weeks, 70% of patients taking TOLT ER 4 mg perceived an improved bladder condition compared to 60% in the TOLT ER 2 mg group, 59% in the OXY ER 5 mg group, and 60% in the OXY ER 10 mg group. Dry mouth was dose dependent with both drugs; however, patients treated with TOLT ER 4 mg reported a significantly lower severity of dry mouth compared with OXY ER 10 mg. Fewer patients withdrew from the TOLT ER 4 mg group (12%) than either the OXY ER 5 mg group (19%) or the OXY ER 10 mg group (21%). Although the findings suggest that TOLT ER 4 mg may have improved clinical efficacy and tolerability to OXY ER 10 mg the open label design of this study makes for a less convincing conclusion.

In the IMPACT (Improvement in patients: assessing symptomatic control with TOLT ER) study, the efficacy of TOLT in improving patients' most bothersome symptoms was assessed (56). It found significant reduction in bothersome symptoms whether it be incontinence, urgency episodes, or micturition frequency. Dry mouth occurred in 10% of patients and constipation in 4%.

Conflicting data exists on the concomitant use of TOLT and pelvic floor muscle training. In a prospective, open study of 139 women with OAB who were randomized to TOLT, bladder training or both, combination therapy was found to be most effective (57). Similarly, a multicenter, single-blind study of 505 patients comparing TOLT alone to TOLT plus bladder training concluded that the effectiveness of TOLT can be augmented with the addition of a bladder training regimen (58). However, a similar multinational RCT including 480 patients concluded that no additional benefit was seen with the addition of pelvic floor muscle exercises to TOLT (59).

Trospium

Trospium is a hydrophilic, quaternary amine with limited ability to cross the blood brain barrier. This should result in minimal cognitive related dysfunction (60). Trospium does not have muscarinic subtype selectivity, and unlike the previous antimuscarinics mentioned, is not metabolized by the CYP enzyme system. It is mainly eliminated unchanged in the urine by renal tubular secretion, and as a result, may affect the urothelial mucosal signaling system as has been shown in the rat (61). Whether this contributes to clinical efficacy in humans remains unknown at this time.

In a multicenter, double-blind RCT the effect of trospium on urodynamic parameters was studied in patients with neurogenic DO secondary to spinal cord injury (SCI) (62). A 20 mg dose was given twice daily for three weeks. An increase in maximum cystometric capacity and compliance, and a decrease in maximal detrusor pressure were seen in the treatment group. A similar study compared the use of trospium and OXY in the treatment of neurogenic DO (63). Both medications appeared to have equal effect, but the patients on trospium had fewer side effects. The effectiveness of trospium in the treatment of non-neurogenic DO has also been well documented. Allousi et al. performed a double blind RCT comparing trospium 20 mg twice daily to placebo in 309 patients (64). At three weeks, urodynamic studies revealed an increase in maximum bladder capacity and volume at first IVC in the trospium group. In a study comparing the efficacy of trospium 20 mg twice daily with TOLT 2 mg twice daily and placebo in 232 patients with DO or mixed urinary incontinence, Jünemann and Al-Shukri found trospium to be significantly more effective in decreasing the frequency of micturition than either TOLT or placebo (65). Additionally, trospium caused a greater reduction in incontinence episodes with a similar rate of dry mouth as TOLT.

A long term tolerability and efficacy study comparing trospium 20 mg twice daily and OXY 5 mg twice daily in 358 patients with DO undergoing treatment for 52 weeks was performed (66). Urodynamics and patient recorded voiding diaries were performed at baseline, 26 weeks, and 52 weeks. Mean maximum cystometric capacity increased in the trospium group by 92 ml at 26 weeks and by 115 ml at 52 weeks. No other significant urodynamic differences were seen between the groups. The micturition diaries indicated a reduction in micturition frequency, incontinence frequency, and a reduction in urgency episodes in both treatment groups. At least one adverse event occurred in the majority of patients: 64.8% in the trospium group and

76.6% in the OXY group. The most common side effect in both groups was dry mouth. Overall, both drugs were comparable in the efficacy in improving urinary symptoms, but trospium had a better benefit-risk ratio than OXY due to better tolerability.

An ER formulation of trospium, 60 mg once daily, has been shown in RCTs to have similar efficacy and side effects as the twice daily preparation (67).

Intravesical installation of trospium was studied with a single center, single blind RCT with 84 patients (68). Since intravesical trospium does not seem to be absorbed, an opportunity exists for treatment with minimal systemic antimuscarinic effects (69). Compared to placebo, intravesical trospium produced a significant increase in maximum bladder capacity and a decrease in detrusor pressure. No improvement in uninhibited bladder contractions was seen. No adverse events were reported but, an increase in residual urine was noted. Trospium has not been reported to have resulted in cognitive dysfunction.

Dual Musculotropic Relaxants-Antimuscarinic Agents
Some agents have been identified that have dual mechanisms of action. They have antimuscarinic activity as well as direct musculotropic relaxant effects on the bladder smooth muscle at a site metabolically distal to the antimuscarinic receptor. It is felt that the clinical effects of these drugs are primarily explained by an antimuscarinic action.

Flavoxate
Flavoxate also has direct inhibitory action on smooth muscle along with very weak anticholinergic properties (70). The drug has also been found to possess moderate calcium antagonistic activity, exhibit local anesthetic properties, and have the ability to inhibit phosphodiesterase (PDE) (71). In rats and in cats there is some evidence that flavoxate may also have central effects on the inhibition of the micturition reflex (72,73).

Clinical studies addressing the efficacy of flavoxate in the treatment of OAB/DO have been mixed. In a double-blind crossover study comparing flavoxate 1200 mg daily with OXY 15 mg daily in 41 women with idiopathic DO, both drugs had similar efficacy with flavoxate having fewer and milder side effects (74). A very small study in the elderly population with non-neurogenic DO showed flavoxate had essentially no effect on cystometric capacity and incontinence (75). Chapple et al. also suggest no beneficial effect of flavoxate in the treatment of idiopathic DO (76). In general, few side effects were reported during treatment. No recent RCTs addressing the efficacy of this drug have been performed.

Oxybutynin
OXY is a moderately potent antimuscarinic agent that has strong independent musculotropic relaxant activity as well as local anesthetic activity (that is likely only important during intravesical administration). It is a tertiary amine that is metabolized primarily by the CYP system into its primary metabolite, N-desethyl-oxybutynin (DEO) (77). The recommended oral adult dose for the IR formulation is 5 mg three or four times daily. An ER once daily oral formulation as well as a transdermal delivery system (TDS) with twice weekly

dosing, and a transdermal gel with once daily dosing is available. Side effects are secondary to nonspecific muscarinic receptor binding.

Initial reports documented success in depressing neurogenic DO (78), and subsequent reports documented success in inhibiting idiopathic DO as well (79). A meta-analysis summarizing 15 RCTs (n = 476) reported a 52% mean reduction in incontinence episodes, a 33% mean reduction in micturition frequency, and a mean overall improvement rate of 74%. This came at the expense of a 70% of patients experiencing an adverse event (80).

Holmes and associates compared the results of OXY and propantheline in a small group of women with DO (37). The experimental design was a randomized crossover trial with a patient regulated variable dose regimen. This kind of dose titration study allows the patient to increase the drug dose to whatever is perceived to be the optimum ratio between clinical improvement and side effects. Of the 23 women in the trial, 14 reported subjective improvement with OXY as opposed to 11 with propantheline. Both drugs significantly increased the maximum cystometric capacity and reduced the maximum detrusor pressure on filling. The only significant objective difference was a greater increase in the maximum cystometric capacity with OXY. The mean total daily dose of OXY tolerated was 15 mg (range 7.5–30 mg) and that of propantheline was 90 mg (range 45–145 mg).

The therapeutic effect of OXY IR is associated with a high incidence of side effects which are often dose limiting (81). The ER form of OXY uses an osmotic system to release the active compound at a controlled rate over a period of 24 hours. As a result there is less absorption in the proximal portion of the gastrointestinal tract and less first pass metabolism. By decreasing the liver metabolite DEO it was thought that fewer side effects, especially dry mouth, would occur, thus improving patient compliance (82). Studies looking at salivary output showed markedly diminished production following administration of OXY IR or TOLT IR with gradual return to normal. In OXY ER group salivary output was maintained at pre-dose levels throughout the day (83). OXY IR and ER have been compared in a multicenter, double-blind RCT of 106 patients, all of whom had previously responded to IR OXY (84). Similar efficacy and similar side effect profiles were noted for both formulations.

As noted above in the OBJECT study, OXY 10 mg ER proved superior to TOLT 2 mg IR twice daily with respect to weekly UUI episodes, total incontinence and frequency (53). The two drugs were equally well tolerated. The follow-up OPERA study compared OXY 10 mg ER to TOLT 4 mg ER and found no significant difference in efficacy between the two drugs (54). The incidence of dry mouth was statistically lower in the TOLT group. One general consensus following this study was that IR formulations of one drug should not be compared to ER formulations of another drug.

Three difference doses of OXY (5, 10, and 15 mg) were compared in a RCT and a significant dose-response relationship for both UUI episodes and dry mouth was found. The greatest patient satisfaction was with the 15 mg dose (85).

Transdermal administration of OXY (OXY-TDS) alters the metabolism of the drug further reducing the production of DEO compared to OXY ER. The 3.9 mg daily dose patch decreased both micturition frequency and incontinence episodes while increasing mean voided volume (86). Dry mouth rate was similar to placebo. In a study comparing OXY-TDS to OXY IR similar reductions in incontinence episodes were found but significantly less dry mouth was seen with OXY-TDS (38% vs. 94% with OXY IR) (87). In a third study, OXY-TDS was compared to placebo and TOLT ER (88). Both drugs had similarly significant reduced daily incontinence episodes and increased voided volume, but TOLT ER was associated with a higher rate of adverse events. The major side effect for OXY-TDS was pruritus at the application site in 14% and erythema in 8.3%. The pharmacokinetics of OXY-TDS were studied using blood and saliva samples in a two way crossover RCT with OXY ER (89). The TDS route of administration resulted in greater systemic availability of drug with minimal metabolism to DEO. As a result, patients had greater salivary output and less dry mouth than when taking OXY ER. However, in a review by Cartwright and Cardozo on the published and presented data they concluded that the good balance between efficacy and tolerability with OXY-TDS was offset by the rate of local skin reaction (90).

Intravesical administration of OXY is a conceptually attractive form of drug delivery, especially for patients who already perform CIC. A specific intravesical formulation of the drug is not available and currently the oral formulation, either liquid or crushed tablet in solution, is delivered by periodic insertion through a catheter. Several nonrandomized, unblinded, and non-placebo controlled studies have demonstrated efficacy of this therapy in a variety of patients with neurogenic bladders showing significant improvements in cystometric capacity, volume at first IVC, bladder compliance, and overall continence (91,92). In a study looking at the pharmacokinetics of intravesical OXY versus oral, it was found that plasma OXY levels following oral administration rose to 7.3 mg/ml within two hours then precipitously dropped to <2 mg/ml at four hours (93). In the intravesical group, plasma levels rose gradually to a peak of 6.2 mg/ml at 3.5 hours and remained between 3 and 4 mg/ml at nine hours. From these data it is unclear whether the intravesically applied drug acted locally or systemically.

In a double-blind RCT in 52 women with DO, patients received once daily intravesical OXY (20 mg in 40 ml sterile water) or placebo for 12 days (94). The results revealed significant differences in first desire to void (from 95 ml pretreatment to 150 ml post treatment), cystometric capacity (205–310 ml), maximum pressure during filling (16–9 cmH$_2$0), daytime frequency (7.5–4), and nocturia (5.1–1.8). Side effects were similar in the treated and placebo groups. For unexplained reasons, 19/23 patients in the treated group continued to have symptomatic relief after termination of the study.

OXY topical gel is a new transdermal formulation which is applied once daily to the abdomen, thigh, shoulder or upper arm area (95). The 1-g application dose delivers approximately 4 mg of drug to the circulation with stable plasma concentrations. In a multicenter RCT, 789 patients (89% women) with urge predominant urinary incontinence were assigned to OXY gel or placebo once daily for 12 weeks. Mean number of UUI episodes, as recorded on three-day voiding diary, were reduced by 3.0 episodes/day versus 2.5 in the placebo arm (p < 0.0001). Urinary frequency was decreases by 2.7 episodes/day and voided volume

increased by 21 ml (vs. 2.0 episodes, p = 0.0017 and 3.8 ml, p = 0.0018 in the placebo group, respectively). Dry mouth was reported in 6.9% of the treatment group versus 2.8% of the placebo group. Skin reaction at the application site was reported in 5.4% of the treatment group versus 1.0% in the placebo arm. It is felt that improved skin tolerability of the gel over the OXY TDS delivery system is secondary to lack of adhesive and skin occlusion. The gel dries rapidly upon application and leaves no residue; person to person transference via skin contact is largely eliminated if clothing is worn over the application site.

Propiverine

Propiverine is a musculotropic smooth muscle relaxant with non-selective antimuscarinic activity. Calcium antagonistic properties have also been found, but the importance of this component for the drug's clinical effects has not been established (96). In an analysis of nine RCTs using propiverine in a total of 230 patients, a 17% reduction in micturition frequency was seen. Additionally, there was a 64 ml mean increase in bladder capacity and a 77% subjective improvement rate. Side effects were found in 14% (97). In a study on patients with neurogenic DO, propiverine was found to increase bladder capacity and decrease maximum detrusor contractions compared to placebo (98). Several comparative studies have confirmed the efficacy of propiverine and suggested that the drug may be equally efficacious in increasing bladder capacity and lowering bladder pressure with fewer side effects than OXY (99,100). A study comparing propiverine 15 mg twice daily to TOLT IR 2 mg twice daily showed comparable efficacy, tolerability, and improvement in HRQL (101). In 2006, Abrams and colleagues presented data that refuted these prior studies (102). In a double-blind, placebo-controlled crossover study comparing propiverine 20 mg daily, propiverine 15 mg three times daily, OXY 5 mg three times daily and placebo, propiverine 20 mg daily was inferior to OXY in reducing IVCs. Additionally, propiverine had a more pronounced effect on gastrointestinal, cardiovascular, and visual function.

A large Japanese study of 1584 patients randomized patients to solifenacin 5 or 10 mg, propiverine 20 mg, or placebo (103). All active treatments showed superiority to placebo in reducing voiding frequency, increasing voided volume, and improving HRQL. Solifenacin 10 mg showed greater reduction in nocturia episodes and urgency episodes, and increased volume voided compared to propiverine 20 mg. Side effects were also greater for the solifenacin 10 mg group with more dry mouth and constipation.

Antimuscarinic drugs are proven efficacious and safe, and are the mainstay of treatment for OAB (15). The continuous evolution and development of newer agents stems from the fact that the ideal agent has yet to be found—one that is LUT selective, easily administered, and relatively inexpensive. This search continues and therapies with different mechanisms of action are currently being studied with great promise. Until then, the lessons we have learned from comprehensive systematic review of the literature include (15):

1. Older drugs such as OXY have high withdrawal rates due to side effects while TOLT ER has consistently favorable tolerability

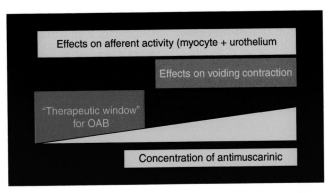

Figure 42.2 Rationale for use of antimuscarinics for treatment of OAB/DO. Blockade of muscarinic receptors at both detrusor and nondetrusor sites may prevent OAB symptoms and DO without depressing the contraction during voiding. *Abbreviations*: OAB, overactive bladder; DO, detrusor overactivity. *Source*: Adapted from Ref. 12.

2. Newer agents such as darifenacin, solifenacin, and fesoterodine provide dose flexibility to allow individual titration for maximal efficacy versus tolerability
3. Once a day dosing appears to be better tolerated and potentially more efficacious in improving symptoms and HRQL

However, head to head studies comparing all of these agents are not available.

Three specific areas of concern with antimuscarinic medication deserve special mention: urinary retention, cognitive impairment, and glaucoma.

In the past there was universal concern regarding the risk of urinary retention when prescribing antimuscarinic drugs. However, as Andersson and Wein (11) and Andersson et al. (12) propose, these drugs are usually competitive antagonists which imply that when there is massive release of ACh during voiding, the effect of the drug should be diminished. If this did not occur, urinary retention would result from inability of the bladder to contract. And in fact, at high doses urinary retention can occur but this is uncommon at the doses typically prescribed for DO (11). Figure 42.2 illustrates our current understanding regarding the dose range used for beneficial effects in OAB/DO, and those needed to produce a significant reduction in the voiding contraction. Monitoring post void residuals (PVRs) in patients with prostatic enlargement or incomplete bladder emptying is still recommended; however, these diagnoses should not be considered as absolute contraindications to the use of antimuscarinics.

More recently, concern over the association of anticholinergics and cognitive impairment has prompted several studies evaluating reaction time, memory, confusion, and other cognitive decrements. In a longitudinal cohort study involving 372 adults age >60 years without dementia at recruitment, the effects of continuous anticholinergic drug use on cognition was assessed (104). Eighty percent of anticholinergic users were classified as having mild cognitive impairment compared with only 35% of non-users. There was no difference between users and non-users in the risk of developing dementia after eight years of follow-up. Other studies in continent elderly volunteers have shown no significant effects on cognition (27).

There are few data available on the cognitive consequences of anticholinergics in patients with dementia. However, cholinesterase inhibitors which are often used to improve cognition in Alzheimer's disease have been shown to precipitate urinary incontinence (105).

Patients with OAB and glaucoma present another therapeutic dilemma for urologists. Both conditions increase in prevalence with age and it has been estimated that the conditions co-exist in approximately 11.6% of female patients (in Japan) (106). The distinction between open angle and narrow angle glaucoma is an important one, and when the answer is unknown referral to an ophthalmologist is imperative. A Japanese study reported that in approximately 75% of patients with glaucoma and OAB, the glaucoma is open angle, and this was felt to confer no additional risk to therapeutic intervention with anticholinergic medication. In the remaining 25% with narrow angle glaucoma, risk was felt to be elevated only if iridotomy has not been performed or has not successfully controlled the disease, reducing the true contraindication rate to approximately 8.3% of patients with OAB. Interestingly, the same study found that 33% of patients did not report glaucoma on their medical intake form. Underestimating the risk of glaucoma can result in blindness, albeit rarely, while overestimating (which often occurs out of fear) can result in denial of the most effective oral agents for the treatment of OAB. Complaints of eye pain, headache, or visual loss following initiation of anticholinergic therapy should be taken seriously and prompt medical advice should be sought (107).

Calcium Antagonists
Calcium channels and free intracellular calcium play a large role in excitation-contraction coupling in striated, cardiac, and smooth muscle (108). Inhibitors of calcium channels have repeatedly been shown to inhibit bladder contraction in vitro (109), suggesting a possible role in the treatment of DO and incontinence; however, only limited clinical studies are available. Common side effects include headache, dizziness, flushing, and peripheral edema. These drugs are contraindicated in patients with poor cardiac conduction and those taking β-blockers (110).

Nifedipine
Nifedipine has been shown to be effective in inhibiting contraction in human and guinea pig bladder muscle (111). It has also been shown to completely block the non-cholinergic portion of contraction in the rabbit bladder (112). These data suggest a potential role for nifedipine in controlling "atropine resistant" contractions, possibly in combination with an antimuscarinic agent. No clinical data is available to support this view.

Nimodipine
A double-blind, crossover RCT of 30 mg of nimodipine versus placebo in 86 patients with DO was performed (113). There was no significant difference in number of incontinent episodes or scores on validated questionnaires in those patients on treatment versus placebo.

Verapamil

Intravesical verapamil was compared to intravesical OXY, intravesical trospium, and placebo in 84 patients with urgency or UUI (114). While OXY and trospium both significantly increased bladder capacity, decreased detrusor pressure, and decreased IVCs, verapamil did not.

There is no agent that will specifically block intracellular calcium release only in the bladder smooth muscle cells. Presently, there is no clinical evidence to support the use of calcium channel inhibitors in the treatment of bladder dysfunction.

Potassium-Channel Openers

Similar to calcium channels, potassium channels also contribute to the membrane potential of smooth muscle cells and as a result affect smooth muscle tone. Potassium channel openers relax various types of smooth muscle, including the detrusor, by increasing potassium efflux (79). Several types of potassium channel openers exist and at least two types, ATP dependant and big calcium activated, have been shown to induce bladder smooth muscle relaxation and reduce spontaneous contractions in human and other mammalian detrusor muscle (115). Potassium channel openers are not specific for the bladder however and are more potent in relaxing other tissues. In particular, potassium channels are expressed in vascular smooth muscle producing side effects on cardiovascular function, with potentially significant lowering of blood pressure (116). Common side effects of this class of drug include headaches, flushing, reflex tachycardia, edema, angina, and hypertrichosis (117).

Chromakalim and Levcromakalim

Chromakalim was evaluated in 16 patients with refractory DO or neurogenic DO who had stopped other drug therapy due to intolerable side effects (118). Six patients (38%) showed a decrease in micturition frequency and an increase in volume voided. Long-term observation was not possible because the drug was withdrawn from the market owing to reported adverse effects of high doses in animal toxicology studies.

Levcromakalim was administered intravenously to six patients with SCI and neurogenic DO (119). An increase in the duration of detrusor contraction was seen but no other effects on urodynamic parameters were appreciated. A significant drop in blood pressure was seen precluding studies at a higher dose.

Pinacidil

Pinacidil is a potassium channel opener that inhibits spontaneous myogenic contractions as well as contractile responses induced by electrical field stimulation and carbachol in isolated human detrusor (120). A double-blind, crossover study in nine patients with DO and BOO failed to show any effects of pinacidil 25 mg daily on symptoms (121). A significant decrease in standing blood pressure with stable heart rate was reported.

ZD0947

A double-blind, placebo-controlled phase II study evaluated the efficacy and safety of ZD0947 at a dose of 25 mg daily for 12 weeks (122). Results showed no improvement in voided volume, micturition frequency, or incontinence episodes.

Despite promising preclinical efficacy data, presently potassium channel openers are not a therapeutic option due to a lack of selectivity for bladder over cardiovascular tissues.

Prostaglandin and Cyclo-oxygenase Inhibitors

Prostaglandins (PGs) can be synthesized from the human bladder and released in response to different types of trauma (123). They appear to cause contraction of bladder muscle but it is unclear if PGs contribute to the pathogenesis of DO. Possible sensitization of sensory afferent nerves by PGs has been suggested by Andersson (79). This would essentially increase the afferent input produced by a given degree of bladder filling contributing to the triggering of IVCs at a small bladder volume. Provided this theory is correct, PG synthesis inhibitors should decrease bladder contractility in response to various stimuli. However, clinical evidence for this is scant. Common side effects include: hypertension, headache, diarrhea, dyspepsia, nausea, gastroesophageal reflux, and arthralgias. These drugs are contraindicated in renal impairment, advanced liver disease, congestive heart failure, and in the peri-operative setting following coronary artery bypass surgery (124).

Flurbiprofen

Flurbiprofen is a PG synthesis inhibitor. A double-blind RCT evaluated the effects of flurbiprofen 50 mg three times daily in women with DO (125). The results showed a favorable effect of the drug on delaying the intravesical pressure rise to a larger volume but did not abolish IVCs. There was a 43% incidence of side effects, primarily nausea, vomiting, headache, and gastrointestinal symptoms.

Indomethacin

A single-blind, cross-over RCT in 32 patients with neurogenic DO compared indomethacin 50 to 100 mg daily to bromocriptine. Results showed symptomatic relief in daytime micturition frequency and nocturia in the indomethacin group. There was no urodynamic data reported. The incidence of side effects was high, occurring in 19 of 32 patients; no patients withdrew from the study.

Numerous PG synthesis inhibitors exist, most of which belong to the category of nonsteroidal anti-inflammatory drugs, but few have been studied in the treatment of DO. Despite the recent rage over cyclo-oxygenase inhibitors in many fields of medicine, no new RCTs in patients with DO have been published in the last decade.

β-Adrenergic Agonists

We have yet to prove whether the sympathetic nervous system plays an active rolling in filling/storage of the bladder in humans; however, the presence of β adrenoceptors (AR) in human bladder muscle prompted many attempts to increase bladder capacity with β adrenergic stimulation. Such stimulation can cause significant increases in the capacity of animal bladders which contain a moderate density of β AR (1). In vitro studies show a strong dose-related relaxant effect of β_2 agonists on the bladder body of rabbits but little effect on the bladder base or proximal urethra. Receptor binding studies suggest that the β AR of the human detrusor are primarily of the β_2

subtype and favorable effects have been reported in patients with DO with the use of selective β_2 agonists (108,126). More recently attention has turned to β_3 AR agonists after real time reverse transcriptase-polymerase chain reaction data revealed a predominant expression of β_3 AR mRNA in human detrusor muscle (127). Common side effects include: tachycardia, hypotension, headache, gastrointestinal effects, nervousness, palpitations, elevated serum glucose and lactate, and decreased serum potassium and calcium. These drugs are contraindicated in patients with cardiac arrhythmias associated with tachycardia (128).

Clenbuterol

Clenbuterol is a selective β_2 agonist. A double-blind, controlled study in women with UUI showed clenbuterol 0.01 mg three times daily had good therapeutic effect in 15 of the 20 patients (129). This drug is not available in the United States.

Terbutaline

Terbutaline, a β_2 agonist, has been reported to have a beneficial clinical effect at an oral dose of 5 mg three times a day (126). In 15 patients evaluated, 12 became subjectively continent. Of the eight patients with documented urodynamic DO, six had stabilization of the detrusor on repeat evaluation. In nine patients, transient side effects including palpitations, tachycardia, or hand tremor occurred.

Selective β_3 Agonists (GW427353: Solabegron, YM178: Acetanilide)

Several selective β_3 AR agonists are being evaluated in human clinical trial for the potential treatment of DO. In isolated human detrusor muscle, GW427353 and YM178 were found to mediate muscle relaxation (130,131). YM178 was evaluated in patients with DO in a RCT versus TOLT and placebo (132). The treatment group experienced a significant reduction in micturition frequency, incontinence episodes, and urgency symptoms, as well as an increase in volume voided. The drug was well tolerated in this study with the most common side effects being headache and gastrointestinal effects. Further studies are needed to determine whether this class of drugs is truly efficacious in the treatment of OAB/DO and whether they are equivalent or superior to currently available alternatives in terms of efficacy, tolerability, and safety.

Antidepressants

Several antidepressants have been found to have beneficial effects in patients with OAB/DO (1). These effects include facilitating urine storage by decreasing bladder contractility and increasing outlet resistance. In general, these agents have two major pharmacologic actions. They have anticholinergic effects both centrally and peripherally, and they block the reuptake of serotonin and noradrenaline (133). The most common side effect include: nausea, followed by dry mouth, dizziness, constipation, insomnia, and fatigue. Tricyclic antidepressants (TCAs) can have cardiotoxic side effects, as well as CNS effects including weakness, Parkinsonian effects, fine tremor, manic or schizophrenic picture, and sedation (133). The use of TCAs in conjunction with monoamine oxidase

inhibitors is contraindicated. In general, the doses given for the treatment of DO are much lower than those prescribed for depression. Whether the same toxicity profile exists for these drugs at the lower dose remains to be seen.

Doxepin

Doxepin is a TCA that has been found to be more potent than other tricyclic compounds with respect to antimuscarinic and musculotropic relaxant activity (134). In a double-blind, crossover RCT of women with IVCs and frequency, urgency, or UUI, found that this agent caused a significant decrease in nighttime frequency and incontinence episodes (135). There was a near significant decrease in urine loss measured by pad weight and in cystometric parameters of first sensation and maximum bladder capacity. Doxepin treatment was preferred by 14 of the 19 patients, while two preferred placebo, and three had no preference. Twelve patients claimed they became continent during treatment.

Duloxetine

Duloxetine is a combined serotonin-norepinephrine re-uptake inhibitor (SNRI) which has been shown to increase both bladder capacity and sphincteric muscle activity during filling and storage in the cat (136). The data to support its role in increasing outlet resistance will be presented later. A RCT on 306 women with OAB looked at the effects of duloxetine 80 mg daily for four weeks, followed by 120 mg daily for eight weeks (137). The duloxetine group showed significant improvement in number of voids and incontinence episodes, voiding interval, and HRQL. No urodynamic indices showed improvement. The product information for this drug contains a black box warning due to increased suicidal thinking and behavior in those taking the drug for psychiatric disorders.

Imipramine

Imipramine is a TCA that has been widely used clinically to treat DO despite no good RCTs to document its effects. Imipramine has prominent systemic anticholinergic effects but only a weak anti-muscarinic effect on bladder smooth muscle (138). The effect of imipramine on noradrenalin reuptake is non-selective, and direct evidence suggesting it occurs in the LUT as well as the brain has been provided (139).

Clinically, imipramine seems to be effective in decreasing bladder contractility and increasing outlet resistance. In a study of elderly patients with DO, imipramine 25 mg nightly was given and increased by 25 mg every three days until either the patient was continent, had side effects or a dose of 150 mg was reached (140). Six of ten patients became continent. In those patients who underwent repeated cystometry, bladder capacity increased by a mean of 105 ml and bladder pressure at capacity decreased by a mean of 18 cmH$_2$0. In our experience, the effects of imipramine on the LUT are often additive to those of antimuscarinic agents; however, it should be noted that the anticholinergic side effects may also be additive. A combination of low dose imipramine and an antimuscarinic or an antispasmodic has been reported as useful for decreasing bladder contractility and detrusor pressure in some neurogenic patients (141). However, serious toxic side effects can occur with therapeutic

428

doses of imipramine, including orthostatic hypotension, ventricular arrhythmias, and prolongation of the QT interval. A proper risk-benefit analysis of imipramine in a good quality clinical trial has not been performed.

Phosphodiesterase Inhibitors
PDE inhibitors were initially prescribed for the treatment of erectile dysfunction (ED) and found incidentally to improve LUT symptoms in men (142). LUT smooth muscle undergoes relaxation in the presence of cyclic adenosine monophosphate (cAMP) and cyclic guanosine monophosphate (cGMP) (143). PDE inhibitors block the degradation of cAMP and cGMP resulting in greater intracellular concentrations. Side effects include: headache, flushing, dyspepsia, vision changes, and myalgias. This class of drug is contraindicated in patients taking nitrates (34).

Sildenafil
A RCT evaluated the effects of sildenafil on ED and LUT symptoms in 189 men. Significant improvements in International Prostate Symptom Score (IPSS) and HRQL were seen (144). In the first RCT looking at sildenafil and voiding dysfunction in women, no significant differences were seen in patients with complete retention, partial retention, or obstructed voiding (145).

Tadalafil
A RCT comparing tadalafil to placebo in 281 men with ED and lower urinary tract symptoms (LUTS) produced clinically meaningful and significant symptomatic improvement in LUTS (146). The drug was well tolerated with mild side effects.

Vardenafil
In another RCT, vardenafil 10 mg twice daily in men with ED and LUTS showed a significant improvement in IPSS and HRQL (147).

Vinpocetine
The PDE-1 inhibitor vinpocetine was evaluated in a multicenter, double-blind RCT in patients with urgency and UUI with urodynamically documented DO who failed anticholinergic therapy (148). The patients received either vinpocetine 20 mg three times daily or placebo. The results showed a significant reduction in micturition frequency in men; however, the remainder of assessed outcomes showed a trend toward improvement without reaching significance. The lack of side effects indicate that the dose delivered may have been too low.

While large scale studies in women using PDE inhibitors for DO have yet to be done, the early data in men suggest a possible role in the treatment of bladder diseases. The mechanism of action to produce this beneficial effect in OAB remains unknown at this time. Few data are available regarding use in women.

Botulinum Toxin
Botulinum toxin (BTX) is a neurotoxin produced by *Clostridium botulinum* and is a potent presynaptic inhibitor of ACh release at the neuromuscular junction of muscle. It is applied directly by cystoscopic injection into the detrusor muscle producing a chemical denervation which is reversible after approximately six months. Intravesical administration allows for high concentrations of the agent to reach the bladder tissue without systemic administration and resultant unsuitable levels in other organs. BTX is considered second line therapy in patients who are refractory to conventional oral antimuscarinic therapy or who do not tolerate it due to systemic side effects.

There are seven subtypes of BTX with subtype A (BTX-A) being the most relevant clinically. BTX-A is available under at least three different trade names, Botox®, Dysport®, and Xeomin®, and it has been found that these formulations are not equivalent. The vast majority of intravesical experience has been with Botox, with no bladder experience reported for Xeomin. Botox appears to be approximately three times more potent than Dysport (149).

The dose and injection protocol for BTX has not been universally agreed upon and several variations exist. In the initial description, 300 Units (U) of BTX-A was diluted in normal saline to a concentration of 10 U/ml. Under direct cystoscopic visualization using a 6F injection needle, 30 injections of 1 ml each were administered to the bladder wall in 30 different locations above the trigone (150). Since that description, several other authors have described varying doses, dilutions, number of sites, and locations (trigone, suburothelial space).

In a prospective, non-randomized trial of 21 patients with neurogenic DO secondary to SCI, 200 to 300 U of BTX-A was administered (150). Seventeen patients were completely continent and had stopped all oral agents for their DO at six weeks follow-up. Urodynamics demonstrated an increase in mean bladder capacity and PVR, and a decrease in maximum voiding pressure.

A large multicenter, non-controlled trial including 231 neurogenic patients, most with SCI, was conducted in Europe (151). Botox 300 U was injected supratrigonally in 30 locations. Follow-up was available on 200 patients and revealed marked improvement with respect to continence in all patients. Urodynamic evaluation 12 weeks after injection revealed significant increases in maximum cystometric capacity, PVR, and compliance. These changes were observed up to 36 weeks after injection. No injection related complications or toxin side effects were reported. This study still represents the largest trial with BTX-A conducted. Several other non-controlled studies have been published confirming these observations (152).

The onset of BTX-A effects is seen within the first two weeks after injection (152). Urgency, nocturia, and frequency have been shown to improve as early as two days after BTX-A injection in neurogenic DO patients (153). The reported duration of BTX-A following the first injection was six to nine months (152) and duration of effect along with beneficial clinical effect after subsequent injections is maintained (154).

In a double-blind RCT including 34 patients with idiopathic DO refractory to antimuscarinics, 200 U of BTX-A was studied (155). Significant improvements in maximum cystometric capacity, frequency, and incontinence episodes were seen at 4 and 12 weeks. Despite clinical improvement, six patients (37.5%) required CIC to empty the bladder. In another RCT, 28 women with refractory idiopathic DO received BTX-A 200 U and

15 received placebo (156). Approximately 60% of the women who received BTX-A reported a clinical response with a mean duration of response of 373 days (compared to 62 days or less for placebo). PVR urine was increased in 43% of women in the treatment group and urinary tract infections occurred in 75% of these women. The duration of retention following the first injection was approximately two months; however, following repeat injection this duration increased to five months.

Given the degree of voiding dysfunction seen after BTX injection in patients with idiopathic DO, dose reductions studies looking at 100 U have been done. In a prospective, non-randomized study including 100 men and women, 100 U of BTX-A was injected in 30 locations (157). At 4 and 12 weeks follow-up, 88% of patients showed significant improvement in bladder function in regard to subjective symptoms, urodynamic parameters, and HRQL. There were four cases of urinary retention.

Side effects of intravesical BTX include: elevated PVR, urinary retention, and urinary tract infection (158)

BTX appears to be a promising therapy in the treatment of neurogenic and idiopathic DO. Further studies are needed to determine optimum dosages, locations, and methods of injection. The case for usage in neurogenic OAB/DO patients on CIC who leak between catheterizations seems clearer than in patients with idiopathic OAB/DO, in whom the PVR issue has yet to be clarified.

Polysynaptic Inhibitors
Baclofen
Baclofen depresses synaptic excitation of motor neurons in the spinal cord and normalizes interneuron activity (159). It has been found useful for the treatment of skeletal spasticity due to a variety of causes, and oral baclofen was tried in patients with idiopathic DO however, its efficacy was poor likely due to the fact that it does not cross the blood brain barrier (160). Intrathecal baclofen has been shown to be useful in some patients with spasticity and bladder dysfunction (161). All patients reported marked symptomatic improvement. Increases in bladder compliance and capacity were seen. Side effects of baclofen include: drowsiness, vertigo, insomnia, weakness, ataxia, slurred speech, and psychiatric disturbances (162).

Other Potential Agents
Estrogen
The hormonally sensitive tissues of the bladder, urethra, and pelvic floor may play a role in voiding mechanisms. Noteworthy scientific work has been done looking at the effects of estrogen and its receptors on the LUT. Two types of estrogen receptors (α and β) have been identified in the trigone of the bladder, urethra, vagina, levator ani muscles, pelvic fascia, and the supporting ligaments (163). In fact, all four layers of the urethra (epithelium, vasculature, connective tissue, and muscle) are estrogen sensitive and thought to play a role in maintaining positive urethral pressure. Menopause causes marked decline in the presence and expression of both α and β-receptor subtypes. Epidemiologic studies have implicated estrogen deficiency, as a result of menopause, in the etiology of voiding symptoms that occur as women age. However, the role of estrogen replacement for the treatment of LUT symptoms remains controversial.

It has been recognized that estrogen therapy has little effect in the management of SUI (this topic will be addressed further below) (164). Estrogen may be of benefit in treatment of irritative voiding symptoms including urgency, frequency, and UUI. It is unclear whether this is the effect of the drug on the reversal of urogenital atrophy or direct action on the LUT. One difficulty in interpreting the available conflicting data on the topic is the use of several difference estrogen preparations, doses, routes of administration, and the inconsistent use of concomitant progesterone. There is good evidence that urogenital atrophy, both the symptoms and cytological changes, can be reversed by treatment with low dose vaginal estrogen.

Estrogen is hypothesized to be able to affect LUT symptoms by several potential mechanisms including: increasing urethral resistance, raising the sensory threshold of the bladder (165), and by promoting relaxation of the bladder via the β_3 AR (166). In the ovariectomized rabbit, estrogen replacement has been shown to decrease muscarinic receptor density thereby diminishing contractile response (167). Estradiol has also been found to reduce the frequency and amplitude of rabbit spontaneous rhythmic detrusor contractions (168).

In the human clinical literature, conflicting data on the efficacy sustained release 17β-estradiol vaginal tablets for urgency and UUI exists. Cardozo et al. performed a RCT in 110 women with urgency, frequency, and UUI (169). After three months of treatment they were unable to show objective evidence of a reduction in urinary frequency or urgency. In a subset of patients with pretreatment urodynamic urgency without DO, visual analog scales post-treatment showed a reduction in urgency symptoms. The authors hypothesized that the symptomatic improvement in this group was likely related to the treatment of their urogenital atrophy. They concluded that "improvement in LUT pathology can not be expected unless it is due to estrogen deficiency." A further RCT on 154 women using the same estrogen preparation showed a significant improvement in subjective frequency, urgency, and urge and SUI. No urodynamic assessment was performed in this study (170).

A systematic review of the effects of estrogen on OAB was performed by Cardozo et al. and identified 11 RCTs with 236 women receiving estrogen and 230 placebo controls (171). Statistically significant improvements in urinary frequency, urgency, number of incontinence episodes, first sensation to void, and bladder capacity were found for patients taking estrogen therapy. Separate analysis for systemic and locally applied estrogen revealed that local therapy, but not systemic, had a significant beneficial effect on all outcome variables. Systemic estrogen did have a beneficial impact on incontinence episodes and first sensation to void.

Major concerns about the use of estrogen must be addressed. Common adverse effects include: anxiety, insomnia, irritability, mood disturbances, melasma, rash, pruritis, breast enlargement, breast pain, increase in high-density lipoprotein cholesterol and triglycerides, glucose intolerance, hot flashes, change in libido, dysmenorrhea, vaginal discharge, and arthralgias. Estrogen is contraindicated in women with hepatic dysfunction. Results of the Women's Health Initiative (WHI) study clearly established a small but significant increase in the risk of breast cancer in estrogen-progestin combination therapy given for >3 years (172). Unopposed estrogen in postmenopausal women increases the risk of endometrial carcinoma by 5 to 15 fold. However, co-administration with progestin eliminates this risk (172). The Heart and Estrogen Replacement Study (HERS) together with results of WHI unequivocally establish that combination estrogen-progestin does not protect against coronary heart disease (172). The risk of thromboembolic disease is clearly elevated in women taking oral estrogens with a history of preexisting cardiovascular disease (172).

The female LUT is greatly influenced by estrogen throughout life. The LUT symptoms that temporally coincide with menopause may or may not be the result of estrogen deficiency. Regardless, estrogen replacement has produced conflicting results in improving symptoms. Most authors believe that urogenital atrophy is the result of estrogen deficiency and responds well to estrogen replacement, especially locally. In some cases irritative urologic symptoms (usually in combination with vaginal symptoms) may result from atrophy and may respond to estrogen therapy (173). At the current time, there is little evidence to support the primary use of estrogen therapy alone for the treatment of OAB symptoms. Further studies are needed to define its role as an adjuvant therapy in the treatment of OAB and perhaps provide a strong argument for primary use. Of great interest would be a study looking at the role of prophylactic estrogen versus that of therapeutic estrogen on LUT symptom development and progression.

Gabapentin
Gabapentin was originally designed as an anticonvulsant, but now has expanded indications for neuropathic pain, anxiety, and sleep disorders (174). In a study of 16 patients with neurogenic DO the efficacy of gabapentin was explored (175). Results showed significant improvement in urodynamic parameters, particularly IVCs, and a reduction in irritative voiding symptoms. No adverse events were recorded. The authors hypothesized that DO may be controlled by modulating the afferent input from the bladder and the excitability of the sacral reflex center. In a second study of 31 patients with refractory OAB, 14 patients reported subjective improvement of their frequency (176). Eight of these patients were still on the drug one year later with persistent efficacy. Adverse effects of gabapentin include: somnolence, dizziness, ataxia, fatigue, diarrhea, tremor, and nystagmus (177). Further studies which include a clarification of the recommended dosages are needed.

NK1-Receptor Antagonists (Aprepitant)
Tachykinins are a class of neuropeptides that includes substance P, neurokinin A, and neurokinin B which function as sensory neurotransmitters. Their respective receptors, NK1, NK2, and NK3, are found in various areas of the brain and spinal cord and may play a role in DO (178). NK1 and NK2 receptor antagonists were administered to rats undergoing awake cystometry and both a dose dependent decrease in detrusor pressure and an increase in bladder capacity were

seen (179). A combination of the two drugs caused an additive effect. In animals with BOO, the antagonists produced urinary retention at a high rate. The authors concluded that NK1 and NK2 receptors may be involved in micturition control.

Aprepitant, an NK1 receptor antagonist used to treat nausea and vomiting in patients on chemotherapy, was found to improve OAB symptoms in a double-blind RCT of 125 postmenopausal women (180). The drug significantly decreased micturition frequency and number of urgency episodes as reported on a 4 to 10 day voiding diary. Despite statistical significance, the clinical significance of these findings is questionable. With respect to micturition frequency, a reduction of 1.3 episodes/day was seen in the treatment group compared to 0.4 episodes/day in the placebo group. Urgency episodes were reduced by 1.8/day in the treatment group and 0.5/day in the placebo group. The mean number of UUI episodes and total urinary incontinence were also reduced in the treatment group (−1.5 vs. −1.1 and −1.5 vs. −1.2, respectively), although not significantly. Aprepitant was well tolerated in this study. The results of this pilot study suggest that NK1 receptor antagonists may hold promise as a novel therapeutic approach to treating OAB. An NK1 antagonist is currently in phase 2 trial for the treatment of OAB. Side effects include: fatigue, nausea, constipation, diarrhea, weakness, hiccups, hypotension, dizziness, dyspepsia, neutropenia, leucopenia, and proteinuria (181).

Tramadol
Tramadol is a widely prescribed analgesic that is centrally acting and has dual mechanisms of action (182). The drug is a weak opioid receptor agonist but its metabolites are nearly as effective as morphine at the opioid receptor. Additionally, the drug and its metabolites inhibit serotonin and noradrenalin reuptake. This drug profile may be particularly useful in the treatment of DO as shown in a RCT with duloxetine (137). Animal studies have shown that tramadol abolishes experimentally induced DO (183). In a double-blind RCT of 76 patients with idiopathic DO, tramadol 100 mg twice daily caused significant reduction in frequency and number of incontinence episodes (184). Urodynamic parameters also showed improvement. Side effects of this drug include: flushing, dizziness, headache, insomnia, somnolence, pruritus, constipation, nausea, vomiting, dyspepsia, hot flashes, diaphoresis, and weakness (185).

Increasing Bladder Capacity/Decreasing Sensory Input
Vanilloids
Relatively recently, the concept of blocking afferent nerves as a mechanism for controlling the micturition reflex has gained momentum as a potential therapeutic target in the treatment of OAB. Afferent blockade would, at least in theory, be more desirable since it would block the micturition reflex rather than blocking the contraction of the detrusor.

There appears to be an upregulation of C-fiber afferent neurons in the bladders of patients with SCI (186), chronic BOO (187), and those with idiopathic DO (188). It has also been found that these upregulated C-fibers, in the bladders of patients with neurogenic DO, have increased expression of the vanilloid receptor, transient receptor potential vanilloid-1 (TRPV1) (189). This receptor naturally responds to noxious stimuli including acidic pH, high temperatures and spicy peppers (190). A number of vanilloids, most notably capsaicin and resiniferatoxin (RTX) can also bind to this receptor creating an inhibitory effect. Side effects of these drugs tend to be local in nature and may include transient burning and stinging, elevated PVR, urinary retention, and urinary tract infections.

BTX

As mentioned above BTX produces a muscular paralysis in the bladder that improves DO. Additionally, BTX-A may decrease levels of neurotrophic agents in the bladder decreasing visceral afferent nerve transmission. Nerve growth factor (NGF), one of these agents, is important in sensory nerve growth, maintenance, and plasticity. Generally, patients with neurogenic DO are found to produce greater levels of NGF in the bladder than controls. A significant decrease in NGF can be detected after intravesical administration of BTX pointing to another possible mechanism whereby BTX acts on the bladder (191).

Capsaicin

Capsaicin binds to TRPV1 and causes depolarization and excitation of sensory nerve fibers followed by a refractory period. Repeated or high dose exposure causes desensitization, inactivating the nerve terminal. Systemic and topical capsaicin produce a reversible anti-nociceptive and anti-inflammatory action after an initially undesirable analgesic effect (192). In a non-controlled study of six patients, intravesical instillation of capsaicin (0.1–10 μM) produced a dose related reduction in first desire to void, bladder capacity, and voiding pressure (193). Five patients reported marked attenuation of symptoms beginning two to three days after instillation and lasting for 4 to 16 days; after that time the symptoms gradually reappeared but were no worse. During instillation patients reported a warm burning sensation in the suprapubic area that was felt in the urethra during voiding. Fowler and colleagues (194) reported considerably higher doses (1 or 2 mmol/l) in 12 patients with SCI and intractable urinary incontinence and two patients with idiopathic DO. Nine patients showed improvement in bladder function lasting for between three weeks and six months. Urodynamics revealed an increase in bladder capacity and a decrease in maximum detrusor pressure. There were no reported complications. In a larger study on 79 patients with five-year follow-up, De Ridder and colleagues found intravesical administration of 1 to 2 mmol/l of capsaicin produced complete continence in 44% of patients, satisfactory improvement in 36%, and failure in 20% (195). Clinical benefit from single instillation lasted three to six months. Other studies have shown no beneficial effects of capsaicin with marked reactive changes of the urothelium (196). Only one RCT has compared capsaicin to 30% ethanol, the vehicle solution (197). The 10 patients randomized to capsaicin had significant decreases in voiding frequency, urinary leakage, and maximum detrusor pressure and significant increase in cystometric capacity. These changes were not seen

in the control group who received the vehicle, 30% ethanol. Side effects consisted primarily of instillation triggered suprapubic pain, urgency, hematuria, and autonomic dysreflexia and were seen in seven patients from each group. The authors concluded that the side effects of capsaicin are attributable to the vehicle. Further studies by the same group showed that 1 mmol/l capsaicin diluted in glucidic solvent produced favorable and similar results as RTX 100 nMol/l diluted in 10% ethanol (198). Neither group experienced significant side effects and the tolerance of the new capsaicin solvent was excellent.

RTX

RTX is an analog of capsaicin that is approximately 1000 times more potent for desensitization, but much less potent for excitation (199). Several small, open label studies showed beneficial effects of RTX with reduction in micturition frequency and incontinence episodes (198). In a double-blind, placebo-controlled trial of RTX in 28 patients with neurogenic DO, a significant decrease in micturition frequency and incontinence episodes, and an increase in bladder capacity were seen (200). In a study comparing RTX to BTX-A in patients with neurogenic DO, both neurotoxins improved bladder capacity and reduced the number of incontinence episodes (201). BTX-A, however, was considered more effective. In 54 patients with idiopathic DO, a RCT showed RTX is effective in improving incontinence (202). Rios and colleagues however were unable to replicate those results in their RCT of 58 patients with idiopathic DO (203). They showed no significant difference between a single dose of RTX 50 nM and placebo. The variability in clinical results may stem from the fact that different origins of RTX and different preparation techniques may cause substantial differences in the amount of drug actually delivered.

Overall, intravesical capsaicin and RTX may be promising therapy for DO and possibly sensory dysfunction of the LUT; however, many problems exist. Optimal dosage, method, and timing of delivery, as well as delivery vehicle remain unclear. TRPV1 antagonists that block rather than desensitize the receptor are entering preliminary clinical trials.

Increasing Outlet Resistance

As mentioned above, decreased outlet resistance may manifest from damage to the smooth or striated sphincter secondary to surgical, obstetric, or other mechanical trauma, or degeneration of innervation with loss of neuronal mass secondary to neurologic disease, aging or trauma (4). In addition, in women it may result from decreased pelvic floor support of the bladder outlet. Clinically, this manifests as effort related or SUI or, when severe, as complete gravitational incontinence. Treatment is aimed at increasing outlet resistance. Outlet resistance, at least as reflected by urethral pressure measurements, does not seem to be clinically affected by anticholinergic therapy.

Alpha-adrenergic Agonists

The bladder neck and proximal urethra contain a preponderance of α-adrenergic receptor sites, which, when stimulated, produce smooth muscle contraction and an increase in maximal urethral pressure (MUP) and maximal urethral closure pressure (MUCP) (1). α-Adrenergic stimulation generally increase outlet resistance to a variable degree but are most often limited by their potential side-effects including blood pressure elevation, anxiety, insomnia, headache, tremor, weakness, palpitations, cardiac arrhythmia, and respiratory difficulties. These agents should be used with caution in patients with hypertension, cardiovascular disease, and hyperthyroidism (204).

Ephedrine

The use of ephedrine to treat SUI was mentioned as early as 1948 (204). This is a non-catecholamine sympathomimetic agent that enhances release of noradrenalin from sympathetic neurons and directly stimulates both α and β-ARs. The oral adult dosage is 25–50 mg four times daily (205). In 38 patients with sphincteric incontinence treated with ephedrine sulfate, 27 reported "good-to-excellent" results. The beneficial effects were most often achieved in those with minimal to moderate incontinence symptoms; little benefit was achieved in patients with severe SUI (205).

Midodrine

Midodrine is a long acting α-adrenergic agonist reported to be useful in the treatment of seminal emission and ejaculation disorders following retroperitoneal lymphadenectomy. Treatment with 5 mg twice a day for four weeks in 20 patients with SUI produced a cure in 1 and improvement in 14. The MUCP rose by 8.3% and the planometric index of the continence area on profilometry increased by 9% (206).

Norfenefrine

Norfenefrine is an α-agonist given as a slow release tablet. In a study on 20 women with SUI treated with norfenefrine, 19 reported reduced urinary leakage with 10 reporting resolution of their incontinence (207). MUCP increased in 16 patients during treatment, the mean rise being 53 to 64 cmH$_2$O. Another study randomized 44 patients with SUI to treatment with norfenefrine (15–30 mg three times daily) or placebo for six weeks duration. Subjective improvement was reported in 12/23 (52%) of the treatment group versus 7/21 (33%) of the placebo group, this difference was not statistically significant. Judged by a stress test, seven patients in each group became continent with 11/23 (48%) of the treatment group improving both subjectively and objectively compared to 5/21 (24%) of the placebo group (p = 0.09).

Phenylpropanolamine

Phenylpropanolamine (PPA) shares the pharmacologic properties of ephedrine and is approximately equal in peripheral potency while causing less central stimulation. It was available in 25 or 50 mg tablets and 75 mg timed-release capsules, and was a component of numerous proprietary mixtures marketed for the treatment of nasal and sinus congestion and appetite suppression (208). After a report that the risk of hemorrhagic stroke was 16 times greater in women <50 years of age who had been taking PPA as an appetite suppressant and three

times higher in women who had been taking the drug for <24 hours as a cold remedy, PPA was removed from the market in the United States (209).

Pseudoephedrine

Pseudoephedrine, a stereoisomer of ephedrine, is used for similar indications and carries similar precautions. The adult dosage is 30 to 60 mg four times a day, and the 30 mg dose is available in the United States without prescription.

A recent Cochrane review evaluated randomized and quazi-RCTs in adults with SUI treated in at least one arm of the trial with an adrenergic agonist drug (210). Twenty-two eligible trials were identified involving 1099 women (there were no controlled trials reporting on the use of these drugs in men). The authors concluded, "there was weak evidence to suggest that use of an adrenergic agonist was better than placebo treatment." They also reported a similar adverse events profile for adrenergic agonists and placebo.

α_2 AR Antagonists

Early data in rats following spinal cord transection suggests a potential role for α_2 antagonists in the treatment of SUI (211). Potential mechanisms of action include CNS inhibition of the release of glutamate, an excitatory neurotransmitter released at nerve terminals to modulate the continence reflex in response to increases in intra-abdominal pressure. Essentially, α_2 antagonists may add to striated sphincter activity by inhibiting an inhibitory action on Onuf's nucleus.

β-Adrenergic Antagonists and Agonists

Theoretically, β-adrenergic antagonists might be expected to "unmask" or potentiate α-adrenergic effect, thereby increasing urethral resistance. The opposite effect may be expected with β-adrenergic agonists with a decrease in urethral pressure, but β-agonists have been reported to increase the contractility of fast-contracting striated muscle fibers and suppress slow-contracting fibers (212).

Clenbuterol

Clenbuterol, a selective β_2-agonist, has been reported to potentiate field stimulation induced contraction of periurethral muscle from the rabbit. This study led to speculation on the drugs ability to treat sphincteric incontinence and in fact, increased urethral pressures were seen with the clinical use of clenbuterol (213). In a RCT comparing clenbuterol to pelvic floor exercises or combined therapy in 61 patients with SUI, efficacy from drug alone was 76.9% versus 52.6% in the exercise group and 89.5% in the combined group (214). Further work is needed to adequately assess the effects of this drug on SUI. This drug is not available in the United States. Side effects include: headache, muscle tremor, insomnia, sweating, increased appetite, palpitations, hypertension, anxiety, and hyperglycemia (215).

Propranolol

Propranolol, a β-antagonist, has been reported to have beneficial effects in the treatment of SUI; however, no RCTs have been performed for this indication. In one study, a dose of

10 mg four times daily (a relatively small dose) was found to be effective, but these results became manifest only after 4 to 10 weeks of treatment (216). This is a difficult phenomenon to explain as cardiac effects of the drug occur rather promptly. Potential side effects, including heart failure and increased airway resistance have limited its acceptance as a therapeutic agent for SUI. Side effects include: bradycardia, hypotension, confusion, depression, dizziness, fatigue, lethargy, insomnia, bronchospasm, constipation, and diarrhea. Propranolol is contraindicated in patients with uncompensated congestive heart failure, severe heart block, and severe asthma or chronic obstructive pulmonary disease (217).

Antidepressants
Duloxetine
Duloxetine, as mentioned above, is a combined SNRI FDA approved in the United States for depression, diabetic neuropathic pain, and generalized anxiety disorder and licensed in the European Union for the treatment of SUI. It has been shown to increase sphincteric muscle activity during the filling/storage phase of micturition with no effect on sphincter function during voiding in a cat model of irritated bladder (218). It was also noted that duloxetine increased bladder capacity, as noted above, probably through a CNS effect. The effects on the sphincter were reversed by α_1-adrenergic and $5HT_2$-serotonergic antagonism, while the effects on the bladder were provoked by serotonin and noradrenaline in the synaptic cleft. Duloxetine is lipophilic, well absorbed, and extensively metabolized (219).

There have been several RCTs documenting the effects of duloxetine in the treatment of SUI. Dmochowski and colleagues enrolled 683 patients in a double-blind RCT comparing duloxetine 40 mg twice daily to placebo (220). There was a 50% decrease in incontinence episodes in the duloxetine group compared to 27% in the placebo group; a significant improvement in HRQL was also seen in the duloxetine group. The improvements with duloxetine were associated with significant increases in the voiding interval (20 min vs. 2 min) compared to placebo. The discontinuation rate was higher in the duloxetine group (24%) than placebo (4%), most frequently due to nausea which was usually transient.

A Cochrane review of the effects of duloxetine on SUI summarizes data from nine RCTs totaling 3060 women (221). Cure rate in the duloxetine 40 mg twice daily group was higher than in the placebo group (10.8% vs. 7.7%, $p = 0.04$). Significant reductions in incontinence episodes and improvement in HRQL and patient global impression of improvement were seen. However, no data was available on sustainability of treatment. The estimated absolute size of effect showed that for every 100 patients treated, three patients were cured. Only one trial reported objective cure data and showed no clear difference between drug and placebo. Adverse events were common (71% vs. 59% in placebo) but were not considered serious. Nausea was the most common complaint and the incidence ranged from 23% to 25% and was the main reason for discontinuation. Other side effects reported were vomiting, constipation, dry mouth, fatigue, dizziness, and insomnia. Across these six trials 17% in the drug group withdrew versus 4% in the placebo arm. The authors conclude that more research is needed to determine whether duloxetine is clinically effective and cost effective compared to the other minimally invasive or more invasive treatment options available. Longer follow-up is currently being acquired to answer the question of whether the drug has sustainable efficacy and safety. Adverse effects are listed on p. 428.

Imipramine
The actions of imipramine have been discussed in further detail above. On a theoretical basis, an increase in urethral resistance might be expected if an enhanced α-adrenergic effect at this level resulted from an inhibition of noradrenalin reuptake. However, imipramine also causes α-adrenergic blocking effects, at least in vascular smooth muscle. Many clinicians have noted improvement in patients treated with imipramine primarily for DO but who had in addition some component of sphincteric incontinence. In a study of 30 women with SUI who were treated with imipramine 75 mg daily for four weeks, 21 women reported continence; the mean MUCP for the group increased from 34.06 to 48.23 cmH_2O (222). There are no RCTs on the use of imipramine for SUI. The safety issues (see pp. 428–9) are potentially significant. Adverse effects are listed in pp. 428–9.

Estrogens
Although estrogens have been recommended for the treatment of incontinence for many years, there remains considerable controversy over the risk-benefit ratio for this purpose. Numerous clinical studies exists however little consistency in methodology or delivered drug make interpretation of the available data problematic. As mentioned in the section above on estrogen treatment for OAB, menopause causes marked decline in the presence and expression of both α- and β-estrogen receptor subtypes. After menopause, urethral pressure parameters normally decrease slightly, and although this change is generally conceded to be related in some way to decreased estrogen levels, it is still largely a matter of speculation whether the actual changes occur in smooth muscle, blood circulation, supporting tissues, or the mucosal seal mechanism (223).

Two meta-analyses have shed some light on the use of estrogen therapy in the treatment of SUI. The Hormones and Urogenital Therapy Committee reviewed 166 articles containing six controlled and 17 uncontrolled trials (165). They were able to show subjective improvement in urinary continence, but when objective urine loss was measured, there was no significant change. Only one study showed an increase in MUCP. In the second meta-analysis, the authors concluded that "published trials do not support estrogen replacement as efficacious therapy for SUI" (224).

In an open comparative crossover RCT in 20 postmenopausal women with SUI, both vaginal estriol suppositories 1mg daily and oral PPA 50 mg twice daily increased the MUCP and the continence area on profilometry (225). PPA was clinically more effective than estriol but not sufficiently so to obtain complete continence. With combined therapy eight patients became completely continent, nine were considerably improved, and only one remained unchanged. Two patients dropped out of the study because of side effects. PPA is no longer on the market, but this study suggests estrogen may have a role in combination therapy with α-agonists.

Secondary analysis of 1525 participants of HERS who were randomly assigned to hormone therapy (n = 768) or placebo (n = 757) revealed greater worsening of incontinence symptoms in the treatment group (39% vs. 27%, p < 0.001). Review of the data from the WHI study on 23,296 postmenopausal women revealed that after one year of use hormone therapy increased all types of urinary incontinence, with SUI being the most common (226).

These women were randomized based on hysterectomy status to estrogen alone, estrogen plus progesterone, or placebo. Estrogen alone, or in combination with progesterone, was shown to increase the risk of incontinence amongst continent women and worsen incontinence in mildly symptomatic women.

A review article by Cardozo concluded that there is no convincing evidence that estrogen improves SUI; however, there is suggestion that vaginal estrogen alleviates urgency, UUI, frequency, nocturia, and dysuria (227). Vaginal estrogen is though to exert this positive effect via improvement in cytological changes secondary to urogenital atrophy (228).

The debate over the use of estrogen runs much deeper than its potential effects on the urinary tract. Impact on cardiovascular disease, osteoporosis, vasomotor symptoms, breast cancer, and other conditions must factor into the risk-benefit analysis. Adverse effects are listed in pp. 430–1.

FACILITATION OF BLADDER EMPTYING

Absolute or relative failure to empty the bladder results from decreased bladder contractility, increased outlet resistance, or both (2). Failure of adequate bladder contractility may result from temporary or permanent alterations in any one of the neuromuscular mechanisms necessary for initiating and maintaining a normal detrusor contraction. In a neurologically normal individual, inhibition of the micturition reflex may be secondary to painful stimuli, especially stimuli from the pelvic and perineal areas, or it may be psychogenic. Some drug therapies may inhibit bladder contractility through neurologic or myogenic mechanisms. Bladder smooth muscle function may be impaired from over distension, severe infection, or fibrosis. Increased outlet resistance is generally secondary to anatomic obstruction but may be secondary to a failure of coordination of smooth or striated sphincter during bladder contraction. Treatment of failure to empty consists of attempts to increase intravesical pressure, to facilitate the micturition reflex, or to decrease outlet resistance—or some combination of the above.

Facilitating Bladder Contraction

Parasympathomimetic Agents

Because a major portion of the final common pathway in physiologic bladder contraction is the stimulation of parasympathetic postganglionic muscarinic cholinergic receptor sites, agents that imitate the actions of ACh might be expected to be effective in treating patients who cannot empty because of inadequate bladder contractility. ACh itself cannot be used for therapeutic purposes because of its actions at central and ganglionic levels

and because of its rapid hydrolysis by acetylcholinesterases and butyrylcholinesterases (229).

Bethanechol Chloride

Many ACh-like drugs exist, but only bethanechol chloride (BC) has a relatively selective action in vitro on the urinary bladder and gut, with little or no nicotinic action (230). In vitro, BC causes a contraction of smooth muscle from all areas of the bladder (231). For more than 60 years BC has been recommended for the treatment of the atonic or hypotonic bladder and it has been reported to be effective in achieving "rehabilitation" or the chronically atonic or hypotonic detrusor (232). When so used, it is recommended that the drug be initially administered subcutaneously in a dose of 5 to 10 mg every four to six hours, along with an intermittent bladder decompression regimen. The patient is asked to try to void 20 to 30 minutes after each dose. When the residual urine volume has decreased to an acceptable level, the dose is gradually decreased and ultimately changed to an oral dose of 50 mg four times daily. In cases of partial bladder emptying, a therapeutic trial with an oral dose of 25 to 100 mg four times daily may be utilized in conjunction with attempted voiding every four hours. BC has also been used to stimulate or facilitate the development of reflex bladder contractions in patients with spinal shock secondary to suprasacral SCI (233).

Although anecdotal success in using BC in patients with voiding dysfunction is reported, there is little or no evidence to support its success in facilitating bladder emptying in series of patients in which the drug was the only variable (234). Short-term studies in which the drug was the only variable have generally failed to demonstrate significant efficacy in terms of urine flow and PVR (235). In a double-blind RCT that looked at the effects of two catheter-management protocols and the effect of BC on post-operative urinary retention following gynecologic urinary incontinence surgery, BC was not at all helpful (236). Although BC is capable of eliciting an increase in bladder smooth muscle tension, as would be expected from studies in vitro, its ability to stimulate or facilitate a coordinated and sustained physiologic bladder contraction in patients with voiding dysfunction has been unimpressive (234). However, due to the paucity of pharmacotherapy to improve bladder emptying, many clinicians continue to use BC in the hope of improving emptying as long as the medication is tolerated without adverse effects by the patient or is contraindicated. The potential side effects of cholinomimetic drugs include flushing, nausea, vomiting, diarrhea, gastrointestinal cramps, bronchospasm, headache, salivation, sweating, and difficulty with visual accommodation (230). Intramuscular and intravenous use can precipitate acute and severe side effects, resulting in acute circulatory failure and cardiac arrest, and is therefore prohibited.

PGs

The reported use of PGs to facilitate emptying is based on the hypothesis that these substances contribute to the maintenance of bladder tone and bladder contractile activity (108). PGE_2 and $PGF_2\alpha$ cause bladder contractile responses in vitro and in vivo. PGE_2 seems to cause a net decrease in urethral smooth muscle tone; $PGF_2\alpha$ causes an increase. The most common side effect reported with PG therapy is diarrhea (237).

PGE_2

Instillation of 0.5 mg PGE_2 into the bladders of 22 women with varying degrees of urinary retention resulted in acute emptying and an improvement in long term emptying over several months in two-thirds of the patients studied (238). In general, a decrease in the volume at which voiding was initiated, an increase in bladder pressure, and a decrease in PVR were seen. Another studied looked at the intravesical use of 1.5 mg of PGE_2 (diluted with 20 ml 0.2% neomycin solution) in patients whose bladder exhibited no contractile activity or in whom bladder contractility was relatively impaired (239). Of 36 patients, 20 showed a strongly positive response, and six showed a weakly positive response; 14 patients were reported to show prolonged beneficial effects. The authors noted that the effects of PGE_2 appeared to be additive or synergistic with cholinergic stimulation in some patients. Other studies have reported no effect of PGE_2 on urinary retention (240), with other suggesting instigation of urinary urgency, reduced bladder capacity, and bladder instability with intravesical PGE_2 (241).

$PGF_2\alpha$

Intravesical installation of 7.5 mg $PGF_2\alpha$ produced reflex voiding in some patients with incomplete suprasacral SCI (242). The favorable response to a single dose of drug, when present, lasted from 1 to 2.5 months. In women undergoing hysterectomy, 16 mg of $PGF_2\alpha$ in 40 ml of saline given intravesically reduced the frequency of urinary retention compared to saline instillation alone (243). The same treatment protocol given to women undergoing other vaginal procedures did not yield these results. Daily intravesical doses of $PGF_2\alpha$ and intravaginal PGE_2 reduced the number of days required for catheterization after SUI surgery compared with a control group receiving intravesical saline (244). Other investigators, however, have reported conflicting or negative results (240).

PGs have a relatively short half-life, and it is difficult to understand how any effects after a single application can last as long as several months. If such an effect does occur, it must be the result of a "triggering effect" on some as yet unknown physiologic or metabolic mechanism. Because of the number of conflicting positive and negative reports with various intravesical preparations, double-blind RCTs would be helpful to determine whether there are circumstances in which PG usage can reproducibly facilitate emptying or treat post-operative retention.

α-Adrenergic Blockers

Studies in cats have demonstrated a sympathetic reflex during bladder filling that promotes urine storage partly by exerting an α-adrenergic inhibitory effect on pelvic parasympathetic ganglionic transmission (245). Some investigators have suggested that α-adrenergic blockage, in addition to decreasing outlet resistance, may facilitate transmission through these ganglia and thereby enhance bladder contractility. Although such an effect may be due solely to an α-adrenergic effect on the outlet, it may be that α-adrenergic blockade can, under

certain circumstances, facilitate the detrusor reflex, through either a direct effect on parasympathetic ganglia or an indirect one.

Opioid Antagonists

Recent advances in neuropeptide physiology and pharmacology have provided new insights into LUT function and its potential pharmacologic alteration. It has been hypothesized that endogenous opioids may exert a tonic inhibitory effect on the micturition reflex at various levels, and agents such as narcotic antagonists may, therefore, offer possibilities for stimulating reflex bladder activity (1).

Naloxone

In one study on 15 patients with SCI, no significant cystometric changes following intravenous naloxone were noted (246). Interestingly, 11 of these patients showed decreased perineal electromyographic (EMG) activity but no associated change in dyssynergia pattern was seen. Although this issue is intriguing, it is of little practical use at present. Side effects of naloxone include precipitating withdrawal in patients addicted to opioids and sedation (247).

Decreasing Outlet Resistance at the Level of the Smooth Sphincter

α-Adrenergic Antagonists

Whether or not one believes that there is significant innervation of the bladder and proximal urethral smooth musculature by postganglionic fibers of the sympathetic nervous system, one must acknowledge the existence of α and β-AR sites in these areas (1). The smooth muscle of the bladder base and proximal urethral contains predominantly α-ARs. The bladder body contains both types, with the β-type being more common.

The implication that α-adrenergic blockade could be useful in certain patients who cannot empty the bladder was first made by Kleeman in 1970 (248). Krane and Olsson were among the first to endorse the concept of a physiologic internal sphincter that is partially controlled by sympathetic stimulation of contractile α-ARs in the smooth musculature of the bladder neck and proximal urethra (249). Furthermore, they hypothesized that some obstructions that occur at this level during detrusor contraction result from an inadequate opening of the bladder neck or an inadequate decrease in resistance in the area of the proximal urethra. They also theorized and presented evidence that α-adrenergic blockade could be useful in promoting bladder emptying in such a patient, one with an adequate detrusor contraction but without anatomic obstruction or detrusor external sphincter dyssynergia (DESD). Many others have subsequently confirmed the utility of α-blockade in the treatment of what is now usually referred to as smooth sphincter or bladder neck dyssynergia or dysfunction. Successful results, usually defined as an increase in flow rate, a decrease in PVR, and an improvement in upper tract appearance can often be correlated with an objective decrease in MUCP.

One would expect such success with α-blockade in treating emptying failure to be least evident in patients with DESD, as reported by Hachen (250). Although most would agree that α-blockers exert their favorable effects on voiding dysfunction primarily by affecting the smooth muscle of the bladder neck and proximal urethra, some information suggests that they may decrease striated sphincter tone as well. Much of the confusion about whether α-blockers have a direct, as opposed to indirect, inhibitory effect on the striated sphincter relates to the interpretation of observations of their effect on urethral pressure and periurethral striated muscle EMG activity in the region of the urogenital diaphragm. It is impossible to tell from pressure tracings alone whether a decrease in resistance in one area of the urethra is secondary to a decrease in smooth or striated muscle activity.

α-Adrenergic blocking agents have also been used to treat both bladder and outlet abnormalities in patients with so-called autonomous bladders (251). These include those with myelodysplasia, sacral or infrasacral SCI, and voiding dysfunction following radical pelvic surgery. Parasympathetic decentralization has been reported to lead to a marked increase in adrenergic innervation of the bladder, resulting in conversion of the usual β-(relaxant) bladder response to sympathetic stimulation to an α-(contractile) response (252). Although the alterations in innervation have been disputed, the alterations in receptor function have not. Koyanagi (253) demonstrated urethral super-sensitivity to α-adrenergic stimulation in a group of patients with autonomous neurogenic bladders, implying that a change had occurred in adrenergic receptor function in the urethra following parasympathetic decentralization. Parsons and Turton (254) observed the same phenomenon but ascribed the cause to adrenergic super-sensitivity of the urethral smooth muscle caused by sympathetic decentralization. Nordling and colleagues (255) described a similar occurrence in women who had undergone radical hysterectomy and ascribed this change to damage to the sympathetic innervation.

The most common adverse effects reported with this class of drugs are orthostatic hypotension, abnormal or retrograde ejaculation, dizziness, diarrhea, thirst, nasal congestion, and headache. Rarely, intraoperative floppy iris syndrome can occur and cause complications of cataract surgery. There is insufficient data to conclude whether there are additive hypotensive effects with concomitant PDE-5 inhibitor use for all α-antagonists. α-Blockers are metabolized primarily by the liver, predominantly via CYP3A4 (256).

Phenoxybenzamine

Phenoxybenzamine (POB) was the α-adrenolytic agent originally used for the treatment of voiding dysfunction; it has blocking properties at both α_1 and α_2 receptor sites. Nordling and colleagues (257) demonstrated that POB and clonidine, both of which pass the blood brain barrier, decreased urethral pressure in the striated sphincteric area but had no effect on EMG activity. They concluded that the effect of clonidine and possibly POB was elicited mostly through centrally induced changes in striated urethral sphincter tonus, and that these agents also had an effect on the smooth muscle component of urethral pressure. POB is capable of increasing bladder compliance thereby increasing storage and decreasing urethral resistance thus facilitating emptying. The initial adult dosage of this agent is 10 mg daily, and the usually daily dose for voiding dysfunction is 10 to 20 mg. After the drug has been

discontinued, the effects may persist for days because the drug irreversibly inactivates α-receptors, and the duration of effect depends on the rate of receptor synthesis (258). Side effects include orthostatic hypotension, reflex tachycardia, nasal congestion, diarrhea, miosis, sedation, nausea, and vomiting.

McGuire and Savastano (259), reported that POB decreased filling cystometric pressure in the decentralized primate bladder. None of these drugs, however, affected the reflex rise in either urethral pressure or EMG activity that was seen during bladder filling, and none decreased the urethral pressure or EMG activity response to voluntary contraction of the pelvic floor striated musculature.

Prazosin

In the cat, Gajewski and colleagues (260), concluded that α-blockers do not influence the pudendal nerve-dependent urethral response through a peripheral action, but prazosin, at least, can significantly inhibit this response at a central level. In 10 healthy female volunteers, Thind and co-workers (261) reported on the effects of prazosin on static urethral sphincter function. They found that function was diminished, predominantly in the midurethral area, and hypothesized that this response was due to a decrease in both smooth and striated sphincter muscle tone, the latter as a result of a reduced somatomotor output from the CNS. α-Adrenergic blockade can also decrease bladder contractility as Jensen (262) reported, with an increase in the "α-adrenergic effect" in bladders characterized as "uninhibited." Short- and long-term prazosin administration increased bladder capacity and decreased the amplitude of contractions. Prazosin is a potent selective α_1 antagonist (258), with a duration of action of four to six hours. Therapy is generally begun in daily divided doses of 2 to 3 mg and can be gradually increased to a maximum daily dose of 20 mg. Side effects are similar to those listed above for POB. Prazosin is contraindicated in patients taking PDE-5 inhibitors.

Terazosin and Doxazosin

Terazosin and doxazosin are two selective postsynaptic α_1-blocking drugs. They have a long plasma half-life enabling their activity to be maintained over 24 hours following a sing dose (263). These drugs are most often used for the treatment of benign prostatic hyperplasia (BPH) in men due to the high α_1-receptor content of the prostate stroma and capsule. Daily doses range from 1 to 10 mg, and is generally given at bedtime. Terazosin is said to have the same affinity for α_1-receptors in genitourinary as in vascular tissue and a four-fold greater selectivity for α_1-receptors than doxazosin.

Swierzewski and colleagues (264) prospectively studied the effects of terazosin on 12 patients with SCI and decreased compliance. All patients were refractory to medical therapy and on CIC. Urodynamic studies were conducted before, during and at the conclusion of four weeks of therapy with 5 mg of terazosin daily. The authors found statistically significant improvements in bladder compliance, "safe bladder volume" and bladder pressure in all patients, with the additional benefits of decreased episodes of both urinary incontinence and autonomic dysreflexia. They speculated that the improvement was due either to a direct effect on the α-receptors of the detrusor or to a central effect, but not to any effects on outlet resistance. Terazosin is contraindicated in patients taking PDE-5 inhibitors.

Tamsulosin and Alfuzosin

Tamsulosin is an α_1-blocking agent that is selective for the α_{1a} and α_{1d}-receptor subtypes over the α_{1b}-subtype (265). It appears to have no significant drug related adverse effects over placebo and has less effect on blood pressure than alfuzosin. The effects of Tamsulosin on resting tone and contractile behavior of the urethra in 11 healthy females was studied using urethral pressure profilometry (266). The drug significantly reduced the mean and MUP in the proximal, middle, and distal thirds of the urethra without any effect on systemic blood pressure. In a study on functional bladder neck obstruction diagnosed by video-urodynamics, 18 women were treated with Tamsulosin 0.4 mg daily for at least 30 days (267). Repeats video-urodynamics were performed with 56% of patients showing improvement in maximum flow, PVR, and symptoms. Tamsulosin 0.2 mg daily was studied in 97 women with chronic voiding symptoms and subnormal uroflow rates (268). After six weeks of treatment, all patients experienced significant improvements in symptoms score, flow rate, and PVR, with 35.1% of the women achieving a >50% reduction in voiding symptom score and >30% increase in maximal flow rate. Only one patient in this study discontinued therapy due to intolerable dizziness. Tamsulosin was also studied in a RCT involving 364 women with OAB (269). No difference was seen in primary or secondary outcome variables. Tamsulosin was well tolerated with 4.7% of women discontinuing treatment due to adverse events. Further, well designed, RCTs are needed to document tamsulosin's effect on the LUT in women.

Recent molecular characterization of the α_1-receptor has led to the recognition, classification and cloning of a number of α_1-receptor subtypes. In the human prostate, there appears to be some tissue specificity in that the majority of the stromal α_1-receptors are of the α_{1a}-subtype (270). A drug selective to the α_{1a}-subtype would be expected to cause fewer undesired effects than the less selective drugs while maintaining clinical efficacy.

Alfuzosin is a new agent that is reported to be a selective and competitive antagonist of α_1-mediated contraction of the bladder base, proximal urethral smooth muscle, and prostate capsule (in men), with efficacy similar to that of prazosin (271). It is said to be more specific for receptors in the genitourinary tract than in the vasculature, raising the possibility that voiding may be facilitated by doses that have minimal vasodilatory effects, thus minimizing postural hypotension. A sustained-release form of the drug, which allows for once daily dosing, is available. In a placebo controlled study (272), it was shown to have no significant incidence of adverse effects above those of placebo. In addition, effects on blood pressure (orthostatic hypotension) were minimal, supporting its selectivity of the LUT over the vasculature.

Silodosin

Silodosin is a very selective α_{1a}-antagonist with minimal α_{1b} binding and therefore minimal cardiovascular side effects. The drug has encouraging phase III data for the treatment of LUT symptoms in men. There is no data available in women.

Agents with α-adrenergic blocking properties have been used in patients with various types of voiding dysfunction including functional outlet obstruction, urinary retention, decreased compliance, and neurogenic and idiopathic DO. Although there remains a paucity of data regarding the use of α-blockers in women, our experience suggests that a trial of such an agent is certainly worth while, because its effect or non-effect should become obvious in a matter of days and the pharmacologic side effects are reversible. However, our results with such therapy for non-BPH related dysfunction have not been spectacular.

Decreasing Outlet Resistance at the Level of the Striated Sphincter

No class of pharmacologic agents selectively relaxes the striated musculature of the pelvic floor. Three different types of drug, all generally characterized as anti-spasticity drugs, have been used to treat voiding dysfunction secondary to outlet obstruction at the level of the striated sphincter: benzodiazepines (diazepam), baclofen, and dantrolene. Diazepam and baclofen act predominantly within the CNS, whereas dantrolene acts directly on skeletal muscle. Although these drugs are capable of providing variable relief in specific circumstances, their efficacy is far from complete, and troublesome muscle weakness, adverse effects on gait and other side-effects limit their overall usefulness. Benzodiazepines and baclofen are thought to exert their effects on the LUT through interactions with inhibitory neurotransmitters in the CNS, γ-aminobutyric acid (GABA) and glycine (273). The specific substrate for spinal cord inhibition consists of the synapses located on the terminals of the primary afferent fibers. GABA is the transmitter secreted by these synapses and activates specific receptors, resulting in a decrease in the amount of excitatory transmitter released by impulses from primary afferent fibers, consequently reducing the amplitude of the excitatory postsynaptic potentials.

Benzodiazepines

Benzodiazepines potentiate the inhibitory actions of GABA at pre- and postsynaptic sites in the brain and spinal cord (274). When pre-synaptic inhibition is augmented, and it is thought that the release of excitatory transmitters from afferent fibers is reduced, thereby diminishing the stretch and flexor reflexes in patients with bladder spasticity. This is a postulated mechanism of action of the muscle relaxant properties of diazepam at least (275). Side effects include non-specific CNS depression, manifested as sedation, lethargy, drowsiness, slowing of thought processes, ataxia, and decreased ability to acquire or store information.

There are few available published papers that provide valuable data on the use of benzodiazepines for treatment of functional obstruction at the level of the striated sphincter. We have not found the recommended oral dose of diazepam effective in controlling the classic type of DESD secondary to neurologic disease. If the cause of incomplete emptying in a neurologically normal patient is obscure, and the patient has what appears urodynamically to be inadequate relaxation of the pelvic floor striated musculature (e.g., occult neuropathic bladder, the Hinman syndrome), a trial of such an agent may we worthwhile. The rationale for its use is either relaxation of the pelvic floor striated musculature during bladder contraction, or that such relaxation removes and inhibitory stimulus to reflex bladder activity. However, improvement under such circumstances may simply be due to the anti-anxiety effect of the drug or to the intensive explanation, encouragement, and modified biofeedback therapy that usually accompanies such treatment in these patients.

Baclofen

Baclofen depresses excitation of motor neurons in the spinal cord and was originally thought to function as a GABA agonist (275). However, its electrophysiologic and pharmacologic profiles differ radically from those of GABA. Because both GABA and baclofen can produce some effects that are insensitive to blockade by classic GABA antagonists, two classes of GABA receptors have been proposed: the $GABA_A$ receptor (the classic receptor) and the $GABA_B$ receptor. Baclofen does not bind strongly or specifically to classic $GABA_A$ receptors but does to the $GABA_B$ receptors in brain and spinal membranes. Accordingly, the primary sites of action of baclofen are the spinal cord and brain. Its effect in reducing spasticity is caused primarily by normalizing interneuron activity and decreasing motor neuron activity (159).

Drug delivery often frustrates adequate pharmacologic treatment, and baclofen is a good example of this. GABA's hydrophilic properties prevent it from crossing the blood brain barrier in sufficient amounts to make it therapeutically useful. Baclofen was developed as a more lipophilic analog of GABA; however, its passage through the barrier is likewise limited, and it has proved to be a generally insufficient when given orally to treat severe somatic spasticity and micturition disorders secondary to neurogenic dysfunction (276). Hachen (250) found that a daily oral dose of 75 mg was ineffective in patients with DESD and traumatic paraplegia, whereas a daily intravenous dose of 20 mg was highly effective. Leyson and associates (235) reported that 73% of their patients with voiding dysfunction secondary to acute and chronic SCI had lower striated sphincter responses and decreased PVRs following baclofen treatment, but only with an average daily oral dose of 120 mg. Intrathecal infusion bypasses the blood brain barrier and cerebrospinal fluid levels 10 times higher than those reached with oral administration are achieved with much lower doses (277). Direct administration into the subarachnoid space by an implanted infusion pump has shown promising results, not only for skeletal spasticity but also for DESD and DO. Nanninga and colleagues (278) reported on such administration to seven patients with intractable bladder spasticity: all patients experienced a general decrease in spasticity and the amount of striated sphincter activity during bladder contraction. The action of baclofen on DO is not unexpected, given its spinal cord mechanism of action, and this inhibition of bladder contractility when the drug is administered intrathecally may, in fact, prove to be its most important benefit.

Potential side effects of baclofen include drowsiness, insomnia, rash, pruritis, dizziness, and weakness. Sudden withdrawal has been shown to provoke hallucinations, anxiety, and tachycardia;

hallucinations due to reductions in dosage during treatment have also been reported (214). Development of tolerance to intrathecal baclofen with a consequent requirement for increasing doses may prove to be a problem with long-term chronic usage. Further studies on the long-term efficacy of intrathecal baclofen specifically on the LUT in patients with neurogenic bladder are anticipated.

Dantrolene

Dantrolene exerts its effect by direct peripheral action on skeletal muscle (279). It is thought to inhibit the excitation induced release of calcium ions from the sarcoplasmic reticulum of striated muscle fibers, thereby inhibiting excitation-contraction coupling and diminishing the mechanical force of contraction. The drug improves voiding function in some patients with classic DESD and was initially reported to be very successful in doing so (280). In adults, the recommended starting dose is 25 mg daily, gradually increasing by increment of 25 mg every four to seven days to a maximum oral dose of 400 mg given in four divided doses. Hackler and colleagues (281) reported improvement in voiding function in approximately half of their patients treated with dantrolene but found that such improvement required oral doses of 600 mg daily. Although no inhibitory effect on bladder smooth muscle seems to occur (282), the generalized weakness that dantrolene can induced is often sufficiently significant to compromise its therapeutic effects.

Potential side effects other than severe muscle weakness include euphoria, dizziness, diarrhea, and hepatotoxicity. Fatal hepatitis has been reported in 0.1% to 0.2% of patients treated with the drug for 60 days or longer and symptomatic hepatitis may occur in 0.5% of patients treated for more than 60 days; chemical abnormalities of liver function are noted in up to 1%. The risk of hepatic injury is two-fold greater in women (107).

BTX

BTX, a potent inhibitor of ACh release at the neuromuscular junction, has been injected directly into the striated sphincter to cause relaxation in the treatment of DESD (283). This application has led to the use of BTX in treating neurogenic and non-neurogenic causes of urethral sphincter hypertonicity which may lead to retention. Injections of 100 units of BTX-A weekly for three weeks can achieve duration of effect averaging six to nine months. Fowler and colleagues (194) used BTX injection in six women with difficulty voiding or urinary retention secondary to abnormal myotonus-like EMG activity in the striated urethral sphincter. Although voiding did not improve in any patient (attributed to the type of repetitive discharge activity present), three patients developed transient SUI, indicating that the sphincter muscle had, indeed, been weakened. Phelan and colleagues (284) performed a prospective study to assess the efficacy of injecting 80 to 100 units of BTX-A into the external sphincter of 13 women and 8 men with voiding dysfunction due to various causes, including DESD, pelvic floor spasticity, and bladder hypocontractility. All patients except one were able to void spontaneously, and all but two were able to discontinue catheterization. Similarly, Kuo injected 50 or 100 units of BTX-A into the urethra of 103 patients (55 women) with chronic urinary retention or

439

severe difficulty urinating (202). The reasons for the LUT voiding dysfunction were quite heterogeneous: DESD, dysfunctional voiding, non-relaxing urethral sphincter, cauda equine lesion, peripheral neuropathy, and idiopathic detrusor underactivity. Subjectively, 39% had "excellent" results and 46% had "significant" improvement. There was a significant decrease in maximum voiding pressure, MUCP and PVR. In a small double-blind RCT, the efficacy of BTX-A was compared with lidocaine (285). This study was performed in 13 patients with DESD secondary to SCI. The injections were performed transperineally. BTX-A was superior to lidocaine, resulting in decreased PVR and MUP. Those treated with BTX-A also had an increase in patient satisfaction. Side effects of BTX were listed in pp. 429–31.

Clonidine

Clonidine is the prototypical α_2-adrenergic receptor agonist. It is considered to be a centrally acting agent with a variety of associated systemic effects including antihypertensive, anti-nociceptive, and antispasmodic effects. Potential effects on relaxation of the external urethral sphincter (EUS) have been reported previously (257). Herman and Wainberg (286) administered oral clonidine (400 mcg) in three divided doses over a 16 hour period under monitored inpatient conditions to five SCI patients with neurogenic DO and quantified effects on the EUS via needle electrodes. They found that clonidine had a profound suppressive effect on volume induced EMG activity in the EUS in four of five patients. The one patient in whom there were only minimal effects on the EUS had received an intrathecal dose of morphine two days before, which the authors feel may have confounded the effects of clonidine in this patient. The authors speculate that the somewhat selective effect of clonidine on the EUS is attributable to postsynaptic suppression of excitatory spinal interneurons (unmasked by the spinal lesion) via the α_2-agonist activity of clonidine. Adverse effects included significant reductions in blood pressure as well as sedative effects. Further clinical studies on the effects of clonidine on the LUT and striated sphincter (as well as its clinical utility) may be limited owing to its significant effects on blood pressure.

CIRCUMVENTING THE PROBLEM
Antidiuretic Hormone-Like Agents
Endogenous production of antidiuretic hormone (ADH) serves two purposes: stimulation of water reabsorption in the renal medulla and contraction of vascular smooth muscle. A genetic or acquired defect in ADH synthesis or secretion results in central diabetes insipidus while a defect in the ADH receptor results in nephrogenic diabetes insipidus. A relative lack in ADH is believed to be important in polyuria, specifically nocturnal polyuria (287).

Desmopressin

The synthetic ADH analog, desmopressin (DDAVP), has been used for the symptomatic relief of refractory nocturnal enuresis in children and adults (288). More recently it has been explored for the treatment of OAB and incontinence. The drug can be administered by oral, parenteral, or intranasal spray and effectively suppresses urine production for 7 to 10 hours.

Several small controlled studies on patients with multiple sclerosis and nocturia have consistently reported efficacy of DDAVP at the risk of asymptomatic or minimally symptomatic hyponatremia (289). Further studies in non-neurologic patients have confirmed the efficacy and determined effective dose regimens for the treatment of nocturia (290). In a phase IIb study on the use of oral DDAVP in the treatment of OAB symptoms a decrease in frequency and urgency episodes was observed. Patients also reported an improvement in HRQL with only mild side effects including headache. No hyponatremia was reported (291). Further studies on DDAVP for the treatment of OAB and incontinence are needed.

Given the safety concerns over hyponatremia, it is recommended that the drug not be given in patients older than 79 years of age or to those with 24 hour urine volumes >28 ml/kg. It is also recommended that serum sodium levels be checked at baseline and at three days and seven days after starting treatment or changing dose (292). General precautions including limiting fluid intake from one hour before the dose until eight hours after, periodic blood pressure measurements, and weight measurements to monitor for fluid overload should be instituted. The original intranasal spray has been withdrawn from the market in several countries due to side effects and unpredictable absorption. Side effects include: headache, hyponatremia, water intoxication, and rhinitis. DDAVP is contraindicated in patients with baseline hyponatremia and moderate to severe renal impairment (293).

Loop Diuretics
Bumetanide
A similar circumventive approach is to give a rapidly acting loop diuretic four to six hours before bedtime. This, of course assumes that the nocturia is not due to obstructive uropathy. A double blind, crossover RCT of this approach using bumetanide 1mg was performed in a group of 14 general practice patients (294). Nocturia episodes per week averaged 17.5; with placebo this decreased to 12 and with drug to 8. Bumetanide was preferred to placebo by 11 of 14 patients. Side effects include hyperuricemia, hypochloremia, hypokalemia, hyponatremia, hyperglycemia, and serum creatinine elevation (295).

REFERENCES
1. Wein AJ, Levin RM, Barrett DM. Voiding function: relevant anatomy, physiology, and pharmacology. In: Duckett JW, Howards ST, Grayhack JT, Gillenwater JY, eds. Adult and Pediatric Urology. St. Louis: Mosby, 1991: 933–99.
2. Wein AJ. Neuromuscular dysfunction of the lower urinary tract. In: Walsh PC, Retik AB, Stamey TA, Vaughan ED, eds. Campbell's Urology, 6th edn. Philadelphia: Saunders, 1992: 573–642.
3. Abrams P, Cardozo L, Fall M, et al. The standardisation of terminology of lower urinary tract function: report from the Standarisation Sub-committee of the International Continence Society. Neurourol Urodyn 2002; 21: 167–78.
4. Wein AJ. Pathophysiology and classification of voiding dysfunction. In: Wein AJ, Kavoussi LR, Novick AC, Partin AW, Peters CA, eds. Campbell-Walsh Urology, 9th edn. Philadelphia: Saunders, 2007: 1973–85.
5. Anderson KE. Pharmacology of lower urinary tract smooth muscles and penile erectile tissues. Pharmacol Rev 1993; 45: 253–308.
6. Anderson KE, Wein AJ. Pharmacology of the lower urinary tract: basis for current and future treatments of urinary incontinence. Pharmacol Rev 2004; 56: 581–631.

7. Jensen D Jr. Pharmacological studies of the uninhibited neurogenic bladder. Acta Neurol Scand 1981; 64: 175–80.

8. Anderson KE, Yoshida M. Antimuscarinics and the overactive detrusor—which is the main mechanism of action? Eur Urol 2003; 43: 1–5.

9. Chess-Williams R. Muscarinic receptors of the urinary bladder: detrusor, urothelial and prejunctional. Auton Autacoid Pharmacol 2002; 22: 133–45.

10. Yoshida M, Miyamae K, Iwashita H, et al. Management of detrusor dysfunction in the elderly: changes in acetylcholine and adenosine triphosphate release during aging. Urology 2004; 63(Suppl 1): 17–23.

11. Andersson KE, Wein AJ. Pharmacologic management of storage and emptying failure. In: Wein AJ, Kavoussi LR, Novick AC, Partin AW, Peters CA, eds. Campbell-Walsh Urology, 9th edn. Philadelphia: Saunders, 2007: 2091–123.

12. Andersson KE, Chapple CR, Cardozo L, et al. Pharmacological treatment of urinary incontinence. In: Abrams P, Cardozo L, Khoury S, Wein AJ, eds. Incontinence, 4th edn. Paris: Health Publication Ltd., 2009: 631–99.

13. Abrams P, Andersson KE. Muscarinic receptor antagonists for overactive bladder. BJU Int 2007; 100: 987–1006.

14. Guay DR. Clinical pharmacokinetics of drugs used to treat urge incontinence. Clin Pharmacokinet 2003; 42: 1243–85.

15. Chapple CR, Khullar V, Gabriel Z, et al. The effects of antimuscarinic treatments in overactive bladder: an update of a systematic review and meta-analysis. Eur Urol 2008; 54: 543–62.

16. Witte LP, Mulder WM, de la Rosette JJ, et al. Muscarinic receptor antagonists for overactive bladder treatment: does one fit all? Curr Opin Urol. 2009; 19: 13–19.

17. Food and Drug Administration (FDA). Enablex (darifenacin) extended-release tablets. [Available from: http://www.fda.gov/cder/foi/label/2008/021513s004lbl.pdf].

18. European Medicines Agency (EMEA). Toviaz 4 mg prolonged-release tablets. [Available from: http://www.emea.europa.eu/humandocs/PDFs/EPAR/toviaz/H-723-PI-en.pdf].

19. Food and Drug Administration (FDA). VESIcare (solifenacin succinate) tablets. [Available from: http://www.fda.gov/cder/foi/label/2008/021518s004lbl.pdf.].

20. Food and Drug Administration (FDA). Detrol tolterodine tartrate tablets. [Available from: http://www.fda.gov/cder/foi/label/2005/020771s013lbl.pdf].

21. Andersson K-E. Antimuscarinics for treatment of overactive bladder. Lancet Neurol 2004; 3: 46–53.

22. Fader M, Glickman S, Haggar V, et al. Intravesical atropine compared to oral oxybutynin for neurogenic detrusor overactivity: a double-blind, randomized crossover trial. J Urol 2007; 177: 208–13.

23. Andersson KE. Potential benefits of muscarinic M3 receptor selectivity. Eur Urol 2002; 1: 23.

24. Haab F, Stewart L, Dwyer P. Darifenacin, an M3 selective receptor antagonist, is an effective and well tolerated once daily treatment for overactive bladder. Eur Urol 2004; 45: 420–9.

25. Chapple CR, Steers W, Norton P, et al. A pooled analysis of three phase III studies to investigate the efficacy, tolerability and safety of darifenacin, a muscarinic M3 selective receptor antagonist, in the treatment of overactive bladder. BJU Int 2005; 95: 993.

26. Cardozo L, Dixon A. Increased warning time with darifenacin: a new concept in the management of urinary urgency. J Urol 2005; 173: 1214.

27. Lipton RB, Kolodner K, Wesnes K. Assessment of cognitive function of the elderly population: effects of darifenacin. J Urol 2005; 173: 493–8.

28. Chapple C, Van Kerrebroeck P, Tubaro A, et al. Clinical efficacy, safety, and tolerability of once-daily fesoterodine in subjects with overactive bladder. Eur Urol 2007; 52: 1204–12.

29. Michel MC. Fesoterodine: a novel muscarinic receptor antagonist for the treatment of overactive bladder syndrome. Expert Opin Pharmacother 2008; 9: 1787–96.

30. Ney P, Pandita RK, Newgreen DT, et al. Pharmacological characterization of a novel investigational antimuscarinic drug, fesoterodine, in vitro and in vivo. BJU Int 2008; 101: 1036–42.

31. Khullar V, Rovner ES, Dmochowski R, et al. Fesoterodine dose response in subjects with overactive bladder syndrome. Urology 2008; 71: 839–43.

32. Kelleher CJ, Tubaro A, Wang JT, et al. Impact of fesoterodine on quality of life: pooled data from two randomized trials. BJU Int 2008; 102: 56–61.

33. Muskat Y, Bukovsky I, Schneider D, Langer R. The use of scopolamine in the treatment of detrusor instability. J Urol 1996; 156: 1989–90.

34. Beermann B, Hellstrom K, Rosen A. On the metabolism of propantheline in man. Clin Pharmacol Ther 1972; 13: 212–20.

35. Blaivas JG, Labib KB, Michalik J, Zayed AA. Cystometric response to propantheline in detrusor hyperreflexia: therapeutic implications. J Urol 1980; 124: 259–62.

36. Thüroff JW, Bunke B, Ebner A, et al. Randomized, double-blind, multi-center trial on treatment of frequency, urgency and incontinence related to detrusor hyperactivity: Oxybutynin versus propantheline versus placebo. J Urol 1991; 16(Suppl 1): 48–61.

37. Holmes DM, Montz FJ, Stanton SL. Oxybutynin versus propantheline in the management of detrusor instability. A patient-regulated variable dose trial. Br J Obstet Gynaecol 1989; 96: 607–12.

38. Wiener LB, Baum NH, Suarez GM. New method for management of detrusor instability: transdermal scopolamine. Urology 1986; 28: 208–10.

39. Ikeda K, Kobayashi S, Suzuki M, et al. M(3) receptor antagonism by the novel antimuscarinic agent solifenacin in the urinary bladder and salivary gland. Naunyn Schmiedebergs Arch Pharmacol 2002; 366: 97–103.

40. Chapple CR, Arano P, Bosch JL, et al. Solifenacin appears effective and well tolerated in patients with symptomatic idiopathic detrusor overactivity in a placebo- and tolterodine-controlled phase 2 dose-finding study. BJU Int 2004; 93: 71–7.

41. Cardozo L, Lisec M, Millard R, et al. Randomized, double-blind placebo controlled trial of the once daily antimuscarinic agent solifenacin succinate in patients with overactive bladder. J Urol 2004; 172(pt 1): 1919–24.

42. Chapple CR, Martinez-Garcia R, Selvaggi L, et al. STAR study group. A comparison of the efficacy and tolerability of solifenacin succinate and extended release tolterodine at treating overactive bladder syndrome: results of the STAR Trial. Eur Urol 2005; 48: 464–70.

43. Kelleher C, Cardozo L, Kobashi K, et al. Solifenacin: as effective in mixed urinary incontinence as in urge urinary incontinence. Int Urogynecol J Pelvic Floor Dysfunct 2006; 17: 382.

44. Wagg A, Wyndaele JJ, Siever P. Efficacy and tolerability of solifenacin in elderly subjects with overactive bladder syndrome: a pooled analysis. Am J Geriatr Pharmacother 2006; 4: 14.

45. Garely AD, Kaufman JM, Sand PK, et al. Symptom bother and health-related quality of life outcomes following solifenacin treatment for overactive bladder: the VESIcare Open-Label Trial (VOLT). Clin Ther 2006; 28: 1935.

46. Brynne N, Stahl MMS, Hallen B, et al. Pharmacokinetics and pharmacodynamics of tolterodine in man: a new drug for the treatment of urinary bladder overactivity. Int J Clin Pharmacol Ther 1997; 35: 287.

47. Nilvebrant L, Sundquist S, Gillberg PG. Tolterodine is not subtype (m1-m5) selective but exhibits functional bladder selectivity in vivo. Neurourol Urodyn 1996; 15: 310–11.

48. Nilvebrant L, Hallen B, Larsson B. Tolterodine-a new bladder selective muscarinic receptor antagonist: preclinical pharmacological and clinical data. Life Sci 1997; 60: 1129–36.

49. van Kerrebroeck P, Kreder K, Jonas U, et al. Tolterodine once daily: superior efficacy and tolerability in the treatment of overactive bladder. Urology 2001; 57: 414–21.

50. Hills CJ, Winter SA, Balfour JA. Tolterodine. Drugs 1998; 55: 813.

51. Xie HG, Kim RB, Wood AJ, et al. Molecular basis of ethnic differences in drug disposition and response. Annu Rev Pharmacol Toxicol 2001; 41: 815–50.

52. Diefenbach K, Jaeger K, Wollny A, et al. Effect of tolterodine on sleep structure modulated by CYP2D6 genotype. Sleep Med 2008; 9: 579–82.

53. Appell RA, Sand P, Dmochowski R, et al. Prospective randomized controlled trial of extended release oxybutynin chloride and tolterodine tartrate in the treatment of overactive bladder: results of the OBJECT study. Mayo Clin Proc 2001; 76: 358–63.

54. Diokno AC, Appell RA, Sand PK, et al. OPERA Study Group. Prospective, randomized, double-blind study of the efficacy and tolerability of the

extended-release formulations of oxybutynin and tolterodine for overactive bladder: results of the OPERA trial. Mayo Clin Proc 2003; 78: 687–95.

55. Sussman D, Garely A. Treatment of overactive bladder with once-daily extended-release tolterodine or oxybutynin: The antimuscarinic clinical effectiveness trial (ACET). Curr Med Res Opin 2002; 18: 177–84.

56. Elinoff V, Bavendam T, Glasser DB, et al. Symptom-specific efficacy of tolterodine extended release in patients with overactive bladder: the IMPACT trial. Int J Clin Pract 2006; 60: 745–51.

57. Song C, Park JT, Heo KO, et al. Effects of bladder training and/or tolterodine in female patients with overactive bladder syndrome: a prospective, randomized study. J Korean Med Sci 2006; 21: 1060–3.

58. Mattiasson A, Blaakaer J, Høye K, et al. Tolterodine Scandinavian Study Group. Simplified bladder training augments the effectiveness of tolterodine in patients with an overactive bladder. BJU Int 2003; 91: 54–60.

59. Millard RJ. Asia Pacific Tolterodine Study Group. Clinical efficacy of tolterodine with or without a simplified pelvic floor exercise regimen. Neurourol Urodyn 2004; 23: 48–53.

60. Todorova A, Vonderheid-Guth B, Dimpfel W. Effects of tolterodine, trospium chloride, and oxybutynin on the central nervous system. J Clin Pharmacol 2001; 41: 636–44.

61. Kim Y, Yoshimura N, Masuda H, et al. Intravesical instillation of human urine after oral administration of trospium, tolterodine, and oxybutynin in a rat model of detrusor overactivity. BJU Int 2006; 97: 400.

62. Stöhrer M, Bauer P, Giannetti BM, et al. Effect of trospium chloride on urodynamic parameters in patients with detrusor hyperreflexia due to spinal cord injuries: a multicenter placebo-controlled double-blind trial. Urol Int 1991; 47: 138–43.

63. Madersbacher H, Stöhrer M, Richter R, et al. Trospium chloride versus oxybutynin: a randomized double blind, multicenter trial in the treatment of detrusor hyperreflexia. Br J Urol 1995; 75: 452–6.

64. Allousi S, Laval K-U, Eckert R. Trospium chloride (Spasmo-lyt) in patients with motor urge syndrome (detrusor instability): a double-blind, randomised, multicentre, placebo-controlled study. J Clin Res 1998; 1: 439–51.

65. Jünemann KP, Al-Shukri S. Efficacy and tolerability of trospium chloride and tolterodine in 234 patients with urge-syndrome: a double-blind, placebo-controlled multicenter clinical trial. Neurourol Urodyn 2000; 19: 488–9.

66. Halaska M, Ralph G, Wiedemann A, et al. Controlled, double-blind, multicenter clinical trial to investigate long-term tolerability and efficacy of trospium chloride in patients with detrusor instability. World J Urol 2003; 20: 392–9.

67. Dmochowski RR, Sand PK, Zinner NR, Staskin DR. Trospium 60 mg once daily (QD) for overactive bladder syndrome: results from a placebo-controlled interventional study. Urology 2008; 71: 449–54.

68. Fröhlich G, Burmeister S, Wiedemann A, Bulitta M. Intravesical instillation of trospium chloride, oxybutynin and verapamil for relaxation of the bladder detrusor muscle. a placebo controlled, randomized clinical test. Arzneimittelforschung 1998; 48: 486–91.

69. Walter P, Grosse J, Bihr AM, et al. Bioavailability of trospium chloride after intravesical instillation in patients with neurogenic lower urinary tract dysfunction: a pilot study. Neurourol Urodyn 1999; 18: 447–53.

70. Ruffmann R. A review of flavoxate hydrochloride in the treatment of urge incontinence. J Intern Med Res 1988; 16: 317–30.

71. Guarneri L, Robinston E, Testa R. A review of flavoxate: pharmacology and mechanism of action. Drugs Today 1994; 30: 91.

72. Oka M, Kimura Y, Itoh Y, et al. Brain pertussis toxin-sensitive G proteins are involved in the flavoxate hydrochloride-induced suppression of the micturition reflex in rats. Brain Res 1996; 727: 91.

73. Kimura Y, Sasaki Y, Hamada K, et al. Mechanisms of suppression of the bladder activity by flavoxate. Int J Urol 1996; 3: 218–27.

74. Milani R, Scalambrino S, Milia R, et al. Double-blind crossover comparison of flavoxate and oxybutynin in women affected by urinary urge syndrome. Int Urogynecol 1993; 4: 3–8.

75. Briggs RS, Castleden CM, Asher MJ. The effect of flavoxate on uninhibited detrusor contractions and urinary incontinence in the elderly. J Urol 1980; 123: 665–6.

76. Chapple CR, Parkhouse H, Gardener C, et al. Double-blind, placebo-controlled, cross-over study of flavoxate in the treatment of idiopathic detrusor instability. Br J Urol 1990; 66: 491–4.

77. Waldeck K, Larsson B, Andersson K-E. Comparison of oxybutynin and its active metabolite, N-desethyl-oxybutynin, in the human detrusor and parotid gland. J Urol 1997; 157: 1093.

78. Thompson I, Lauvetz R. Oxybutynin in bladder spasm, neurogenic bladder and enuresis. Urology 1976; 8: 452–4.

79. Andersson K-E. Current concepts in the treatment of disorders of micturition. Drugs 1988; 35: 477–94.

80. Thüroff JW, Chartier E, Corcus J, et al. Medical treatment and medical side effects in urinary incontinence in the elderly. World J Urol 1998; 16(Suppl 1): S48–61.

81. Baigrie RJ, Kelleher JP, Fawcett KP, et al. Oxybutynin: is it safe? Br J Urol 1988; 62: 319.

82. Gupta SK, Sathyan G. Pharmacokinetics of an oral once-a-day controlled-release oxybutynin formulation compared with immediate-release oxybutynin. J Clin Pharmacol 1999; 39: 289–96.

83. Chancellor MB, Appell RA, Sathyan G, et al. A comparison of the effects on saliva output of oxybutynin chloride and tolterodine tartate. Clin Ther 2001; 23: 753.

84. Anderson R, Mobley D, Blank B, et al. Once daily controlled versus immediate release oxybutynin chloride for urge urinary incontinence. J Urol 1999; 161: 1809–12.

85. Corcos J, Casey R, Patrick A, et al. Uromax Study Group. A double-blind randomized dose-response study comparing daily doses of 5, 10 and 15 mg controlled-release oxybutynin: balancing efficacy with severity of dry mouth. BJU Int 2006; 97: 520–7.

86. Dmochowski RR, Davila GW, Sinner NR, et al. Efficacy and safely of transdermal oxybutynin in patients with urge and mixed urinary incontinence. J Urol 2002; 168: 580–6.

87. Davila GW, Daugherty CA, Sanders SW. A short-term, multi-center, randomized double-blind dose titration study of the efficacy and anticholinergic side effects of transdermal compared to immediate release oral oxybutynin treatment of patients with urge urinary incontinence. J Urol 2001; 166: 150–1.

88. Dmochowski RR, Davila GW, Sinner NR, et al. Comparative efficacy and safety of transdermal oxybutynin and oral tolterodine versus placebo in previously treated patients with urge and mixed urinary incontinence. Urology 2003; 62: 237–42.

89. Appell RA. Efficacy and safety of transdermal oxybutynin in patients with urge and mixed urinary incontinence. Curr Urol Rep 2003; 4: 343.

90. Cartwright R, Cardozo L. Transdermal oxybutynin: sticking to the facts. Eur Urol 2007; 51: 907–14.

91. Connor JP, Betrus G, Fleming P, et al. Early cystometrograms can predict the response to intravesical instillation of oxybutynin chloride in myelomeningocele patients. J Urol 1994; 151: 1045–7.

92. Szollar SM, Lee SM. Intravesical oxybutynin for spinal cord injury patients. Spinal Cord 1996; 34: 284–7.

93. Madersbacher H, Jilg G. Control of detrusor hyperreflexia by the intravesical instillation of oxybutynin hydrochloride. Paraplegia 1991; 29: 84–90.

94. Enzelsberger H, Helmer H, Kurz C. Intravesical instillation of oxybutynin in women with idiopathic detrusor instability: a randomized trial. Br J Obstet Gynaecol 1995; 102: 929–39.

95. Staskin DR, Dmochowski RR, Sand PK, et al. Efficacy and safety of oxybutynin chloride topical gel for overactive bladder: a randomized, double-blind, placebo controlled, multicenter study. J Urol 2009; 181: 1764–72.

96. Haruno A. Inhibitory effects of propiverine hydrochloride on the agonist-induced or spontaneous contractions of various isolated muscle preparations. Arzneimittelforschung 1992; 42: 815–17.

97. Thuroff JW, Chartier-Kastler E, Corcus J, et al. Medical treatment and medical side effects in urinary incontinence in the elderly. World J Urol 1998; 16(Suppl): S48.

98. Stöhrer M, Madersbacher H, Richter R, et al. Efficacy and safety of propiverine in SCI patients suffering from detrusor hyperreflexia—a double-blind, placebo-controlled clinical trial. Spinal Cord 1999; 37: 196–200.

99. Stöhrer M, Mürtz G, Kramer G, et al. Propiverine compared to oxybutynin in neurogenic detrusor overactivity—results of a randomized, double-blind, multicenter clinical study. Eur Urol 2007; 51: 235.

100. Madersbacher H, Halaska M, Voigt R, et al. A placebo-controlled, multicentre study comparing the tolerability and efficacy of propiverine and oxybutynin in patients with urgency and urge incontinence. BJU Int 1999; 84: 646.

101. Jünemann KP, Halaska M, Rittstein T, et al. Propiverine versus tolterodine: efficacy and tolerability in patients with overactive bladder. Eur Urol 2005; 48: 478–82.

102. Abrams P, Cardozo L, Chapple C. Comparison of the efficacy, safety, and tolerability of propiverine and oxybutynin for the treatment of overactive bladder syndrome. Int J Urol 2006; 13: 692–8.

103. Yamaguchi O, Marui E, Kakizaki H. Randomized, double-blind, placebo- and propiverine-controlled trial of the once-daily antimuscarinic agent solifenacin in Japanese patients with overactive bladder. BJU Int 2007; 100: 579–87.

104. Ancelin ML, Artero S, Portet F, et al. Non-degenerative mild cognitive impairment in elderly people and use of anticholinergic drugs: longitudinal cohort study. BMJ 2006; 332: 455–9.

105. Hashimoto M, Imamura T, Tanimukai S, et al. Urinary incontinence: an unrecognised adverse effect with donepezil. Lancet 2000; 356: 568.

106. Kato K, Furuhashi K, Suzuki K, et al. Overactive bladder and glaucoma: a survey at outpatient clinics in Japan. Int J Urol 2007; 14: 595–7.

107. Fink AM, Aylward GW. Buscopan and glaucoma: a survey of current practice. Clin Radiol 1995; 50: 160–4.

108. Andersson KE. Pharmacology of lower urinary tract smooth muscles and penile erectile tissues. Pharmacol Rev 1993; 45: 253–308.

109. Frazier EP, Peters SL, Braverman AS. Signal transduction underlying the control of urinary bladder smooth muscle tone by muscarinic receptors and beta-adrenoceptors. Naunyn Schmiedebergs Arch Pharmacol 2008; 377: 449–62.

110. Abernethy DR, Schwartz JB. Calcium-antagonist drugs. N Engl J Med 1999; 341: 1447.

111. Forman A, Andersson K, Henriksson L, et al. Effects of nifedipine on the smooth muscle of the human urinary tract in vitro and in vivo. Acta Pharmacol Toxicol 1978; 43: 111–18.

112. Husted S, Andersson K, Sommer L, et al. Anticholinergic and calcium antagonistic effects of terodiline in rabbit urinary bladder. Acta Pharmacol Toxicol 1980; 46(Suppl 1): 20–30.

113. Naglie G, Radomski SB, Brymer C, et al. A randomized, double-blind, placebo controlled crossover trial of nimodipine in older persons with detrusor instability and urge incontinence. J Urol 2002; 167(2 Pt 1): 586–90.

114. Fröhlich G, Burmeister S, Wiedemann A, et al. Intravesical instillation of trospium chloride, oxybutynin and verapamil for relaxation of the bladder detrusor muscle. A placebo controlled, randomized clinical test. Arzneimittelforschung 1998; 48: 486–91.

115. Andersson KE. Clinical pharmacology of potassium channel openers. Pharmacol Toxicol 1992; 70: 244–54.

116. Shieh C-C, Brune ME, Buckner SA, et al. Characterization of a novel ATP-sensitive K+ channel opener, A-251179, on urinary bladder relaxation and cystometric parameters. Br J Pharmacol 2007; 151: 467.

117. Klabunde RE. Potassium-channel openers. Cardiovascular Pharmacology Concepts, 2007.

118. Nurse DE, Restorick JM, Mundy AR. The effect of cromakalim on the normal and hyper-reflexic human detrusor muscle. Br J Urol 1991; 68: 27–31.

119. Komersova K, Rogerson JW, Conway EL, et al. The effect of levcromakalim (BRL 38227) on bladder function in patients with high spinal cord lesions. Br J Clin Pharmacol 1995; 39: 207–9.

120. Fovaeus M, Andersson KE, Hedlund H. The action of pinacidil in isolated human bladder. J Urol 1989; 141: 637–40.

121. Hedlund H, Mattiasson A, Andersson KE. Effects of pinacidil on detrusor instability in men with bladder outlet obstruction. J Urol 1991; 146: 1345–7.

122. Chapple CR, Patroneva A, Raines SR. Effect of an ATP-sensitive potassium channel opener in subjects with overactive bladder: a randomized, double-blind, placebo-controlled study (ZD0947IL/0004). Eur Urol 2006; 49: 879–86.

123. Downie JW, Karmazyn M. Mechanical trauma to bladder epithelium liberates prostanoids which modulate neurotransmission in rabbit detrusor muscle. J Pharmacol Exp Ther 1984; 230: 445–9.

124. Mattia C, Coluzzi F. COX-2 inhibitors: pharmacological data and adverse effects. Minerva Anestesiol 2005; 71: 461–70.

125. Cardozo L, Stanton SL, Robinson H, et al. Evaluation of flurbiprofen in detrusor instability. Br Med J 1980; 2: 281–2.

126. Lindholm P, Lose G. Terbutaline (Bricanyl) in the treatment of female urge incontinence. Urol Int 1986; 41: 158–60.

127. Michel MC, Vrydag W. Alpha1-, alpha2- and beta-adrenoceptors in the urinary bladder, urethra and prostate. Br J Pharmacol 2006; 147(Suppl 2): S88–119.

128. Sears MR, Lötvall J. Past, present and future—beta2-adrenoceptor agonists in asthma management. Respir Med 2005; 99: 152–70.

129. Grüneberger A. Treatment of motor urge incontinence with clenbuterol and flavoxate hydrochloride. Br J Obstet Gynaecol 1984; 91: 275–8.

130. Biers SM, Reynard JM, Brading AF. The effects of a new selective beta3-adrenoceptor agonist (GW427353) on spontaneous activity and detrusor relaxation in human bladder. BJU Int 2006; 98: 1310–14.

131. Takasu T, Ukai M, Sato S, et al. Effect of (R)-2-(2-aminothiazol-4-yl)-4′-{2-[(2-hydroxy-2-phenylethyl)amino]ethyl} acetanilide (YM178), a novel selective beta3-adrenoceptor agonist, on bladder function. J Pharmacol Exp Ther 2007; 321: 642–7.

132. Chapple CR, Yamaguchi O, Ridder A, et al. Clinical proof of concept study (Blossom) shows novel b3 andrenoceptor agonist YM178 is effective and well tolerated in the treatment of symptoms of overactive bladder. Eur Urol Suppl 2007; 7: 239 (abstract 674).

133. Hollister LE. Current antidepressants. Annu Rev Pharmacol Toxicol 1986; 26: 23–37.

134. Bigger J, Giardino E, Perel JE. Cardiac antiarrhythmic effect of imipramine hydrochloride. N Engl J Med 1977; 296: 206–8.

135. Lose G, Jorgensen L, Thunedborg P. Doxepin in the treatment of female detrusor overactivity: a randomized, double-blind crossover study. J Urol 1989; 142: 1024–6.

136. Thor KB, Katofiasc MA. Effects of duloxetine, a combined serotonin and norepinephrine reuptake inhibitor, on central neural control of lower urinary tract function in the chloralose-anesthetized female cat. J Pharmacol Exp Ther 1995; 274: 1014–24.

137. Steers WD, Herschorn S, Kreder KJ, et al. Duloxetine compared with placebo for treating women with symptoms of overactive bladder. BJU Int 2007; 100: 337–45.

138. Olubadewo J. The effect of imipramine on rate detrusor muscle contractility. Arch Int Pharmacodyn Ther 1980; 145: 84–94.

139. Foreman MM, McNulty AM. Alterations in K(+)-evoked release of 3H-norepinephrine and contractile responses in urethral and bladder tissues induced by norepinephrine reuptake inhibition. Life Sci 1993; 53: 193–200.

140. Castleden CM, George CF, Renwick AG, et al. Imipramine—a possible alternative to current therapy for urinary incontinence in elderly. J Urol 1981; 125: 318–20.

141. Raezer DM, Benson GS, Wein AJ, et al. The functional approach to the management of the pediatric neuropathic bladder: a clinical study. J Urol 1977; 117: 649–54.

142. Sairam K, Kulinskaya E, McNicholas TA, et al. Sildenafil influences lower urinary tract symptoms. BJU Int 2002; 90: 836–9.

143. Andersson KE. Pathways for relaxation of detrusor smooth muscle. Adv Exp Med Bio 1999; 462: 241–52.

144. McVary KT, Monnig W, Camps JL Jr, et al. Sildenafil citrate improves erectile function and urinary symptoms in men with erectile dysfunction and lower urinary tract symptoms associated with benign prostatic hyperplasia: a randomized, double-blind trial. J Urol 2007; 177: 1071.

145. Datta SN, Kavia RB, Gonzales G, et al. Results of double-blind placebo-controlled crossover study of sildenafil citrate (Viagra) in women suffering from obstructed voiding or retention associated with the primary disorder of sphincter relaxation (Fowler's Syndrome). Eur Urol 2007; 51: 495–7.

146. McVary KT, Roehrborn CG, Kaminetsky JC, et al. Tadalafil relieves lower urinary tract symptoms secondary to benign prostatic hyperplasia. J Urol 2007; 177: 1401–7.

147. Stief CG, Porst H, Neuser D, et al. A randomised, placebo-controlled study to assess the efficacy of twice-daily vardenafil in the treatment of lower urinary tract symptoms secondary to benign prostatic hyperplasia. Eur Urol 2008; 53: 1236–44.

148. Truss MC, Stief CG, Uckert S, et al. Phosphodiesterase 1 inhibition in the treatment of lower urinary tract dysfunction: from bench to bedside. World J Urol 2001; 19: 344–50.

149. Nitti VW. Botulinum toxin for the treatment of idiopathic and neurogenic overactive bladder: state of the art. Rev Urol 2006; 8: 198–208.

150. Schurch B, Schmid DM, Stöhrer M. Treatment of neurogenic incontinence with botulinum toxin A. N Engl J Med 2000; 342: 665.

151. Reitz A, Stöhrer M, Kramer G, et al. European experience of 200 cases treated with botulinum-A toxin injections into the detrusor muscle for urinary incontinence due to neurogenic detrusor overactivity. Eur Urol 2004; 45: 510–15.

152. Dmochowski R, Sand PK. Botulinum toxin A in the overactive bladder: current status and future directions. BJU Int 2007; 99: 247–62.

153. Kalsi V, Gonzales G, Popat R, et al. Botulinum injections for the treatment of bladder symptoms of multiple sclerosis. Ann Neurol 2007; 62: 452–7.

154. Reitz A, Denys P, Fermanian C, et al. Do repeat intradetrusor botulinum toxin type a injections yield valuable results? Clinical and urodynamic results after five injections in patients with neurogenic detrusor overactivity. Eur Urol 2007; 52: 1729–35.

155. Sahai A, Khan MS, Dasgupta P. Efficacy of botulinum toxin-A for treating idiopathic detrusor overactivity: results from a single center, randomized, double-blind, placebo controlled trial. J Urol 2007; 177: 2231–6.

156. Brubaker L, Richter HE, Visco A, et al. Pelvic Floor Disorders Network. Refractory idiopathic urge urinary incontinence and botulinum A injection. J Urol 2008; 180: 217–22.

157. Schmid D, Sauermann P, Werner M, et al. Experience with 100 cases treated with botulinum-A toxin injections in the detrusor muscle for idiopathic overactive bladder syndrome refractory to anticholinergics. J Urol 2006; 176: 177–85.

158. Duthie J, Wilson DI, Herbison GP. Botulinum toxin injections for adults with overactive bladder syndrome. Cochrane Database Syst Rev 2007; (3): CD005493.

159. Milanov IG. Mechanisms of baclofen action on spasticity. Acta Neurol Scand 1991; 85: 304–10.

160. Taylor MC, Bates CP. A double-blind crossover trial of baclofen—a new treatment for the unstable bladder syndrome. Br J Urol 1979; 51: 504–5.

161. Bushman W, Steers WD, Meythaler JM. Voiding dysfunction in patients with spastic paraplegia: urodynamic evaluation and response to continuous intrathecal baclofen. Neurourol Urodyn 1993; 12: 163–70.

162. See S, Ginzburg R. Skeletal muscle relaxants. Pharmacotherapy 2008; 28: 207–13.

163. Gebhardt J, Richard D, Barrett T. Expression of estrogen receptor isoforms alpha and beta in messenger RNA in vaginal tissue of premenopausal and postmenopausal women. Am J Obstet Gynecol 2001; 185: 1325–30.

164. Robinson D, Cardozo LD. The role of estrogens in female lower urinary tract dysfunction. Urology 2003; 62(4 Suppl 1): 45–51.

165. Fantl JA, Cardozo L, McClish DK. Estrogen therapy in the management of urinary incontinence in postmenopausal women: a meta-analysis. First report of the Hormones and Urogenital Therapy Committee. Obstet Gynecol 1994; 83: 12–18.

166. Matsubara S, Okada H, Shirakawa T, et al. Estrogen levels influence beta-3-adrenoceptor-mediated relaxation of the female rat detrusor muscle. Urology 2002; 59: 621–5.

167. Batra S, Andersson KE. Oestrogen-induced changes in muscarinic receptor density and contractile responses in the female rabbit urinary bladder. Acta Physiol Scand 1989; 137: 135–41.

168. Shenfield OZ, Blackmore PF, Morgan CW, et al. Rapid effects of estriol and progesterone on tone and spontaneous rhythmic contractions of the rabbit bladder. Obstet Gynecol 1998; 71: 823–8.

169. Cardozo LD, Wise BG, Benness CJ. Vaginal oestradiol for the treatment of lower urinary tract symptoms in postmenopausal women—a double-blind placebo-controlled study. J Obstet Gynaecol 2001; 21: 383–5.

170. Eriksen PS, Rasmussen H. Low-dose 17 beta-estradiol vaginal tablets in the treatment of atrophic vaginitis: a double-blind placebo controlled study. Eur J Obstet Gynecol Reprod Biol 1992; 44: 137–44.

171. Cardozo L, Lose G, McClish D, et al. A systematic review of the effects of estrogens for symptoms suggestive of overactive bladder. Acta Obstet Gynecol Scand 2004; 83: 892–7.

172. Loose DS, Stancel GM. Estrogens and progestins. In: Brunton LL, Lazo JS, Parker KL, eds. Goodman and Gilman's The Pharmacological Basis of Therapeutics. New York: The McGraw-Hill Companies, 2006: 1541–72.

173. Robinson D, Cardozo L. Overactive bladder in the female patient: the role of estrogens. Curr Urol Rep 2002; 3: 452–7.

174. Striano P, Striano S. Gabapentin: a Ca2+ channel alpha 2-delta ligand far beyond epilepsy therapy. Drugs Today (Barc) 2008; 44: 353–68.

175. Carbone A, Palleschi G, Conte A, et al. Gabapentin treatment of neurogenic overactive bladder. Clin Neuropharmacol 2006; 29: 206–14.

176. Kim YT, Kwon DD, Kim J, et al. Gabapentin for overactive bladder and nocturia after anticholinergic failure. Int Braz J Urol 2004; 30: 275–8.

177. Sills GJ. The mechanisms of action of gabapentin and pregabalin. Curr Opin Pharmacol 2006; 6: 108–13.

178. Lecci A, Maggi CA. Tachykinins as modulators of the micturition reflex in the central and peripheral nervous system. Regul Pept 2001; 100: 1–18.

179. Gu BJ, Ishizuka O, Igawa Y, et al. Role of supraspinal tachykinins for micturition in conscious rats with and without bladder outlet obstruction. Naunyn Schmiedebergs Arch Pharmacol 2000; 361: 543–8.

180. Green SA, Alon A, Ianus J, et al. Efficacy and safety of a neurokinin-1 receptor antagonist in postmenopausal women with overactive bladder with urge urinary incontinence. J Urol 2006; 176(6 Pt 1): 2535–40; discussion 2540.

181. Kris MG, Hesketh PJ, Somerfield MR, et al. American Society of Clinical Oncology Guideline for Antiemetics in Oncology: Update 2006. J Clin Oncol 2006; 24: 2931–47.

182. Reeves RR, Burke RS. Tramadol: basic pharmacology and emerging concepts. Durgs Today (Barc) 2008; 44: 827–36.

183. Pehrson R, Andersson KE. Tramadol inhibits rat detrusor overactivity caused by dopamine receptor stimulation. J Urol 2003; 170: 272–5.

184. Safarinejad MR, Hosseini SY. Safety and efficacy of tramadol in the treatment of idiopathic detrusor overactivity: a double-blind, placebo-controlled, randomized study. Br J Clin Pharmacol 2006; 61: 456–63.

185. Dayer P, Collart L, Desmeules J. The Pharmacology of Tramadol. Drugs 1994; 47(Suppl 1): 3–7.

186. de Groat WC, Kruse MN, Vizzard MA, et al. Modification of urinary bladder function after spinal cord injury. Adv Neurol 1997; 72: 347–64.

187. Chai TC, Gray ML, Steers WD. The incidence of a positive ice water test in bladder outlet obstructed patients: evidence for bladder neural plasticity. J Urol 1998; 160: 34–8.

188. Silva C, Ribeiro MJ, Cruz F. The effect of intravesical resiniferatoxin in patients with idiopathic detrusor instability suggests that involuntary detrusor contractions are triggered by C-fiber input. J Urol 2002; 168: 575–9.

189. Brady CM, Apostolidis AN, Harper M, et al. Parallel changes in bladder suburothelial vanilloid receptor TRPV1 and pan-neuronal marker PGP9.5 immunoreactivity in patients with neurogenic detrusor overactivity after intravesical resiniferatoxin treatment. BJU Int 2004; 93: 770–6.

190. Pingle SC, Matta JA, Ahern GP. Capsaicin receptor: TRPV1 a promiscuous TRP channel. Handb Exp Pharmacol 2007; 179: 155–71.

191. Giannantoni A, Di Stasi SM, Nardicchi V, et al. Botulinum-A toxin injections into the detrusor muscle decrease nerve growth factor bladder tissue levels in patients with neurogenic detrusor overactivity. J Urol 2006; 175: 2341–4.

192. Maggi CA. Capsaicin and primary afferent neurons: from basic science to human therapy? J Auton Nerv Syst 1991; 33: 1–14.

193. Maggi CA, Barbanti G, Santicioli P. Cystometric evidence that capsaicin-sensitive nerves modulate the afferent branch of micturition reflex in humans. J Urol 1989; 142: 150–4.

194. Fowler CJ, Beck RO, Gerrard S, et al. Intravesical capsaicin for treatment of detrusor hyperreflexia. J Neurol Neurosurg Psychiatry 1994; 57: 169–73.

195. De Ridder D, Chandiramani V, Dasgupta P, et al. Intravesical capsaicin as a treatment for refractory detrusor hyperreflexia: a dual center study with long-term followup. J Urol 1997; 158: 2087–92.

196. Petersen T, Nielsen JB, Schrøder HD. Intravesical capsaicin in patients with detrusor hyper-reflexia—a placebo-controlled cross-over study. Scand J Urol Nephrol 1999; 33: 104–10.

197. de Sèze M, Wiart L, Joseph PA, et al. Capsaicin and neurogenic detrusor hyperreflexia: a double-blind placebo-controlled study in 20 patients with spinal cord lesions. Neurourol Urodyn 1998; 17: 513–23.

198. de Sèze M, Wiart L, de Sèze MP, et al. Intravesical capsaicin versus resiniferatoxin for the treatment of detrusor hyperreflexia in spinal cord injured patients: a double-blind, randomized, controlled study. J Urol 2004; 171: 251–5.

199. Szallasi A, Blumberg PM. Vanilloid receptors: new insights enhance potential as a therapeutic target. Pain 1996; 68: 195–208.

200. Silva C, Silva J, Ribeiro MJ, et al. Urodynamic effect of intravesical resiniferatoxin in patients with neurogenic detrusor overactivity of spinal origin: results of a double-blind randomized placebo-controlled trial. Eur Urol 2005; 48: 650–5.

201. Giannantoni A, Di Stasi SM, Stephen RL, et al. Intravesical resiniferatoxin versus botulinum-A toxin injections for neurogenic detrusor overactivity: a prospective randomized study. J Urol 2004; 172: 240–3.

202. Kuo HC, Liu HT, Yang WC. Therapeutic effect of multiple resiniferatoxin intravesical instillations in patients with refractory detrusor overactivity: a randomized, double-blind, placebo controlled study. J Urol 2006; 176: 641–5.

203. Rios LA, Panhoca R, Mattos D Jr, et al. Intravesical resiniferatoxin for the treatment of women with idiopathic detrusor overactivity and urgency incontinence: a single dose, 4 weeks, double-blind, randomized, placebo controlled trial. Neurourol Urodyn 2007; 26: 773–8.

204. Rashbaum M, Mandelbaum CC. Non-operative treatment of urinary incontinence in women. Am J Obstet Gynecol 1948; 56: 777.

205. Diokno AC, Taub M. Ephedrine in treatment of urinary incontinence. Urology 1975; 5: 624–5.

206. Kiesswetter H, Hennrich F, Englisch M. Clinical and pharmacologic therapy of stress incontinence. Urol Int 1983; 38: 58–63.

207. Lose G, Lindholm D. Clinical and urodynamic effects of nofenefrine in women with stress incontinence. Urol Int 1984; 39: 298–302.

208. Hoffman BB, Lefkowitz RJ. Catecholamines and sympathomimetic drugs. In: Gilman AG, Rall TW, Nies AS, Taylor P, eds. Goodman and Gilman's The Pharmacological Basis of Therapeutics, 8th edn. New York: Pergamon Press, 1990: 187–220.

209. Kernan WN, Viscoli CM, Brass LM, et al. Phenylpropanolamine and the risk of hemorrhagic stroke. N Engl J Med 2000; 343: 1826.

210. Alhasso A, Glazener CMA, Pickard R, et al. Adrenergic drugs for urinary incontinence in adults. Cochrane Database for Syst Rev 2005; (3): Art. No. CD001842.

211. Furuta A, Asano K, Egawa S, et al. Role of alpha2-adrenoceptors and glutamate mechanisms in the external urethral sphincter continence reflex in rats. J Urol 2009; 181: 1467–73.

212. Fellenius E, Hedberg R, Holmberg E, Waldbeck B. Functional and metabolic effects of terbutaline and propranolol in fast and slow contracting skeletal muscle in vitro. Acta Physiol Scand 1980; 109: 89–95.

213. Kishimoto T, Morita T, Okamiyou Y. Effect of clenbuterol on contractile response in periurethral striated muscle of rabbits. Tohoku J Exp Med 1991; 165: 243–5.

214. Ishiko O, Ushiroyama T, Saji F, et al. Beta(2)-adrenergic agonists and pelvic floor exercises for female stress incontinence. Int J Gynaecol Obstet 2000; 71: 39–44.

215. Hoffman RJ, Hoffman RS, Freyberg CL, et al. Clenbuterol ingestion causing prolonged tachycardia, hypokalemia, and hypophosphatemia with confirmation by quantitative levels. J Toxicol Clin Toxicol 2001; 39: 339–44.

216. Gleason D, Reilly R, Bottaccini M, Pierce MJ. The urethral continence zone and its relation to stress incontinence. J Urol 1974; 112: 81–8.

217. Lexi-Comp I. Propranolol: Drug Information. Up to Date; 1978–2009.

218. Thor KB, Katofiasc MA. Effects of duloxetine, a combined serotonin and norepinephrine reuptake inhibitor, on central neural control of lower urinary tract function in the chloralose-anesthetized female cat. J Pharmacol Exp Ther 1995; 274: 1014–24.

219. Fraser MO, Chancellor MB. Neural control of the urethra and development of pharmacotherapy for stress urinary incontinence. BJU Int 2003; 91: 743–8.

220. Dmochowski RR, Miklos JR, Norton PA, et al. Duloxetine Urinary Incontinence Study Group. Duloxetine versus placebo for the treatment of North American women with stress urinary incontinence. J Urol 2003; 170(4 Pt 1): 1259–63.

221. Mariappan P, Alhasso A, Ballantyne Z, et al. Duloxetine, a serotonin and noradrenaline reuptake inhibitor (SNRI) for the treatment of stress urinary incontinence: a systematic review. Eur Urol 2007; 51: 67–74.

222. Gilja I, Radej M, Kovacic M, et al. Conservative treatment of female stress incontinence with imipramine. J Urol 1984; 132: 909–11.

223. Rud T. Urethral pressure profile in continent women from childhood to old age. Acta Obstet Gynecol Scand 1980; 59: 331–5.

224. Sultana CJ, Walters MD. Estrogen and urinary incontinence in women. Maturitas 1994; 20: 129–38.

225. Beisland HO, Fossberg E, Moer A. Urethral sphincteric insufficiency in postmenopausal females: treatment with phenylpropanolamine and estriol separately and in combination. Urol Int 1984; 39: 211–16.

226. Hendrix SL, Cochrane BB, Nygaard IE, et al. Effects of estrogen with and without progestin on urinary incontinence. JAMA 2005; 293: 935–48.

227. Cardozo L. Role of oestrogens in the treatment of female urinary incontinence. J Am Geriatr Soc 1990; 38: 326–8.

228. Robinson D, Cardozo LD. The role of estrogens in female lower urinary tract dysfunction. Urology 2003; 62(4 Suppl 1): 45–51.

229. Brown JH, Taylor P. Muscarinic receptor agonists and antagonists. In: Brunton LL, Lazo JS, Parker KL, eds. Goodman and Gilman's The Pharmacological Basis of Therapeutics, 11th edn. New York: The McGraw-Hill Companies, 2006: 183–200.

230. Taylor P. Cholinergic agonists. In: Gilman AG, Rall TW, Nies AS, Taylor P, eds. Goodman and Gilman's The Pharmacological Basis of Therapeutics, 8th edn. New York: Pergamon Press, 1990: 122–30.

231. Raezer DM, Wein AJ, Jacobowitz DM. Autonomic innervation of canine urinary bladder. Cholinergic and adrenergic contributions and interactions of sympathetic and parasympathetic systems in bladder function. Urology 1973; 2: 211–21.

232. Sonda LP, Gershon C, Diokno AC. Further observations on the cystometric and uroflowmetric effects of bethanechol chloride on the human bladder. J Urol 1979; 122: 776–7.

233. Perkash I. Intermittent catheterization and bladder rehabilitation in spinal cord injury patients. J Urol 1975; 114: 230–3.

234. Finkbeiner AE. Is bethanechol chloride clinically effective in promoting bladder emptying? J Urol 1985; 134: 443–9.

235. Sporer A, Leyson J, Martin B. Effects of bethanechol chloride on the external urethral sphincter in spinal cord injury patients. J Urol 1978; 120: 62–6.

236. Farrell GA, Webster RD, Higgins LM, et al. Duration of postoperative catheterization : a randomized double blind trial comparing two catheter management protocols and the effect of bethanechol chloride. Int Urogynecol J 1990; 1: 132.

237. Aly A. Prostaglandins in clinical treatment of gastroduodenal mucosal lesions: a review. Scand J Gastroenterol Suppl 1987; 137: 43–9.

238. Bultitude MI, Hills NH, Shuttleworth KE. Clinical and experimental studies on the action of prostaglandins and their synthesis inhibitors on detrusor muscle in vitro and in vivo. Br J Urol 1976; 48: 631–7.

239. Desmond AD, Bultitude MI, Hills NH, et al. Clinical experience with intravesical prostaglandin E2. A prospective study of 36 patients. Br J Urol 1980; 52: 357–66.

240. Delaere KP, Thomas CM, Moonen WA, et al. The value of intravesical prostaglandin E2 and F2 alpha in women with abnormalities of bladder emptying. Br J Urol 1981; 53: 306–9.

241. Schüssler B. Comparison of the mode of action of prostaglandin E2 (PGE2) and sulprostone, a PGE2-derivative, on the lower urinary tract in healthy women. A urodynamic study. Urol Res 1990; 18: 349–52.

242. Vaidyanathan S, Rao MS, Mapa MK, et al. Study of intravesical instillation of 15(S)-15 methyl prostaglandin F2-alpha in patients with neurogenic bladder dysfunction. J Urol 1981; 126: 81–5.

243. Jaschevatzky OE, Anderman S, Shalit A, et al. Prostaglandin F2 alpha for prevention of urinary retention after vaginal hysterectomy. Obstet Gynecol 1985; 66: 244–7.

244. Koonings PP, Bergman A, Ballard CA. Prostaglandins for enhancing detrusor function after surgery for stress incontinence in women. J Reprod Med 1990; 35: 1–5.

245. de Groat WC. Anatomy and physiology of the lower urinary tract. Urol Clin North Am 1993; 20: 383–401.

246. Wheeler JSJ, Robinson CJ, Culkin DJ, et al. Naloxone efficacy in bladder rehabilitation of spinal cord injury patients. J Urol 1987; 137: 1202–5.

247. Lexi-Comp I. Naloxone: Drug Information. Up to Date; 1978–2009.

248. Kleeman FJ. The physiology of the internal urinary sphincter. J Urol 1970; 104: 549–54.

249. Krane RJ, Olsson CA. Phenoxybenzamine in neurogenic bladder dysfunction. II. Clinical considerations. J Urol 1973; 110: 653–6.

250. Hachen HJ. Clinical and urodynamic assessment of alpha-adrenolytic therapy in patients with neurogenic bladder function. Paraplegia 1980; 18: 229–40.

251. Norlen L. Influence of the sympathetic nervous system on the lower urinary tract and its clinical implications. Neurourol Urodyn 1982; 1: 129–33.

252. Sundin T, Dahlström A, Norlén L. The sympathetic innervation and adrenoreceptor function of the human lower urinary tract in the normal state and after parasympathetic denervation. Invest Urol 1977; 14: 322–8.

253. Koyanagi T. Further observation on the denervation supersensitivity of the urethra in patients with chronic neurogenic bladders. J Urol 1979; 122: 348–52.

254. Parsons K, Turton M. Urethral supersensitivity and occult urethral neuropathy. Br J Urol 1980; 52: 131–7.

255. Nordling J, Meyhoff HH, Hald T, et al. Urethral denervation supersensitivity to noradrenaline after radical hysterectomy. Scand J Urol Nephrol 1981; 15: 21–4.

256. Westfall TCWD. Adrenergic agonists and antagonists. In: Brunton LL, Lazo JS, Parker KL, eds. Goodman and Gilman's The Pharmacological Basis of Therapeutics. New York: The McGraw-Hill Companies, 2006: 237–96.

257. Nordling J, Meyhoff HH, Hald T. Sympatholytic effect on striated urethral sphincter. A peripheral or central nervous system effect? Scand J Urol Nephrol 1981; 15: 173–80.

258. Hoffman BB, Lefkowitz RJ. Adrenergic receptor agonists. In: Gilman AG, Rall TW, Nies AS, Taylor P, eds. Goodman and Gilman's The Pharmacological Basis of Therapeutics, 8th edn. New York: Pergamon Press, 1990: 221–43.

259. McGuire E, Savastano J. Effect of alpha adrenergic blockage and anticholinergic agents on the decentralized primate bladder. Neurourol Urodyn 1985; 4: 139–42.

260. Gajewski J, Downie JW, Awad SA. Experimental evidence for a central nervous system site of action in the effect of alpha-adrenergic blockers on the external urinary sphincter. J Urol 1984; 132: 403–9.

261. Thind P, Lose G, Colstrup H, et al. The effect of alpha-adrenoceptor stimulation and blockade on the static urethral sphincter function in healthy females. Scand J Urol Nephrol 1992; 26: 219–25.

262. Jensen D Jr. Pharmacologic studies of the uninhibited neurogenic bladder. Acta Neurol Scand 1981; 64: 145–74.

263. Taylor SH. Clinical pharmacotherapeutics of doxazosin. Am J Med 1989; 87(Suppl 2A): 2S–11S.

264. Swierzewski SJ 3rd, Gormley EA, Belville WD, et al. The effect of terazosin on bladder function in the spinal cord injured patient. J Urol 1994; 151: 951–4.

265. Chapple C, Wyndaele JJ, Nordling J, et al. European Tamsulosin Study Group. Tamsulosin, the first prostate selective α1a adrenoceptor antagonist. A meta-analysis of two randomized placebo-controlled, multicentre studies in patients with benign prostatic obstruction (symptomatic BPH). Eur Urol 1996; 29: 155–67.

266. Reitz A, Haferkamp A, Kyburz T, et al. The effect of tamsulosin on the resting tone and the contractile behaviour of the female urethra: a functional urodynamic study in healthy women. Eur Urol 2004; 46: 235–40.

267. Pischedda A, Pirozzi Farina F, Madonia M, et al. Use of alpha1-blockers in female functional bladder neck obstruction. Urol Int 2005; 74: 256–61.

268. Chang SJ, Chiang IN, Yu HJ. The effectiveness of tamsulosin in treating women with voiding difficulty. Int J Urol 2008; 15: 981–5.

269. Robinson D, Cardozo L, Terpstra G, et al. Tamsulosin Study Group. A randomized double-blind placebo-controlled multicentre study to explore the efficacy and safety of tamsulosin and tolterodine in women with overactive bladder syndrome. BJU Int 2007; 100: 840–5.

270. Lepor H, Tank R, Kobayashi S, et al. Localization of the α1a-adrenoceptor in the human prostate. J Urol 1995; 154: 2096–9.

271. Buzelin JM, Herbert M, Blondin P, The PRAZALF group. Alpha-blocking treatment with alfuzosin in symptomatic benign prostatic hyperplasia: comparative study with prazosin. Br J Urol 1993; 72: 922–7.

272. Buzelin JM, Roth S, Geffriaud-Ricouard C, et al., ALGEBI Study Group. Efficacy and safety of sustained-release alfuzosin 5 mg in patients with benign prostatic hyperplasia. Eur Urol 1997; 31: 190–8.

273. Bloom FE. Neurohumoral transmission and the central nervous system. In: Gilman AG, Rall TW, Nies AS, Taylor P, eds. Gooman and Gilman's The Pharmacological Basis of Therapeutics, 8th edn. New York: Pergamon Press, 1990: 244–68.

274. Lader M. Clinical pharmacology of benzodiazepines. Annu Rev Med 1987; 38: 19–28.

275. Davidoff RA. Antispasticity drugs: mechanisms of action. Ann Neurol 1985; 17: 107–16.

276. Kums JJM, Delhaas EM. Intrathecal baclofen infusion in patients with spasticity and neurogenic bladder disease. Preliminary results. World J Urol 1991; 9: 153–6.

277. Penn RD, Savoy SM, Corcose DE. Intrathecal baclofen for severe spinal spasticity. N Engl J Med 1989; 320: 1517–21.

278. Nanninga J, Kaplan P, Lal S. Effects of phentolamine on peripheral muscle EMG activity in paraplegia. Br J Urol 1977; 49: 537–9.

279. Cedarbaum JM, Schleifer LS. Drugs for Parkinson's disease spasticity, and acute muscle spasms. In: Gilman AG, Rall TW, Nies AS, Taylor P, eds. Goodman and Gilman's The Pharmmacological Basis of Therapeutics, 8th edn. New York: Pergamon Press, 1990: 463–84.

280. Murdock MM, Sax D, Krane RJ. Use of dantrolene sodium in external sphincter spasm. Urology 1976; 8: 133–7.

281. Hackler R, Broecker B, Klein F, et al. A clinical experience with dantrolene sodium for external urinary sphincter hypertonicity in spinal cord injured patients. J Urol 1980; 124: 78–81.

282. Zinner N, Gittelman M, Harris R, et al., Trospium Study Group. Trospium chloride improves overactive bladder symptoms: a multicenter phase III trial. J Urol 2004; 171(pt 1): 2311–15.

283. Dykstra DD, Sidi AA. Treatment of detrusor-striated sphincter dyssynergia with botulinum A toxin. Arch Phys Med Rehabil 1990; 71: 24–6.

284. Phelan MW, Franks M, Somogyi GT. Botulinum toxin urethral sphincter injection to restore bladder emptying in men and women with voiding dysfunction. J Urol 2001; 165: 1107–10.

285. de Sèze M, Petit H, Gallien P. Botulinum A toxin and detrusor sphincter dyssynergia: a double blind lidocaine-controlled study in 13 patients with spinal cord disease. Eur Urol 2002; 42: 56–62.

286. Herman RM, Wainberg MC. Clonidine inhibits vesico-sphincter reflexes in patients with chronic spinal lesions. Arch Phys Med Rehabil 1991; 72: 539–45.

287. Matthiesen TB, Rittig S, Nørgaard JP, et al. Nocturnal polyuria and natriuresis in male patients with nocturia and lower urinary tract symptoms. J Urol 1996; 156: 1292–9.

288. Nørgaard JP, Rittig S, Djurhuus JC. Nocturnal enuresis: an approach to treatment based on pathogenesis. J Pediatr 1989; 114(4 Pt 2): 705–10.

289. Valiquette G, Herbert J, Maede-D'Alisera P. Desmopressin in the management of nocturia in patients with multiple sclerosis. A double-blind, crossover trial. Arch Neurol 1996; 53: 1270–5.

290. Hashim H, Abrams P. Desmopreesin for the treatment of adult nocturia. Therapy 2008; 5: 667–83.

291. Hashim H, Malmberg L, Graugaard-Jensen C. Desmopressin, as a "designer-drug," in the treatment of overactive bladder syndrome. Neurourol Urodyn 2009; 28: 40–6.

292. Rembratt A, Riis A, Norgaard JP. Desmopressin treatment in nocturia; an analysis of risk factors for hyponatremia. Neurourol Urodyn 2006; 25: 105–9.

293. Lexi-Comp I. Desmopressin: Drug information. Up to Date; 1978–2009.

294. Pedersen PA, Johansen PB. Prophylactic treatment of adult nocturia with bumetanide. Br J Urol 1988; 62: 145–7.

295. Lexi-Comp I. Bumetanide: Drug information. Up to Date; 1978–2009.

43 Peripheral Neuromodulation
John Heesakkers and Michael van Balken

INTRODUCTION

Neurostimulation of the lower urinary tract could theoretically be used to treat as well stress urinary incontinence or incontinence caused by detrusor overactivity. Several attempts have been made to reinforce the urinary sphincter by stimulation of the pudendal nerve and pelvic floor muscles. In fact the idea of treating stress urinary incontinence by pudendal stimulation was the embarkment for modern neuromodulation of the lower urinary tract. Moore tried to achieve this by using surface electrodes (1). It was concluded, however, that for these kinds of experiments the applied current has to be very high in order to have sphincter contraction. This is very painful to the patient so in this way this technique can not be put in clinical practice. Apart from this, the results were also disappointing, therefore attempts to treat stress urinary incontinence were abandoned. However, the results of neuromodulation of the pelvic nerves on detrusor overactivity and overactive bladder (OAB) were appealing. This has incurred all developments that are ongoing at the moment.

Electrical stimulation or neuromodulation of nerves of the lower urinary tract has been studied and tried extensively over the years. The best known and best documented technique is sacral nerve stimulation (SNS) by means of an implantable pulse generator. Percutaneous tibial nerve stimulation (PTNS) is the most extensive documented way of nerve stimulation away from the sacral nerves. Other sites and ways of stimulation have been explored and tested as well, but the published data are scarce and there is a huge variety in applied techniques.

The explorations to elucidate the best technique of electrical stimulation are based on three important concepts. First, it is easier to apply stimulation in a less invasive way. For this reason transcutaneous stimulation with surface electrodes or stimulation probes suit best. Secondly, the way of stimulation should be in an area that is the least intimate in order to be acceptable for the majority of patients. This makes sacral dermatomes or legs appropriate areas for stimulation. The third reason is that it should be practical to apply. Continuous stimulation is therefore less ideal and discontinuous stimulation is easier. Combining these ideal features the best way of stimulation is probably the use of surface electrodes applied at a remote spot away from the urogenital region in a discontinuous matter. This chapter mainly deals with posterior tibial nerve stimulation because it is best documented in a standardized way. Other ways of peripheral nerve stimulation are also mentioned with some examples of technique and outcome without trying to give a complete overview. Invasive techniques, like SNS and pudendal nerve stimulation, and the application of stimulation probes usually used in a physiotherapy setting, or not discussed.

WAYS OF PERIPHERAL NEUROMODULATION

The nerves that innervate the lower urinary tract originate from the lumbar, sacral, and coccygeal segmental nerves from L2 to S4 (Fig. 43.1). Afferent and efferent fibers from these segmental sacral roots merge in the periphery outside the spinal cord. After merging they leave as combined nerves that have lost their segmental innervation pattern. The sciatic nerve is a merger of fibers from L4 to S3. The posterior tibial nerve is a part of the sciatic nerve. The pudendal nerve is a merger of fibers from the sacral roots S3 to S5. The dorsal genital (penile and clitoral) nerves are the beginning of the afferent pathways of the pudendal nerve.

Peripheral neuromodulation has been attempted via one of the involved nerves like the dorsal genital nerve, the posterior tibial nerve, or the common peroneal nerve, by the overlying skin or by stimulating the dermatomes that are innervated by the same nerve as the ones that innervate the lower urinary tract organs.

SACRAL DERMATOMES

Stimulation of the sacral dermatomes is a valid and practical option to apply stimulation for influencing the lower urinary tract. Stimulation adhesives can be stuck on the skin whereafter the stimulation can start for some time. The most appropriate sacral dermatome is the S3 dermatome. It covers the suprapubic region and the intermediate part of the gluteal area.

Fall was the first to publish on suprapubic transcutaneous stimulation twice a day for 15 to 30 minutes during one to six months in a group of nine interstitial cystitis (IC) patients who also suffered from detrusor overactivity (2). He observed good results especially on pain and voiding frequency. In a randomized trial Soomro et al. performed suprapubic stimulation by means of surface electrodes for up to six hours/day during six weeks (3). They compared this technique to the effect of oxybutinin in 43 patients with proven detrusor overactivity. They observed subjective improvements in both groups and conclude that the medication group did better. On the other hand Fjorback et al. did not see any acute urodynamic effects with dermatome stimulation in a group of neurogenic patients (4).

DORSAL CLITORAL OR PENILE NERVE

Stimulation of the afferent dorsal clitoral nerve and dorsal penile nerve has been studied fairly extensively. The conclusion by most authors is that it is effective clinically as well as urodynamically. Nakamura and Sakurai published on 22 male patients with complaints of OAB dry and OAB wet of unknown origin (5). They used surface electrodes with continuous stimulation. The reported outcome showed four cured patients. Transcutaneous electrical stimulation was applied to the penis

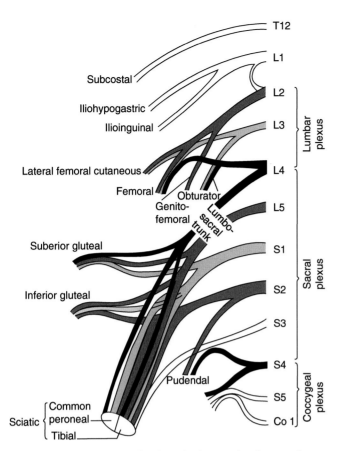

Figure 43.1 The organization of the lower lumbar, sacral, and coccygeal nerve plexus, the merger of the various roots and the most important nerves that branches from the merge nerve plexus.

in 22 patients complaining of frequency, urgency, and/or urge incontinence. Urodynamic parameters improved in 10 of 22 patients. Opisso et al. performed automatic stimulation and patient controlled genital stimulation to suppress detrusor overactivity in 17 patients with neurogenic diseases (6). They observed that patient controlled genital nerve stimulation is as effective as automatic controlled stimulation to treat neurogenic detrusor overactivity.

Goldman et al. showed a reduction in OAB symptoms with dorsal genital nerve stimulation in 21 women with OAB wet complaints (7). The women underwent percutaneous placement of an electrode during one week with urodynamic and clinical control. About 50% reported more than 50% reduction in incontinence episodes. Eighty-one percent of the subjects with severe urgency experienced more than 50% improvement. The authors did not find a relationship between the acute effects of stimulation on cystometry and the clinical results during home use.

TIBIAL NERVE STIMULATION

There is an ancient Chinese custom to perform acupuncture of the leg. With this technique, developed in China over 5000 years ago, the "energetic harmony" of the urogenital tract might be restored through the stimulation of specific points like SP-6 or Sanyinjiao point. With this type of acupuncture, most likely nerve stimulation of the common peroneal nerve or the posterior tibial nerve area is performed and effects on the pelvic organs as well as the spleen are obtained. When electrical current is applied to the acupuncture needle the technique is called electrical acupuncture. This is considered the same as peripheral neuromodulation. The fundamental feature of neuromodulation is that nerves are stimulated and not energy pathways or other routes that do not have any anatomical substrate. Nerve stimulation ideally has an efferent motor effect and an afferent sensory effect. Stimulation of posterior tibial nerve results in great toe flexion or fanning of the toes. The sensory effect is a radiation tickling sensation of the foot sole. McGuire was the first to explore tibial nerve stimulation in 1983 (8). He performed transcutaneous posterior tibial nerve stimulation in 15 patients with detrusor overactivity because of a neurological disease.

PTNS

Inspired by this previous work by McGuire, Marshall Stoller started research on PTNS as a neuromodulative treatment in lower urinary tract dysfunction. After initial testing in pig-tailed monkeys (9), PTNS was later investigated in humans with promising results (10).

PTNS is performed in patients placed in the supine position with the soles of the feet together and the knees abducted and flexed ("frog-position"). A 34 gauge stainless steel needle is inserted approximately 3 to 4 cm, about three fingerbreadths cephalad to the medial malleolus, between the posterior margin of the tibia and soleus muscle. A stick-on electrode is placed on the same leg near the arch of the foot. The needle and electrode are connected to a low voltage (9 V) stimulator (Urgent PC®, Uroplasty Inc, Minnetonka, Minnesota, U.S.A.) with an adjustable pulse intensity of 0 to 10 mA, a fixed pulse width of 200 µsec and a frequency of 20 Hz. The amplitude is slowly increased until the large toe starts to curl or toes start to fan. If the large toe does not curl or pain occurs near the insertion site, the stimulation device is switched off and the procedure is repeated. If the large toe curls or toes start to fan stimulation is applied at an intensity well tolerated by the patient. If necessary the amplitude can be increased during the session. In general, patients undergo 12 weekly outpatient treatment sessions, each lasting 30 minutes. If a good response occurs the patient is offered recurrent discontinuous treatment (11).

Most of what is known regarding the mechanisms of action of neuromodulation was found by studying SNS. In chronic pelvic pain the working mechanism is believed to be a gate-control mechanism (12). Neuromodulation is thought to restore the control at the spinal segmental gate as well as at supraspinal sites such as the brainstem and limbic system nuclei. The same goes for OAB syndrome, where a gate-control mechanism may also play a part. Neuromodulation is suggested to treat OAB complaints by restoring the balance between inhibitory and excitatory control systems, peripherally as well as centrally (13). For example, neuromodulation at the sacral level is believed amongst others to inhibit spinal tract neurons, and to inhibit neurons involved in spinal segmental reflexes as well as postganglionic and primary afferent pathways (14). In case of voiding disorders, theories as direct afferent pudendal nerve stimulation resulting in a direct change of pelvic floor behavior (15), a rebound phenomenon (16), suppression of the guarding reflexes (17), and retuning of the L and M regions or "on-off" switch mechanism in the brainstem (18) have been suggested.

The observation that the maximum effect of neuromodulation is not immediately attained is an indication that neuromodulation induces learning changes of the neural system and therefore of neural plasticity. The carry-over effect may be caused by negative modulation of excitatory synapses in the central micturition reflex pathway (19).

Mechanisms of action of PTNS supposedly are the same as in SNS, but research about this subject is yet to be performed.

Since the introduction of PTNS in 1999 (10) several studies have been performed that evaluated its effectiveness in mostly patients with OAB syndrome and in nonobstructive urinary retention.

Almost all studies on OAB used micturition diaries and general and/or disease specific quality of life questionnaires to measure the effects of PTNS (20–24). Subjective success was found in 59% to 64% of patients (20,21). Depending on the definition used, objective success, that is most of the time an over 50% decrease in incontinence episodes and/or micturition frequency, was found in 47% to 56% of patients (21,22), a percentage that may go up to approximately 70% if only 25% improvement was aimed for (21,23).

With regard to chronic nonobstructive urinary retention, studies have shown subjective success in 58% to 59% of patients, with success defined as patients request for continuation of treatment to maintain the obtained results (20,25). More objective outcome measures improved over 50% in 41% of patients. Although in those patients post void residuals decreased to <100 cm^3, or even to 0 cm^3, none of them dared to stop catheterizations entirely. Beside micturition and catheterization parameters, significant improvements were seen in general and disease specific quality of life measures (25).

In studies on PTNS for the treatment of refractory chronic pelvic pain as the main complaint only very modest results were shown: a subjective response was seen in 42% of all patients, the objective response (mean visual analogue scale (VAS) for pain decreased >50%) varied between 21% and 60% of cases (26,27). Although these results in chronic pelvic pain are not very substantial, they are in concordance with the results of other neuromodulation techniques.

Although rather objective parameters, especially from voiding diaries, can be obtained, urodynamic studies may provide more robust data on the effectiveness of PTNS. There is a difference, however, between urodynamic effects during stimulation as compared to urodynamic data when they are performed after a series of PTNS sessions. When acute PTNS is performed as soon as detrusor overactivity occurs during urodynamics, the suppressive effects, at least in neurological patients, are contradicting (4,28,29). This is different for a series of PTNS sessions. In a study on patients with symptoms related to OAB syndrome treated with PTNS for twelve weeks, a reduction in the number of urinary leakage episodes of 50% or more per 24 hours could be obtained in 56% (30). Frequency/volume chart data and quality of life scores improved significantly. Of the participants with pre- and post-treatment urodynamic data, only a few showed complete resolution of detrusor

overactivity. Nevertheless, increments in cystometric bladder capacity and in volume at detrusor overactivity were significant. Subjects without detrusor overactivity at baseline appeared 1.7 times more prone to respond to PTNS. The more the bladder overactivity was pronounced, the less these patients responded to PTNS (area under the receiver operating characteristic curve 0.64).

In a study about patients with chronic voiding dysfunction enrolled in a comparable prospective trial, objective success was obtained in 41% of patients (31). Detrusor pressure at maximal flow, cystometric residuals, and various bladder indices (bladder contractility index and bladder voiding efficiency) improved significantly for all patients. Patients with minor voiding dysfunction were more prone to notice success (OR: 0.7).

It can be concluded that PTNS not only results in clinical, but also in more objective urodynamic changes over time. In OAB patients PTNS increases cystometric capacity and delays the onset of, but not resolves detrusor overactivity. In patients with voiding disorders PTNS improves parameters regarding more effective bladder emptying.

In SNS, the result of percutaneous nerve evaluation (PNE) prior to definitive implantation is the most important prognostic factor for success. Efforts to establish other predictive parameters proved not to be very successful. Therefore, at present, most is expected from refining the PNE technique. For example, age, duration of complaints, number and kind of former treatments, indication for neuromodulation therapy, and different neurostimulation parameters were not predictive for treatment outcome (32–34). Although some studies suggest the opposite (32,35) gender similarly seems not to influence treatment outcome (33,34). The only factor rather consistently reported to predict poor treatment outcome is the history or presence of psychological disorders or poor mental health (34,36,37). For PTNS little data are available. Studies on urodynamic changes by PTNS suggest that if voiding dysfunction is not too severe or, in case of OAB, detrusor overactivity is absent, patients are more likely to have a successful treatment outcome (30,31). All above mentioned clinical parameters for predicting SNS outcome were also tested in 132 patients treated with PTNS, but proved of no significance as well (38). Even a history of sexual or physical abuse did not alter PTNS treatment outcome. However, a low total score at baseline in the SF-36 general quality of life questionnaire proved to be predictive for not obtaining objective nor subjective success. Especially patients with a low SF-36 Mental Component Summary were prone to fail neuromodulation therapy. These patients also scored worse on disease-specific quality of life questionnaires, although they had no different disease severity compared to patients with good mental health.

Apart from evaluating which patients may be best suited to start therapy, it is also important to evaluate how, if possible, positive results can be sustained. Although Klingler et al. (22) seemed to suggest otherwise, it is now well known that once positive treatment outcome has been obtained, a maintenance program is needed to avoid recurrence of complaints. In a recent study the necessity of maintenance therapy was evaluated by means of a six week break of therapy in successfully treated PTNS patients, leading to over 50% worsening of main symptoms in almost all patients. Restarting PTNS afterwards improved complaints to the level present before the break (39).

These results have implications beyond the basic idea that maintenance therapy is indispensable to keep up positive clinical results. Obviously, such maintenance programs put great strains on caregivers and hospital facilities. Each patient that is put on a maintenance schedule will visit the outpatients department at least 20 to 30 times per annum. This issue was prompted to develop a prototype of an implantable device that allows a patient to perform self-stimulation at home as frequently as the individual situation requires (40). In prospect, this implantable device should lessen the burden on medical professionals and institutions.

PTNS is a minimally invasive, easily accessible neuromodulation technique and has proven its benefit in OAB and non obstructive urinary retention. Regretfully, in chronic pelvic pain its benefits seem only modest. Although a placebo controlled study is currently being performed, there is now quite some "circumstantial" evidence for its efficacy, including animal studies (41,42) and studies with urodynamic data (30,31). When PTNS becomes a more established treatment modality, no doubt other indications will be explored. Subject of further investigation most likely will be children, neurologic patients, and patients with fecal incontinence.

Almost all research done on PTNS used the same stimulation protocol: PTNS was performed in 10 to 12 weekly sessions, each lasting for 30 minutes. Stimulation parameters were preset and rather fixed and every time only one needle was inserted. It may be well anticipated that changes in treatment scheme and/or stimulation parameters could lead to a different, possibly even superior outcome. The same goes for bilateral instead of unilateral therapy.

Compared to the once-a-week protocol, an accelerated scheme of three to four times a week for example seems not to significantly influence treatment outcome, although there are some conflicting reports on its effect on the necessity of maintenance therapy afterwards (22,39). On the other hand, it is obvious that an accelerated scheme has the advantage of achieving clinical results faster (43). Regarding stimulation parameters, it is rather widely agreed that pulse intensity in neuromodulation should be set at a well tolerable level. However, although for PTNS the stimulation frequency is set at 20 Hz, the stimulation frequency has been varied in the different neuromodulation techniques from 5 to 20 Hz, but even frequencies up to 150 Hz are reported. As it is suggested that frequency is optimal at more unpleasantly low levels (5–6 Hz) (44), studies on PTNS with pulse frequencies below 20 Hz may produce interesting results. The same goes for changes in pulse duration, in PTNS set at 0.2 msec, but in other techniques also up to 0.5 or even over 1 msec.

Apart from research on stimulation scheme and parameters, it is also interesting to evaluate the possible beneficial effect of stimulating both legs at the same time. At least in sacral neuromodulation there is some evidence that bilateral stimulation may improve results not so much in relieving symptoms better than unilateral stimulation once successful, as well in improving the chance that patients react at all (45–47). Obviously, a positive outcome of bilateral stimulation in PTNS would also need a solution with regard to a possible implantable device.

If a subcutaneous implant for chronic tibial nerve stimulation is readily experimentally and commercially available, by analogy with sacral neuromodulation additional efforts should be undertaken to refine the pre-implant testing phase in order to decrease the amount of unnecessarily treated patients. This will eventually be the way PTNS directions should be heading: a readily available subcutaneous implantable device, easily controllable by patients themselves in flexible, individualized treatment schemes.

REFERENCES

1. Moore T, Schofield PF. Treatment of stress incontinence by maximum perineal electrical stimulation. Br Med J 1967; 3: 150–1.
2. Fall M, Carlsson CA, Erlandson BE. Electrical stimulation in interstitial cystitis. J Urol 1980; 123: 192–5.
3. Soomro NA, Khadra MH, Robson W, Neal DE. A crossover randomized trial of transcutaneous electrical nerve stimulation and oxybutynin in patients with detrusor instability. J Urol 2001; 166: 146–9.
4. Fjorback MV, van Rey FS, van der Pal F, et al. Acute urodynamic effects of posterior tibial nerve stimulation on neurogenic detrusor overactivity in patients with MS. Eur Urol 2007; 51: 464–70.
5. Nakamura M, Sakurai T. Bladder inhibition by penile electrical stimulation. Br J Urol 1984; 56: 413–15.
6. Opisso E, Borau A, Rodríguez A, Hansen J, Rijkhoff NJ. Patient controlled versus automatic stimulation of pudendal nerve afferents to treat neurogenic detrusor overactivity. J Urol 2008; 180: 1403–8.
7. Goldman HB, Amundsen CL, Mangel J, et al. Dorsal genital nerve stimulation for the treatment of overactive bladder symptoms. Neurourol Urodyn 2008; 27: 499–503.
8. McGuire EJ, Zhang SC, Horwinski ER, Lytton B. Treatment of motor and sensory detrusor instability by electrical stimulation. J Urol 1983; 129: 78–9.
9. Stoller ML, Copeland S, Millard AR, et al. The efficacy of acupuncture in reversing unstable bladder in pig-tailed monkeys. [abstract 2]. J Urol 1987; (Suppl 137): 104A.
10. Stoller ML. Afferent nerve stimulation for pelvic floor dysfunction. [abstract 62]. Eur Urol 1999; 35(Suppl 2): 16.
11. Govier FE, Litwiller S, Nitti V, et al. Percutaneous afferent neuromodulation for the refractory overactive bladder: results of a multicenter study. J Urol 2001; 165: 1193–8.
12. Alo K, Holsheimer J. New trends in neuromodulation for the management of neuropathic pain. Neurosurgery 2002; 50: 690–703.
13. Schmidt R. Advances in genitourinary neurostimulation. Neurosurgery 1986; 19: 1041–4.
14. Peeren F, Hoebeke P, Everaert K. Sacral nerve stimulation: Interstim® therapy. Expert Rev Med Devices 2005; 2: 253–8.
15. Goodwin R, Swinn M, Fowler C. The neurophysiology of urinary retention in young women and its treatment by neuromodulation. World J Urol 1998; 16: 305–7.
16. Schultz-Lampel D, Jiang C, Lindstrom S, et al. Experimental results on mechanisms of action on electrical neuromodulation in chronic urinary retention. World J Urol 1998; 16: 301–4.
17. van Balken MR, Vergunst H, Bemelmans BL. The use of electrical devices for the treatment of bladder dysfunction: a review of methods. J Urol 2004; 172: 846–51.
18. Bemelmans BL, Mundy A, Craggs M. Neuromodulation by implant for treating lower urinary tract symptoms and dysfunction. Eur Urol 1999; 36: 81–91.
19. van der Pal F, Heesakkers JP, Bemelmans BL. Current opinion on the working mechanisms of neuromodulation in the treatment of lower urinary tract dysfunction. Curr Opin Urol 2006; 16: 261–7.
20. van Balken MR, Vandoninck V, Gisolf KW, et al. Posterior tibial nerve stimulation as neuromodulative treatment of lower urinary tract dysfunction. J Urol 2001; 166: 914–18.
21. Vandoninck V, van Balken MR, Agro EF, et al. Posterior tibial nerve stimulation in the treatment of urge incontinence. Neurourol Urodyn 2003; 22: 17–23.

22. Klingler HC, Pycha A, Schmidbauer J, et al. Use of peripheral neuromodulation of the S3 region for treatment of detrusor overactivity: a urodynamic-based study. Urology 2000; 56: 766–71.

23. Govier FE, Litwiller S, Nitti V, et al. Percutaneous afferent neuromodulation for the refractory overactive bladder: results of a multicenter study. J Urol 2001; 165: 1193–8.

24. Ruiz BC, Pena OX, Martinez PC, et al. Peripheral afferent nerve stimulation for treatment of lower urinary tract irritative symptoms. Eur Urol 2004; 45: 65–9.

25. Vandoninck V, van Balken MR, Finazzi Agro E, et al. Posterior tibial nerve stimulation in the treatment of idiopathic nonobstructive voiding dysfunction. Urology 2003; 61: 567–72.

26. van Balken MR, Vandoninck V, Messelink EJ, et al. Percutaneous tibial nerve stimulation as neuromodulative treatment of chronic pelvic pain. Eur Urol 2003; 43: 158–63.

27. Kim SW, Paick JS, Ku JH. Percutaneous posterior tibial nerve stimulation in patients with chronic pelvic pain: a preliminary study. Urol Int 2007; 78: 58–62.

28. Kabay SC, Yucel M, Kabay S. Acute effect of posterior tibial nerve stimulation on neurogenic detrusor overactivity in patients with multiple sclerosis: urodynamic study. Urology 2008; 71: 641–5.

29. Kabay SC, Kabay S, Yucel M, Ozden H. Acute urodynamic effects of percutaneous posterior tibial nerve stimulation on neurogenic detrusor overactivity in patients with Parkinson's disease. Neurourol Urodyn 2009; 28: 62–7.

30. Vandoninck V, van Balken MR, Finazzi Agro E, et al. Percutaneous tibial nerve stimulation in the treatment of overactive bladder: urodynamic data. Neurourol Urodyn 2003: 22: 227–32.

31. Vandoninck V, van Balken MR, Finazzi Agro E, et al. Posterior tibial nerve stimulation in the treatment of voiding dysfunction: urodynamic data. Neurourol Urodyn 2004; 23: 246–51.

32. Janknegt RA, Hassouna MM, Siegel SW, et al. Long-term effectiveness of sacral nerve stimulation for refractory urge incontinence. Eur Urol 2001; 39: 101–6.

33. Koldewijn EL, Rosier PF, Meuleman EJ, et al. Predictors of success with neuromodulation in lower urinary tract dysfunction: results of trial stimulation in 100 patients. J Urol 1994; 152: 2071–5.

34. Weil EH, Ruiz-Cerda JL, Eerdmans PH, et al. Clinical results of sacral neuromodulation for chronic voiding dysfunction using unilateral sacral foramen electrodes. World J Urol 1998; 16: 313–21.

35. Bosch JL, Groen J. Disappointing results of neuromodulation in men with urge incontinence due to detrusor instability. Neurourol Urodyn 1997; 16: 347–9.

36. Spinelli M, Bertapelle P, Cappellano F, et al. Chronic sacral neuromodulation in patients with lower urinary tract symptoms: results from a national register. J Urol 2001; 166: 541–5.

37. Rosier PF, Meuleman EJ, Debruyne FM. Quality of life of patients with lower urinary tract dysfunction after treatment with sacral neuromodulation. Neurourol Urodyn 1997; 16: 483–4.

38. van Balken MR, Vergunst H, Bemelmans BL. Prognostic factors for successful percutaneous tibial nerve stimulation. Eur Urol 2006; 49: 360–5.

39. Van der Pal F, van Balken MR, Heesakkers JP, et al. Percutaneous tibial nerve stimulation (PTNS) in the treatment of refractory overactive bladder syndrome: is maintenance treatment a necessity? BJU Int 2006; 97: 547–50.

40. Van der Pal F, van Balken MR, Heesakkers JP, et al. Implant driven tibial nerve stimulation in the treatment of refractory overactive bladder syndrome: 12-month follow up. Neuromodulation 2006; 9: 163–71.

41. Chang CJ, Huang ST, Hsu K, et al. Electroacupuncture decreases c-fos expression in the spinal cord induced by noxious stimulation of the rat bladder. J Urol 1998; 160: 2274–9.

42. Van der Pal F, Heesakkers JP, Debruyne FM, et al. Modulation of the micturition reflex in an anesthetized cat through percutaneous stimulation of the tibial nerve. Eur Urol 2005; (Suppl 4): 193.

43. Finazzi Agro E, Campagna A, Sciobica F, et al. Posterior tibial nerve stimulation: is the once-a-week protocol the best option? Minerva Urol Nefrol 2005; 57: 119–23.

44. Fall M, Lindstrom S. Electrical stimulation. A physiologic approach to the treatment of urinary incontinence. Urol Clin North Am 1991; 18: 393–407.

45. Hohenfellner M, Schultz-Lampel D, Dahms S, et al. Bilateral chronic sacral neuromodulation for treatment of lower urinary tract dysfunction. J Urol 1998; 160: 821–4.

46. Scheepens WA, De Bie RA, Weil EH, et al. Unilateral versus bilateral sacral neuromodulation in patients with chronic voiding dysfunction. J Urol 2002; 168: 2046–50.

47. Van Kerrebroeck EV, Scheepens WA, de Bie RA, et al. European experience with bilateral sacral neuromodulation in patients with chronic lower urinary tract dysfunction. Urol Clin North Am 2005; 32: 51–7.

44 Sacral Neuromodulation in the Treatment of Female Overactive Bladder Syndrome and Non-obstructive Urinary Retention

JLH Ruud Bosch

INTRODUCTION

Female voiding dysfunctions such as those related to overactive bladder syndrome and non-obstructive urinary retention often are refractory to conservative management including drug therapy, behavioral therapy, pelvic floor muscle exercises, biofeedback, non-invasive neuromodulation, and intermittent self-catheterization. Sacral nerve neuromodulation has proved to be valuable in these situations (1). In 2007, the Food and Drug Administration approved sacral neuromodulation for treatment of refractory urge urinary incontinence in the United States. Subsequently, approval was also granted for the treatment of urge-frequency syndrome and for non-obstructive urinary retention.

The precise mode of action of neuromodulation is unknown. Its effects can be explained by modulation of reflex pathways at the spinal cord level (1,2). However, there are now studies that indicate that supraspinal pathways are involved as well (3). Experimental work in animals, human volunteers, and patients has revealed that at least two mechanisms are important: activation of efferent nerve fibers to the striated urethral sphincter reflexively causes detrusor relaxation, and activation of afferent nerve fibers causes inhibition of the voiding reflex at a spinal and/or supraspinal level.

Tanagho and Schmidt, who introduced sacral neuromodulation, adhered to the first theory (4). In agreement with this theory, Shafik has shown that electrical stimulation of the external urethral sphincter in human volunteers is able to inhibit detrusor contraction (5). Studies supporting the second theory are those in which the dorsal clitoral or dorsal penile nerve, both purely afferent branches of the pudendal nerve, were electrically stimulated. This induced a strong inhibition of the micturition reflex and detrusor hyperreflexia (6–8). Thus, pudendal nerve afferents seem to be particularly important for the inhibitory effect on the voiding reflex. Pudendal afferent activity mapping during neurosurgical procedures of the sacral nerve roots has shown that the S1, S2, and S3 roots contribute 4%, 60.5%, and 35.5%, respectively, of the overall pudendal afferent activity (9). In spite of the fact that S2 carries more pudendal afferents, the S3 spinal nerve is the preferential site for lead implantation in conjunction with sacral neuromodulation using the Interstim device. S3 stimulation in comparison to S2 stimulation causes less undesired excitation of efferent fibers that innervate leg muscles. For this reason S2 stimulation would be unacceptable for patients with intact neural pathways to the lower extremities. However, it has also been shown that pudendal afferent distribution is confined to a single level (i.e., S2) in 18% of the subjects (9). A lack of effect of S3 stimulation can therefore be expected in

some subjects and direct pudendal nerve stimulation may be more effective in these cases.

Experimental work in spinalized rats showed that neuromodulation reduced the degree of hyperreflexia as well as the expression of the *c-fos* gene after bladder instillation with acetic acid (10). C-fos protein is expressed in the spinal cord after irritation of the lower urinary tract; this expression is mainly mediated by afferent C fibers. This shows that inhibition of afferent C fiber activity may be one of the underlying mechanisms of neuromodulation.

Paradoxically, neuromodulation also works in patients with urinary retention in the absence of anatomical obstruction. It has been postulated that neuromodulation interferes with the increased afferent activity arising from the urethral sphincter, restoring the sensation of bladder fullness and reducing the inhibition of the detrusor muscle contraction (11).

Detailed assessment of the sensory and motor response during lead placement seems to be important for long-term success (12). This is now possible with a two-stage procedure using tined lead placement under local anesthesia. A two-stage implant has also been shown to reduce the reoperation rate (13).

It is clear that the mechanisms of action of neuromodulation are still debated, but stimulation of afferent pathways seems to play a crucial role.

CLINICAL APPLICATION OF SACRAL NERVE NEUROMODULATION

Sacral nerve neuromodulation (InterStim therapy) differs from other types of neuromodulation by its continuous stimulation and close nerve contact. Its characteristic feature is the implantation of a pulse generator and an electrode lead stimulating one of the sacral nerves, mostly S3. Patients only undergo a permanent implantation if the preceding percutaneous nerve evaluation (PNE) test is successful, or if the effects of the first stage of a two-stage implantation are favorable. In the first stage lead implantation (FS2S), only the definitive electrode is implanted but not the implantable pulse generator (IPG). A test-stimulation, either PNE or FS2S, still is the only way by which candidates for a permanent implant can be identified. When testing the S3 nerves, a true negative PNE response of about 20% can be expected based on the fact that pudendal afferents are confined to the S2 level only in 18% of the subjects (9).

Test Stimulation

At present, the only way to determine whether a patient is a candidate for implantation is a PNE test or a staged implantation.

Attempts to identify factors predicting the success of sacral nerve stimulation (SNS) have largely failed (14,15). However, in a multivariate logistic regression model, failure to respond to the test-stimulation was associated with no previous surgery for intervertebral disk prolapse, longer duration of symptoms before IPG implant (longer than seven months), neurogenic bladder (vs. no neurology), and non-obstructive urinary retention (vs. urinary incontinence), but not to patient age (16). However, the odds ratios in this study were too low to justify the exclusion from testing of some patient categories. Furthermore, psychological factors seem to play an important role (17,18); experienced implanters know that this constitutes an important determinant of their personal bias in the assessment of the result of a test stimulation.

Patients in whom the symptoms of the voiding dysfunction are reduced by more than 50% during testing may receive the permanent implant. Established indications for this treatment are urge incontinence, urge-frequency syndrome, and non-obstructive urinary retention.

The percentage of urge incontinence patients responding to traditional test stimulation (PNE) was in the order of 61% to 76% in reports of early adopters of this technique (17). More recent reports of success percentages of PNE are somewhat lower and in the order of 50% (19). This discrepancy may have more relation to factors associated with the selection of patients than to the technique of PNE itself. Recent experience with the two-stage implant using a tined lead has resulted in a higher implantation rate of 77% to 90% in patients with various indications (12,20–22). Based on their experience with PNE-testing or two-stage testing before tined lead implantation, Van Voskuilen et al. (23) concluded that there is an approximately 20% false negative rate of PNE testing only; however, in this report the authors had a much lower positive PNE response rate (20%) than the 54% in a previous report from the same institution (14). One explanation for this difference might be the fact that previously, PNE negative patients were subjected to more trials: i.e., 25% of the PNE responders underwent more than one PNE-session.

Only a well designed randomized controlled study between PNE and FS2S can confirm whether this is truly due to a better performance of the test. Borawski et al. conducted a randomized study (21) to compare PNE and FS2S; they concluded that the response rate to FS2S was about twice as high as that to traditional PNE. Because of the nature of these procedures, this unfortunately was a non-blinded study subjected to the bias and preconceived expectations of the investigator(s) performing the tests. Actually, the study was prematurely closed (sample size not achieved) after a non-planned interim analysis that was surprisingly based on an "impression" of the investigators that was not at variance with the expected/postulated outcomes of the two approaches on which the initial power calculation was based. Additionally, five of the seven non-responders in the PNE-group did not cross over to FS2S and the two women who did cross over did not qualify for a permanent implant, suggesting some unidentified bias in this study.

Interestingly, a report on the results of sacral neuromodulation from a Swiss registry showed that only 59 of 80 patients (74%) who tested successfully with traditional PNE went on to

a permanent implant without further evaluation, as compared to 32 of 33 patients (97%) who tested successfully with the definitive lead (FS2S) (24). This suggests that for some reason, either the patient or the investigator was not convinced by the positive PNE-result. Of the 21 successful PNE-patients who did not immediately proceed to permanent implant, 11 were additionally tested with the definitive lead before implantation was finally performed, but 10 others refused an implant for "personal reasons." One wonders which investigator and/or patient bias towards the testing methods has been at play in this group.

It is clear that it remains difficult to eliminate personal investigator biases that surround the interpretation of test stimulation results, even in a randomized study design. And maybe this kind of personal view and interaction with the patient is necessary to filter out those individuals who are unsuitable for this type of treatment (like patients with a psychiatric problem) before a point from which return is difficult, has been reached. Weil et al. have previously shown that a poor result after permanent implantation is found in 82% of patients with a history of psychological/psychiatric problems as opposed to 28% of patients without this kind of history (18). In summary, although there seems to be widespread expert opinion that FS2S is better than PNE, there is no solid evidence for this. FS2S is probably considered superior because it results in a higher implantation rate. However, a higher implantation rate after testing is only acceptable if the "additional" patients that are identified with FS2S over PNE, i.e., the presumed false-negatives of PNE, have at least the same long term outcome as the presumed true positives of PNE. Unfortunately, there are as yet no studies that have looked at this issue. In the randomized study of Borawski et al., none of the presumed false negatives of PNE went on to a permanent implant in spite of the availability of FS2S, which at least questions the false negative status of these patients (21). Obviously, a higher implantation rate is also associated with increased costs.

Clinical Results of Permanent Implantation

Multiple case series and several randomized controlled studies of sacral neuromodulation have been reported. However, a completely satisfactory picture cannot yet be drawn in spite of 10 to 15 years of follow-up in some series. Basically, there are two problems with follow-up data of sacral neuromodulation: If complete follow-up of all implanted patients is available, the follow-up duration is usually short; however, if (average) follow-up is longer, the percentage of patients that is accounted for is usually low. If those who are lost to follow-up are not in some way included in the final analysis, the reported success rates will be over optimistic. Furthermore, the estimated complication or revision rates will be too low. An additional problem which makes the comparison of different series somewhat difficult is the variable interpretation of the ">50%-improvement-over-baseline-equals-success" criterion. For example, in urge incontinence, some investigators would call a result successful only if a >50% decrease in pad use *and* leaking episodes per day is achieved, while others would be satisfied if there is a >50% decrease in pad use *or* leaking episodes per day. Furthermore, some implanters have challenged the ">50%" success criterion and have stated that >80% improvement is more relevant to the patient (25).

Refractory Urge Urinary Incontinence
The results of several case series with a total of 115 patients with urge incontinence who were treated early in the experience with sacral neuromodulation have been summarized: After a follow-up duration of about one to three years, approximately 50% of urge incontinence patients without neurogenic causes demonstrate a more than 90% improvement in their incontinence after the permanent implant; 25% demonstrate a 50% to 90% improvement; and another 25% demonstrate a <50% improvement (17).

In two comparative multicenter studies involving patients with refractory urge incontinence and urgency-frequency, respectively, half of the patients in whom the PNE test was successful were implanted (14,26). Implantation was delayed for six months in the remaining patients, who received standard medical treatment and comprised the control group. The stimulation groups demonstrated significantly better symptomatic results than the control groups at six months follow-up.

In two different studies, longer term results have been reported: after three-year (27) and five-year (28) follow-up, respectively, a more than 50% reduction in leaking episodes per day was found in 52.8% and 59% of the implanted patients, respectively. Furthermore, 46% and 22.2% were considered dry after three and five years, respectively (27,28).

An analysis of a nation-wide Swiss registry revealed that 27 of 71 implanted patients with urge urinary incontinence failed (38%) after a median follow-up of 24 months. Furthermore, 25% of patients were dry based on zero pad use, but another 25% of the 71 patients needed three or more pads after a median follow-up of 24 months (24).

One group has reported less good results. These authors reported on the long-term experience (mean follow-up 6.5 years) in a total of 52 implanted patients of which 41 were available for evaluation. Of these, six belonged to the urge incontinence group. Persistent improvement was found in one of six, only (29).

In 45 patients with a mean follow-up of 47 months, Bosch and Groen reported that the success rate dropped to about 80% and 65% after 1 and 1.5 years, respectively, but subsequently remained relatively constant through the fifth year (30).

Recently the five-year results of a post approval study of the original randomized controlled MDT-103 study, were reported. Of the 96 patients with urge incontinence, five-year follow-up diaries were available from 54 patients (eight patients had been explanted); and of these, 58% and 61% still had successful outcomes concerning the number of leaks per day and the number of pads used per day, respectively. In this evaluation, success was defined as >50% improvement of *selected* voiding diary parameters as compared to base line. The percentage of patients who were dry is not reported and the number of patients not accounted for in this analysis indicates that the results should be interpreted with caution (31).

The studies with a long-term follow-up deal with patients that were implanted with a non-tined lead. It is hoped that the currently-used, minimally invasive tined lead implantation, will result in a more precise positioning of the electrode, less lead dislocation, and better long-term results.

The mid-term outcome of patients implanted with the tined lead seems to be comparable with the outcomes achieved in patients implanted with the original lead design. In patients with refractory urge urinary incontinence who were implanted with the tined lead, Van Voskuilen et al. (23) reported a treatment failure rate of 32.4% (95% CI: 17–56%) at three years. However, the adverse events rates with the tined lead seem to be less than with the original lead.

Sutherland et al. reported on their 11-year experience in 104 patients. In this population, 47.1% of the leads were tined (32). The 104 patients in the analysis represent only 44% of the implanted patients between 1993 and 2004. The reasons for not consenting are unknown for what seems to be an exceptionally high percentage of patients not consenting (56%) to a retrospective chart analysis. Nevertheless, a 53% adverse event rate was reported. Notably, the adverse event rates associated with tined and non-tined leads were 28% and 73%, respectively. However, the follow-up duration was different. The following statements in the manuscript are important in this respect: First, the study period ran from 12/1993 until 12/2004; second, there was an approximately fifty-fifty tined versus non-tined lead distribution and thirdly, tined leads were used after 2002. From these statements we can deduce that the average follow-up of the tined lead versus the non-tined lead group is approximately 1 to 1.5 years versus 5 to 5.5 years. This difference in follow-up time can at least partly explain the difference in adverse event rates.

A worrying aspect of most sacral neuromodulation series is the finding that a certain percentage of patients who respond well to PNE will fail to show a beneficial response immediately after the implantation. One would hope that a two-stage procedure with prolonged testing would decrease the number of early failures after an implant. In the study of Everaert et al. (33), 42 patients who all had responded successfully to a traditional PNE test were randomized between a one-stage and two-stage procedure. Failure was reported in 7 of 21 and 3 of 21 from the one-stage and two-stage group, respectively. Unfortunately, there was no statistically significant difference in the number of early failures between the one-stage and the two-stage group.

Urge-Frequency Syndrome
In the urge-frequency group Siegel et al. (27) reported that two years post implantation, 56% of the patients showed a more than 50% reduction in voiding frequency. After an average follow-up of 69.8 months, Van Voskuilen et al. reported "good results" in 63.6% of 107 implanted patients with overactive bladder symptoms (34). Elhilali et al. reported persistent improvement in 10 of 22 (45%) urge-frequency patients after an average follow-up of 6.5 years (29).

Recently the five-year results of a post approval study of the original randomized controlled MDT-103 study were reported. Success was defined as >50% improvement of selected voiding diary parameters as compared to base line. Of the 25 patients with urge frequency syndrome, five-year follow-up diaries were available from 11 patients (seven patients had been explanted) and 40% and 56% of these still had successful outcomes concerning the number of voids per day and the average volume voided per micturition, respectively (31).

Non-obstructive Urinary Retention
Sacral nerve neuromodulation for the treatment of non-obstructive urinary retention is another established indication. Jonas et al. reported that 68 of 177 retention patients responded to traditional PNE with a greater than 50% improvement. Of the implanted patients 69% eliminated catheterization at six months follow-up and an additional 14% had a greater than 50% reduction in catheterization volume. At 18 months follow-up catheterization was completely eliminated in 58% of 24 evaluable patients (35). Swinn et al. reported a 68% success rate to PNE in 38 women, mostly with Fowler's syndrome (11). The same group reported their long-term results in 26 implanted women. After a mean follow-up of 37 months, 17 of 26 (65%) women voided spontaneously without the need for self-catheterization (36).

The five-year results of a post approval study of the original randomized controlled MDT-103 study were recently reported. Success was defined as >50% decrease in the number of catheterizations per day as compared to base line. Of the 31 patients with non-obstructive urinary retention, five-year follow-up diaries were available from 22 patients (one patient had been explanted) and 58% of these still had successful outcomes concerning the number of catheterizations per day. The percentage of patients who did not have to catheterize at all was not reported (31).

Kessler and Fowler reviewed the results of sacral neuromodulation for urinary retention and found that the success rate of a permanent implant ranged between 55% and 100% after a follow-up duration of 43 and 15 months, respectively (37). Furthermore, the long-term success rate after four to six years ranged between 71% and 76% in several well-documented series; the percentage of patients not needing to catheterize at all is not reported.

Interstitial Cystitis
Several authors performed permanent implantations of the InterStim® device for treatment of patients with interstitial cystitis. Mixed results have been reported with S3 sacral nerve stimulation. Some investigators report good results with up to 75% improvement in symptoms (13,38,39), including a 20% "cure" rate (38). Follow-up in these studies was relatively short and ranged between 5.6 and 14 months. Berman et al. could not confirm these results (40). In 13 patients that were implanted with the Interstim device, only 2 (25%) were pleased or delighted with the results. Elhilali et al. reported that of four patients with interstitial cystitis with intractable pelvic pain, only one was improved after a mean follow-up of 6.5 years (29).

Adverse Events
The necessity to reposition the electrode after migration is the most frequently reported complication, occurring in about 20% of the patients (14,30). Some patients complained of pain at the site of the pulse generator, which resolved after repositioning. Pain in the leg can often be solved by reduction of the stimulation amplitude. Van Voskuilen et al. reported a reoperation rate of 48.3% (excluding pulse generator replacements) after an average follow-up of 64.2 months (34). Dasgupta et al. reported an overall adverse events rate of 51.6% (36). Siegel et al. reported adverse events for 219 Interstim implanted patients (27). The majority of events observed were: pain at stimulator site (15.3%), new pain (9%), pain at lead site (5.4%), suspected lead migration (8.4%), infection (6.1%), transient electric shock (5.5%), and adverse changes in bowel function (3%).

Displacement of the electrode during the PNE test may give a falsely negative result. Janknegt et al. therefore repeated the test by placing a permanent electrode and an extension cable in patients in whom displacement was suspected and connected those to an external pulse generator (41). The permanent pulse generator was placed at a later stage if the patient demonstrated a good response (which was true in 8 out of 10 patients). The two-stage implant has now become the standard particularly since the introduction of a minimally invasive technique for the placement of a tined lead (22). The pulse generator was traditionally placed in a lower abdominal pocket. Buttock placement has the advantage that the patient needs not to be repositioned during operation and saves about one hour operative time; this has become the standard now (42).

CONCLUDING REMARKS
Neuromodulation is a valuable treatment option for patients with an overactive bladder syndrome (either OAB-wet or OAB-dry) and non-obstructive urinary retention and should be considered before applying a more invasive operation such as a bladder augmentation. However, the durability of the initial success is probably overrated in most of the published reports. The published reoperation rate approaches 50% after an average follow-up of five years (34). Unfortunately, the true cost-benefit ratio of this expensive type of treatment is not known (25).

No parameters predictive of success have been identified. The determination of reliable selection criteria would be a major step forward. A better understanding of the mechanism of action might contribute considerably to this goal. Discouraging is the high surgical revision rate with the implantable systems. This adds to the costs of this type of treatment which are already very high. The high costs do not encourage the use of these devices in an earlier stage of the disease, which may be preferable over the treatment of desperate cases only. However, some technical advances such as the use of the tined lead, the two-stage implant, and the minimally invasive technique seem to have decreased the necessity for revision. Little is known about the outcome of the "additional" patients that are identified with FS2S, as compared to PNE. More data of the treatment results in these presumed false negatives to traditional PNE testing are eagerly awaited.

REFERENCES

1. Bemelmans BL, Mundy AR, Craggs MD. Neuromodulation by implant for treating lower urinary tract symptoms and dysfunction. Eur Urol 1999; 36: 81–91.
2. Fall M, Lindström S. Electrical stimulation. A physiologic approach to the treatment of urinary incontinence. Urol Clin North Am 1991; 18: 393–407.
3. Blok BFM, Groen J, Bosch JLHR, et al. Different brain effects during chronic and acute sacral neuromodulation in urge incontinent patients with implanted neurostimulators. BJU Int 2006; 98: 1238–43.
4. Tanagho EA, Schmidt RA. Electrical stimulation in the clinical management of the neurogenic bladder. J Urol 1988; 140: 1331–9.
5. Shafik A. A study of the continence mechanism of the external urethral sphincter with identification of the voluntary urinary inhibition reflex. J Urol 1999; 162: 1967–71.
6. Vodusek DB, Light JK, Libby JM. Detrusor inhibition induced by stimulation of pudendal nerve afferents. Neurourol Urodyn 1986; 5: 381–9.
7. Craggs M, Edhem I, Knight S, et al. Suppression of normal human voiding reflexes by electrical stimulation of the dorsal penile nerve. [abstract 239]. Eur Urol 1998; 33(Suppl 1): 60.
8. Shah N, Edhem I, Knight S, et al. Acute suppression of provoked detrusor hyperreflexia by electrical stimulation of dorsal penile nerve. [abstract 240]. Eur Urol 1998; 33(Suppl 1): 60.
9. Huang JC, Deletis V, Vodusek DB, Abbott R. Preservation of pudendal afferents in sacral rhizotomies. Neurosurgery 1997; 41: 411–15.
10. Wang Y, Hassouna MM. Neuromodulation reduces c-fos gene expression in spinalized rats: a double-blind randomized study. J Urol 2000; 163: 1966–70.
11. Swinn MJ, Kitchen ND, Goodwin RJ, Fowler CJ. Sacral neuromodulation for women with Fowler's syndrome. Eur Urol 2000; 38: 439–43.
12. Cohen BL, Tunuguntla HS, Gousse A. Predictors of success for first stage neuromodulation: motor versus sensory response. J Urol 2006; 175: 2178–81.
13. Peters KM, Carey JM, Konstadt DB. Sacral neuromodulation for the treatment of refractory interstitial cystitis: outcomes based on technique. Int Urogynecol J 2003; 14: 223–8.
14. Weil EHJ, Ruiz-Cerdá JL, Eerdmans PHA, et al. Sacral root neuromodulation in the treatment of refractory urinary urge incontinence: a prospective randomized clinical trial. Eur Urol 2000; 37: 161–71.
15. Koldewijn EL, Rosier PFWM, Meuleman EJH, et al. Predictors of success with neuromodulation in lower urinary tract dysfunction: results of trial stimulation in 100 patients. J Urol 1994; 152: 2071–5.
16. Scheepens WA, Jongen MMGJ, Nieman FHM, et al. Predictive factors for sacral neuromodulation in chronic lower urinary tract dysfunction. Urology 2002; 60: 598–602.
17. Bosch JLHR. Sacral neuromodulation in the treatment of the unstable bladder. Curr Opin Urol 1998; 8: 287–91.
18. Weil EHJ, Ruiz-Cerdá JL, Eerdmans PHA, et al. Clinical results of sacral neuromodulation for chronic voiding dysfunction using unilateral sacral foramen electrodes. World J Urol 1998; 16: 313–21.
19. Spinelli M, Sievert K-D. Latest technologic and surgical developments in using Interstim TM therapy for sacral neuromodulation: impact on treatment success and safety. Eur Urol 2008; 54: 1287–96.
20. Spinelli M, Giardello G, Gerber M, et al. New sacral neuromodulation lead for percutaneous implantation using local anesthesia: description and first experience. J Urol 2003; 170: 1905–7.
21. Borawski KM, Foster RT, Webster GD, Amundsen CL. Predicting implantation with a neuromodulator using two different test stimulation techniques: a prospective randomized study in urge incontinent women. Neurourol Urodyn 2007; 26: 14–18.
22. Spinelli M, Giardello G, Arduini A, Van den Hombergh U. New percutaneous technique of sacral nerve stimulation has high initial success rate: preliminary results. Eur Urol 2003; 43: 70–4.
23. Van Voskuilen AC, Oerlemans DJAJ, Weil EHJ, et al. Medium-term experience of sacral neuromodulation by tined lead implantation. BJU Int 2007; 99: 107–10.
24. Kessler TM, Buchser E, Meyer S, et al. Sacral neuromodulation for refractory lower urinary tract dysfunction: results of a nationwide registry in Switzerland. Eur Urol 2007; 51: 1357–63.
25. Reynolds WS, Bales GT. RE: [van Kerrebroeck PEV, van Voskuilen AC, Heesakkers JPFA, et al. Results of sacral neuromodulation therapy for urinary voiding dysfunction: outcomes of a prospective, worldwide clinical study. J Urol 2007; 178: 2029–34.]. J Urol 2008; 179: 2483–4.
26. Hassouna MM, Siegel SW, Lycklama à Nijeholt AAB, et al. Sacral neuromodulation in the treatment of urgency-frequency symptoms: a multicenter study on efficacy and safety. J Urol 2000; 163: 1849–54.
27. Siegel SW, Catanzaro F, Dijkema H, et al. Long-term results of a multicenter study on sacral nerve stimulation for treatment of urinary urge incontinence, urgency-frequency and retention. Urology 2000; 56(6A Suppl): 87–91.
28. Bosch R, Groen J. Complete 5-year follow-up of sacral (S3) segmental nerve stimulation with an implantable electrode and pulse generator in 36 consecutive patients with refractory detrusor overactivity incontinence. Neurourol Urodyn 2002; 21: 390–1.
29. Elhilali MM, Khaled SM, Kashiwabara T, et al. Sacral neuromodulation: long-term experience of one center. Urology 2005; 65: 1114–17.
30. Bosch JLHR, Groen J. Sacral nerve neuromodulation in the treatment of patients with refractory motor urge incontinence: long-term results of a prospective longitudinal study. J Urol 2000; 163: 1219–22.
31. van Kerrebroeck PEV, van Voskuilen AC, Heesakkers JPFA, et al. Results of sacral neuromodulation therapy for urinary voiding dysfunction: outcomes of a prospective, worldwide clinical study. J Urol 2007; 178: 2029–34.
32. Sutherland SE, Lavers A, Carlson A, et al. Sacral nerve stimulation for voiding dysfunction: one institution's 11-year experience. Neurourol Urodyn 2007; 26: 19–28.
33. Everaert K, Kerkhaert W, Caluwaerts H, et al. A prospective randomized trial comparing the 1-stage with the 2-stage implantation of a pulse generator in patients with pelvic floor dysfunction selected for sacral nerve stimulation. Eur Urol 2004; 45: 649–54.
34. Van Voskuilen AC, Oerlemans DJAJ, Weil EHJ, et al. Long term results of neuromodulation by sacral nerve stimulation for lower urinary tract symptoms: a retrospective single center study. Eur Urol 2006; 49: 366–72.
35. Jonas U, Fowler CJ, Chancellor MB, et al. Efficacy of sacral nerve stimulation for urinary retention: results 18 months after implantation. J Urol 2001; 165: 15–19.
36. Dasgupta R, Wiseman OJ, Kitchen N, Fowler CJ. Long-term results of sacral neuromodulation for women with urinary retention. BJU Int 2004; 94: 335–7.
37. Kessler TM, Fowler CJ. Sacral neuromodulation for urinary retention. Nat Clin Pract Urol 2008; 5: 657–66.
38. Caraballo R, Bologna RA, Lukban J, Whitmore KE. Sacral nerve stimulation as a treatment for urge incontinence and associated pelvic floor disorders at a pelvic floor center: a follow-up study. Urology 2001; 57(6 Suppl 1): 121.
39. Comiter CV. Sacral neuromodulation for the symptomatic treatment of refractory interstitial cystitis: a prospective study. J Urol 2003; 169: 1369–73.
40. Berman N, Itano J, Gore J, et al. Poor results using sacral nerve stimulation (Interstim) for treating pelvic pain patients. [abstract 365]. J Urol 2003; 169(4 Suppl): 94.
41. Janknegt RA, Weil EHJ, Eerdmans PHA. Improving neuromodulation technique for refractory voiding dysfunctions: two-stage implant. Urology 1997; 49: 358–62.
42. Weil E, Scheepens W, Nilkamal J, van Kerrebroeck P. Buttock placement of the implantable pulse generator: a new technique for sacral nerve modulation. [abstract 129]. Eur Urol 2000; 37(Suppl 2): 33.

45 Pessaries and Devices: Nonsurgical Treatment of Pelvic Organ Prolapse and Stress Urinary Incontinence

Catherine S Bradley

INTRODUCTION

Pessaries, or devices placed in the vagina to support the uterus or vaginal walls, have been used for thousands of years to treat pelvic organ prolapse (POP). Hippocrates documented the use of pomegranates soaked in vinegar as vaginal pessaries, and ring pessaries made of wood, cork, silver, and gold were described in the early 1700s (1,2). In the 19th century, the development of pessaries made out of vulcanized rubber allowed safer long-term use (2). Pessaries remained the treatment of choice for POP through the early 1900s when over 100 types of pessaries were available, but their use declined in the following decades as developments in aseptic techniques and anesthesia made surgical correction more feasible.

Recently, interest in pessaries as a noninvasive treatment option for POP and stress urinary incontinence (SUI) has again increased, although opinions on pessary use and pessary training continue to vary widely among clinicians. In a 2000 survey of American Urogynecologic Society members, most (77%) reported using pessaries as first-line therapy for prolapse, but some (12%) offered pessaries only to women who were not surgical candidates (3). In a similar 2001 survey of American gynecologists, 86% reported prescribing pessaries for prolapse, but most received minimal training in pessary use and few believed pessaries were an effective treatment for SUI (4).

Many experts now recommend pessaries as a long-term treatment option for any woman with POP and SUI seeking non-surgical therapy, not just for women for whom surgery is not an option (5). However, evidence on the effectiveness of pessaries remains limited.

PESSARIES FOR POP

Pessaries used for treating POP can be loosely grouped into supportive and space-occupying pessaries. Supportive pessaries (Fig. 45.1) are held in place by levator muscle tone, while space-occupying pessaries (Fig. 45.2) keep prolapse reduced by filling the vagina. Most pessaries today are made from medical-grade silicone, which is non-allergenic, non-toxic, and latex-free. This material does not absorb odors, and it can be sterilized and lasts for several years.

Effectiveness of Treatment

Prospective research on the effectiveness of pessaries for POP treatment is sparse. In fact, in 2005 the third International Consultation on Incontinence identified an "urgent need" for randomized controlled trials focusing on the effectiveness of pessaries as well as on aspects of pessary management (6). In 2007, Cundiff et al. (7) published the first randomized trial

focusing on pessary therapy for POP (the PESSRI study). This multi-center randomized crossover trial compared outcomes of women with symptomatic POP treated with two common types of pessaries. Women were randomized to initial treatment with a ring with support pessary or with a Gellhorn pessary. After three months of treatment, participants were fitted and treated with the other type of pessary. The primary outcome was change in prolapse symptoms, assessed using validated questionnaires. Ninety-two percent of the participants were successfully fit with at least one pessary, and 60% continued the pessary therapy for three months (no differences seen between pessary types). Using a strict criterion for defining clinically-significant improvement in quality of life scores, both pessaries were found to be equally effective in decreasing POP-related symptom bother as well as bother from obstructive and irritative urinary and colo-rectal symptoms (7).

Three small prospective cohort studies (n = 80–203) also demonstrated significant improvements in pelvic floor symptoms when POP was treated with a pessary (8–10). Fernando et al. (8) studied 203 patients in a U.K. urogynecology clinic who agreed to pessary treatment for POP. Seventy-five percent were successfully fit with a pessary and 48% continued use through a four-month follow-up appointment. Using a validated symptom questionnaire, the women continuing pessary use at four months reported improvements in all or most general prolapse and urinary symptoms and in a few defecatory symptoms. A small subgroup (n = 36) who were sexually active also had improved sexual frequency and satisfaction compared to baseline (8).

In a similar U.S. study, Clemons et al. (10) followed 100 consecutive urogynecology patients with symptomatic POP who agreed to a pessary trial. Seventy-three were successfully fit with a pessary. At two months, vaginal bulge and pressure symptoms had nearly resolved (bulge 90% to 3%; pressure 49% to 3%). In women with baseline urinary symptoms, stress incontinence, urge incontinence, and voiding difficulty improved (in 45%, 46%, and 53%, respectively). However, among women without urinary symptoms at baseline, 21% developed new stress incontinence symptoms. Only six women (8%) were dissatisfied with their pessary at two months, and dissatisfaction was associated with new stress incontinence symptoms (10). After 12 months, 43% of the original cohort continued to use their pessary (11).

Komesu et al. (9) prospectively enrolled 80 urogynecology patients who were successfully fitted with pessaries for POP and used a validated symptom questionnaire to compare symptom outcomes between women continuing and discontinuing pessary use. Of 64 women with follow-up data, 56%

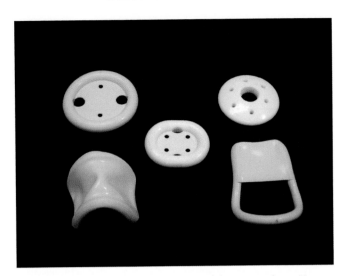

Figure 45.1 Support pessaries used to treat pelvic organ prolapse. *Top row:* (*left*) ring with support (Milex Inc, Chicago, Illinois, U.S.A.); (*right*) Shaatz (Mentor Corp., Santa Barbara, California, U.S.A.). *Middle row:* oval with support (Mentor). *Bottom row:* (*left*) Gehrung (Milex); (*right*) Hodge (Milex).

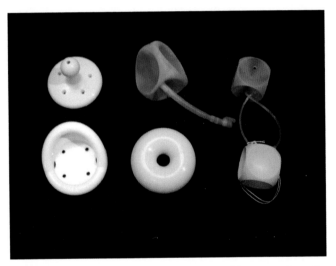

Figure 45.2 Space-occupying pessaries used to treat pelvic organ prolapse. *Top row:* (*left*) Gellhorn (Mentor Corp., Santa Barbara, California, U.S.A.); (*middle*) inflatoball (Milex Inc, Chicago, Illinois, U.S.A.); (*right*) cube with drainage holes (Mentor). *Bottom row:* (*left*) Marland; (*middle*) donut; (*right*) cube (all three by Milex).

continued pessary use after 6 to 12 months. The most commonly reported reasons for discontinuing use were difficulty retaining the pessary and discomfort. While both groups showed improvements in prolapse and bladder symptom scores after 6 to 12 months, the pessary continuation group showed significantly more improvement than those that discontinued use. A two-month prolapse symptom score improvement of >50% was found to best predict continuation of pessary use (area under the curve = 0.77) (9).

In summary, research published to date suggests that pessary therapy for POP will improve or resolve most prolapse symptoms and many bladder symptoms. The development of new stress incontinence occurs in a minority of patients, but it is associated with pessary discontinuation. Most women interested in pessary treatment can be successfully fitted with a

pessary, and 40% to 60% will continue use for greater than 6 to 12 months.

Pessary Fitting

Rates of successful pessary fitting in the literature range from 41% to 92%, with variable definitions used for success (7,8,12–14). Often, more than one visit and the use of two or more pessaries are required for fitting. Among 1216 POP and UI patients referred to a pessary clinic, Hanson et al. (14) initially fitted 1043 (86%) with a pessary, but only 744 (62%) continued to wear the pessaries for >1 month. Half of the patients required two or more visits for fitting and a median of two pessaries were tried. Clemons et al. (13) successfully fitted 73% of POP patients with a pessary that was defined as a successful fit and planned continued use of the pessary after a one-week follow-up visit. Thirty percent of patients required two visits and on average two pessaries were tried per visit to achieve a successful fit.

Patient characteristics that predict a successful pessary fitting are inconsistent across studies (8,12–14). Age, POP stage, and the type of support defect (e.g., anterior, posterior, or apical) are not associated with fitting failure. In several studies, prior hysterectomy and prior reconstructive surgery were more common in those with pessary fitting failure (8,12,14). Possible anatomic predictors include a wide introitus (>4 fingerbreadths) and short vaginal length (<7 cm) (13). Among postmenopausal women, use of vaginal estrogen therapy may increase fitting success rates (14).

Pessary types used for POP vary among published reports. Most pessary providers report tailoring their choice of pessary to specific support defects (3), but this practice is based on limited evidence. Conventional wisdom states that support pessaries will be more successful in women with milder degrees of POP, while space-occupying pessaries may be required in women with advanced POP and in those with a wide genital hiatus or a weak perineal body (15). In support of this assertion, one study found that only 36% of women with Stage IV prolapse were able to be fit with a support pessary, compared to 80% of women with Stages II and III prolapse (p < 0.001) (13). However, in the PESSRI clinical trial all women were treated sequentially with both ring and Gellhorn pessaries, and fitting success rates were high (92%) and did not differ by pessary type (7).

Many published protocols use the ring or ring with support pessary as a first choice pessary in all patients because of its ease of use, and reserve other pessary types (most often Gellhorn, donut, or cube pessaries) for women unable to retain or to be comfortably fitted with a ring (8,13,16,17). In fact, 64% to 70% of POP patients can be fit successfully with a size 3, 4, or 5 ring pessary (13,16).

The Iowa Pessary Protocol

Given the few published studies on pessary management, much of clinical practice related to pessaries is based on clinical experience and expert opinion. Here we present the pessary protocol used at the University of Iowa Urogynecology Clinic.

Prior to fitting a pessary, we treat most women that demonstrate vaginal atrophy for six weeks with vaginal estrogen therapy, as this may increase the likelihood of a successful pessary fitting (14). Similar to other reported protocols (8,13,16), we begin by trying to fit a ring or ring with support pessary, as these pessaries are easy for providers to fit and for patients to self-manage. If unable to successfully fit a ring pessary, we next try a Gellhorn pessary. Our experience mirrors reports in the literature that >90% of women with POP can be fit with one of these two pessaries types (13). If unable to fit either a ring or Gellhorn pessary, other types (commonly a donut or cube) are tried.

An appropriately fitting pessary should fill the vagina, but allow the clinician's finger to easily sweep between the pessary and the vaginal wall. After finding a pessary with a good fit, we instruct women to do vigorous activity in the clinic area (such as brisk walking and straining) to ensure that the pessary is retained in the vagina and is comfortable. We also ask that women attempt to void with the pessary in place before leaving the office. In postmenopausal patients without contra-indications to hormonal therapy, low-dose vaginal estrogen is often prescribed. In most cases, patients are scheduled for an initial follow-up appointment within two weeks. Women fitted with a cube pessary are asked to return sooner (after two to three days) because of an increased risk of vaginal erosions (16), which in our experience may occur rapidly.

At each subsequent pessary appointment, patients are first examined with the pessary in place to ensure correct fit and placement in the vagina. The pessary is then removed and washed. The vagina is examined for signs of excessive discharge, irritation, or erosions. Careful inspection of all vaginal surfaces is essential to identify erosions. We recommend turning the speculum 90° to visualize the anterior and posterior surfaces carefully. After an initial two-week and three-month check, we examine women who manage their own pessary yearly.

In contrast to reports from some centers (13,16), we find the majority of women can be instructed to remove and replace their pessaries at home. We recommend that women remove the pessary once or twice weekly, leave it out overnight, and then reinsert it in the morning. When removed, the pessary is simply washed with warm water. Women rarely encounter excessive or malodorous vaginal discharge using this approach. If women are unable or unwilling to remove the pessary at home, they are seen at regular intervals in the office for pessary removal and examination. In these patients, we gradually increase the office visit interval after the initial follow-up visit to a maximum interval of three months. Women who develop increasing vaginal discharge or erosions over shorter intervals will need more frequent follow-up.

Visiting nurses can be an invaluable resource for women unable to care for the pessary on their own. They are often able to visit the woman at home, remove the pessary in the evening and return in the morning to replace it. Excessive or foul-smelling discharge, increased discomfort, or vaginal bleeding signals a need to arrange medical follow-up.

PESSARIES AND DEVICES FOR SUI
Supportive pessaries are also used for treating SUI. Pessaries used to treat incontinence frequently have a knob that is placed under the urethra (Fig. 45.3). Some of the most commonly used incontinence pessaries include the incontinence dish (with or without support and the incontinence ring with knob (with or without support) (inset, Fig. 45.3), but other types (e.g., Hodge with knob), are also available. Clinical protocols for fitting and following patients with incontinence pessaries are similar to those used in patients who use pessaries for POP (described above). In addition to pessaries, other vaginal and urethral devices may be used to

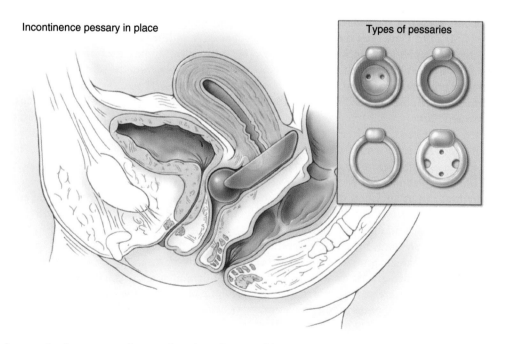

Incontinence pessary in place

Types of pessaries

Figure 45.3 Pessary placement for the treatment of stress urinary incontinence and (inset) commonly-used incontinence pessaries (*clockwise from top left:* an incontinence dish with support, an incontinence dish without support, an incontinence ring with support and knob, and an incontinence ring without support). *Source:* Adapted from Ref. 18.

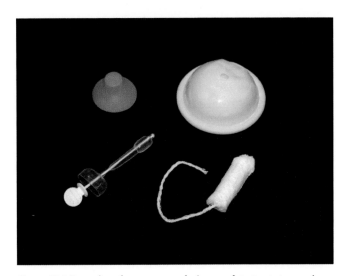

Figure 45.4 Examples of non-pessary devices used to treat stress urinary incontinence. *Top row:* (*left*) urethral suction cap (Apple/Insight Medical Corp., Bolton, Massachusetts, U.S.A.; currently not available); (*right*) contraceptive diaphragm. *Bottom row:* (*left*) urethral insert (Rochester Medical, Inc., Stewartville, Minnesota, U.S.A.); (*right*) menstrual tampon.

treat SUI, including tampons, diaphragms, disposable vaginal devices, and urethral inserts and caps. Examples of non-pessary devices either currently available or recently marketed in the United States that may improve continence are shown in Figure 45.4.

Mechanism of Action

Small prospective studies of incontinence pessaries have demonstrated positive changes in urethral function and support measures using urodynamic tests and dynamic magnetic resonance imaging (MRI) (19–21). In 12 women who underwent urodynamic studies with and without a Smith Hodge pessary, the pessary increased urethral functional length and static and dynamic urethral closure pressures and reduced urodynamic stress incontinence (USI) (19). Flow rates did not decrease, and voided and postvoid volumes were unchanged with the pessary, suggesting that urethral obstruction did not occur. Maximal urethral closure pressures also increased in 33 women with SUI after placement of an incontinence dish, and urethral straining angles decreased (20).

A recent study used urodynamics and dynamic MRI in 15 women to assess changes associated with incontinence dish pessaries (21). All women had USI before pessary placement, but only three had USI after placement of the dish. At urodynamics, maximal urethral closure pressures did not increase (as seen in previous studies), but functional urethral length did increase. Contrary to prior findings (19), maximal flow rates decreased and detrusor pressures increased, suggesting increased urethral resistance, although postvoid volumes were not elevated. MRI findings included greater bladder neck elevation, increased urethral length, decreased urethral funneling with cough, and smaller (more acute) posterior urethrovesical angles following pessary placement (21). These studies together suggest that pessaries may reduce SUI by stabilizing the proximal urethra and urethrovesical junction, thereby facilitating pressure transmission to the proximal urethra. Increasing urethral resistance and elevation of the bladder neck may also help restore continence.

Effectiveness—Incontinence Pessaries

Most studies evaluating the use of incontinence pessaries are small or retrospective. Nygaard (22) performed a small, randomized clinic-based study of 18 women who completed three standardized aerobics sessions, wearing either a Hodge with support pessary, a large menstrual tampon, or no device. Both devices significantly decreased urine loss (measured with a pad test) during exercise when compared to the control session. The tampon achieved continence in 8 of 14 women while the pessary did in 5 of 14 women. Better outcomes were seen with both devices in women who had milder urine loss (22).

In a retrospective study, 119 (63%) of 190 women offered incontinence pessary treatment for stress or mixed urinary incontinence chose to undergo a pessary fitting and most (89%) were successfully fit (23). Of those successfully fit with a pessary, 55% used the pessary for at least six months (median duration 13 months, range 6–30 months). Most women who discontinued use did so within one to two months. A second retrospective study of incontinence pessary use had very similar results (24). Of 100 women, 86% were successfully fit with a pessary and continued use after an initial two week follow-up appointment. After an average follow-up time of 11 months (range 2–42 months), 59% of the women continued use of the pessary.

In contrast to these findings, in a small prospective study, only 16% of 38 women fit with an incontinence ring with support pessary chose to continue use out to one year (25). In the few that continued use, the pessary resulted in fewer leaking episodes and 9 (24%) were subjectively "dry."

In a recent study of 32 women, a novel bell-shaped self-positioning incontinence pessary (Uresta, EastMed, Inc., Halifax, Nova Scotia, Canada) was found to significantly improve urinary symptoms as well as diary-recorded leaking episodes and urinary pad weights (26). Similar to the larger retrospective studies described above, 50% of women beginning the study chose to continue use of the pessary for SUI treatment after 12 months.

Overall, these studies suggest that most women who are interested can be successfully fit with an incontinence pessary, and about half of those women find it an acceptable long-term therapy. However, study findings remain limited by the lack of control or comparison groups. A 2006 Cochrane review of vaginal and intraurethral incontinence devices found that there was insufficient evidence to recommend any specific pessary or device or to show that mechanical devices are better than other forms of treatment (27). In response to the lack of evidence in this area, the National Institutes of Health Pelvic Floor Disorders Network is conducting a multi-center randomized clinical trial of non-surgical therapy in 450 women with stress-predominant urinary incontinence. Participants are randomized to incontinence pessary, behavioral therapy with pelvic muscle training or a combined treatment arm (28). Results from this trial will provide much needed information about the relative efficacy and satisfaction seen with incontinence pessaries compared to other nonsurgical therapies for SUI.

Effectiveness—Other Vaginal and Urethral Devices

The vaginal contraceptive diaphragm has been shown to decrease SUI symptoms with success rates of 40% and 75% in two small, short-term studies (29,30). Placement of a menstrual tampon has similar moderate levels of success (57% continent during use) in treating exercise-induced incontinence (22).

A vaginal bladder neck prosthesis [Introl (Uromed Corp., Needham, Massachusetts, U.S.A.); no longer commercially available] was specially designed to elevate and support the urethrovesical junction. This ring-shaped device had two blunt prongs intended to support either side of the urethra, mimicking anatomic results of a cystourethropexy. Early studies of the device demonstrated continence rates as high as 83% (31), but in later studies success rates were lower and withdrawal rates were high, largely due to sizing and fitting problems and discomfort with insertion and removal. In one series of 65 patients, 60% withdrew from the study before four weeks (32).

Other vaginal incontinence devices have been studied, particularly in Europe and Australia. The reusable Contiform device (Contiform International, Australia), shaped like a large hollow tampon, is inserted behind the pubic bone to support the proximal urethra (33). The device, made from non-allergenic thermoplastic rubber, can be reused for 30 to 60 days. This device was designed to be easily fitted and self-managed by patients. In an initial prospective study of 59 women offered Contiform therapy, 12% could not be fit or were unable to insert and remove the device by themselves (33). Among the 69% who completed the three-week trial, urine leakage was reduced by a median of 72% overall, but only 20% were continent. Recently, an additional size of the device was made available, and in a subsequent study, 54% of women who completed the short-term trial were dry (34).

Single-use, disposable vaginal devices are available for treating SUI in several countries outside the United States. Two polyurethrane foam tampons have been marketed, one shaped like a menstrual tampon [Contrelle Continence Tampon (Colopast, Humlebaek, Denmark)] and one a clam-shaped tampon [Conveen Continence Guard (also Coloplast)]. A randomized, multi-center cross-over trial of 94 women compared the two disposable tampon-like devices for treatment of stress-predominant urinary incontinence (35). Both devices significantly improved symptoms over a five-week period, but the Contrelle Continence Tampon had slightly better outcomes, with 48% of participants subjectively continent and 36% improved. Two-thirds of the patients preferred the Contrelle device to the Conveen device, perhaps because of greater ease of use.

A novel disposable vaginal device was recently described, consisting of a flexible resin core surrounded by a porous nylon mesh (ConTIPI Ltd., Caesaria, Israel), intended to provide urethral support similar to a tension-free suburethral sling. When this device was used by 60 women with severe SUI, 85% had a ≥70% reduction of urine loss on daily pad weights. In the 50 women who completed the four-week trial, 92% were subjectively continent (36).

Urethral inserts and external urethral occlusive devices function as mechanical barriers to prevent urinary leakage. These devices require highly motivated and manually dexterous patients as the devices must be removed to urinate and then replaced after each void. These devices may be used episodically during exercise or other activities. Studies suggest they have lower overall success rates than seen for some of the vaginal devices, partly because of higher dropout rates (37).

Urethral inserts are sterile, single-use inserts placed into the urethra by the patient and held in place by an inflated balloon at the bladder neck. Such inserts are appropriate for women with relatively pure stress incontinence, no history of recurrent urinary tract infections, and no serious contraindications to bacteriuria (e.g., artificial heart valves). Two urethral inserts have been available in the United States, including the Reliance Urinary Control Insert (UroMed, Inc., Needham, Massachusetts, U.S.A.) and the FemSoft Urethral insert (Rochester Medical, Inc., Stewartville, Minnesota, U.S.A.). At this time, only the FemSoft insert is commercially available. Multi-center studies demonstrate high rates of continence with the inserts in place (80–95%) and high rates of satisfaction in women that continue use, but overall results are limited by high withdrawal rates and frequent adverse events (38,39). In 112 women using a urethral insert, 57% continued use for one year and had a >50% reduction in frequency of incontinence episodes (39). Among women using a urethral insert over an average follow-up time of 15 months, 1.2 devices on average were used per day and the inserts were worn for a median of 5.7 hours per day (39).

External urethral occlusive devices fit over the external urethral meatus and are held in place by adhesive or gentle suction. Several types of these have been marketed in the United States [Miniguard (UroMed, Inc., Needham, Massachusetts, U.S.A.), FemAssist (Apple/Insight Medical Corp., Bolton, Massachusetts, U.S.A.), CapSure Shield (Bard, Covington, Georgia, U.S.A.)], but are no longer commercially available. These devices have fewer reported side effects than the urethral inserts, but reported continence rates are lower. Short-term studies of external urethral occlusive devices demonstrate significant improvements in subjective and objective outcomes and continence rates of 40% to 50% in women with SUI (40–42). Patient acceptability of this type of device appears to be highly variable. In two one-month trials of a urethral suction cap, completion rates were 57% and 62% (40,42), but in a three-month study of the same occlusive device, only 5% of participants completed the study, the majority withdrawing for reasons most often related to dissatisfaction with the device (43).

ADVERSE EVENTS

Adverse events related to pessary use are uncommon and generally minor, although published data in this area is sparse. Frequent removal and care of a pessary may prevent most pessary problems (15). Vaginal discharge, odor, and vaginal infections may occur in pessary users, but these are infrequent reasons for discontinuing use (16,23). Vaginal erosions have been reported to occur in 5% to 10% of women treating POP and/or SUI with a pessary (11,14,16). Erosions may be more common in women with hypoestrogenic vaginal changes and in those using a cube pessary. In one case series, erosions developed in five of six women using cube pessaries, but in only 3 of 101 women using ring pessaries (16).

More serious complications related to pessaries can also occur, but these appear to be rare and typically are seen in patients with a "neglected" pessary (44). A recent literature review identified 39 cases of major complications, including 8 vesicovaginal fistulas, 5 other urologic complications, 4 rectovaginal fistulas, 3 other bowel complications, and 19 impacted pessaries (44). Sixty percent of these complications required operative management. Only 2 of the 39 occurred in women who received appropriate clinical follow-up, again supporting the importance of careful pessary management by providers and patients.

Adverse events associated with the use of disposable vaginal devices for SUI are typically mild, and most often include vaginal spotting, irritation, and discomfort (35,36). Such local side effects may decrease over time, perhaps because patients become more skilled at device placement. In a four-week trial of a disposable vaginal device, 52% of patients reported adverse events (most often discomfort and spotting) in week 1 compared to 5% in week 4 of device use (36). Vaginal infections (e.g., candidiasis), asymptomatic bacteriuria, and cystitis are less frequently reported (36). Two of nineteen women who used a disposable vaginal device over a one-year period had an uncomplicated urinary tract infection, and none had vaginitis (45).

Urethral devices, especially urethral inserts, have higher rates of adverse events than the vaginal devices. The most commonly reported complications include urinary tract infections, hematuria, and urethral and/or bladder irritation and discomfort (38,39). These complications appear to occur most often in the first month of device use, and generally resolve simply with treatment or temporary suspension of device use. In a long-term study of a urethral insert, symptomatic cystitis occurred in 10.5% of participants during the first month of use, but in only 2% to 3% in subsequent months (39). Rarely (1–3% of users), a urethral insert may migrate into the proximal urethra or bladder and an endoscopic procedure may be required for its retrieval. Two cases of urethral mucosal prolapse occurred among 62 women during a one-month trial of a urethral suction cap device, and both resolved spontaneously after discontinuing use of the device (40).

CONCLUSION

Pessaries and other devices are an important non-surgical treatment option for both POP and SUI. Current research supports that most women with an interest in pessary treatment can be successfully fit with a pessary, and about 50% of women who are successfully fit will continue pessary use for a year or longer. Urethral inserts and occlusive devices are also effective, but their use is limited by more frequent adverse effects and the intensive patient effort required for use. Careful pessary and device management and follow-up is essential to minimize side effects and avoid complications. Clinical trials comparing pessary treatment with other non-surgical and surgical treatments and long-term studies of both effectiveness and adverse events associated with pessaries and devices are needed.

REFERENCES

1. Shah SM, Sultan AH, Thakar R. The history and evolution of pessaries for pelvic organ prolapse. Int Urogynecol J Pelvic Floor Dysfunct 2006; 17: 170–5.
2. Vierhout ME. The use of pessaries in vaginal prolapse. Eur J Obstet Gynecol Reprod Biol 2004; 117: 4–9.
3. Cundiff GW, Weidner AC, Visco AG, et al. A survey of pessary use by members of the American urogynecologic society. Obstet Gynecol 2000; 95(6 Pt 1): 931–5.
4. Pott-Grinstein E, Newcomer JR. Gynecologists' patterns of prescribing pessaries. J Reprod Med 2001; 46: 205–8.
5. ACOG Committee on Practice Bulletins—Gynecology. ACOG Practice Bulletin No. 85: Pelvic organ prolapse. Obstet Gynecol 2007; 110: 717–29.
6. Wilson PD, Berghmans B, Hagen S, et al. Adult conservative management. In: Abrams P, Cardozo L, Khoury S, Wein A, eds. Incontinence. London: Health Publication Ltd., 2005: 855–964.
7. Cundiff GW, Amundsen CL, Bent AE, et al. The PESSRI study: symptom relief outcomes of a randomized crossover trial of the ring and Gellhorn pessaries. Am J Obstet Gynecol 2007; 196: 405.e1.
8. Fernando RJ, Thakar R, Sultan AH, et al. Effect of vaginal pessaries on symptoms associated with pelvic organ prolapse. Obstet Gynecol 2006; 108: 93–9.
9. Komesu YM, Rogers RG, Rode MA, et al. Pelvic floor symptom changes in pessary users. Am J Obstet Gynecol 2007; 197: 620.e1.
10. Clemons JL, Aguilar VC, Tillinghast TA, et al. Patient satisfaction and changes in prolapse and urinary symptoms in women who were fitted successfully with a pessary for pelvic organ prolapse. Am J Obstet Gynecol 2004; 190: 1025–9.
11. Clemons JL, Aguilar VC, Sokol ER, et al. Patient characteristics that are associated with continued pessary use versus surgery after 1 year. Am J Obstet Gynecol 2004; 191: 159–64.
12. Mutone MF, Terry C, Hale DS, et al. Factors which influence the short-term success of pessary management of pelvic organ prolapse. Am J Obstet Gynecol 2005; 193: 89–94.
13. Clemons JL, Aguilar VC, Tillinghast TA, et al. Risk factors associated with an unsuccessful pessary fitting trial in women with pelvic organ prolapse. Am J Obstet Gynecol 2004; 190: 345–50.
14. Hanson LA, Schulz JA, Flood CG, et al. Vaginal pessaries in managing women with pelvic organ prolapse and urinary incontinence: patient characteristics and factors contributing to success. Int Urogynecol J Pelvic Floor Dysfunct 2006; 17: 155–9.
15. Weber AM, Richter HE. Pelvic organ prolapse. Obstet Gynecol 2005; 106: 615–34.
16. Wu V, Farrell SA, Baskett TF, et al. A simplified protocol for pessary management. Obstet Gynecol 1997; 90: 990–4.
17. Handa VL, Jones M. Do pessaries prevent the progression of pelvic organ prolapse? Int Urogynecol J Pelvic Floor Dysfunct 2002; 13: 349–51; discussion 352.
18. Rogers RG. Clinical practice. Urinary stress incontinence in women. N Engl J Med 2008; 358: 1029–36.
19. Bhatia NN, Bergman A, Gunning JE. Urodynamic effects of a vaginal pessary in women with stress urinary incontinence. Am J Obstet Gynecol 1983; 147: 876–84.
20. Noblett KL, McKinney A, Lane FL. Effects of the incontinence dish pessary on urethral support and urodynamic parameters. Am J Obstet Gynecol 2008; 198: 592.e1.
21. Komesu YM, Ketai LH, Rogers RG, et al. Restoration of continence by pessaries: magnetic resonance imaging assessment of mechanism of action. Am J Obstet Gynecol 2008; 198: 563.e1.
22. Nygaard I. Prevention of exercise incontinence with mechanical devices. J Reprod Med 1995; 40: 89–94.
23. Donnelly MJ, Powell-Morgan S, Olsen AL, et al. Vaginal pessaries for the management of stress and mixed urinary incontinence. Int Urogynecol J Pelvic Floor Dysfunct 2004; 15: 302–7.
24. Farrell SA, Singh B, Aldakhil L. Continence pessaries in the management of urinary incontinence in women. J Obstet Gynaecol Can 2004; 26: 113–17.

25. Robert M, Mainprize TC. Long-term assessment of the incontinence ring pessary for the treatment of stress incontinence. Int Urogynecol J Pelvic Floor Dysfunct 2002; 13: 326–9.

26. Farrell SA, Baydock S, Amir B, et al. Effectiveness of a new self-positioning pessary for the management of urinary incontinence in women. Am J Obstet Gynecol 2007; 196: 474.e1.

27. Shaikh S, Ong EK, Glavind K, et al. Mechanical devices for urinary incontinence in women. Cochrane Database Syst Rev 2006; 3: CD001756.

28. Richter HE, Burgio KL, Goode PS, et al. Non-surgical management of stress urinary incontinence: ambulatory treatments for leakage associated with stress (ATLAS) trial. Clin Trials 2007; 4: 92–101.

29. Realini JP, Walters MD. Vaginal diaphragm rings in the treatment of stress urinary incontinence. J Am Board Fam Pract 1990; 3: 99–103.

30. Suarez GM, Baum NH, Jacobs J. Use of standard contraceptive diaphragm in management of stress urinary incontinence. Urology 1991; 37: 119–22.

31. Davila GW, Ostermann KV. The bladder neck support prosthesis: a non-surgical approach to stress incontinence in adult women. Am J Obstet Gynecol 1994; 171: 206–11.

32. Moore KH, Foote A, Burton G, et al. An open study of the bladder neck support prosthesis in genuine stress incontinence. BJOG 1999; 106: 42–9.

33. Morris AR, Moore KH. The Contiform incontinence device—efficacy and patient acceptability. Int Urogynecol J Pelvic Floor Dysfunct 2003; 14: 412.

34. Allen W, Leek H, Izurieta A, et al. Update: the "Contiform" intravaginal device in four sizes for the treatment of stress incontinence. Int Urogynecol J Pelvic Floor Dysfunct 2008; 19: 757.

35. Thyssen H, Bidmead J, Lose G, et al. A new intravaginal device for stress incontinence in women. BJU Int 2001; 88: 889–92.

36. Ziv E, Stanton SL, Abarbanel J. Efficacy and safety of a novel disposable intravaginal device for treating stress urinary incontinence. Am J Obstet Gynecol 2008; 198: 594.e1.

37. Vierhout ME, Lose G. Preventive vaginal and intra-urethral devices in the treatment of female urinary stress incontinence. Curr Opin Obstet Gynecol 1997; 9: 325–8.

38. Staskin D, Bavendam T, Miller J, et al. Effectiveness of a urinary control insert in the management of stress urinary incontinence: early results of a multicenter study. Urology 1996; 47: 629–36.

39. Sirls LT, Foote JE, Kaufman JM, et al. Long-term results of the FemSoft urethral insert for the management of female stress urinary incontinence. Int Urogynecol J Pelvic Floor Dysfunct 2002; 13: 88–95; discussion 95.

40. Versi E, Griffiths DJ, Harvey MA. A new external urethral occlusive device for female urinary incontinence. Obstet Gynecol 1998; 92: 286–91.

41. Brubaker L, Harris T, Gleason D, et al. The external urethral barrier for stress incontinence: a multicenter trial of safety and efficacy. Obstet Gynecol 1999; 93: 932.

42. Moore KH, Simons A, Dowell C, et al. Efficacy and user acceptability of the urethral occlusive device in women with urinary incontinence. J Urol 1999; 162: 464.

43. Tincello DG, Adams EJ, Bolderson J, et al. A urinary control device for management of female stress incontinence. Obstet Gynecol 2000; 95: 417–20.

44. Arias B, Ridgeway B, Barber M. Complications of neglected vaginal pessaries: case presentation and literature review. Int Urogynecol J Pelvic Floor Dysfunct 2008; 19: 1173.

45. Thyssen H, Lose G. Long-term efficacy and safety of a disposable vaginal device (continence guard) in the treatment of female stress incontinence. Int Urogynecol J Pelvic Floor Dysfunct 1997; 8: 130.

Lynette E Franklin

INTRODUCTION

The history of catheterization to empty the bladder dates back to approximately 1000 BC. Records from India attest to the use of tubular objects made from iron, gold, silver, and wood and lubricated with liquid butter to drain the bladder and manage urethral strictures. Chinese records from the 100 BC time period, record use of lacquered onion leaves to provide hollow instruments to empty the bladder (1). In China in 30 AD, urinary retention was managed with lead and bronze pipes. These devices were smoother, as compared to other devices, and had a more manageable size that functioned both for men and women's needs. Catheters have also been found in Pompeii, preserved in the lava from the eruption of Vesuvius (2). The early devices were rigid and did not provide the user with a continuous drainage system. Urinary catheterization was revolutionized with the advent of rubber technology. In the mid-19th century, Auguste Nelaton produced catheters that were portable, flexible, and reusable. Eventually this flexibility allowed for indwelling catheters that could be secured with tape, external device or sutures. Hence, the advent of the modern indwelling urinary catheter was realized.

Urosepsis was a common almost invariably fatal problem in the early years of catheterization usage. The introduction of antiseptics, beginning with Lister, followed by the use of antibiotic therapies decreased mortality associated with this therapy and provided better outcomes overall. In 1966, the Stoke Mandeville National Spinal Injuries Center introduced sterile technique for catheterization which provided more options for people requiring catheterizations (1). Shortly after the sterile technique introduction, Lapides pioneered the clean intermittent self-catheterization (CISC) technique after one of his patients reused a catheter that had been dropped, without resterilization, without untoward consequences to the patient's bladder system.

Catheters for bladder care continue to change and evolve whilst providing patients with more options for comfort, ease, and safe usage.

CATHETERS

Goals of Catheterization

Catheterization of the bladder may be indicated for in the long and short term. The goals may be quite different in different situations. When considering the selection, one must consider the overall goal of therapy. These goals may include one or more of the following:

- *Temporary emptying of the bladder*: This includes the maintenance of bladder drainage during periods of acute or sudden urinary retention such as that during or following surgical procedures.

- *Long-term emptying of the bladder*: Chronic bladder dysfunction, and urinary retention such as that due to bladder underactivity or bladder outlet obstruction not amenable to treatment.

- *Intravesical instillation therapy and treatment*: Instillation of medications or solutions into the bladder to treat underlying diseases such as bladder cancer, interstitial cystitis, or infection.

- *Incontinence management*: To divert urine into a containment device to reduce skin exposure to moisture for goals of wound healing, patient/caregiver respite, and palliative care.

- *Studies*: Radiographic and urodynamic studies may require intubation of the bladder to instill radiographic contrast agents, or measure bladder pressures

- *Monitoring*: Measurement of urine output in the acutely ill or post-operative patient.

- *Testing*: Catheterization can be utilized to obtain accurate post void residual measurement or acquire an uncontaminated urine specimen for laboratory analysis.

Urethral Catheterization

Definition

Urethral catheterization is the passage of a tube through the urethral os into the bladder to drain the bladder of urine. This process may be done on an intermittent basis or as a permanent indwelling arrangement. Intermittent catheterization may be chronic or a one-time event for an acute patient care need, for example, urinary retention or drug administration. Indwelling catheterization is the passage and anchoring of a catheter for an extended period of time. The catheter is not immediately removed but is stabilized to the skin through an anchoring device such as a leg strap (1).

Designs and Materials

Catheters have evolved as new materials are developed and patient demands dictate market need. Choice of materials and design allows the best catheter to be employed. There is not one catheter that does all, but the variety currently available permits patients and care providers the opportunity to choose the best catheter for the specific need of the patient. However, depending on the location of practice and the macroeconomic environment, third party payers may at times dictate the catheter used (Table 46.1).

Size and Length

Catheters are sized in the standardized measurement developed by J.F.B Charriere. This so called French scale is based on

Table 46.1 Catheter Types

Material	Definition	Pros	Cons	Best use
Silicone elastomer-coated latex	A coating of chemically bonded silicone adhered to a latex catheter	• Reduces contact of latex to the urethra in the latex sensitive patient • Reduces incidence of insertion trauma, urethritis and encrustation	• More rigid • Elastic coating may dissolve over time exposing patient to latex	• Short term usage • Patients with latex sensitivity
Red rubber-latex	• A latex catheter that is soft allowing for flexibility • Latex is a natural product that is a yellowish brown in color	• Flexible allowing for easy insertion especially for short term usage • Low Cost	• Latex based; contraindicated in patients with latex allergies • Becomes brittle after repeated usage • Swells with absorption of fluid thereby decreasing diameter of lumen and increasing outside diameter. • Some toxicity with mucosal tissue resulting in stricture and inflammation	• Short term usage as in CISC • For patients without allergies to latex
PVC	A firm catheter made from a plastic polymer that has had plasticizer added to soften and increase flexibility	• Becomes soft and pliable at body temperature	• Limited utility as indwelling catheters, since encrustation is common with >1 week usage • Has been debated as to safety with exposure to liquid over long periods of time, i.e., may break down	• CISC
Hydrophilic coated catheters	A plastic polymer catheter with a coating of PVP: PVP and salt. When exposed to water this outer coating becomes very lubricated and slippery	• Easier insertion and withdrawal resulting in a minimization of urethral trauma • Safer for allergy prone patients as no latex is present • Reduction in the amount of catheter associated UTIs (5)	• Only one time use • May be difficult for some patients to manipulate secondary to the very slick nature of the catheter • Some packaging includes water to activate, may be difficult to break seal or may become broken early, causing problems for patient with clean up • Expensive	• Long term usage for CISC
Silicone	An inert product that is clear or white in color	• Inexpensive • Thin walled tube with larger lumen • Catheters more compatible with lining of the urethra	• Rigid and uncomfortable—increasing risk for bypassing and bladder spasms • Balloons tend to form cuffs when deflated making removal difficult	Long term usage, patients with allergies to other products
Silver alloy	Silver ions, bactericidal and non-toxic to humans, are used to coat the catheter on the outside, inner lumen or both	• Some evidence that catheter related UTI (CAUTI) are reduced from between 3.3% and 35.5% per year • Potential reduction in the rate of asymptomatic bacteriuria with short term use	• More research needed to know full extent of CAUTI reduction • Expensive	CISC, indwelling or SPT
Antibiotic impregnated	Catheter coated with minocycline, rifampicin, and nitrofurazone	• May reduce CAUTI (2)	• Expensive	Long or short-term catheterization

Abbreviations: CISC, clean intermittent self catheterization; PVC, polyvinyl chloride; PVP, polyvinyl pyrrolidone; SPT, suprapubic tube; UTI, urinary tract infection.

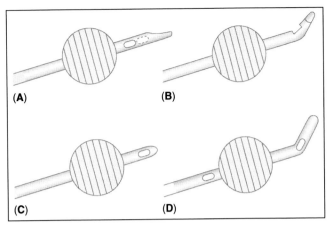

Figure 46.1 Catheter tips: (**A**) whistle; (**B**) Tiemann; (**C**) round; (**D**) Roberts.

the metric system where the external circumference is measured in millimeters. This measurement referred to as either French gauge (Fg or Fr) or Charriere (Ch) and is approximately equal to three times the external diameter. Thus a 30 Fr catheter is 10 mm in diameter. In women, the size of catheter used most often is between 14 Fr and 16 Fr. However, at times a larger diameter may be indicated. For an indwelling catheter, a retention balloon is needed; the balloon should be inflated properly to the correct size. If under inflated, there can be distortion of the catheter tip, and over inflation can risk balloon rupture. Correct selection of catheter size is important to decrease pain and discomfort with insertion of the catheter. Generally, the smallest, softest catheter that is sufficient to fulfill the clinical indication for catheterization is used. At times, selection of a larger catheter may be necessary for a variety of indications including hematuria drainage.

Catheter lengths, for intermittent catheterization, are measured in the imperial or metric system. Long or male length is 42 cm or 16″. This length is not however gender specific and in fact a longer catheter may be beneficial for obese women with large perineal skin folds. Female or short length is 6″ or 26 cm. Shorter pediatric length catheters are also available. The choice of length used should meet the needs of the patient and/or caregivers taking into consideration the patient's habitus, preference, and dexterity. Generally, indwelling catheters are a standard long length of 42 cm.

Various catheter tips are available. Catheter tips differ in order to facilitate insertion and drainage of the bladder in a variety of clinical scenarios (Fig. 46.1).

Indwelling Vs. Clean Intermittent Catheterization Vs. Suprapubic

Patient Selection

Although health professionals may be very comfortable with the practice of long term catheterization the lay person may experience high degrees of anxiety when approached with this modality. Varying responses including fear, anxiety, and revulsion can be exhibited in the patient who is attempting to assimilate not only the diagnosis of the underlying urinary tract problem, but also the prospect of caring for oneself with a foreign object.

General criteria to evaluate if a woman should be managed with a chronic versus intermittent catheter should be reviewed with the patient, and her caregivers if applicable. Evaluation should include but not be limited to:

- *Motivation*: This is the ability of the patient to review goals and incorporate a desired outcome into her treatment plan. Acceptable levels of self involvement in continence care will differ between patients and an assessment of such will help develop the best treatment plan for her.
- *Dexterity*: This is the combination of the ability of the patient to properly position herself for catheterization, and the ability to self access her perineal area and the precision and ability of her upper arm extremities movement to separate and locate the urethral os either visually or by tactile sense. The degrees of dexterity will dictate independence with respect to urinary tract management. If a caregiver is willing to provide self catheterization services, then he or she will need to have a similar skill set.
- *Bladder capacity*: The low pressure storage capacity of the bladder should be adequate such that if intermittent catheterization is recommended, there can be a reasonable time interval between catheterizations so that urinary storage pressures are maintained in a safe range, urinary incontinence is minimized, and upper urinary tract integrity is maintained.
- *Adequate mental capacity*: The woman should have the cognitive capacity to independently care for herself, follow directions for self care or, alternatively, allow a caregiver to complete care with minimal stress to the patient and/or caregiver.
- *Health care beliefs*: The choice of management is ultimately a decision made to effectively control the woman's condition. Her understanding of the condition coupled with social, religious, personal, and economic beliefs and responsibilities should be considered as these may or may not lead to successful implementation of a given strategy.

Despite adequate planning and informed consent, problems with a catheterization method can arise after implementation has been enacted. These problems need to be identified and addressed in a time efficient manner to decrease potential adverse outcomes. Such issues include (1):

- *Psychological issues*: Implementation may require the assistance of a trained counselor or mental health expert to overcome fear, depression, and/or anger about the current adaption.
- *Visual problems*: Although initially visualization of the urethral os may be assisted with the use of a mirror, the continual use of a mirror may be cumbersome and awkward especially when catheterizing away from home. Teaching patients to use manual location of the urethral opening in relation to the vagina can be beneficial to prevent this problem.

Table 46.2 General Guidelines for Clean Intermittent Self Catheterization

1. Gather supplies
2. Wash hands and perineum with soap and water
3. Separate labia and locate the urethral os with the non-dominant hand.
4. Pass the lubricated catheter into the urethra until urine passage is achieved
5. Once the bladder is drained slowly advance the catheter approximately 5 cm further to fully drain the bladder, then slowly remove the catheter

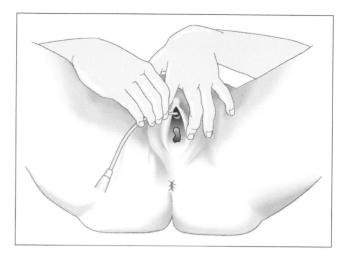

Figure 46.2 Self-catheterization by a woman.

• *Dexterity changes*: Due to aging, illness, or other factors, anatomical or functional factors can change throughout the course of a woman's illness, altering her ability to continue in the mode of catheterization initially chosen. Under these circumstances, physical and occupational health services can help provide devices that may maintain or re-establish dexterity in otherwise difficult situations. These professionals are also experts with upper and lower limb aids to assist with adduction or abduction which may provide access to the urethral os. Also, these professionals may provide additional therapy that may be initiated to decrease other co morbidities that impede dexterity such as range of motion exercises for those individuals with arthritis.

Technique of CISC

The first self catheterization will set the tone for the woman to become confident and self sufficient in self care. The environment should be calm, prepared, and unrushed, to assist her in achieving maximum benefit from the lesson. As an adult learner, it is best that she demonstrate the catheterization as opposed to watching the health care provider do it (3).

Many manufacturers provide written and visual material to review with patients. It is prudent to review with the patient the anatomy and physiology of the urinary tract system prior to introduction of the catheter to prevent any misconceptions of passage and potentially decrease anxiety. Written materials in the patient's native language should be given if possible to further increase knowledge acquisition.

Once the supplies are gathered, positioning the patient in a semi-reclining position with good lighting will aid her in seeing the urethral orifice with a mirror. Prior to attempting the initial catheterization, it is important to review her preexisting knowledge, goals, and consider any limitations. These considerations will help to tailor the lesson to provide successful outcomes.

Using a touchless system with an attached drainage bag may be beneficial in the early stages of learning. This technique decreases the concerns regarding spillage of urine out of the catheter and generally decreases anxiety and embarrassment. As the woman gains mastery of CISC, her positioning may change and her ability to direct the fluid becomes easier without added appliances. Table 46.2 provides general instructions for CISC (Fig. 46.2).

Indwelling Catheters

A catheter may be placed that is retained with a fluid balloon. The catheter is placed through the urethral os into the bladder using sterile technique. The balloon is inflated with sterile water according to the manufacture's guidelines. Generally, the balloon holds between 5 cm³ and 30 cm³ of fluid. Saline and contrast should not be used to inflate the balloon. These fluids may crystallize in the balloon port, clogging it, and prevent balloon deflation and catheter removal. The bladder can be maintained in a decompressed state with use of a drainage bag, or may be intermittently drained with a plug. The catheter should be changed every four to six weeks.

Suprapubic Catheters

A suprapubic tube (SPT) is an indwelling catheter that is surgically or percutaneously placed through the abdominal wall directly into the bladder. It is secured in this location using the same balloon mechanism as a urethral catheter. This type of drainage system avoids urethral catheterization. Approximately one month after initial placement, a well healed epithialized tract is formed maintaining a patent opening for simplified office based catheter changes. These tubes are indicated for patients who are unwilling or unable to manage urethral indwelling catheters or clean intermittent catheterization, and for those individuals who have urethral disease precluding placement of a urethral catheter (e.g., severe urethral stricture disease). SPTs may be temporary as for example in patients who have recently had pelvic surgery and bladder decompression must be maintained temporarily postoperatively. This therapy is not optimal for the patient who is willing and able to perform CISC. As described later, indwelling tubes (urethral and suprapubic) are associated with complications which are much less likely than with CISC.

SPTs are usually placed electively in the operating room in sensate patients. Under anesthesia, a catheter is passed directly into bladder via a stab incision through the abdomen 2 to 4 cm cephalad to the symphysis pubis. The catheter is exchanged in the office or in the patient's residence every four to six weeks. A well epithialized tract develops through the abdomen wall into the bladder allowing for simple catheter changes. When

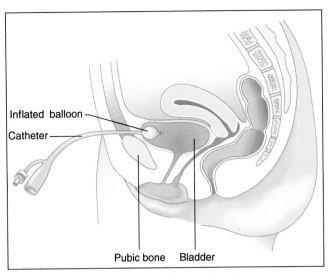

Figure 46.3 Position of suprapubic catheter.

counseling a patient about the possibility of this catheterization type, acknowledgment and discussion about altered body image are essential. Many patients will find it difficult to accept a permanent foreign body protruding from their abdomen, identifying concerns of "normal function loss," changes in sexual practices, and leakage. Although warranted concerns, quality of life indicators may actually improve when patients have been converted from urethral to a suprapubic catheters especially in patients who are dependent on wheelchairs or who are sexually active (Fig. 46.3) (4).

Catheter Associated Problems

Infection/Hematuria/Trauma

The most prevalent type of hospital acquired infection are urinary tract infections (UTIs), with 80% of infections being associated with indwelling catheters (5). Women are more susceptible to catheter associated UTI as compared to men (6). Infection is related to several potential mechanisms of entry of bacteria: insertion technique, cross contamination with staff care, or retrograde flow from drainage bags.

UTI symptoms in patients with catheters are often atypical. Upon insertion of the catheter, bacterial biofilms will begin to develop within 24 hours. These bacterial colonies are found on the device surface, and they will not necessarily result in an infection. Patients with catheters often have bacteriuria, presence of bacteria in normally sterile urine. Bacteria will be present in the bladder within 2 to 10 days of insertion, but not necessarily result in an infection (6). After 30 days of an indwelling catheter, virtually all patients have bacteriuria due to colonization. This colonization of bacteria may not be eliminated with antibiotic use. It is important to differentiate colonization from infection. An infection is an immunological activation in response to a foreign body such as a microorganism. Colonization is a symbiotic growth of bacteria in the body that has does not result in activation of the body's immune system (7).

Newman (6) has outlined signs and symptoms of UTI in nursing home residents with catheters to include two of the following:

- Fever (>38° C) or chills
- New flank pain or suprapubic pain or tenderness

- Change in character of urine (smell, blood, etc.) OR lab report of new hematuria or pyuria
- Worsening mental or functional status
- Local findings of obstruction, leakage mucosal trauma, or hematuria

If a UTI is suspected with an indwelling catheter, or in a patient who self catheterizes, the specimen needs to be obtained from a new catheter insertion. The catheter is changed and the urine is obtained from the bladder through the new tube. This prevents a sample of the catheter biofilm being collected and is more representative of the bladder flora.

Multiple other complications may result from catheter usage (8). Long term catheter usage may result in the formation of bladder stones. Hematuria may result from the trauma of insertion, the trauma of removal, or trauma with sudden traction on the tube itself. Trauma from insertion or removal without deflating the balloon can cause urethra injury, tearing, or subsequent stricture. Removal of the catheter inadvertently, is common among women with dementia or those prone to falls, those who strain for bowel movements or when excessive tension is suddenly placed on the catheter (6). Securing the catheter to the leg can aid in decreasing the movement of the catheter and friction on the perineal skin, and potentially reducing bladder spasms. In addition, secure placement of the bag probably reduces intravesical trauma thus reduces gross hematuria. Devices to secure catheters are available in a variety of forms including self adhesives, Velcro closures, latex leg straps, and abdominal belts. There has not been consensus established as to the most beneficial location for placement of the securement device, but rather to place it to provide maximum functioning for the women wearing the catheter (6). Fistula, traumatic hypospadius, and bladder cancer are also complications associated with catheter usage. Stop-orders, written orders to discontinue catheters in hospitalized patients when justified indications ceased, did not show a decrease in urinary tract infections, but did reduce duration of inappropriate catheter usage (9).

Complications specific to suprapubic catheterization are similar to those complications listed for other types of catheters (3). In addition, placement of a SPT may result in bowel injury, vascular injury, and soft tissue infection.

The Joanna Briggs Institute (10) developed a best practice paper on short term catheter removal based on a review on current research. These authors recommend for practice the following three strategies for removal of short term indwelling urethral catheters, defined as insertion for a period from 1 to 14 days:

1. Timing of removal when appropriate should be at midnight.
2. Duration of catheterization should be as brief as possible, and medically appropriate following pelvic surgery. Early catheter removal results in a reduced risk for UTI and a shorter hospital stay, but also carries with it a greater risk of voiding problems.
3. Placing and removing a clamp from the tube to "retrain the bladder," a technique known as clamping, prior to the removal of the catheter has limited degree of effectiveness in facilitating a successful voiding trial.

Leakage

Pericatheter leakage should always be investigated. Causes for pericatheter leakage include UTIs, stones, malignancy, bladder spasms, poor drainage due to clogging, urethral erosion, and a number of other causes. A careful physical examination and history along with gentle irrigation will be able to differentiate between several of these entities. Careful assessment of the patient and the system should be conducted to evaluate for easily reversible factors such as tubing kinks and poor catheter drainage. The addition of an antimuscarinic agent may treat leakage associated with bladder spasms. Before prescribing these medications other causes of pericatheter leakage should be considered and investigated when appropriate.

Table 46.3 Recommendations for Bag Cleaning (6)

1. Rinse bag with lukewarm water
2. Vigorously agitate clean water in the collection system twice
3. Pour a diluted solution of bleach (1:10 parts water) on drainage port, sleeve, cap and connector. Also pour in bag and agitate for 30 seconds, drain and allow to air dry. The bag should always be rinsed with soap and water after using any disinfectant

Drainage Bags

Before the advent of drainage bags, indwelling urinary catheters were drained into non-sterile open systems. Ascending bacterial infections occurred very commonly in this setting. Subsequently closed drainage systems with non-return valves were developed that reduced the incidence of ascending bacteria from the bag to the person. Drainage bags range in collection volumes of 250 to 1000 ml. These bags can be fastened to the bed, the leg, or abdomen. Volume selection may be changed based on need. For example, larger systems are convenient for overnight use, and smaller leg bags may be used discreetly during the day. These can be washed and reused for months at a time. Recommendations for bag cleaning are listed in Table 46.3. Minimal disruption of the closed system should be maintained to reduce infection risk. Strict adherence to a hand washing prior to manipulation should also be maintained.

Manufacturers have developed various systems for the ambulatory and bed-restricted patient. These bags can be maintained in a dependent position using straps, buttons, Velcro, and hooks. The goal is to keep the bag in a dependent position so that urine will flow freely and from the patient into the bag and not in the opposite direction (Fig. 46.4).

Drainage Valves

To facilitate emptying the catheter and/or the bag, various spigots and valves have been developed. These devices come in

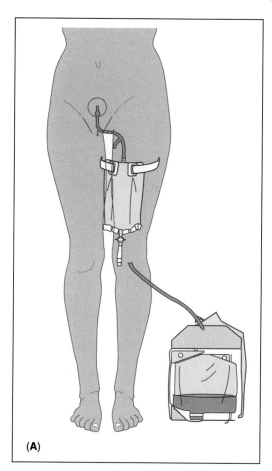

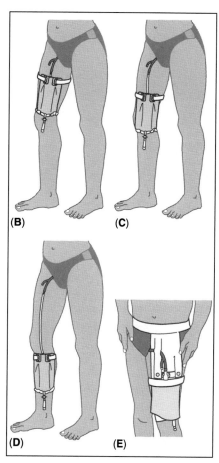

Figure 46.4 Leg bags and lengths. (**A**) Closed drainage system with a night bag attached to the leg bag; note the short female catheter. (**B–E**) Different lengths of leg bags, ranging from 350 to 750 ml in capacity, and suspensory systems: (**B**) short-tube bag; (**C**) medium-tube bag; (**D**) long-tube bag; (**E**) alternative method of suspension.

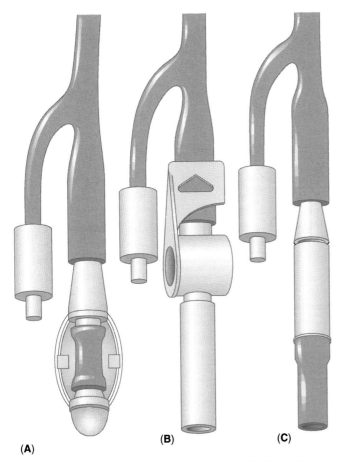

(A) (B) (C)

Figure 46.5 Examples of catheter valves: (**A**) EMS Medical; (**B**) Bard Flip-Flo; (**C**) Sims Portex Uro-Flo.

a variety of sizes that attach directly to the bag or may be inserted into the catheter. These systems provide a non continuous drainage system which allows increased freedom for the patient to perform activities of daily living without a bag. When deciding if a valve is an appropriate adaptation for a patient, one must also consider the selection process as listed earlier: motivation, dexterity, level of mental capacity, and bladder functioning/capacity (Fig. 46.5) (11).

PADS AND PANTS
Pads
Urinary incontinence can be managed by absorbent products that are either known as "body-worn" or for the protection of furniture. Body worn systems are defined as those which are placed in undergarments. The goal of these products is to contain the urine. Other functions may include odor protection, skin protection, and avoidance of stained outer garments. Currently pads are available in reusable/washable or single-use/disposable products. Geographic location, will partially dictate the availability of different products. In some countries, pads are considered medical devices and are allocated by the government health care system, whereas, in other countries, these products are available over the counter and consumption is consumer driven. There are very few studies which directly compare these products with respect to efficacy, safety, or cost, and international standards do not exist.

Product design is based on numerous factors. These factors include gender and amount of fluid to be absorbed. Female products are designed to absorb urine that drains into the middle of the undergarment. The capacity of the product's absorption is dependent on fiber arrangement and type. Urinary incontinence pads are designed to absorb and/or contain urine and are not interchangeable with products designed to absorb menstrual waste. This is an important differentiation that should be emphasized to the patient (12).

Urine collection pads are designed to collect the urine from the surface of the pad and wick it away to an inner core away from the perineal skin. Currently, there is no standardization as to capacity, or quality of product used in incontinence pads. Newman et al. (6) recommend some standardization for evaluation to include:

1. Re-wet value: This value reflects the dryness of a product after subsequent wetting of the product when the measurement is taken at the skin level. Lower re-wet values represent drier product performance.
2. Rate of acquisition: This is the speed at which a product is able to absorb a set volume of liquid.
3. Total absorbent capacity: This measurement would help delineate the differences in absorption between products that are designed for light, medium, and heavy absorbency.

Pads are fairly uniform in their construction. Typically, there is (*i*) a securement layer which is an adhesive strip or strap, (*ii*) a waterproof layer to protect garments, (*iii*) a fluff layer to absorb the fluid, and (*iv*) a top mesh layer to wick away the fluid from the skin. Technological advances have improved the saturation point of disposables with the addition of superabsorbent polymer (SAP). This polymer is added to the middle layer of the pad's fluff layer, in a powder form. This hydrocolloid material changes from a powder into a gel that wicks away urine from the pad's surface. Urine leakage outside the pad is decreased as the SAP can absorb 70 times its original weight while maintaining a relatively small particle size of 1 to 2 mm.

Reusable products are made from fibers such as rayon or polyester. These options are attractive to users in that they can be used repeatedly and may provide more stability for the user. As compare to pads secured with an adhesive, these products are less likely to shift allowing for a more secure feeling of placement. The absorbant pad is fixed into the undergarment and does not lend itself to shifting from the perineal area as a disposable or removable product potentially could. They also provide the user with a more flexible quiet system without the inclusion of plastic.

Urinary leakage can be quantified per episode (6) as:

- Light 0 to 50 ml
- Moderate 50 to 200 ml
- Severe >300 ml

The importance of quantifying urinary leakage is that it allows the consumer to choose the smallest product for maximum benefit. It also helps health care providers know the extent of urinary leakage per episode (Table 46.4).

Table 46.4 Pads for Undergarments

Pad type	Description	Pros	Cons
Perineal pads	Discreet options for women with light to moderate incontinence. Available in disposable and reusable products, these pads adhere to the underwear of the patient to provide body formed protection. Generally rectangular shaped with some differences to accommodate larger volumes, i.e., gathered edges, width changes to accommodate larger volumes	• Self adhesive strips provide use of preexisting undergarments • Convenient: easily carried in purses to provide ease of change when out of the home environment • Pads stay in place although can be reused in the event a leakage accident does not occur • May contain built in deodorant • "Booster systems" can be used with other products to increase absorptive capacity	• Expensive • May be difficult for manually dexterity challenged patient to position
Undergarments	Form fitting pads that are attached with elasticized, Velcro or button fasteners.	• Provides protection moderate to severe protection from urine leakage. • Available in various shapes that accommodates application in supine, sitting and standing positioning. • Soft external backing provides comfort and air exchange	• Often bulky and cumbersome • May not be as discreet when applied under from fitting clothing • Storage of multiple garments requires large area, more inconvenient to transport when travelling
Protective underwear	Disposable product that is pulled on, as with the cloth counter part, but can be ripped off at the side to provide ease of removal	• Moderate to severe leakage protection • Option to provide security especially with women who may attempt to remove device when disoriented or demented • Available in systems that provide active patients to continue activities such as swimming	Bulky, difficult to change with patient who has limited mobility or who is bed bound
Adult brief	Disposable product similar to the child's diaper, provides protection with self adhesive tabs that can be refastened and repositioned	• Moderate to severe urinary incontinence containment • Positioning ease especially with the patient who is bed bound	• Expensive • Bulky • Can become disheveled with frequent position changes and transfers
Pad and pant systems	Combination products using mesh or knit pants with disposable inserts for moderate incontinence	• Allows for self toileting between changes without removal of all clothing, option for ambulatory patient • Adaptations for lingerie and nightgown options provide for apparel during intimate moments	Inconvenience while travelling, as inserts can be bulky and nondiscreet

Generally, when choosing a pad product, the woman and or care giver should evaluate the goals of treatment. Reviewing leakage quantity, type (urine, feces, menses), and timing may dictate changes in the padding system throughout the day and night. Typically, discreet protection coupled with ease of use while maintaining a reasonable cost, will provide a product that is beneficial to meet identified goals (Fig. 46.6) (11).

Pads for Beds and Chairs
Designed similarly to undergarment pads, these pads can be placed on furniture to provide protection. Many of these products have non slip backing to maintain positioning under the patient. Disposable products have lost favor to the reusable products (Fig. 46.7).

Economical and Environmental Issues
In recent years, global knowledge about so called "green" choices have influenced consumers on their choice of products. The reusable pad is often thought of as a more environmentally friendly alternative but considerations must be given to the by-product wastes of reuse including energy expenditures, and cleaning product run off. The downsides of disposable products include biodegradability, landfill versus incineration disposal of waste by-products, and manufacturing expenditures. Economically both types of products have their advantages and disadvantages. The initial cost for the reusable product is usually higher and then one must consider the cost of maintaining this product with washing, drying, and convenience for the patient and the caregiver. Ultimately, the

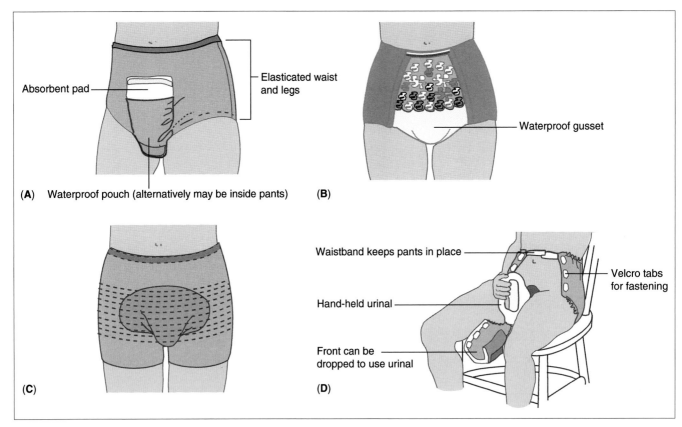

Figure 46.6 Pouch pads and pants: (**A**) pouch pants; (**B**) stretch pants with waterproof gusset; (**C**) stretch pants for use with plastic-backed pad; (**D**) drop-front pants.

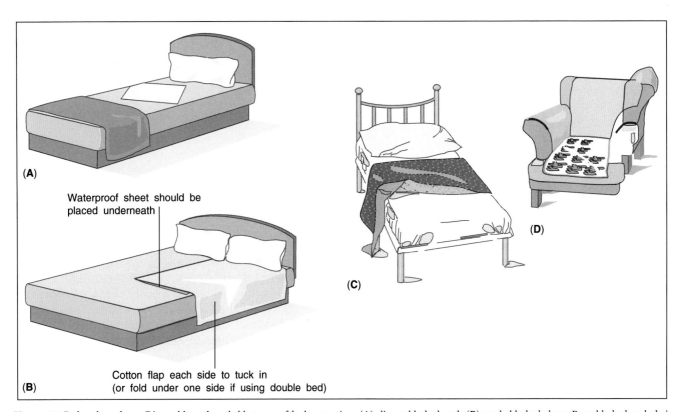

Figure 46.7 Bed pad products. Disposable and washable types of bed protection: (**A**) disposable bed pad; (**B**) washable bed sheet. Reusable bed and chair protection: (**C**) reusable bed pad; (**D**) reusable chair pad.

decision for the product used will be dependent on resources available to the patient.

Skin Care

The skin is the largest organ in the human body and it has multiple functions to perform. It does these functions best when it is healthy and intact. Prevention of skin breakdown, especially in the patient with incontinence, will minimize future problems such as pain, infection, and non-healing wounds.

Skin pH

Skin has a natural acid mantle which is a protective layer and usually maintains a pH between 4.3 and 5.9. When this pH is maintained, the integrity of the skin is maximized thus decreasing the risk of infection, breakdown, and problems associated with these maladies. When a patient is incontinent, the chronic exposure to urine and/or cleaning products, can change the pH to a more alkaline environment which promotes transepidermal water loss, and barrier break down. Many commercially available cleansers are now produced which remove the incontinence debris from the perineal skin, while maintaining the normal pH. Traditionally, commercially available soaps do not offer this option and actually will slowly raise the pH of the skin with repeated usage. It is therefore recommended, that patients requiring frequent cleaning during the day invest in pH balanced cleansers. These are typically more expensive initially, but the long term benefits will promote skin health. This point is especially sensitive for patients with dual fecal and urinary incontinence. When mixed, these substances produce urea, which further increases the alkalinity. In the presence of an alkaline environment, digestive enzymes that have not been activated, will become activated outside of the gastrointestinal tract, thereby prompting further skin breakdown (3).

Skin Barriers Vs. Treatments

Many commercially available products are now available for protection of the perineal skin. Prevention prior to breakdown is by far the easiest way to keep skin intact and decrease further complications such as infection, pain and pressure damage. Urine barriers include dimethicone, petrolateum, and skin barrier products (e.g., Cavlion Spray, 3M, St. Paul, Minnesota, U.S.A.). These products when used prophylactically provide a physical barrier between the skin and the effluence. This barrier repels the fluid away from the skin, thus maintaining the acid mantle and decreasing maceration changes and breakdown in the epidermal layer of skin. In the presence of stool, a zinc oxide based barrier provides additional protection as it has the properties to repel stool effluence and maintain skin integrity. Once applied, these products do not need to be removed from the skin but cleansed and reapplied after each incontinent episode to maintain sufficient barrier protection.

Cutaneous candidiasis is also common in the patient with incontinence. Typically, candidiasis is not a microorganism that is found in the perineal skin area, but can easily be deposited to this area from the gastrointestinal tract. When provided the right environment, (a moist, dark, location in an immunocompromised host), candidiasis can rapidly reproduce causing a topical cutaneous candidiasis. Treatment topically may include miconazole or clotrimazole in ointment, powder or cream form. Treatment is usually initiated with empirical therapy when identification by observation is made. Cutaneous candidiasis is identified as a reddened rash with a confluent erythema with satellite lesions around the border. There may also be evidence of tiny fluid filled vesicles or macules that have been opened as a result of friction from shear of clothing and pads (3).

AIDS AND APPLIANCES
Toileting Aids
Commodes

To provide access to a toilet, when a lavatory is not available or easily accessible, many free standing commodes are available. These have such features as raised seats, adjustable legs, and chemical emptying devices. This provides women with options to facilitate access and support independent toileting (Fig. 46.8).

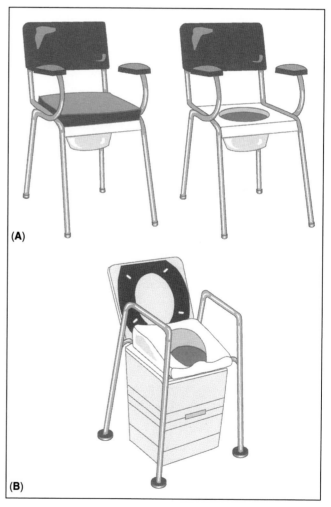

Figure 46.8 Toilet aids.

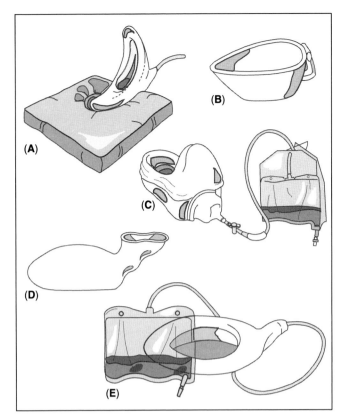

Figure 46.9 Female urinals: (**A**) bridge urinal with U-shaped cushion; (**B**) St Peter's boat; (**C**) female urinal connected to drainage bag; (**D**) swan-neck urinal; (**E**) pan-type urinal connected to drainage bag.

Urinals for Females

Although available, these products are not used frequently. They do have some function in providing urination for the continent patient who is not a candidate for catheter management, yet does not want pads, or many not be able to get to the toilet, such as a women in rehabilitation for hip surgery (Fig. 46.9).

Odor Control

A good hygiene program includes adequate skin protection and control of odor. Women with incontinence tend to shower more, and use additional perfumes, creams, and deodorants to conceal leakage (13). Many women will use scented laundry detergents, which in fact may contribute to dermatitis problems as these perfumes can cause an allergic dermatitis.

Assessment to control odor should include (13):

- History of devices used and current hygiene practices
- Difficulties maintaining hygiene and odor control
- Perineal assessment (skin, prolapsed, hemorrhoids, dermatitis)
- Allergies

Odor control can be accomplished by removal of the offending fluid. Also keeping the urine in an acidic state through fluid intake, the urine smell will be decreased. Various sprays are commercially available to mask the odor, without harming the skin.

REFERENCES

1. Wilson MCR. Clean intermittent catheterization and self catheterization. Br J Nurs 2008; 17: 1140–6.
2. Schumm K, Lam TBL. Types of urethral catheters for management of short-tem voiding problems in hospitalized adults: a short version Cochrane review. Neurourol Urodyn 2008; 27: 738–46.
3. Doughty DB. Urinary and Fecal Incontinence, 2nd edn. St. Louis: Mosby, 2000.
4. Pellatt GC, Geddis T. Neurogenic continence. Part 2: neurogenic bladder management. Br J Nurs 2008; 17: 904–12.
5. Lo E, Nicolle L, Classen D, et al. Strategies to prevent catheter-associated urinary tract infections in acute care hospitals. Infect Control Hosp Epidemiol 2008; 29: S41–50.
6. Newman DK. The indwelling urinary catheter: principles for best practice. J Wound Ostomy Continence Nurs 2007; 34: 655–61.
7. Up to Date. Urinary tract infection associated with indwelling bladder catheters [homepage on the internet], 2009 [cited 13 March 2009]. [Available from: http://www.utdol.com/online/content/topic.do?topicKey=uti_infe/2922&view=print.]
8. MedlinePlus Medical Encyclopedia [homepage on the Internet]. Bethesda, MD: US National Library, 2009 [cited 20 March 2009]. [Available from: http://www.nlm.nih.gov/medlineplus/ency/article/003981.htm.]
9. Loeb M, Hunt D, O'Hallorn K, et al. Stop orders to reduce inappropriate urinary catheterization in hospitalized patients: a randomized controlled trial. J Gen Intern Med 2008; 23: 816–20.
10. Joanna Briggs Institute. Removal of short-term indwelling urethral catheters. Nurs Stand 2008; 22: 42–5.
11. Newman DK, Wein AJ. Urinary Incontinence, 2nd edn. Baltimore: Health Professionals Press, 2009.
12. The Simon Foundation for Continence. About Incontinence [homepage on internet], 2009 [cited 13 March 2009]. [Available from: http://www.simonfoundation.org/About_Incontinence.html.]
13. Wallis P, McKenzie S, Griffiths S, et al. What now? Helping clients live positively with urinary incontinence [booklet on the internet]. Queensland, Australia: Australian Government, Department of Health and Ageing, 2007 [cited 20 March 2009]. [Available from: http://www.bladder-bowel.gov.au/doc/HelpingClients.pdf.]

APPENDIX: RESOURCES

International Agencies

The International Continence Society offers extensive lists on their webpage, www.icsoffice.org, about international agencies. Many of these agencies provide information on incontinence and resource to professional and lay persons about available products and guidelines for use within the said country's health care system.

Continence Organizations

Australia

Continence Foundation of Australia Ltd
Website: www.contfound.org.au/

Austria

Medizinische Gesellschaft für lnkontinenzhilfe Österreich
Website: www.inkontinenz.at

Belgium

U-Control vzw (Belgian association for incontinence)
Website: www.sosincontinence.org

Canada

The Canadian Continence Foundation
Website: www.continence-fdn.ca/

Czech Republic
Inco Forum
Website: www.inco-forum.cz

Denmark
Kontinensforeningen (The Danish Association of Incontinent People)
Website: www.kontinens.dk/

France
Association d'Aide aux Personnes Incontinentes
Website: www.aapi.asso.fr
Femmes Pour Toujours
Website: www.femsante.com

Germany
Deutsche Kontinenz Gesellschaft e.V.
Website: www.gih.de
Women's Health Coalition
Website: http://www.w-h-c.de

Hong Kong
Hong Kong Continence Society
Email: emfleung@ha.org.hk

Hungary
Inko Forum
Website: www.inkoforum.hu

India
Indian Continence Foundation
Website: www.indiancontinencefoundation.org/

Indonesia
Indonesian Continence Society
Email: urogyn@centrin.net.id

Israel
The National Centre for Continence
Website: welcome.to/continence

Italy
Fondazione Italiana Continenza
(The Italian Continence Foundation)
Website: http://www.continenza-italia.org/
Associazione Italiana Donne Medico (AIDM)
Website: www.donnemedico.org
The Federazione Italiana INCOntinenti (FINCO)
Website: www.finco.org

Japan
Japan Continence Action Society
Website: www.jcas.or.jp

Korea
Korea Continence Foundation
Website: www.kocon.or.kr

Malaysia
Continence Foundation (Malaysia)
Email: lohcs@medicine.med.um.edu.my

Mexico
Asociacion de Enfremadades Uroginecologicas
Website: www.asenug.org

Netherlands
Pelvic Floor Netherlands
Website: www.pelvicfloor.nl
Pelvic Floor Patients foundation(SBP) (Netherlands)
Website: www.bekkenbodem.net
Vereniging Nederlandse Incontinentie, Verpleegkundigen (V N I V)
Website: www.vniv.nl/

New Zealand
New Zealand Continence Association Inc
Website: www.continence.org.nz/

Norway
NOFUS (Norwegian Society for Patients with Urologic Diseases)
Website: www.nofus.noPhillipines
Continence Foundation of the Phillipines
email: dtbolong@pacific.net

Poland
NTM "Incontinence—To live a Normal Life"
(The Polish Continence Organization)
Website: www.ntm.pl

Singapore
Society for Continence (Singapore)
Website: http://sfcs.org.sg

Slovakia
Slovakia Inco Forum
Website: www.incoforum.sk

Spain
Associacion Nacional de Ostomizados e Incontinentes (ANOI)
Website: www.coalicion.org

Sweden
SINOBA—Föreningen för kunskap om urininkontinens och blåsproblem
Website: www.sinoba.se
Swedish Urotherapists
Tel: (46) 31 50 26 39

Switzerland
Schweizerische Gesellschaft für Blasenschwäche
Website: www.inkontinex.ch

Taiwan
Taiwan Continence Society
Website: www.tcs.org.tw

Thailand
Email: ravkc@mahidol.ac.th

United Kingdom
Association for Continence Advice (ACA)
Website: www.aca.uk.com/
The Continence Foundation
Website: www.continence-foundation.org.uk
Enuresis Resource and Information Centre (ERIC)
Website: www.eric.org.uk/
InconTact
Website: www.incontact.org/

Royal College of Nursing Continence Care Forum
Tel: (44) 020 7409 3333

United States of America
The Simon Foundation for Continence
Website: www.simonfoundation.org/
National Association for Continence
Website: www.nafc.org/
International Foundation for Functional Gastrointestinal Disorders
Website: www.iffgd.org/ and www.aboutincontinence.org
Society of Urologic Nurses and Associates (SUNA)
Website: www.suna.org
Wound Ostomy & Continence Nurses
Website: www.wocn.org

47 The Overactive Bladder

Rob Jones and Marcus Drake

INTRODUCTION

The term overactive bladder (OAB) syndrome was formally adopted in 2002. It is defined by the International Continence Society (ICS) as urinary urgency, usually with frequency and nocturia, in the absence of proven infection or other obvious pathology (1). As such, OAB is a clinical diagnosis derived from a symptom complex centered on urinary urgency, and not upon confirmatory urodynamic evaluation. This represents an important shift in emphasis from previous terminology, with significant implications for patient management.

The personal and socio-economic burden of OAB is considerable. OAB is highly prevalent within society and, while not life-threatening, it is associated with a significant adverse effect on quality of life (QoL), sleep quality, and emotional well being (2,3). OAB has been proposed to have a greater negative effect on health-related quality of life (HRQoL) than diabetes mellitus, hypertension, asthma, or depression (4,5). The estimated economic cost attributable to OAB in the United States was estimated at $12 billion per anum in 2003 (6). The real cost may be greater, due to indirect or intangible costs (e.g., falls and fractures in the elderly, or loss of earnings). Growing awareness of the scale and impact of OAB has driven recent advances in our understanding of the assessment, pathophysiology, and management of this common and challenging condition.

TERMINOLOGY

As with many conditions, understanding and research in the field of urinary incontinence may be hampered by the use of a variety of different terms to describe the same, or similar, conditions. In addition these terms may be used to describe the patients' symptoms, the results of diagnostic tests, or both. The term "unstable bladder" was previously generally used to describe both patients with involuntary detrusor contractions during bladder filling on cystometry and also patients presenting with urgency and frequency, who were often treated without urodynamic evaluation. In addition there were potential misconceptions and negative connotations for patients being labeled as in some way "unstable." To make matters worse, the terms "urge syndrome" and "urgency/frequency syndrome" were also in use as synonyms, compounding the lack of clarity and consistency.

The term OAB was originally proposed by Wein and Abrams in 2000 (7). The definition is based on urgency, the complaint of a "sudden compelling desire to pass urine that is difficult to defer." This symptom is usually associated with increased daytime urinary frequency and nocturia (waking at night to pass urine), and may be associated with urge incontinence (urine leakage accompanied or immediately preceded by urgency). OAB patients are often further sub-classified as OAB wet and OAB dry, on the basis of the presence or absence of associated urge incontinence. The terms urge and urgency are currently under scrutiny; the term urgency incontinence is increasingly being used to replace urge incontinence as being more linguistically exact (8).

The term detrusor overactivity (DO) was adopted by the ICS as the corresponding urodynamic observation, replacing the term detrusor instability. DO is identified on filling cystometry as either phasic or terminal DO. Phasic DO, a characteristic waveform of detrusor pressure rise during filling cystometry, may be either spontaneous or provoked; it may or may not lead to urinary incontinence (detrusor overactivity incontinence, DOI). Terminal DO is a single involuntary detrusor contraction occurring at cystometric capacity, which cannot be suppressed, and may also be associated with incontinence. Neurogenic DO (NDO) is the term used to describe DO in the presence of a relevant neurologic condition. Idiopathic DO (IDO) has no defined cause and is therefore a diagnosis of exclusion.

Although the symptom of urgency incontinence is suggestive and predictive of the urodynamic observation of DO, a substantial proportion of patients with OAB turn out not to have DO. When correlating symptoms and urodynamic results in over 1000 patients, DO was only demonstrated in 69% of men and 44% of women complaining of urgency (9). Conversely, asymptomatic detrusor contractions are frequently seen during filling cystometry in patients without urgency, particularly on ambulatory studies. Turner Warwick's famous observation that the bladder is "an unreliable witness" appears to apply to this patient group and particularly so in women.

EPIDEMIOLOGY

Prevalence of OAB has only been fully clarified in recent years, as previous epidemiological studies focused primarily on the prevalence of urinary incontinence (10,11). In recent population-based studies, storage urinary symptoms have been reported in 17.4% of women in Europe over the age of 40 (5) and 16.9% women in the United States over the age of 18 (3). The overall male prevalence was only slightly lower in both studies. This equates to around 49 million people in Europe and 33 million people in United States with OAB. Prevalence increases with age in both sexes, increasing to 41% of men and 31% of women over the age of 75 (5); this is an important observation, since the aged population is expected to expand significantly over the next 25 years according to projected population growth.

The EPIC study (12) is the largest population-based study to quantify lower urinary tract symptoms according to the current ICS definitions, and hence provides the most precise estimate of OAB prevalence. In 58,139 adults aged 18 or over in Canada, Germany, Italy, Sweden and UK, OAB was reported by 11.8% of the population (12.8% of women and 10.8% of men). Under the age of 60, OAB was more common in women and over the age of 60 it was more common in men. Of women with OAB, 49.2% were incontinent (OAB-wet), compared to 28.7% of men.

Although OAB symptoms are so common in the population, discussions about them are often avoided by those suffering from them. Only 60% of individuals with storage urinary symptoms seek help and only 27% receive treatment (5). There appears to be a clear relationship between the severity of symptoms and the likelihood of reporting these to a healthcare provider. Reasons for delay in seeking advice include acceptance of symptoms as being a normal part of ageing, particularly in older patients, and the inherent fear that surgery is the only treatment. Embarrassment and reluctance to discuss the problem with the general practitioner are very common, and may be more so in women if the general practitioner is male. One-fifth of women consult a doctor within one year of symptoms becoming troublesome, a third delay for up to five years, and a quarter wait for more than five years (13). As a result, there is undoubtedly a large hidden population of patients with untreated OAB.

PHYSIOLOGY AND PATHOPHYSIOLOGY

The scientific focus in explaining the basis of urgency incontinence symptoms has previously been on DO, which can be evaluated urodynamically and provides an objective and demonstrable abnormality, relevant in both the clinical setting and in animal models. Two main hypotheses have for some time underpinned the understanding of the motor aspects of DO. The first arise from the long-standing recognition of the crucial role of the pontine brain stem, and more recently the midbrain, in determining the transition between the two phases of the micturition cycle. When sufficient bladder volume is reached, or under volitional command from the frontal cortex, a complex comprising the periaqueductal grey and the pontine micturition center (PMC) will switch the lower urinary tract from storage to voiding. As a consequence, the bladder contracts and the bladder outlet opens, allowing urinary flow. The overarching regulatory control intuitively leads one to assume that lower urinary tract problems may derive from alterations in the neural regulatory circuits (14). This neurogenic dysfunction could derive from alterations in the balance of excitation and inhibition or from re-organisation of reflexes. Certainly, such changes do appear to be critical in urinary incontinence in many clinical situations. However, it is clear that detrusor muscle itself shows significant changes in its properties in DO (15). Receptors on the surface of the smooth muscle are altered in response to various physiological challenges, for example partial denervation. As a consequence, the muscle can become abnormally excitable, a feature which has been established in animal models of bladder outlet obstruction-induced DO. In addition, the abnormal excitation can spread over an excessive distance in these individuals, so a substantial proportion of the bladder wall can contract simultaneously, hence giving rise to overactive detrusor contractions. The increased excitability and abnormal propagation of excitation, perhaps as a consequence of partial denervation, underpins the myogenic hypothesis of DO (15).

In contrast to DO, the emphasis in OAB syndrome is shifted away from the motor side towards the sensations which patients find most bothersome. Changes in the afferent nerves could in theory give rise to excessive sensory information coming from the lower urinary tract (16). The afferent nerves within the bladder wall are surprisingly complex and can express a range of transmitters and receptors. Furthermore, nearby cell types could contribute to the generation of sensory information; the urothelium itself and nearby interstitial cells both represent interesting possibilities for modulating the sensitivity of sensory nerve function (17). Finally, other chemical mediators released within the vicinity of the afferent nerves, could alter transmission of sensory activity. Alteration in sensory nerve sensitivity, such that a greater degree of sensory information is transmitted from the bladder than would be expected for a given bladder volume, underpins the afferent hypothesis of OAB (16).

The motor and afferent arms converge in the integrative peripheral autonomy hypothesis (18), which focuses on interactions between different cell types in the bladder wall. It describes the presence of localized contractions in the normal bladder and exaggerated localized activity in models of OAB, asserting that such change is a result of increased excitability not only in the muscle but also in the other relevant cell types (interstitial cells and ganglia). Furthermore, excitation can propagate through various cellular channels, including muscle-to-muscle communication (as in the myogenic hypothesis), interstitial cell networks, intramural nerve trunks or waves of excitation through the urothelium. Widespread propagation of abnormal excitation will give rise to DO, while increased localized distortion will stimulate the sensory nerves and underpin urgency. The relative balance of localized excitability and wider propagation may explain why some people report significant urgency but are not found to have DO on urodynamic testing, while other people have significant urodynamic DO but relatively little in the way of symptoms associated with it.

The very latest scientific insights derive from evaluating cerebral and psychological responses to stimuli being conveyed from the lower urinary tract (19). Functional brain imaging techniques such as functional MRI can look at patterns of brain activation and definite changes in brain activity had been found in people with urinary tract symptoms (20). This field is relatively new and difficult to study but certainly represents an interesting area for future research.

PATIENT ASSESSMENT

OAB is a clinical diagnosis, and an assessment algorithm from the Fourth International Consultation on Incontinence (21) gives recommendations for initial basic clinical assessment, which may typically begin in primary care. In addition to a careful history and physical examination, minimum investigations should include urinalysis (to exclude infection, blood, and glucosuria) and a bladder diary. Post void residual measurement is particularly indicated when voiding symptoms are present or where impaired bladder emptying is suspected (e.g., co-existing neurological disease).

In addition to characterizing the nature and severity of lower urinary tract symptoms (including associated stress incontinence or voiding symptoms), history should exclude associated visible hematuria or other symptoms suggestive of organic bladder pathology. The differential diagnosis of OAB is extensive (Table 47.1). An account should be taken of the patient's lifestyle including caffeine and alcohol consumption, as alteration of fluid intake may have significant impact on symptoms.

Symptoms suggesting vaginal wall prolapse, neurological disease, bowel, and sexual dysfunction should be sought specifically, including urinary incontinence related to sexual intercourse. Comorbid conditions should be recorded, in particular a history of diabetes mellitus, congestive cardiac failure, previous pelvic surgery, and neurological disease (e.g., Parkinson's disease or stroke). Coexisting medication may well be relevant, particularly in elderly patients in whom

Table 47.1 Differential Diagnosis of Overactive Bladder (OAB)

• Polyuria due to polydipsia
• Bacterial cystitis
• Bladder cancer
• Bladder stones
• Atrophic vaginitis
• Vaginal prolapse
• Chronic urinary retention
• Interstitial cystitis or painful bladder syndrome
• Nocturnal polyuria
• Drugs (e.g., diuretics)

Table 47.2 Drugs Potentially Affecting Continence

• Anticholinergics
• Diuretics
• Alpha and beta-adrenergic agonists and antagonists
• Calcium channel antagonists
• Anti-parkinsonian
• Antidepressants
• Antipsychotics
• Opiates
• Sedatives

polypharmacy is common (Table 47.2). A cognitive and functional assessment may also be necessary in older women.

As the adverse effects of OAB relate principally to QoL, an assessment of bother or impact on daily activities has fundamental importance in management decisions. There is a relationship, although not a strong one, between symptom severity and the perception of the degree of bother: 14% of women with mild incontinence have been found to be worried by their storage symptoms, compared with 24% with moderate and 29% with severe incontinence (22). Sleep interruption due to nocturia and the unpredictable nature of urgency mean that these symptoms impact QoL most strongly (4,23). Validated condition-specific QoL tools have been developed (e.g., ICIQ-OAB, OAB-q).

Bladder Diary

An invaluable adjunct to patient history, this allows more accurate quantification of daytime urinary frequency and nocturia, functional bladder capacity, fluid intake, nocturnal urine output, and an assessment of patient compliance with treatment. A three day chart is recommended for routine assessment (21), and will typically show frequent small volume voids throughout the day and night in patients with OAB. More detailed charts include incontinence and urgency episodes and pad usage though increasing complexity or duration is known to reduce patient compliance. Exclusion of nocturnal polyuria (>33% daily urine output voided overnight in patients over the age of 65, or >20% in patients under the age of 65) is only possible by frequency-volume charts, which are therefore an essential component in the evaluation of nocturia.

Urodynamics

As OAB is a symptomatic diagnosis, the role of urodynamic studies in diagnosis is limited. Urodynamic assessment is an interactive test aiming to reproduce symptoms and provide an explanation for them to guide patient management (Figure 47.1).

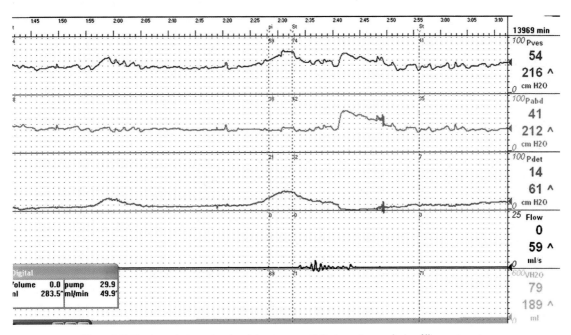

Figure 47.1 Urodynamic trace showing detrusor overactivity incontinence during filling cystometry.

Over-reliance on urodynamic traces, without referring back to the patient's history or reproduction of symptoms during the test, results in reduced diagnostic sensitivity of the test and risk of erroneous diagnosis such as underreporting of DO. In particular, failure of cystometry to demonstrate an isovolumetric pressure rise does not mean that the detrusor muscle did not contract. If the urethral resistance is reduced by intrinsic urethral sphincter deficiency, or by a (patho) physiologic relaxation of the urethra, then an isotonic contraction occurs and results in a decrease in volume rather than an increase in pressure.

These limitations aside, urodynamic evaluation may be useful for specific patient groups. While the majority of untreated and uncomplicated patients can begin management on the basis of clinical assessment alone, urodynamic evaluation is usually indicated in more complex cases or where invasive treatment is being contemplated. These patients might include those failing to respond to pharmacotherapy, those with suspected bladder outlet obstruction or incomplete bladder emptying, coexisting vaginal prolapse, neurological disease, or previous lower urinary tract surgery.

The blue trace shows pressure measured in the bladder and the red line shows that in the rectum (abdominal pressure). The green line represents the difference between the two ("detrusor pressure"), calculated by subtracting red from green. At two minutes, the detrusor pressure goes up, signifying DO. At two minutes and thirty seconds, it happens again, and this time there is urine flow, that is,, DO incontinence. At two minutes and forty seconds, both bladder and abdominal pressure increase slightly, as the patient contracts her pelvic floor to resist the DO.

TREATMENT
Lifestyle Changes
All women with OAB should be managed conservatively in the first instance and a multidisciplinary approach is important. Many patients benefit greatly from simple advice regarding fluid balance and to minimize tea, coffee, and alcohol intake. Fluid intake can be estimated from the frequency volume chart and fluid restriction, including restriction of water-containing foods, may have significant symptomatic benefit (24). Where caffeine intake is high, a staged reduction in intake may be better tolerated and more realistic for the patient. Significant continence benefits can sometimes be achieved by quite limited weight loss in obese patients, though benefit may relatively greater for those with stress urinary incontinence (25); the U.K. National Institute of Health and Clinical Excellence Guidelines on managing urinary incontinence in women recommends advising weight loss in women with a body mass index of 30 or greater.

Behavioral Therapy
Bladder retraining is considered a first line therapy in OAB, whether or not patients are incontinent. Bladder retraining involves consistent incremental voiding regimes, aiming to restore central cortical control. In simple terms, this is allowing the various centers of the brain which feed into the PMC to suppress the dominant stimuli that precipitate detrusor contraction. Different schedules for bladder retraining are described, including prompted voiding, timed voiding, habit retraining, and bladder drill. Bladder drill involved an intensive and regimented protocol performed during an inpatient stay of 7 to 10 days (26). Although effective, this may not be compatible with modern healthcare systems and most patients are managed on an outpatient basis with incremental increases in their voiding interval. Bladder retraining appears to have benefits similar to those of drug therapy to date, and may have greater long-term benefit. Bladder retraining is often used in combination with antimuscarinic pharmacotherapy and level 1 evidence supports this approach (27).

Pelvic floor muscle training may be used successfully by patients with OAB to suppress urgency episodes, DO, and urgency incontinence episodes (28). The effectiveness of bladder retraining in combination with pelvic floor muscle training in comparison to either bladder or pelvic floor training alone is as yet unclear and further investigation is warranted.

PHARMACOTHERAPY
Antimuscarinic Agents
Most women with troublesome OAB will require drug therapy, and antimuscarinic therapy remains the mainstay of conservative treatment, provided non-drug-based treatment has been tried. All currently available agents are associated with anticholinergic side effects, limiting long term compliance, such as dry mouth, constipation, blurred vision, and cognitive effects (29,30). In addition a significant minority of patients fails to respond adequately. For some of the drugs available, clinical use is based on open studies rather than randomized controlled trials and the placebo effect in trials of OAB is known to be large (29). The clinical efficacy and safety of antimuscarinic agents has been reviewed in large meta-analyses (29,30). As the profiles of the agents differ, pharmacotherapy should be individually tailored to each patient according to efficacy, tolerability, co-morbidity, and patient lifestyle.

The number of antimuscarinic agents available for contemporary use has increased recently, along with extended release (ER) formulations and alternative delivery routes, and enhanced bladder or M3 receptor selectivity and once daily dosing have been used in attempting to improve acceptability to patients. ER formulations have a smoother pharmacokinetic profile and appear to have benefits over immediate release (IR) formulations in terms of efficacy and tolerability (29). Other than increasing cystometric capacity, studies with antimuscarinic agents have failed to demonstrate consistent urodynamic effects, yet clear benefit has been demonstrated in terms of frequency, urgency, and incontinence episodes (29). The 4th ICI has produced an expert consensus on available drugs based upon level of evidence and grade of recommendation (21). Table 47.3 shows currently used antimuscarinic agents receiving grade A ICI recommendation, based upon level 1 evidence. The ICS recommends the use of validated HRQoL assessments in trials of antimuscarinic agents, and HRQoL benefits have been demonstrated for darifenacin, fesoterodine, transdermal oxybutynin, propiverine ER, solifenacin, tolterodine ER and IR, and trospium (30).

Table 47.3 Antimuscarinic Agents Recommended for Use in OAB (21)

Name	Preparation and dose	Strengths and limitations
• Darifenacin	• 7.5–15 mg	• Highest M3 receptor selectivity (in vitro) • Dose escalation possible • Once daily dosing
• Fesoterodine	• 4–8 mg	• Active metabolite 5-hydroxymethyltolterodine (5-HMT) • Dose escalation possible • Once daily dosing
• Oxybutynin	• IR 2.5 mg bd–5 mg qds • ER 5–20 mg od • Transdermal 36 mg twice weekly	• Most commonly prescribed agent worldwide • IR relatively cheap but limited by side effects • ER once daily dosing • Dose escalation possible • Transdermal avoids metabolite N-desethyloxybutynin (reducing side effects) but causes pruritis in 15%
• Propiverine	• IR 15 mg od–qds • ER 30 mg od	• Mixed antimuscarinic (no muscarinic receptor selectivity) and calcium antagonist action • Most commonly prescribed agent in Germany, Austria, and Japan
• Solifenacin	• 5–10 mg od	• M3 receptor selectivity (in vitro) • Dose escalation possible • Once daily dosing
• Tolterodine	• IR 1–2 mg bd • ER 4 mg od	• Bladder selectivity (over salivary gland) • ER once daily dosing
• Trospium	• 20 mg bd	• Quaternary amine with low lipophilicity, limited CNS side effects • Low risk of drug interactions • No muscarinic receptor selectivity

Abbreviations: bd, twice daily; ER, extended release; IR, immediate release; OAB, overactive bladder; od, once daily; qds, four times daily.

Desmopressin

Desmopressin, a vasopressin analogue, has an established role in treating pediatric nocturnal enuresis and has also been approved for nocturia in multiple sclerosis and nocturnal polyuria (31). In addition to improving nocturia in patients with OAB, recent evidence suggests desmopressin may allow patients to effectively control daytime OAB symptoms (32), including incontinence (33). Although generally well tolerated, hyponatremia is recognized in a minority of patients; serum sodium should be closely monitored and it is recommended the treatment be avoided in patients aged 80 or over and those with a 24 hour urine output >28 ml/kg (34).

Estrogen

Estrogen has an important physiological effect in the lower urinary tract and estrogen deficiency has been implicated in the pathogenesis of several conditions, including OAB (35). Although there is currently no evidence to support the use of estrogen replacement in the management of urinary incontinence (21), there appears to be benefit in relieving symptoms of OAB and topical administration may be most appropriate (35).

BOTULINUM TOXIN A

Botulinum toxin A (BT-A), a 150-kDa neurotoxin produced by *Clostridium botulinum*, is able to cleave proteins within nerve terminals preventing acetylcholine release at the presynaptic membrane. Although this effect has been harnessed successfully in the management of refractory NDO, and more recently IDO, the precise mechanism of action(s) on BT-A on motor and sensory bladder function remains unclear (36). Multiple injections are given into the detrusor muscle throughout the bladder under cystoscopic guidance, generally avoiding the trigone. The development of new nerve terminals and synaptic contacts allows recovery of function, the effect is therefore temporary. Repeated injections are required in most patients and although the duration of response varies between studies, efficacy appears to be maintained for around six months for patients with IDO (37).

Level 1 evidence for the efficacy of BT-A in IDO is lacking (21,38), but more studies are emerging. Recent small randomized placebo controlled trials (39,40) have demonstrated benefit in both clinical and urodynamic outcomes. Urinary retention is the commonest complication of BT-A, and although complete acute retention is uncommon, around 20% of patients with IDO (and the majority of patients with NDO) will develop high postvoid residuals and need to self-catheterize (41). Several questions remain to be answered including optimal dose, concentration, number of injections and means of administration, and not least clarification of the therapeutic mechanism. Currently this agent remains unlicensed for use in DO, though rapid acceptance of the treatment has seen widespread use in routine practice. The results of several large multi-center placebo controlled trials are awaited, so regulatory approval has yet to be obtained.

NEUROMODULATION AND NERVE STIMULATION

Stimulation of the S3 nerve root sacral nerve stimulation by an implanted electrical pulse generator can provide effective relief from DO (42). A period of temporary percutaneous nerve root stimulation is performed to assess clinical response prior to insertion of a permanent stimulator. The stimulator is a small electrical pulse generator, approximately the same size as a cardiac pacemaker, and is usually implanted in the upper outer quadrant of the buttock. Around 80% of patients with a positive test stimulation experience >50% reduction in incontinence at six months (43) though this efficacy may not be maintained in the long term (44). Complications most commonly reported are implant site or lead site pain (25%), lead migration (16%), bowel dysfunction (6%), and the need for explantation (9%) (43). Patients need expert assessment and support, adding to the costs of treatment. Although not suitable for routine management therefore, sacral neuromodulation appears to be effective and safe for a well selected minority with refractory DO, and its role may increase in the future as the technological development of generators and implant leads progresses.

Intermittent percutaneous stimulation of the tibial nerve above the medial malleolus has been described for the management of OAB (45). The technique shows promise in small uncontrolled studies of patients with refractory IDO (45–47), and it can be considered as a primary treatment for OAB. It appears that treatment must be continued for clinical efficacy to be maintained (48). Recent studies have demonstrated suppression of DO, based objective improvements in urodynamic parameters, in patients with NDO (49,50). The technique shows considerable promise and requires further evaluation before introduction into routine practice.

SURGERY
Augmentation Cystoplasty
Enterocystoplasty aims to create a low pressure reservoir by increasing bladder capacity and reducing filling pressure (51). The most commonly used technique is the clam ileocystoplasty (52) in which the bladder in split in a coronal or sagittal plane and a patch of detubularized ileum is sutured into the defect. It is indicated in patients with severe refractory IDO or NDO with a low functional bladder capacity or in patients with high bladder filling pressures endangering the upper tracts (usually in the presence of neurological disease). Good or moderate long-term outcome has been reported in 92% of patients with NDO but only 58% of those with IDO (53). Preoperative consideration should be given to co-existing urethral dysfunction on video-urodynamic studies, as some patients with NDO may also require insertion of an artificial urinary sphincter cuff.

Postoperative complications include a significant risk of postoperative difficulty with bladder emptying, secondary to a failure to generate adequate voiding pressures. In the long-term most patients (and nearly all neuropathic patients) need to self catheterize to empty their augmented bladder adequately (53). Creation of a continent catheterizable stoma (using the Mitrofanoff principle) is an option in patients unable or unwilling to catheterize via the urethra. Bowel complications are common, particularly in patients with IDO (54). Mucus production by the ileal segment may cause problems, and there is a significant risk of urinary infections and stones. Electrolyte and acid-base balance may become disturbed, resulting in a metabolic acidosis, though this is usually subclinical in adults. Rupture of the augmented bladder is a life-threatening complication that may occur in up to 10% of patients, particularly those with neurological sensory dysfunction (55). Malignant change rarely occurs within the ileal segment; many of the reported cases have followed chronic cystitis due to conditions such as tuberculosis (56). The number of patients with IDO undergoing enterocystoplasty appears to have reduced sharply following the widespread introduction of BT.

Autoaugmentation
Detrusor myectomy was developed in an attempt to reduce the risks associated with augmentation cystoplasty (57). This procedure involves excising the detrusor muscle over the dome of the bladder, leaving the bladder epithelium intact, thereby creating a pseudodiverticulum and increasing bladder capacity. Around 80% of patients with IDO have successful outcome in the medium term but nearly half have to self-catheterize (58). Bladder capacity is increased to a lesser degree compared to augmentation cystoplasty but with the advantage of avoiding bowel complications.

Urinary Diversion
Selected patients with disabling intractable incontinence may be best served by urinary diversion, most commonly via an ileal conduit. This may be appropriate if the bladder becomes severely contracted due to severe long-term DO. In this situation, the management of a urinary stoma may be more acceptable to the patient than constantly changing incontinence pads and washing wet underwear. In addition to the risk of stoma complications, it is now recognized that there is a significant long term risk to upper tract function following ileal conduit formation, due to renal scarring, infection, and stones (59); these risks must be weighed up against the potential benefits, particularly in younger patients.

FUTURE THERAPIES
There are a variety of central and peripheral pathways identified as potential therapeutic targets in OAB (21).

Central targets include:

- γ-aminobutyric acid (GABA)–an inhibitory neurotransmitter in the central nervous system (CNS) (e.g., baclofen, a GABA agonist)
- Serotonin and noradrenaline–may underlie effect of imipramine
- μ opioid receptor–limited evidence with tramadol suggests potential therapeutic effect

Peripheral targets include:

- β3 adrenergic receptors–agonists relax human smooth muscle and several agents are currently under clinical evaluation
- Sensory nerves (C fibers)–resiniferotoxin causes desensitization via vanilloid transient receptor potential (trp-V) receptors, and agents addressing vanilloid receptors are in development
- Vitamin D receptors–agonists may inhibit up-regulated Rho kinase pathway in DO

From a surgical perspective, minimally invasive (laparoscopic and robotic) bladder augmentation has recently been described in small numbers of patients (60,61). These initial results and any potential benefits over open surgery need further confirmation before a clear role for these new techniques can be established. The first report of autologous bladder augmentation using tissue bio-engineering has recently been published (62), and development is ongoing.

CONCLUSION
OAB is a common disorder affecting the QoL of millions of women worldwide; unfortunately it is often easier to diagnose

than to treat. Management remains unsatisfactory in many patients as behavioral modification is often overlooked and drug therapy with anticholinergic medication is commonly associated with side effects. Selective agents have been introduced, increasing the therapeutic options available. Surgical intervention is associated with significant morbidity and only appropriate for a minority of patients refractory to, or intolerant of, conservative therapies. BT has made ground in the clinical setting prior to regulatory approval; scientific data remains limited and long term effect is unknown. Increasing general awareness and decreased tolerance of urinary incontinence over the last 10 to 15 years has helped to raise the profile of OAB, and pathophysiological advances have indicated new potential therapeutic pathways. The next 10 years promise to be as exciting as the last, with a real opportunity to improve symptoms and QoL for patients.

REFERENCES

1. Abrams P, Cardozo L, Fall M, et al. The standardisation of terminology of lower urinary tract function: report from the Standardisation Subcommittee of the International Continence Society. Neurourol Urodyn 2002; 21: 167–78.
2. Chiaffarino F, Parazzini F, Lavezzari M, Giambanco V. Impact of urinary incontinence and overactive bladder on quality of life. Eur Urol 2003; 43: 535–8.
3. Stewart WF, Van Rooyen JB, Cundiff GW, et al. Prevalence and burden of overactive bladder in the United States. World J Urol 2003; 20: 327–36.
4. Kobelt G, Kirchberger I, Malone-Lee J. Review. Quality-of-life aspects of the overactive bladder and the effect of treatment with tolterodine. BJU Int 1999; 83: 583–90.
5. Milsom I, Abrams P, Cardozo L, et al. How widespread are the symptoms of an overactive bladder and how are they managed? A population-based prevalence study. BJU Int 2001; 87: 760–6.
6. Hu TW, Wagner TH, Bentkover JD, et al. Estimated economic costs of overactive bladder in the United States. Urology 2003; 61: 1123–8.
7. Abrams P, Wein A. Introduction: overactive bladder and its treatments. Urology 2000; 55(5A): 1–2.
8. Abrams P. Reviewing the ICS 2002 terminoloy report: the ongoing debate. Neurourol Urodyn 2006; 25: 293.
9. Hashim H, Abrams P. Is the bladder a reliable witness for predicting detrusor overactivity? J Urol 2006; 175: 191–4; discussion 194–5.
10. Brocklehurst JC. Aging of the human bladder. Geriatrics 1972; 27: 154 passim.
11. Yarnell JW, Voyle GJ, Richards CJ, Stephenson TP. The prevalence and severity of urinary incontinence in women. J Epidemiol Community Health 1981; 35: 71–4.
12. Irwin DE, Milsom I, Hunskaar S, et al. Population-based survey of urinary incontinence, overactive bladder, and other lower urinary tract symptoms in five countries: results of the EPIC study. Eur Urol 2006; 50: 1306–14; discussion 1314–5.
13. Norton PA, MacDonald LD, Sedgwick PM, Stanton SL. Distress and delay associated with urinary incontinence, frequency, and urgency in women. BMJ 1988; 297: 1187–9.
14. de Groat WC. Integrative control of the lower urinary tract: preclinical perspective. Br J Pharmacol 2006; 147(Suppl 2): S25–40.
15. Brading AF, Turner WH. The unstable bladder: towards a common mechanism. Br J Urol 1994; 73: 3–8.
16. Andersson KE. Mechanisms of disease: central nervous system involvement in overactive bladder syndrome. Nat Clin Pract Urol 2004; 1: 103–8.
17. Wiseman OJ, Fowler CJ, Landon DN. The role of the human bladder lamina propria myofibroblast. BJU Int 2003; 91: 89–93.
18. Drake MJ, Mills IW, Gillespie JI. Model of peripheral autonomous modules and a myovesical plexus in normal and overactive bladder function. Lancet 2001; 358: 401–3.
19. Mayer EA, Naliboff BD, Craig AD. Neuroimaging of the brain-gut axis: from basic understanding to treatment of functional GI disorders. Gastroenterology 2006; 131: 1925–42.
20. Griffiths D, Tadic SD, Schaefer W, Resnick NM. Cerebral control of the bladder in normal and urge-incontinent women. Neuroimage 2007; 37: 1–7.
21. Abrams P, Cardozo L, Khoury S, Wein A. Incontinence. 4th International Consultation on Incontinence. Paris: Health Publications Ltd, 2009.
22. Lagro-Janssen TL, Smits AJ, Van Weel C. Women with urinary incontinence: self-perceived worries and general practitioners' knowledge of problem. Br J Gen Pract 1990; 40: 331–4.
23. Coyne KS, Zhou Z, Bhattacharyya SK, et al. The prevalence of nocturia and its effect on health-related quality of life and sleep in a community sample in the USA. BJU Int 2003; 92: 948–54.
24. Swithinbank L, Hashim H, Abrams P. The effect of fluid intake on urinary symptoms in women. J Urol 2005; 174: 187–9.
25. Subak LL, Wing R, West DS, et al. Weight loss to treat urinary incontinence in overweight and obese women. N Engl J Med 2009; 360: 481–90.
26. Frewen WK. A reassessment of bladder training in detrusor dysfunction in the female. Br J Urol 1982; 54: 372–3.
27. Alhasso AA, McKinlay J, Patrick K, Stewart L. Anticholinergic drugs versus non-drug active therapies for overactive bladder syndrome in adults. Cochrane Database Syst Rev 2006; (4): CD003193.
28. Burgio KL, Goode PS, Locher JL, et al. Behavioral training with and without biofeedback in the treatment of urge incontinence in older women: a randomized controlled trial. JAMA 2002; 288: 2293–9.
29. Novara G, Galfano A, Secco S, et al. A systematic review and meta-analysis of randomized controlled trials with antimuscarinic drugs for overactive bladder. Eur Urol 2008; 54: 740–63.
30. Chapple CR, Khullar V, Gabriel Z, et al. The effects of antimuscarinic treatments in overactive bladder: an update of a systematic review and meta-analysis. Eur Urol 2008; 54: 543–62.
31. Cvetkovic RS, Plosker GL. Desmopressin: in adults with nocturia. Drugs 2005; 65: 99–107; discussion 108–9.
32. Hashim H, Malmberg L, Graugaard-Jensen C, Abrams P. Desmopressin, as a designer-drug, in the treatment of overactive bladder syndrome. Neurourol Urodyn 2009; 28: 40–6.
33. Robinson D, Cardozo L, Akeson M, et al. Antidiuresis: a new concept in managing female daytime urinary incontinence. BJU Int 2004; 93: 996–1000.
34. Rembratt A, Riis A, Norgaard JP. Desmopressin treatment in nocturia; an analysis of risk factors for hyponatremia. Neurourol Urodyn 2006; 25: 105–9.
35. Robinson D, Cardozo LD. The role of estrogens in female lower urinary tract dysfunction. Urology 2003; 62(4 Suppl 1): 45–51.
36. Drake MJ. Mechanisms of action of intravesical botulinum treatment in refractory detrusor overactivity. BJU Int 2008; 102(Suppl 1): 11–6.
37. Schmid DM, Sauermann P, Werner M, et al. Experience with 100 cases treated with botulinum-A toxin injections in the detrusor muscle for idiopathic overactive bladder syndrome refractory to anticholinergics. J Urol 2006; 176: 177–85.
38. Duthie J, Wilson DI, Herbison GP, Wilson D. Botulinum toxin injections for adults with overactive bladder syndrome. Cochrane Database Syst Rev 2007; (3): CD005493.
39. Sahai A, Khan MS, Dasgupta P. Efficacy of botulinum toxin-A for treating idiopathic detrusor overactivity: results from a single center, randomized, double-blind, placebo controlled trial. J Urol 2007; 177: 2231–6.
40. Brubaker L, Richter HE, Visco A, et al. Refractory idiopathic urge urinary incontinence and botulinum A injection. J Urol 2008; 180: 217–22.
41. Shaban AM, Drake MJ. Botulinum toxin treatment for overactive bladder: risk of urinary retention. Curr Urol Rep 2008; 9: 445–51.
42. Schmidt RA, Jonas U, Oleson KA, et al. Sacral nerve stimulation for treatment of refractory urinary urge incontinence. Sacral nerve stimulation study group. J Urol 1999; 162: 352–7.
43. Brazzelli M, Murray A, Fraser C. Efficacy and safety of sacral nerve stimulation for urinary urge incontinence: a systematic review. J Urol 2006; 175(3 Pt 1): 835–41.
44. Elhilali MM, Khaled SM, Kashiwabara T, Elzayat E, Corcos J. Sacral neuromodulation: long-term experience of one center. Urology 2005; 65: 1114–7.

45. Govier FE, Litwiller S, Nitti V, Kreder KJ, Jr., Rosenblatt P. Percutaneous afferent neuromodulation for the refractory overactive bladder: results of a multicenter study. J Urol 2001; 165: 1193–8.

46. Amarenco G, Ismael SS, Even-Schneider A, et al. Urodynamic effect of acute transcutaneous posterior tibial nerve stimulation in overactive bladder. J Urol 2003; 169: 2210–5.

47. van der Pal F, van Balken MR, Heesakkers JP, et al. Correlation between quality of life and voiding variables in patients treated with percutaneous tibial nerve stimulation. BJU Int 2006; 97: 113–6.

48. van der Pal F, van Balken MR, Heesakkers JP, Debruyne FM, Bemelmans BL. Percutaneous tibial nerve stimulation in the treatment of refractory overactive bladder syndrome: is maintenance treatment necessary? BJU Int 2006; 97: 547–50.

49. Kabay SC, Kabay S, Yucel M, Ozden H. Acute urodynamic effects of percutaneous posterior tibial nerve stimulation on neurogenic detrusor overactivity in patients with Parkinson's disease. Neurourol Urodyn 2009; 28: 62–7.

50. Kabay SC, Yucel M, Kabay S. Acute effect of posterior tibial nerve stimulation on neurogenic detrusor overactivity in patients with multiple sclerosis: urodynamic study. Urology 2008; 71: 641–5.

51. Bramble FJ. The treatment of adult enuresis and urge incontinence by enterocystoplasty. Br J Urol 1982; 54: 693–6.

52. Mundy AR, Stephenson TP. Clam ileocystoplasty for the treatment of refractory urge incontinence. Br J Urol 1985; 57: 641–6.

53. Hasan ST, Marshall C, Robson WA, Neal DE. Clinical outcome and quality of life following enterocystoplasty for idiopathic detrusor instability and neurogenic bladder dysfunction. Br J Urol 1995; 76: 551–7.

54. N'Dow J, Leung HY, Marshall C, Neal DE. Bowel dysfunction after bladder reconstruction. J Urol 1998; 159: 1470–4; discussion 1474–5.

55. Gough DC. Enterocystoplasty. BJU Int 2001; 88: 739–43.

56. Lane T, Shah J. Carcinoma following augmentation ileocystoplasty. Urol Int 2000; 64: 31–2.

57. Cartwright PC, Snow BW. Bladder autoaugmentation: partial detrusor excision to augment the bladder without use of bowel. J Urol 1989; 142: 1050–3.

58. Kumar SP, Abrams PH. Detrusor myectomy: long-term results with a minimum follow-up of 2 years. BJU Int 2005; 96: 341–4.

59. Neal DE. Complications of ileal conduit diversion in adults with cancer followed up for at least five years. Br Med J (Clin Res Ed) 1985; 290: 1695–7.

60. El-Feel A, Abdel-Hakim MA, Abouel-Fettouh H, Abdel-Hakim AM. Laparoscopic augmentation ileocystoplasty: results and outcome. Eur Urol 2009; 55: 721–7.

61. Al-Othman KE, Al-Hellow HA, Al-Zahrani HM, Seyam RM. Robotic augmentation enterocystoplasty. J Endourol 2008; 22: 597–600; discussion 600.

62. Atala A, Bauer SB, Soker S, Yoo JJ, Retik AB. Tissue-engineered autologous bladders for patients needing cystoplasty. Lancet 2006; 367: 1241–6.

48 Neurologic Disorders
Ricardo R Gonzalez, David W Goldfarb, Renuka Tyagi, and Alexis E Te

INTRODUCTION
Neural control of voiding involves complex interactions between the central and peripheral nervous systems, the bladder, and urethral sphincter. Neurologic disorders can affect this system in multiple levels, resulting in a disruption in the bladder's ability to store or empty urine. This chapter will systematically review the characteristic voiding dysfunctions as they relate to various disease states.

VOIDING FUNCTION AND DYSFUNCTION
The bladder's ability to store and empty urine is under neurologic control. Therefore, any neurologic abnormality can result in voiding dysfunction. In general, neurologic lesions either cause loss of function (i.e., areflexia or denervation) or result in unopposed reflex "overactivity," i.e., detrusor overactivity (DO) or hyperreflexia, now called neurogenic DO (1). The effects of neurologic lesions can be broadly divided into two groups: those that cause areflexia (which usually results in failure to empty) and those that cause overactivity (which affects the ability to store urine). Neurologic lesions can also affect urethral sphincter function, resulting in loss of the usual coordination between the two structures, a condition termed detrusor–sphincter dyssynergia (DSD).

To some extent, the anatomic level of neurologic injury can predict the type of dysfunction. The three gross anatomic distinctions that predict effect on voiding function are cerebral (suprapontine), spinal (suprasacral), or peripheral (infrasacral). These levels will serve as a structure by which to examine different neurologic disorders and their voiding effects later in this chapter. Table 48.1 summarizes characteristic dysfunctions that result from known levels of injury as adapted from Wein (2).

Voiding dysfunction includes failure to store and/or empty urine, and can be categorized by the three broad urodynamic categories listed below. Cerebral lesions above the pons usually result in DO with intact sphincter coordination. Suprasacral spinal (i.e., upper motor neuron) lesions result in DO with a variable effect on sphincter coordination. Injuries involving the sacral cord or cauda equina result in lower motor lesions and detrusor areflexia (DA), with or without sphincter denervation (1). However, neurologic lesions can be multiple or incomplete in nature, resulting in a mixed pattern of voiding dysfunction not predicted by anatomic location (3–5).

DO with Synergistic External Sphincteric Function
Incomplete and non-traumatic spinal lesions tend to result in DO with synergistic external sphincter function. Similarly, in patients with lesions above the pons, DO is not associated with loss of sphincteric coordination because the lesion is above the level where detrusor contraction is coordinated with reflex urethral relaxation. Typical causes of DO with preserved synergistic sphincteric function include cerebrovascular disease, Parkinson's disease, and some cases of multiple sclerosis (MS) (1,6). Exaggerated detrusor contractions that occur after suprasacral trauma may be explained by any of the following three mechanisms:

- loss of the inhibitory impulse transmission;
- emergence of primitive alternative micturition pathways; and
- from the collateral sprouting of new neural pathways (7).

Medical management of the resulting DO can usually be achieved with oral or intravesical anticholinergic therapy (see chap. 47). However, when DO persists despite medical therapy, intravesical botulism toxin instillation, augmentation cystoplasty, or sacral neuromodulation may be used to manage DO resulting in urge incontinence (8).

DO with Detrusor–Sphincter Dyssynergia
Suprasacral spinal cord injury (SCI) above the pons can disrupt the coordinated voiding reflex between the bladder and external sphincter. This can lead to DO with simultaneous contraction of the striated urethral sphincter (9,10). This is known as DSD, typical causes of which are SCI and MS (11–13). Identifying DSD is crucial because there is a 50% or greater chance of developing urologic complications within five years of the onset of DSD (14–16), particularly vesicoureteral reflux and upper tract damage due to the elevation in intravesical pressure (usually when the pressure is chronically above 40 cmH$_2$O) (17). Successful management of DO with DSD involves treating both aspects of the condition. As described above, managing DO involves decreasing detrusor activity medically or surgically to allow low-pressure urinary storage. Effective control of intravesical pressure with the anticholinergic therapy can stabilize and even reverse upper tract dilation with DO (18). Management of DSD includes clean intermittent catheterization (CIC) to bypass the sphincteric obstruction or by disruption of the urinary sphincter (e.g., pharmacologically with botulinum toxin or mechanically with an intraurethral stent or surgical ablation) (19,20), which may render the patient incontinent. Pharmacologic treatments are usually temporary while mechanical disruption is a more permanent solution. Continuous drainage with an indwelling urethral catheter should be avoided, given the well-characterized complications of infection, urolithiasis, tissue erosion, loss of detrusor compliance, and urothelial cancers. In addition, in those patients with normal sensation, the catheter may be uncomfortable, particularly where there is urethral spasm (DSD). If a long-term catheter is required, then a suprapubic approach is preferable as it reduces the risk of infection and

Table 48.1 Neuromuscular Dysfunction of the Lower Urinary Tract

Defect	Detrusor activity	Compliance	Smooth sphincter/ bladder neck	Striated sphincter	Notes
Cerebral (suprapontine)					
Cerebrovascular accident	DO	N	S	S, possible LOC	Possible decreased sensation of lower urinary tract events
Brain tumor	DO	N	S	S	Possible decreased sensation of lower urinary tract events
Cerebral palsy	DO	N	S	S, D (25%), LOC	
Parkinson's disease	DO, IDC	N	S	S, bradykinesia	
Shy–Drager syndrome	DO, IDC	N, D	O	S	Possible denervation of striated sphincter
Multiple sclerosis	DO, IDC	N	S	S, D (30–65%)	Dyssynergia figures refer to percentage of those with DO
Spinal cord injury					
Suprasacral injury	DO	N	S	D	Smooth sphincter may be dyssynergic if lesion above T7
Sacral injury	DA	N, possible D	CNR, possible O	F	
Autonomic hyperreflexia	DO	N	Ds	D	
Myelodysplasia	DA, DO	N, possible D	O	F	Findings variable. Striated sphincter often denervated
Tabes dorsalis, pernicious anemia	IDC, DA	N, I	S	S	Primary problem is loss of sensation; detrusor may become decompensated from chronic overdistension
Disk disease	DA	N	CNR	S	Striated sphincter may be denervated with fixed tone
Peripheral					
Radical pelvic surgery	IDC, DA	D, N	O	F	
Diabetes	IDC, DA, DO	N, I	S	S	Sensory and motor neuropathy. DO predominates

Abbreviations: CNR, competent, not relaxing; D, decreased; DA, detrusor areflexia; DO, detrusor overactivity; Ds, dyssynergic; F, fixed tone; I, increased; IDC, impaired detrusor contractility; LOC, loss of (voluntary) control; N, normal; O, open (incompetent at rest); S, synergic.

can improve sexual function (21). It should be noted that DSD is a functional outlet obstruction and therefore cannot be treated safely by condom catheterization or crede/valsalva voiding alone.

Detrusor Areflexia

In patients with lumbosacral or peripheral nerve lesions, such as myelodysplasia, cauda equina injury, and diabetes mellitus, DA with high or low bladder compliance may develop (1). DA is characterized by the absence of a detrusor contraction, usually resulting in low pressure urinary storage with failure to empty. Impaired detrusor contraction and DA tend to result with sacral and low lumbar injuries. However, certain upper motor neuron lesions can also result in DA, especially if clinical or subclinical sacral lesions (e.g., coexistent traumatic injury) are present (22). CIC is the standard treatment for DA (23). Because upper tract damage varies directly with increasing time at or above the critical 40 cmH_2O pressure, diminished compliance requires the use of anticholinergic agents or surgical bladder augmentation to establish urinary storage under acceptable pressure (24).

CONDITIONS OF THE BRAIN AFFECTING THE URINARY TRACT
Cerebrovascular Accident

Cerebrovascular accident (CVA)—stroke—is defined as the acute onset of a focal neurologic deficit, usually caused by an occlusive event such as an atherosclerotic thrombus, or hemorrhage. Over 500,000 CVAs occur annually in the United States. One-third are fatal, another third necessitate long-term nursing care, and a third allow patients to return home close to their prior level of functioning (25). The effects of CVA on the function of the lower urinary tract are variable, depending on the location of the neural injury, its size, and etiology (26). Additionally, because CVAs occur predominantly in the elderly population, evaluation, and management are often confounded by coexisting stress incontinence, dementia, and voiding dysfunction from impaired contractility attributable to aging and peripheral neuropathy (25).

Clinical and Urodynamic Features

Clinically, patients may experience a range of voiding complaints from urinary retention, urgency, and frequency, and/or incontinence. Neural arcs above the pontine level—where most non-fatal CVAs occur—serve to inhibit micturition. Thus, injury in this area decreases inhibitory control over detrusor function, most often resulting in DO (27).

While DO is the most common long-term urologic problem following a CVA, a significant number of newly affected patients initially develop urinary retention. This retention occurs as a result of "cerebral shock" and may last for a period of several weeks and is much like the classic acontractile bladder "spinal shock" phase that immediately follows a SCI (28). During the first month after CVA, the incidence of incontinence is as high has 70%. It is however usually transient, and in many patients is due to immobility and dependency subsequent to paralysis or disrupted cognition (29).

As recovery ensues, patients most commonly experience urinary urgency, with the incidence of incontinence reported to be as high as 51% within a year of injury. Urinary incontinence may also result from limitations in cognitive function and mobility resulting from neural injury (30), known as functional incontinence.

Although urethral sphincter function is usually preserved, urinary incontinence results from uninhibited detrusor contractions (31). Patients with lesions above the level of the pons characteristically maintain synergetic activity of the sphincter with detrusor contractions (26). However, patients with suprapontine lesions may purposely increase sphincteric activity during an uninhibited detrusor contraction to avoid urge incontinence. This guarding reflex—termed overactive bladder (OAB) type 3 or pseudodyssynergia—may be confused with true dyssynergia by those not familiar with the interpretation of urodynamic studies (32). As long as urethral sphincter activity remains coordinated with detrusor contraction, intra-vesical pressure should remain physiologic, and therefore preserve the function of the urinary tracts.

Evaluation of the stroke patient can be riddled with challenges. Difficulties include obtaining an adequate history, technical difficulty with performing studies, and interpreting urodynamic studies given coexisting findings incidental to aging or co-morbidities (25). However, careful neurologic examination and urodynamic evaluation are crucial when assessing the stroke patient who presents for evaluation of voiding dysfunction.

Parkinson's Disease

Parkinson's disease affects men and women equally, primarily in the sixth and seventh decades of life, and it increases in prevalence with advancing age (33). It occurs with a prevalence of 0.1% in the United States, making it one of the most frequent neurologic entities causing voiding dysfunction (34). Pathologically, the pigmented neurons in the substantia nigra and locus ceruleus in the brainstem degenerate. Systemic clinical features of tremor, bradykinesia, and muscular rigidity are probably due to focal dopamine deficiency in these areas, as well as the caudate nucleus, putamen, and globus pallidus (35). The typical urodynamic findings of patients with Parkinson's disease include DO, sphincter bradykinesia, and impairment of relaxation of the striated muscle component of the urethral sphincter muscle (1,34).

Clinical and Urodynamic Features

Up to 75% of patients with Parkinson's disease experience some degree of voiding dysfunction (36,37). Irritative symptoms of urinary frequency, urgency, and urge incontinence are reported by 57% of patients with Parkinson's disease. Voiding disturbance may also be troublesome, with 23% of patients experiencing obstructive symptoms including hesitancy, incomplete emptying, or urinary retention; 20% have mixed symptoms (35). However, voiding dysfunction associated with Parkinson's disease in female patients is complex and not always congruent with symptoms (34).

Table 48.2 Clinical and Urodynamic Features of Parkinson's Patients by Severity of Symptoms

Parkinson's severity	Urge	Urge incontinence	Detrusor overactivity	Bladder capacity (ml)
Mild	5/14	0	6/14	380
Moderate	14/14	2	10/14	290
Severe	9/9	4	9/9	260

Source: Data from Ref. 41.

Urodynamic evaluation reveals DO in up to 90% of patients, with sporadic electrical activity of the sphincter during uninhibited detrusor contractions in 61% (6). The classic finding is sphincteric bradykinesia where there is a delay in relaxation of the external sphincter at the onset of volitional micturition (38). In a study of 17 women with Parkinson's disease, stress urinary incontinence was identified in 50% (39). Impaired detrusor contractility is a much less frequent urodynamic finding in the patient with Parkinson's (40). Managing prostatic obstruction surgically in a Parkinson's patient can be difficult. In the general population, the risk of incontinence after transurethral prostatectomy is <2%; however, this risk in the Parkinson's patient may be as high as 20% (38).

More recent attempts to correlate clinical disease states with urodynamic findings have revealed that increasing Parkinson's disease stage results in worsening urge incontinence, DO, and decreasing bladder capacity (41). Holligar et al. (41) studied 37 idiopathic parkinsonian patients with a mean age of 65 years. Symptoms were classified as mild, moderate, or severe; mild symptoms were unilateral in nature, moderate involved exacerbated bilateral symptoms and deteriorating balance, and severe symptoms required the use of assistance with daily activities and/or ambulation. Table 48.2 summarizes the significant findings. As parkinsonian symptoms worsen, so do clinical and urodynamic parameters. This suggests that bladder function may worsen progressively with advancing disease.

Neurologic evaluation is crucial to evaluate bladder function and to guide appropriate therapy. Urodynamics with simultaneous electromyography is the most sensitive available tool to investigate the nature of voiding dysfunction (34). The goals of proper management are to improve symptoms and protect the upper urinary tracts. Treatment of the patient with L-dopa can significantly improve symptoms; however, anticholinergic therapy can be added to suppress uninhibited detrusor contractions.

Shy–Drager Syndrome (Multiple System Atrophy)

Shy and Drager described a neurologic syndrome of autonomic nervous system dysfunction characterized by orthostatic hypotension, anhydrosis, erectile dysfunction, extrapyramidal symptoms, and poor urinary and fecal control (42). Shy–Drager syndrome is also known as multiple system atrophy (MSA), and it is considered one of the "Parkinson plus" syndromes of movement disorders (34). The mean age of onset is 55 years, with a male predominance of 2 or 3:1 (43). MSA results in the symmetrical degeneration of neurons and associated fibers of motor and extrapyramidal systems, including the cerebellum and brainstem (44). Disease progression usually results in death 7 to 20 years after the onset of neurologic symptoms (43).

The difference in neuropathologic lesion location and number between patients explains the variance in urodynamic findings between Parkinson's patients and those with MSA. Unlike Parkinson's patients, MSA patients tend to have worse lower urinary tract dysfunction, characterized by poor bladder contractility, and pelvic floor electromyography findings, suggesting that almost 50% demonstrate peripheral denervation (34). The resulting incontinence is probably caused by DO and some element of paralysis of the external sphincter (45). Blaivas has demonstrated an open bladder neck during cystography, further indicative of peripheral sympathetic dysfunction (45). Thus, MSA affects sympathetic, parasympathetic, and the somatic nervous systems—compared to the relatively more defined idiopathic Parkinson's disease—and thorough neurologic evaluation is invaluable in separating and characterizing these different disease entities (34). The combination of detrusor dysfunction and sphincter denervation does *not* support the surgical management of symptoms; currently recommended treatment is therefore that of a combination of intermittent catheterization and medical therapy, including anticholinergics and desmopressin (42,46).

Brain Neoplasms

The majority of patients with intracranial neoplasms often maintain control over urinary tract function (1). Similar to CVAs, alterations in lower urinary tract function will tend to relate directly to the area of the brain affected, rather than the type of neoplasm. For example, compression by tumor or degeneration of neural arcs above the pontine level—such as the superior aspects of the frontal lobe (47) and frontoparietal areas (48) that inhibit detrusor activity—would induce DO with synergetic sphincter function (26,49).

Dementia

Dementia is the loss of thought and reason that results from deterioration and atrophy of both gray and white matter in the brain, particularly of the frontal lobes (1). Although usually associated with conditions such as head injury, hydrocephalus, encephalitis, syphilis, Alzheimer's, Pick's, and Creutzfeldt–Jakob diseases, the etiology of neuronal degeneration associated with dementia is poorly understood (35).

The most common urinary symptom is incontinence, with a reported prevalence as high as 90% (50). However, the cause of incontinence remains unclear; it is not known whether detrusor dysfunction or, more likely, a defect in cognitive function (functional incontinence) is responsible for the lack of social continence in patients with dementia. In one report, 71% of elderly patients with cognitive impairment showed DO; however, 65% of those with no impairment demonstrated DO by the same criteria. Therefore, the incontinence associated with dementia is not likely due to DO (51). It has been demonstrated that neurogenic incontinence (DO) is more common in multi-infarct and Lewy body disease dementia, while functional incontinence is more prevalent in Alzheimer's disease due to cognitive decline and decreased motivation (52).

Aging, Cognitive Decline, and Conflicting Medication Effects

In both men and women, the prevalence of OAB and incontinence increases significantly with advancing age (53). The impact of OAB can adversely impact quality of life. This includes psychological burden, and an increased risk of falls, fractures, skin infections, and urinary tract infections (UTIs). In fact, the onset of bladder symptoms is often the deciding factor in transitioning from community to residential-based care. The mainstay of treatment for OAB is antimuscarinic therapy; however, caution is warranted in the elderly population when using these drugs. Anticholinergic side effects include both peripheral nervous system symptoms like dry mouth and constipation, and central nervous system symptoms like cognitive impairment, blurry vision, and sleep disturbances. The central nervous system interactions can be the rate limiting step in treatment if the patient is already beginning to experience cognitive decline. In a population of patients that have had a lifetime to accrue lengthy medication regimens, consideration should also be given to drug–drug interactions. With regard to side effect profiles and pharmacokinetics in the elderly, trospium chloride may be better tolerated than other antimuscarinics including, oxybutynin, tolterodine, and solifenacin (54).

The mainstay of treatment for cognitive decline in the aging patient is central cholinergic stimulation (55). Cholinesterase inhibitors slow the breakdown of synaptic acetylcholine and prolong its ability stimulate post-synaptic receptors. The three drugs commonly used are rivastigmine, donepezil, and galantamine. While these drugs are designed to target central nervous system cholinergic pathways, associated peripheral nervous system effects include muscle cramps, weakness, cardiorespiratory events, and urinary incontinence. Cholinergic treatment increases OAB symptoms and has even been shown to lead to an incidence of 8% of urge urinary incontinence in those on donepezil (56) studies have demonstrated less peripheral cholinergic side effects and less drug–drug interactions in rivastigmine compared to donepezil and galantamine (57).

Clearly there is a delicate balance when managing OAB and risking cognitive side effects, as well as when treating dementia and risking OAB side effects. In cognitively-vulnerable populations like the elderly and demented, medical management should consider the use of selective agents with the safest side effect profile and least pharmacokinetic interactions.

Multiple Sclerosis

MS is the most common disabling neurologic disorder affecting people between 20 and 50 years of age (58). It is characterized by focal inflammatory and demyelinating lesions of the nervous system, affecting mainly those living in the temperate climates. Prevalence is estimated at 1/1000 in Americans, 2/1000 Northern Europeans, and 20 to 40/1000 in first-degree relatives of patients with MS (58–60). In approximately 60% of patients, the disease is initially manifested by exacerbations and remissions. The clinical course of MS can be acute, progressive, chronic, and/or benign (61).

Neurologic dysfunction is caused by demyelinating plaques of the white matter of the brain and spinal cord, especially the posterior and lateral columns of the cervical cord, which serve as pathways for neurologic control over vesical and urethral function (62). These plaques are caused by an autoimmune response and attach to the central nervous system myelin, leading to a loss of salutatory conduction, and conduction velocity in axonal pathways (58).

Clinical and Urodynamic Features

Voiding dysfunction is experienced by 90% of patients with MS (63). Interestingly, a change in bladder function is the presenting complaint in at least 10% of MS patients (64). These include not only frequency, urgency, and urge incontinence, but also urinary hesitancy, intermittency, and poor urinary stream. The nature of voiding dysfunction is most dependent on the location of the plaque formation, such as intracranial, suprasacral, or sacral cord plaques.

Urodynamically, the most frequent pattern seen is DO, which is observed in 50% to 99% of patients (58,63,65,66). DSD is also documented in up to 50% of patients with DO (13,67,68). Of patients with symptoms suggestive of obstruction, 73% had DA (69). DA is seen in 20% to 30% of patients, most of whom usually strain to void (70). Hypocontractility may be related to cerebellar plaque involvement, lack of cortical facilitatory input, or sacral cord involvement. Some evidence suggests that DA is a temporary condition that may progress to DO in 57% to 100% (69). Although these patients may be managed effectively with an intermittent catheterization program, periodic video urodynamic re-evaluation is essential to ensure protection of the upper urinary tract (71). Given the waxing and waning nature of MS, re-evaluation is especially important because the neurourologic status of the patient with MS may change over time. Having said that, DSD revealed on urodynamic evaluation rarely remits (69).

Optimal management of lower urinary tract dysfunction is based on the avoidance of indwelling catheters and minimizing intravesical storage pressure while assuring low pressure urinary drainage (71). Urinary storage pressure is minimized with anticholinergic medications, or augmentation cystoplasty if medical therapy is ineffective (72). Unfortunately, sphincterotomy is not an option for women, and many women with neuropathic bladder dysfunction are treated in the community with indwelling urethral or suprapubic catheters (1). However, early experience using botulinum toxin injections into the sphincter for the treatment of DSD is limited but growing, and may eventually prove to be a therapeutic option (73,74).

CONDITIONS OF THE SPINAL CORD AFFECTING THE URINARY TRACT

The degree of voiding dysfunction associated with spinal cord conditions is related to the process of the condition itself, the area of the spinal cord affected, the severity of neurologic impairment, and coexisting pelvic floor pathology. Neurologic injury, which can involve parasympathetic, sympathetic, and somatic nerve fibers, can result in a complex array of signs and symptoms. Urodynamic investigation of those with neurologic impairment is essential as it provides objective information regarding the nature and extent of the effect on lower urinary tract function. Such information is invaluable in adequate patient management.

Spinal Cord Injury

Neurogenic lower urinary tract dysfunction resulting from SCI is an excellent model for understanding neurourologic dysfunction. The principles of urologic evaluation and management of traumatic SCI patients are applicable to those with other spinal cord pathology (19). The estimated annual incidence of SCI reaches 40 new injuries per million population in the United States, or approximately 11,000 new cases per year—with a prevalence of approximately 247,000 persons. (75). With 85% of injuries occurring at or above the T12 level (76), the reported neurologic level and the extent of the lesion of SCI at hospital discharge reveal 34.3% of patients with incomplete quadriplegia and 25.1% with complete paraplegia; 22.1% of patients develop complete quadriplegia and 17.5% incomplete paraplegia (75). Historically, the most common cause of death in SCI patients had been secondary renal failure; however, improved medical assessment and management has led to dramatic shifts in the causes of death (1). Nonetheless, lower urinary tract dysfunction following SCI is frequent and may result in infection, urolithiasis, upper tract failure, and lower urinary tract symptoms.

Clinical and Urodynamic Features

Characteristics of voiding dysfunction after SCI are dependent on the stage of recovery, i.e., spinal shock, recovery, and stable phases (1).

Immediately following spinal cord trauma, *spinal shock* occurs. This phase characteristically presents with flaccid paralysis and absence of reflex activity below the level of the lesion. Voiding symptoms typically include urinary retention due to DA that may last for months. The DA usually resolves weeks to a few months following the SCI with resumption of reflex detrusor activity. While in acute retention, patients should be managed with a regime of intermittent catheterization.

The *recovery* phase follows spinal shock and is marked by the return of reflex detrusor activity. This phase is noted clinically by the appearance of new incontinence, autonomic dysreflexia (AD), or lower extremity spasticity. The neurologic level of the SCI often corresponds to the resulting type of lower urinary tract dysfunction (Figs. 48.1 and 48.2). Performing urodynamic testing at this time is key to understand the pathophysiology of their condition (77,78). With cervical or thoracic spinal cord lesions, the most common outcome will be DO with DSD. Sacral spinal cord injuries are commonly associated with DA, although this may also be seen with higher level lesions. Injuries of the lumbar spine are more difficult to predict, with lower urinary tract dysfunction ranging from DO with DSD, or DO with sphincter deficiency, to DA.

The final phase following SCI is labeled the *stable* phase and by definition is the period characterized by the absence of additional neurologic recovery or change in urodynamic pattern (1). Although the pattern of voiding pathology remains stable, there can be an increase in the severity of the dysfunction, and/or a continued loss of compliance. Therefore, it is critical to continue periodic evaluation of lower urinary tract function and surveillance of the upper urinary tract for further sequellae.

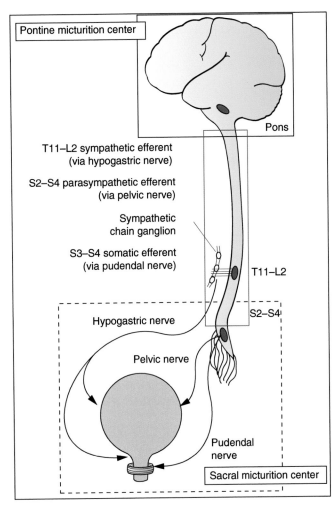

Figure 48.1 Innervation of the lower urinary tract. The control of micturition and continence arise at three levels: suprapontine (thin line box), spinal (thick line box), and peripheral/infrasacral (dashed box). Each level contains distinct nerve fibers with complex interplay between all levels.

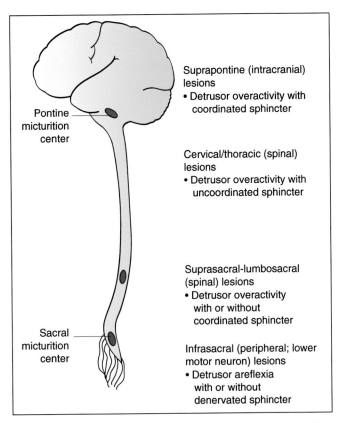

Figure 48.2 Urodynamic outcome following complete denervating injury. Outcomes are dependent on level and extent of injury. Incomplete or partial lesions may lead to variation in urodynamic findings.

The level of spinal lesion and its relationship to lower urinary tract dysfunction has been documented and evaluated in 489 consecutive patients presenting with SCI (79). In 104 patients with cervical SCI, 15% (16 patients) had DA. In the remaining 85% (88 patients), involuntary detrusor contractions were documented, with 65% (57 of 88) exhibiting concurrent DSD. All 87 thoracic SCI patients were found to have DO, and 90% of them exhibited concurrent DSD. Lumbar SCI was found to have the least predictable urodynamic patterns, with 40% having DA, 30% with DO, and 30% with DO with DSD. In the sacral SCI cohort, 12% of patients had normal urodynamic studies, while 64% of patients had DA.

Brown–Sequard Syndrome

Hemitransection of the spinal cord results in this rare, but well-documented condition with pathognomonic findings for a SCI (80,81). The classic presentation of this syndrome—provided that it results from a single spinal lesion—is ipsilateral hemiparesis (pyramidal tract) of the leg with contralateral loss of superficial sensation (spinothalamic tract) and ipsilateral loss of deep sensation (dorsal tract). The variable presentation that results

in either motor or sensory symptoms depends upon the plane of the lesion.

Clinical and Urodynamic Features

Voiding symptoms are variable among these patients. Those presenting with more severe motor deficits (i.e., intramedullary diseases) are more likely to have symptoms ranging from urinary retention to filling phase symptoms such as frequency and urge incontinence (82). However, there is no relationship between voiding symptoms and the laterality of the lesion or concurrent sensory disturbances (82–84). There is also a paucity of publications reporting urodynamic studies in these patients with findings that are concordant with voiding symptom severity. The most frequent urodynamic findings in symptomatic patients tend to be DO and DA (82,85). Because the relationship between the spinal lesion and resulting voiding symptoms is variable, thorough neurologic examination paired with urodynamic evaluation are key in managing symptoms and protecting the upper tracts of each patient.

Autonomic Dysreflexia

AD, is a well-defined syndrome of acute excessive sympathetic output which occurs in patients with spinal cord injuries, most commonly above the T6 level. This condition is associated with an uncontrolled spinal reflex mechanism from afferent visceral (or other noxious) stimulus below the level of the lesion, resulting in, if not managed appropriately, a life-threatening hypertension. The most common cause is stimulation of the lower

Table 48.3 Innervation of the Lower Urinary Tract

	Spinal cord level	Function
Afferent		
Nociceptors	S2–S4	Initiation of micturition
Sensory	S2–S3	Perineal sensation
Efferent (autonomic)		
Sympathetic (hypogastric nerve)	T11–L2	Sphincter contraction, bladder relaxation
Parasympathetic (pelvic nerve)	S2–S4	Bladder contraction
Somatic (pudendal nerve)	S3–S4	External sphincter contraction

urinary tract, with 75% to 85% of cases precipitated by bladder distension (86). Other triggers including infection, urethral distension, instrumentation, stones, and testicular torsion.

At presentation, the symptoms associated with AD generally include a bilateral pounding headache, with diaphoresis above the level of the spinal lesion, nasal congestion, malaise, nausea, and visual blurring. The signs observed commonly are flushed sweaty skin above the level of the lesion with cool, pale skin below that level. The main finding is elevation of the blood pressure with reflex bradycardia—which in a post-SCI patient may mean that readings of 120/80 mmHg are elevated, as base pressures in these patients are often in the 90/60 mmHg range (1). The labile hypertension associated with the AD response can result in intracranial hemorrhage and death (87). Early recognition of the syndrome is critical, with initiation of management immediately (88). If AD does not reverse with bladder decompression, pharmacologic management with oral nifedipine, nitroglycerine ointment, or IV nitruprusside should be initiated.

Intervertebral Disk Disease
Voiding dysfunction is a well-established complication of lumbar intervertebral disk herniation, resulting from displacement of any intervertebral disks into the spinal canal. Herniated disks occur in a variety of disease processes including degenerative disease and trauma. The symptoms resulting from the displacement will be dependent on the level of the lesion, the extent of the displacement, and the type of neural injury, which may involve parasympathetic, sympathetic, and/or somatic nerve fibers (Table 48.3). The combination of these factors will result in a complex combination of signs and symptoms.

Nerve conduction will be compromised in cases of acute compression. At the level of the sacrum this can result in DA from impaired autonomic outflow to the detrusor. If there is additional interference of somatic outflow at the pudendal nerve, concomitant intrinsic sphincteric deficiency may occur (89). The most frequent site of lumbar disk herniation is the L4–L5 and L5–S1 intervertebral spaces, which can result in cauda equina syndrome (90,91). The characteristic symptoms and signs in this syndrome include lower back pain, obstructive voiding symptoms with or without incontinence, sensory loss at the perineum, sensory loss of the lateral foot (S1–S2 dermatome), and absence of the bulbocavernosus reflex (92).

Disruption from gradual degenerative disk displacement may result in hyperexcitability of sensory and motor fibers, with symptoms including irritative urinary frequency and urgency with DO (93). Urodynamic testing should be an integral part of the evaluation of all patients with incomplete lumbosacral spinal injuries (1).

Ankylosing Spondylitis
A rare inflammatory disease of the spine, ankylosing spondylitis results in fusion of the joints, and ligamentous calcification. This disease predominantly affects men, with deleterious effects on neurologic function generally occurring following spinal cord compression, caused by either atlantoaxial subluxation or trauma to the rigid spine (94–96).

The most common neurogenic lower urinary tract dysfunction caused by ankylosing spondylitis results in a cauda equina syndrome with impaired detrusor contractility (94). More severe cases may result in DA, and sphincteric activity may also be compromised as neuropathy progresses. Surgical decompression following neurologic impairment has met with varying success (97).

Guillain–Barré Syndrome
Guillain–Barré syndrome is an inflammatory demyelinating polyneuropathy, usually arising following an infectious episode that primarily affects the peripheral nervous system, with some effect on the nerve roots (98–100). Although recovery is a hallmark of Guillain–Barré syndrome, 85% of patients sustain persistent neurologic deficits (101). In severe cases, progression continues to affect central nervous, respiratory, and autonomic function, often including urinary retention (102).

Lower urinary tract dysfunction is present in 6% to 40% of patients diagnosed with Guillain–Barré syndrome (103). Symptoms include detrusor and sphincter motor and sensory deficits consistent with variation in the combination of nerves affected during the course of Guillain–Barré syndrome (104,105). Urodynamic studies on Guillain–Barré patients have revealed DA, impaired bladder sensation, and occasionally DO; it is not known whether these findings are accounted for by either central nervous system involvement or the timing of the urodynamic study (105,106).

Tabes Dorsalis
Tabes dorsalis (locomotor ataxia) is an uncommon form of neurosyphilis affecting <5% of those with syphilis worldwide. This condition results in a demyelination of the dorsal columns in the spinal cord (107–109). Progression of sacral root and dorsal column degeneration results in advancing stages of disease, and ultimately is manifested urologically with the development of urinary retention (110).

Classic descriptions of the effects of tabes dorsalis on voiding discuss the prevalence of DA; however, more recent studies suggest that DO may occur (108). It is postulated that involvement of the conus medullaris or cauda equina predisposes to a poorly compliant areflexic bladder, and that suprasacral lesions are responsible for the DO in these cases (111). These patients can be managed effectively with treatment of the primary infection with antibiotics and an intermittent catheterization program (112).

Acquired Immune Deficiency Syndrome

Voiding dysfunction in patients with AIDS of variable etiologies have been documented in recent studies (113–115). The most common cause of lower urinary tract dysfunction is simple cystitis, which is more likely to result from opportunistic organisms than in non-AIDS patients. This is because of the multiplicity of medical co-morbidities and the susceptibility of these patients to opportunistic infections. As a result, complete urologic assessment is critical in the evaluation of any complaints suggesting voiding dysfunction, especially as up to 40% of patients with AIDS have associated neurologic dysfunction (116,117).

Neurologic pathologies in AIDS patients which can lead to voiding dysfunctions include toxoplasmosis [reported in 14% of AIDS patients with neurologic disease (117)], neoplasms of the central nervous system, lymphoma, systemic lymphoma with central nervous system involvement, and Kaposi's sarcoma (118–120).

Urodynamic Evaluation

Findings following urodynamic evaluation in patients with AIDS are variable and may include DA, DO, DO with DSD, or non-neurologic bladder outlet obstruction (117,121). In the study by Hermieu et al., the onset of lower urinary tract disturbance represented a poor prognostic indicator, as 44% of these patients died within 24 months of evaluation (121).

Tropical Spastic Paraparesis

Tropical spastic paraparesis is a condition of progressive paraparesis and back pain, most likely induced by infection with the retrovirus human T-cell lymphotrophic virus type 1 (122). This clinical entity is caused by meningomyelitis with demyelinization and axonal loss, which can involve the corticospinal tracts (123). There is significant voiding dysfunction associated with this syndrome, with urinary hesitancy, urgency, and incontinence found in up to 60% of patients (122).

Urodynamic Evaluation

Studies of affected patients have revealed a predominance of DO, often with impaired contractility at voiding, and less frequently DA (124,125). Despite variable presentations, the lower urinary tract dysfunction can precipitate upper tract deterioration; therefore, urodynamic evaluation is recommended in all patients with acquired immune deficiency syndromes with voiding symptoms (116).

Transverse Myelitis

Transverse myelitis is a rare inflammatory condition of the spinal cord which may affect children or adults in an acute or progressive fashion (126,127). The entire thickness of the cord is involved, including both the gray and white matter, with the diagnosis made following elimination of spinal cord compression and the absence of other neurologic disease (128). Affected individuals may suffer from persistent neurologic deficits, most commonly urologic, although complete recovery may occur within 3 to 18 months (127,129).

Urodynamic Evaluation

Lower urinary tract dysfunction in these patients usually presents as either urinary retention or incontinence. A recent study showed the outcomes with predominant DO, DO with DSD, and less frequently DA (130). These urodynamic findings often persisted despite complete neurologic recovery.

Lyme Disease

Lyme borreliosis is caused by the spirochete *Borrelia burgdorferi*, which has demonstrated the ability to invade numerous body tissues, including the central and peripheral nervous systems and the bladder (1). Although initially associated with urinary retention, symptoms of urinary urgency, urge incontinence, and nocturia may occur at any time during the disease process (131). Patients with Lyme disease may present with DA or DO (132). Although the disease may respond to a two-week course of antimicrobial therapy (133), those with relapsing and remitting symptoms may require long-term administration of antimicrobials (134).

Herpes Zoster

Reactivation of persistent varicella virus from a dorsal root ganglion will result in episodes of Herpes zoster (135). During such episodes, symptoms primarily include sensory disturbances such as pain and paresthesia, although paralytic complications do rarely occur (136).

Infrequently, the virus reactivation includes the autonomic nerves of the bladder, with resultant irritative voiding symptoms such as dysuria and frequency. In cases involving the afferent neurons of the sacral micturition reflex arc, somatic, and visceral motor neuropathy can occur, and urinary retention may ensue (137,138). The course of the viral infection is usually self-limiting, with spontaneous recovery typically occurring within several months (1,139).

Poliomyelitis

Following a WHO resolution in 1988, great strides have been made in the eradication of poliomyelitis worldwide, with only 11 countries currently affected with endemic polio (140). Poliomyelitis results in destruction of the gray matter of the anterior horn cells and selective destruction of large-diameter fast-conducting motor neurons (141). Polio is essentially a pure motor neuropathy with sensory function usually preserved (142). Urinary retention may occur in up to 40% of patients, depending on disease severity. Patients with post-polio syndrome may manifest an increased incidence of irritative lower urinary tract symptoms, although studies on this issue are incomplete (1).

Urodynamic evaluation reveals DA when testing affected individuals, with bladder sensation and anal sphincter function remaining intact (143).

Tethered Cord Syndrome and Short Filum Terminale

The tethered cord syndrome results from impediment of the cephalad migration of the conus medullaris, and may result from a short filum terminale, intraspinal lipoma, or fibrous adhesions resulting from the surgical repair of spinal dysraphism (144,145). The syndrome is classically diagnosed in children, especially during adolescence, but rarely the process may occur in adulthood (146,147). Lower urinary tract dysfunction is common in this syndrome and, in otherwise

asymptomatic children, urodynamic abnormalities may be the basis for surgical intervention (148).

Urodynamic Evaluation
DA has been reported in 60% of patients, although recovery of lower tract function approached 60% with surgical release of the cord (146). Similarly, DO has also been reported (149). In another series, 22% of patients with tethered cords had DO; all improved following spinal surgery (150). Early and aggressive neurosurgical correction is therefore indicated (151).

CONDITIONS OF THE PERIPHERAL NERVOUS SYSTEM AFFECTING THE URINARY TRACT
Pelvic Plexus Injury
The major sympathetic and parasympathetic innervation of the lower urinary tract follows the branching array of the pelvic plexus. These nerve fibers can be disrupted during complicated pelvic surgical procedures, or following pelvic fracture, with resultant lower urinary tract dysfunction. Sympathetic (thoracolumbar) nerves promote urine storage by relaxing the detrusor muscle and relaxing the bladder outlet. Parasympathetic (sacral) nerves stimulate detrusor contraction. If the primary injury affects the parasympathetic nerve fibers, generally there is impaired detrusor contractility, although DA may occur in severe instances (1). Similarly, in cases involving predominately sympathetic innervation, the resultant symptoms usually include intrinsic sphincter deficiency with stress urinary incontinence. Study of patients with voiding dysfunction following major pelvic surgery has shown resolution of symptoms in six months for up to 80% of affected patients (152).

Abdominoperineal Resection
Abdominoperineal resection (APR) for rectal cancer almost invariably results in the disruption of the pelvic plexus, with both cadaveric and operative dissection of the plexus pathway demonstrating its susceptible nature during rectal resection (153,154). The courses of the pelvic nerves are as follows:

- from the inferior hypogastric plexus, it has multiple branches forming a web-like complex within the endopelvic fascial sleeve, some of which innervate the bladder detrusor;
- a main branch traveling inferolateral to the rectum remains deep to the fascia of the levator ani muscle and courses to the external urinary sphincter;
- at the level of the bladder neck in females, this pelvic nerve branch sends direct branches to the urinary sphincter (154).

As a result of this course, this has been associated with significant lower urinary tract dysfunction as an operative complication (155). The reported rate of urinary retention following APR ranges from 25% to 90%, with UTI frequently being associated (156,157).

Prior studies reveal evidence of sympathetic denervation in 100%, parasympathetic denervation in 38%, and pudendal denervation in 54% of patients postoperatively (1). The postoperative voiding dysfunction is usually transitory, although sphincteric insufficiency may be permanent (158). Post-APR urinary retention is best managed by clean intermittent self-catheterization.

Radical Hysterectomy
A similar effect on the lower urinary tract is seen from radical hysterectomy as in APR due to the similar dissection necessitated during the operation and bilateral pelvic lymphadenectomy. However, the location of the plexus inferolateral to the rectum reduces the disruption of the parasympathetic nerve fibers during hysterectomy, and the extent of pericervical dissection (e.g., "nerve-sparing" approach) does not appear to affect the postoperative urinary symptom complex (159). Persistent postoperative lower urinary tract dysfunction is best managed with a combination of anticholinergic therapy to decrease intravesical storage pressure and catheterization for retention, with most oncologists leaving the patients catheterized for a minimum of one week postoperatively.

Diabetic Cystopathy
Diabetes mellitus is the most prevalent medical condition resulting in sensory neurogenic lower urinary tract dysfunction affecting 2% of the U.S. population. (1,160,161). Voiding symptoms generally develop at least 10 years after the onset of the disease, as a result of one of three types of neuropathy: peripheral neuropathy, mononeuritis multiplex, and autonomic neuropathy (45,162). Metabolic abnormalities of Schwann cell function result in segmental demyelination and subsequent axonal degeneration, impairing nerve conduction (163,164).

Clinical and Urodynamic Features
Diabetes contributes significantly to voiding dysfunction in women (165). Urinary frequency is a common symptom, and this can result from impaired sensation and/or DO. Traditionally, gradual development of impaired bladder sensation is believed to be the first sign, usually associated with other sensory impairment consistent with peripheral neuropathy. Decreased sensation leads to increased intervoiding intervals which cause an increase in bladder capacity. Eventually the bladder may become overstretched, impairing contractility, and leading to incomplete emptying (166). Subsequently, symptoms associated with traditional "diabetic cystopathy" may include urinary hesitancy, slowing of the urine stream, and decreasing urinary frequency (165,167). These symptoms may progress to include a sensation of incomplete emptying or even urinary dribbling from overflow incontinence (165,168).

When questioned, up to 50% of unselected diabetes mellitus patients have subjective evidence of traditional diabetic cystopathy. The urodynamic evaluation, however, suggests alterations in lower urinary tract function in only 27% to 85% of these patients (168,169). Urodynamic studies frequently reveal impaired bladder sensation, increased cystometric bladder capacity, decreased detrusor contractility, an impaired urine flow, and an elevated post-void residual urine volume (45). However, more recent studies suggest that DO rather than the "traditional diabetic cystopathy" may be the most common observed voiding dysfunction in patients with diabetes. Kaplan and Te reported on another group of patients with diabetes referred because of voiding symptoms. Of this group, 55% were found to have DO, 23% impaired detrusor contractility, 10% DA, and 11% "indeterminate findings." In the 42 patients in this group with sacral cord neurologic signs, 50% had impaired detrusor contractility, and 24% had DA (170). In addition, poor diabetic control will contribute to urgency and frequency as a result of decreased warning time from impaired sensation and polyuria from the elevated glucose.

Upper tract changes depend upon the duration and severity of the disease process, as well as the effect on intravesical pressure. The effect of diabetes-induced lower urinary tract dysfunction on the upper urinary tract is difficult to determine because of the other effects of diabetes on renal function (1). When managing patients with diabetic cystopathy, preservation of renal function is paramount. A direct effect of diabetes on renal microvasculature, combined with upper tract obstructive changes resulting from diabetic cystopathy, put the diabetic kidneys at great risk. A timed voiding schedule is effective in those with impaired contractility, while intermittent catheterization is reserved for those who experience greater difficulty with emptying. Anticholinergic therapy may be effective for those with DO or impaired bladder compliance (161).

CONCLUSIONS

While neurologic conditions are frequently associated with lower urinary tract dysfunction, clinicians often overlook neurologic etiologies during workup and treatment of voiding dysfunctions. A high index of suspicion should be maintained where the severity of symptoms is disproportionately high or in rapid onset of symptoms. A brief neurologic examination at the time of presentation of new patients—or during urodynamic—should be considered as a standard for good practice. Management of voiding dysfunction in patients with neurological comorbities requires consideration of functional disabilities and other medications.

REFERENCES

1. Jung SY, Chancellor MB. Neurological disorders. In: Cardozo L, Staskin D, eds. Textbook of Female Urology and Urogynaecology. London: Martin Dunitz, 2001.
2. Wein AJ. Neuromuscular dysfunction of the lower urinary tract and its management. In: Walsh PC, Retik AB, Stamey TA, Vaughan ED, eds. Campbell's Urology. Philadelphia: Saunders, 2003.
3. Weiss DJ, Fried GW, Chancellor MB, et al. Spinal cord injury and bladder recovery. Arch Phys Med Rehabil 1996; 77: 1133–5.
4. Shenot PJ, Rivas DA, Watanabe T, et al. Early predictors of bladder recovery and urodynamics after spinal cord injury. Neurourol Urodyn 1998; 17: 25–9.
5. Watanabe T, Vaccaro AR, Kumon H, et al. High incidence of occult neurogenic bladder dysfunction in neurologically intact patients with thoracolumbar spinal injuries. J Urol 1998; 159: 965–8.
6. Berger Y, Blaivas JG, DeLaRocha ER, Salinas J. Urodynamic findings in Parkinson's disease. J Urol 1987; 138: 836–8.
7. de Groat WC, Kawatani M. Neural control of the urinary bladder: possible relationship between peptidergic inhibitory mechanisms and detrusor instability. Neurourol Urodyn 1985; 4: 285–300.
8. Karsenty G, Denys P, Amarenco G, et al. Botulinum toxin A (Botox) intradetrusor injections in adults with neurogenic detrusor overactivity/neurogenic overactive bladder: a systematic literature review. Eur Urol 2008; 53: 275–87. [Epub 2007 Oct 16].
9. Blaivas JG. The neurophysiology of micturition: a clinical study of 550 patients. J Urol 1982; 127: 958–63.
10. McGuire EJ, Brady S. Detrusor–sphincter dyssynergia. J Urol 1979; 121: 774–9.
11. Anderson RU. Urodynamic patterns after acute spinal cord injury: association with bladder trabeculation in male patients. J Urol 1983; 129: 777–9.
12. Ruutu M. Cystometrographic patterns in predicting bladder function after spinal cord injury. Paraplegia 1985; 23: 243–52.
13. Goldstein I, Siroky MB, Sax DS, Krane RJ. Neurourologic abnormalities in multiple sclerosis. J Urol 1982; 128: 541–5.
14. Blaivas JG, Barbalias GA. Detrusor–external sphincter dyssynergia in men with multiple sclerosis: an ominous urologic condition. J Urol 1984; 131: 91–4.
15. Borges P, Hackler RH. The urologic status of the Vietnam War paraplegic: a 15-year prospective follow-up. J Urol 1982; 127: 710–11.
16. Lloyd K. New trends in urologic management of spinal cord injured patients. Central Nervous System Trauma 1986; 3: 3–11.
17. McGuire EJ, Woodside JR, Borden TA. Prognostic value of urodynamic testing in myelodysplasia patients. J Urol 1981; 126: 205.
18. McGuire EJ. Urodynamic evaluation after abdominal–perineal resection and lumbar intervertebral disc herniation. Urology 1975; 6: 63–70.
19. Chancellor MB, Rivas DA, Ackman D. Multicenter trials of Urolume™ endourethral Wallstent® prosthesis for the urinary sphincter in spinal cord injured men. J Urol 1994; 152: 924–30.
20. Phelan MW, Franks M, Somogyi GT, et al. Botulinum toxin urethral sphincter injection to restore bladder emptying in men and women with voiding dysfunction. J Urol 2001; 165: 1107–10.
21. Rutkowski SB, Middleton JW, Truman G, et al. The influence of bladder management on fertility in spinal cord injured males. Paraplegia 1995; 33: 263.
22. Tosi L, Righetti C, Terrini G, Zanette G. Atypical syndromes caudal to the injury site in patients following spinal cord injury. A clinical, neurophysiological and MRI study. Paraplegia 1993; 31: 751–6.
23. Lapides J, Diokno AC, Silber SJ, Lowe BS. Clean, intermittent self-catheterization in the treatment of urinary tract disease. J Urol 1972; 107: 458.
24. Staskin D, Nehra A, Siroky M. Hydroureteronephrosis after spinal cord injury: effects of lower urinary tract dysfunction on upper tract anatomy. Urol Clin North Am 1991; 18: 309–16.
25. Marinkovic SP, Badlani G. Voiding and sexual function after cerebrovascular accidents. J Urol 2001; 165: 359–70.
26. Tsuchida S, Noto H, Yamaguchi O, Itoh M. Urodynamic studies on hemiplegic patients after cerebrovascular accident. Urology 1983; 21: 315–18.
27. Redding MJ, Winter SW, Hochrein SA. Urinary incontinence after unilateral hemispheric stroke: a neurologic epidemiologic perspective. J Neurorehabil 1987; 1: 25–31.
28. Blaivas JG, Chancellor MB. Cerebrovascular accidents and other intracranial lesions. Practical Neurology—Genitourinary Complications in Neurologic Disease. Boston: Butterworth-Heinemann, 1995: 119–25.
29. Blaivas J, Chancellor M, et al. Cerebral vascular accident, Parkinson's disease and other supra spinal neurologic disorders. In: Atlas of Urodynamics, 2nd edn. Malden, MA: Blackwell Publishing, 2007: 152.
30. Borrie MJ, Campbell AJ, Caradoc-Davies TH, Spears GFS. Urinary incontinence after stroke: a prospective study. Age Aging 1986; 15: 177–81.
31. Brocklehurst JC, Andrews K, Richards B, et al. Incidence and correlates of incontinence in stroke patients. J Am Geriatric Soc 1985; 33: 540–2.
32. Siroky MB, Krane RJ. Neurologic aspects of detrusor–sphincter dyssynergia, with reference to the guarding reflex. J Urol 1982; 127: 953–7.
33. Yahr MD. Parkinson's disease—overview of its current status. Mt Sinai J Med 1977; 44: 183–91.
34. Dmochowski RR. Female voiding dysfunction and movement disorders. Int Urogynecol J 1999; 10: 144–51.
35. Staskin DR. Intracranial lesions that affect lower urinary tact function. In: Krane RJ, Siroky MB, eds. Clinical Neuro-urology, 2nd edn. Boston: Little, Brown, 1991: 345–51.

36. Antel JP, Arnason BW. Demyelinating diseases. In: Wilson JD, Braunwald EB, Isselbacher KJ, eds. Harrison's Principles of Internal Medicine. New York: McGraw-Hill, 1991: 2038–65.

37. Pavlakis AJ, Siroky MB, Goldstein I, Krane RJ. Neurourologic findings in Parkinson's disease. J Urol 1983; 129: 80–3.

38. Blaivas J, Chancellor M, Verhaaren M, Weiss J. Cerebral vascular accident, Parkinson's disease and other supra spinal neurologic disorders. In: Atlas of Urodynamics, 2nd edn. Malden, MA: Blackwell Publishing, 2007: 153.

39. Kahn Z, Starr P, Bhola A. Urinary incontinence in female Parkinson's disease patients. Urology 1989; 33: 486–9.

40. Blaivas JG, Chancellor MB. Parkinson's disease. Practical Neurourology—Genitourinary Complications in Neurologic Disease. Boston: Butterworth-Heinemann, 1995: 139–47.

41. Holligar S, Wenning GK, Kiss G, et al. The natural history of voiding dysfunction in patients with idiopathic Parkinson's disease. J Urol 1997; 157: 1378.

42. Wulfsohn MA, Rubenstein A. The management of Shy–Drager syndrome with propantheline and intermittent self-catheterization: a case report. J Urol 1981; 126: 122–3.

43. Abyad A. Shy–Drager syndrome: recognition and management. J Am Board Fam Pract 1995; 8: 325–30.

44. Lockhart JL, Webster GD, Sheremata W, et al. Neurogenic bladder dysfunction in the Shy–Drager syndrome. J Urol 1981; 126: 119–21.

45. Blaivas JG. Neurologic dysfunctions. In: Yalla SV, McGuire EJ, El-Badawi A, Blaivas JG, eds. Neurourology and Urodynamics: Principles and Practice. New York: Macmillan, 1988; 343–57.

46. Beck RO, Betts CD, Fowler CJ. Genitourinary dysfunction in multiple system atrophy: clinical features and treatment in 62 cases. J Urol 1994; 151: 1336–41.

47. Hald T, Bradley WE. The Urinary Bladder: Neurology and Dynamics. Baltimore: Williams and Wilkins, 1982: 48–50, 157–9.

48. Kahn Z, Hertanu J, Yang WC, et al. Predictive correlation of urodynamic dysfunction and brain injury after cere-brovascular accident. J Urol 1981; 126: 86–8.

49. Yalla SV, Fam BA. Spinal cord injury. In: Krane RJ, Siroky MB, eds. Clinical Neuro-urology, 2nd edn. Boston: Little, Brown, 1991: 319–22.

50. Skelly J, Flint AJ. Urinary incontinence associated with dementia. J Am Geriatr Soc 1995; 43: 286–94.

51. Resnick NM, Yalla SV, Laurino E. The pathophysiology of urinary incontinence among institutionalized elderly persons. N Engl J Med 1989; 320: 1421–2.

52. Sakakibara R, Uchiyama T, Yamanishi T, Kishi M. Dementia and lower urinary dysfunction: with a reference to anticholinergic use in elderly population [Review]. Int J Urol 2008; 15: 778–88. [Epub 2008 Jul 14].

53. Stewart WF, Van Rooyen JB, Cundiff GW, et al. Prevalence and burden of overactive bladder in the United States. World J Urol 2003; 20: 327–36. [Epub 2002 Nov 15].

54. Staskin DR. Overactive bladder in the elderly: a guide to pharmacological management. Drugs Aging 2005; 22: 1013–28.

55. Sakakibara R, Uchiyama T, Yamanishi T, Kishi M. Dementia and lower urinary dysfunction: with a reference to anticholinergic use in elderly population [Review]. Int J Urol 2008; 15: 778–88. [Epub 2008 Jul 14].

56. Pratt R. Results of clinical studies with donepezil in vascular dementia. Presented at the 2nd International Congress on Vascular Dementia, Salzburg, Austria, January 24–27, 2002.

57. Inglis F. The tolerability and safety of cholinesterase inhibitors in the treatment of dementia. Int J Clin Pract Suppl 2002; 127: 45–63.

58. Litwiller SE, Frohman EM, Zimmern PE. Multiple sclerosis and the urologist. J Urol 1999; 161: 743–57.

59. Ebers GC, Sandivick AD, Risch NJ; and the Canadian Collaborative Study Group. A genetic basis for familial aggregation in multiple sclerosis. Nature 1995; 377: 150–5.

60. Poser CM. The epidemiology of multiple sclerosis: a general overview. Ann Neurol 1994; 36: S180–93.

61. McFarlin DE, McFarland HF. Multiple sclerosis. N Engl J Med 1982; 307: 1183–8.

62. Nathan PW, Smith NC. The centrifugal pathway for micturition with the spinal cord. J Neurol Neurosurg Psychiatry 1958; 21: 177–86.

63. McGuire EJ, Savastano JA. Urodynamic findings and long-term outcome management of patients with multiple sclerosis-induced lower urinary tract dysfunction. J Urol 1984; 132: 713–15.

64. Carr L. Lower urinary tract dysfunction due to multiple sclerosis. Can J Urol 2006; 13(Suppl 1): 2–4.

65. Blaivas JG, Bhimani G, Labib KB. Vesicourethral dysfunction in multiple sclerosis. J Urol 1979; 122: 342–7.

66. Awad SA, Gajewski JB, Sogbein SK, et al. Relationship between neurological and urological status in patients with multiple sclerosis. J Urol 1984; 132: 499–502.

67. Weinstein MS, Cardenas DD, O'Shaughnessy EJ, Catanzaro ML. Carbon dioxide cystometry and postural changes in patients with multiple sclerosis. Arch Phys Med Rehabil 1988; 69: 923–7.

68. Sirls LT, Zimmern PE, Leach GE. Role of limited evaluation and aggressive medical management in multiple sclerosis: a review of 113 patients. J Urol 1994; 151: 946–50.

69. Blaivas JG, Bhimani G, Labib KB. Vesicourethral dysfunction in multiple sclerosis. J Urol 1982; 127: 342–8.

70. Gonor SE, Carroll DJ, Metcalfe JB. Vesical dysfunction in multiple sclerosis. Urology 1985; 25: 429–31.

71. Chancellor MB, Blaivas JG. Multiple sclerosis. Practical Neurourology—Genitourinary Complications in Neurologic Disease. Boston: Butterworth-Heinemann, 1995: 127–37.

72. Fowler CJ, van Kerrebroeck PEV, Nordenbo A, van Poppel H. Treatment of lower urinary tract dysfunction in patients with multiple sclerosis. J Neurol Neurosurg Psychiatry 1992; 55: 986–9.

73. Dykstra DD, Sidi AA. Treatment of detrusor–sphincter dyssynergia with botulinum A toxin: a double-blind study. Arch Phys Med Rehabil 1990; 71: 24–6.

74. Smith CP, Chancellor MB. Emerging role of botulinum toxin in the management of voiding dysfunction. J Urol 2004; 171: 2128–37.

75. National Spinal Cord Injury Statistical Center. Online. [Available from: www.spinalcord.uab.edu].

76. Watanabe T, Rivas DA, Chancellor MB. Urodynamics of spinal cord injury. Urol Clin North Am 1996; 23: 459–73.

77. Kaplan SA, Chancellor MB, Blaivas JG. Bladder and sphincter behavior in patients with spinal cord lesions. J Urol 1991; 146: 113.

78. Weld KJ, Dmochowski RR. Association of level of injury and bladder behavior in patients with post-traumatic spinal cord injury. Urology 2000; 55: 490–4.

79. Kaplan SA, Chancellor MB, Blaivas JG. Bladder and sphincter behavior in patients with spinal cord lesions. J Urol 1991; 146: 113–17.

80. Brown-Sequard CE. De la transmission des impressions sensitives par la moelle epiniere. Comptes Rendures des Seances et Memoires de la Societe de Biologie 1849; 1: 192–4.

81. Brown-Sequard CE. Lectures on the physiology and pathology of the central nervous system and on the treatment of organic nervous affections; lecture 1, on spinal hemiplegia. Lancet 1868; 2: 593–6, 659–62, 755–7, 821–3.

82. Sakakibara R, Hattori T, Uchiyama T, Yamanishi T. Urinary dysfunction in Brown–Sequard syndrome. Neurourol Urodyn 2001; 20: 661–7.

83. Inatomi Y, Itoh Y, Fujii N, Nakanishi K. The spinal cord descending pathway for micturition: analysis in patients with spinal cord infarction. J Neurol Sci 1998; 157: 154–7.

84. Koehler PJ, Endtz LJ. The Brown–Sequard syndrome: true or false? Arch Neurol 1986; 43: 921–4.

85. Kaplan SA, Chancellor MB, Blaivas JG. Bladder and sphincter behavior in patients with spinal cord injury. J Urol 1991; 146: 113–17.

86. Lindan R, Joiner E, Freehafer A, Hazel C. Incidence and clinical features of autonomic dysreflexia in patients with spinal cord injury. Paraplegia 1980; 18: 285–92.

87. Rivas DA, Chancellor MB, Huang B, Salzman SK. Autonomic dysreflexia in a rat model of spinal cord injury and the effect of pharmacologic agents. Neurourol Urodyn 1995; 14: 141–52.

88. Blackmer J. Rehabilitation medicine: autonomic dysreflexia. CMAJ 2003; 169: 931–5.

89. Malloch JD. Acute retention due to intervertebral disc prolapse. Br J Urol 1965; 37: 578–85.

90. O'Flynn KJ, Murphy R, Thomas DG. Neurogenic bladder dysfunction in lumbar intervertebral disc prolapse. Br J Urol 1992; 69: 38–40.

91. Scott PJ. Bladder paralysis in cauda equina syndrome from disc prolapse. J Bone Joint Surg 1965; 47: 224–7.

92. Goldman HB, Appell RA. Voiding dysfunction in women with lumbar disc prolapse. Int Urogynecol J 1999; 10: 134–8.

93. Jones DL, Moore T. The types of neuropathic bladder dysfunction associated with prolapsed lumbar intervertebral discs. Br J Urol 1973; 45: 39–43.

94. Russell ML, Gordon DA, Ogryzlo MA, McPhedran RS. The cauda equina syndrome of ankylosing spondylitis. Ann Int Med 1973; 78: 551–4.

95. Haddad FS, Sachdev JS, Bellapravalu M. Neuropathic bladder in ankylosing spondylitis with spinal diverticula. Urology 1990; 35: 313–16.

96. Garza-Mercado R. Traumatic extradural hematoma of the cervical spine. Neurosurgery 1989; 24: 410–14.

97. Tyrrell PNM, Davies AM, Evans N. Neurological disturbances in ankylosing spondylitis. Ann Rheumatic Dis 1994; 53: 714–17.

98. Guillain G, Barré JA, Strohl A. Sur un syndrome de radiculo-névrite avec hyperalbuminose du liquode céphalo-rachidien sans réaction cellulaire: remarques sur les caractéres cliniques et graphiques des réflexes tendineux. Bulletins et Mémoires de la Société Médicale des Hôpitaux de Paris 1916; 40: 1462–70.

99. Asbury AK, Arnason BG, Adams RD. The inflammatory lesion in idiopathic polyneuritis: its role in pathogenesis. Medicine 1969; 48: 173–215.

100. Haymaker W, Kernohan JW. The Landry–Guillain–Barré syndrome: clinicopathologic report of fifty fatal cases and a critique of the literature. Medicine 1949; 28: 59–65.

101. Ng KKP, Howard RS, Fish DR, et al. Management and outcome of severe Guillain–Barré syndrome. Q J Med 1995; 88: 243–50.

102. Ropper AH. The Guillain–Barré syndrome. N Engl J Med 1992; 326: 1130–6.

103. Truax B. Autonomic disturbance in the Guillain–Barré syndrome. Semin Neurol 1984; 4: 462–8.

104. Kogan BA, Solomon MH, Diokno AC. Urinary retention secondary to Landry–Guillain–Barré syndrome. J Urol 1981; 126: 643–4.

105. Sakakibara R, Hattori T, Kuwabara S, et al. Micturitional disturbance in patients with Guillain–Barré syndrome. J Neurol Neurosurg Psychiatry 1997; 63: 649–53.

106. Wheeler JS, Siroky MB, Pavlakis A, Krane RJ. The urodynamic aspects of the Guillain–Barré syndrome. J Urol 1984; 131: 917–19.

107. Wheeler JS Jr, Culkin DJ, O'Hara RJ, Canning JR. Bladder dysfunction and neurosyphilis. J Urol 1986; 136: 903–5.

108. Berger JR, Sabet A. Infectious myelopathies. Semin Neurol 2002; 22: 133–42.

109. Garber SJ, Christmas TJ, Rickards D. Voiding dysfunction due to neurosyphilis. Br J Urol 1990; 66: 19–21.

110. Harper JM, Politano VA, Schwarcz B. The FTA–ABS test in the diagnosis of the neurogenic bladder. J Urol 1967; 97: 862–3.

111. Hattori T, Yasuda K, Kita K, Hirayama K. Disorders of micturition in tabes dorsalis. Br J Urol 1990; 65: 497–9.

112. Chancellor MB, Blaivas JG. Infectious neurologic diseases. Practical Neurourology—Genitourinary Complications in Neurologic Disease. Boston: Butterworth-Heinemann, 1995: 179–85.

113. Khan Z, Singh VK, Yang WE. Neurogenic bladder in AIDS. Urology 1992; 40: 289–91.

114. Hermieu JF, Delmas V, Boccon-Gibod L. Micturition disturbances and human immunodeficiency virus infection. J Urol 1996; 156: 157–9.

115. Kane CJ, Bolton DM, Connolly JA, Tanagho EA. Voiding dysfunction in human immunodeficiency virus infections. J Urol 1996; 155: 523–6.

116. Lange DJ, Britton CB, Younger DS, Hays AP. The neuromuscular manifestations of human immunodeficiency infections. Arch Neurol 1988; 45: 1084–8.

117. Levy RM, Bredesen DE, Rosenblum ML. Neurological manifestations of acquired immunodeficiency syndrome: experiences at UCSF and review of the literature. J Neurosurg 1985; 62: 475–95.

118. Snider WD, Simpson DM, Aronyk KE. Primary lymphoma of the nervous system associated with acquired immunodeficiency syndrome [letter]. N Engl J Med 1983; 308: 45.

119. Levy RM, Pons VG, Rosenblum ML. Intracerebral-mass lesions in the acquired immunodeficiency syndrome (AIDS) [letter]. N Engl J Med 1983; 309: 1454.

120. Levy RM, Pons VG, Rosenblum ML. Central nervous system mass lesions in the acquired immunodeficiency syndrome (AIDS). J Neurosurg 1984; 61: 9–16.

121. Hermieu JF, Delmas V, Boccon-Gibod L. Micturition disturbances and human immunodeficiency virus infection. J Urol 1996; 156: 157–9.

122. Cruickshank JK, Rudge P, Dalgleish AG. Tropical spastic paraparesis and human T-cell lymphotrophic virus type 1 in the United Kingdom. Brain 1989; 112: 1057–90.

123. Montgomery RD, Cruickshank JK, Robertson WB. Clinical and pathological observations on Jamaican neuropathy. A report of 206 cases. Brain 1964; 87: 425–40.

124. Eardley I, Fowler CJ, Nagendran K, et al. The neurourology of tropical spastic paraparesis. Br J Urol 1991; 68: 598–603.

125. Yamashita H, Kumazawa J. Voiding dysfunction: patients with human T-lymphotropic-virus-type-1-associated myelopathy. Urol Int 1991; 47(Suppl 1): 69–71.

126. Dunne K, Hopkins IJ, Shield LK. Acute transverse myelopathy in childhood. Dev Med Child Neurol 1986; 28: 198–204.

127. Lipton HL, Teasdall RD. Acute transverse myelopathy in adults. Arch Neurol 1973; 28: 252–7.

128. Adams RD, Victor M. Principles of Neurology, 3rd edn. New York: McGraw–Hill, 1985: 673–702.

129. Ropper AH, Poskanzer DC. The prognosis of acute and subacute transverse myelopathy based on early signs and symptoms. Ann Neurol 1978; 4: 51–9.

130. Kalita J, Shah S, Kapoor R, Misra UK. Bladder dysfunction in acute transverse myelitis: magnetic resonance imaging and neurophysiological and urodynamic correlations. J Neurol Neurosurg Psychiatry 2002; 73: 154–9.

131. Chancellor MB, Dato VM, Yang J. Lyme disease presenting as urinary retention. J Urol 1990; 143: 1223–4.

132. Chancellor MB, McGinnis D, Shenot PJ, et al. Urinary dysfunction in Lyme disease. J Urol 1993; 149: 26–30.

133. Steere AC, Green J, Schoen RT, et al. Successful penicillin therapy of Lyme arthritis. N Engl J Med 1985; 312: 869–74.

134. Rahn DW, Malawista SE. Lyme disease: recommendations for diagnosis and treatment. Ann Intern Med 1991; 114: 472–81.

135. Weller TH. Varicella and herpes zoster: a perspective and overview. J Infect Dis 1992; 166(Suppl 1): S1–6.

136. Thomas JE, Howard FM. Segmental zoster paresis—a disease profile. Neurology 1972; 22: 459–66.

137. Izumi AK, Dewards J Jr. Herpes zoster and neurogenic bladder dysfunction. J Am Med Assoc 1973; 224: 1748–9.

138. Straus SE, Ostrove JM, Inchauspe G. Varicella zoster virus infections. Biology, natural history, treatment, and prevention. Ann Intern Med 1988; 109: 438–9.

139. Rosenfeld T, Price MA. Paralysis in herpes zoster. Aust N Z J Med 1985; 15: 712–16.

140. Centers for Disease Control and Prevention (CDC). Progress toward poliomyelitis eradication—poliomyelitis outbreak in Sudan, 2004. MMWR Morb Mortal Wkly Rep 2005; 54: 97–9.

141. Hodes R. Selective destruction of large motor-neurons by poliomyelitis virus: I. Conduction velocity of motor nerve fibers of chronic poliomyelitis. J Neurophysiol 1949; 12: 257–66.

142. So YT, Olney RK. AAEM case report #23: acute paralytic poliomyelitis. Muscle Nerve 1991; 14: 1159–64.

143. Bors E, Comarr AE. Neurologic Urology. Baltimore: University Park Press, 1971.

144. Pang D, Wilberger JE Jr. Tethered cord syndrome in adults. J Neurosurg 1982; 57: 32–47.

145. Al-Mefty O, Kandzari S, Fox JL. Neurogenic bladder and the tethered spinal cord syndrome. J Urol 1979; 179: 112–15.

146. Kondo A, Kato K, Kanai S, Sakakibara T. Bladder dysfunction secondary to tethered cord syndrome in adults: is it curable? J Urol 1986; 135: 313–16.

147. Adamson AS, Gelister J, Hayward R, Snell ME. Tethered cord syndrome: an unusual case of adult bladder dysfunction. Br J Urol 1993; 71: 417–21.

148. Meyrat BJ, Tercier S, Lutz N, et al. Introduction of a urodynamic score to detect pre- and postoperative neurological deficits in children with a primary tethered cord. Childs Nerv Syst 2003; 19: 716–21.

149. Kondo A, Kato K, Sakakibar T, et al. Tethered cord syndrome: cause for urge incontinence and pain in lower extremities. Urology 1992; 40: 143–6.

150. Hellstrom WJG, Edwards MSB, Kogan BA. Urological aspects of the tethered cord syndrome. J Urol 1986; 135: 317–20.

151. Fukui J, Kaizaki T. Urodynamic evaluation of tethered cord syndrome including tight filum terminale. Urology 1980; 16: 539–52.

152. Blaivas JG, Chancellor MB. Cauda equina and pelvic plexus injury. Practical Neurourology—Genitourinary Complications in Neurologic Disease. Boston: Butterworth-Heinemann, 1995: 155–63.

153. Mundy AR. An anatomical explanation for bladder dysfunction following rectal and uterine surgery. Br J Urol 1982; 54: 501–4.

154. Hollabaugh Jr RS, Steiner MS, Sellers KD, Samm BJ, Dmochowski RR. Neuroanatomy of the pelvis: implications for colonic and rectal resection. Dis Colon Rectum 2000; 43: 1390–7.

155. Marshal VF, Pollack RS, Miller C. Observations on urinary dysfunction after excision of the rectum. J Urol 1946; 55: 409–21.

156. Fowler JW, Bremner DN, Moffat LEF. The incidence and consequences of damage to the parasympathetic nerve supply to the bladder after abdominoperineal resection of the rectum for carcinoma. Br J Urol 1978; 50: 95–8.

157. Petrelli NJ, Nagel S, Rodriguez-Bigas M, Piedmonte M, Herrera L. Morbidity and mortality following abdominoperineal resection for rectal adenocarcinoma. Am Surg 1993; 59: 400–4.

158. Blaivas JG, Barbalias GA. Characteristics of neural injury after abdominoperineal resection. J Urol 1983; 129: 84–7.

159. Querleu D, Narducci F, Poulard V, et al. Modified radical vaginal hysterectomy with or without laparoscopic nerve-sparing dissection: a comparative study. Gynecol Oncol 2002; 85: 154–8.

160. Wetterhall SF, Olson DR, DeStefano F, et al. Trends in diabetes and diabetic complications, 1980–1987. Diabetes Care 1992; 15: 960–7.

161. Chancellor MB, Blaivas JG. Diabetic neurogenic bladder. Practical Neurourology—Genitourinary Complications in Neurologic Disease. Boston: Butterworth-Heinemann, 1995: 149–54.

162. Frimodt-Moller C, Hald T. A new method for quantitative evaluation of bladder sensibility. Scand J Urol Nephrol 1972; 15: 134–5.

163. Faerman I. Autonomic nervous system and diabetes: histological and histochemical study of the autonomic nerve fibers of the urinary bladder in diabetic patients. Diabetes 1973; 22: 225–37.

164. Thomas PK, Lascelles RG. The pathology of diabetic neuropathy. Q J Med 1978; 35: 449–57.

165. Lee WC, Wu HP, Tai TY, et al. Effects of diabetes on female voiding behavior. J Urol 2004; 172 : 989–92.

166. Blaivas J, Chancellor M, Verhaaren M, Weiss J. Spinal Cord Injury, Multiple sclerosis and Diabetes Mellitus. In: Atlas of Urodynamics, 2nd ed. Malden, MA: Blackwell Publishing, 2007: 169.

167. Clark CMJ, Lee DA. Prevention and treatment of the complications of diabetes mellitus. N Engl J Med 1995; 332: 1210–17.

168. Appel RA, Whiteside HV. Diabetes and other peripheral neuropathies affecting lower urinary tract function. In: Krane RJ, Siroky MB, eds. Clinical Neurourology, 2nd ed. Boston: Little, Brown, 1991: 365–73.

169. Ueda T, Yoshimura N, Yoshida O. Diabetic cystopathy: relationship to autonomic neuropathy detected by sympathetic skin responses. J Urol 1997; 157: 580–4.

170. Kaplan SA, Te AE, Blaivas JG. Urodynamic findings in patients with diabetic cystopathy. J Urol 1995; 153: 342–3.

497

INTRODUCTION

One of the core aims of the clinical and urodynamic assessment of women with symptoms of pelvic floor dysfunction is to screen for the presence of voiding dysfunction (VD), i.e., abnormally slow and/or incomplete micturition (1). Clinical assessment may provide limited, generally non-specific, information with two screening urodynamic tests, uroflowmetry, and a postvoid residual (PVR) measurement of much greater value. Uroflowmetry or the measure of urine flow over time allows the simple and non-invasive analysis of the normality or otherwise of urine flow whilst the complementary measurement of PVR will indicate the completeness or otherwise of micturition.

Abnormal urine flow rates or patterns or high PVRs in women will generally require the further investigation of voiding cystometry in order to determine the cause. Pressure and flow analysis will assist the discrimination between the presence of one of the two main causes of abnormally slow urine flow or abnormally high PVRs, i.e., bladder outflow obstruction and a hypotonic or atonic bladder.

It is important clinically to diagnose or eliminate the diagnosis of VD in women presenting for assessment of symptoms of pelvic floor dysfunction. Surgical treatment of urodynamic stress incontinence (USI) and drug treatment of detrusor overactivity (DO) both have the potential to cause VD. Pre-existing VD will prejudice these treatments, leading to the possibility of acute or chronic retention.

The subsequent discussion will focus on women not presenting with existing neurological disorders known to be associated with VD.

CLINICAL ASSESSMENT

Symptoms of VD should be included in a comprehensive history in women presenting with symptoms of pelvic floor dysfunction. The Standardization and Terminology Committees of the International Continence Society (ICS) and the International Urogynecological Association (IUGA) (1) have suggested the following definitions for "voiding and postmicturition symptoms."

- *Voiding and postmicturition symptoms*: A departure from normal sensation or function, experienced by a woman during or following the act of micturition.
- *Hesitancy*: Complaint of a delay in initiating micturition.
- *Slow stream*: Complaint of a urinary stream perceived as slower compared to previous performance or in comparison with others.
- *Intermittency*: Complaint of urine flow that stops and starts on one or more occasions during voiding.
- *Straining to void*: Complaint of the need to make an intensive effort (by abdominal straining, valsalva, or suprapubic pressure) to either initiate, maintain, or improve the urinary stream.

- *Spraying (splitting) of urinary stream*: Complaint that the urine passage is a spray or split rather than a single discrete stream.
- *Feeling of incomplete (bladder) emptying*: Complaint that the bladder does not feel empty after micturition.
- *Need to immediately re-void*: Complaint that further micturition is necessary soon after passing urine.
- *Post-micturition leakage*: Complaint of a further involuntary passage of urine following the completion of micturition.
- *Position-dependent micturition*: Complaint of having to take specific positions to be able to micturate spontaneously or to improve bladder emptying, e.g., leaning forwards or backwards on the toilet seat or voiding in the semi-standing position.
- *Dysuria*: Complaint of burning or other discomfort during micturition. Discomfort may be intrinsic to the lower urinary tract or external (vulvar dysuria).
- *(Urinary) Retention*: Complaint of the inability to pass urine despite persistent effort.

These symptoms are mostly non-specific and not diagnostic in themselves though the symptoms of hesitancy, a poor stream, and straining to void have been more commonly linked to an abnormally slow urine flow rate or a high PVR (2).

Of the various clinical signs, that of uterine and/or vaginal prolapse, particularly if higher stage, can be associated with a diagnosis of VD by a urethral "kinking effect." Atrophic vaginal changes might be an indicator that atrophic urethral changes might be present causing a possible "stenotic" effect.

HISTORY OF UROFLOWMETRY

The first attempt to obtain an objective measurement of the urine flow rate was made in 1897 by Rehfisch (3) using a poorly detailed method employing an air displacement principle (4). Ballenger et al. (5) felt that the cast distance of urinary stream (voiding distance) might be a useful clinical guide to the presence of prostatic disease.

Drake (6) made the first accurate measurements of urine flow. He used a spring balance; a pen that wrote on a kymograph was attached to one end, and a receptacle for the voided volume was attached to the other end. By rotating the kymograph drawn at a known speed, Drake obtained a trace of voided urine volume against time. He calculated the maximum urine flow rate by a measurement of the steepest part of the volume-time curve. It is evident from his description that the apparatus was relatively crude and difficult to use. Furthermore, urine flow rates had to be calculated from volume-time data. Drake's flowmeter was never produced commercially. Kaufman (7) commercially produced a modification of Drake's flowmeter that was more refined but similarly made no direct recording of flow rate.

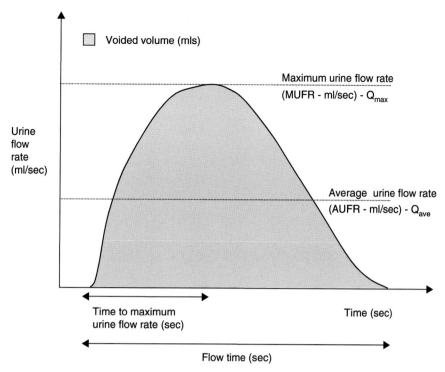

Figure 49.1 Urine flow rates (IUGA/ICS definitions).

The advent of electronics in medical instrumentation allowed the mass production of accurate and reliable recording devices. Von Garrelts (8) designed the first of the electronic urine flowmeters, which consisted of a tall urine-collecting cylinder with a pressure transducer in the base. The pressure transducer measured the pressure exerted by an increasing column of urine as the patient voided. Since a direct relationship existed between the volume voided and the pressure recorded, Von Garrelts was able to produce a direct recording of urine flow rate by electronic differentiation with time.

In 2010, it is 33 years since it was determined that uroflowmeters of acceptable accuracy were available (9). The current accuracy of modern uroflowmeters is around ±2% to 5%, despite the fact that a variety of different physical principles are currently used. Regular calibration of the uroflowmeter is required to maintain accuracy.

DEFINITION OF URINE FLOW RATE MEASUREMENTS

In any field of scientific measurement, it is important that all workers use standardized terminology. Urine flow rates are measured in milliliters per second (ml/sec). Figure 49.1 denotes the definitions for urine flow rate measurements as suggested by the Standardization and Terminology Committees of ICS and IUGA (1):

- *Urine flow*: Voluntary urethral passage of urine which may be:
  - ○ *Continuous*: No interruption to flow.
  - ○ *Intermittent*: Flow is interrupted.
- *Flow rate*: Volume of urine expelled via the urethra per unit time. It is expressed in ml/sec.
- *Voided volume (ml)*: Total volume of urine expelled via the urethra.

- *Maximum (urine) flow rate (MUFR—ml/sec)–Q_{max}*: Maximum measured value of the flow rate correcting for artifacts.
- *Flow time (sec)*: The time over which measurable flow actually occurs.
- *Average (urine) flow rate (AUFR—ml/sec)–Q_{ave}*: Voided volume divided by the flow time. It may be calculated from the area beneath the flow time curve.
- *Voiding time (sec)*: This is the total duration of micturition, i.e., includes interruptions. When voiding is completed without interruption, voiding time is equal to flow time.
- *Time to maximum flow (sec)*: This is the elapsed time from the onset of urine flow to maximum urine flow.

METHODS OF URINE FLOW RATE MEASUREMENT

Numerous physical principles have been employed over the years in an attempt to develop what Backman (10) and Von Garrelts and Strandell (11) would see as an ideal uroflowmeter:

1. high level of accuracy at different voided volumes and urine flow rates;
2. easy to read and rapidly available permanent tracings;
3. unobtrusive and not distracting to the patient by appearance or sound;
4. easy to clean.

There have been many methods used for urine flow measurement, from measuring the time to void a given volume through audiometric and radioisotopic methods to even include high-speed cinematography. The most common method has been that of Drake (6) modified by Von Garrelts and Strandell (11)—the measurement of urine weight.

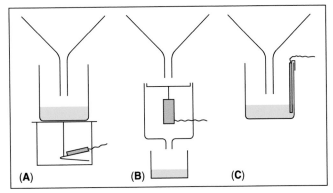

Figure 49.2 Urine flowmeters (**A**) weight transducer (**B**) rotating disc (**C**) capacitance (dipstick).

In addition, flowmeters have been produced that use the principles of air displacement, differential resistance to gasflow, electromagnetism, photo-electricity, electrical capacitance, and a rotating disc.

Flowmeters employing the principles of weight transduction, a rotating disc, and a capacitance transducer are the best known and the most completely tested and validated of the flowmeters available.

The weight transducer type of flowmeter weighs the voided urine and by differentiation with time produces an "on-line" recording of urine flow rate:

$$FR = dV/dt$$

where dV is the change in volume of urine over change in time, dt.

The rotating disc flowmeter depends on a servometer maintaining the rotation of the disc at a constant speed. Urine hits the disc, and the extra power required to maintain the speed is electronically converted into a measurement of flow rate.

The capacitance flowmeter is the simplest of the three flowmeters. This flowmeter consists of a funnel leading urine into a collecting vessel. The transducer is in the form of a dipstick made of plastic and coated with metal, which dips into the vessel containing the voided urine.

All three types of flowmeter perform accurately and efficiently. For clinical purposes, the measured and indicated flow rate should be accurate to within ±5% over the clinically significant flow rate range (12). The capacitance (dipstick) flowmeter is the least expensive to buy and has the advantage of no moving parts, which means mechanical breakdowns are eliminated. Rotating disc flowmeters have the advantage of not requiring priming with fluid. Automatic start and stop facilities in some modern flowmeters assist by minimizing patient and staff involvement during the uroflowmetry (Fig. 49.2).

CLINICAL MEASUREMENT OF URINE FLOW RATES

The environment for patient flow rate recording is of considerable importance. Female patients usually void in circumstances of almost complete privacy. It is essential in the clinical situation that every effort is made to make the patient feel comfortable and relaxed. If these requirements are ignored, psychological factors are introduced and a higher proportion of patients will fail to void in a representative way. Ideally, all free uroflowmetry studies should be performed in a completely private uroflowmetry room/toilet, lockable from the inside and out of hearing range of other staff and patients. As crouching over a toilet seat causes a 21% reduction in the average urine flow rate (13), patients should be encouraged to sit to void. When video studies are combined with pressure-flow recordings in a radiology department, up to 30% of women may fail to void.

Patients should be encouraged to attend for uroflowmetry with their bladder comfortably full. It is desirable that the measured urine flow rates should be for a voided volume within the patient's normal range. This range can be determined if, in the week before the flow study, the patient completes a frequency-volume chart (urinary diary). On this chart, the patient enters the volumes of fluid consumed and the volumes of urine voided. Recent nomograms, however, provide normal reference ranges for urinary flow rates over a wide range of voided volumes. There is generally no need for multiple uroflowmetry in most women. Abnormal or unusual flow curves and urinary flow rates however, merit repeating the study.

URINE FLOW RATES IN NORMAL (ASYMPTOMATIC) WOMEN

The maximum and average urinary flow rates are the two most important uroflowmetry parameters. They are both numerical representations of the urine flow curve. The clinical usefulness of urine flow rates had been attenuated by the lack of absolute values defining normal limits (14). As urinary flow rates are known to have a strong dependence on voided volume (6,15); these normal limits need to be over a wide range of voided volumes, ideally in the form of nomograms.

Studies on normal values for urinary flow rates in women include those of Peter and Drake (16), Scott and McIhlaney (17), Backman (18), Susset et al. (19), Walter et al. (20), Drach et al. (15), Bottacini and Gleason (21), Fantl et al. (22), and Rollema (23). Data and/or statistical analysis in these studies has not allowed effective nomogram construction. Study restrictions have included small patient numbers (19–23); the use of outmoded or less well-evaluated equipment (15–16) and the incompleteness of data at lower voided volumes (15,18) due in part to the inaccuracy of some equipment at lower voided volumes (15).

In a 1989 study, Haylen et al. (24) studied 249 female volunteers (aged 16 to 63 years), all of whom were deemed normal by denying specific urinary symptomatology, underwent uroflowmetry studies. Each women voided once in a completely private environment over a calibrated rotating disc-type uroflowmeter; 46 voided on a second occasion. The maximum and average flow rates of the first voids were compared with the respective voided volumes. By using statistical transformations of both voided volumes and urine flow rates, relationships between the two variables were obtained. This allowed the construction of nomograms, which, for ease of interpretation, have been displayed in centile form (Fig. 49.3A & B).

Very recently, Barapatre et al. (25) produced nomograms using the data of 343 healthy Indian women. The results, after elimination of "abnormal" data, were much slower urine flow rates overall than those in the Liverpool nomograms and an age dependency of urine flow rates, not normally noted in

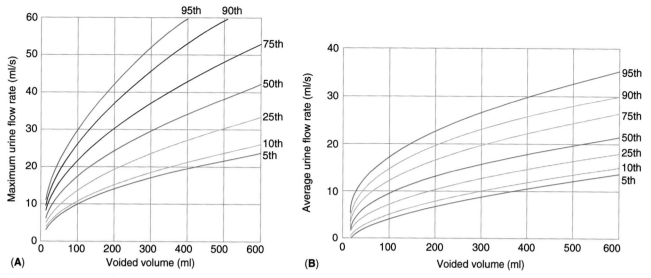

Figure 49.3 (**A**) Liverpool maximum urine flow rate nomogram for women. Equation: ln(MUFR) = 0.511 + 0.505 × ln(Voided volume). Root mean square error = 0.340. (**B**) Liverpool average urine flow rate nomogram for women. Equation: Square root(AUFR) = –0.921 + 0.869 × ln(Voided volume). Root mean square error = 0.640. *Source*: From Refs. 24 and 28.

asymptomatic women (15,22,24,26). As noted later, their median centiles in asymptomatic women were slower than studies using the Liverpool nomograms in symptomatic women.

Traditional "cut-off" values for normal urine flow rates have been used with due scientific analysis of their accuracy or value. The maximum urine flow rate has been most studied. Recommended lower limits of normality range between 12 and 20 ml/sec. Most commonly, a minimum rate of 15 ml/sec is quoted for the same parameter if at least 150 ml (or sometimes 200 ml) has been voided. The practice of artificially imposing minimum limits for the voided volume is difficult to justify (27) and often impractical. Women with certain states of lower urinary tract dysfunction, those in whom the flow rate might be most important, may not be able to hold 200 ml. It has been demonstrated that only 45% voided volumes are over 200 ml and 55% are over 150 ml making interpretation of fixed urine flow rates valid (28). Because of the strong dependency of urine flow rates on voided volume a normal urine flow rate at 200 ml may not also be normal at 400 ml.

CLINICAL FACTORS INFLUENCING URINE FLOW RATES IN NORMAL (ASYMPTOMATIC) WOMEN
Voided Volume
The use of nomograms overcomes the dangers of referencing flow rates to any one voided volume. A maximum flow rate of 15 ml/sec might fall just within the fifth centile curve at 200 ml voided volume, though well below the same curve at 400 ml. The median voided volume of 171 ml and 175 ml in the above series (24,28) again highlights the need for normal reference ranges to include data at lower voided volumes.

Both the maximum and average urine flow rates in the above study were found to have a strong and essentially equal dependence on voided volume. The clinical use of either flow rate is equally valid. However, the centile lines onto which the maximum and average urine flow rates respectively fall for the same voided volume (centile rankings) are not interchangeable in

an individual instance, due to wide variations in urine flow patterns. The closer the urine flow pattern comes to the "ideal" flow time curve seen in Figure 49.1, the more chance there will be that the centile rankings for the maximum and average urine flow rates are the same.

No systematic deterioration of either flow rate at higher voided volumes was discernible from this population study. The same may not be true for an individual.

Age and Parity
Drach et al. (15), Fantl et al. (22) and Haylen et al. (24) found no significant age dependence of urinary flow rates in normal women, unlike the findings of Barapatre et al. (25). The same studies also found that there was no significant effect of parity on urine flow rates in normal women. This was not tested by Barapatre et al. (25).

Repeated Voiding
There was a remarkable consistency in the centile rankings of the paired first and second voids in the study of Haylen et al. (24). This consistency is further witnessed in the multiple voids from a single 25-year-old normal female volunteer (Figure 49.4). Fantl et al. (22) found no significant difference between the first and up to the sixth void in the sixty women he tested. This was not tested by Barapatre et al. (25). Clinically, in the majority of normal women, the centile rankings of successive voids will not differ widely. It is uncertain, at present, whether this is also true for women with lower urinary tract dysfunction. As suggested previously, abnormal or unusual flow rates or curves merit repeating the study.

Presence of a Catheter
The above nomograms refer to free flowmetry voids; they are not applicable where a pressure of other catheter is present in the urethra. All urethral catheters can be expected to have the effect of decreasing urinary flow rates for the equivalent voided volume. Part of this reduction is physical obstruction

501

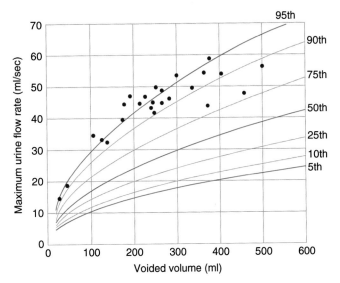

Figure 49.4 Maximum urine flow rates from a large number of voids by a single 25-year-old female volunteer superimposed on the respective Liverpool nomogram.

	Symptomatic		Asymptomatic	
	1999 (31)	1990 (30)	1989 (24)	2009 (25)
Median centile maximum urine flow rate (MUFR)	32	31	50	15
Median centile average urine flow rate (AUFR)	26	26	50	

with pressure catheters varying from 6 FG (microtranducer) to 10 FG (water-filled). By necessity, potentially unfavorable environmental and psychological factors are introduced when catheterization flowmetry is performed. Ryall and Marshall (29) suggested that the reduction is maximum urinary flow rate caused by the fine (diameter = 2 mm) urethral catheter used in their study of 147 symptomatic men was of the order of several milliliter per second. Though small, this reduction was enough to change the diagnostic categorization of one-third of their subjects.

Normal Male Vs. Normal Female Urine Flow Rates

Female urine flow rates are higher than those of men (10,15,24). Female maximum urine flow rates are on average 0.19 times greater than those of young men and 0.39 times greater than the older men (24). Urethral length (4 cm vs. 20 cm) should account for all the intersex difference (10,24).

URINE FLOW RATES IN WOMEN WITH SYMPTOMS OF PELVIC FLOOR DYSFUNCTION

Between 1958 and 1990, there were four studies on urine flow rates in symptomatic women (those with symptoms of pelvic floor dysfunction), three of which were small (15,16,21). The other study (30) was limited to the effect of final urodynamic diagnosis on urine flow rates. Three studies indicated that symptomatic women had slower urine flow rates than normal women with one study (15) showing no difference. In 1999, Haylen et al. (31) completed a study of 250 women who were consecutive referrals for urogynecological assessment with symptoms of pelvic floor dysfunction. The flow data for these women were converted to centiles from the Liverpool nomograms for the following analyses of their median values.

A Comparison of the Urine Flow Rates of Symptomatic and Asymptomatic Women

Table 49.1 shows that the median centiles of the maximum and average urine flow rates of the urogynecology (symptom-

atic) patients were significantly reduced from those of the asymptomatic population. There was close agreement between the studies with the 1990 study (30) performed in a different country to the 1999 study (31).

As noted, Barapatre et al.'s (25) 2009 study gives results for urine flow rate centiles in asymptomatic women far slower than equivalent studies in either asymptomatic or symptomatic women.

Effect of the Presence of Genital Prolapse on Urine Flow Rates in Symptomatic Women

A generally progressive decline in the maximum and average urine flow rates (median centiles) of symptomatic women (31) with increasing grades of genital prolapse was noted. The most significant decline occurred in the presence of uterine prolapse closely followed by cystocoele and enterocoele. Recent unpublished data (Haylen et al.), however, would suggest the significance of this may be lost in multivariate analysis of a much larger cohort (1140) of symptomatic women.

Effect of Prior Hysterectomy on Urine Flow Rates in Symptomatic Women

A significant decline in the urine flow rates (31) of symptomatic women (median centiles) in the presence of a prior hysterectomy. The effect was the same with both vaginal and abdominal hysterectomy. The flow rates for those symptomatic women without prior hysterectomy was found to be the same as that for the asymptomatic female population. Further analysis suggests that in women with both prior hysterectomy and intercurrent genital prolapse, there is a cumulative decline in urine flow. Recent unpublished data (Haylen et al.), however, would suggest the significance of this may be lost in multivariate analysis of a much larger cohort of symptomatic women.

Effect of Age and Parity on Urine Flow Rates in Symptomatic Women

Unlike asymptomatic women, there is a significant effect of age on the maximum and average urine flow rates (30,31) in symptomatic women. Recent unpublished data (Haylen et al.) suggests that age is the main association of abnormally slow urine flow rates in a large cohort of symptomatic women. Parity was not found to be a significant factor in either this or the 1999 study (31).

Table 49.2 Effect of Final Urodynamic Diagnosis on the Urine Flow Rates of Symptomatic Women

Diagnosis	Number	MUFR	AUFR
Urodynamic Stress incontinence (USI)	107	48	40
Detrusor overactivityity (DO)	14	38	32
Voiding dysfunction (VD)	7	1	6
USI + DO	39	34	32
USI + VD	22	3	2
DO + VD	14	3	2
USI + VD + DO	10	4	7
Normal	7	70	52

Abbreviations: MUFR, median centile maximum urine flow rate; AUFR, median centile average urine flow rate.

Effect of Final Urodynamic Diagnosis on the Urine Flow Rates of Symptomatic Women

Median urine flow rate centiles of the urogynecology patients separated according to the final urodynamic diagnosis are given in Table 49.2. All categories of diagnoses have their median centiles under those for the normal female population (50 by definition).

VD appears to be the diagnosis for which urine flow rates might have the best discriminatory ability. Further analysis shows that the *10th centile of the Liverpool nomogram* (28,30,31) for the maximum urine flow rate has the best discriminatory ability (sensitivity 81%, specificity 92%) with respect to diagnosing the presence or absence of the final diagnosis of VD, either as a solitary or a mixed diagnosis.

Recent unpublished data on a large cohort of symptomatic women again showed the highest urine flow rate centiles in women with USI and DO and the lowest in women with VD.

OTHER FACTORS INFLUENCING URINE FLOW RATES

Urine flow depends on the relationship between the bladder and urethra during voiding. The situation during voiding is the antithesis of the situation required for continence. Continence depends on intraurethral pressure being higher than intravesical pressure. For voiding to occur intravesical pressure must exceed intraurethral pressure.

Einhorning (32) and later Asmussen and Ulmsten (33) showed clearly that before any rise in intravesical pressure, a fall in intraurethral pressure occurred. This suggests that the urethra actively relaxes during voiding rather than being passively "blown open" by the detrusor contraction. Soon after the urethra has relaxed and pelvic floor descent has occurred, the detrusor contracts. The detrusor normally contrives to contract until the bladder is empty, producing a continuous flow curve. Many women void by urethral relaxation alone with minimal or no detrusor involvement. This method of voiding is common in women with USI.

Changes in intra-abdominal pressure also influence urine flow. Some women appear to void entirely by increasing intra-abdominal pressure, that is, by contraction of the diaphragm and anterior abdominal wall muscles.

It follows from this discussion that the urine flow may differ from normal as a result of abnormalities of the urethra or the detrusor.

Urethral Factors

Anatomical Factors

The urethra may be abnormally narrow, or the urethra may not be straight. The narrowest part of the urethra, as shown by video studies of voiding, is usually the midzone. However, the urethra may become narrowed and the most common site is at the external meatus associated with oestrogen deficiency in the post-menopausal women. Bladder neck obstruction in the female is extremely rare (34). The female urethra is usually straight, and deviation from this state is most common in anterior vaginal wall prolapse and higher degrees of uterine and vaginal vault prolapse. Data above point to a possible adverse effect of such prolapse on urine flow rates.

Pathological Factors

Unusual congenital conditions such as urethral duplication, urethral diverticula, or urethral cysts may obstruct voiding. Infective lesions as in urethritis or infected paraurethral cysts may lead to voiding difficulties. Post-traumatic strictures and urethral neoplasms will have a similar effect. Intravaginal abnormalities, such as prolapse or foreign bodies, may also obstruct micturition.

Functional Factors

Abnormal urethral behavior during voiding may lead to alteration in the urine flow rate recording. Urethral closure may be due to contraction of the intraurethral striated muscle or to contraction of the pelvic floor. In the neurologically abnormal patient, contraction of the intraurethral striated muscle with or without the pelvic floor is known as detrusor sphincter dyssynergia. In the nervous and anxious but neurologically normal patient, the urethra may be closed by pelvic floor contraction.

Detrusor Factors

Contractility

It is well known that when neurological disease occurs, bladder behavior may be altered. However, in patients with no neurological disease, poor detrusor contractility may be responsible for a slow flow rate. Such patients may have UTI or urinary retention. These patients have normal urethral function as judged by pressure profilometry or radiology. Their reduced flow rates are secondary to a weak and poorly sustained detrusor contraction. A proportion of this clinical group go on to demonstrate classical neurological disease such as multiple sclerosis.

Innervation

Normal detrusor behavior depends on normal innervation. Bladder contractions are preserved if the sacral reflex arc is intact even when the upper motor neurons are damaged. However, if the sacral reflex arc is damaged, bladder contractions are generally absent. The only form of contractile activity possible when the lower motor neuron is damaged is locally mediated—the "autonomous" bladder. The urine flow rates produced by the abnormally innervated bladder are usually reduced and interrupted.

Pathological Factors

Although little specific literature on the subject exists, it is evident that gross disease of the detrusor will result in abnormal urine flow rates. The fibrosis resulting from irradiation, tuberculosis, cystitis, or interstitial cystitis is likely to impair detrusor contractility.

URINARY FLOW PATTERNS

Urine flow curves are complementary to flow rates in the assessment of voiding. Because flow curves cannot be numerically represented (except by urine flow rates), they are less useful for clinical comparisons than flow rates. Several patterns of flow curves can however be recognized.

Normal

The normal flow trace (Fig. 49.5A and B) shows a symmetrical peak with maximum flow rate generally achieved within five seconds of the beginning of voiding. The maximum flow rate is generally 1.5 to 2 times the average flow rate.

A low normal (suboptimal) flow trace (Fig. 49.6A) shows no symmetrical peak. Maximum flow rate, somewhere between the 5th and 25th centile, occurs early, then the flow trails off. An abdominal strain pattern (Fig. 49.6B) shows the influence of generally intermittent abdominal strain during the void. The manifests itself as irregular moderately fast accelerations in maximum urine flow. A high takeoff pattern (Fig. 49.6C) shows a very rapid acceleration to a high maximum flow rate. A higher incidence of such traces has been noted in both men and women with detrusor instability.

Abnormal–Continuous Flow

Urine flow curves reflected in flow rates below the fifth centile may generally be regarded as abnormal; abnormality can be suspected in those curves with flow rates between the 5th and 10th centile.

A reduced flow rate may be due either to a urethral obstruction or to a poor detrusor contraction (Fig. 49.7A and B). It is necessary to perform full pressure flow studies (voiding cystometry) to demonstrate the cause of a reduced urine flow rate.

Abnormal–Interrupted Flow

An abdominal pressure voiding pattern (Fig. 49.8A) is where abdominal straining provides the pressure behind the voiding. Little detrusor activity is present. Irregular interrupted peaks of flow is the result. Maximum urine flow rate is more than twice the average urine flow rate.

A voluntary sphincter contraction urine flow pattern (Fig. 49.8B) occurs as the anxious nervous patient closes her distal urethral sphincter mechanism. Flow rate may decrease or stop. Characteristically, the rate of change of flow rate is rapid, indicating sphincter closure. The fluctuations due to detrusor underactivity would be much slower than those seen here.

Detrusor sphincter dyssynergia is an involuntary phenomenon in which the expected coordination of the detrusor contraction and urethral relaxation is lost. Despite an effective detrusor contraction, the urethral mechanism remains closed for longer periods of time (up to several minutes). Detrusor sphincter dyssynergia may result in a large residual urine together with upper tract dilatation and renal failure and is often associated with repeated infection. Detrusor sphincter dyssynergia only occurs in neurologically abnormal patients, most classically in high spinal cord trauma. The flow rate produced by detrusor sphincter dyssynergia (Fig. 49.8C) is usually reduced and always interrupted.

PVR MEASUREMENT
Definition

The PVR is defined as the volume of urine remaining in the bladder at the completion of micturition (1).

Clinical Relevance

The PVR is a key marker of bladder function in terms of emptying ability. An abnormally high PVR, if confirmed by repeat measurement confirms the presence of VD. Voiding cystometry is needed to assist in determining the cause.

Accuracy of PVR Measurement

The accuracy of PVR measurement has not matched other urodynamic variables such as pressure and flow. Subsequent

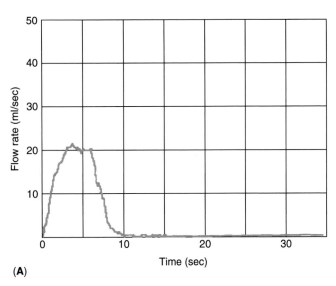

(A)

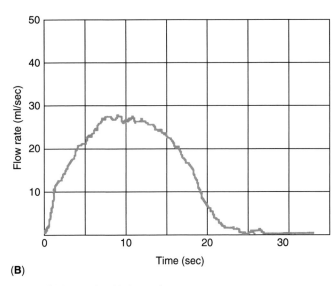

(B)

Figure 49.5 Normal flow curve for voided volume of (**A**) 121 ml and (**B**) 345 ml.

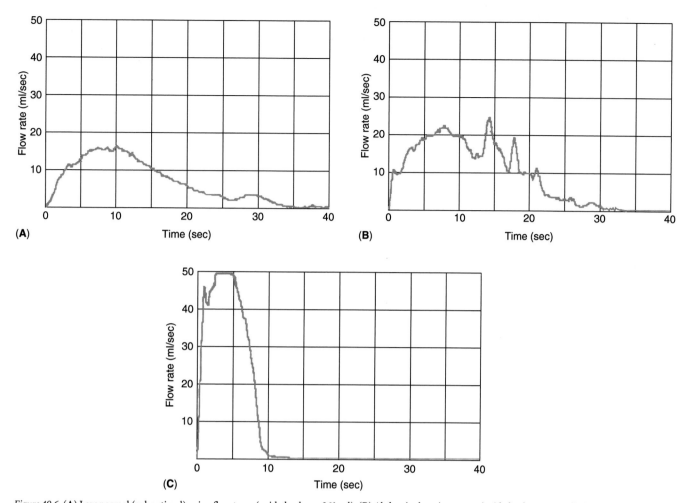

Figure 49.6 (**A**) Low normal (suboptimal) urine flow trace (voided volume 261 ml). (**B**) Abdominal strain pattern (voided volume 353 ml). (**C**) High takeoff urine flow pattern (voided volume 336 ml).

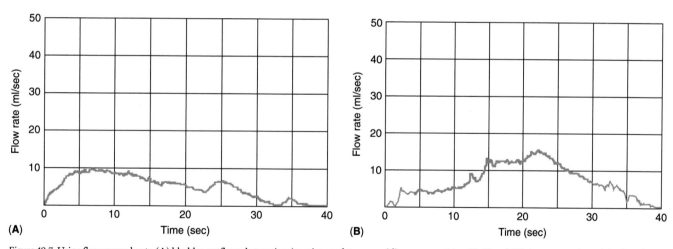

Figure 49.7 Urine flow curve due to (**A**) bladder outflow obstruction (maximum detrusor voiding pressure 54 cmH$_2$O) and (**B**) detrusor underactivity (maximum detrusor voiding pressure 15 cmH$_2$O).

discussion will show that best accuracies are around ±25% for methodologies, usually ultrasound, involving immediate measurement (within 60 sec). Those techniques (usually catheterization) involving delayed measurement can lead to errors, generally overestimation of many hundred percent.

Diuresis Factor

The main source of error in PVR measurement is the additional renal input into bladder volume from the delay in PVR measurement following micturition leading to an overestimation. Two factors can be multiplied to determine this input: (*i*)

505

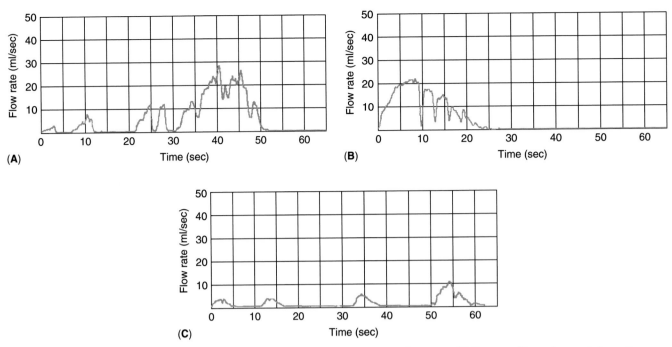

Figure 49.8 (**A**) Abdominal pressure voiding pattern. (**B**) Voluntary sphincter contraction urine flow pattern. (**C**) Detrusor sphincter dyssynergia flow pattern.

the diuresis (ml/min) occurring at the time this can be 1 to 14 ml/min (35,36), and (*ii*) the duration of the delay (min) between completion of micturition and PVR measurement (if the latter is by urethral catheterization, the end-point of the delay is the completion of bladder drainage). If both are excessive, the overestimation can be marked.

PVR Measurement by Catheterization

Urethral catheterization, the traditional approach to PVR measurement, is most vulnerable to the *diuresis factor*, as it takes 4.5 minutes minimum in studies (35,36) from the completion of micturition to the completion of bladder drainage using a catheter. Other factors are relevant as well.

Catheter Factor

For PVR measurement by urethral catheterization, the use of a catheter which incompletely drains the bladder will lead to an underestimation of the true PVR. A short plastic catheter (particularly a 14 FG though a 12 FG is probably also adequate), will make sure (36,37) that whatever PVR is present will be completely drained (under 1 ml post-catheterization bladder volume). A 14 FG Foley urethral catheter will leave, on average, 77 ml of post-catheterization bladder volume (36,37). Smaller Foley catheters than 14 FG can be expected to have an even higher post-catheterization bladder volume.

It is a quoted practice to enhance the drainage of a Foley catheter by suction drainage using a syringe. Whilst there is weak evidence that this might be helpful (38), the efficacy of this technique has not been proven. Similarly, small bore urodynamic filling catheters have been used to drain the bladder, though this may be relatively slow, thus increasing the delay in collection. There are no published data to confirm their efficacy in bladder drainage.

Measurement Apparatus Factor

Presuming the PVR collection occurs without delay, a catheter with known efficacy in bladder drainage is used and there is no PVR spillage, one has to rely on the accuracy of the measuring apparatus used which might have variable and often inappropriate (for the volume) and inaccurate calibration.

PVR Measurement by Ultrasound

Accuracy

Ultrasound techniques of known accuracy offer the best prospects of minimizing the above inaccuracies in PVR measurement, cost considerations allowing. The benefits of ultrasound for PVR measurement (known accuracy, reduced time, and patient trauma) need to be added to the increasing array of other indications for ultrasound in urogynecology [bladder neck assessment and intercurrent lower urinary tract and pelvic floor pathology, etc. (39)] when equipment costs are being considered. With ultrasound, all women with any PVR have the opportunity of a second attempt to reduce or clear this volume. This might avoid the need for subsequent repeat PVR measurements if surgery was being contemplated in a patient with an abnormally high PVR measured using urethral catheterization.

Abdominal Ultrasound

The use of this modality to measure bladder volumes dates back to 1967 (40). Different formulae have been used generally, using three bladder diameters, height, width, and depth [generally multiplied by a constant, with 0.625 commonly used (41)]. Results have been variable and conflicting (41) with accuracies limited by the variability in bladder shape and filling (42). Accuracies in most published series are around 21% to 25% (40–42). The key limitation of transabdominal ultrasound is the distance between the abdominal wall and the bladder, with fat (obesity), gas, and bone (shadowing of the pubis) potential impediments to the transmission of the sound beam. Smaller bladder volumes (under 100 ml) have been cited as more difficult to quantify with false negatives occurring under 50 ml (41). Advances in ultrasound technology will have improved visualization over time.

Transvaginal Ultrasound
This modality, first reported in 1989 (43), involves the calculation of bladder volumes using two bladder dimensions in the sagittal plane. It has been shown to provide accurate and validated (44) measurements of PVRs from 0 to 175 ml with superior visualization of PVR under 30 ml, where around 80% to 90% of PVR appear likely to occur (45,46). Accuracy is 24% (overall) and 15% (volumes 50 ml and over). Under 50 ml, the accuracy rises to 55%. Transrectal ultrasound was also reported in 1989 (47), using similar methodology to that for transvaginal ultrasound with a mean accuracy of 16%. Although its calibration was done only in men, it is possible to measure PVRs in women accurately using this modality. The accuracy of transperineal (translabial) ultrasound in PVR measurement needs to be researched. This modality is already used widely in urogynecology (39), with perhaps less specialized probes than used with transvaginal or transrectal ultrasound.

Doppler Planimetry
This alternate form of abdominal ultrasound has gained popularity in measuring PVRs. Commercial application had started in 1986 (48) with an early report in 1996 (49). The systems are small and portable with the technique for use quickly learned. Cross-sectional planes of the bladder are measured at 15° angular increments with the computer software constructing a 3-dimensional model of the bladder from which volume is determined. This form of PVR assessment has been shown to be accurate within 15% of bladder volumes as measured by urethral catheter within the range 0 to 999 ml (48,49). Reported limitations on its use are serious abdominal scars, uterine prolapse, and pregnancy (49,50) with false positives in cases of pelvic cysts (51).

Overall correlation of more recent models of doppler planimetry, the BME-150A (S & D Medicare Co, Seoul, Korea), and BladderScan BVI 3000 (Diagnostic Ultrasound Co., Bothell, WA, USA) with catheterized bladder volumes (12 FG latex rubber urethral catheter) were 0.92 and 0.94 respectively with a mean difference from true residual volume of 7.8 ml and 3.6 ml (52). Whilst both scanners were reported (52) to have good accuracy at low bladder volumes, like previous studies, exact sensitivities and accuracies for volumes under 100 ml have not been reported. Both types of bladder scanners do not have the other applications of conventional transabdominal, transvaginal, and transperineal ultrasound.

PVR Measurement by Other Methods
Not discussed here are those other possible methods of PVR assessment such as abdominal palpation and bimanual pelvic examination, which are imprecise. Radiology and radionucleotide scans have not gained favor as these techniques are more invasive, carry additional risks and also impractical in the settings outlined.

NORMAL AND ABNORMAL PVRS AND URINARY RETENTION
PVRs in Asymptomatic Women
Using transvaginal ultrasound (45) within 60 seconds of micturition, the upper limit of normal PVR (95th centile) is 30 ml. In a study with measurement delayed to up to 10 minutes, an upper limit of normal of 100 ml has been quoted (53).

PVRs in Symptomatic Women
Using transvaginal ultrasound (31,46), the upper limit of normal (87th centile) is 30 ml. Other studies quote higher figures of 50 ml (54), 100 ml (55), and 150 ml (56). All of the latter studies (54–56) used urethral catheterization with the post-micturitional delay in PVR measurement was (*i*) up to 10 minutes (55) and (*ii*) untimed (54,56).

Prevalence of Immediate PVRs in Symptomatic Women
In a recent study of 1140 women presenting with symptoms of pelvic floor dysfunction (46), Haylen et al. showed that the prevalence of the different immediate (measured by transvaginal ultrasound within 60 seconds of voiding) PVRs was: *0 to 10 ml–76%; 11 to 30 ml–5%; 31 to 50 ml–5%; 51 to 100 ml–8%; over 100 ml–6%; over 200 ml–2%.*

Combining the data from studies 31 and 46, *an upper limit of normal for PVRs (immediate measurement) in symptomatic women of 30 ml* is suggested.

Associations of Immediate PVRs in Symptomatic Women
The prevalence of PVRs over 30 ml was shown to increase significantly with *age* (p < 0.001) and *higher grades of prolapse* (p < 0.001). A PVR over 30 ml is associated with a significantly higher risk of *recurrent UTI* (p < 0.001). There is an inverse relationship between a PVR over 30 ml and the symptom of stress incontinence (p = 0.018) and the final diagnosis of USI (p < 0.001).

Acute Retention of Urine
This is defined as a generally (but certainly not always) painful, palpable, or percussable bladder, when the patient is unable to pass any urine when the bladder is full (1).

Chronic Retention of Urine
This defined as a non-painful bladder, where there is a chronic high PVR. From Haylen et al.'s study (51), 200 ml might be a reasonable "cut-off" for chronic retention.

FINAL DIAGNOSIS OF VD
Diagnosis of VD
As stated in the introduction, VD is defined as abnormally slow and/or incomplete micturition. This implies an abnormally slow urine flow rate and/or an abnormally high PVR. There should be confirmation by repeat measurement. Pressure–flow studies are indicated to evaluate the cause of any VD. Some possible causes are (*i*) detrusor underactivity, (*ii*) acontractile detrusor, and (*iii*) bladder outflow obstruction (1).

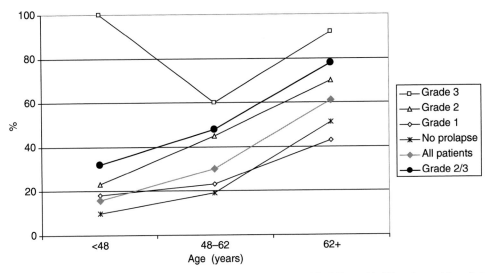

Figure 49.9 The relationship of VD-1 to age for (i) all patients; (ii) patients with grade 0 prolapse (final diagnosis); (iii) patients with grade 1 prolapse; (iv) patients with grade 2 prolapse; (v) patients with grade 3 (3–4) prolapse. *Abbreviation*: VD, voiding dysfunction.

Prevalence of VD

Depending on definition, VD has a prevalence of 14% (57) to 39% (58), and over 40% (54) the middle figure making it either the third or fourth most common urodynamic diagnosis (after USI, pelvic organ prolapse, and possibly DO).

Criteria for Diagnosis of VD

The only validated criteria to date are: (*i*) A urine flow rate under the 10th centile of the Liverpool nomogram; and/or (*ii*) An immediate PVR over 30 ml. Alternate suggested criteria of a PVR over 50 ml and a maximum urine flow rate under 15 ml/min require validation. More studies are required employing PVR criteria by urethral catheterization.

Associations of the Diagnosis of VD

The study of Haylen et al. (58) determined the following associations using the validated criteria in the above section. VD-1 uses the maximum urine flow rate; VD-2 uses the average urine flow rate.

- *Age*: There was a significant increase in the prevalence of VD with age (VD-1, VD-2: p < 0.001) (Fig. 49.9).
- *Parity*: There was a lesser but still significant increase with parity (VD-1, p = 0.010; VD-2, p = 0.014).
- *Presenting symptoms*: Symptoms of voiding difficulty (p < 0.001) and prolapse (p < 0.001) were significantly linked to VD-1, VD-2 with the symptom (p < 0.001) and sign (p <0.001) of stress incontinence significantly linked to NON VD-1, NON VD-2 (absence of voiding difficulty).
- *Prior hysterectomy*: There was a significant relationship of voiding difficulty to prior hysterectomy (VD-1, p = 0.006; VD-2, p = 0.053) and prior continence surgery (VD-1, p = 0.008; VD-2, p = 0.010), respectively. There was a greater increase in VD-1, VD-2 with vaginal hysterectomy compared with abdominal hysterectomy but the difference didn't reach significance.

- *Menopause*: Data initially showed that menopausal women on combined oestrogen/progesterone therapy had significantly less voiding difficulty than those not taking hormone replacement therapy. However, this effect was lost when age was taken into account.
- *Prolapse*: There is a significant relationship of voiding difficulty to increasing grades of uterine prolapse, anterior vaginal wall (cystocoele), posterior vaginal wall (rectocoele), and vaginal vault (enterocoele), respectively (p < 0.001 for VD-1 and VD-2 for all types of prolapse). Much of the relationship would be due to a PVR rather than a urine flow rate effect.
- *Retroverted uterus*: Relationship between the retroverted uterus and voiding difficulty was non-significant (p = 0.250).
- *Recurrent UTI*: There was no significant relationship between voiding difficulty [VD-1 (p = 0.213), VD-2 (p = 0.213)] and recurrent UTI. The strong relationship of PVRs and recurrent UTI noted above is not continued when urine flow rates are added to make the diagnosis of VD (urine flow rates appearing to have no significant association with recurrent UTI).

INDICATIONS TO SCREEN FOR VD

Uroflowmetry and a PVR measurement should be regarded as appropriate screening tests for VD in all women with symptoms of pelvic floor dysfunction.

Abnormal urine flow studies in female patients are less common than in male patients. This is because in the male patient a high proportion of lower urinary tract problems are related to bladder outflow obstruction. In the female, the incidence of outflow obstruction is low, whereas the incidence of incontinence and associated abnormalities of bladder behavior is high.

Urine flow studies and a PVR are preliminary to cystometry that is necessary to define the urodynamic abnormality responsible for the symptom complex of frequency, nocturia, urgency and urge incontinence. Anticholinergic medications will exacerbate any tendency towards urinary retention in patients with the combined diagnoses of DO and VD.

Urine flow studies and a PVR are an important preoperative investigation in women awaiting surgery USI. Assuming USI has been urodynamically proven, a normal urine flow rate and PVR reassures the surgeon that longterm VD are much less likely to follow the operation to cure the stress incontinence. Since effective surgery usually results in an increase in urethral resistance, in women with poor pre-operative flow rates, incomplete emptying or even persistent failure to void may follow surgery (59,60)]. Therefore, urine flow studies, with or without pressure flow studies (61), are to be recommended before surgery.

Voiding problems in patients with neuropathic lower urinary tract dysfunction consists of three main types. Patients may experience incontinence as a result of bladder instability. The main problem may be the failure to empty the bladder because of a poorly sustained detrusor contraction. Detrusor sphincter dyssynergia may prevent an effective detrusor contraction from emptying the bladder with the consequent possible complications of recurrent infections or renal failure. Urine flow studies may suggest the origin of the problems experienced by this group of patients, although video-pressure-flow studies are desirable in almost every case.

ACKNOWLEDGEMENTS

The contribution of Professor Paul Abrams to earlier chapters co-authored with the current author on uroflowmetry is acknowledged.

REFERENCES

1. Haylen BT, Freeman R, De Ridder D, et al. An International Urogynecological Association (IUGA)—International Continence Society (ICS) joint report on the terminology for female pelvic floor dysfunction. Int Urogynecol J 2010; 21: 5–26.
2. Haylen BT. Screening for voiding difficulties in women. MD Thesis. University of Liverpool. 1988: 105.
3. Rehfisch E. Ueben den mechanismus des harnblasenverschlusses under der harnentkerung. Virchow Arch Path Anat 1897; 150: 1111–51.
4. Ryall RL, Marshall VR. Measurement of urinary flow rate. Urology 1983; 22: 556–64.
5. Ballenger EG, Elder OF, McDonald HP. Voiding distance decrease as important early symptom of prostatic obstruction. South. Med. J 1932; 25: 863.
6. Drake WM. The uroflowmeter: an aid to the study of the lower urinary tract. J. Urol 1948; 59: 650–8.
7. Kaufman J. A new recording uroflowmeter: a simple automatic device for measuring voiding velocity. J. Urol 1957; 78: 97–102.
8. Von Garrelts B. Analysis of micturition: a new method of recording the voiding of the bladder. Acta Chir. Scand 1956; 112: 326.
9. Rowan D, McKenzie AL, McNee SG, Glen ES. A technical and clinical evaluation of the Disa uroflowmeter. Brit J Urol 1977; 49: 285–93.
10. Backman K-A, Von Garrelts B. Apparatus for recording micturition. Acta Chir Scand 1963; 126: 167–71.
11. Von Garrelts B, Strandell P. Continuous recording of urinary flow rate. Scand J Urol Nephrol 1972; 6: 224–7.
12. Rowan D, James ED, Kramer AEJL, et al. Urodynamic equipment: technical aspects. International Continence Society working party on urodynamic equipment. J Med Engin Techn 1987; 11: 57–64.
13. Moore KH, Richmond DH, Sutherst JR, et al. Crouching over the toilet seat: prevalence among British gynaecological outpatients and its effect upon micturition. Brit J Obstet Gynaecol 1991; 98: 569–72.
14. Marshall VR, Ryall RI, Austin ML, Sinclair GR. The use of urinary flow rates obtained from voided volumes less than 150 ml in the assessment of voiding ability. Brit J Urol 1983; 55: 28–33.
15. Drach GW, Ignatoff J, Layton T. Peak urine flow rate: observations in female subjects and comparison to male subjects. J Urol 1979; 122: 215–19.
16. Peter WP, Drake WM, Jr. Uroflowmetric observations in gynecologic patients. JAMA 1958; 166: 721–4.
17. Scott R, McIhlaney JG. Voiding rate in normal adults. J Urol 1961; 128: 429–32.
18. Backman K-A. Urinary flow during micturition in normal women. J Urol 1965; 137: 497–9.
19. Susset JG, Picker P, Kretz M, Jorest R. Clinical evaluation of uroflowmeters and analysis of normal curves. J Urol 1973; 109: 874–8.
20. Walter S, Olesen KP, Nordberg J, Hald T. Bladder function in urologically normal middle aged females. Scand J Urol Nephrol 1979; 13: 249–58.
21. Bottacini MR, Gleason DJ. Urodynamic norms in women: normals versus stress incontinents. J Urol 1980; 124: 659–61.
22. Fantl JA, Smith PJ, Schneider V, Hurt, et al. Fluid weight uroflowmetry in women. Am J Obstet Gynec 1982; 145: 1017–24.
23. Rollema HJ, Griffiths DJ, Jones U. Computer-aided uroflowmetry. Normal values in healthy women and applications in gynaecological patients. Proc Int Cont Soc London 1985; 210–11.
24. Haylen BT, Ashby D, Sutherst JR, et al. Maximum and average urine flow rates in normal male and female populations—the Liverpool nomograms. Brit J Urol 1989; 64: 30–8.
25. Barapatre Y, Agarwal MM, Singh SK, et al. Uroflowmetry in healthy women: Development and validation of flow-volume and corrected flow-age nomograms. Neurol Urodyn 2009; 28: 1003–9.
26. Jorgen B, Klaus M. Uroflowmetry. Urol Clin North Am 1996; 23: 237–42.
27. Ryall RL, Marshall VR. Normal peak urinary flow rate obtained from small voided volumes can provide a reliable assessment of bladder function. J Urol 1982; 127: 484–7.
28. Haylen BT, Yang V, Logan V. Uroflowmetry: its current clinical utility in women. Int Urogynecol J 2008; 19: 899–903.
29. Ryall RL, Marshall VR. The effect of a urethral catheter on the measurement of maximum urinary flow rate. J Urol 1982; 128: 429–32.
30. Haylen BT, Parys BT, Anyaegbunam WI, et al. Urine flow rates in male and female urodynamic patients compared with the Liverpool Nomograms. Brit J Urol 1990; 65: 483–7.
31. Haylen BT, Law MG, Frazer MI, Schulz S. Urine flow rates and residual urine volumes in urogynaecology patients. Int Urogynecol J 1999; 10: 378–81.
32. Einhorning G. Simultaneous recording of intravesical and intraurethral pressure. Acta Chir Scand Suppl. 1961; 276: 1–68.
33. Asmussen M, Ulmsten U. Simultaneous urethrocystometry with a new technique. Scand J Urol Nephrol 1976; 10: 7–11.
34. Turner-Warwick R, et al. A urodynamic view of the clinical problems associated with bladder neck dysfunction and its treatment by endoscopic incision and trans-trigonal posterior prostatectomy. Br J Urol 1973; 45: 44–59.
35. Haylen BT, Frazer MI, Sutherst JR, Ashby D. The accuracy of measurement of residual urine volumes in women by urethral catheterization. Brit J Urol 1989; 63: 152–4.
36. Haylen BT, Lee J. The accuracy of post-void residual measurement in women. Int Urogynecol J 2008; 19: 603–6.
37. Haylen BT, Frazer MI, MacDonald JH. Assessing the effectiveness of different urinary catheters in emptying the bladder: an application of transvaginal ultrasound. Brit J Urol 1989; 64: 353–6.

38. Stoller ML, Millard RJ. The accuracy of catheterized residual urine. J Urol 1989; 141: 15–16.

39. Tunn R, Schaer G, Peschers U, et al. Updated recommendations on ultrasonography in urogynecology. Int Urogynecol J 2005; 16: 236–41.

40. Holmes JH. Ultrasonic studies of the bladder. J Urol 1967; 97: 684–91.

41. Hakenberg OW, Ryall RL, Langlois SL, Marshall VR. The estimation of bladder volume by sonocystography. J Urol 1983; 130: 249–52.

42. Keily EA, Hartnell GG, Gibson RN, Williams G. Measurement of bladder volume by real-time ultrasound. Brit J Urol 1987; 60: 33–5.

43. Haylen BT, Frazer MI, Sutherst JR, West CR. Transvaginal ultrasound in the assessment of bladder volumes in women. Preliminary report. Br J Urol 1989; 64: 149–51.

44. Haylen BT. Verification of the accuracy and range of transvaginal ultrasound in measuring bladder volumes in women. Brit J Urol 1989; 64: 350–2.

45. Haylen BT. Residual urine volumes in a normal female population: application of transvaginal ultrasound. Br J Urol 1989; 64: 347–9.

46. Haylen BT, Lee J, Logan V, et al. Immediate postvoid residuals in women with symptoms of pelvic floor dysfunction. Obstet Gynecol 2008; 111: 1305–12.

47. Haylen BT, Parys BT, West CR. Transrectal ultrasound in the measurement of residual urine volumes in men. Neurourol Urodyn 1989; 8: 327–8.

48. Teng C-H, Huang Y-H, Kuo B-J, Bih L-I. Application of portable ultrasound scanners in the measurement of post-void residual urine. J Nurs Res 2005; 13: 216–23.

49. Coombes GM, Millard RJ. The accuracy of portable ultrasound scanning in the measurement of postvoid residual urine volume. J Urol 1996; 152: 2083–5.

50. Goode PS, Locher JL, Bryant RL, et al. Measurement of postvoid residual urine with portable transabdominal bladder ultrasound scanner and urethral catheterization. Int Urogynaecol J 2000; 11: 296–300.

51. Teng C-H, Huang Y-H, Kuo B-J, Bih L-I. Application of portable ultrasound scanners in the measurement of post-void residual urine. J Nurs Res 2005; 13: 216–23.

52. Choe JH, Lee JY, Lee K-S. Accuracy and precision of a new portable ultrasound scanner, the BME-150A, in residual urine volume measurement: a comparison with the bladderscan BV1 3000. Int Urogynecol J 2007; 18: 641–4.

53. Gehrich A, Stany MP, Fischer JR, et al. Establishing a mean postvoid residual volume in asymptomatic perimenopausal and postmenopausal women. Obstet Gynecol 2007; 110: 827–30.

54. Costantini E, Mearini E, Pajoncini C, et al. Uroflowmetry in female voiding disturbances. Neurourol Urodyn 2003; 22: 569–73.

55. Lukacj ES, DuHamel E, Menefee SA, Luber KM. Elevated postvoid residual in women with pelvic floor disorders: Prevalence and associated risk factors. Int Urogynecol J 2006; 18: 397–400.

56. Dwyer PL, Desmedt E. Impaired bladder emptying in women. Aust NZ J Obstet Gynaecol 1994; 34: 73–8.

57. Massey JA, Abrams PH. Obstructed voiding in the female. Brit J Urol 1988; 61: 36–9.

58. Haylen BT, Krishnan S, Schulz S, et al. Has the true prevalence of voiding difficulty in urogynecology patients been underestimated? Int Urogynecol J 2007; 18: 53–6.

59. Stanton SL, Cardozo L, Chaudhury N. Spontaneous voiding after surgery for urinary incontinence. Br J Obstet Gynaecol 1978; 83: 149–52.

60. Dawson T, Lawton V, Adams E, Richmond D. Factors predictive of post-TVT voiding dysfunction. Int Urogynecol J 2007; 18: 1297–1302.

61. Groutz A, Blaivas JG, Chaikin DC. Bladder outflow obstruction in women: Definition and characteristics. Neurourol Urodyn 2000; 19: 213–20.

50 Pathophysiological Mechanisms of Chronic Pelvic Pain
Ursula Wesselmann

INTRODUCTION

Chronic pelvic pain syndromes belong to the category of visceral pain. Pelvic pain is a debilitating problem that can significantly impair the quality of life of a woman. Patients with chronic pelvic pain are usually evaluated and treated by gynecologists, urologists, gastroenterologists, and internists. Although these patients seek medical care because they are looking for help to alleviate their pelvic discomfort and pain, in clinical practice much emphasis has been placed on finding a specific etiology and specific pathologic markers for pelvic disease. These patients typically undergo many diagnostic tests and procedures. However, often the examination and workup remain unrevealing and no specific cause of the pain can be identified. In these cases, it is important to recognize that pain is not only a symptom of pelvic disease, but that the patient is suffering from a chronic pelvic pain syndrome, where "pain" is the prominent symptom of the chronic visceral pain syndrome.

This chapter will focus on the neurobiology of chronic nonmalignant pelvic pain, a chronic visceral pain syndrome. Knowledge of the neurophysiologic characteristics of visceral pain will guide the physician in making a diagnosis of chronic pelvic pain and in differentiating it from the lump diagnosis of idiopathic pain (1). A basic understanding of neurobiology is paramount to gain further insights into the mechanisms of the pelvic pain disorders and to develop effective clinical management strategies for patients presenting with these syndromes.

DEFINITIONS OF CHRONIC PELVIC PAIN

Definitions are important if a body of reliable information which will eventually lead to a better understanding of the pathophysiology of chronic pelvic pain is to be built up in scientific literature (2). At present, one of the major problems of research into chronic pelvic pain is the lack of agreed definitions, which would allow comparison between studies. On the other hand, the lack of understanding of the pathophysiologic mechanisms of the pelvic pain syndromes makes it difficult to decide on criteria to define chronic pelvic pain conditions.

There is no generally accepted definition of chronic pelvic pain. The International Association for the Study of Pain (IASP) defines chronic pelvic pain without obvious pathology as chronic or recurrent pelvic pain that apparently has a gynecologic origin but for which no definitive lesion or cause is found (3). However, the IASP definition for pelvic pain has not been widely used in the literature (4). This definition implies absence of pathology, which might not necessarily be the case, and it also excludes cases where pathology is present although not necessarily the cause of pain. In fact, the relationship of pain to the presence of pathology is often unclear in women with chronic pelvic pain.

More recently, several medical societies have taken a lead in revising the definition of chronic pelvic pain. The International Continence Society has defined "pelvic pain syndrome" as the occurrence of persistent or recurrent episodic pelvic pain associated with symptoms suggestive of lower urinary tract, sexual, bowel, or gynecologic dysfunction in the absence of proven infection or other obvious pathology (5). The European Association of Urology has suggested extending this definition by considering two subgroups based on the presence or absence of well-defined conditions that produce pain (6). In the gynecologic literature, chronic pelvic pain is often referred to as pelvic pain in the same location for at least six months. The American College of Obstetricians and Gynecologists has proposed the following definition (7):

Chronic pelvic pain is non-cyclic pelvic pain of six or more months' duration that localizes to the anatomic pelvis, anterior abdominal wall at or below the umbilicus, the lumbosacral back, or the buttocks and is of sufficient severity to cause functional disability or lead to medical care. A lack of physical findings does not negate the significance of a patient's pain, and normal examination results do not preclude the possibility of finding pelvic pathology.

EPIDEMIOLOGY OF CHRONIC PELVIC PAIN

Chronic pelvic pain is a common condition. Epidemiologic data from the United States showed that 14.7% of women in their reproductive years reported chronic pelvic pain (8). Extrapolating to the total female population gave an estimated 9.2 million chronic pelvic pain sufferers in the United States alone. Analysis of a large primary care database from the United Kingdom demonstrated that the annual prevalence rate of chronic pelvic pain in women is 38/1000, which is comparable to the prevalence rate of asthma (9). Diagnoses related to the urinary or gastrointestinal tracts were more common than gynecologic causes (10). Irritable bowel syndrome (IBS) accounts for 12% of primary care visits and 28% of gastroenterological practice (11). While prevalence estimates vary widely, it has been suggested that somewhere between 450,000 (12) and one million people (13) in the United States suffer from interstitial cystitis (IC) or IC-like conditions. Using the Nurses' Health Study (NHS) I and II cohort as a study population the prevalence of IC in NHS II was reported as 67/100,000 and in NHS I as 52/100,000 (14). Recent preliminary data from the Rand IC Epidemiology Study reported at the 2009 American Urological Association Meeting showed a prevalence of women over 18 years of age in the United States who have symptoms compatible with painful bladder syndrome of 3.4 to 7.9 million, significantly higher than previous estimates (http://www.urotoday.com/49/browse_categories/icpbsbps/aua_2009_infectioninflammation_of_genitourinary_tract_ interstitial_cystitis_moderated_poster_session_highlights. html; accessed June 21, 2009). A recent WHO systematic review of the prevalence of chronic pelvic pain assessing the world-wide literature found, that the rate for dysmenorrhea was 16.8% to 81%, for dyspareunia 8% to 21.8% and for non-cyclic pelvic pain 2.1% to 24% (15). Not surprisingly the study found that there were few studies on chronic pelvic from less developed countries, and the variation of rates of chronic pelvic pain worldwide was due to variable study quality. Importantly, wherever valid data were available, a high disease burden of pelvic pain was documented. Despite a high prevalence of pain, many women never had the condition diagnosed (16). Populations at risk of having chronic pelvic pain seem to be women with a history of pelvic inflammatory disease, endometriosis, IC, IBS, obstetric history, previous abdominopelvic surgery, musculoskeletal disorders, and physical and sexual abuse (7).

INNERVATION OF THE PELVIS

Over the last 20 years, the basic neurobiology of the pelvis, despite the complexity of this region of the body, has come to be a reasonably well-developed discipline (17). This section provides an overview of the innervation of the pelvis, which is a prerequisite to understanding the functional mechanisms that might play a role in the neuropathology of chronic pelvic pain. It is important to note that this summary attempts to derive as much information as possible from investigations involving humans although some generalizations are necessarily taken from animal studies, recognizing that much research in this field is in its infancy.

In general, the pelvis and the pelvic floor are innervated by both divisions of the autonomic nervous system (the sympathetic and parasympathetic), as well as by the somatic and sensory nervous systems. In a broad anatomic view, dual projections from the thoracolumbar and sacral segments of the spinal cord carry out this innervation, converging primarily into discrete peripheral neuronal plexuses before distributing nerve fibers throughout the pelvis (Fig. 50.1). Interactive neuronal pathways routing from higher origins in the brain through the spinal cord add to the complexity of neuronal regulation in the pelvis.

The nomenclature of the various plexuses, ganglia, and nerves in the pelvic cavity (19) is varied and sometimes confusing, presenting designations from both Nomina Anatomica (1977) and clinical usage (20). In this chapter the anatomic nomenclature is provided, and the clinical usage is given in brackets: superior hypogastric plexus (presacral nerve), hypogastric plexus (hypogastric nerve), inferior hypogastric plexus (pelvic plexus), and pelvic splanchnic nerve (pelvic nerve).

Within the pelvis, the inferior hypogastric plexus (pelvic plexus) is regarded as the major neuronal integrative center. This plexus is located retroperitoneally adjacent to each lateral aspect of the rectum, with interconnections between the left and right inferior hypogastric plexuses at the posterior aspect of the rectum. It innervates multiple pelvic organs, including the urinary bladder, proximal urethra, distal ureter, rectum, and internal anal sphincter, as well as genital and reproductive tract structures (21). The anterior part of the inferior hypogastric plexus, associated with the distal extent of the hypogastric plexus (hypogastric nerve), is referred to as the paracervical ganglia in females (22).

The inferior hypogastric plexus receives sympathetic and parasympathetic input. Sympathetic nerves originate in the thoracolumbar segments of the spinal cord (T10-L2) and condense into the superior hypogastric plexus (presacral nerve) located just inferior to the aortic bifurcation. Preganglionic efferents originate largely in the intermediolateral cell column whereas afferents have their cell bodies located in dorsal root ganglia of these segments. Nerve fibers project from the superior hypogastric plexus as paired hypogastric plexuses (hypogastric nerves) and fuse distally before diverging bilaterally into branches destined for the inferior hypogastric plexuses. Additional sympathetic innervation to pelvic organs may involve preganglionic nerves, which synapse on post-ganglionic nerves originating in sympathetic chain ganglia; these postganglionic nerves join sacral nerves and course to their destinations via pelvic somatic neuronal pathways (23). Parasympathetic preganglionic nerve efferents are thought to arise from cell bodies of the sacral parasympathetic nucleus located in the sacral spinal cord (S2–S4) and fuse as the pelvic splanchnic nerve (pelvic nerve) before entering the inferior hypogastric plexus (24). Parasympathetic afferents have cell bodies located in the S2–S4 dorsal root ganglia and course also within the pelvic splanchnic nerve. In addition to its parasympathetic efferent and afferent component, the pelvic splanchnic nerve also receives postganglionic axons from the caudal sympathetic chain ganglia (25).

Somatic efferent and afferent innervation to the pelvis is generally understood to involve the sacral nerve roots (S2–S4) and their ramifications. Somatic efferents arise within Onuf's nucleus situated in the ventral horn of the S2–S4 spinal cord, and afferents reach the dorsal horn with their cell bodies in dorsal root ganglia of these segments (26). Central projections of somatic afferents overlap with pelvic nerve afferents within the spinal cord, which theoretically allows coordination of somatic and visceral motor activity (23). The sacral nerve roots emerge from the spinal cord forming the sacral plexus, from which the pudendal nerve diverges (S2–S3). The pudendal nerve also receives postganglionic axons from the caudal sympathetic chain ganglia.

Nociception and pain arising from within the pelvis and pelvic floor involve diverse neuronal mechanisms. In general, sensations from the pelvic viscera are conveyed within the sacral afferent parasympathetic system, with a far lesser afferent supply from thoracolumbar sympathetic origins (27). Receptive fields in the perineum are understood to be carried out primarily by sensory–motor discharges associated with pudendal nerve afferents (27,28). While the interactions of sensory afferents are quite complex, likely possibilities by which these pathways exert effects on autonomic efferent function include mediatory effects on spinal cord reflexes and modulatory effects on efferent release in peripheral autonomic ganglia and in peripheral organs. These neural structures in the periphery comprise the first of numerous relays of sensory neurons, which transmit painful sensations from the abdominal/pelvic cavity to the brain.

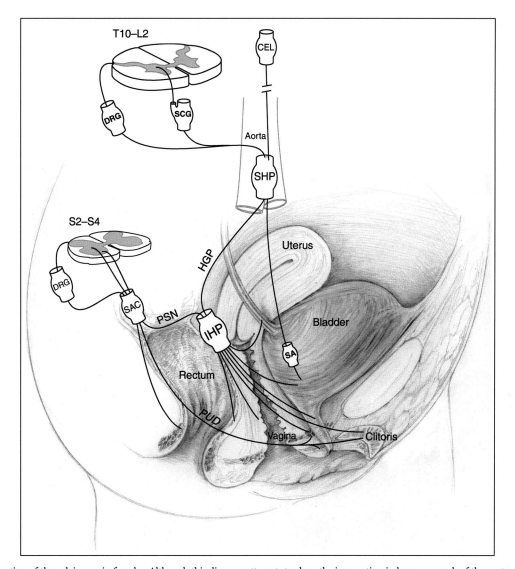

Figure 50.1 Innervation of the pelvic area in females. Although this diagram attempts to show the innervation in humans, much of the anatomic information is derived from animal data. *Abbreviations*: CEL, celiac plexus; DRG, dorsal root ganglion; HGP, hypogastric plexus; IHP, inferior hypogastric plexus; PSN, pelvic splanchnic nerve; PUD, pudendal nerve; SA, short adrenergic projections; SAC, sacral plexus; SCG, sympathetic chain ganglion; SHP, superior hypogastric plexus. *Source*: Reproduced from Ref. (18) with permission of the International Association for the Study of Pain.

Traditionally it was thought that ascending pathways for visceral and other types of pain were mainly the spinothalamic and spinoreticular tracts. However, three previously undescribed pathways that carry visceral nociceptive information have been discovered: the dorsal column pathway, the spino(trigemino)-parabrachio-amygdaloid pathway, and the spino-hypothalamic pathway (29). Specifically, the dorsal column pathways play a key role in the processing of pelvic pain, and neurosurgeons have successfully used punctate midline myelotomy to relieve pelvic pain due to cancer (30). In addition, descending facilitatory influences may contribute to the development of maintenance of hyperalgesia, thus contributing to the development of chronic pelvic pain (31).

DIFFERENCES BETWEEN VISCERAL AND SOMATIC PAIN
Persistent pain of visceral origin is a much greater clinical problem than that from skin, but the overwhelming

focus of experimental work on pain mechanisms relates to cutaneous sensation. Until relatively recently, it was often assumed that concepts derived from cutaneous studies could be transferred to the visceral domain. However, there are several reasons to believe that the neural mechanisms involved in pain and hyperalgesia of the skin are different from the mechanisms involved in painful sensations from the viscera (32,33). In contrast to somatic pain, visceral pain cannot be evoked from all viscera and is not always linked to visceral tissue injury (see "Visceral Nociceptors and Sensitization," below). In addition, visceral pain tends to be diffuse and poorly localized, whereas somatic pain can be localized exactly. This is due to the fact that the visceral innervation is not as dense as the somatic innervation and that there is an extensive divergence in the central nervous system (CNS). Further, visceral pain can be referred to other visceral structures and somatic structures of the same segmental level (see "Referred Visceral Pain Mechanisms," below).

Visceral Nociceptors and Sensitization

The existence of visceral nociceptors has been debated for a long time. This is partially due to the difficulty of defining and applying physiologically relevant noxious stimuli to the viscera. Research in animal models of visceral pain has shown that several types of sensory receptor exist in most internal organs, and that different pain states are mediated by different neurophysiologic mechanisms (34). Acute, brief visceral pain appears to be triggered initially by the activation of high-threshold visceral afferents and by the high-frequency bursts that these stimuli evoke in intensity coding afferent fibers, which are afferents with a range of responsiveness in the innocuous and noxious ranges. However, more prolonged forms of visceral stimulation, including those leading to hypoxia and inflammation of the tissue, result in sensitization of high-threshold receptors and the bringing into play of previously unresponsive afferent fibers (silent nociceptors; see below). This increased afferent activity enhances the excitability of central neurons and leads to the development of persistent pain states. In addition, a special class of C-fiber nociceptors—mechano-insensitive or "silent" nociceptors—has been found in nearly all tissues. They were first described in an animal model of experimental arthritis (35) and subsequently in animal models of visceral pain (36). Silent afferents are activated only in the presence of tissue damage or inflammation. Following release of injury products, these previously silent receptors are activated by a wide range of thermal and mechanical stimuli and may also have a background discharge.

Referred Visceral Pain Mechanisms

There are two components of visceral pain, both of which were described more than 100 years ago (37); "true visceral pain" (deep visceral pain arising from inside the body) and "referred visceral pain" (pain that is referred to segmentally related somatic and also other visceral structures). Secondary hyperalgesia usually develops at the referred site (38). A number of explanations have been offered for the existence of referred pain (33). An initial model for interpreting referred pain was based on the idea of viscerosomatic convergence occurring in primary afferent fibers, with multiple branches innervating both viscera and somatic structures. This hypothesis is unlikely, since few branching axons have been found in animal studies. In addition, the hypothesis does not explain the time delay in the evolution of referred pain.

Another suggested mechanism for referred pain is that visceral and somatic primary neurons converge onto common spinal neurons. This is the convergence–projection theory. There is considerable experimental evidence for this hypothesis. It offers a ready explanation for the segmental nature of referred pain, but does not address explicitly the issue of hyperalgesia in the referred zone. To interpret "referred pain with hyperalgesia," two main theories have been proposed, which are not mutually exclusive. The first is known as the convergence-facilitation theory. It proposes that the abnormal visceral input would produce an irritable focus in the relative spinal cord segment, thus facilitating messages from somatic structures. The second theory postulates that the visceral afferent barrage induces the activation of a reflex arc whose afferent branch is presented by visceral afferent fibers and the efferent branch by somatic efferents and sympathetic efferents toward the somatic structures (muscle, subcutis, and skin). The efferent impulses towards the periphery would then sensitize nociceptors in the parietal tissues of the referred area, thus resulting in the phenomenon of hyperalgesia.

When examining and treating a woman with chronic pelvic pain it is important to consider both aspects of the pain syndrome (true and referred pain), including the pain deep in the pelvic cavity and pain referred to somatic structures (lower back and legs) and other visceral organs. Considering the concept of referred visceral pain will allow the physician to look at the global picture of visceral dysfunction, rather than "chasing" one aspect of the visceral pain syndrome out of context.

COMORBIDITIES AND PELVIC PAIN

Careful clinical history and examination show, that patients with pelvic pain often suffer from "more than one pain." These clinical observations are supported by epidemiological studies. Data from the Interstitial Cystitis Data Base Study (39) show that 93.6 % of the patients enrolled with a diagnosis of IC reported having some pain in some part of their body. Of the patients having pain, 80.4%, 73.8%, 65.7%, and 51.5% reported having pain in their lower abdomen, urethra, lower back, and vaginal area, respectively. There is substantial overlap observed between chronic pelvic pain and other abdominal and urogenital symptoms (16,40,41). These observations could be explained pathophysiologically by referred visceral pain mechanisms to other visceral and somatic areas with overlapping spinal cord projections. In addition, there is increasing clinical and epidemiological evidence of the co-occurrence of chronic pelvic pain conditions with chronic pain syndromes in other "non-pelvic" body areas (e.g., fibromyalgia), raising the question of systemic alterations of pain modulatory mechanisms in this patient population (42). Thus, research efforts to elucidate the pathophysiological mechanisms of pelvic pain have recently shifted from an organ-based approach to a more global approach (http://www3.niddk.nih.gov/fund/other/UrologicPainSynd/; accessed July 30, 2008).

PHARMACOLOGIC ASPECTS

Despite the fact that it is a very common chronic pain syndrome, very little is known about effective pharmacologic treatment for chronic pelvic pain (43–45). Pharmacological pain management is empirical only. Often drugs are used to alleviate chronic pelvic pain, which have shown efficacy for the treatment of chronic neuropathic pain states (45). Very few drugs have been specifically approved for the treatment of chronic pelvic pain syndromes. An example is Elmiron (pentosan polysulfate sodium), which is indicated for the relief of bladder pain or discomfort associated with IC. Controlled clinical trials are desperately needed to design improved pharmacologic treatment strategies.

The principal guidelines for pharmacologic pain management for chronic pelvic pain are similar to the pharmacologic treatment of other chronic pain states. Although clinical trials and case reports on the pharmacologic management of chronic pain syndromes provide general guidelines as to which drug to

514

choose, currently we have no method to predict which drug is most likely to alleviate pain in a given patient. The goal of pharmacotherapy is to find a medication that provides significant pain relief with minimal side effects. It is important that the patient understands the limitations of this "trial and error" method of prescribing drugs. Adequate trials should be performed for each drug prescribed and only one drug should be titrated at a time, otherwise it is not possible to assess the effects of a certain drug on pain scores. The starting dose should always be the smallest available and titration should occur at frequent intervals, guided by pain scores, and side effects. This requires frequent contact between the patient and the pain clinic during the titration period. It is important for the patient and the physician to understand that some side effects actually improve as the patient continues to take the drug for several weeks. If these side effects are not intolerable, the patient should be guided through this period.

Since epidemiologic data have confirmed the widespread existence of chronic pelvic pain in the female population in the last 15 years, there is growing interest in the pharmaceutical industry to expand basic science and clinical research efforts for this underserved patient population. Several receptor targets have been identified in the pelvis and urogenital tract, which might play a role in pelvic pain (46). The mammalian transient receptor potential (TRP) family consists of six different classes. They play a role in sensing mechanisms throughout the body. TRPV1, TRPV2, TRPV4, TRPM8, and TRPA1 have been identified in the urogenital tract so far (47–49). Pharmacological interventions targeting these ion channels might provide a new opportunity for painful bladder syndrome and other chronic pelvic pain syndromes (47,50,51). Prostaglandins are synthesized in response to tissue injury by cyclooxygenase. They sensitize sensory fibers to mechanical and thermal stimuli and contribute to spinal processing of visceral pain (52). Cytokines and other neuroactive substances associated with inflammation also have a clear role in visceral inflammatory pain states. N-methyl D-aspartate (NMDA) receptors are expressed in primary afferents and in dorsal horn neurons. Intrathecal application of NMDA and non-NMDA receptor antagonists significantly attenuate visceral hypersensitivity in behavioral models, and spinal application of NMDA agonists increases the magnitude and duration of visceral pain responses (53,54). ATP is released from all tissue types when there is tissue damage. In visceral tissue, ATP binds ionotropic puringergic (P2X) receptors. P2X3 receptors are specific for nociceptors and P2X receptor antagonists attenuate colonic afferent activity (55–57). ATP, released from bladder urothelium, binds P2X3 receptors on bladder afferents increasing bladder contraction and micturition (58,59). This also increases bladder afferent activity resulting in pain. P2X3 knockout mice have urinary bladder hyporeflexia with increased voiding volume and decreased voiding frequency and decreased inflammatory pain (60,61). The corticotropin releasing factor (CRF) receptor is involved in the stress response, activating the hypothalamic–pituitary–adrenal (HPA) and sympatho-adrenal axes. Women with chronic pelvic pain demonstrate HPA axis alterations similar to patients with other stress-related bodily disorders (62). Enhanced pelvic responses

to stressors have been demonstrated in CRF-overexpressing mice (63). Opioids constitute a major class of analgesics to treat visceral pain. Nociceptin–orphanin receptor agonists have been used in preclinical models of pelvic pain with promising potential for therapeutic effects. This anti-hyperalgesic effect does not involve a CNS site of action (64). In summary, modulation of visceral nociceptive pathways can occur at peripheral, spinal, and supraspinal sites. There is a concerted effort underway to develop target-specific visceral analgesics for the treatment of chronic pelvic pain (65). A key issue for the success of future clinical trials will be improved patient phenotyping to identify subgroups of patients with chronic pelvic pain, based on aspects such as clinical symptoms, quantitative sensory testing parameters, biomarkers, and co-morbid conditions.

CLINICAL IMPLICATIONS

Treating patients with chronic pelvic pain remains a significant clinical challenge. Given the many co-morbidities observed in this patient population, it will be important to identify which patients will be at risk to develop other chronic pain syndromes and to design strategies for early intervention. As the pathophysiologic mechanisms of visceral pain explored in basic science research provide an explanation for some of the clinical phenomena observed in patients, additional, revived, and new concepts of chronic pelvic pain have emerged:

1. a spectrum of different insults might lead to chronic pelvic pain;
2. different underlying pathogenic pain mechanisms may require different pain treatment strategies for patients presenting with pelvic pain; and
3. multiple different pathogenic pain mechanisms may coexist in the same patient presenting with chronic pelvic pain, requiring several different pain treatment strategies (perhaps concomitantly) to treat visceral pain successfully (44).

These are very exciting times for the field of pelvic pain, since pelvic nociceptive pathways are being identified and pharmacological compounds are being discovered to modulate visceral nociceptive pathways. There is hope that these advances in research of the neurobiology of pelvic pain will translate into better clinical pain management options in the near future.

ACKNOWLEDGMENTS
Ursula Wesselmann is supported by NIH grants DK066641 (NIDDK), HD39699 (NICHD, Office of Research for Women's Health), and the National Vulvodynia Association.

REFERENCES
1. Wesselmann U. Guest editorial: pain—the neglected aspect of visceral disease. Eur J Pain 1999; 3: 189–91.
2. Wesselmann U, Baranowski AP. Classifications and definitions of urogenital pain. In: Baranowski AP, Abrams P, Fall M, eds. Urogenital Pain in Clinical Practice. . New York: Informa Healthcare, 2008: 3–15.
3. Merskey H, Bogduk N. Classification of Chronic Pain. Seattle: IASP Press, 1994.
4. Campbell F, Collett BJ. Chronic pelvic pain. Br J Anaesth 1994; 73: 571–3.

5. Abrams P, Cardozo L, Fall M, et al. The standardisation of terminology of lower urinary tract function: report from the Standardisation Sub-committee of the International Continence Society. Neurourol Urodyn 2002; 21: 167–78.

6. Fall M, Baranowski AP, Fowler CJ, et al. EAU guidelines on chronic pelvic pain. Eur Urol 2004; 46: 681–9.

7. ACOG Practice Bulletin No. 51. Chronic pelvic pain. Obstet Gynecol 2004; 103: 589–605.

8. Mathias SD, Kuppermann M, Liberman RF, et al. Chronic pelvic pain: prevalence, health-related quality of life, and economic correlates. Obstet Gynecol 1996; 87: 321–7.

9. Zondervan KT, Yudkin PL, Vessey MP, et al. Prevalence and incidence of chronic pelvic pain in primary care: evidence from a national general practice database. Br J Obstet Gynaecol 1999; 106: 1149–55.

10. Zondervan KT, Yudkin PL, Vessey MP, et al. Patterns of diagnosis and referral in women consulting for chronic pelvic pain in UK primary care. Br J Obstet Gynaecol 1999; 106: 1156–61.

11. Hahn B, Yan S, Strassels S. Impact of irritable bowel syndrome on quality of life and resource use in the United States and United Kingdom. Digestion 1999; 60: 77–81.

12. Slade D, Ratner V, Chalker R. A collaborative approach to managing interstitial cystitis. Urology 1997; 49: 10–13.

13. Jones CA, Nyberg LM. Epidemiology of interstitial cystitis. Urology 1997; 49(Suppl 5A): 2–9.

14. Curhan GC, Speizer FE, Hunter DJ, et al. Epidemiology of interstitial cystitis: a population based study. J Urol 1999; 161: 549–52.

15. Latthe P, Latthe M, Say L, et al. WHO systematic review of prevalence of chronic pelvic pain: a neglected reproductive health morbidity. BMC Public Health 2006; 6: 177.

16. Zondervan KT, Yudkin PL, Vessey MP, et al. Chronic pelvic pain in the community—symptoms, investigations, and diagnoses. Am J Obstet Gynecol 2001; 184: 1149–55.

17. Burnett AL, Wesselmann U. History of the neurobiology of the pelvis. Urology 1999; 53: 1082–9.

18. Wesselmann U, Burnett AL, Heinberg LJ. The urogenital and rectal pain syndromes. Pain 1997; 73: 269–94.

19. Dail WG. Autonomic innervation of male reproductive genitalia. In: Maggi CA, ed. Nervous Control of the Urogenital System. Chur, Switzerland: Harwood Academic, 1993: 69–101.

20. Baljet B, Drukker J. The extrinsic innervation of the pelvic organs in the female rat. Acta Anat (Basel) 1980; 107: 241–67.

21. Burnstock G. Innervation of bladder and bowel. In: Bock G, Whelan J, eds. Neurobiology of Incontinence. Ciba Foundation Symposium. Chichester: Wiley, 1990: 2–26.

22. Janig W, McLachlan EM. Organization of lumbar spinal outflow to distal colon and pelvic organs. Physiol Rev 1987; 67: 1332–404.

23. McKenna KE, Nadelhaft I. The organization of the pudendal nerve in the male and female rat. J Comp Neurol 1986; 248: 532–49.

24. Nadelhaft I, Booth AM. The location and morphology of preganglionic neurons and the distribution of visceral afferents from the rat pelvic nerve: a horseradish peroxidase study. J Comp Neurol 1984; 226: 238–45.

25. de Groat WC. Neurophysiology of the pelvic organs. In: Rushton DN, ed. Handbook of Neuro-urology. New York: Marcel Dekker, 1994: 55–93.

26. Lincoln J, Burnstock G. Autonomic innervation of the urinary bladder and urethra. In: Maggi CA, ed. Nervous Control of the Urogenital System. Chur, Switzerland: Harwood Academic, 1993: 33–68.

27. Jänig W, Koltzenburg M. Pain arising from the urogenital tract. In: Maggi CA, ed. Nervous Control of the Urogenital System. Chur, Switzerland: Harwood Academic, 1993: 525–78.

28. de Groat WC, Booth AM, Yoshimura N. Neurophysiology of micturition and its modification in animal models of human disease. In: Maggi CA, ed. Nervous Control of the Urogenital System. Chur, Switzerland: Harwood Academic, 1993: 227–90.

29. Cervero F, Laird JMA. Visceral pain. Lancet 1999; 353: 2145–8.

30. Willis WD, Westlund KN. The role of the dorsal column pathway in visceral nociception. Curr Pain Headache Rep 2001; 5: 20–6.

31. Gebhart GF. Descending modulation of pain. Neurosci Biobehav Rev 2004; 27: 729–37.

32. Gebhart GF. Visceral nociception: consequences, modulation and the future. Eur J Anesthesiol 1995; 12: 24–7.

33. McMahon SB, Dmitrieva N, Koltzenburg M. Visceral pain. Br J Anaesth 1995; 75: 132–44.

34. Cervero F, Jänig W. Visceral nociceptors: a new world order? Trends Neurosci 1992; 15: 374–8.

35. Schaible HG, Grubb BD. Afferent and spinal mechanisms of joint pain. Pain 1993; 55: 5–54.

36. Häbler HJ, Jänig W, Koltzenburg M. A novel type of unmyelinated chemo-sensitive nociceptor in the acutely inflamed urinary bladder. Agents Actions 1988; 25: 219–21.

37. Head H. On disturbances of sensation with special reference to the pain of visceral disease. Brain 1893; 16: 1–113.

38. Giamberardino MA, Vecchiet L. Experimental studies on pelvic pain. Pain Reviews 1994; 1: 102–15.

39. Simon LJ, Landis JR, Erickson DR, et al. The interstitial cystitis data base study: concepts and preliminary baseline descriptive statistics. Urology 1997; 49(Suppl 5A): 64–75.

40. Alagiri M, Chottiner S, Ratner V, et al. Interstitial cystitis: unexplained associations with other chronic disease and pain. Urology 1997; 49(Suppl 5A): 52–7.

41. Chung MK, Chung RR, Gordon D, Jennings C. The evil twins of chronic pelvic pain syndrome: endometriosis and interstitial cystitis. JSLS 2002; 6: 311–14.

42. Clauw DJ, Schmidt M, Radulovic D, et al. The relationship between fibromyalgia and interstitial cystitis. J Psychiatr Res 1997; 31: 125–31.

43. Wesselmann U. Chronic pelvic pain. In: Turk DC, Melzack R, eds. Handbook of Pain Assessment. New York: Guilford Press, 2001: 567–78.

44. Wesselmann U. A call for recognizing, legitimizing and treating chronic visceral pain syndromes. Pain Forum 1999; 8: 146–50.

45. Chong MS, Hester J. Pharmacotherapy for neuropathic pain with special reference to urogenital pain. In: Baranowski AP, Abrams P, Fall M, eds. Urogenital Pain in Clinical Practice. New York: Informa Healthcare, 2008: 427–39.

46. Wesselmann U, Baranowski PA, Börjesson M, et al. Emerging therapies and novel approaches to visceral pain. Drug Discov Today: Ther Strategies 2009. In press.

47. Everaerts W, Gevaert T, Nilius B, et al. On the origin of bladder sensing: Tr(i)ps in urology. Neurourol Urodyn 2008; 27: 264–73.

48. Mukerji G, Yiangou Y, Corcoran SL, et al. Cool and menthol receptor TRPM8 in human urinary bladder disorders and clinical correlations. BMC Urol 2006; 6: 6.

49. Mukerji G, Yiangou Y, Agarwal SK, et al. Transient receptor potential vanil-loid receptor subtype 1 in painful bladder syndrome and its correlation with pain. J Urol 2006; 176: 797–801.

50. Lashinger ES, Steiginga MS, Hieble JP, et al. AMTB, a TRPM8 channel blocker: evidence in rats for activity in overactive bladder and painful bladder syndrome. Am J Physiol Renal Physiol 2008; 295: F803–10.

51. Araki I, Du S, Kobayashi H, et al. Roles of mechanosensitive ion channels in bladder sensory transduction and overative bladder. Int J Urol 2008; 15: 681–7.

52. Svensson CI, Yaksh TL. The spinal phospholipase-cyclooxygenase-prostanoid cascade in nociceptive processing. Annu Rev Pharmacol Toxicol 2002; 42: 553–83.

53. Rice AS, McMahon SB. Pre-emptive intrathecal administration of an NMDA receptor antagonist(AP-5) prevents hyper-reflexia in a model of persistent visceral pain. Pain 1994; 57: 335–40.

54. McRoberts JA, Coutinho SV, Marvizon JC, et al. Role of peripheral N-methyl-D-aspartate (NMDA) receptors in visceral nociception in rats. Gastroenterology 2001; 120: 1737–48.

55. Brierley SM, Carter R, Jones W 3rd, et al. Differential chemosensory function and receptor expression of splanchnic and pelvic colonic afferents in mice. J Physiol 2005; 567(Pt 1): 267–81.

56. Wynn G, Rong W, Xiang Z, et al. Puringergic mechanisms contribute to mechanosensory transduction in the rat colorectum. Gastroenterology 2003; 125: 1398–1409.

57. Page AJ, Martin CM, Blackshaw LA, et al. Vagal mechanoreceptors and chemoreceptors in mouse stomach and esophagus. J Neurophysiol 2002; 87: 2095–2103.

58. Rong W, Spyer KM, Burnstock G. Activation and sensitisation of low and high threshold afferent fibers mediated by P2X receptors in the mouse urinary bladder. J Physiol 2002; 541(Pt 2): 591–600.

59. Pandita RK, Andersson KE. Intravesical adenosine triphosphate stimulates the micturition reflex in awake, freely moving rates. J Urol 2002; 168: 1230–4.

60. Cockayne DA, Hamilton SG, Zhu QM, et al. Urinary bladder hyporeflexia and reduced pain-related behaviour in P2X3-deficient mice. Nature 2000; 407: 1011–15.

61. Burstock G. Purinergic P2 receptors as targets for novel analgesics. Pharmacol Ther 2006; 110: 433–54.

62. Heim C, Ehlert U, Hanker JP, et al. Abuse-related posttraumatic stress disorder and alterations of the hypothalamic-pituitary-adrenal axis in women with chronic pelvic pain. Psychosom Med 1998; 60: 309–18.

63. Million M, Wang L, Stenzel-Poore MP, et al. Enhanced pelvic responses to stressors in female CRF-overexpressing mice. Am J Physiol Regul Intergr Comp Physiol 2007; 292: R1429–38.

64. Agostini S, Eutamene H, Broccardo M, et al. Peripheral anti-nociceptive effect of nociceptin/orphanin FQ in inflammation and stress-induced colonic hyperalgesia in rats. Pain 2009; 141: 292–9.

65. Hobson AR, Aziz Q. Modulation of visceral nociceptive pathways. Curr Opin Pharm 2007; 7: 593–97.

51 Painful Bladder Syndrome/Interstitial Cystitis
Edward J Stanford and Candice Hinote

DEFINITION

Interstitial cystitis (IC) is a chronic bladder pain disorder mainly affecting women with no known etiology. IC is most consistently defined by symptoms of urinary frequency, urgency, and pain in the absence of urinary infection or other identified pathology. The most recent international definition is an unpleasant sensation (pain, pressure, discomfort), perceived to be related to the urinary bladder, associated with lower urinary tract symptoms of more than six months duration, in the absence of infection or other identifiable causes (1). Unfortunately, it remains a diagnosis of exclusion and hence there are no specific diagnostic physical signs, urologic findings, or laboratory tests that clearly diagnose IC (2,3). Past definitions used to describe gross anatomic changes on cystoscopy and mast cell characteristics from bladder biopsies coined the terms classic or ulcerative IC and non-ulcerative IC (4).

Most recently the term painful bladder syndrome (PBS)/IC has been commonly used together and these describe a chronic pelvic pain (CPP) condition with episodic pelvic pain involving the lower urinary tract, bowel, pelvic floor, or gynecologic organs. The International Continence Society defines PBS as suprapubic pain related to bladder filling, with increased daytime and night-time frequency in the absence of proven urinary infection, and other obvious pathology (5). The European Society for the study of IC (ESSIC) and the European Association of Urology define bladder pain syndrome (BPS) by pain in the bladder area increasing with bladder filling, urinary frequency, and nocturia. Pain may radiate to referred areas such as the groin, vagina, clitoris, rectum, sacrum, and pelvic floor, and may be relieved by voiding (6). Included in this definition is pelvic pain syndrome which refers to commonly associated gynecologic pain conditions such as endometriosis, irritable bowel syndrome (IBS), vulvar pain, and pelvic floor pain. The ESSIC further defines BPS as type 1 with no obvious pathology on biopsy or cystoscopy; type 2 shows histological changes on biopsy but no changes at cystoscopy; and type 3 in which obvious cystoscopic changes are seen.

HISTORICAL PERSPECTIVES

As early as 1836, Dr. Philip Syng Physick and his student Dr. Joseph Parrish are credited with describing the constellation of symptoms associated with IC: frequency, urgency, dysuria, and pelvic pain, referring to the disease entity as tic douloureux of the bladder. At that time, the major differential diagnosis was a bladder stone. The term IC first appeared in a textbook in 1886 by a New York Gynecologist A.J.C. Skene but became known due to the work of Guy Hunner from 1914 to 1918, in which he described the erythematous lesions called Hunner's ulcers. The diagnosis of these characteristic lesions then fell into disrepute until the 1960s, which was probably the result of the poor quality of the optical instruments available in the early 20th century. Cystoscopic diagnosis was therefore historically based until 1987 the National Institutes of Diabetes and Digestive and Kidney Diseases (NIDDK) of the National Institutes of Health established diagnostic criteria based on patient symptoms and cystoscopic findings under anesthesia (7) (Table 51.1). However, these criteria have now been largely abandoned in favor of symptom based diagnosis.

PATHOGENESIS OF IC

The exact pathogenesis of PBS/IC remains unknown and it is difficult to summarize the events leading to the ultrastructural changes seen on tissue specimens of the bladder. IC is multifactorial and involves structural, neurologic, immune, and endocrine processes (8,9).

Currently, the most plausible explanation appears to be that the protective urothelial barrier is disrupted allowing urinary caustic substances (primarily potassium) to stimulate urothelial, detrusor, and perivesical nerves leading to pain and the associated symptoms of urgency and frequency. Alternatively, an insult to the bladder may lead to an inflammatory response. Mast cell degranulation of histamines and other molecules appears to play a key role causing neurogenic inflammation. The episodic symptoms of IC and the association of autoimmune disorders such as systemic lupus erythematous and Sjogren's syndrome may indicate a genetic component and an abnormal immune response as a potential cause.

Bladder Epithelium/Glycosaminoglycan (GAG) Layer

Bladder biopsies of patients with IC may show denuded epithelium, ulceration, and submucosal inflammation none of which are pathognomonic for IC (10). In the healthy, non-IC bladder, the urothelium is impermeable due in part to a mucus layer consisting primarily of GAGs, chondroitin sulfate, and hyaluronate sodium. Protamine sulfate has been used to damage the urothelial barrier in animal and human studies (11,12). A defective bladder mucus lining leads to a dysfunctional uroepithelium with increased permeability through which the bladder is exposed to urine solutes such as allergens, chemicals, drugs, toxins, potassium, and bacteria. The GAG layer protects the urothelium from caustic solutes stored in the bladder and prevents bacteria from adhering to the urothelial surfaces (13). According to this mechanism a defective GAG layer and permeable urothelium will allow urinary potassium to depolarize nerves in the urothelium, detrusor, and perivesical area leading to urgency, frequency, and pain. There are several studies that lend support to this disease process. One study demonstrated that urea absorption is increased in IC patients compared to normal controls supporting the concept of a permeable or "leaky" urothelium (14). Exposure of the bladder

Table 51.1 National Institute of Diabetes and Digestive and Kidney Diseases Criteria for Interstitial Cystitis Research Studies

Both of the following are required:

(1) Bladder pain or urinary urgency
(2) Classic Hunner's ulcer or glomerulations (≥10/quadrant, in ≥3 quadrants) after distention under anesthesia

Any of the following are exclusions:

(1) Awake bladder capacity of >350 cc fluid
(2) Absence of intense urge at bladder volume 150 cc fluid
(3) Involuntary bladder contractions on urodynamics
(4) Symptom duration of <9 months
(5) Absence of nocturia
(6) Symptoms relieved by antimicrobials, urinary antiseptics, anticholinergics, or antispasmodics
(7) Voiding <8 times/day while awake
(8) Bacterial cystitis or prostatitis within the past three months
(9) Bladder or ureteral calculi
(10) Vaginitis or active genital herpes
(11) Uterine, cervical, vaginal, or urethral cancer
(12) Urethral diverticulum
(13) Cyclophosphamide or any type of chemical cystitis, tuberculosis cystitis, or radiation cystitis
(14) Benign or malignant bladder tumors
(15) Age <18 years

epithelium to potassium due to a defective mucus layer may be one source of the pain experienced by IC patients. Repeated exposure to potassium leads to inflammation, mast cell degranulation, and sensory nerve depolarization. For this reason the potassium sensitivity test (PST) (see "Diagnosis") was designed to identify IC patients by recreating their pelvic pain in an awake office setting (15). It has been shown that urine is critical in causing bladder inflammation across a permeable urothelium (16). Treatment to replenish the GAG layer increases urinary potassium compared to creatinine levels indicating a decrease in urothelial permeability (17). The role of the bladder epithelium in IC is further supported by the success of heparinoid compounds in the treatment of IC (18). Heparin and pentosan polysulfate sodium (PPS) are exogenous GAGs used to repair the antiadherence effect of the mucus lining of the bladder (19). Additionally, an assessment of total sulfated GAGs normalized to urine creatinine found elevated levels in patients with moderate to severe IC but there is no way to know if such an elevation is due to loss from the epithelium or increased production of glycoproteins. Urinary GAG has been found to be lower in feline IC compared to controls (20).

Neurogenic Inflammation

Ultrastructural changes in the bladder show vascular lesions of the intrinsic microcirculation, degenerative and regenerative neural changes, muscular edema, and disruption of the urothelial surface umbrella cells. In contrast to the theory that a leaky urothelium leads to an inflammatory condition, these changes suggest that neurogenic inflammation may trigger a process leading to a leaky urothelium and mast cell activation (21).

Bladder mucosal and submucosal biopsies have not been shown to be helpful in establishing the diagnosis of IC (22). Due to the heterogeneity of IC patients, early attempts to subgroup IC patients based on mast cell content on biopsies were unsuccessful (23). However, in contrast to normal bladders, there are a higher number of activated mast cells with increased histamine content in the bladders of patients with IC (24–27). Detrusor mastocytosis is found in both classic and nonulcerative IC with higher counts seen in the detrusor of classic IC biopsies (28). It appears that in IC mast cells migrate and concentrate in the detrusor and lamina propria (29). In contrast to transitional cell carcinoma in which mastocytosis is also noted, the mast cells are not activated on histologic analysis (30). In IC, when stimulated, the mast cells degranulate to release histamines stimulating vasoactive and nociceptive substances within the detrusor and suburothelium (31,32). Electron microscopy reveals that over 90% of mast cells in PBS/IC patients are activated to varying degrees (33). Mast cells can be activated by acetylcholine and substance P (SP) (34). In human IC bladder biopsies, SP containing nerve fibers are increased in the submucosa in juxtaposition to activated mast cells but not in the detrusor (35). Another finding of note is that in chronic IC patients, there are significantly more nerve fibers within the suburothelium and detrusor muscle. The number of nerve fibers, mast cells, and histamines appear to correlate (25).

Women have a higher incidence of inflammatory disorders (36). An endocrine component of IC is suggested since women with PBS and IC often complain of a cyclic flare up of their symptoms. One explanation is that mast cells in female IC patients express high affinity estrogen receptors. Therefore, degranulation during the luteal phase of the menstrual cycle may be related to hormonal changes (37). Progesterone inhibits mast cell degranulation which may explain why IC symptoms are suppressed during pregnancy in most women (38). Mast cells appear to be a predominant factor in several painful disorders including IBS (39), endometriosis (40), fibromyalgia (41), vulvar vestibulitis (42), and possibly migraines.

DIAGNOSIS

At present, there is no internationally agreed upon criteria for diagnosing IC (1). Historically, cystoscopic findings were considered imperative to making a diagnosis however this misdiagnosed up 60% of patients. Current definitions using symptom based diagnosis will potentially miss up to 30% of patients. Symptom questionnaires are useful in screening patients but they are not sensitive enough to diagnose IC patients.

Cystoscopy

The original descriptions of patients with IC involved cystoscopic findings of vascular changes. It was felt that multiple petechial hemorrhages (Fig. 51.1), called glomerulations, seen on redistention of the bladder during cystoscopy under anesthesia were a hallmark of IC (43). The finding of Hunner's ulcers was described as classic IC and glomerulations as nonclassic IC. These diagnostic criteria were the mainstay of IC diagnosis for many years. In order to standardize inclusion criteria in IC research, the NIDDK established criteria based on observations made during cystoscopic hydrodistention under

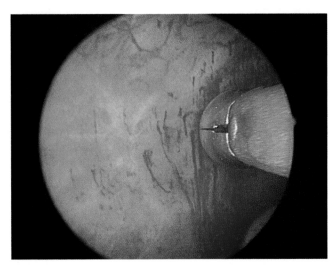

Figure 51.1 Cystoscopy showing petechial hemorrhage.

Table 51.2 PUF Score/PST Correlations

PUF score	Positive PST (%)
0–4	1.9
5–9	55
10–14	74
15–19	76
20+	91

Abbreviations: PUF, pelvic pain, urgency, and frequency; PST, potassium sensitivity test.
Source: From Refs. 55, 69.

anesthesia (Table 51.1). Although the NIDDK criteria were established for research purposes they became accepted criteria in the diagnosis of IC for the general population. Only recently have these criteria been challenged due to their poor correlation with biopsy findings, symptoms, and treatment outcomes.

There are several issues related to using cystoscopy to diagnose PBS/IC. Hunner's ulcers are found in <10% of patients (44). There are no accepted criteria for identifying glomerulations after hydrostatic bladder dilation under general anesthesia, which are found in only 50% of IC patients. The etiology of glomerulations is proposed to be related to increased angiogenic and endothelial growth factors in the bladder (45,46). Glomerulations are reported in patients with IC although they may be seen in the bladders of patients without IC making their presence inconclusive as for diagnosis (47). Therefore, the lack of Hunner's ulcers or glomerulations on cystoscopy does not exclude the diagnosis of BPS/PBS/IC (48).

Symptom Questionnaires

The lack of diagnostic criteria led many clinicians to rely on the NIDDK criteria to diagnose IC although such use was never intended. The purpose of the NIDDK criteria was to provide a homogenous study population. Researchers have long pointed out that the exclusion criteria they employed would easily lead to the underdiagnosis of IC by as many as 60% (49) to 90% (50). Many clinicians have suggested that cystoscopy is necessary to rule out bladder carcinoma and other bladder pathology. In the absence of significant risk factors the incidence of bladder carcinoma is quite low. Hematuria may prompt a cystoscopic evaluation however, microscopic hematuria is found in up 24% of IC patients and should be considered an incidental finding unless the patient has risks factors for bladder carcinoma (51).

CPP is defined as continuous pain for over three months or cyclic pain for six months or more localized to the pelvis, low back, or buttocks sufficient enough to lead to disability or medical care (52). It is well known that woman with IC will seek care from multiple physicians for several years before they are correctly diagnosed with IC (53,54). IC patients often present to the gynecologist with symptoms of dyspareunia and symptom flares associated with menstrual cycles (55). CPP accounts for 10% of visits to gynecologists, 20% of laparoscopies, and 10% to 20% of hysterectomies (56).

Currently, the diagnosis of PBS/IC is based on patient symptoms of urgency, frequency, and pain with sterile urine (5). However, this definition may lack sensitivity and may fail to identify over one-third of patients (44). Therefore, screening questionnaires are useful in screening patients. There are three validated questionnaires available to screen and assess PBS/IC patients: the pelvic pain, urgency, frequency (PUF) questionnaire (55); the IC symptom and problem index (ICSI, ICPI) known also as the O'Leary—Sant questionnaire (57); and the University of Wisconsin Scale (58).

The PUF questionnaire (55) is a 35 point symptom scale. There is a strong correlation between PUF scores and positive PST results. The PUF correlates poorly with cystoscopic findings (59). There is no standard cutoff PUF score diagnostic of IC however a score of >10 is associated with positive PST in 74% and in 91% with a score of >19 (Table 51.2). It appears that patients with IC and concomitant disorders have higher PUF scores and tend to present at a younger age compared to patients with IC alone (unpublished data). The University of Wisconsin IC Scale (UW-IC) is a scale that identifies seven IC symptoms (discomfort, pain, nocturia, daytime frequency, sleep disturbance, urgency, and burning). Reports of its use are limited. The O'Leary—Sant ICSI and ICPI scale has been widely used in research trials. Comparisons of these questionnaires shows that there is a strong correlation between the three instruments (60,61). One study comparing the UW-IC, ICSI, and ICPI showed that the diagnosis of PBS/IC correlated with questionnaire findings of urgency, nocturia, pain, and frequency (60). Comparison of the PUF with ICSI/ICPI demonstrated that the PUF may be more sensitive in screening the general population (62). Whether the questionnaires can be used to diagnose IC is unlikely.

Potassium Sensitivity Test

The diagnosis of PBS/IC based on clinical symptoms, urodynamics, cystoscopy, bladder biopsies, and urinary markers all have shortcomings in proving the diagnosis of IC (63). Cystoscopic diagnosis may miss up to 60% of patients with symptoms suggestive of PBS/IC while a diagnosis based on symptoms may fail to identify up one-third. Human and animal studies have shown that a likely etiology of PBS/IC is a defective GAG layer resulting in a permeable urothelium.

Table 51.3 Potassium Sensitivity Test

Empty bladder after cleansing urethra

Place a small urethral catheter (e.g., 8 Fr pediatric feeding tube)

Instill slowly 40 cc sterile water

Record the level of urgency and pain on a 0–5 point scale to establish a baseline

Urgency

| 0 | 1 | 2 | 3 | 4 | 5 |

Pain

| 0 | 1 | 2 | 3 | 4 | 5 |

Leave catheter in place and empty the bladder

Instill slowly up to 40 cc of a dilute KCl solution (20 cc KCl 40 mEq/L in 80 cc water)

Record the level of urgency and pain on a 0–5 point scale

Urgency

| 0 | 1 | 2 | 3 | 4 | 5 |

Pain

| 0 | 1 | 2 | 3 | 4 | 5 |

A change or difference of 2 points between the water test and the KCl test is considered positive

If the patient suffers acute or severe discomfort or urgency—stop instilling the KCl and empty the bladder

Consider instilling 40,000 U heparin with 20 cc 2% lidocaine or 0.5% bupivicaine

Table 51.4 Markers

Potential urinary markers of IC

Antiproliferative factor—inhibits the growth of normal bladder epithelial cells

Epidermal growth factor—may decrease inward potassium current in normal bladder urothelium

Interleukins-6 (IL-6)—may have a positive correlation with nocturia in IC patients. Correlates with mononuclear inflammation. IL-2, IL-6, and IL-8 decrease after BCG vaccine

IGF binding protein-3

Glycoprotein-51—lower in IC patients and may distinguish IC patients from controls

Eosinophil cationic protein—may correlate with mast cell density. Decrease with subcutaneous heparin

1,4-Methylimidazole acetic acid—may correlate with mast cell density

Nitric oxide synthase—increase with L-arginine treatment

Cyclic guanosine monophosphate—increase with L-arginine treatment

Prostaglandin E2—decrease after bladder distention

Kallikrein—decrease after bladder distention

Neutrophil chemotactic activity—decrease after DMSO

Uroplakin may be involved in increased permeability of the urothelium

Tryptophan

Tryptase

Abbreviations: IC, Interstitial cystitis; BCG, bacillus Calmette Guerin; DMSO, dimethyl sulfoxide; IGF, insulin-like growth factor.

The ability of the PST to diagnose PBS/IC is based upon the theory that normal urinary levels of potassium, which range from 40 to 140 mEq/L are capable of depolarizing nerves due to the defective lining of the bladders of IC patients (64). It was proposed, therefore, that instilling a dilute potassium solution could mimic bladder symptoms in those patients with a GAG defect. In patients who meet NIDDK diagnostic criteria the PST is positive in up to 80% (65).

The PST identifies the bladder as the source of bladder pain by the intravesical administration of dilute (0.4 M) KCl (Table 51.3). The PST has been shown to diagnose up to 90% of IC patients with a low false positive rate. No correlation has been found between the PST and cystoscopic findings, which is not surprising given that studies show only 10% of patients with IC have positive cystoscopic findings (66).

Several studies support the role of potassium in the symptoms of PBS/IC patients and therefore the role of the PST. Parsons et al. demonstrated that instilling a 0.4 M solution of KCl intravesically provoked symptoms in 70% of patients with clinical IC and 4.5% of controls (67). A study looking at women presenting to gynecologic clinics for evaluation of CPP of presumed gynecologic origin found that 85% of these patients had a positive PST (68). A follow up study revealed similar findings with 81% of women with CPP testing positive for the bladder pain during the PST (69). In this study, the PUF questionnaire was used. Controls all had a PUF score of <4 and 0% tested positive during the PST (55). Treatment with PPS which acts to replace the GAG layer reversed a positive PST in treated patients (70). As opposed to the commonly held belief that women with CPP suffer more commonly from endometriosis and pain from reproductive organs, these studies demonstrated that the bladder may be a likely source of chronic pain in the majority of women. The importance of these studies has been largely overlooked however they show that the PST is unique in that it allows an awake patient to respond to a provocative test and to identify the source of their pain. One criticism of the PST is that other bladder conditions with sensory or urothelial inflammation can test positive such as radiation cystitis, some patients with overactive bladder, and acute urinary tract infection (UTI) (13).

Markers

Although many potential urinary markers have been studied, to date no urinary markers or proteins found to be abnormal in IC patients are in clinical use (Table 51.4). The roles of the identified markers and proteins are largely unknown. At present, urine markers do not predict or correlate with cystoscopic or bladder biopsy findings in IC patients (71). It is hoped that eventually a protein marker will find clinical utility and will help identify IC patients based on urine samples. Urinary markers found to be altered in IC patients include epidermal growth factor (EGF) (72), heparin-binding (HB)-EGF, cyclic guanosine monophosphate, insulin-like growth factor binding protein-3 (73), interleukin-6 (73), glycoprotein 51 (74), uroplakin (75), Tamm-Horsfall protein (76), and chondroitin sulfate. Glycoprotein 51 is secreted by the transitional epithelium of the genitourinary tract. Chondroitin sulfate is a component of the GAG layer (77).

Antiproliferative factor (APF) protein is a toxic, low-molecular-weight molecule that inhibits the growth of normal bladder epithelial cells found in the urine of 94% of patients with IC and only 9% of controls (78,79). The action of APF is thought to regulate HB-EGF leading to an inhibition of regeneration of damaged or denuded urothelial cells (80). APF may be related to increased purinergic or adenosine triphosphate signaling leading to increased bladder pain (75). It was shown that APF levels decreased after hydrodistention but the decline was not associated with improved symptom scores (81). Both APF and glycoprotein-51 distinguish IC patients from normal controls with minimal overlap (82). To date, glycoprotein-51 and APF are not in clinical use.

Neural Changes

IC is a CPP condition that is often not recognized early due to other confusable disorders that also cause pelvic pain. It is important to recognize that the nerve signals from the uterus, bladder, colon, and pelvic floor converge along the same neural pathways in the spinal cord. Under normal conditions, afferent alpha–delta fibers respond to passive distension during bladder filling and active contraction. Silent poorly myelinated or unmyelinated C-fibers are insensitive to bladder filling under normal conditions. However, C-fibers do respond to noxious stimulus to the urothelium. The cell bodies of these fibers are in the dorsal root ganglia of S2–S3 and T11-L2. Efferent nerve signals from the lower urinary tract receive involve both sympathetic and parasympathetic nerves. Stimulation of the pelvic nerves (parasympathetic pelvic plexus) causes contraction of the detrusor resulting in bladder emptying and relaxation of the bladder neck and urethra. Sympathetic nerves (T11–T12, L1–L2) arise from the inferior mesenteric ganglia and hypogastric nerve or pass through the paravertebral chain to enter the pelvic nerves at the bladder base and urethra.

A commonly held model of the neurologic alterations associated with IC is that chronic neural stimulation leads to upregulation of spinal nerves. The presence of c-Fos proteins is evidence of both peripheral and central neural upregulation in IC (83). Nociceptive and sensory signals travel through sympathetic (T10–T12) and parasympathetic (S2–S4) branches merging in the pelvic ganglion and continue to the dorsal horn of the spinal cord where signals from various organs may be received. This convergence can lead to conflicting signals whereby nonpainful stimuli are perceived as painful, a phenomenon referred to as visceroviseral hyperalgesia. In the gate control theory, afferent neural impulses are modified by spinal and cortical signals altering the level of firing of the afferent nerves in some way so that pain impulses from the bladder could result in the sensation of pain anywhere in the pelvis masking the bladder as the source of the pain (84). A hyperalgesic state could also result from repeated assault of the bladder epithelium with noxious stimuli. Substances responsible for nociception are located in primary afferent nociceptors. When sensory fibers are stimulated they release both an afferent and an efferent signal, which then stimulates the primary afferent nociceptor C-fibers and causes neurogenic inflammation by the release of neuropeptides. Thirty to eighty percent of visceral afferents are silent. With prolonged stimulation, these silent afferents become active with prolonged stimulation. The spinal cord receives afferent input influenced by somatic input which is referred to as viscerosomatic convergence. Afferent activation of pelvic nerves may influence the efferent output to another organ which is known as cross-talk.

Visceral cross-sensitization can occur. Rat studies show that neurons receiving nociceptive input from convergent input to common dorsal root ganglion (DRG) from inflamed pelvic organs (85).

Physiological neurogenic inflammation is an adaptive response providing injured tissue with more substrates for rebuilding, causing plasma extravasation for transport, and to dilute concentrations of bacteria and toxins and activating an immunological response. Chronic inflammation leads to increased excitability of nociceptive C-fibers in rat models (86). The role of neurogenic inflammation in IC is supported by an increase in levels of SP found in the urine of IC patients. ATP mediates excitation of small diameter sensory neurons during bladder distention via purinergic receptors. The normal bladder contracts due to muscarinic cholinergic nerve activation. In the IC bladder and other inflammatory bladder conditions however non-cholinergic activation via purinergic receptors may occur (87).

CONCOMITANT DISORDERS

It is becoming increasingly evident that it is imperative for physicians who treat CPP and IC patients to attempt to diagnose all of the potential causes of the chronic pain. The etiology of IC is multifactorial therefore concomitant or confusable diseases are common due to the interaction of neural, immune, and endocrine factors involved in IC and other chronic pain conditions. Most IC patients are women with a ratio between 5:1 and 9:1. Most women present to a primary provider and historically to many different physicians and receive many procedures and treatments before a diagnosis of IC is given and appropriate treatment is started. The problem with this approach is that there may be multiple potential pain sources or pain generators in women (50) and failure to recognize them leads to neural upregulation and refractory pain.

Many women with CPP are given a diagnosis of endometriosis. Unfortunately, biopsy-proven endometriosis is found in only 33% of women with CPP (56). Studies have shown that endometriosis coexists with IC in between 45% and 75% (50,88). Vulvar pain, primarily vulvar vestibulitis co-exists in approximately 20% (50). IBS is a diagnosis of exclusion also affecting mainly women. Up to 27% of IC patients report symptoms or a diagnosis of IBS compared to a prevalence of 2.9% in the general population. Other commonly found concomitant pain disorders found more commonly in women with IC include OAB (20%) (89), migraines (up to 20%) (90), and fibromyalgia.

IC is associated with several other chronic pain and autoimmune disorders including fibromyalgia (91,92), systemic lupus, Sjogren's syndrome (93), migraines, and depression (94). Fibromyalgia lacks confirmatory diagnostic tests and varies in its presentation. IC and fibromyalgia are also associated with IBS and migraines, all of which may share mast cells activation in common (95).

It is common for IC patients to be treated with an anticholinergics for OAB although it has been shown that only about 24% of patients with IC have urodynamically proven detrusor spasms. IC patients are often diagnosed as having recurrent UTI and are treated with repeated courses of antibiotics.

Disease flares may be mistaken for recurrent UTIs. It has been shown that only about 7% of IC patients have an actual history of recurrent bacteremia (96,97).

An infectious etiology was first considered for IC due to the similarity between the clinical presentation of IC and UTIs (98). Both result in dysuria, frequency, and nocturia and, like UTIs, IC occurs predominantly in women rather than men. IC patients are more likely to have a history of UTIs than controls. UTIs have been shown to cause damage to the bladder epithelium and abnormal bladder epithelium is common to IC patients. Despite these similarities, no infectious agent has been identified that causes IC and it has been shown that only about 7% of IC patients have an actual history of recurrent bacteremia (97,98).

TREATMENTS

Three is a considerable lack of evidence supporting many of the treatments offered to patients with IC. One study (99) found that hydrodistention (61%), intravesical medication (40%), and urethral dilation (26.5%) were the most common therapeutic procedures given to IC patients. Patients reported some improvement in 24% to 45%, no effect in 27% to 49%, and worsening in 26% to 30%. The majority of patients reported that medications improved their condition compared to surgical procedures.

Oral

Pentosan Polysulfate

A presumed etiology of IC is dysfunction of the protective GAG layer of the urothelium. In the early 1980s, PPS, a synthetic, heparin-like, sulfated polysaccharide that is excreted into the urine was introduced to treat IC (100). PPS appears to work by re-establishing the protective GAG layer in the bladder and may have an anti-inflammatory effect by stabilizing mast cells (101,102). It is most often used orally but can be instilled intravesically. Currently PPS is the only approved oral preparation used to treat IC. One study (103) using cystoscopic diagnostic criteria, urodynamic findings, and bladder biopsies did not show a treatment effect for PPS compared to placebo. Several trials, randomized and retrospective, have shown PPS to more effective than placebo in improving patient symptoms at doses ranging from 300 to 900 mg/day (104–106). A meta-analysis found that PPS was effective in treating pain, urgency, and frequency but not nocturia (107). PPS alone or in combination with hydroxyzine or amitriptyline have been shown to be cost efficient therapies for IC due to decreased physician visits, emergency room visits, and operative procedures (Stanford AJOG 2008).

Amitriptyline/Antidepressants

Amitriptyline is a tricyclic antidepressant that inhibits synaptic reuptake of serotonin and norepinephrine and has been well studied in patients with pelvic pain. It decreases nociception at the spinal cord, brain, and thalamus. The usual dose is 25 mg (range 10–150 mg; maximum dose 300 mg daily) with higher doses causing anticholinergic side effects such as dry mouth, constipation, and sedation. Animal data shows that amitriptyline may inhibit histamine release from mast cells (108).

One trial demonstrated that in patients meeting NIDDK criteria, amitriptyline was more effective than placebo in improving pain, urgency, frequency, and functional bladder capacity however the response rate was only 64% (109). At higher doses, patient compliance was decreased due to side effects. In an open label study of 25 patients who failed hydrodistension and intravesical dimethyl sulfoxide (DMSO) there was a 50% reduction in pain and daytime frequency, but not nocturia at a dose of 75 mg at bedtime over three weeks (89).

A non-tricyclic antidepressant, duloxetine (titrated to 40 mg b.i.d. for five weeks) studied in 48 women with IC found no significant improvement of symptoms (110). In a database analysis, antidepressants other than amitriptyline were not effective in decreasing the cost of care of IC patients (93).

Histamine Receptor Antagonists

Antihistamine therapy, particularly hydroxyzine, is commonly used to treat IC symptoms. It has been shown that activated bladder mast cells are found close to SP containing nerve endings in IC. Since histamine release may contribute to IC symptoms, select H-1 receptor antagonists (hydroxyzine pamoate or hydrochloride) may have some benefit in treating IC through anxiolytic, sedative, anticholinergic actions as well as by stabilizing mast cells. In vitro rat studies have shown that hydroxyzine suppresses carbachol-induced mast cell activation. In contrast, diphenhydramine had no effect on rat bladder mast cell activation (111). Using NIDDK selection criteria, a pilot study did not show a favorable response to hydroxyzine (112). An open-label study showed only a modest effect (40%) on decreasing visual analog scores in IC patients. The therapeutic effect increased to (65%) in patients with allergies (113). Similarly, cromolyn sodium, an inhaled antihistamine used in asthma, does not appear to be effective in treating IC however data is lacking. In a small group of refractory IC patients, the H2-receptor antagonist cimetidine, showed some benefit (114,115). Based on the current evidence, hydroxyzine or cimetidine may be considered in the treatment of IC patients however the therapeutic effect is modest at best.

Misoprostol

Misoprostol is an oral prostaglandin E1 analogue that has gastrointestinal protective and uterotonic actions. It has been studied in the treatment of IC based on its effect on immune pathways. An open-labeled study using a dose of 600 μm/day found improvement of symptoms in 56% of IC patients at three months and 48% at nine months reported sustained improvement. Misoprostol may be cytoprotective to the bladder (116).

Cyclosporine (117)

Cyclosporine is an immunosuppressive agent used in organ transplant patients to inhibit T-cell activation and cytokine release. At a dose of 2.5 to 5 mg/kg/day for three to six months there was a decrease in urinary frequency and bladder pain with an increased voided volume. Symptom relief was not long-term and returned in most patients treated (117).

L-Arginine and Nitric Oxide (NO)

NO is synthesized from L-arginine, a semi-essential amino acid, by isoenzymes called NO synthase (118). NO production has been shown to be a neurotransmitter in the lower urinary tract, a marker for inflammatory disorders in the bladder, and has a physiologic role in overactive bladder and IC/PBS (119) with higher levels of NO found in the bladders of patients with IC/PBS (120). Oral L-arginine increases NO synthase activity. It appears that interstitial cells, nerve fibers, and transitional epithelium are targets of NO in the bladder.

One study found that L-arginine increased NO synthase activity at 1.5 gm daily given for six months. Urinary voiding discomfort, lower abdominal pain, vaginal/urethral pain, and daytime and nighttime frequency were decreased (121). Followup studies have failed to demonstrate significant clinical responses to L-arginine compared to placebo (122). L-arginine (2.4 g/day) versus placebo given for one month after a two week washout period was given to 16 patients with IC/PBS. Side effects of severe headaches, night sweats, and flushing were found and were not associated with significant decreases in voided volume, frequency, or nocturia (123). NO may serve as a marker on inflammation and L-arginine increases NO synthase activity; however, a clinical response is not associated with L-arginine therapy.

Suplatast Tosilate

Suplatast tosilate is an immunoregulator that suppresses cytokine production in helper T cells, immunoglobulin E synthesis, chemical mediator release from mast cells, and eosinophilic recruitment. Treatment with 300 mg/day for one year in 14 patients with IC increased bladder capacity and decreased urinary urgency, frequency, and lower abdominal pain (124).

Quercetin

Chondroitin sulfate and quercetin have anti-inflammatory properties and may inhibit mast cell activiation. Limited studies on IC patients meeting NIDDK criteria have shown significant improvement in ICSI and ICPI scores (125).

Intravesical Treatment

Intravesical treatment for IC includes bladder instillations and detrusor injections. A Cochrane Database review found 9 trials involving 616 participants and reported that resiniferatoxin (RTX), DMSO, bacillus Calmette Guerin, oxybutynin, and urinary alkinalization were largely unsuccessful in treating IC/PBS (126).

Heparin

Heparin is a sulfated polysaccharide thought to emulate the GAG layer of the bladder. Heparin has been used to treat IC symptoms alone and in combination with lidocaine (1% and 2%), alkinalized lidocaine, bupivicaine, DMSO, methylprednisolone, oral medications, and neuromodulation (Table 51.5). Overall, heparin, which acts as a GAG layer substitute, is effective in treating the symptoms of IC. ATP release is increased in IC urothelium. One potential mechanism of action of heparin is to block activated ATP release in stretched urothelial cells (127). Heparin also appears to stabilize mast cells. Improvement in symptom scores, nocturia, first sensation of filling,

Table 51.5 Heparin Intravesical Instillation

Have patient empty the bladder
Cleanse urethra
Insert a small urethral catheter (e.g., 8 Fr pediatric feeding tube)
Empty the bladder of residual urine
Instill 40,000 U heparin mixed with 8 mL 2% lidocaine and 3 mL 8.4% sodium bicarbonate
Can mix with 0.5% bupivicaine—do not alkalinize bupivicaine
Remove catheter
Have patient hold the heparin in her bladder for 20 minutes or longer

cystometric capacity, and a reversal of a positive PST has been shown (128).

Heparin has been studied in various doses. Mixing 10,000 U with 10 mL of sterile water given three times per week for three months was effective in 56% (129). Heparin can be administered with alkalinized lidocaine to offer some immediate pain management (130,62). Subcutaneous heparin (5000 IU/day to 5000 IU 2–3 times/week) showed a clinical effect lasting up one year (131).

Dimethyl Sulfoxide

DMSO is a solvent with anti-inflammatory, analgesic, and muscle relaxing properties (132). It does not appear to inhibit mast cell degranulation. Currently it is the only approved intravesical treatment for IC/PBS. The traditional regimen is to instill a 50% solution (RIMSO 50) one to two times weekly for a period of four to eight week although this varies considerably and the actual therapeutic dose has not been determined (133). DMSO is often combined with other medications such as corticosteroids and heparin. Randomized studies on DMSO are not possible due to the strong odor produced after instillation. In a prospective study, DMSO was shown to decrease pain and urinary frequency in ulcerative IC/PBS but did not affect functional bladder capacity (134). Its use in treating IC has a traditional basis and may be of therapeutic value in classic ulcerative patients (135).

Botulinum Toxin A (BTX-A)

BTX-A is used for pelvic pain and bladder disorders such as neurogenic detrusor overactivity, pelvic floor spasticity, and detrusor–sphincter dyssynergia. The mechanism of action of BTX-A is to irreversibly inhibit the release of the neurotransmitter acetylcholine however the long-term effects are limited by the formation of new neuromuscular junctions. Studies looking at BTX-A in IC patients are limited by data from a small number of patients refractory to traditional treatments and from only a few institutions (136). The effects of BTX-A on the bladder are to decrease pain and bladder contractions. There is an anti-nociceptive affect as shown by decreased visual analog scores in patients. The mechanism may be due to blocking bladder afferent nerve fibers. calcitonin gene-related peptide (CGRP) found in rat bladder afferent nerves is decreased after treatment with BTX-A (137). Bladder mucosal biopsies show increased nerve growth factor levels in IC patients which is decreased to the level of control patients after BTX-A (138).

In clinical use, 100 to 200 U in 20 mL of 0.9% saline injected submucosally in the trigone and lateral walls of the bladder has been shown to decrease visual analog scores and urinary frequency (daytime and nighttime) (139) while increasing cystometric and functional bladder capacity (140). Subjective improvement is seen in 87% of IC/PBS patients however the effects appear to diminish within six months. In a recent study on the utility of BTX-A injections on 13 patients with IC, the ICSI, and ICPI mean scores improved by 71% and 69%, respectively. Urinary frequency, nocturia, and pain were all significantly decreased, however long term results were not reported (141). The effect of BTX-A alone may not be as effective as BTX-A combined with bladder hydrodistention but further study is needed.

Capsaicin/RTX

Capsaicin is a vanilloid that acts by decreasing the temperature necessary for the activation of transient receptor potential vanilloid-1 (TRPV-1). Nociceptive signals are transmitted by C-fibers. Capsaicin desensitizes the TRPV-1 channels inactivating the C-fibers leading to decreased bladder pain (142). The terminal nerve endings are desensitized resulting in decreased pain sensation. A study of 36 patients with IC who received capsaicin 10 μmol/L two times a week for a month versus placebo showed significant decrease in urinary frequency, nocturia, and pain with capsaicin treatment. Urgency was not improved. Decreased pain was reported at both the one month and six month interval.

RTX is a more potent analogue of capsaicin that has also been studied as a potential treatment for IC. In a small, randomized study, patients with hypersensitive disorder of the lower urinary tract were given either placebo or 10 nmol/L of RTX and evaluated for improvement of symptoms at 30 days and 3 months. At both 30 days and 3 months, patients receiving RTX reported improvement in urinary frequency and nocturia although the improvement was less marked at the three month interval. There was also a significant decrease in pain at 30 days (143). A multicenter trial in which a single dose of RTX (50 mL of 0.01 , 0.05, and 0.1 m, or placebo) did not show improvement in urgency, frequency, nocturia, or average voided volume at 12-weeks followup (144). Both capsaicin and RTX therapy may result is severe discomfort limiting its use in certain patients (145,146).

Corticosteroids

Corticosteroids have been studied in the treatment of refractory IC/PBS patients usually by suburothelial injections or injections into Hunner's ulcers under endoscopic control. Oral prednisone (25 mg daily for 1–2 months) was shown to decrease pain and ICSI/ICPI scores in small group of chronic severe IC/PBS patients (144). A prospective study on Hunner's ulcer subtype IC/PBS using 10 mL of triamcinolone acetonide (40 mg/mL) injected suburothelially and into the ulcers resulted in a therapeutic decrease in PUF scores (147).

A small study showed that oral prednisone (up to 25 mg daily for 1–2 months) resulted in decreased pain and a modest decrease in the ICPI/ICSI in patients with refractory ulcerative IC (148).

Chlorpactin

The mechanism of action of chlorpactin is uncertain. A small study measuring urinary levels of CGRP were measured before and after treatment with chlorpactin. No statistically significant response was found. Chlorpactin may act by desensitizing nerve terminals in the bladder (149).

Systemic Therapy

Montelukast

Montelukast, a leukotriene D receptor antagonist used as an antiashmatic agent. In a small study it was found to significantly reduce the symptoms of urinary frequency, nocturia, and pain daily use for three months. These IC patients all had detrusor mastocytosis as well, which may account for the effectiveness of treatment with Montelukast (150).

Gene Therapy

Preproenkephalin (PPE) is a precursor of enkephalin opioids (151). Herpes simplex virus (HSV)-PPE (replication-defetive HSV) injected in the bladder wall are taken up at afferent nerve terminals and specifically transported to lumbosacral dorsal root ganglia which contain bladder afferent neurons. The PPE transgene is expressed in transfected DRG neurons suppressing bladder nociceptive responses induced by intravesical capsaicin (137).

Surgical Treatment

Hydrodilation

Hydrodistension of the bladder has been used for years to treat the symptoms of IC. It has been shown to have short-term effects in controlling IC symptoms (152). Hydrodistention causes release of ATP from urothelial cells activates purinergic receptors.

Neurostimulation

Sacral nerve neuromodulation has been shown to be effective in decreasing urgency, frequency, pain (153), and narcotic requirements in IC patients (154). Urinary marker activity (HB-EGF and APF) are changed towards normal in response to sacral neuromodulation (155). Limited trials are available, however, its use in refractory patients particularly patients with predominant symptoms of frequency or pain related to bladder filling appear to respond favorably.

Laser

Neodymium:yttrium aluminum garnet laser cystoscopic ablative therapy has been studied in a scant number of patients. Patients refractory to medical therapy had significant improvement in pain, urgency, frequency, and nocturia. Repeat treatments were necessary in nearly half with no reported complications (156).

Pediatric IC

Pediatric IC is similar in presentation to adult IC and is treated much the same. The predominant symptoms include frequency and abdominal pain (157). Similar to older patients, IC is associated may be associated with concomitant

Table 51.6 Treatments

Oral treatment		Intravesical treatment		Surgical treatment	
Pentosan polysulfate	R	Pentosan polysulfate	R	Hydrodistention	N
Amitriptyline	R	Heparin	R	Sacral neurostimulation	R
Hydroxyzine	R	Hyaluronic acid	U	Peripheral neurostimulation	U
Cimetidine	U	Chondroitin sulfate	U	Acupuncture	U
Antibiotics	N	Dimethyl sulfoxide	N	Nerve blockade	N
Prostaglandins	N	Bacillus Calmette Guerin	N	Bladder augmentation	N
Corticosteroids	N	Chlorpactin	N	Cystectomy	N
L-arginine	N	Capsaicin	U		
Cyclosporine A	U	Resiniferatoxin	U		
Duloxetine	N				
Oxybutynin	U				
Tolteridine	N				
Gabapentin	N				
Suplatast tosilate	N				
Quercetin	R				
Analgesics	U				

Abbreviations: R, recommended; U, unsure, further research needed; N, use not supported.

endometriosis (158) and the workup should be the same as for older adult patients (159).

Cystoplasty

Bladder augmentation and cystectomy with urinary diversion have been used to treat severe cases of IC with mixed results. These surgical treatments are used sparingly and their success is questionable. Intestinal exposure to urine causes inflammation and possible fibrosis. It has been reported in IC patients who have undergone diversion that inflammatory changes consistent with bladder changes seen in IC (160). After bladder augmentation histologic changes resembling those of IC in which mast cells infiltrate the intestinal graft used to augment the bladder in PBS/IC patients have been reported (161) (Table 51.6).

REFERENCES

1. Hanno P, Dmochowski R. Status of international consensus on interstitial cystitis/bladder pain syndrome/painful bladder syndrome: 2008 snapshot. Neurourol Urodyn 2009; 28: 274–86.
2. Theoharides TC, Whitmore K, Stanford E, Moldwin R, O'Leary MP. Interstitial cystitis: bladder pain and beyond. Expert Opin Pharmacother 2008; 9: 2979–94.
3. Warren JW, Langenberg P, Greenberg P, et al. Sites of pain from interstitial cystitis/painful bladder syndrome. J Urol 2008; 180: 1373–7.
4. Peeker R, Enerbäck L, Fall M, Aldenborg F. Recruitment, distribution and phenotypes of mast cells in interstitial cystitis. J Urol 2000; 163: 1009–15.
5. Abrams P, Cardozo L, Fall M, et al. The standardisation of terminology of lower urinary tract function: report from the Standardisation Sub-committee of the International Continence Society. Am J Obstet Gynecol 2002; 187: 116–26.
6. van de Merwe JP, Nordling J, Bouchelouche P, et al. Diagnostic criteria, classification, and nomenclature for painful bladder syndrome/interstitial cystitis: an ESSIC proposal. Eur Urol 2008; 53: 60–7.
7. Gillenwater JY, Wein AJ. Summary of the National Institute of Arthritis, Diabetes, Digestive and Kidney Diseases Workshop on Interstitial Cystitis, National Institutes of Health, Bethesda, Maryland, August 28–29, 1987. J Urol 1988; 140: 203–6.
8. Burkman R. Chronic pelvic pain of bladder origin? Epidemiology, pathogenesis and quality of life. J Reprod Med 2004; 49: 225–9.
9. Sant GR. Etiology, pathogenesis and diagnosis of interstitial cystitis. Rev Urol 2002; 4: S9–15.
10. Lynes WL, Flynn SD, Shortliffe LD, Stamey TA. The histology of interstitial cystitis. Am J Surg Pathol 1990; 14: 969–76.
11. Niku SD, Stein PC, Scherz HC, Parsons CL. A new method for cytodestruction of bladder epithelium using protamine sulfate and urea. J Urol 1994; 152: 1025–8.
12. Chuang YC, Chancellor MB, Seki S, et al. Intravesical protamine sulfate and potassium chloride as a model for bladder hyperactivity. Urology 2003; 61: 664–70.
13. Parsons CL, Greenberger M, Gabal L, Bidair M, Barme G. The role of urinary potassium in the pathogenesis and diagnosis of interstitial cystitis. Urology 1998; 159: 1862–6.
14. Parsons CL, Lilly JD, Stein P. Epitelial dysfunction in nonbacterial cystitis (interstitial cystitis). J Urol 1991; 145: 732–5.
15. Parsons CL. Potassium sensitivity test. Tech Urol 1996; 2: 171–3.
16. Soler R, Bruschini H, Freire MP, et al. Urine is necessary to provoke bladder inflammation in protamine sulfate induced urothelial injury. J Urol 2008; 180: 1527–31.
17. Parsons CL, Greene RA, Chung M, Stanford EJ, Singh G. Abnormal urinary potassium metabolism in patients with interstitial cystitis. J Urol 2005; 173: 1182–5.
18. Parsons CL. Successful downregulation of bladder sensory nerves with combination of heparin and alkalinized lidocaine in patients with interstitial cystitis. Urology 2005; 65: 45–8.
19. Parsons CL, Mulholland SG, Anwar H. Antibacterial activity of bladder surface mucin duplicated by exogenous glycosaminocan (heparin). Infect Immun 1979; 24: 552–7.
20. Buffington CA, Blaisdell JL, Binns SP Jr, Woodworth BE. Decreased urine glycosaminoglycan excretion in cats with interstitial cystitis. J Urol 1996; 155: 1801–4.
21. Elbadawi AE, Light JK. Distinctive ultrastructural pathology of nonulcerative interstitial cystitis: new observations and their potential significance in pathogenesis. Urol Int 1996; 56: 137–62.
22. Larsen S, Thompson SA, Hald T, et al. Mast cells in interstitial cystitis. Br J Urol 1982; 54: 283–6.
23. Holm-Bentzen M, Jacobsen F, Nerstrøm B, et al. Painful bladder disease: clinical and pathoanatomical differences in 115 patients. J Urol 1987; 138: 500–2.
24. Kastrup J, Hald T, Larsen S, Neilsen VG. Histamine content and mast cell count of detrusor muscle in patients with interstitial cystitis and other types of chronic cystitis. Br J Urol 1983; 55: 495–500.
25. Lundeberg T, Liedberg H, Nordling L, et al. Interstitial cystitis: correlation with nerve fibres, mast cells and histamine. Br J Urol 1993; 71: 427–9.
26. Pang X, Cotreau-Bibbo MM, Sant GR, Theoharides TC. Bladder mast cell expression of high affinity oestrogen receptors in patients in interstitial cystitis. Br J Urol 1995; 75: 154–61.
27. Sant GR, Kempuraj D, Marchand JE, Theoharides TC. The mast cell in interstitial cystitis: role in pathophysiology and pathogenesis. Urology 2007; 69(Suppl 4): 34–40.
28. Theoharides TC, Kempuraj D, Sant GR. Mast cell involvement in interstitial cystitis: a review of human and experimental evidence. Urology 2001; 57(6 Suppl 1): 47–55.
29. Aldenborg F, Fall M, Enerbäck L. Proliferation and transepithelial migration of mucosal mast cells in interstitial cystitis. Immunology 1986; 58: 411–16.
30. Sant GR, Theoharides TC. The role of the mast cell in interstitial cystitis. Urol Clin North Am 1994; 21: 41–53.

31. Theoharides TC, Sant GR. Bladder mast cell activation in interstitial cystitis. Semin Urol 1991; 9: 74–87.

32. Christmas TJ, Rode J. Characteristics of mast cells in normal bladder, bacterial cystitis and interstitial cystitis. Br J Urol 1991; 68: 473–8.

33. Letourneau R, Sant GR, el-Mansoury M, Theoharides TC. Activation of bladder mast cells in interstitial cystitis. Int J Tissue React 1992; 14: 307–12.

34. Theoharides TC, Pang X, Letourneau R, Sant GR. Interstitial cystitis: a neuroinnumoendocrine disorder. Ann NY Acad Sci 1998; 840: 619–34.

35. Pang X, Marchand J, Sant GR, Kream RM, Theoharides TC. Increased number of substance P positive nerve fibers in interstitial cystitis. Br J Urol 1995; 75: 744–50.

36. Bjorling D, Wang Z. Estrogen and neuroinflammation. Urology 2001; 57(6 Suppl 1): 40–6.

37. Pang X, Cotreau-Bibbo MM, Sant GR, Theoharides TC. Bladder mast cell expression o high affinity oestrogen receptors in patients with interstitial cystitis. Br J Urol 1995; 75: 154–61.

38. Vasiadi M, Kempuraj D, Boucher W, Kalogeromitros D, Theoharides TC. Pregesterone inhibits mast cell secretion. Int J Immunopathol Pharmacol 2006; 19: 787–94.

39. Pang X, Boucher W, Triadafilopoulos G, Sant GR, Theoharides TC. Mast cell and substance P-positive nerve involvement in a patient with both irritable bowel syndrome and interstitial cystitis. Urology 1996; 47: 436–8.

40. Kempuraj D, Papadopoulou N, Stanford EJ, et al. Increased numbers of activated mast cells in endometriosis lesions positive for corticotrophin-releasing hormone and urocortin. Am J Reprod Immunol 2004; 52: 267–75.

41. Lucas HJ, Brauch CM, Settas L, Theoharides TC. Fibromyalgia—new concepts of pathogenesis and treatment. Int J Immunopathol Pharmacol 2006; 19: 5–10.

42. Chaim W, Meriwether C, Gonik B, Qureshi F, Sobel JD. Vulvar vestibulitis subjects undergoing surgical intervention: a descriptive analysis and histopathological correlates. Eur J Obstet Gynecol Reprod Biol 1996; 68: 165–8.

43. Messing EM, Stamey TA. Interstitial cystitis: early diagnosis, pathology, and treatment. Urology 1978; 12: 381–92.

44. Warren JW, Meyer WA, Greenberg P, et al. Using the International Continence Society's definition of painful bladder syndrome. Urology 2006; 67: 1138–42.

45. Tamaki M, Saito R, Ogawa O, Yoshimura N, Ueda T. Possible mechanisms inducing glomerulations in interstitial cystitis: relationship between endoscopic findings and expression of angiogenic growth factors. J Urol 2004; 172: 945–8.

46. Kiuchi H, Tsujimura A, Takao T, et al. Increased vascular endothelial growth factor expression in patients with bladder pain syndrome/interstitial cystitis: its association with pain severity and glomerulations. BJU Int 2009. [Epub ahead of print].

47. Waxman JA, Sulak PF, Kuehl TJ. Cystoscopic findings consistent with interstitial cystitis in normal women undergoing tubal ligation. J Urol 1998; 160: 1663–7.

48. Evans RJ, Stanford EJ. Current issues in the diagnosis of painful bladder syndrome/interstitial cystitis. J Reprod Med 2006; 51(Suppl 3): 241–52.

49. Hanno P, Landis JR, Matthews-Cook Y, Kusek J, Nyberg L Jr. The diagnosis of interstitial cystitis revisited: lessons learned from the National Institutes of Health Interstitial Database Study. J Urol 1999; 161: 553–7.

50. Stanford EJ, Koziol J, Feng A. The prevalence of interstitial cystitis, endometriosis, adhesions, and vulvar pain in women with chronic pelvic pain. J Minim Invasive Gynecol 2005; 12: 43–9.

51. Stanford EJ, Mattox TF, Parsons JK, McMurphy C. Prevalence of benign microscopic hematuria among women with interstitial cystitis: implications for evaluation of genitourinary malignancy. Urology 2006; 67: 946–9.

52. American College of Obstetricians and Gynecologists Committee on Practice Bulletins—Gynecology: chronic pelvic pain. Obstet Gynecol 2004; 103: 586–605.

53. Ottem DP, Teichman JM. What is the value of cystoscopy with hydrodistension for interstitial cystitis? Urology 2005; 66: 494–9.

54. Curhan GC, Speizer FE, Hunter DJ, Curhan SG, Stampfer MJ. Epidemiology of interstitial cystitis: a population based study. J Urol 1999; 161: 549–52.

55. Parsons CL, Dell J, Stanford EJ, et al. Increased prevalence of interstitial cystitis: previously unrecognized urologic and gynecologic cases identified using a new symptom questionnaire and intravesical potassium sensitivity. Urology 2002; 60: 573–8.

56. Howard FM. Chronic pelvic pain. Obstet Gynecol 2003; 101: 594–611.

57. O'Leary MP, Sant GR, Fowler FJ Jr, Whitmore KE, Spolarich-Kroll J. The interstitial cystitis symptom index and problem index. Urology 1997; 49(Suppl 5A): 58–63.

58. Goin JE, Olaleye D, Peters KM, et al. Psychometric analysis of the University of Wisconsin interstitial cystitis scale: implications for use in randomized clinical trials. J Urol 1998; 159: 1085–90.

59. Brewer ME, White WM, Klein FA, Klein LM, Waters WB. Validity of pelvic pain, urgency, and frequency questionnaire in patients with interstitial cystitis/painful bladder syndrome. Urology 2007; 70: 646–9.

60. Sirinian E, Azevedo K, Payne CK. Correlation between 2 interstitial cystitis symptom instruments. J Urol 2005; 173: 835–40.

61. Kushner L, Moldwin RM. Efficiency of questionnaires used to screen for interstitial cystitis. J Urol 2006; 176: 587–92.

62. Moldwin RM, Evans RJ, Stanford EJ, et al. Rational approaches to the treatment of patients with interstitial cystitis. Urology 2007; 69: 73–81.

63. Sant GR, Hanno PM. Interstitial cystitis: current issues and controversies in diagnosis. Urology 2001; 57(6 Suppl 1): 82–8.

64. Parsons CL, Zupkas P, Parsons JK. Intravesical potassium sensitivity in patients with interstitial cystitis and urethral syndrome. Urology 2001; 57: 428–33.

65. Sun ZQ, Qian WQ, Xie DS, Song JD. The study of diagnosis and treatment of interstitial cystitis. Zhonghua Wai Ke Za Zhi 2005; 43: 659–61.

66. Gergiore M, Liandier F, Naud A, Lacombe L, Fradet Y. Does the potassium stimulation test predict cystometric, cystoscopic outcome in interstitial cystitis? J Urol 2002; 168: 556–7.

67. Parsons CL, Stein PC, Bidair M, Lebow D. Abnormal sensitivity to intravesical potassium in interstitial cystitis and radiation cystitis. Neurourol Urodyn 1994; 13: 515–20.

68. Parsons CL, Bullen M, Kahn BS, Stanford EJ, Willems JJ. Gynecologic presentation of interstitial cystitis as detected by intravesical potassium sensitivity. Obstet Gynecol 2001; 98: 127–32.

69. Parsons CL, Dell J, Stanford EJ, et al. The prevalence of interstitial cystitis in gynecologic patients with pelvic pain, as detected by intravesical potassium sensitivity. Am J Obstet Gynecol 2002; 187: 1395–400.

70. Parsons CL, Forrest J, Nickel JC, et al. Elmiron Study Group. Effect of pentosan polysulfate therapy on intravesical potassium sensitivity. Urology 2002; 60: 939; author reply 939–40.

71. Erickson DR, Tomaszewski JE, Kunselman AR, et al. Urine markers do not predict biopsy findings or presence of bladder ulcers in interstitial cystitis/painful bladder syndrome. J Urol 2008; 179: 1850–6.

72. Sun Y, Chen M, Lowentritt BH, et al. EGF and HB-EGF modulate inward potassium current in hyman bladder urothelial cells from normal and interstitial cystitis patients. Am J Physiol Cell Physiol 2007; 292: C106–14.

73. Erickson ER, Xie SX, Bhavanandan VP, et al. A comparison of multiple urine markers for interstitial cystitis. J Urol 2002; 167: 2461–9.

74. Byrne DS, Sedor JF, Estojak J, et al. The urinary glycoprotein GP51 as a clinical marker for interstitial cystitis. J Urol 1999; 161: 1786–90.

75. Graham E, Chai TC. Dysfunction of bladder urothelium and bladder urothelial cells in interstitial cystitis. Curr Urol Rep 2006; 7: 440–6.

76. Neal DE Jr, Dilworth JP, Kaack MB. Tamm-Horsfall autoantibodies in interstitial cystitis. J Urol 1991; 145: 37–9.

77. Sand PK. Proposed pathogenesis ofpainful bladder syndrome/interstitial cystitis. J Reprod Med 2006; 51: 234–40.

78. Keay S, Kleinberg M, Zhang CO, Hise MK, Warren JW. Bladder epithelium cells from patients with interstitial cystitis produce an inhibitor of heparin-binding epidermal growth factor-like growth factor production. J Urol 2000; 164: 2112–18.

79. Keay SK, Zhang CO, Shoenfelt J, et al. Sensitivity and specificity of anti-proliferative factor, heparin-binding epidermal growth factor-like growth factor, and epidermal growth factor as urine markers for interstitial cystitis. Urology 2001; 57(6 Suppl 1): 9–14.

80. Rashid HH, Reeder JE, O'Connell MJ, et al. Interstitial cystitis antiproliferatie factor (APF) as a cell-cycle modulator. BMC Urol 2004; 4: 3.

81. Erickson DR, Kunselman AR, Bentley CM, et al. Changes in urine markers and symptoms after bladder distention for interstitial cystitis. J Urol 2007; 177: 556–60.

82. Erickson DR. Urine markers of interstitial cystitis. Urology 2001; 57(Suppl 1): 15–21.

83. Nazif O, Teichman JM, Gebhart GF. Neural upregulation in interstitial cystitis. Urology 2007; 69(4 Suppl): 24–33.

84. Stanford EJ, Dell JR, Parsons CL. The emerging presence of interstitial cystitis in gynecologic patients with chronic pelvic pain. J Urol 2006; 69: 53–9.

85. Chaban VV. Visceral sensory neurons that innervate both uterus and colon express nociceptive TRPv1 and P2X3 receptors in rats. Ethn Dis 2008; 18(2 Suppl 2): S2-20–4.

86. Yoshimura N, deGroat WC. Increased excitability of afferent neurons innervating rat urinary bladder after chronic bladder inflammation. J Neurosci 1999; 19: 4644–53.

87. Andersson KE, Hedlund P. Pharmacologic perspective on the physiology of the lower urinary tract. Urology 2002; 60(5 Suppl 1): 13–20.

88. Paulson JD, Delgado M. The relationship between interstitial cystitis and endometriosis in patients with chronic pelvic pain. JSLS 2007; 11: 175–81.

89. Hanno PM, Buehler J, Wein AM. Use of amityiptiline in the treatment of interstitial cystitis. J Urol 1989; 141: 846–8.

90. Theoharides TC, Sant GR, el-Mansoury M, et al. Activation of bladder mast cells in interstitial cystitis: a light and electron microscopic study. J Urol 1995; 153(3 Pt 1): 629–36.

91. Warren JW, Howard FM, Cross RK, et al. Antecedent nonbladder syndromes in case-control study of interstitial cystitis/painful bladder syndrome. Urology 2009; 73: 52–7. [Epub 2008 Nov 8].

92. Clauw DJ, Schmidt M, Radulovic D, et al. The relationship between fibromyalgia and interstitial cystitis. J Psychiatr Res 1997; 31: 125–31.

93. van de Merwe JP, Yamada T, Sakamoto Y. Systemic aspects of interstitial cystitis, immunology and linkage with autoimmune disorders. Int J Urol 2003; 10(Suppl): S35–8.

94. Clemens JQ, Meenan RT, O'Keeffe Rosetti MC, Kimes TA, Calhoun EA. Case-control study of medical comorbidities in women with interstitial cystitis. J Urol 2008; 179: 2222–5.

95. Lucas HJ, Brauch CM, Settas L, Theoharides TC. Fibromyalgia—new concepts of pathogenesis and treatment. Int J Immunopathol Pharmacol 2006; 19: 5–10.

96. Stanford E, McMurphy C. There is a low incidence of recurrent bacteriuria in painful bladder syndrome/interstitial cystitis patients followed longitudinally. Int Urogynecol J Pelvic Floor Dysfunct 2007; 18: 551–4.

97. Irwin P, Samsudin A. Reinvestigation of patients with a diagnosis of interstitial cystitis: common things are sometimes common. J Urol 2005; 174: 584–7.

98. Porru D, Politano R, Gerardini M, et al. Different clinical presentation of interstitial cystitis syndrome. Int Urogynecol J Pelvic Floor Dysfunct 2004; 15: 198–202.

99. Hill JR, Isom-Batz G, Panagopoulos G, Zakariasen K, Kavaler E. Patient perceived outcomes of treatments used for interstitial cystitis. Urology 2008; 71: 62–6.

100. Parsons CL, Schmidt JD, Pollen JJ. Successful treatment of interstitial cystitis with sodium pentosanpolysulfate. J Urol 1983; 130: 51–3.

101. Anderson VR, Perry CM. Pentosan polysulfate: a review of its use in the relief of bladder pain or discomfort in interstitial cystitis. Drugs 2006; 66: 821–35.

102. Chiang G, Patra P, Letourneau R, et al. Pentosan polysulfate inhibits mast cell histamine secretion and intracellular calcium ion levels: an alternative explanation of its beneficial effect in interstitial cystitis. J Urol 2000; 164: 2119–25.

103. Holm-Bentzen M, Jacobsen F, Nerstrom B, et al. A prospective double-blind clinically controlled multicenter trial of sodium pentosanpolysulfate in the treatment of interstitial cystitis and related painful bladder disease. J Urol 1987; 138: 503–7.

104. Mulholland SG, Hanno PM, Parsons CL, Sant GR, Staskin DR. Pentosan polysulfate dosium for therapy of interstitial cystitis. A double-blind placebo-controlled clinical study. Urology 1990; 35: 552–8.

105. Parsons CL, Benson G, Childs SJ, et al. A quantitatively controlled method to study prospectively interstitial cystitis and demonstrate the efficacy of pentosanpolysulfate. J Urol 1993; 150: 845–8.

106. Nickel JC, Barkin J, Forrest J, et al. Randomized, double-blind, dose-ranging study of pentosan polysulfate sodium for interstitial cystitis. Urology 2005; 65: 654–8.

107. Hwang P, Auclair B, Beechinor D, Diment M, Einarson TR. Efficacy of pentosan polysulfate in the treatment of interstitial cystitis: a meta-analysis. Urology 1997; 50: 39–43.

108. Ferjan I, Erjavec F. Characteristics of the inhibitory effect of tricyclic antidepressants on histamine release from rat peritoneal mast cells. Inflamm Res 1996; 45(Suppl 1): S17–18.

109. Van Ophoven A, Pokupic S, Heinecke A, Hertle L. A prospective, randomized, placebo controlled, double-blind study of amityiptiline for the treatment of interstitial cystitis. J Urol 2004; 172: 533–6.

110. Van Ophoven A, Hertle L. The dual serotonin and noradrenaline reuptake inhibitor duloxetine for the treatment of interstitial cystitis: results of an observational study. J Urol 2007; 177: 552–5.

111. Minogiannis P, El-Mansoury M, Betances JA, Sant GR, Theoharides TC. Hydroxyzine inhibits neurogenic bladder mast cell activation. Int J Immunopharmacol 1998; 20: 553–63.

112. Sant GR, Propert KJ, Hanno PM, et al. Interstitial Cystitis Clinical Trials Group. A pilot clinical trial of oral pentosan polysulfate and oral hydroxyzine in patients with interstitial cystitis. J Urol 2003; 170: 810–15.

113. Theoharides TC, Sant GR. Hydroxyzine therapy for interstitial cystitis. Urology 1997; 49(Suppl 5A): 108–10.

114. Seshadri P, Emerson L, Morales A. Cimetidine in the treatment of interstitial cystitis. Urology 1994; 44: 614–16.

115. Dasgupta P, Sharma SD, Womack C, Blackford HN, Dennis P. Cimetidine in painful bladder syndrome: a histopathological study. BJU Int 2001; 88: 183–6.

115. Kelly JD, Young MR, Johnson SR, et al. Clinical response to an oral prostaglandin analogue in patients with interstitial cystitis. Eur Urol 1998; 34: 53–6.

117. Forsell T, Ruutu M, Isoniemi H, Ahonen J, Alfthan O. Cyclosporine in severe interstitial cystitis. J Urol 1996; 155: 1591–3.

118. Fathian-Sabet B, Bloch W, Klotz T, et al. Localization of constitutive nitric oxide synthase isoforms and the nitric oxide target enzyme soluble guanylyl cyclase in the human bladder. J Urol 2001; 165: 1724–9.

119. Ho MH, Bhatia NN, Khorram O. Physiologic role of nitric oxide and nitric oxide synthase in female lower urinary tract. Curr Opin Obstet Gynecol 2004; 16: 423–9.

120. Birder LA, Wolf-Johnston A, Buffington CA, et al. Altered inducible nitric oxide synthase expression and nitric oxide production in the bladder of cats with feline interstitial cystitis. J Urol 2005; 173: 625–9.

121. Smith SD, Wheeler MA, Foster HE Jr, Weiss RM. Improvement in interstitial cystitis scores during treatment with oral L-arginine. J Urol 1997; 158(3 Pt 1): 703–8.

122. Korting GE, Smih SD, Wheeler MA, et. al. A randomized double blind trial of oral L-arginine for treatment of interstitial cystitis. J Urol 1999; 161: 558–65.

123. Cartledge JJ, Davies AM, Eardley I. A randomized double-blind placebo-controlled crossover trial of the efficacy of L-arginine in the treatment of interstitial cystitis. BJU Int 2000; 85: 421–6.

124. Ueda T, Tamaki M, Ogawa O, et al. Improvement of interstitial cystitis symptoms and problems that developed during treatment with IPD-1151T. J Urol 2000; 164: 1917–20.

125. Theoharides TC, Sant GR. A pilot open label study of Cystoprotek in interstitial cystitis. Int J Immunopathol Pharmacol 2005; 18: 183–8.

126. Dawson TE, Jamison J. Intravesical treatments for painful bladder syndrome/interstitial cystitis. Cochrane Database Syst Rev 2007; 4: CD006113.

127. Sun Y, Chai TC. Effects of dimethyl sulphoxide and heparin on stretch activated ATP release by bladder urothelial cells from patients with interstitial cystitis. BJU Int 2002; 90: 381–5.

128. Kuo JC. Urodynamic results of intravesical heparin therapy for women with frequency urgency syndrome and interstitial cystitis. J Formos Med Assoc 2001; 5: 309–14.

129. Parsons CL, Housley T, Schmidt JD, et al. Treatment of interstitial cystitis with intravesical heparin. Br J Urol 1994; 73: 504–7.

130. Parsons CL. Successful downregulation of bladder sensory nerves with combination of heparin and alkalinized lidocaine in patients with interstitial cystitis. Urology 2005; 65: 45–8.

131. Lose G, Jespersen J, Frandsen B, Højensgård JC. Subcutaneous heparin in the treatment of interstitial cystitis. Scand J Urol Nephrol 1985; 19: 27–9.

132. Shiga KI, Hirano K, Nishimura J, et al. Dimethyl sulphoxide relaxes rabbit detrusor muscle by decreasing the Ca²⁺ sensitivity of the contractile apparatus. Br J Pharmacol 2007; 151: 1014–24.

133. Melchior D, Packer CS, Johnson TC, Kaefer M. Dimethyl sulfoxide: does it change the functional properties of the bladder wall? J Urol 2003; 170: 253–8.

134. Peeker R, Haghsheno MA, Homang S, Fall M. Intravesical bacillus Calmette–Guerin and dimethyl sulfoxide for treatment of classic and nonulcer interstitial cystitis: a prospective, randomized double-blind study. J Urol 2000; 164: 1912–15.

135. Rossberger J, Fall M, Peeker R. Critical appraisal of dimethyl sulfoxide treatment for interstitial cystitis: discomfort, side effects and treatment outcome. Scand J Urol Nephrol 2005; 39: 73–7.

136. Smith CP, Somogyi GT, Chancellor MB. Emerging role of botulinum toxin in the treatment of neurogenic and non-neurogenic boiding dysfunction. Curr Urol Rep 2002; 3: 382–7.

137. Chuang YC, Yoshimura N, Juang CC, Chiang PH, Chancellor MB. Intravesical botulinum toxin A administration produces analgesia against acetic acid induced bladder pain responses in rats. J Urol 2004; 172 (4 Pt 1): 1529–32.

138. Liu HT, Kuo HC. Intravesical botulinum toxin A injections plus hydrodistension can reduce nerve growth factor production and control bladder pain in interstitial cystitis. Urology 2007; 70: 463–8.

139. Giannantoni A, Porena M, Costantini E, et al. Botulinum A toxin intravesical injection in patients with painful bladder syndrome: 1-year followup. J Urol 2008; 179: 1031–4.

140. Kuo JC, Chancellor MB. Comparison of intravesical botulinum toxin type A injections plus hydrodistention with hydrodistention alone for the treatment of refractory interstitial cystitis/painful bladder syndrome. BJU Int 2009. [Epub ahead of print].

141. Smith CP, Radziszewski P, Borkowski A, et al. Botulinum toxin A has antinociceptive effects in treating interstitial cystitis. Urology 2004; 64: 871–5.

142. Gunthorpe MJ, Benham CD, Randall A, et al. The diversity in the vanilloid (TRPV) receptor family of ion channels. Trends Pharmacol Sci 2002; 23: 183–191.

143. Lazzeri M, Beneforti P, Spinelli M, et al. Intravesical resiniferatoxin for the treatment of hypersensitive disorder of the lower urinary tract: a randomized placebo controlled study. J Urol 2000; 164: 676–9.

144. Payne CK, Mosbaugh PG, Forrest JB, et al. ICOS RTX Study Group (resiniferatoxin treatment for interstitial cystitis). Intravesical resiniferatoxin for the treatment of interstitial cystitis: a randomized, double-blind, placebo controlled trial. J Urol 2005; 173: 1590–4.

145. Lazzeri M, Beneforti P, Benaim G, et al. Intravesical capsaicin for treatment of severe bladder pain: a randomized placebo controlled study. J Urol 1996; 156: 947–52.

146. Peng CH, Kuo HC. Multiple intravesical instillations of low-dose resiniferatoxin in the treatment of refractory interstitial cystitis. Urol Int 2007; 78: 78–81.

147. Cox M, Klutke JJ, Klutke CG. Assessment of patient outcomes following submucosal injection of triamcinolone for treatment of Hunner's ulcer subtype interstitial cystitis. Can J Urol 2009; 16: 4536–40.

148. Soucy F, Gregoire M. Efficacy of prednisone for severe refractory ulcerative interstitial cystitis. J Urol 2005; 173: 841–3.

149. Kreder K, Lugtendorf S, Knopf, KA, et al. Chlorpactin instillation releases calcitonin gene-related peptide in interstitial cystitis patients. Urology 2001; 57: 128–9.

150. Bouchelouche K, Nordling J, Hald T, et al. The cysteinyl leukotriene D4 receptor antagonist montelukast for the treatment of interstitial cystitis. J Urol 2001; 166: 1734–7.

151. Yoshimura N, Franks ME, Sasaki K, et al. Gene therapy of bladder pain with herpes simplex virus (HSV) vectors expressing preproenkephalin (PPE). Urology 2001; 57(6 Suppl 1): 116.

152. Ottem DP, Teichman JM. What is the value of cystoscopy with hydrodistension for interstitial cystitis. Urology 2005; 66: 494–9.

153. Caraballo R, Bologna RA, Lukban J, Whitmore KE. Sacral nerve stimulation as a treatment for urge incontinence and associated pelvic floor disorders at a pelvic floor center: a follow-up study. Urology 2001; 57(Suppl 6A): 121.

154. Peters KM, Konstandt D. Sacral neuromodulation decreases narcotic requirements in refractory interstitial cystitis. BJU Int 2004; 93: 777–9.

155. Chai TC, Zhang C, Warren JW, Keay S. Percutaneous sacral third nerve root neurostimulation improves symptoms and normalizes urinary HB-EGF levels and antiproliferative activity in patients with interstitial cystitis. Urology 2000; 55: 643–6.

156. Rofeim O, Hom D, Freid RM, Moldwin RM. Use of the neodymium: YAG laser for interstitial cystitis: a prospective study. J Urol 2001; 166: 134–6.

157. Sea J, Teichman JM. Paediatric painful bladder syndrome/interstitial cystitis: diagnosis and treatment. Drugs 2009; 69: 279–96.

158. Rackow BW, Novi JM, Arya LA, Pfeifer SM. Interstitial cystitis is a etiology of chronic pelvic pain in young women. J Pediatr Adolesc Gynecol 2009; 22: 181–5.

159. Shear S, Mayer R. Development of glomerulations in younger women with interstitial cystitis. Urology 2006; 68: 253–6.

160. MacDermott JP, Charpied GL, Tesluk H, Stone AR. Recurrent interstitial cystitis following cystoplasty: fact or fiction? J Urol 1990; 144: 37–40.

161. Kisman IK, Lycklama à Nijeholt AA, van Krieken JH. Mast cell infiltration in intestine used for bladder augmentation in interstitial cystitis. J Urol 1991; 146: 1113–14.

52 Lower Urinary Tract Infections—Simple and Complex

James Gray and Dudley Robinson

INTRODUCTION

Cystitis is the clinical term used to describe inflammation of the urinary bladder, which occurs in response to lower urinary tract infection (UTI). It describes the inflammatory response to microbiologic invasion of the lower urinary tract and includes the clinical symptoms of urinary frequency, urgency, and dysuria.

Lower UTI may be acute, chronic or recurrent as well as being simple or complex. Infection is characterized by large numbers of microorganisms and leukocytes in the urine. The natural history is dependent on the type and virulence of the urinary pathogen, resistance to antimicrobial agents, and host defences.

Diagnosis in the majority of simple cases is based on clinical symptoms, preferably together with laboratory confirmation through urine dipstick testing, microscopy, and/or culture. Recurrent or complex lower UTIs may require additional investigations such as imaging of the upper urinary tracts and testing for fastidious microorganisms.

Overall, the principles of management are to identify the causative organism and, based on the results of urine culture and sensitivity, to administer an appropriate antimicrobial agent for an appropriate length of time. In those women with recurrent or complex infections, specific strategies may need to be developed to treat the infection adequately.

An understanding of the natural history and pathogenesis of lower UTI can facilitate both primary prevention, through reduction or modification of associated risk factors, and secondary prevention by directing cost-effective screening of women who have an increased susceptibility to UTI.

This chapter examines the epidemiology, etiology, and pathogenesis of UTIs, and reviews the management of women presenting with both simple and complex lower UTI.

PREVALENCE

Lower UTI is one of the most common clinical diagnoses in developed countries, accounting for eight million consultations a year in the United States (1,2) and between 1% and 6% of visits to general practitioners in the United Kingdom. Other than in the elderly, UTI is more common in women than in men. Approximately 50% of women will develop a urinary infection during their lifetime (3), the prevalence being 5% per year.

DEFINITIONS

Bacteriuria

The term bacteriuria means the presence of bacteria in urine. In health urine in the bladder is sterile. However, voided urine has to pass through the distal urethral and introitus that may not be sterile. Thus detection of bacteriuria in a voided urine

sample does not always indicate that bacteria were present and multiplying in urine in the bladder. The clinician must therefore assess whether the presence of bacteria in urine represents true bacteriuria, or contamination of the urine during or after collection.

Significant Bacteriuria

The concept of significant bacteriuria was developed by Kass and colleagues in the mid-1950s, on the premise that quantitative culture could help distinguish between the presence of bacteria causing infection by multiplying in the urine and bacteria introduced as contaminants from the urethra or introitus during voiding of a midstream sample of urine (MSU). Based on the fact that most UTIs are caused by *Escherichia coli* and related Gram-negative bacteria that multiply rapidly in urine, significant bacteriuria was defined as a microbial count of >100,000 cfu/ml (4), although even using this criterion a single culture has up to a 20% chance of representing contamination only (5). Following the widespread adoption of quantitative urine cultures, it was noted that 20% to 40% of women with symptoms of acute UTI have bacterial counts of <100,000 cfu/ml. Further evidence that UTI can be associated with bacterial counts of <100,000 cfu/ml stems from observations that the species of bacteria isolated from these women are the same as those from women with higher bacterial counts; bacteria can be isolated from urine samples collected directly from the bladder (e.g., by catheterization or suprapubic aspiration), and symptoms often respond to antimicrobial therapy.

Some studies have reported that bacterial counts as low as 100 cfu/ml can be associated with symptoms. However, up to 10% of asymptomatic women have bacterial counts of this magnitude in urine. As the bacterial count increases within the range 100 to 100,000 cfu/ml, the greater the association with symptoms and in the magnitude of pyuria (6,7). Thus there is no reliable cut-off for bacteriuria to be considered significant, but the importance of bacterial counts of <100,000 cfu/ml should be assessed in the light of symptoms and pyuria. There are several possible explanations for the finding of low level bacteriuria in symptomatic UTI, including concurrent use of antimicrobials, production of very dilute urine, or the representation of an early phase of the infection (8).

Asymptomatic Bacteriuria (ASB)

This is the term used to describe the condition when there is confirmed bacteriuria but the patient remains asymptomatic (9). It is found in approximately 5% of young women and increases with age, reaching a prevalence of 22% to 43% in elderly women. In general, it is not thought to be of clinical significance except in certain clinical circumstances such as

Table 52.1 Risk Factors for Recurrent Urinary Tract Infection

- Lower urinary tract obstruction and chronic retention of urine
- Bladder stones or intravesical foreign bodies
- Trauma
- Enterovesical and vesicovaginal fistulae
- Urethral diverticulae
- Malformations of the urinary tract
- Cystocele
- Vesicoureteric reflux
- Infected paraurethral glands
- Contraceptive diaphragm use

Table 52.2 Conditions Associated with Complicated Lower Urinary Tract Infection

1. Structural
   - Urolithiasis
   - Malignancy
   - Ureteric stricture
   - Urethral stricture
   - Bladder diverticulae
   - Renal cysts
   - Fistulae
   - Urinary diversions
2. Functional
   - Neurogenic bladder
   - Vesicoureteric reflux
   - Voiding difficulties (incomplete bladder emptying)
3. Foreign bodies
   - Indwelling catheter
   - Ureteric stent
   - Nephrostomy tube
4. Other
   - Diabetes mellitus
   - Pregnancy
   - Renal failure
   - Renal transplant
   - Immunosuppression
   - Multidrug resistance
   - Hospital-acquired (nosocomial) infection

pregnancy, instrumentation of the lower urinary tract, and renal transplant patients. It is more likely to be present in those patients with a chronic indwelling catheter (10).

Recurrent UTI

This is the term used to describe a symptomatic infection which follows the resolution of a previous UTI, generally after treatment. It occurs in up to 26% of women within six months of their first UTI (6) and in 48% of women who have had a previous infection (7). The ratio of recurrent lower UTI to pyelonephritis has been estimated to range between 18:1 (8) to 28:1 (11). Overall, approximately 20% to 40% of women who experience a UTI develop recurrent infections (12) and 10% to 15% of women over the age of 60 complain of frequent recurrences (13).

Recurrent infection may be due to relapse of the original organism or to reinfection with the same or a different organism. Relapse is defined as recurrence of bacteriuria with the same organism within seven days of treatment and implies failure to eradicate the infection. In contrast, if bacteriuria is absent after treatment for 14 days or longer, and it is then followed by recurrence of infection with the same or a different organism, this is considered to represent reinfection. Risk factors for recurrent infection are shown in Table 52.1. Around 80% to 90% of recurrent infections are due to reinfections, with one-third being with the same organism (11).

While recurrent infections are relatively common in adult women, they are rarely accompanied by upper tract dysfunction such as reflux, renal scarring, or renal hypertension.

Complicated Lower UTI

This describes infections that are related to other conditions (Table 52.2). These are important because there may be an increased likelihood of ascending infection and/or bacteremia, and the causative microorganisms are more likely to be antibiotic-resistant. One of the most common forms of complicated UTI is related to the use of catheterization. The incidence of bacteriuria associated with an indwelling urinary catheter is 3% to 10% per day, duration of catheterization being the most important risk factor for infection. While fewer than 5% of catheter-associated UTIs result in bacteremia, they are nevertheless a significant cause of morbidity, and they are also an important reservoir of antibiotic-resistant bacteria in hospitals and nursing homes.

Although pregnant women are not at greater risk of ASB, unless such women are treated, there is an increased risk of perinatal complications such as premature delivery and developing a symptomatic infection and pyelonephritis in later pregnancy. for this reason all women should be offered routine screening for ASB early in pregnancy

PATHOGENESIS

The urinary tract is usually sterile above the level of the distal urethra although bacteria do gain access to the bladder, generally from neighboring sites. The fecal–perineal–urethral route of infection is well documented. E. coli is the main causative organism, with the rectal flora serving as the main reservoir (14). Other sites include the bowel, perineum, vaginal vestibule, urethra, and paraurethral tissues.

Ascending infection along the urethra is the most commonly occurring symptom, and may be spontaneous or facilitated by sexual intercourse or catheterization. Meatal colonization occurs, mediated by fimbriae and specific receptor proteins in the epithelial cells in the region of the external meatus. The periurethral area is heavily colonized with bacteria, and these ascend the urethra to enter the bladder and adhere to the urothelium (15).

The method of entry is not fully understood although it has been proposed that bacteria may reflux into the bladder following a void, may ascend against the urinary stream because of turbulent flow, or may milk back into the bladder (16).

However, these factors alone do not necessarily stimulate infection within the bladder and it has been demonstrated that even virulent organisms require some degree of host susceptibility (17). Consequently, it would appear that there is a relationship between host factors (determining susceptibility) and the characteristics of urinary pathogens to invade and colonize the bladder, which affect the course and severity of the disease (18).

In addition, infection may also be via lymphatic spread or blood-borne on rare occasions.

HOST DEFENCES

The bladder has a number of mechanisms to resist infection. The most important is the hydrokinetic or "washout" effect in which diuresis and voiding dilute the bacterial load and wash away infecting organisms. In one study, 40% of women with bacteriuria became free of infection spontaneously within 12 months (19) while a further study demonstrated that the urine of 80% of women with simple infections became sterile on placebo alone (20). Consequently, the risk of infection will depend on the size and multiplication rate of the organism in addition to the urinary residual, urine flow rate, and frequency of voiding.

Antimicrobial Factors

The mechanism by which uroepithelial cells of the bladder resist ascending infection remains poorly understood although it has been demonstrated that activation of uroepithelial cell defense and suppression of bacterial growth depend on direct contact between the two. The composition of urine within the bladder may also have an effect on bacterial growth with extremes of urine pH, high osmolality, and high urea concentration tending to be protective, which is why historically urine has been used as an antiseptic. Urea is the principal antibacterial electrolyte in urine, and its effect is also modulated by concentration and the pH (21).

Epithelial Factors

The bladder mucosa is also thought to have a bactericidal action although the cells themselves are not phagocytic. In addition, it has been postulated that nitric oxide may have a role in bladder wall inflammation and host defense. Nitric oxide produced locally in the bladder has a cytotoxic effect and may contribute as a host defense mechanism within the bladder. Levels of nitric oxide have been found to be 30 to 50 times higher in all types of cystitis when compared to controls (22). In addition, natural killer cells have been shown to be activated in inflamed urothelium, with increased cytolytic activity enhancing the immunologic defense mechanisms of the bladder (23). The bladder also produces a surface secretion of mucus preventing bacterial adhesion to the bladder wall (24).

Immunologic Factors

Secretory immunoglobulin A (IgA) is synthesized by plasma cells within the lamina propria of the bladder wall and hence provides a degree of humoral immunity. In addition, a significant proportion of IgA originates in the urethra and this may help prevent ascending infection (25). Secretory IgA has also been shown to prevent microbial invasion by disrupting bacterial adherence (26) and that production of IgA may be deficient in women with recurrent UTI (27).

Tamm–Horsfall Protein

Tamm–Horsfall protein, a mucoprotein shed from the renal tubular cells and excreted in the urine, has been demonstrated in concentrated urine by electrophoresis (28). This uromucoid protein can bind and trap E. coli, thus providing a natural defense mechanism (29). Levels of antibodies to this protein have been shown to be significantly higher in women with pyelonephritis and vesicoureteric reflux although less is known about the response in uncomplicated lower UTI (30,31).

ROLE OF THE ORGANISM

Uropathogens have the ability to survive and multiply in the bladder as well as being able to adhere to the bladder epithelium. These unique qualities make them particularly virulent in the lower urinary tract.

Adherence

The ability of bacteria to adhere to the urothelium of the lower urinary tract is an important initial step in the pathogenesis of lower UTI. This is supported by the findings of one study in which those women with recurrent UTIs had increased receptivity of urothelial cells for bacteria and increased frequency of vaginal colonization and subsequent infection when compared to a control population (32). Adherence of the organism to the bladder wall triggers an acute inflammatory response by the activation of cytokines. These in turn stimulate the production of an intracellular adhesion molecule, which, by leukocyte adhesion, causes migration of cells to the point of infection (33). These events inadvertently prevent the organism from being "washed out" and, by increasing their nutrient supply, they divide more efficiently.

Uropathogen Structure

The structure of bacteria is also known to be important when considering virulence and pathogenicity. Members of the family Enterobacteriaceae possess an antigenic structure which promotes an antibody immune response and this contributes to the invasiveness and virulence of these bacteria. The outer cell membrane contains O antigens which, together with endotoxins, initiate the immune response in the bladder wall by stimulating cytokine production (34). Capsular (K) antigens on the surface of the bacteria help to inhibit phagocytosis and the actions of IgA and IgG in the urothelium.

Pili and fimbriae are found on the outer membrane of uropathogenic bacteria and promote binding using an adhesion molecule on their tip. This is responsible for the binding of the bacterium to the surface of the epithelial cells within the bladder wall. P-fimbriae mediate adherence to the glycolipids in the urothelium (35) while Type I fimbriae confer the ability to adhere to the mucus layer within the bladder. In addition, some uropathogens are able to break down bladder mucin and invade the urothelium beneath, and this has been associated with the development of recurrent infections (36).

RISK FACTORS FOR UTI

In general, host factors rather than bacterial virulence are probably the most important contributors to lower UTI. These

Table 52.3 Congenital Risk Factors for Urinary Tract Infection

1. Bladder
   - Vesicoureteric reflux
   - Ectopic ureters
   - Obstructive megaureter
2. Pelvis
   - Pelvic–ureteric junction obstruction
3. Central nervous system
   - Meningomyelocele
   - Tethered cord syndrome

Table 52.4 Acquired Risk Factors for Urinary Tract Infection

1. Traumatic
   - Surgery (urinary diversion, clam cystoplasty)
   - Sexual intercourse
   - Sexual abuse
   - Foreign bodies (catheters, stents)
   - Contraceptive diaphragm
2. Inflammatory
   - Vulvourethritis
   - Chronic inflammation (Tuberculosis, syphilis, schistosomiasis)
   - Interstitial cystitis
   - Radiotherapy
   - Fistula
3. Metabolic
   - Calculi
   - Diabetes mellitus
4. Drugs
   - Cyclophosphamide
   - Tiaprofenic acid
5. Anatomic
   - Cystocele
   - Urethral diverticulum
6. Functional
   - Detrusor hypotonia
   - Detrusor dyssynergia
   - Constipation
7. Malignancy
   - Bladder tumors
   - Other pelvic tumors (cervix, uterus, ovary)

predisposing factors can be considered in terms of congenital anomalies (Table 52.3) and acquired causes (Table 52.4).

Age

Among children the incidence of UTI is highest in the first year of life, with a gradual decrease to the lowest rate at 11 to 15 years of age. In children there is a strong association between recurrent infection and non-neurogenic bladder dysfunction, with one study of urodynamic studies revealing a 44% incidence of detrusor overactivity (37).

The incidence of UTI increases in young adult women, where sexual activity is an important contributory factor, and increases again in old age. The increasing prevalence of lower UTI in old age is most likely to be multifactorial in nature, and is associated with the presence of concomitant systemic disease, increasing immobility, fecal and urinary dysfunction, and instrumentation of the urinary tract. Acute cystitis has been found to be one of the most commonly acquired infections in nursing home residents and is often the most frequent cause for admission to hospital (38).

Obesity

At present there is little evidence to suggest a link between obesity and lower UTI. In a large study assessing the factors influencing the rate of first referral for urinary infection in 17,032 women, the risk of first infection declined with age, was higher in nulliparous than in parous women, and was higher in the non-obese compared to the obese (39). Several studies have shown that obese patients are more at risk of developing UTIs after surgery than non-obese patients (40).

Behavioral Factors

There is considerable evidence to suggest that behavioral factors such as voiding habits, diet, clothing, and use of soaps and bubble baths may be associated with the development of UTIs. The use of tampons as opposed to sanitary towels has been associated with an increased risk of infection (41).

There is also a strong association with sexual intercourse, with 75% to 90% of women relating infections to sexual intercourse (42,43). Furthermore, the frequency of intercourse has also been shown to be a significant risk factor (44) and certain strains of E. coli may be transmitted between partners (45).

Contraceptive usage has also been implicated in the development of UTIs. The contraceptive diaphragm and spermicide creams have been found to be positively associated with the risk of developing UTIs (46). This may be due to the effect of intermittent urethral obstruction for six to eight hours following intercourse or, alternatively, due to changes in the vaginal flora. In one large study, the main increase in risk in current diaphragm users occurred during the first 24 months when overall rates were two to three times higher in users than non-users (44).

Instrumentation of the Urinary Tract

The incidence of lower UTI following urethral catheterization is approximately 5%, and a patient has only a 50% probability of remaining free of infection for four days following catheterization (47). Following catheter removal the bacteriuria will resolve spontaneously in around a third of cases (48). Suprapubic catheterization provides an alternative method of long- or short-term bladder drainage and is associated with lower infection rates. In a meta-analysis of studies comparing suprapubic to urethral catheterization following vaginal surgery, the incidence of bacteriuria ranged from 12.5% to 44.5% in the suprapubic group compared to 37.2% to 50.7% in the urethral group (49). The suprapubic route also has the advantage that it allows women to void with the catheter in situ and have post-void residuals checked without the need for repeated catheterization. Finally, the rate of UTI following cystoscopy is approximately 7.5% without interventions (50). As a result, clinicians are increasingly being encouraged to use a single dose of antibiotic prophylaxis such as gentamicin.

Voiding Dysfunction

Incomplete emptying of the bladder is an important cause of UTI in women (51). Voiding dysfunction in women is predominantly secondary to detrusor failure or hypotonia although it may also be associated with detrusor–sphincter dyssynergia or outflow obstruction secondary to a pelvic mass, significant urogenital prolapse, surgery or urethral stricture. In addition, urodynamic studies have shown that, with increasing age, there is a significant increase in post-void residual and a decrease in urinary flow rates, voided volume, and bladder capacity (52). This would suggest that voiding function deteriorates with age and may be partly responsible for the increased incidence of UTI in the elderly.

Vesicoureteric Reflux

During a detrusor contraction, if the vesicoureteric valves are incompetent, vesicoureteric reflux may occur. When the detrusor relaxes again, stagnant urine drains back from the upper renal tracts into the bladder which predisposes to infection. In a review of 200 girls with recurrent lower UTI, 43% demonstrated vesicoureteric reflux, whereas in those with only one episode of infection the corresponding rate was 36% (53). These findings would suggest that failure to institute appropriate investigations in children may mean that potentially severe urinary tract abnormalities remain undetected.

CAUSATIVE ORGANISMS

Gram-negative coliform bacilli of the family Enterobacteriaceae are the most common cause of UTI, accounting for over 80% of cases. *E. coli* is the predominant species in both community and hospital infections, but more antibiotic-resistant species such as Klebsiella and Enterobacter are more common in the latter. Antibiotic-resistant non-coliform Gram-negative bacilli such as *Pseudomonas aeruginosa* and *Acinetobacter* species occur almost exclusively in hospital-acquired infections. Among Gram-positive bacteria, *Staphylococcus saprophyticus* is an important cause of UTI in sexually active women. Other coagulase-negative staphylococci, and *S. aureus*, are more commonly hospital associated. Fastidious bacteria that can only be isolated on enriched culture media, including *Streptococcus pneumoniae* and *Haemophilus influenzae*, are an occasional cause of UTI in primary care. Bacteria that require special detection techniques, such as the cell wall deficient mycoplasma (including *Ureaplasma urealyticum*) and the obligate intracellular pathogen *Chlamydia trachomatis*, are also recognized causes of lower urinary tract symptoms.

UTI can also be caused by microorganisms other than bacteria. Lower UTI due to candida species is most common in patients with urinary catheters. Cystitis due to viruses such as polyoma and adenoviruses occasionally occurs in immunocompromised patients, especially those who have undergone renal or bone marrow transplantation.

Hospital- vs. Community-Acquired Infections

Community-acquired infections differ from those originating from within the hospital environment (54) (Table 52.5) where Klebsiella, Staphylococcus, and Pseudomonas are more prevalent.

Table 52.5 Common Uropathogens in Primary Care and Hospital Practice

Species	Percentage of isolates in UTI in:	
	Primary care	Hospital practice
Escherichia coli	70–90	30–60
Proteus mirabilis	5–10	5–10
Klebsiella–Enterobacter spp.	1–5	10–20
Enterococcus spp.	1–5	5–10
Staphylococcus spp.	5–15	5–10
Pseudomonas aeruginosa	<1	5–10
Candida spp.	<1	1–10
Other	7.4	1–10

Abbreviation: UTI, urinary tract infection.

CLINICAL SYMPTOMS

Women with lower UTIs typically complain of symptoms of cystitis, these being dysuria, suprapubic discomfort, frequency, and nocturia. There may also be associated microscopic or macroscopic hematuria. Of these women, approximately 30% will also have an upper UTI which may present as loin pain and tenderness (55). However, only around half of patients in general practice with the typical symptoms of frequency, dysuria, and suprapubic pain are found to have bacteriuria (54). In the elderly, UTIs may present with atypical symptoms such as confusion and falls (56), whereas young children may present with general malaise and pyrexia. Consequently, symptoms and signs may be unreliable, and in complicated cases or in recurrent infections, it may be necessary to perform investigations to localize the site of infection within the urinary tract (57).

INVESTIGATIONS

In primary care the diagnosis of UTI is often made on clinical grounds, preferably supported by point-of-care dipstick urinalysis (see below). This approach is reasonable for women and children aged three years or older with uncomplicated non-recurrent UTIs in whom the etiologic agents and local antibiotic sensitivity patterns can be predicted with reasonable accuracy. There are several reasons why primary care physicians may elect not to send samples to the laboratory, including the advantages of completing the consultation at a single visit, and the fact that urine samples can deteriorate during transport to the laboratory. Urine examination in suspected UTI can include tests of urine for non-specific markers of urinary infection, as well as tests to establish the microbial etiology and antimicrobial susceptibilities.

Point-of-Care Diagnosis

It is now common practice to investigate urine samples by dipstick testing using test strips that detect leukocyte esterase (LE) (produced by segmented neutrophils) and nitrite (produced by most uropathogens by reduction of urinary nitrates). In some primary care settings a positive result is used to confirm UTI, and samples are not sent to the laboratory. In other

Table 52.6 Urine Dip Testing Strategies for Symptomatic Adults and Children Aged Three Years or Older

Both leukocyte esterase and nitrite are positive	The patient should be regarded as having UTI and antibiotic treatment should be started
Leukocyte esterase is negative and nitrite is positive	Antibiotic treatment should be started if the urine test was carried out on a fresh sample of urine. A urine sample should be sent for culture. Subsequent management will depend upon the result of urine culture
Leukocyte esterase is positive and nitrite is negative	Send urine sample for microscopy and culture. Do not commence empiric antibiotic treatment for UTI unless there is good clinical evidence of UTI
Both leukocyte esterase and nitrite are negative	The patient should not be regarded as having UTI. Antibiotic treatment for UTI should not be started, and a urine sample should not be sent for culture

Abbreviation: UTI, urinary tract infection.

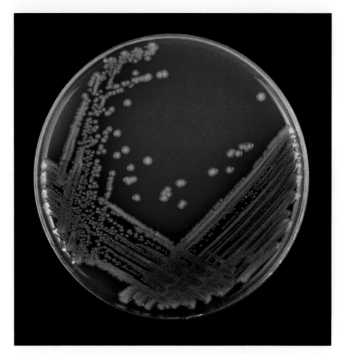

Figure 52.1 *Escherichia coli* growing on blood agar.

settings, a negative dipstick test may be used to exclude UTI, avoiding the need to send urine samples to the laboratory. The interpretation of different patterns of dipstick test results are shown in Table 52.6. Dipstick testing performs less well for specific patient groups. In screening pregnant women for ASB, the sensitivity may be as low as 33.3% (44,45), probably because women with ASB often have low level or absent pyuria. In patients with urinary symptoms associated with low bacterial counts, nitrite testing is of little value, meaning that the sensitivity of combined LE and nitrite testing may be as low as 25% (41). Although dipstick testing has been reported to be useful in a urodynamics clinic (49), it is probably inadvisable to use it as a replacement for culture in specialist urology or urogynecology clinics.

Microbiologic Investigation

In the laboratory, urine samples are conventionally investigated by microscopy and culture. Microscopy is mainly used to detect and quantify leukocytes. Gram staining is sometimes useful where there is a clinical need to establish the diagnosis urgently, because the presence of bacteria can be confirmed, and it may be possible to presumptively identify the causative microorganisms on the basis of the Gram stain appearance.

Different species of bacteria have differing growth requirements. Media used to culture urine routinely (e.g., cysteine lactose electrolyte deficient (CLED), blood, and MacConkey agars) are selected to optimize growth of common uropathogens. Figure 52.1 illustrates *E. coli*, the most common uropathogen, growing on blood agar. These standard urine culture media do not support the growth of fastidious microorganisms that are occasional causes of UTI. Consideration should be given to further investigation of culture-negative urine samples from women with significant pyuria, especially if this is confirmed on a second sample. However, in the authors' experience there is little value in further investigating such samples unless the white cell count exceeds 100 per high powered field and anti-

Table 52.7 Laboratory Investigations of Sterile Pyuria

Sample required	Microorganisms	Test method
MSU	Fastidious bacteria (e.g., *Streptococcus pneumoniae, Haemophilus influenzae*)	Culture on enriched media, (e.g., chocolate agar)
MSU	Mycoplasmas, Ureaplasmas	Mycoplasma culture system
Three early morning urine samples	*Mycobacterium tuberculosis*	Mycobacterial culture
First pass urine or urethral, vaginal or endocervical swab	*Chlamydia trachomatis*	Nucleic acid amplification technique
MSU	Adenoviruses, Polyomaviruses	Specialist virologic investigations

Abbreviation: MSU, midstream sample of urine.

bacterial substances are absent from the urine. There is a wide range of potential pathogens that require different detection methods (Table 52.7) and have different epidemiologic and clinical risk factors. Liaison between the requesting clinician and the laboratory is essential to ensure optimal investigation.

Further Investigations

In the majority of women with simple acute cystitis there is no need for further investigation. However, some cases (Table 52.8) warrant further investigation in order to exclude an underlying cause.

In those women who have recurrent or complicated urinary infections, renal function should be assessed with serum creatinine, urea, and electrolytes.

Table 52.8 Indications for Investigation of Lower Urinary Tract Infection

- Children
- Proven recurrent urinary tract infection
- Adults with a childhood history of urinary tract infection
- Hematuria
- Persistent infection
- Failure to respond to antibiotic therapy

Table 52.9 Aims of Treatment

- Symptomatic relief
- Clinical cure
- Microbiologic cure
- Detection of predisposing factors
- Prevention of upper urinary tract involvement
- Management of recurrence
- Prevention of recurrence

In specific cases it may be helpful to exclude atypical infections (*Mycoplasma hominis, Ureaplasma urolyticum,* and *Chlamydia trachomatis*). The usual history is of a woman suffering repeated cystitis episodes which improve with antibiotics, but symptoms return as soon as antibiotics are stopped. Often there have been repeated MSUs which demonstrate a sterile pyuria but no growth on culture.

While it is generally accepted that assessment of the upper urinary tract is not mandatory in all women with UTI (58), consideration should be given to further investigation in those patients with a history of recurrent or complex infections.

Ultrasound of the renal tract will exclude causes such as hydronephrosis or calculi and a postmicturition scan will rule out a significant urinary residual. A pelvic ultrasound should be performed to exclude the possibility of a pelvic mass which may affect voiding function and therefore predispose to UTI.

The upper tracts can also be imaged using MR or CT urography (59). These modalities have largely replaced intravenous urograms (IVU), although the latter still involves exposure to ionizing radiation. An IVU has not been shown to influence treatment in the majority of cases (60). Renal imaging may be useful in women with demonstrated upper urinary tract abnormalities in order to detect or confirm obstructed drainage from the kidney and also to determine differential function between the left and right kidneys or upper and lower poles unilaterally. Dimercaptosuccinic acid (DMSA) scans are generally not indicated in women with acute pyelonephritis where there is a rapid response to antimicrobial therapy, but may be considered when the course of the infection is complicated or protracted (61). Mercaptoacetyl triglycine and technetium-labeled diethyltriaminepentaacetic acid may also be considered in order to exclude both upper urinary tract obstruction and renal scarring.

Women with a history suggestive of voiding dysfunction should be investigated initially using non-invasive tests to determine urinary flow rate and residual urine.

Women complaining of recurrent UTI should undergo cystourethroscopy and bladder biopsy to exclude an intravesical lesion such as a bladder tumor and also anomalies such as diverticulae and calculi. A bladder biopsy may show evidence of chronic follicular or interstitial cystitis. Microscopic or frank hematuria should also be considered as an indication for cystoscopy.

Those who also complain of other lower urinary tract symptoms should be investigated using videocystourethrography in order to exclude underlying detrusor overactivity, bladder or urethral diverticulae, and vesicoureteric reflux.

TREATMENT

Management of lower UTI is aimed at treating the current infection and preventing further recurrences (Table 52.9).

General Measures—Prophylaxis

Primary prevention consists of general advice regarding hygiene, fluid intake, and frequency of voiding. In women complaining of recurrent infections related to sexual intercourse, postcoital voiding should be encouraged. They should also be advised to avoid using a diaphragm or condoms with nonoxynol-9 as both of these may increase the risk of recurrent infection. Appropriate advice regarding bladder emptying such as timed voiding or double voiding may also help those with voiding difficulties. Should these not be successful, then intermittent self-catheterization or a long-term suprapubic catheter may be required.

General Measures—Treatment

Patients with cystitis should be encouraged to increase their fluid intake in order to achieve a short voiding interval and a high flow rate which will help to dilute and flush out the infecting organism. Symptomatic relief may be provided by using potassium citrate preparations. With such measures spontaneous remission of symptoms may occur in up to 40% of women (62).

Cranberry juice has also been shown to reduce infections in women with recurrent lower UTIs (63). Regular intake of at least 300 ml/day has been associated with a reduced risk of UTIs. The incidence of bacteriuria in those taking cranberry juice was 42% of that in the control group; they were also found to be four times more likely to clear bacteria spontaneously (64). Cranberry juice is thought to act by reducing bacterial adherence to the bladder wall.

ANTIMICROBIALS

When treating UTIs, an antimicrobial that has an appropriate spectrum of activity, achieves a high concentration within the urinary tract, and has a low risk of promoting the emergence or spread of antibiotic resistance should be selected (Table 52.10). The latter is an especially important consideration as recognition of the association between antimicrobial use and *Clostridium difficile* has increased. Many of the antibiotics that were most commonly used to treat UTIs now have to be used with caution, either because resistance rates amongst uropathogens are high (as in the case of amoxicillin and trimethoprim) or because of the association with *C. difficile* (as in the case of cephalosporins and quinolones). Where the pathogen is known, narrow spectrum therapy can be used.

Table 52.10 Choice of Antimicrobial Agent

- Specificity for the urinary tract
- High levels of drug in the urine
- Broad spectrum of activity
- Safe and efficacious
- Rapid and complete absorption
- Minimal effect on normal bowel reservoir and vaginal flora
- Bactericidal for known pathogens

Broader spectrum therapy may be necessary for empiric treatment, especially for hospital-associated infections, but in such cases consideration should be given to switching to a narrower spectrum agent once the pathogen has been identified. Ideally, drugs should be reliably absorbed after oral administration, safe, and well-tolerated.

Undue emphasis is often placed on the distinction between bactericidal and bacteriostatic antibiotics. In most cases it makes no difference to outcome. However, bactericidal antibiotics are preferred on theoretical grounds for patients with immunodeficiencies. Of the antibiotics commonly used to treat UTIs, the β-lactam antibiotics, and aminoglycosides and fluoroquinolones are the most reliably bactericidal.

Individual Antibiotics

Amoxicillin

Amoxicillin is a derivative of ampicillin that has a similar antibacterial spectrum, but is better and more reliably absorbed. These drugs are no longer recommended as first line empiric therapy for UTIs because of the high prevalence of resistance amongst Enterobacteriaceae.

Co-amoxiclav is a combination of amoxicillin and clavulanic acid that inhibits the β-lactamase enzymes produced by many amoxicillin-resistant bacteria. Co-amoxiclav has a spectrum of antibacterial activity that is often unnecessarily broad for treating UTIs. Although co-amoxiclav use has been associated with *C. difficile* the association may be less strong than with cephalosporins. Co-amoxiclav has therefore superseded second generation cephalosporins in many hospitals, but it should still be used with caution, especially in the elderly.

Piperacillin-Tazobactam

This is a combination of piperacillin (an anti-pseudomonal penicillin) and tazobactam (a β-lactamase inhibitor). It has an antibacterial spectrum that is similar to co-amoxiclav, together with activity against *Pseudomonas aeruginosa*. It appears to be much less likely to select for *C. difficile* than the broad-spectrum cephalosporins, and has largely superseded their use in many hospitals.

Cephalosporins

First generation cephalosporins have a spectrum of activity that encompasses most community-associated uropathogens. However, they are not active against enterococci, Enterobacter and Pseudomonas, and therefore may be less suitable for use in complex UTIs. Although serum levels of first generation cephalosporins are poor after oral administration, they appear in high concentrations in urine.

For treating UTIs the newer and more expensive second generation oral cephalosporins offer little or no benefits over the earlier (and cheaper) cephalosporins. Use of broad-spectrum cephalosporins has been strongly associated with *C. difficile*, especially third generation cephalosporins given to the elderly.

Carbapenems

These are expensive very broad-spectrum β-lactam antibiotics that are for intravenous use only. Their main use in treating UTIs is in treating infections with extended-spectrum β-lactamase (ESBL) producing Gram-negative bacteria, including strains that are resistant to other antibiotic classes such as the fluoroquinolones and aminoglycosides. Meropenem and imipenem with cilastatin are the most commonly used carbapenems for hospital in-patients. Ertapenem is another carbapenem antibiotic. Unlike meropenem and imipenem with cilastatin it has no useful anti-pseudomonal activity, but it has a longer half-life, permitting once daily administration so that it can be used for out-patient therapy of infections with multiplt-resistant bacteria such as ESBL producers.

Trimethoprim

Trimethoprim is now widely used as first line empiric therapy for UTIs; however, resistance is increasing, even in the community. Trimethoprim is best avoided in pregnancy (especially first trimester), because of the theoretical risk of teratogenicity.

Co-trimoxazole is a mixture of trimethoprim and sulfamethoxazole, which rarely offers any benefits over trimethoprim but has a higher risk of side effects. The U.K. Committee for Safety of Medicines recommends that co-trimoxazole should be used only where there is good bacteriologic evidence of benefit over trimethoprim.

Tetracyclines

Tetracyclines have a spectrum of activity that covers most uropathogens, including atypical microorganisms. Other than doxycycline and minocycline, they are excreted mainly in the urine. However, they are little used for treating UTIs because widespread use of tetracyclines in the past was associated with rapid emergence of resistance.

Tetracyclines are deposited in growing bones and teeth, and are contraindicated in pregnancy, breastfeeding women, and children aged <12 years.

Fluoroquinolones

Fluoroquinolones such as ciprofloxacin, ofloxacin, and norfloxacin are predominantly active against Gram-negative bacteria. They are the only orally available drugs with activity against *P. aeruginosa*.

Because high drug concentrations occur in urine, they may be effective in UTIs due to Gram-positive bacteria, although they are not the recommended first line therapy for these infections. They are contraindicated in pregnancy, and recommended for use in children only where there is no alternative. Fluoroquinolones may have contributed to the spread of the new *C. difficile* strain 027 in the United Kingdom, although data are conflicting.

Nalidixic acid is an older quinolone antibiotic that is inactive against *P. aeruginosa*, and is now little used.

Nitrofurantoin
Nitrofurantoin appears in high concentrations in urine, but serum and tissue levels are subtherapeutic. It is therefore only useful for treating lower UTIs. Because it has a complex mode of action, acquired resistance to nitrofurantoin is uncommon. In particular, nitrofurantoin is often the only oral therapeutic option for UTIs with ESBL-producing bacteria.

Nitrofurantoin is notoriously associated with nausea, but this can often be contained by taking the drug with food. Nitrofurantoin is safe during pregnancy, but is contraindicated at term because of the risk of causing neonatal hemolysis.

Aminoglycosides
Amoniglycosides such as gentamicin and amikacin have been used to treat serious infections, especially with Gram-negative bacteria, for several decades. The later introduction of broad-spectrum cephalosporins and fluoroquinolones offered an apparently safer alternative to the aminioglycosides and their use declined. However, aminoglycosides appears to be much less likely to promote *C. difficile*, and they are experiencing a renaissance as a treatment for serious infections. Once-daily administration are now generally used, being as effective and with less risk of toxicity than traditional three times daily regimens.

Azithromycin
Azithromycin is a macrolide-like antibiotic that is not excreted in the urine, nor does its spectrum of activity encompass most common uropathogens. However, it is effective in treating genital chlamydial infections after single dose therapy, and there are anecdotal reports that longer courses of treatment have been successful in treating refractory urogenital mycoplasma infections.

Antibiotic Resistance
Antibiotic resistance in bacteria causing UTI is a growing problem both in hospitals and in the community. Amoxicillin resistance is now prevalent in *E. coli* and other Enterobacteriaceae, and resistance to trimethoprim is increasing. Most isolates in the community remain susceptible to cephalosporins and co-amoxiclav, although this is not the case in hospitals where cephalosporinase-producing species such as Enterobacter are more common. The recent emergence and spread of plasmid-borne ESBLs that confer resistance to penicillins and cephalosporins in Enterobacteriaceae and other Gram-negative bacteria present a growing problem. The genes encoding these enzymes are readily transferred between species and are frequently associated with genes conferring resistance to other antibiotic classes, such as quinolones and aminoglycosides. Community-acquired UTIs with ESBL-producing bacteria that are resistant to all oral antibiotics are already being encountered, and pose real therapeutic difficulties.

There may be some local variation in antibiotic resistance patterns amongst uropathogens. Table 52.11 summarizes the activity of oral antibiotics against common uropathogens.

Duration of Antibiotic Therapy
Compliance with therapy may be improved by using shorter courses of antimicrobial therapy or ideally by using a single dose regimen. This also has the advantage of reducing the effect on fecal and vaginal flora and thus reduces the risk of *C. difficile*, However, a large number of studies have assessed the use of single dose therapy and found it not to be as effective as a short-term (3 day) regimen (65). There is also a risk of selecting resistance in the surviving bacteria.

There is no evidence to show that protracted courses are more effective in uncomplicated lower UTIs in adult women (66).

Estrogens
Estrogen therapy has been shown to increase vaginal pH and reverse the microbiologic changes that occur in the vagina following the menopause (67). Initial small uncontrolled studies using oral or vaginal estrogens in the treatment of recurrent UTI appeared to give promising results (68,69); unfortunately, this has not been supported by larger randomized trials. Several studies have been performed examining the use of oral and vaginal estrogens although these have had mixed results.

Kjaergaard and colleagues (70) compared vaginal estriol tablets with placebo in 21 postmenopausal women over a five-month period and found no significant difference between the two groups. However, a subsequent randomized, double-blind, placebo-controlled study assessing the use of estriol vaginal cream in 93 postmenopausal women during an eight-month period did reveal a significant effect (71).

Kirkengen et al. randomized 40 postmenopausal women to receive either placebo or oral estriol and found that although initially both groups had a significantly decreased incidence of recurrent infections, after 12 weeks estriol was shown to be significantly more effective (72). These findings, however, were not confirmed subsequently in a trial of 72 postmenopausal women with recurrent UTIs randomized to oral estriol or placebo. Following a six-month treatment period and a further six-month follow-up, estriol was found to be no different from placebo (73).

More recently, a randomized, open, parallel-group study assessing the use of an estradiol-releasing silicone vaginal ring (Estring) in postmenopausal women with recurrent infections has been performed which showed the cumulative likelihood of remaining infection free was 45% in the active group and 20% in the placebo group (74). Estring was also shown to decrease the number of recurrences per year and to prolong the interval between infection episodes.

Antimicrobial Prophylaxis
Antimicrobials may be used as prophylaxis for recurrent UTIs. Short- and long-term low-dose prophylaxis as well as intermittent and postcoital therapy may be used depending

Table 52.11 Expected Antibiotic Susceptibilities of Common Uropathogens

Species	Amoxicillin	First generation cephalosporins	Second generation cephalosporins	Co-amoxiclav	Trimethoprim	Fluoroqui-nolones	Nitrofurantoin	Tetracyclines
Escherichia coli	++	+++	+++	+++	++	+++	+++	++
Proteus	++	+++	+++	+++	++	+++	−	++
Klebsiella	−	++	+++	+++	++	+++	+++	++
Enterobacter	−	−	−	−	++	+++	+++	++
Pseudomonas aeruginosa	−	−	−	−	−	+++	−	−
Streptococci	+++	+++	+++	+++	++	−	+++	+++
Enterococci	++	−	−	++	++	−	++	++
Staphylococcus saprophyticus	++	+++	+++	+++	++	++	+++	+++
Other coagulase-negative staphylococci	+	+	+	+	+	++	++	
S. aureus (meticillin-sensitive; MSSA)	−	+++	+++	+++	+++	++	+++	+++
S. aureus (meticillin-resistant; MRSA)	−	−	−	−	++	+	+++	++
Mycoplasmas	−	−	−	−	−	++	−	++
Chlamydia trachomatis	−	−	−	−	−	++	−	+++

Abbreviations: +++, >90% isolates sensitive; ++, 51% to 90% isolates sensitive; +, 10% to 50% isolates sensitive; −, <10% isolates sensitive.

on the clinical situation. The most effective drugs include norfloxacin, nitrofurantoin, and trimethoprim. In addition, cephalexin may be used as effective prophylaxis against recurrent infections in sexually active women. Overall prophylactic therapy has been shown to reduce recurrence rates by up to 95% when compared to placebo, with reinfection rates being reduced from two to three per patient year to 0.1 to 0.4 per patient year (75).

The idea of single dose treatment of simple (recurrent) infections in susceptible women at a time of increased risk has given rise to some clinicians using antibiotics on an as needed basis in women with recurrent infections, rather than low dose continual therapy.

COMPLEX LOWER UTI
Lower UTI in Pregnancy
ASB occurs in 4% to 7% of pregnancies (76). It is associated with the development of acute cystitis, pyelonephritis, preterm labor, and low birth weight. The prevalence of bacteriuria in the first trimester of pregnancy is 5% to 6%, similar to that in non-pregnant women (77). If untreated, up to 30% of women will develop acute cystitis although this can be reduced to 3% with effective treatment (78). Recurrent infections may also be a problem following delivery in women who have had bacteriuria in pregnancy, occurring in up to 25% of cases (79).

The increased susceptibility to lower UTI in pregnancy may be due to the effects of incomplete bladder emptying and chronic residual urine secondary to the weight of the gravid uterus. Progesterone is also known to increase stasis in the urinary tract by causing ureteric relaxation which will also increase the risk of ascending infections. In addition, bacterial growth is also increased in pregnancy, the bacterial count of *E. coli* being twice that in non-pregnant women (80).

During pregnancy, more serious UTIs follow untreated silent bacteriuria in 25% of women (81). There is also an increased risk of developing pyelonephritis in pregnancy and, of these women, up to 20% may develop serious complications such as septic shock (82). Several authorities have suggested that there may be an association between positive urine cultures for group B streptococci and chorioamnionitis and preterm delivery (83), although this remains unproven. However, an association has been reported between elevated levels of urinary antibacterial antibodies and bacterial antigens and preterm delivery, suggesting that a local inflammatory response to urogenital infection may be important in stimulating preterm labor (84). Treatment of ASB in early pregnancy has been shown to reduce preterm delivery.

Treatment
The treatment of ASB in pregnancy will lead to a decrease in the risk of cystitis and pyelonephritis, and has been shown to be cost effective (85). Treatment of bacteriuria prevents up to 80% of cases of pyelonephritis and has been shown to be effective in the reduction of preterm labor (86). Surprisingly

however, there is little evidence that women with ASB in early pregnancy require to be re-screened later in pregnancy.

When treating lower UTIs in pregnancy, penicillins and cephalosporins have been shown to be safe in the first and second trimesters (87). Trimethoprim, since it is a folate antagonist, should be avoided in the first trimester although may be used safely in late pregnancy (88). Conversely, nitrofurantoin is safe in early pregnancy but should be avoided around term when it may cause neonatal hemolytic anemia (89).

There is little agreement on the duration of therapy for ASB in pregnancy. Although single dose regimens have been investigated (90) the shortest course of therapy that appears promising is three days, and even here it is recommended that a follow-up culture be undertaken after around 10 days to ensure microbial clearance. Many clinicians still prefer to use conventional treatment courses of 7 to 10 days.

Lower UTIs in the Elderly

Following the menopause there is a fall in endogenous estrogen levels, resulting in a decrease in lactobacilli colonization of the vagina, a rise in vaginal pH, and a subsequent increase in colonization with uropathogenic bacteria. Bacteriuria has a low predictive value for identifying febrile UTIs in the elderly (91).

Persistent bacteriuria has been shown to be common in non-catheterized nursing home residents, with little evidence that it is associated with significant morbidity (92). In part this is because bacteriuria with low virulence Gram-positive bacteria such as enterococci, coagulase-negative staphylococci, and group B streptococci is more common in this age group (93). Consequently, ASB, although very common in the elderly, need not be treated (94). However, it is important to recognize that UTI in the elderly can be associated with systemic symptoms and signs such as fever, confusion, nausea, and vomiting without localizing urinary tract symptoms.

With regard to symptomatic infection, the aim of antimicrobial treatment is the relief of symptoms rather than achieving long-term sterility of urine, and it should be noted that the elderly are less likely to be cured by shorter courses of therapy (95). Antibiotics must be used with particular care in the elderly because of the risk of *C. difficile*.

Lower UTIs in Children

The U.K. National Institute for Health and Clinical Excellence recently published evidence-based guidance on the diagnosis and management of UTIs in children (96). These guidelines recommend that a first lower UTI in children aged three months or older require less intensive investigation and treatment than has been previously recommended. Infants aged six months or under should always be investigated in view of the potential for subsequent renal scarring and other sequelae; otherwise investigations such as renal tract ultrasound, DMSA, and micturating cystograms are required only for atypical or recurrent infection (96).

It is difficult to obtain good quality clean-catch urine samples from children. Perhaps partly for this reason low bacterial counts, the absence of pyuria or a finding of sterile pyuria are not uncommon in the course of acute or chronic cystitis and

should not be regarded as insignificant (97). In cases of doubt, techniques to obtain urine directly from the bladder, such as suprapubic aspiration or in-out catheterization may be required.

The difficulties and inconsistencies in managing UTIs in children are exemplified by a large follow-up study of 57,432 children under the age of 15 years and 7143 children under two years, where it was found that infection is often under diagnosed and, after a confirmed infection, only a minority of children received imaging for complications and microbiology follow-up to assess cure (98).

The frequency of vesicoureteric reflux in babies born to women with a history of the condition is significantly higher than in the general population. Because the condition is not usually diagnosed in children until it is complicated by an ascending UTI screening of newborn babies at risk of familial reflux has been suggested (99). However, the clinical and cost effectiveness of this intervention has not been evaluated, and it is certainly not common practice.

Treatment

Much of the risk of developing complications following lower UTIs in children is related to the delay in diagnosis and treatment, and also the lack of suitable imaging. When first diagnosed with a UTI 5% of children will already have renal scarring (100), As children get older the risk of new scarring reduces and after the fourth birthday the risk is almost zero (101). Consequently, efforts to reduce the incidence and severity of renal scarring following cystitis in infancy and childhood should be directed towards rapid diagnosis and early effective treatment.

When considering the treatment of children with lower UTIs the choice of antimicrobial should be based on local multidisciplinary guidance and the results of urine culture and sensitivity. A three day course of antibiotics is sufficient (102). Antibiotic prophylaxis should be given when performing a micturating cystogram.

Catheterization

The frequency of catheter-acquired infection increases with the duration of catheterization and the failure to maintain a closed drainage system. Consequently, it is not uncommon that infections with multiple organisms occur in women with long-term indwelling catheters (103). Using interventions such as topical antimicrobials, disinfectants added to the urinary drainage bag, antimicrobial coatings for catheters, or antimicrobial irrigation does not decrease the incidence of catheter-associated infections (104). There is evidence that catheters impregnated with silver alloy may reduce the risk of UTIs (105). U.K. evidence-based guidelines for preventing infections associated with short-term urethral catheters have been published (106).

Bacteriuria should be expected in women with long-term catheterization and, if asymptomatic, treatment is generally not justified as it is unlikely to give a microbiological cure, and risks selecting for antibiotic-resistant microorganisms. It is common practice to collect a urine sample for culture at the time of catheter removal, and to treat any infection

documented at that time. However, the value of this approach has been questioned. Given that bacteriuria will be common at the time of catheter removal, it is probably more rational to collect a urine sample 24 hours or more after catheter removal if there is clinical suspicion of infection at that time.

As an alternative to long-term catheterization, the technique of clean intermittent self-catheterization (CISC) may be considered in women who are able to learn the technique. Bacteriuria occurs in up to 61% of women performing long-term CISC although the incidence of significant cystitis is approximately 6% (107). Overall, the incidence of infection was 10.3 per 1000 patient days of CISC during early follow-up and 13.6 per 1000 patient days of CISC over an average of 22 months (108). Evidence, however, would suggest that the use of prophylactic antibiotics does not improve the outcome in women performing CISC and should not be used.

CONCLUSION

Lower UTI is common in women of all ages. Rigid adherence to Kass's criteria and the use of standard urine culture techniques lead to significant under diagnosis of UTI. The continuing emergence and spread of antibiotic-resistant bacteria presents a growing challenge in treating UTI, with options for oral therapy in particular becoming more limited. Liaison between clinicians and their microbiology laboratory is essential to facilitate the diagnosis and management of UTI.

REFERENCES

1. Griebling TL. Urologic diseases in America project: trends in resource use for urinary tract infections in women. J Urol 2005; 173: 1281–7.
2. Foxman B. Epidemiology of urinary tract infection:incidence, morbidity and economic costs. Dis Mon 2003; 49: 53–70.
3. Asscher AW. Urinary tract infections. J R Coll Physicians Lond 1981; 15: 232–8.
4. Kass EH. Asymptomatic infections of the urinary tract. Trans Assoc Am Phys 1956; 69: 56–64.
5. Kass EH. The role of asymptomatic bacteriuria in the pathogenesis of pyelonephritis. In: Quinn EL, Kass EH, eds. Biology of Pyelonephritis. Boston: Little Brown, 1960: 399–406.
6. Foxman B. Recurring urinary tract infection: incidence and risk factors. Am J Public Health 1990; 80: 331–3.
7. Ikaheimo R, Siitonen A, Heiskanen T, et al. Recurrence of urinary tract infection in a primary care setting: analysis of a 1 year follow up of 179 women. Clin Infect Dis 1996; 22: 91–9.
8. Stamm WE, McKevitt M, Roberts PL, White NJ. Natural history of recurrent urinary tract infections in women. Rev Infect Dis 1991; 13: 77–84.
9. Nicolle LE. Asymptomatic bacteriuria: review and discussion of the IDSA guidelines. Int J Antimicrob Agents 2006; 28(Suppl 1): S42–8.
10. Raz R. Asymptomatic bacteriuria. Clinical significance and management. Int J Antimicrob Agents 2003; 22(Suppl 2): 45–7.
11. Brauner A, Jacobson SH, Kuhn I. Urinary Escherichia coli causing recurrent infections—a prospective follow-up of biochemical phenotypes. Clin Nephrol 1992; 38: 318–23.
12. Mabeck CE. Treatment of uncomplicated urinary tract infection in non-pregnant women. Postgrad Med J 1972; 48: 69–75.
13. Romano JM, Kaye D. UTI in the elderly: common yet atypical. Geriatrics 1981; 36: 113–5.
14. Yamamoto S, Tsukamato T, Terai A, et al. Genetic evidence supporting the faecal–perineal–urethral hypothesis in cystitis caused by Escherichia coli. J Urol 1997; 157: 1127–9.
15. Kallenius G, Svenson S, Hulberg H, et al. P-fimbriae of pyelonephrogenic Escherichia coli: significance for reflux and renal scarring—a hypothesis. Infections 1983; 11: 73–6.

16. O'Grady F, Cattell WR. Kinetics of urinary tract infection II. The bladder. Br J Urol 1966; 38: 156–62.
17. Schlager TA, Whittam TS, Hendley JO, et al. Comparison of expression of virulence factors by Escherichia coli causing cystitis and Escherichia coli colonising the periurethra of healthy girls. J Infect Dis 1995; 172: 772–7.
18. Wisinger DB. Urinary tract infection. Current management strategies. Postgrad Med 1996; 100: 229–36.
19. Asscher A, Sussman M, Waters W, et al. The clinical significance of asymptomatic bacteriuria in the non-pregnant woman. J Infect Dis 1969; 120: 17–21.
20. Mabeck CE. Uncomplicated urinary tract infections in women. Proc R Soc Med 1971; 3: 31–5.
21. Schegel J, Cuellar J, O'Dell R. Bactericidal effects of urea. J Urol 1961; 86: 819–21.
22. Lundberg JO, Ehern I, Jansson O, et al. Elevated nitric oxide in the urinary bladder in infectious and non–infectious cystitis. Urology 1996; 48: 700–2.
23. Natsis K, Toliou T, Stravoravdi P, et al. Natural killer cell assay within bladder mucosa of patients bearing transitional cell carcinoma after interferon therapy: an immunohistochemical and ultrastructural study. Int J Clin Pharmacol Res 1997; 17: 31–6.
24. Parsons C, Pollen J, Anwar H, et al. Antibacterial activity of bladder surface mucin duplicated in the rabbit bladder by exogenous glycosaminoglycans (sodium pentosampolysulphate). Infect Immun 1980; 27: 876–81.
25. Burdon D. Immunoglobulins of the urinary tract: discussion on a possible role in urinary tract infection. In: Brumfitt W, Asscher A, eds. Urinary Tract Infection. London: Oxford University Press, 1973: 148–58.
26. Tomasi TB. Mechanisms of immune regulation at mucosal surfaces. Dev Infect Dis 1983; 5: 5784–92.
27. Riedasch G, Heck P, Rauterberg E, et al. Does low urinary IgA predispose to urinary tract infection? Kidney Int 1983; 23: 759–63.
28. Jenkins MA. Clinical application of capillary electrophoresis to unconcentrated human urine proteins. Electrophoresis 1997; 18: 1842–6.
29. Tamm I, Horsfall F. Mucoprotein derived from human protein which reacts with influenza, mumps and newcastle disease viruses. J Exp Med 1952; 95: 71–97.
30. Jelakovic B, Benkovic J, Cikes N, et al. Antibodies to Tamm-Horsfall protein subunit prepared in vitro in patients with acute pyelonephritis. Eur J Clin Chem Clin Biochem 1996; 34: 315–7.
31. Hanson LA, Fasth A, Jodal U. Autoantibodies to Tamm-Horsfall protein, a tool for diagnosing the level of urinary tract infection. Lancet 1976; 1: 226–8.
32. Kozody NL, Harding GK, Nicolle LE, et al. Adherence of Escherichia coli to epithelial cells in the pathogenesis of urinary tract infection. Clin Invest Med 1985; 8: 121–5.
33. Roberts JA. Factors predisposing to urinary tract infections in children. Pediatr Nephrol 1996; 10: 517–22.
34. Svanborg-Eden C, Korhonen T, Lettler R, Marild S. Pathogenic aspects of bacterial adherence in urinary tract infections. In: Losse H, Asscher A, Lison A, eds. Pyelonephritis, vol IV: Urinary Tract Infection. Stuttgart: Thieme, 1980: 54–9.
35. Domisgue G, Roberts H, Laucirica R, et al. Pathogenic significance of P-fimbriated Escherichia coli in urinary tract infections. J Urol 1985; 133: 983–9.
36. Brooks H, O'Grady F, McSherry M, Cattell W. Uropathogenic properties of Escherichia coli in recurrent urinary tract infection. J Med Microbiol 1980; 13: 57–68.
37. Qvist N, Neilsn KK, Kristensen ES, et al. Detrusor instability in children with recurrent urinary tract infections and/or enuresis. II. Treatment. Urol Int 1986; 41: 199–201.
38. Yoshikawa TT, Norman DC. Approach to fever and infection in the nursing home. J Am Geriatr Soc 1996; 44: 74–82.
39. Vessey MP, Metcalf M, McPhersen K, Yeates D. Urinary tract infection in relation to diaphragm use and obesity. Int J Epidemiol 1987; 16: 441–4.
40. Bamgbade OA, Rutter TW, Nafiu OO, Doije P. Post-operative complicationsin obese and non-obese patients. World J Surg 2007; 31: 556–60.

41. Foxman B, Frerichs R. Epidemiology of urinary tract infection: II. Diet, clothing and urination habits. Am J Public Health 1985; 75: 1314–7.

42. Nicolle LE, Harding GM, Preiksatis J, Ronald AR. The association of urinary infection with sexual intercourse. J Infect Dis 1982; 146: 579–83.

43. Leibovici L, Alpert G, Laor A, et al. Urinary tract infection and sexual activity in young women. Arch Int Med 1987; 147: 345–7.

44. Hooton T, Scholes D, Hughes J. A prospective study of risk factors for symptomatic urinary infection in young women. N Engl J Med 1996; 335: 468–74.

45. Foxman B, Zhang L, Tallman P, et al. Transmission of uropathogens between sex partners. J Infect Dis 1997; 175: 989–92.

46. Foxman B, Chi J. Health behaviour and urinary tract infections in college-aged women. J Clin Epidemiol 1990; 43: 329–37.

47. Maizels M, Schaeffer A. Decreased incidence of bacteriuria associated with periodic instillations of hydrogen peroxide into the urethral catheter drainage bag. J Urol 1980; 123: 841–5.

48. Harding GKM, Nicolle LE, Ronald AR, et al. How long should catheter acquired urinary tract infection in women be treated? A randomised controlled study. Ann Intern Med 1991; 114: 713–9.

49. Schiotz HA. Urinary tract infection after vaginal repair surgery. Int Urogynecol J 1992; 3: 185–90.

50. Clark KR, Higgs MJ. Urinary infection following outpatient flexible cystoscopy. Br J Urol 1990; 66: 503–5.

51. Hansoon S, Hyalmas K, Jodal V, Sixt R. Lower urinary tract dysfunction in girls with untreated asymptomatic or covert bacteriuria. J Urol 1990; 143: 313–5.

52. Madersbacher S, Pycha A, Schatzl G, et al. The ageing lower urinary tract: a comparative urodynamic study of men and women. Urology 1998; 51: 206–12.

53. Baker R, Barbaris HT. Comparative results of urological evaluation of children with initial and recurrent urinary tract infections. J Urol 1976; 116: 503–5.

54. Mond NC, Percival A, Williams JD, Brumfitt W. Presentation, diagnosis and treatment of urinary tract infections in general practice. Lancet 1965; 1: 514–6.

55. Kurowski K. The women with dysuria. Am Fam Phys 1998; 57: 2155–64; 2169–70.

56. Yoshikawa TT, Norman DC. Approach to fever and infection in the nursing home. J Am Geriatr Soc 1996; 44: 74–82.

57. Pollock H. Laboratory techniques for detection of urinary tract infections and assessment of value. Am J Med 1983; 75: 79–84.

58. Fowler J, Pulaski E. Excretory urography cystography and cystoscopy in the evaluation of women with urinary tract infections. N Engl J Med 1981; 304: 462–5.

59. Silverman SG, Leyendecker JR, Amis ES, Jr. What is the current role of CT urography and MR urography in the evaluation of the urinary tract. Radiology 2009; 250: 309–23.

60. Mogensen P, Hansen LK. Do intravenous urography and cystoscopy provide important information in otherwise healthy women with recurrent urinary tract infection? Br J Urol 1983; 55: 261–3.

61. Bailey RR, Lynn KL, Robson RA, Smith AH, Maling TMJ, Turner JG. DMSA renal scans in adults with acute pyelonephritis. Clin Nephrol 1996; 46: 99–104.

62. Froom J. The spectrum of urinary tract infections in family practice. J Fam Pract 1980; 11: 385–91.

63. Jepson RG, Craig JC. Cranberries for preventing urinary tract infections. Cochrane Database Sys Rev 2008; (1): CD001321. DOI: 10.1002/14651858. CD001321.pub4.

64. Foxman B, Geiger AM, Palin K, Gillespie B, Koopman JS. First time urinary tract infection and sexual behaviour. Epidemiology 1995; 6: 162–8.

65. Warren J, Abruityn E, Hebel SR, et al. Guidelines for antimicrobial treatment of uncomplicated acute bacterial cystitis and pyelonephritis in women. Clinical Infectious Disease 1999; 29: 745–58.

66. Lutters M, Vogt-Ferrier NB. Antibiotic duration for treating uncomplicated, symptomatic lower urinary tract infections in elderly women. Cochrane Database Sys Rev 2008; (3):: CD001535. DOI: 10.1002/14651858. CD001535.pub2.

67. Brandberg A, Mellstrom D, Samsioe G. Low dose oral oestriol treatment in elderly women with urogenital infections. Acta Obstet Gynaecol Scand 1987; 140: 33–8.

68. Parsons CL, Schmidt JD. Control of recurrent urinary tract infections in postmenopausal women. J Urol 1982; 128: 1224–6.

69. Privette M, Cade R, Peterson J, et al. Prevention of recurrent urinary tract infections in postmenopausal women. Nephron 1988; 50: 24–7.

70. Kjaergaard B, Walter S, Knudsen A, et al. Treatment with low dose vaginal oestradiol in postmenopausal women. A double blind controlled trial. Ugeskr Laeger 1990; 152: 658–9.

71. Az R, Stamm WE. A controlled trial of intravaginal oestriol in postmenopausal women with recurrent urinary tract infections. N Engl J Med 1993; 329: 753–6.

72. Kirkengen AL, Anderson P, Gjersoe E, et al. Oestriol in the prophylactic treatment of recurrent urinary tract infections in postmenopausal women. Scand J Primary Health Care 1992; 10: 139–42.

73. Cardozo LD, Benness C, Abbott D. Low dose oestrogen prophylaxis for recurrent urinary tract infections in elderly women. Br J Obstet Gynaecol 1998; 105: 403–7.

74. Eriksen B. A randomised, open, parallel-group study on the preventative effect of an oestradiol-releasing vaginal ring (Estring) on recurrent urinary tract infections in postmenopausal women. Am J Obstet Gynecol 1999; 180: 1072–9.

75. Nicolle LE, Ronald AR. Recurrent urinary tract infections in adult women: diagnosis and treatment. Infect Dis Clin North Am 1987; 1: 793–806.

76. Smaill F. Asympotmatic bacteriuria in pregnancy. Best Prac Res Clin Obstet Gynaecol 2007; 21: 439–50.

77. Kass EH. Bacteriuria and pyelonephritis of pregnancy. Arch Intern Med 1960; 105: 194–8.

78. Whalley PJ. Bacteriuria of pregnancy. Am J Obstet Gynecol 1967; 97: 723–38.

79. Gower P, Haswell B, Sidaway M, et al. Follow-up of 164 patients with bacteriuria of pregnancy. Lancet 1968; 1: 990–4.

80. Roberts A, Beard R. Some factors affecting bacterial invasion of the bladder during pregnancy. Lancet 1965; 1: 1133–6.

81. Cunningham FG, Lucas MJ. Urinary tract infections complicating pregnancy. Baillières Clin Obstet Gynaecol 1994; 8: 353–73.

82. Millar LK, Cox SM. Urinary tract infections complicating pregnancy. Infect Dis Clin North Am 1997; 11: 13–26.

83. Anderson BL, Simhan HN, Simons KM, Wiesenfeld HC. Untreated asymptomatic group B streptococcal bacteriuria early in pregnancy and chorioamnionitis at delivery. Am J Obstet Gynecol 2007; 196: 524.e1–5.

84. McKenzie H, Donnet ML, Howice PW, et al. Risk of preterm delivery in pregnant women with group B streptococcal urinary infections or urinary antibodies to group B and E coli antigens. Br J Obstet Gynaecol 1994; 101: 107–13.

85. Villar J, Bergsjo P. Scientific basis for the content of routine antenatal care. I. Philosophy, recent studies and power to eliminate or alleviate adverse maternal outcomes. Acta Obstet Gynaecol Scand 1997; 76: 1–14.

86. Kiningham RB. Asymptomatic bacteriuria in pregnancy. Am Fam Phys 1997; 47: 1232–8.

87. Gerstner G, Muller G, Nahler G. Amoxicillin in the treatment of asymptomatic bacteriuria in pregnancy. A single dose of 3g amoxicillin versus a 4 day course of 3 doses 750mg amoxicillin. Gynecol Obstet Invest 1989; 27: 84–7.

88. Locksmith G, Duff P. Preventing neural tube defects: the importance of periconceptual folic acid supplements. Obstet Gynaecol 1998; 91: 1027–34.

89. Harris RE. Antibiotic therapy of antepartum urinary tract infections. J Int Med Res 1980; 8(Suppl. 1): 40–4.

90. Lumbiganon P, Villar J, Laopaiboon M, et al. One-day compared with 7-day nitrofurantoin for asymptomatic bacteriuria in pregnancy: a randomized controlled trial. Obstet Gynecol 2009; 113: 339–45.

91. Nicolle LE, Orr P, Duckworth H, et al. Gross hematuria in residents of long term care facilities. Am J Med 1993; 94: 611–8.

92. Eberle CM, Winsemius D, Garibaldi RA. Risk factors and consequences of bacteriuria in non-catheterised nursing home residents. J Gerontol 1993; 48: M266–71.

93. Nicolle LE. Topics in long term care: urinary tract infection in long term care facilities. Infect Control Hosp Epidemiol 1993; 14: 220–5.

94. Wood CA, Abrutyn E. Optimal treatment of urinary tract infections in elderly patients. Drugs Aging 1996; 9: 352–62.

95. Nicolle LE. Urinary tract infections in the elderly. J Antimicrob Chemother 1994; 33(Suppl. A): 99–109.

96. CG54 Urinary tract infection in children: NICE Guideline.22 August 2007.

97. Pead L, Maskell R. Study of urinary tract infection in children in one health district. Br Med J 1994; 309: 631–4.

98. Jadresic L, Cartwright K, Cowie N, et al. Investigation of urinary tract infection in children. Br Med J 1993; 307: 761–4.

99. Scott JE, Swallow V, Coulthard MG, et al. Screening of newborn babies for familial ureteric reflux. Lancet 1997; 350: 396–400.

100. Asscher A, McLachlan M, Jones R, et al. Screening for asymptomatic urinary tract infection in schoolgirls. A two centre feasibility study. Lancet 1973; 2: 1–4.

101. Vernon SJ, Coulthard MG, Lambery HJ, et al. New renal scarring in children who at age 3 and 4 years had had normal scans with dimercaptosuccinic acid: follow up study. Br Med J 1997; 315: 905–8.

102. Michael M, Hodson EM, Craig JC, Martin S, Moyer VA. Short versus standard duration oral antibiotic therapy for acute urinary tract infection in children. Cochrane Database Sys Rev 2003; (1): CD003966. DOI: 10.1002/14651858.CD003966.

103. Grahn D, Normal DC, White ML, et al. Validity of urinary catheter specimen for diagnosis of urinary tract infection in the elderly. Arch Intern Med 1985; 145: 1858–60.

104. Nicolle LE. Prevention and treatment of urinary catheter related infections in older patients. Drugs Aging 1994; 4: 379–91.

105. Schumm K, Lam TBL. Types of urethral catheters for management of short-term voiding problems in hospitalised adults. Cochrane Database Sys Rev 2008; (2): CD004013. DOI: 10.1002/14651858.CD004013. pub3.

106. Pellowe C, Pratt RJ, Loveday HP, et al. The EPIC project: Updating the evidence base fornational evidence-based guidelines for preventing healthcare associated infections in NHS hospitals in England. A report with recommendations. Br J of infection control 2004; 5: 10.

107. National Institute on Disability and Rehabilitation Research Consensus Statement, Jan 27–29 1992. The prevention and management of urinary tract infections among people with spinal cord injuries. J Am Paraplegia Soc 1992; 15: 194–204.

108. Rhame F, Perkash I. Urinary tract infections occurring in recent spinal cord injury patients on intermittent catheterisation. J Urol 1979; 122: 669–73.

53 Vaginitis

James Gray and Andrew Hextall

INTRODUCTION

Vaginitis may present with a number of different complaints including vaginal soreness, discharge, pruritus, and dyspareunia. Although many women will present acutely others will have attempted to treat their symptoms for some time with over the counter preparations. Often they will present a diagnostic challenge which may require a team approach. Infection is the most common cause of vaginitis but other non-infective processes, including a number of dermatological conditions, can produce similar symptoms. However, most women and their doctors use the term vaginitis synonymously with infection and they assume that all vulvovaginal irritation or itching, especially when accompanied by abnormal secretions, is caused by infection (1).

There are a large number of causes of vaginitis and treatment will usually depend on the underlying etiology. Often clinical assessment and investigation will reveal more than one problem highlighting the need sometimes for joint clinics involving a gynecologist, dermatologist, and genito-urinary medicine physician with back up of laboratory based staff. While acute infections usually respond quickly to anti-microbiol therapy for many patients vaginitis runs a chronic course which may be resistant to initial therapy.

VAGINAL ECOSYSTEM

An understanding of the normal environment is helpful in identifying abnormal conditions and directing appropriate therapy. The normal vaginal flora is complex, consisting of a wide range of microbial species that associate in a stable way with the vaginal epithelium. A change in the environmental conditions provided by the vaginal epithelium as a result of endogenous or exogenous influences can lead to changes in the population densities of microbial species, such that formerly commensal microorganisms become pathogenic, resulting in vaginal symptoms (2,3). This is the pathogenic mechanism underlying bacterial vaginosis. Vaginitis can also result from the acquisition of new pathogens, such as *Trichomonas vaginalis*, that are not part of the normal vaginal flora.

The estrogen status of the vagina has an important role in determining the vaginal flora. In the prepubertal state (from six weeks postpartum), the vagina is thin and hypoestrogenic. The pH of the vagina is more than 4.7, and culture shows a variety of organisms as shown in Table 53.1.

From puberty to the menopause, increased levels of estrogen stimulate and thicken the vaginal epithelium. The glycogen content of the epithelial cells increases and the pH decreases to <4.5. This encourages the growth of lactobacilli, which comprise more than 95% of the bacteria in the normal vagina (4). This is achieved by the lactobacilli interfering with other bacterial adherence mechanisms and competition for available energy sources. Several mechanisms have been proposed as to why lactobacilli have a protective effect against infective vaginitis, including the production of lactic acid, hydrogen peroxide, and bacterial toxins.

Patients with vaginitis often complain of vaginal discharge. It is important to understand the characteristics of a healthy vaginal discharge in order to differentiate it from the abnormal. Healthy vaginal discharge is slate gray to white in color. It is homogenous, may be thick or thin, and is odorless. The pH varies from 3.8 to 4.6 (4). On microscopy, the squamous epithelial cells are mature and clear, WBCs are absent, and the dominant bacterial morphotype is the lactobacilli (5). The physiologic discharge does not adhere to the vaginal walls and is not usually associated with other symptoms (6). Vaginal discharge varies over the menstrual cycle. Stress increases the rate of vaginal desquamation and thus the amount of discharge (7). Hormonal contraception and pregnancy are associated with increased vaginal discharge (8). Hence the "normal" discharge may vary and it is important to reassure the patient that a discharge, while troublesome, may not be abnormal.

EPIDEMIOLOGY

It is difficult to obtain accurate figures since vaginitis is not a notifiable disease and many women will self-diagnose and obtain over-the-counter (OTC) treatment. Vaginitis is said to be the most common reason for gynecologic consultation in the United States and accounts for approximately 10 million visits annually (9). Up to 90% of vaginitis cases may be secondary to one of three infections: bacterial vaginosis, candidiasis, and trichomoniasis (3). The roles of other microorganisms as a cause of vaginitis are less clear. Gonorrhea and chlamydial infection may present with vaginal discharge, but the site of infection is cervical, rather than vaginal. Genital herpes can also present with vaginal symptoms. *Streptococcus pyogenes* (group A streptococcus) may cause up to 5% of cases of vaginitis (10), but there is little evidence that other bacteria cause vaginal discharge other than occasionally as opportunistic pathogens. Vaginal discharge is a common presenting complaint in primary care, being present in one woman in 10 presenting to her general practitioner (11). National figures in the United States show that 40% to 50% of patients with vaginal symptoms have bacterial vaginosis, 20% to 25% have vulvovaginal candidiasis, and 15% to 20% have trichomoniasis (12). Other studies indicate that up to 30% of women with vaginal symptoms go without a diagnosis (13).

The incidence of vaginitis is greater in the more humid, subtropical countries (14).

Table 53.1 Normal Vaginal Flora

• Lactobacillus
• Staphylococcus
• Streptococcus
• Escherichia
• Enterococcus
• Corynebacterium
• Diphtheroids
• Klebsiella
• Bacteroides
• Proteus
• Peptostreptococcus
• Prevotella
• Eubacterium
• Fusobacterium
• Clostridium

CAUSES OF VAGINITIS

1. Infective
   A) Common
      Bacterial vaginosis
      Candidiasis
      T. vaginalis
   B) Less common
      S. pyogenes
      Gonorrhea
      Chlamydia
      Herpes simplex
      Human papilloma virus
      Entamoeba histolytica
      Enterobius vermicularis
      Giardia lamblia
2. Non-infective
   Atrophic vaginitis
   Desquamative inflammatory vaginitis (DIV)
      (e.g., lichen planus)
   Poor hygiene
   Foreign body (e.g., retained tampon)
   Allergic vulvovaginitis
   Psychosomatic [may have history of sexual abuse (15)]
   Idiopathic
   Lactobaccillosis

Women presenting with vaginitis may be found to also have a number of other problems including:

• vulval skin conditions (e.g., lichen sclerosis) which may cause ulcers/erosions;
• vulval pain syndromes (e.g., vulvodynia or vestibulodynia);
• geniito-urinary prolapse;
• fistula;
• cervicitis;
• endometrial polyp; and
• Carcinoma-vulval/vaginal/cervical.

EVALUATION OF VAGINAL SYMPTOMS

A detailed history is essential in order to arrive at a proper diagnosis and adequately address any associated concerns (16).

Common symptoms of vaginitis include vaginal soreness, pain, or burning often associated with a discharge. Some women find it difficult to describe the exact site of their problem with many unable to differentiate between a problem in the vulva or vagina. Further questioning may reveal a generalized skin problem and soreness in the mouth may point to a mucocutaneous condition such as lichen planus.

Sexually active women are at an increased risk of vaginitis because the presence of semen in the vagina may increase the pH and thereby allow proliferation of pathogenic anaerobic bacteria (9). It is well known that the risk of vaginitis and all sexually transmitted diseases (STDs) is increased in women with multiple sexual partners. A thorough history of the patient's sexual activity is essential. A sexual history may indicate the need to investigate for STDs or may highlight domestic violence issues. It will provide a better understanding of the chronicity of a patient's symptoms, their relationship with sexual activity, and their impact on sexual self-image (16).

Vaginitis is common in postmenopausal women and may co-exist with genito-urinary prolapse and incontinence. Unexpected vaginal bleeding will usually require investigation to exclude a sinister cause (17).

In view of the large number of possible causes of vaginitis it is often valuable to see women in a specialized joint clinic with clinicians from a number of backgrounds present to aid each other and the patient with diagnosis and treatment options. A checklist for history-taking is provided in Table 53.2.

PELVIC EXAMINATION

Vaginitis is frequently, but not invariably, accompanied by inflammatory changes in the vulva, vestibule, and cervix (18). Pelvic examination should be undertaken systematically, starting from the vulva. The vagina should be examined for signs of edema, erythema, excoriation, fissures, scaling, peripheral satellite pustules, ulcers, atrophic signs, etc. The cervix should be visualized for abnormal features such as a "strawberry cervix" and it should be noted whether discharge is from the cervix or the vagina. The presence of discrete, punctuate, bright red hemorrhagic macules, and papules on the cervix produces the classic but non-specific strawberry cervix in trichomoniasis. Retained tampons or other foreign bodies may sometimes be found on examination. Bimanual examination for adnexal tenderness and masses should be part of the evaluation.

Assessment of the skin or mouth may be undertaken, often with the help of a dermatologist, if there is a suspician of generalized skin disorder which may also be affecting the vagina.

INVESTIGATIONS

Symptoms and signs are non-specific; therefore a diagnosis made by history and examination alone may be unreliable. In primary care and reproductive health settings, where diagnostic facilities are not immediately available, it may be possible to diagnose some cases of vaginitis on the basis of the presence of classical symptoms and clinical examination. In one recent study this approach (including determination of vaginal pH) had a sensitivity of over 85% for diagnosis of bacterial vaginosis (19). However, in the hospital setting full investigation is always indicated. With a standardized approach to the evaluation of vaginal symptoms, a cause can be identified in most cases.

Table 53.2 Symptom Checklist

1. Duration and severity of symptoms
2. Vaginal discharge
   - Quantity
   - Color: clear, white, gray, green, yellow
   - Consistency: thin, thick, curd-like
   - Purulent or not
   - Presence of odor
3. Associated symptoms and location of these symptoms (e.g., vulva, deep vagina, or introitus)
   - Pruritus
   - Soreness
   - Irritation
   - Pain
   - Burning
   - Lump or swelling suggestive of prolapse
   - Bleeding
   - Superficial dysuria
   - Superficial dyspareunia
   - Lower abdominal pain
   - Vulvar symptoms
4. History of dermatological problems
5. Soreness in the mouth
6. History of chemicals which have come into contact with the perineum (e.g., perfumed soaps)
7. Past treatment and response (e.g., any use of over-the-counter medication?)
8. Menstrual history and variation of symptoms with menstrual cycle
9. Obstetric history
10. Sexual history
    - Number of sexual partners (if appropriate)
    - Frequency of sexual practice
    - Contraception (e.g., use of condoms, spermicides, intrauterine contraceptive device, etc.)
11. Cervical smear history
12. Medical history
    - History of diabetes, lupus, AIDS
    - Thyroid disease or other autoimmune disorder (17)
13. Drug history (e.g., systemic antibiotics, steroids)
14. History of allergies
15. History of smoking

Table 53.3 Investigations to Diagnose the Different Types of Vaginitis

Investigation	Description
Vaginal pH	Normal 3.5–4.6
Whiff test	Release of a fishy odor after a drop of 10% potassium hydroxide (KOH) is placed on the secretion is a positive "whiff test," diagnostic of bacterial vaginosis
Microscopy	Wet mount: epithelial cells, WBCs, lactobacilli, yeasts, trichomonads, clue cells
	KOH slide: KOH lyses epithelial cells, WBCs, and yeast cells; hyphae are seen more easily
Gram stain	Can be used to diagnose bacterial vaginosis and candidiasis; trichomonads are more difficult to identify
Culture and polymerase chain reaction based tests	Performed when microscopy is negative, or in recurrent or resistant cases
Endocervical swabs	Obtained for Chlamydia and Gonococcus in all sexually active women since the presence of vaginal discharge is poorly correlated with the presence of infection (8)
Other specific tests	Herpes cultures should be obtained in the presence of ulceration
	Tests to rule out allergens (see "Allergic Vulvovaginitis")
	Blood tests to detect antibodies when HIV or syphilis is suspected

On microscopy, the normal vaginal superficial cell is large with a small nucleus. At times of hypoestrogenism (postmenopausally or postnatally) or infection, parabasal cells are found which are smaller and oval shaped with a large nucleus. A ratio of WBCs and epithelial cells of more than 1:1 is suggestive of an infection (16).

Microscopy is central to the diagnosis of bacterial vaginosis. Candidiasis and trichomoniasis can also be diagnosed by microscopy, although the sensitivity of microscopy for diagnosis of these infections is not high: Further investigations may be required to exclude these diagnoses. Culture is the next diagnostic step although nucleic acid amplification techniques are likely to supersede culture, as the range of pathogens detectable by commercially-available tests expands.

The investigations outlined in Table 53.3 may be used to diagnose different types of vaginitis but their use will vary, depending on the availability of resources, staffing, equipment, expertise, time, etc.

SPECIFIC CAUSES OF VAGINITIS
Bacterial Vaginosis

Bacterial vaginosis is the most common cause of abnormal discharge in women of childbearing age (23), but is often underdiagnosed and incorrectly managed as thrush. Reported prevalences range from 5% in asymptomatic women in the United Kingdom (24) to over 50% of asymptomatic women in African countries (25). The prevalence is appreciable in women who have sex with women (26), among whom other infections associated with sexual activity are relatively uncommon.

Bacterial vaginosis represents a disruption in the vaginal ecosystem. There is an overgrowth of bacterial vaginosis-associated

Checking the vaginal pH at the time of examination can be helpful, although results must always be interpreted in the context of the clinical history and other findings. Infective causes of increased pH include bacterial vaginosis, trichomoniasis, and infection secondary to foreign bodies. Other causes of an elevated pH include DIV, hypoestrogenism, menses, heavy cervical mucus, and pregnancy with ruptured membranes. Semen, vaginal douches, and intravaginal medication can also increase the vaginal pH; note also that lubricating gel used on the speculum can affect the recorded pH.

A vaginal swab should ideally be collected from the middle third of the vagina, the anterior fornix or lateral vaginal wall. Swabs from the posterior fornix may not be representative of true vaginal pH and microscopic findings may also be difficult to interpret (16). Self-collected low vaginal swabs have been shown to be acceptable for diagnosing sexually-transmitted infections, such as chlamydial infection or gonorrhea, when sensitive nucleic amplification detection tests are used (20,21). However, such swabs are less reliable for diagnosing vaginal infections (22).

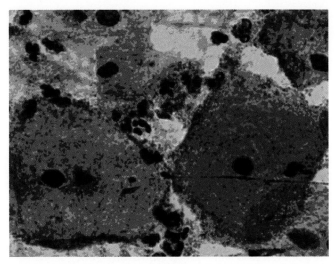

Figure 53.1 Bacterial vaginosis is typified by the presence of coccoid bacteria which adhere in large numbers to squamous cells. These are known as "clue cells." Magnification ×600. *Source:* Courtesy of Mr. Malcolm Mackie, Clinical Cytologist, William Harvey Hospital, Ashford, U.K.

bacteria (predominantly anaerobes) leading to replacement of hydrogen peroxide-producing lactobacilli. On microscopy this is seen as a shift from normal lactobacilli-dominated flora, together with normal numbers of WBCs and the presence of clue cells. These are squamous epithelial cells with a fine granular cytoplasm and indistinct borders due to adherent coccobacilli (Fig. 53.1), and are seen in more than 90% of patients with bacterial vaginosis (4).

Contributory factors and management of bacterial vaginosis are outlined in Table 53.4.

Vulvovaginal Candidiasis

The most common cause of vulvovaginal candidiasis is *Candida albicans*. This accounts for 80% to 90% of cases (Fig. 53.2); non-*albicans Candida* species account for the other 20% (30). Non-*albicans Candida* species are important because they appear to be becoming more common, and resistance to anti-fungal drugs (especially the azoles) is more common, making infections more difficult to treat. Between 20% and 40% of women who have positive cultures are asymptomatic (8). It is

Table 53.4 Contributory Factors and Management of Bacterial Vaginosis

Factor	Description
Causes	Overgrowth of BVAB, including *Gardenerella vaginalis*, *Mycoplasma hominis*, Mobilincus sp., Prevotella sp., Peptostreptococcus sp., Bacteroides sp., etc.
Transmission	Not directly sexually transmitted, but prevalence is higher in women who are sexually active. Importantly, increases susceptibility to HIV transmission
Risk factors	Smoking Intrauterine contraceptive device Vaginal douching Orogenital sex
Signs and symptoms	Increased vaginal discharge which presents as a thin white, homogenous coating on the walls of the vagina Itching and irritation may be present but dysuria and dyspareunia are rare Offensive fishy odor due to volatilization of bacterial amines (produced by anaerobic metabolism following exposure to alkaline substances such as KOH and semen) 50% are asymptomatic (16) Inflammatory signs are absent
Diagnosis	Examination of Gram-stained vaginal smears using Hay/Ison or Nugent's criteria are the most widely used diagnostic methods (23). The Hay/Ison method is easier, and has been shown to have comparable accuracy. Both scoring systems classify appearances as normal, intermediate, or bacterial vaginosis. Intermediate flora is regarded as a transient state, from which around 50% of women will progress to develop the full criteria of BV. Amsel's criteria still regarded by many as the gold standard test, but assessment is more cumbersome: at least three out of four of the following criteria should be present for the diagnosis to be confirmed: (*i*) thin, white, homogenous discharge; (*ii*) clue cells on microscopy; (*iii*) pH > 4.5; (*iv*) fishy odor on addition of 10% KOH Cultures are not useful because *G. vaginalis* can be isolated from up to 50% of women without bacterial vaginosis Bacterial vaginosis may be incidentally diagnosed on cervical cytology [sensitivity and specificity 55% and 98%, respectively (27)]
Treatment	There is a lack of evidence for benefit of treating all asymptomatic cases, but treatment is recommended for asymptomatic cases before some surgical procedures (see below) *Recommended regimens:* Metronidazole 400–500 mg p.o. b.i.d. for 5–7 days or metronidazole 2 g p.o. single dose *Alternatives:* intravaginal metronidazole gel (0.75%) o.d. for 5 days; intravaginal clindamycin cream (2%) o.d. for 7 days; clindamycin 300 mg b.i.d. for 7 days. The cure rate with any of these regimens is 70–80% Lactobacillus recolonization (via yoghurt or capsules) shows promise for the treatment of bacterial vaginosis with little potential for harm (28)
Complications	*Obstetric:* Premature labor [40% elevated risk of having preterm infants with low birth weight (29)], premature rupture of membranes, chorioamnionitis, postpartum endometritis *Gynecologic:*[a] post-termination infections, post-hysterectomy vaginal cuff infections, pelvic inflammatory disease, urinary tract infection, postoperative infections, mucopurulent cervicitis

[a]Screening and treatment with metronidazole results in a significant reduction in these morbidities.
Abbreviation: BVAB, bacterial vaginosis-associated bacteria.

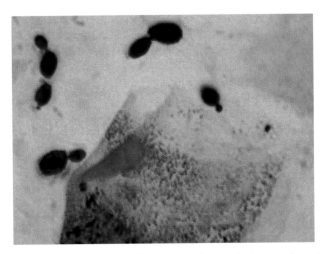

Figure 53.2 Candidiasis. Magnification ×1000. Gram-stained smear of a vaginal swab showing budding yeast cells.

estimated that 75% of adult women will suffer at least one episode of vulvovaginal candidiasis during their lifetime (31). However, accurate figures are difficult to obtain, firstly due to the availability of OTC medication, and secondly to the assumption of candidiasis by clinicians prescribing without microbiologic confirmation (prospectively or retrospectively).

The frequent use of OTC preparations has also increased the likelihood that women will come to medical attention with inadequately treated infections (6). This, along with the widespread use of oral azole antifungal drugs (especially in immunocompromised patients, including those with HIV disease), are likely contributors to the increasing emergence of antifungal resistance (4). The contribution of sexual transmission to vulvovaginal candidiasis is currently poorly defined. In general risk factors for sexually-acquired infections, including number of male sexual partners, are not associated with vaginal candidiasis. However, practices such as receptive anal and oral sex do appear to be associated with vulvovaginal candidiasis (32). There is also evidence of sexual transmission in women who have sex with women (33).

Contributory factors and management of vulvovaginal candidiasis are outlined in Table 53.5.

Table 53.5 Contributory Factors and Management of Vulvovaginal Candidiasis

Factor	Description
Risk factors	Immunocompromise (e.g., diabetes, AIDS)
	Medications (e.g., topical steroids, immunosuppressants, systemic antibiotics, oral contraceptives)
	Pregnancy—increased hormone levels affect the glycogen content which favors the growth of yeast
	A warm, moist environment, and local maceration favor the growth of yeast (e.g., obesity, incontinence, tight-fitting clothing, synthetic underwear)
	Use of diaphragm, spermicide, or intrauterine contraceptive device
	Orogenital sex and frequency of sexual activity (34)
	Any condition causing pruritus—scratching, lichenification, hyperkeratosis, and maceration create a favorable environment for Candida so candidiasis and dermatosis coexist
Symptoms	Pruritus [present in 70–90% (13)]
	Cheesy discharge
	Soreness
	Superficial dysuria
	Superficial dyspareunia
Signs	Edema
	Erythema
	Cheesy discharge which is adherent to vaginal walls
	Excoriation
	Fissuring
	Satellite lesions
Diagnosis	Clinical, but symptoms and signs are non-specific
	Investigations: pH is 4.0–4.5; saline microscopy [sensitivity to detect pseudohyphae ranges from 40% to 60% (35)]; increased polymorphonuclear neutrophils are present; KOH slide [sensitivity is 70% (35)]; Gram stain may detect 65–68% of symptomatic cases (36, 37)
	Culture: Sabouraud's media should be considered where microscopy is inconclusive, or in recurrent cases
	Latex agglutination tests show no advantage over microscopy (38)
Treatment	Both vulva and vagina should be treated simultaneously
	All topical and oral azole (e.g., clotrimazole vaginal cream and pessary) therapies give a 80–90% cure rate in acute cases; nystatin gives a 70–90% cure rate (39)
	Topical therapies: Clotrimazole pessary 500 mg stat/200 mg for three nights/100 mg for six nights; nystatin pessary (100,000 units) 1–2 for 14 nights
	Oral therapy: Fluconazole 150 mg given as a single dose
	Lactobacillus recolonization (via yoghurt or capsules) shows promise for the treatment of yeast vaginitis with little potential for harm (28)

Note: Pregnant women should be treated with topical agents for at least seven days. Oral azole antifungal therapy should not be used (4).

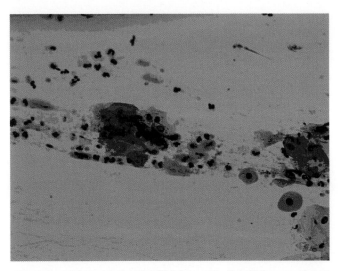

Figure 53.3 Trichomoniasis. Magnification ×100. Unicellular pear-shaped organism 8 to 20 mm in diameter. Appears pale green–gray, often with eosinophilic granules and contains an oval vesicular nucleus. Inflammatory changes are usually pronounced. The single flagellum is not observed in cervical smears. *Source*: Courtesy of Mr. Malcolm Mackie, Clinical Cytologist, William Harvey Hospital, Ashford, U.K.

Recurrent Candidiasis

Recurrent candidiasis is defined as four or more episodes of symptomatic candidiasis in a year; its prevalence is <5% of healthy women of reproductive years (38). The most common cause is incomplete eradication as demonstrated by strain typing (40). In addition, 30% to 50% of women with recurrent candidiasis will be recolonized with Candida within one month of a short-term treatment (41). Drug resistance is less of a factor than with recurrent bacterial infections (42). Risk factors need to be addressed where identified; for example, women who develop post-antibiotic candidiasis should be treated with prophylactic antifungals.

The usual recommended treatment regimen comprises induction with fluconazole 150 mg every 72 hours for three doses, followed by a maintenance dose of 150 mg once weekly for six months. Alternative maintenance regimens include fluconazole 50 mg daily, itraconazole 50 to 100 mg daily or a clotrimazole 500 mg pessary weekly for six months. There is no evidence to support the use of alternative treatments such as use of probiotics or tea tree oil.

Trichomoniasis

Trichomoniasis is caused by the protozoan *T. vaginalis*. It is a relatively unusual cause of vaginal discharge in the United Kingdom (8). *T. vaginalis* is a flagellated protozoan which causes multifocal infection (Fig. 53.3). Apart from vaginitis, it also affects the paraurethral ducts, urethra, Bartholin's glands, and Skene's glands. Infection co-exists in one or more of these sites in up to 90% of vaginal infections, but infection at these sites without accompanying vaginitis is uncommon. Trichomoniasis is associated with a shift in the vaginal flora away from the normal lactobacillus-predominant flora in a majority of cases, and approximately a third meets the diagnostic criteria for frank bacterial vaginosis (43).

Contributory factors and management of trichomoniasis are outlined in Table 53.6.

Allergic Vulvovaginitis

Allergic causes of vulvovaginitis are often overlooked. The vaginal mucosa is able to show an allergic response similar to that seen in the skin, nose, eyes, and lungs. A type 1 IgE-mediated allergic reaction is caused by house dust, latex, foods, semen, *C. albicans*, spermicides, condoms, etc. Type 4 contact and or irritant dermatitis can occur due to K–Y jelly, pads, tampons, deodorants, soaps, vaginal sprays, bubble bath, laundry detergents, textile dyes, etc. (49).

Contributory factors and management of allergic vulvovaginitis are outlined in Table 53.7.

Atrophic Vaginitis

Hormonal changes following the menopause can lead to a number of changes in estrogen sensitive tissues and the vagina is no exception. Typical symptoms of atrophic vaginitis include dryness, soreness, and dyspareunia. Often vaginal symptoms will co-exist with urinary tract problems such as frequency, urgency, and nocturia (50). Atrophic vaginitis may occur following several years of estrogen deficiency and can be exacerbated by the ageing process. The condition can also be present in women on systemic hormone replacement therapy (HRT).

Hypo-estrogenism leads to vaginal atrophy characterized by pallor, loss of rugal folds, petechiae, and occasional eccymoses. Lack of estrogen gives rise to thin vaginal epithelium which lacks glycogen. This change encourages overgrowth of non-acidophilic coliform organisms and loss of lactobacillus species. The vaginal pH is >5.5. Saline microscopy shows the presence of parabasal or intermediate cells (immature cells) with or without leukocytes (Fig. 53.4). Recent work has suggested changes in estrogen receptor expression and levels may be implicated in the etiology of chronic atrophic vaginitis (51).

Local application of estrogen into the vagina is often more acceptable to women than systemic HRT. Creams, pessaries, tablets, and the estradiol releasing ring appear to be equally effective for the symptoms of vaginal atrophy (52). However, women appear to favor the estrogen releasing ring for ease of use.

Often a long-term maintenance regimen is used to prevent recurrence but a break from therapy after three months, or the use of progestogens to prevent endometrial hyperplasia is usually advised for those women with a uterus.

Vaginal Disease due to Increased Levels of Lactobacilli

Increased levels of lactobacilli can cause a thick discharge (similar to Candida) and inflammatory symptoms such as burning, pruritus, superficial dysuria, and dyspareunia. Inflammatory signs are absent on examination and pH is <4.5 (more acidic). On microscopy, there is an abundance of lactobacilli but no increased levels of WBCs.

Two types of vaginosis are described: cytolytic vaginosis and lactobacillus vaginosis.

Cytolytic Vaginosis

This represents an abnormal increase in lactobacilli and is associated with desquamation of squamous epithelial cells (53) as a result of the increased acidity. Treatment aims to

Table 53.6 Contributory Factors and Management of Trichomoniasis

Factor	Description
Other manifestations	Urinary tract infection, Bartholin's gland infection
Transmission	Usually sexually transmitted
	Screening for other sexually transmitted infections, and notification and treatment of all other sexual partners is important
	It is occasionally acquired non-venerally (4)
Risk factors	Multiple sexual partners
	Smoking
	Intrauterine contraceptive device
	History of other sexually transmitted diseases
	Non-use of barrier or oral contraception
Complications	Associated with preterm delivery and low birth weight infants (4)
	May enhance HIV transmission
	Vaginitis emphysematosa is an uncommon condition in which gas-filled blebs occur in vaginal wall (44)
	Vaginal cuff cellulitis can occur after hysterectomy (4)
	Post-abortal infection is less common (4)
	Infection of the upper genital tract is rare (4)
Symptoms	Vaginal discharge (note that classical frothy yellow/green discharge is only present in 30% of cases)
	Pruritus, vaginal irritation, burning, and soreness
	Lower abdominal pain
	Bleeding
	Superficial and internal dysuria (4)
	Superficial dyspareunia
	Offensive odor
	Between 10% and 50% are asymptomatic (45)
	Men are usually asymptomatic but can present with urethral discharge and symptoms of urethritis
Signs	Frothy yellow discharge
	Vulvitis
	Vaginitis
	Strawberry cervix [present in 2% (45)]
Diagnosis	Microscopy (wet mount) will diagnose 60–70% of cases (44)
	Flagellate motile protozoans and increased levels of WBCs are seen
	Culture will diagnose 95% of cases (45)
	Cervical cytology: trichomonads have sometimes been reported; sensitivity is between 50% and 60% (4)
	With nucleic acid amplification techniques, sensitivities, and specificities approaching 100% have been reported: (46,47) these tests are beginning to become commercially available
	With a pH > 4.5, a positive whiff test is not unusual
Treatment	Oral treatment is required because topical treatment does not reach paraurethral ducts and organisms sequestered within the urethra (48)
	Recommended regimens: Metronidazole 2 g p.o. single dose or metronidazole 400–500 mg p.o. b.i.d. for 5–7 days
Treatment failure	Consider possibilities of non-compliance with treatment; reinfection
	Diagnosis should be reconfirmed by wet preparation or culture
	Metronidazole resistance is a very uncommon reason for treatment failure: susceptibility testing is not routinely available
	Dose and duration of metronidazole therapy is increased (29)
	Alternative agents such as tinidazole can be tried in metronidazole-resistant cases

bring the pH to 3.8 to 4.5. Alkalinization with sodium bicarbonate can relieve symptoms, and therapy is continued until symptoms resolve.

Lactobacillus Vaginosis

This putative condition presents as recurrent vaginal discharge and discomfort occurring 7 to 10 days before menses. An association with recent azole antifungal therapy has also been reported. Elongated lactobacilli are present on microscopy with no signs of cytolysis (54). Treatment with doxycycline or co-amoxiclav for two weeks has been reported to be effective in achieving both clinical and microbiological cures.

Desquamative Inflammatory Vaginitis

DIV is an uncommon but disabling condition whose causation and natural history remain largely unknown. It is not a diagnosis in itself but a clinical description which may be associated with a range of mucocutaneous disorders such as lichen planus, pemphigus vulgaris, and pemphigoid (55). It can be a local manifestation of a systemic illness such as systemic lupus erythematosus (4). It can present at any stage of reproductive life, but may be found in an increased incidence in the perimenopausal phase (56).

Patients complain of increased purulent vaginal discharge, severe dyspareunia, discomfort, and irritation.

Table 53.7 Contributory Factors and Management of Allergic Vulvovaginitis

Factor	Description
Risk factors	Sexual intercourse: IgE mediated disease caused by semen, change in pH, microscopic abrasions due to inadequate lubrication, etc. are all risk factors
	Exaggerated personal hygiene: cleansing agents or vaginal douching are significant risk factors
	Styles of clothing such as tight jeans or lycra underwear
Symptoms	Pruritus
	Burning
	Non-odorous vaginal discharge
	Dyspareunia
Signs	Often localized to mucocutaneous margins of vaginal introitus and fourchette but can also affect labia, perineum, and clitoris
	Erythema
	Excoriation
	Lichenification
	Fissuring
Diagnosis	Infection, systemic disease, and vulvar dermatosis should be excluded: (49)
	• Vulvodynia and vulvovestibulitis should be considered
	• Total and specific IgE antibodies to these allergens
	• Specific IgE antibodies in vaginal secretions
	• Total eosinophil counts in vaginal secretions
	• Patch test in cases of contact dermatitis—refer to dermatology if considering allergy
	• Vaginal provocation tests
Treatment	Avoid risk factors
	Avoid allergens (e.g., perfumed soaps) and replace with an emmolient
	Oral antihistamines may be effective for type 1 allergic reactions
	Local cromolyn sodium (a mast cell stabilizer) can improve symptoms
	Immunotherapy and desensitization can be effective

Depending on the cause, the vulva can appear normal (unless associated with a mucocutaneous disorder such as lichen planus when there may be erosions or blistering), but the vagina shows erythematous areas. There may be superficial erosions of the vaginal mucosa, which are characteristic of this condition (4). The vaginal pH is often elevated to >4.6. There is no odor when the vaginal secretions are mixed with 10% KOH. The secretion shows increased numbers of WBCs and immature squamous epithelial cells. Vaginal biopsies are often unhelpful and must be taken from a non-ulcerated area adjacent to an erosion with review by a specialist dermatopathologist.

It has been described as a sterile inflammatory vaginitis (54). No microorganism has been clearly associated with this disease (56).

Treatment is difficult, and relates to the underlying cause if known, though there is some response to topical steroid foam and 2% clindamycin cream (4,18,55).

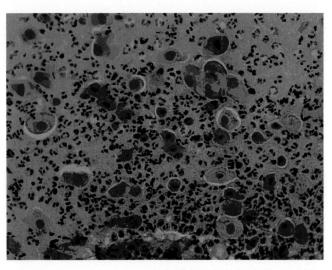

Figure 53.4 A postmenopausal smear which shows parabasal squamous cells. Magnification ×200. *Source*: Courtesy of Mr. Malcolm Mackie, Clinical Cytologist, William Harvey Hospital, Ashford, U.K.

Chronic Vaginitis

It is important that the clinician understands the emotional state of the patient suffering with chronic vaginitis which for many women is a long term condition lasting for over 12 months (57,58). She is often frustrated, depressed, and develops a sense of despair. There is often strain in personal relationships.

Thorough evaluation is needed, and the clinician must reassess the diagnosis before proceeding with further therapy. Further investigations such as culture are needed and other differential diagnoses should be considered.

Sometimes stopping treatment may even be helpful to ascertain if any remaining symptoms are iatrogenic.

There may be a small increased risk of the development of cancer in women with erosive lichen planus (59) suggesting the need for long term surveillance particularly for those resistant to therapy.

CONCLUSION

Vaginitis is the most common cause for gynecologic consultation but has too often been ignored by the medical community or regarded as a minor annoyance to women. Patients who present with vaginitis deserve a thorough evaluation of their symptoms. Vaginitis can have an impact on the physical, emotional, sexual, and social well-being of a patient. This is particularly true in patients with chronic vaginitis.

Trichomoniasis is a sexually transmitted infection and therefore has important implications.

Diagnosis and treatment of bacterial vaginosis prevents complications such as pelvic inflammatory disease and premature labor. Although infection is the commonest cause of vaginitis, other non-infectious, inflammatory causes should not be forgotten.

REFERENCES
1. Edwards L. The diagnosis and treatment of infectious vaginitis. Dermatol Ther 2004; 17: 102–10.
2. Hammill HA. Normal vaginal flora in relation to vaginitis. Obstet Gynecol Clin North Am 1989; 16: 329–36.

3. Egan M, Lipsky MS. Vaginitis: case reports and brief review. AIDS Patient Care STDS 2002; 16: 367–73.

4. McCormack WM. Vulvovaginitis and cervicitis. In: Mandell G, Bennett J, Dolin R, eds. Principles and Practice of Infectious Diseases. Amsterdam: Elsevier, 2005: 357–69.

5. Faro S. Vaginitis: diagnosis and management. Int J Fertil Menopausal Stud 1996; 41: 115–23.

6. Carr PL, Felsenstein D, Freidman RH. Evaluation and management of vaginitis. J Gen Intern Med 1998; 13: 335–46.

7. Friedrich EG. Vaginitis. Am J Obstet Gynecol 1985; 152: 247–51.

8. French P. Sorting out vaginal discharge. Trends Urol Gynaecol Sexual Health 2004; 9: 22–7.

9. Kent HL. Epidemiology of vaginitis. Am J Obstet Gynecol 1991; 165(4 Pt 2): 1168–76.

10. Bruins MJ, Damoiseaux RA, Ruijs GJ. Association between group A beta-haemolytic streptococci and vulvovaginitis in adult women: a case-control study. Eur J Clin Microbiol Infect Dis 2009; 28: 1019–21.

11. O'Dowd TC, Bourne N. Inventing a new diagnostic test for vaginal infection. Br Med J 1994; 309: 40–2.

12. Mulley AG. Approach to the patient with vaginal discharge. In: Goroll AH, Mulley AG, eds. Primary Care Medicine: Office Evaluation and Management of the Adult Patient. Philadelphia: Lippincott Williams and Wilkins, 2000: 702–7.

13. Anderson MR, Klink K, Cohrssen A. Evaluation of vaginal complaints. JAMA 2004; 291: 1368–79.

14. Morison L, Ekpo G, West B, et al. Bacterial vaginosis in relation to menstrual cycle, menstrual protection method, and sexual intercourse in rural Gambian women. Sex Transm Infect 2005; 81: 242–7.

15. Hammill HA. Unusual causes of vaginitis (excluding trichomonas, bacterial vaginosis, Candida albicans). Obstet Gynecol Clin North Am 1989; 16: 337–45.

16. Nyirjesy P. Vaginitis in the adolescent patient. Pediatr Clin North Am 1999; 46: 733–45.

17. Breijer MC, Timmermans A, van Doorn HC, et al. Diagnostic strategies for postmenopausal women. Obstet Gynecol Int 2010; 2010: 850812. Epub 2010 Feb 4.

18. Sobel JD. Vulvo-vaginitis in healthy women. Compr Ther 1999; 25: 335–46.

19. Lascsar RM, Devakumar H, Jungmann E, et al. Is vaginal microscopy an essential tool for the management of women presenting with vaginal discharge? Int J STD AIDS 2008; 19: 859–60.

20. Garrow SC, Smith DW, Harnett GB. The diagnosis of Chlamydia, gonorrhoea, and trichomonas infections by self obtained low vaginal swabs, in remote northern Australian clinical practice. Sex Transm Infect 2002; 78: 278–81.

21. Fang J, Husman C, DeSilva L, Chang R. Peralta L. Evaluation of self-collected vaginal swab, first void urine, and endocervical swab specimens for the detection of Chlamydia trachomatis and Neisseria gonorrhoeae in adolescent females. I Pediatr Adolesc Gynecol 2008; 21: 355–60.

22. Kashyap B, Singh R, Bhalla P, Arora R, Aggarwal A. Reliability of self-collected versus provider-collected vaginal swabs for the diagnosis of bacterial vaginaosis. Int J STD AIDS 2008; 19: 510–13.

23. Clinical Effectiveness Group. National Guideline for the management of bacterial vaginosis. Association for Genitourinary Medicine and the Medical Society for the Study of Venereal Diseases, 2001. [Available from: www.bashh.org/guidelines/2002/bv_0601.pdf].

24. Akinbiyi AA, Watson R, Feyi-Waboso P. Prevalence of Candida albicans and bacterial vaginosis in asymptomatic pregnant women in South Yorkshire, United Kingdom. Outcome of a prospective study. Arch Gynecol Obstet 2008; 278: 463–6.

25. Paxton LA, Sewankambo N, Gray R, et al. Asymptomatic non-ulcerative genital tract infections in a rural Ugandan population. Sex Transm Infect 1998; 74: 421–5.

26. Marrazzo JM, Koutsky LA, Eschenbach DA, et al. Characterization of vaginal flora and bacterial vaginosis in women who have sex with women. J Infect Dis 2002; 185: 1307–13.

27. Davis J, Connor E, Clarke P, et al. Correlation between cervical cytologic results and Gram stain as diagnostic tests for bacterial vaginosis. Am J Obstet Gynecol 1997; 177: 532–5.

28. Van Kessal K, Assefi N, Marrazzo J, Eckert L. Common complementary and alternative therapies for yeast vaginitis and bacterial vaginosis: a systematic review. Obstet Gynecol Survey 2003; 58: 351–8.

29. Haefner HK. Current evaluation and management of vulvo-vaginitis. Clin Obstet Gynaecol 1999; 42: 184–95.

30. Spinillo A, Capuzzo E, Gulminetti R, et al. Prevalence of and risk factors for fungal vaginitis caused by non-albicans species. Am J Obstet Gynecol 1997; 176: 138–41.

31. Sobel JD. Epidemiology and pathogenesis of recurrent vulvovaginal candidiasis. Am J Obstet Gynecol 1985; 1523: 924–35.

32. Bradshaw CS, Morton AN, Garland SM, et al. Higher-risk behavioural practices associated with bacterial vaginosis compared with vaginal candidiasis. Obstet Gynecol 2005; 106: 105–14.

33. Bailey JV, Benato R, Owen C, Kavanagh J. Vulvovaginal candidiasis in women who have sex with women. Sex Transm Dis 2008; 35: 533–6.

34. Geiger AM, Foxman B. Risk factors for vulvovaginal candidiasis: a case-control study among university students. Epidemiology 1996; 7: 182–7.

35. Sobel JD. Vaginitis. N Engl J Med 1997; 337: 1896–903.

36. Emmerson J, Gunputrao A, Hawkswell J, et al. Sampling for vaginal candidiasis: how good is it? Int J STD AIDS 1994; 5: 356–8.

37. Sonnex C, Lefort W. Microscopic features of vaginal candidiasis and their relation to symptomatology. Sex Transm Infect 1999; 75: 417–19.

38. Clinical Effectiveness Group. National guidelines on the management of vulvo-vaginal candidiasis. 2001. [Available from: www.bashh.org/guidelines/2002/candida_0601.pdf].

39. Reef SE, Levine WC, McNeil MM, et al. Treatment options for vulvovaginal candidiasis: 1993. Clin Infect Dis 1995; 20(Suppl 1): S80–90.

40. Vazquez JA, Sobel JD, Demetriou R, et al. Karyotyping of Candida albicans isolates obtained longitudinally in women with recurrent vulvovaginal candidiasis. J Infect Dis 1994; 170: 1566–9.

41. Horowitz BJ, Glaquinta D, Ito S. Evolving pathogens in vulvovaginal candidiasis: implications for patient care. J Clin Pharmacol 1992; 32: 248–55.

42. Fong TW, Bannatyne RM, Wong P. Lack of in vitro resistance of Candidiasis albicans to ketoconazole, itraconazole and clotrimazole in women treated for recurrent vaginal candidiasis. Genitourin Med 1993; 69: 44–6.

43. Hillier SL, Krohn MA, Nugent RP, et al. Characteristics of three vaginal flora patterns assessed by Gram stain among pregnant women. Am J Obstet Gynecol 1992; 166: 938–44.

44. Josey WE, Campbell WG Jr. Vaginitis emphysematosa. A report of four cases. J Reprod Med 1990; 35: 974–7.

45. Wolner-Hanssen P, Krieger JN, Stevens CE, et al. Clinical manifestations of vaginal trichomoniasis. JAMA 1989; 264: 571–6.

46. Madico G, Quinn TC, Rompalo A, McKee KT Jr, Gaydos CA. Diagnosis of trichomonas vaginalis infection by PCR using vaginal swab samples. J Clin Micobiol 1998; 36: 3205–10.

47. Mayto H, Gilman RH, Calderon MM, et al. 18S ribosomal DNA-based PCR for the diagnosis of trichomonas vaginalis. J Clin Microbiol 2000; 38: 2683–7.

48. Clinical Effectiveness Group. National guideline on the management of trichomonas vaginalis. 2001. Online. [Available from: www.bashh.org/guidelines/2002/tv_0601.pdf].

49. Moraes PS, Taketomi EA. Allergic vulvo-vaginitis. Ann Allergy Asthma Immunol 2000; 85: 253–65.

50. Hextall A. Oestrogens and lower urinary tract function. Maturitas 2000; 36: 83–92.

51. Taylor AH, Guzail M, Al_Azzawi F. Differential expression of oestrogen receptor isoforms and androgen receptor in the normal vulva and vagina compared with vulval lichen scleosus and chronic vaginitis. Br J Dermatol 2008; 158: 319–28.

52. Suckling J, Lethaby A, Kennedy R. Local estrogen for vaginal atrophy in postmenopausal women. Cochrane Database Syst Rev 2006; 4: CD001500.

53. Cibley LJ. Cytolytic vaginosis. Am J Obstet Gynecol 1991; 165: 1245–9.

54. Horowitz BJ, Mardh PA, Nagy E, Rank EL. Vaginal lactobacillosis. Am J Obstet Gynecol 1994; 170: 857–61.

55. Murphy R. Desquamative inflammatory vaginitis. Dermatol Ther 2004; 17: 47–9.

56. Sobel JD. Desquamative inflammatory vaginitis: a new subgroup of purulent vaginitis responsive to topical 2% clindamycin therapy. Am J Obstet Gynecol 1994; 171: 1215–20.

57. Nyirjesy P, Peyton C, Weitz MV, et al. Causes of chronic vaginitis:analysis of a prospective database of affected women. Obstet Gynecol 2006; 108: 1185–91.

58. Cooper SM, Wojnarowska F. Influence of treatment of erosive lichen planus of the vulva on its prognosis. Arch Dermatol 2006; 142: 289–94.

59. Kennedy CM, Peterson LB, Galask RP. Erosive vulvar lichen planus: a chort at risk for cancer? J Reprod Med 2008; 53: 781–4.

54 Pregnancy and Childbirth and the Effect on the Pelvic Floor
Charlotte Chaliha

INTRODUCTION

Over the past few decades the consequences of childbirth on the physical and psychological well-being of a woman have been well recognized. MacArthur et al. (1), in a postal survey of 11,701 women 13 months to 9 years after delivery, found that 47% experienced at least one or more health problems within three months of delivery. These included backache, headache, hemorrhoids, depression, and bowel and bladder symptoms that persisted for a minimum of six weeks. Glazener et al. (2) questioned 1249 women about their postnatal symptoms on three occasions after childbirth; 85% of women experienced one new symptom during the first eight weeks and 76% reported one or more health problems persisting for up to 18 months. Sleep and Grant (3) reported that 15% of women experience dyspareunia up to three years after a normal vaginal delivery and up to 8% experience perineal pain 12 weeks after a normal vaginal delivery (4). Perineal pain can occur even without perineal trauma and women who sustain anal sphincter damage have significantly greater pain ratings at seven weeks after delivery compared to those with lesser degrees of perineal trauma (5). It is also known that both urinary and fecal incontinence have a significant negative impact on quality of life and sexual function particularly if both are present (6,7). However, although health problems seem to be common after childbirth, it appears women often do not seek medical attention (1).

Urinary and/or fecal incontinence and genital prolapse are considered to be inevitable sequelae of a vaginal birth. One in every three women will experience incontinence during her lifetime and, of these, up to 65% will recall that it began either during pregnancy or after childbirth (8). Clinical and epidemiologic studies strongly indicate that women who undergo a vaginal delivery are at higher risk of subsequent incontinence than nulliparas and those who undergo cesarean section. This is most likely related to the detrimental impact of vaginal delivery on the pelvic floor (9–15). Furthermore, it appears that the first vaginal delivery is the time when women sustain the most significant damage (13,16). However the effects of mode of delivery with increasing parity is less certain.

There are many studies showing a relationship between vaginal delivery and mechanical and neurologic damage to the pelvic floor which is related to the development of urinary or anal incontinence or both (16–19). There may also be women at increased predisposition to pelvic floor trauma, and thus incontinence and prolapse, due to an inherent weakness of collagen within the pelvic floor fascia (20–22).

This chapter focuses on the effect of pregnancy and childbirth on the pelvic floor and discusses the possible mechanisms by which pelvic floor damage may occur and its long-term sequelae.

MECHANISMS OF INJURY TO THE PELVIC FLOOR

There are several mechanisms of pelvic floor injury: direct muscle trauma, nerve injury, and connective tissue damage disrupting the urethral and anal sphincters and their support (Fig. 54.1).

Direct Perineal Trauma

Direct perineal trauma from perineal laceration and episiotomy is a well-known complication of vaginal delivery. Episiotomy is one of the commonest surgical interventions and was traditionally advocated to decrease perineal damage. The largest review of use of episiotomy (23) found that it reduces anterior perineal laceration but not pelvic floor damage, urinary or fecal incontinence, or protect the newborn from intracranial trauma.

The long-term sequlae of perineal injuries include pain, dyspareunia, fistulae, and anal incontinence (16,24–26). The incidence of lacerations involving the anal sphincter has been reported as 0% to 6.4% when an episiotomy has not been performed, 0.2% to 23.9% after a midline episiotomy, and 0% to 9% after a mediolateral episiotomy (26). There does not, however, seem to be a significant association between episiotomy and the development of urinary incontinence (27).

Severity and frequency of postpartum dyspareunia has been related to perineal trauma and obstetric instrumentation, with a quicker resumption of sexual activity in those with an intact perineum versus those women who have had a spontaneous laceration or episiotomy (25,28).

Muscle Trauma

Anatomic and functional changes to the pelvic floor may occur secondary to pelvic floor distension during descent of the fetal head and maternal expulsive efforts during the active second stage of labor. Peschers et al. (29) evaluated pelvic floor strength by means of palpation, perineometry, and perineal ultrasound, and found that pelvic floor muscle strength was significantly decreased after vaginal delivery compared to cesarean section at three to eight days postpartum. However, at 6 to 10 weeks postpartum there was no significant difference from antenatal values except for a lower intravaginal pressure in nulliparous women. Therefore, although pelvic strength is impaired shortly after vaginal birth, it recovers in most women within two months after the first pregnancy.

A longer-term study, evaluating pelvic floor strength at one year postpartum using perineometry, found no difference between degree of perineal trauma and subsequent muscle strength (30). However, another large study of 519 women evaluated at three months postpartum using symptom assessment and vaginal perineometry, found that the women who had sustained an episiotomy had lower pelvic floor strength

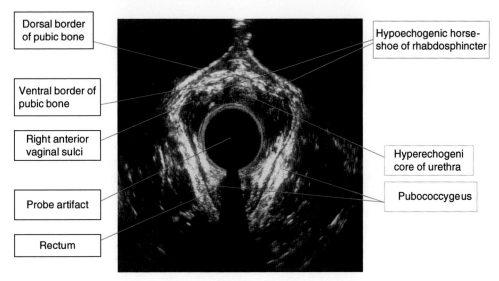

Dorsal border of pubic bone

Ventral border of pubic bone

Right anterior vaginal sulci

Probe artifact

Rectum

Hypoechogenic horse-shoe of rhabdosphincter

Hyperechogeni core of urethra

Pubococcygeus

Figure 54.1 Ultrasound of the pelvic floor.

and more perineal pain and dyspareunia than those with intact perineums or first and second degree lacerations. There was no difference in symptoms of urinary and anal incontinence (31).

Nerve Damage

The pudendal nerve is susceptible to compression and damage at the point where it curves round the ischial spine and enters the pudendal canal enclosed in a tight fibrous sheath. Nerve damage has been shown to occur in patients with a history chronic of straining on defecation who show increased pudendal nerve terminal motor latencies (32). Childbirth-induced denervation injuries of the pubococcygeus and external sphincter muscles may occur by a similar mechanism and have been reported after 42% to 80% of vaginal deliveries (17,18).

THE LOWER URINARY TRACT IN PREGNANCY AND AFTER DELIVERY

Lower urinary tract symptoms are very common in pregnancy. Several large epidemiologic studies have assessed the prevalence of urinary symptoms in pregnancy, most focusing on the symptom of stress incontinence. Most of these symptoms may be a consequence of the normal anatomic and physiologic changes that occur in pregnancy however superimposed on these changes may be further pathologic changes as a consequence of tissue damage, either from pregnancy or labor, resulting in persistent symptoms. The distinction between normal physiologic changes and transient or permanent pathophysiology is often not clear and may be a continuum.

Anatomic and Physiologic Changes

The urinary tract undergoes both structural and functional changes during pregnancy and after delivery. These changes may be specific in response to pregnancy and in some women may be compounded by pathologic changes that persist after delivery.

In normal pregnancy, the kidneys increase by 1 cm in length due to an increase in vascular volume and the volume of the interstitial space. Dilatation of the ureters is a well-known phenomenon in pregnancy and hydroureter is noted in

approximately 90% of pregnant women by the third trimester. This dilatation is more marked on the right compared to the left side, probably related to the relative dextrorotation of the uterus. There is a 40% to 50% increase in glomerular filtration rate and a 60% to 80% increase in the effective renal plasma flow (33). As a result, plasma creatinine, urea, and urate values are lower than the normal range for non-pregnant women.

The bladder is passively drawn upwards and anteriorly as the uterus enlarges, resulting in lengthening of the urethra (34). The urethral mucosa becomes more hyperemic and congested in pregnancy in response to the increase in circulating estrogen levels. The detrusor muscle also hypertrophies in response to estrogen. After delivery, cystoscopy of the bladder shows changes such as mucosal congestion, submucosal hemorrhage, and capillary oozing, especially around the bladder neck, trigone, and ureteric orifices. These changes have been seen in association with a decrease in bladder sensation and tone (35) and are most marked in those who underwent vaginal delivery (36).

Studies assessing bladder capacity have revealed conflicting results, with most early studies using simple cystometry only. Muellner (37) reported an increase in bladder capacity to an average of 1300 ml in the third trimester due to bladder hypotonia, with a return to normal values postpartum. However, other investigators found no change in bladder capacity in the first trimester and a reduced bladder capacity in the third trimester in association with increased detrusor irritability rather than bladder hypotonia (38). Dual channel cystometry studies have found that all urodynamic variables, such as first sensation and maximum bladder capacity, are lower in pregnancy and postpartum compared to a non-pregnant population and this may account for symptoms of frequency, nocturia, and urgency (39,40).

PREGNANCY AND URINARY SYMPTOMS
Frequency and Nocturia

Frequency and nocturia are among the commonest and earliest symptoms to develop in pregnancy. Normal non-pregnant women void between four to six times per day, and rarely at night. Using a definition of frequency as at least seven day-time voids and one night-time void, Francis (38) studied the voiding habits in 400 healthy women during and after an uncomplicated pregnancy and compared them with 50 healthy non-pregnant patients of a similar age. Frequency was reported by 59% in early pregnancy, 61% in mid-pregnancy, and 81% in late pregnancy. Parboosingh and Doig (41), defining nocturia as at least three night-time voids, questioned 873 healthy antenatal patients and found that nearly 66% experienced nocturia by the third trimester. Cutner et al. (42) assessed lower urinary tract symptoms in 47 women undergoing termination of pregnancy at 6 to 15 weeks' gestation, and found that 40% complained of frequency and 23% of nocturia. The cause of frequency was not related to bladder capacity or the effect of posture, but due to the polydypsia and polyuria of pregnancy (32).

Both fluid intake and output rise rapidly in the first trimester, remaining constant until the third trimester, when a decrease in sodium excretion leads to a decrease in output. Despite this, frequency persists related to the pressure on the bladder by the uterus. Cutner (43) found that there was a correlation between the maximum voided volumes and first sensation to void and maximum bladder capacity, which was in turn related to the presence of low compliance. There was no correlation between the maximum voided volumes and diurnal frequency and nocturia. Parboosingh and Doig (44) measured mean urine flow and solute excretion in 24-hour and overnight collections in 100 normal and non-pregnant women. An increase in sodium excretion was the major reason for increased night-time voiding as well as the mobilization of dependent edema at night in the recumbent position.

Voiding Difficulties

Urinary hesitancy may be found in up to 27% of patients in the first two trimesters (44). Fischer and Kittel (45) assessed flow rates in 290 women during pregnancy and found that there was a significant increase in peak flow rates in the second and third trimesters compared to controls and early pregnancy, but these higher flow rates were associated with larger voided volumes. Cutner (43) assessed flow rates in pregnancy, adjusting for volume voided, and found no difference in women complaining of hesitancy, or incomplete emptying, compared to pregnant women with normal voiding.

Urinary retention can occur in pregnancy associated with the enlargement of a retroverted uterus with subsequent entrapment of the fundus below the sacral promontory (46). Other causes include an enlarging fibroid or a pelvic mass. This retention usually resolves by 16 weeks' gestation as the uterus grows out of the pelvis, and can be managed in the interim with either bladder drainage or intermittent self-catheterization. Alternatively, manual reduction of the uterus can be performed or a Hodge pessary may be inserted to maintain uterine position and relieve the obstruction on the bladder neck.

Postpartum urinary retention is common, with a reported incidence of 1.7% to 17.9% (47). Risk factors include a first labor, instrumental delivery epidural analgesia, and a longer duration of labor (>800 min) (48–50). The bladder can take

up to eight hours to regain sensation after the last top-up of an epidural (51). Overdistension of the bladder may occur during this period, leading to permanent detrusor dysfunction.

Urinary Incontinence

Incontinence is a common symptom associated with pregnancy and has been reported in up to 85% of women (38,52–54). The risk of urinary incontinence increases with increasing gestation. Francis (38) found that in the first trimester of pregnancy 16% of women complained of stress incontinence and 34% in the second half of pregnancy. Stanton et al. (55) assessed the prevalence of both stress and urge incontinence at 32 weeks' gestation and found an incidence of 36% and 13%, respectively.

Viktrup and Lose (53) interviewed 305 primiparae and found that 39% had stress incontinence before, during or after pregnancy, and 7% developed de novo stress incontinence after delivery. The association with these obstetric risk factors was lost by three months postpartum and only 3% had incontinence at one year. However, in a subsequent follow-up study of the original cohort of 278 women, they reported a prevalence of stress incontinence of 30% at five years. In those without symptoms after the first delivery the incidence was 19%; however, in those who reported stress incontinence three months after first delivery there was a 92% risk of having stress incontinence five years later (13,56). A prospective cohort study of 949 women undertaken to find risk factors for postpartum stress incontinence at three months, found that urinary incontinence was experienced by 22.3% before pregnancy, 65.1% during the third trimester, and 31.1% after delivery (27). New onset urinary incontinence was more common in parous compared to nulliparous women. Postpartum urinary incontinence was independently associated with incontinence prior to pregnancy and beginning during pregnancy, even amongst those having a caesarean section. This study highlights the high proportion of women who suffer from urinary incontinence as 15.4% of nulliparae had prepregnancy incontinence. It confirms previous data that has found that the presence of antenatal and prepregancy stress incontinence seems to increase the risk of future stress incontinence (57–59).

The pattern of development of incontinence during pregnancy, with rapid postpartum recovery followed by a steady decline of continence over time, suggests a dual mechanism of nerve and tissue damage. The evidence regarding the contribution of obstetric factors to the development of stress incontinence is conflicting. The data are unclear whether it is pregnancy or delivery itself that is the major contributor to postpartum incontinence. Some investigators have found a relationship with the duration of the second stage of labor (60–62) and birth weight (1). Conversely, other investigators have not found a significant correlation between stress incontinence and fetal head circumference (63,64), second stage of labor (1,52,61,65) or birth weight (63–66). However, most of these studies are relatively small population studies that differ widely in their questioning techniques and definition of stress incontinence. The largest community-based epidemiological study of incontinence (EPINCONT study) (14) assessed 15,307 women who were younger than 65 years and were

grouped according to obstetric history into those who were nulliparous, delivered only by cesarean section or only had a history of vaginal deliveries. The authors reported that in the nulliparous group the prevalence of any incontinence was 10.1%, with a prevalence of 15.9% in the cesarean section group and 21.0% in the vaginal delivery group. Thus pregnancy itself rather than delivery may also be an etiological factor in the development of urinary incontinence.

The effect of epidural analgesia is unclear. Epidural analgesia has been reported to be more protective than pudendal block against postpartum stress incontinence (63); however, this was not established by other authors who have found a higher incidence of stress incontinence in those who received epidural analgesia than those who did not (65). Jackson et al. (62) found that the incidence of stress incontinence increased in women delivered with epidural analgesia, especially if the second stage of labor was longer than 120 minutes.

Changes in the Lower Urinary Tract and Pelvic Floor Related to the Development of Incontinence

The exact etiologic mechanism of stress incontinence is unclear and probably multifactorial, related to nerve damage and/or physiologic and structural changes of the lower urinary tract.

Functional Changes

Iosif and Ulmsten (67) compared urethral pressure profile measurements in pregnant women with stress incontinence with continent healthy women from an earlier study (3). They found that the absolute urethral length increased by an average of 6.7 mm and the functional urethral length by 4.8 mm. The maximum urethral closure pressure increased to 93 cmH_2O at 38 weeks and then dropped to pre-pregnancy values of 69 cmH_2O postpartum. These changes were not seen in women complaining of incontinence, and are postulated to be a mechanism whereby continence is maintained despite an increase in intravesical pressure in pregnancy. This corresponds with other studies that have shown evidence of low urethral pressure in non-pregnant women with stress incontinence (68,69). This increase in urethral closure pressure may be the result of an increase in urethral sphincter volume from increased blood flow. There is also an increase in the amplitude of vascular pulsations recorded from the urethral wall, especially in the first 16 weeks of pregnancy, which may be related to an increase in blood volume in pregnancy. Pregnant women with urodynamic stress incontinence showed a decrease in the amplitude of vascular pulsations in the periurethral plexus compared to continent women, suggesting that this affects urethral closure pressure (70). Three-dimensional imaging of the urethral sphincter after vaginal delivery shows a reduction in sphincter volume which has been implicated in the development of stress incontinence (71, 72).

Cystometry in pregnancy has been performed by several workers. Chaliha et al. (40) found a high prevalence of urodynamic stress incontinence and detrusor overactivity. This was 8.7% and 8.1% respectively in the antenatal period and 5.0% and 6.8%, respectively, postpartum. The mean values for urodynamic variables in the third trimester and postpartum were lower than values defined in a non-pregnant population and

Table 54.1 Urodynamic Values (Sitting and Standing Cystometry) and Urodynamic Diagnoses Before and After Delivery

Urodynamic variable	Antenatal values*	Postnatal values*
Sit FDV (ml)	111 (70)	148 (83)
Sit SDV (ml)	188 (91)	217 (94)
Sit MXCC (ml)	301 (146)	299 (114)
Stand FDV (ml)	96 (69)	139 (90)
Stand SDV (ml)	167 (102)	209 (105)
Stand MXCC (ml)	239 (136) ($n = 125$)	271 (123) ($n = 118$)
MVP (cmH_2O)	38 (22) ($n = 153$)	32 (17) ($n = 157$)
Peak flow rate (ml/sec)	28 (16.3)	23 (14)
Urodynamic stress incontinence	14 (9%)	8 (5%)
Detrusor overactivity	13 (8%)	11 (7%)

* $n = 161$. *Source*: Data from Ref. 40.
Abbreviations: FDV, first desire to void; MVP, maximum voiding pressure; MXCC, maximum cystometric capacity; SDV, strong desire to void.

not related to obstetric or neonatal variables (Table 54.1). However, despite the high prevalence of symptoms in this study, there was poor correlation between symptoms and urodynamic findings, which agrees with data in non-pregnant women (73). These observed changes in bladder function were consistent with a pressure effect of a gravid uterus and not related to mode of delivery or neonatal factors.

Nerve Damage

Patients with urodynamic stress incontinence have been shown to have abnormal conduction in the perineal branch of the pudendal nerve which innervates the periurethral striated muscle and pubococcygeus muscle (74,75). Several workers have also demonstrated injury to the nerve supply after childbirth. However, these studies often do not relate objective damage to symptoms. Snooks et al. (17) found prolongation of pudendal nerve terminal motor latencies 48 to 72 hours after delivery in 42% of those delivered vaginally but not those delivered by cesarean section. The degree of pudendal nerve damage was greater in multiparous women and correlated with the use of forceps and a longer second stage of labor. In 60% of these women, pudendal nerve latency had returned to normal at two months postpartum. The authors suggested that vaginal delivery results in pudendal nerve damage, probably through a combination of direct trauma and traction injury during delivery, and this may be involved in the development of stress incontinence. However, this study was not prospective and included multiparous women who may have sustained prior nerve damage. Furthermore, it looked at innervation of the striated anal sphincter which may not actually reflect striated urethral sphincter innervation, and there was a poor correlation between abnormal latencies and symptoms. Using concentric needle electromyography and pudendal nerve conduction tests, Allen et al. (18) found evidence of denervation injury in 80% of women after delivery. Those women with a long (active) second stage of labor (>56.7 min) and a large baby (>3.41 kg) showed a greater degree of nerve damage.

Electromyography of the right and left pubococcygeus muscle has shown that childbirth induces both qualitative as well as quantitative changes such that sphincter weakness was due not only to loss of motor units but also asynchronous activity in those that remained (76).

Structural Changes

Ultrasound studies have shown changes in bladder neck position and the urethral sphincter in relation to delivery. Peschers et al. (77) evaluated bladder neck position and mobility using perineal ultrasound at eight weeks postpartum. Bladder neck position was significantly lower and bladder neck mobility increased after vaginal delivery compared with women who had an elective cesarean section and nulligravid controls. Meyer et al. (78) noted a significant increase in bladder neck mobility after vaginal delivery in primiparae; however, bladder neck position was only lowered after forceps delivery.

Alterations in the urethral sphincter closure mechanism have previously been described in association with stress incontinence (79). Toozs-Hobson et al. (80) investigated 156 primigravid women in the third trimester and at six weeks and six months postpartum using a combination of transvaginal and transperineal ultrasound to measure the levator hiatus, and bladder neck mobility at rest, maximum strain, and maximum valsalva. Urethral sphincter volume was calculated using a three-dimensional imaging probe. They found that vaginal delivery was related to an increased bladder neck mobility and larger levator hiatus with both antenatal and postpartum mobility greater in women who delivered vaginally. The urethral sphincter was smaller post delivery independent of mode of delivery. These results are interesting but their long-term consequences unclear as the findings were not related to symptoms. The authors postulated that the larger sphincter volume in pregnancy was a function of the tissue and hormonal effects of pregnancy. In addition, the finding that women delivered by cesarean section showed less pelvic floor distensability may suggest that this itself may predispose them to their mode of delivery due to inherent differences in pelvic floor tissues. This supports previous observations that increased bladder neck mobility is associated with vaginal delivery (81).

There may be a group of women at an inherent increased risk of developing incontinence due to abnormalities in collagen (82), as the collagenous component of the connective tissue contributes to structural support of the bladder neck. In pregnancy, the tensile properties of the connective tissue are reduced, with a reduction in total collagen content and increase in glycosaminoglycans (83). Changes in collagen may result in greater mobility of the bladder neck resulting in stress incontinence. In a study of 116 primigravidae, perineal ultrasound was used to assess bladder neck mobility. Women with antenatal bladder neck mobility >5 mm on linear movement (equivalent to >10° rotation) were found to be at higher risk of developing postpartum stress incontinence. Approximately 50% of this group reported stress incontinence at three months postpartum (84).

ANAL SPHINCTER MORPHOLOGY DURING PREGNANCY AND AFTER DELIVERY

Sultan et al. (85) examined 20 women before and after a cesarean section and found that pregnancy did not have any significant effect on anal sphincter morphology and function. Further studies show that it is vaginal delivery that leads to structural and functional changes to the anal sphincter.

FECAL INCONTINENCE

Fecal incontinence is a distressing social handicap and vaginal delivery is a major etiologic factor (16,86,87). MacArthur et al. (19) investigated the prevalence of postnatal fecal symptoms in a postal questionnaire study of 906 women 10 months after delivery and reported that 36 women (4%) developed de novo fecal incontinence. Six of these women became incontinent after an emergency cesarean section but none after an elective cesarean section. This estimate for fecal incontinence is conservative, as it did not enquire about incontinence of flatus that is probably more common and has been reported to be as high as 26% at nine months after delivery in one study of 349 primiparous women (88).

Fecal incontinence is especially common after anal sphincter rupture, with a reported prevalence of 16% to 47% (89–92). Tetzschner et al. (64) assessed the long-term impact of obstetric anal sphincter rupture on the frequency of urinary and anal incontinence. At two to four years postpartum, 42% of the 94 women in their study had anal incontinence, 32% had urinary incontinence, and 18% had both urinary and anal incontinence. Despite the high number of women with incontinence, only a few had sought medical advice.

Changes in the Anal Canal and Pelvic Floor Related to Anal Incontinence

The etiology of postpartum anal incontinence is complex and both nerve and mechanical trauma have been implicated.

Nerve Damage

Denervation injury of the pelvic floor may occur from traction and straining during vaginal delivery, similar to the mechanism of nerve damage reported in patients with chronic constipation which may result in anorectal incontinence (93). In 80% of women with idiopathic anorectal incontinence there is histological evidence of denervation of the striated pelvic floor muscle, particularly the puborectalis and external anal sphincter muscles (94–96). Serial measurements of pudendal nerve terminal motor latencies in patients with idiopathic anorectal incontinence show progressive damage from recurrent stretch injury during straining at stool (97).

This mechanism of strain-induced damage may occur during vaginal delivery. Denervation injuries of the pubococcygeus and external sphincter muscles have been reported after 42% to 80% of vaginal deliveries (17,18). The presence of neuropathy has been found to be related to the length of the second stage of labor, size of the baby, and instrumental delivery (98). Sultan et al. (99) investigated pudendal nerve function before and after delivery, and found that pudendal nerve terminal motor latencies were significantly prolonged, especially on the left side, which the authors postulated could be due to the unequal traction from the fetal head on the two sides of the pelvic floor during descent down the birth canal. However, no relationship between abnormal neurophysiology and symptoms of anal incontinence was shown.

Sensory nerve function may also be affected by nerve damage. The anal canal has a greater variety of afferent nerve endings than the rectum. These allow the detection of differences in touch, temperature, and pain in the anal canal. The rectum has a configuration of nerve plexuses that serve as specialized sensory receptors for distension for perception of fullness, urgency to defecate, and pain (100,101).

It is believed that sensory information is critical to the preservation of continence and in patients with fecal incontinence there is a significant reduction in the ability to perceive electrical and other forms of stimulation (102–105). In pregnancy, however, the role of anal sensation is unclear as deficits in anal canal sensation appear to be transient and unrelated to the development of incontinence (106–108).

Anal Sphincter Trauma

The incidence of anal sphincter damage varies between 0.5% and 2.5% in centers where mediolateral episiotomy is practiced and 7% in units performing midline episiotomies (64,109,110). The use of anal endosonography has enabled accurate visualization of the sphincters, thus providing strong direct evidence of the much higher incidence of previously unrecognized occult anal sphincter trauma after delivery and its importance in the pathophysiology of anal incontinence (16,111,112) (Figs. 54.2–54.4).

Sultan et al. (16) investigated 202 pregnant women six weeks before delivery using anal endosonography, manometry, perineometry, and pudendal nerve terminal motor latencies. These tests were repeated in 150 of these women six weeks after delivery and then in the 32 women with abnormal findings (defects on endosonography or prolonged pudendal nerve terminal motor latencies) at six months after delivery. Ten of the 79 primiparous women (13%) and 11 of the 48 multiparous women (23%) who delivered vaginally had anal incontinence or fecal urgency when studied six weeks after delivery. Twenty-eight of the 79 primiparous women (35%) had a sphincter defect on endosonography at six weeks; the defect persisted in all 22 women studied at six months. Of the 48 multiparous women, 19 (40%) had a sphincter defect before delivery and 21 (44%) afterward. None of the 23 women who underwent cesarean section had a new sphincter defect after delivery. The use of forceps was the single independent factor associated with anal sphincter damage and there was a strong correlation with the presence of defects and the development of symptoms. This suggests that it is the first vaginal delivery that is the most important factor for damage to the anal sphincters.

Forceps delivery results in more trauma to the anal sphincters and is associated with a higher incidence of defecatory symptoms than a ventouse delivery. Anal sphincter defects were seen in 81% of those who had a forceps delivery compared to 24% of those who had a ventouse delivery and 36% of controls (112).

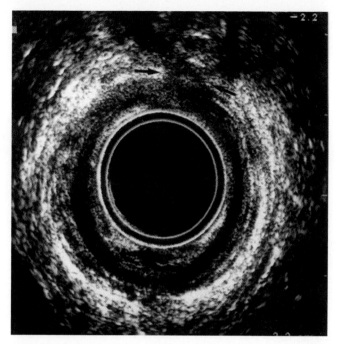

Figure 54.2 Two-dimensional image of the anal sphincter, demonstrating an external sphincter defect (arrows). The external sphincter appears hyperechoic surrounding the hypoechoic external sphincter.

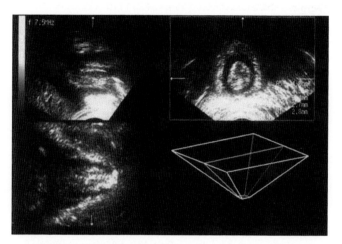

Figure 54.3 Three-dimensional image of an intact anal sphincter.

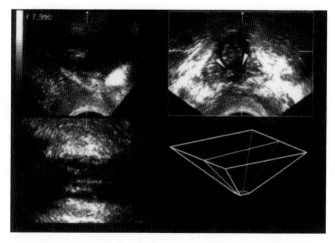

Figure 54.4 Three-dimensional image of internal and external sphincter trauma.

559

Table 54.2 Sphincter Defects and Symptoms: Meta-Analysis of Studies Reporting Obstetric Sphincter Damage

Reference	Total	No. of women for meta-analysis		No. with sphincter defect		Symptomatic defect (%)	Postpartum fecal incontinence but no new sphincter tear (%)	Follow-up rate (%)
		Primip	Multip	Primip	Multip			
Sultan et al. (13)	127	79	48	28	2 new (19 old)	20.4 (10 of 49)	1.3 (1 of 78)	100
Abramovitz et al. (114)	202	96	106	25	14 new	23.1 (9 of 39)	6.7 (11 of 163)	100
Varma et al. (115)	120	78	42	9	6 old and new	0	0	71.6
Fynes et al. (116)	118	59	59	20	2 new	68.2 (15 of 22)	0 (0 of 96)	100
Faltin et al. (117)	150	150	0	42	0	36.6 (15 of 41)	6.8 (7 of 103)	96
Overall	717				167 new and old, all women	32.5 (49 of 151)	4.3 (19 of 440)	

Source: Data from Ref. 113.
Abbreviations: Multip, multiparae; Primip, primiparae.

Subsequent studies have looked at the incidence of anal sphincter injury using endoanal ultrasound and meta-analysis of five of these studies reveals a 26.9% incidence of anal sphincter injury in primiparous women and an 8.5% incidence of new sphincter defects in multiparous women. Overall, 29.7% of women with anal sphincter defects were symptomatic though 3.4% of women experienced postpartum fecal incontinence without a sphincter defect (Table 54.2) (113–117).

The use of episiotomy and its relationship to anal sphincter injury is unclear. Poen et al. (118) reported that the use of a mediolateral episiotomy was associated with fewer third-degree tears. Sultan et al. (109) in a retrospective study of women who had sustained third-degree tears, reported that almost half of these women had undergone an episiotomy. The use of midline episiotomies, favored in the United States, has been strongly associated with third-degree tears, with those women having midline episiotomies 50 times more likely to sustain a third-degree tear (119). This is reflected in the three-fold increased risk of fecal incontinence following midline episiotomy versus a spontaneous perineal laceration (120).

The degree of anal sphincter trauma may also be related to occurrence of symptoms. A questionnaire study of 208 women 13 years after vaginal delivery found that 25% of women after fourth degree tears, and 11.5% after third degree tears complained of anal incontinence of gas or liquid or solid stool (121). In another American study of 2858 primiparous women delivered vaginally 19% were known to have sustained third or fourth degree tears (122).

Although this study was limited in that it was questionnaire based and retrospective, it highlighted the high prevalence of anal sphincter tears which may be a reflection of the practice of midline episiotomy performed in the United States. The incidence of worse bowel control was ten times higher in those with fourth degree lacerations versus third-degree lacerations which is not surprising as both the internal and external sphincter are then compromised and as such cannot compensate so easily for loss of function in the other. The urgency associated with internal sphincter damage may also exacerbate loss of bowel control to a greater degree. Another observation was that more than 50% reported new onset urinary incontinence indicating that similar risk factors pertaining to anal sphincter trauma may relate to damage and loss of function of the urethral continence mechanism.

There may also be an inherent predisposition to anal sphincter trauma as there are racial difference in incidence of trauma which is highest in Asian women compared to white women and with black women having the lowest incidence (123,124). Further evidence of a genetic predisposition due to tissue types comes from a telephone survey of women who had undergone an instrumental delivery. This study reported that those with a history of joint hypermobility (a marker for collagen weakness) had an increased risk of postpartum anal incontinence (125).

Despite obvious injury to the anal sphincters, symptoms of anal incontinence may not occur for some time after delivery. Bek et al. (126) found that in women who experienced transient anal incontinence after a complete tear, 39% had a relapse of symptoms after the next vaginal delivery. The major long-term problem seen in these women was incontinence of flatus. Fynes et al. (116) in a study of women undergoing a second vaginal delivery, with a history of occult sphincter injury or transient fecal incontinence after their first delivery, found that there was a significant risk of these women having persistent fecal incontinence. Full thickness anal sphincter disruption was the most significant risk factor in the development of fecal incontinence after a second vaginal delivery.

CHILDBIRTH AND PROLAPSE

Genital prolapse occurs as a consequence of weakness of the fibromuscular supports of the pelvic organs. The etiology is multifactorial but childbirth has been implicated as a major factor. It is far commoner in parous women, with 50% of parous women having some degree of genital prolapse, of which 10% to 20% are symptomatic. In contrast, only 2% of symptomatic prolapse is found to occur in nulliparous women. The risk of prolapse is higher with increasing parity (127).

The mechanism of prolapse is unclear. Pathologic and electrophysiological studies have shown that significant pelvic nerve denervation and reinnervation are associated with stress incontinence and prolapse. However, there are also collagenous changes in the pelvic floor which are related to ageing, childbirth, and endogenous hormone changes which may also predispose to prolapse and stress incontinence (128–131).

During vaginal delivery the combination of distension by the fetal head and pressure of maternal expulsive efforts stretching the pelvic floor may lead to functional and anatomic alterations in the muscles, nerves, and the connective tissue of the pelvic floor and anal canal. Trauma to the pelvic floor may also lead to repair with weaker collagen and so predispose to incontinence and prolapse. Prolapse is noted to be more common in women after a vaginal delivery compared to after a cesarean section (132,133). Using the pelvic organ prolapse quantification (POPQ) examination, O'Boyle et al. found that the 23 nulliparous pregnant women had an increased POPQ stage compared to 21 non-pregnant controls (134). An increase in POPQ stage is also seen after vaginal delivery and this correlates well with increased mobility of the bladder base and neck (135). These studies suggest that both pregnancy and delivery are important etiologic factors for the development of pelvic organ prolapse.

The use of magnetic resonance imaging (MRI) and ultrasound has provided greater insight into pelvic floor dysfunction. Changes in levator hiatus have been shown to be related to urogenital prolapse and surgery for prolapse has been associated with a reduction in the size of the urogenital hiatus (136,137). This suggests that a more distensible levator hiatus is associated with risk of pelvic organ prolapse. MRI has previously shown abnormalities in the levator ani in women with stress incontinence and prolapse (138). In an MRI study in nulliparous women and women after their first vaginal birth, 20% of primiparous women had a visible defect in the pubovisceral or iliococcygeal portion of the levator ani muscle. These defects were not seen in nulliaparae. Those women with urinary incontinence were more likely to have a defect in the levator muscle. In another study it was noted that increasing levator trauma was found in those with a longer second stage of labor (139).

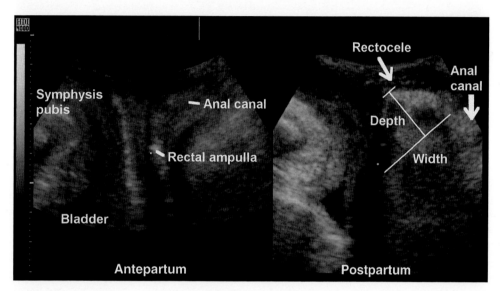

Figure 54.5 Comparison of posterior compartment imaging (midsagittal plane) in the third trimester (*left*) and three months postpartum (*right*) on maximal valsalva manoeuvre. The anorectal junction appears normal on the left. On the right there is a rectocele, with a depth of about 2 cm, filled with stool. *Source*: Reproduced from Ref. 140 with permission and by courtesy of HP Dietz.

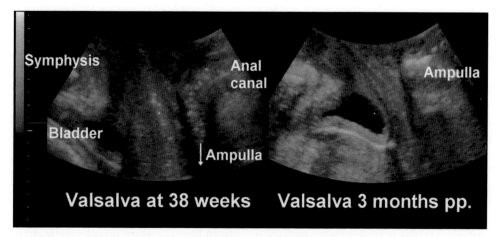

Figure 54.6 Comparison of posterior compartment imaging (midsagittal plane) in the third trimester (*left*) and three months postpartum (*right*), on maximal valsalva. The anorectal junction is normal on the left. The right image shows increased bladder descent and perineal mobility, resulting in displacement of the rectal ampulla below the synphysis pubis. There is no actual rectocele, that is, no defect of the rectobaginal septum shown in Figure 54.5. *Source*: Reproduced from Ref. 140 with permission and by courtesy of HP Dietz.

561

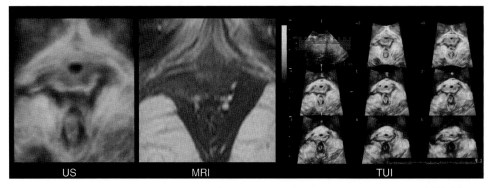

Figure 54.7 Unilateral avulsion on ultrasound, MR, and tomographic ultrasound. *Source*: Courtesy of HP Dietz.

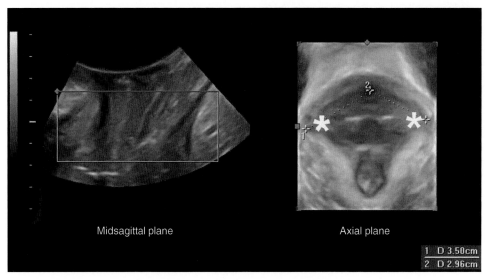

Figure 54.8 Typical bilateral avulsion injury seen in primiparous patient (forceps) as seen in the axial plane (right image). The defects are indicated by *. *Source*: Reproduced from Ref. 142 with permission and by courtesy of HP Dietz.

These defects are thought to be either due to avulsion of the muscles from their origin or as a result of denervation; however, whatever the possible mechanism, it is clear that such damage to the levator "plate" leads to a decrease in muscular support of the pelvic organs and an increase in the load carried by connective tissue and fascia. These muscular injuries may themselves relate to stress incontinence or predispose to weakening of fascial and connective tissue supports resulting in stress incontinence.

Pelvic floor ultrasound has been an increasingly useful tool for revealing changes in levator anatomy related to parity. Using translabial ultrasound Dietz et al. in a study of 68 nulliparous women during the third trimester and two to six months postpartum found that vaginal delivery resulted in an increased prevalence and size of a true rectoceles (defects in the rectovaginal septum). These defects were associated with symptoms of POP and obstructed defecation (140,141). However, rectoceles were also seen in those after cesarean section, so pregnancy itself may affect the integrity of the rectovaginal septum. In another study by this group, vaginal delivery was noted to be associated with avulsion of the levator ani from the pelvic side wall in one third of women. There was also a weak but significant association between avulsion injury and de novo stress incontinence (142) (Figs. 54.5–54.8).

CONCLUSIONS

The development of pelvic floor disorders such as urinary and fecal incontinence and genital prolapse have been associated with pregnancy and vaginal delivery. Over the last two decades histology, imaging, and physiology techniques have revealed mechanisms of injury to the pelvic floor which include direct muscle trauma, disruption of connective tissue support and denervation with the time of greatest risk of damage at the first vaginal delivery.

In recent years, there has been an ongoing debate regarding the protective effect of an elective cesarean section in reducing the risk of pelvic floor disorders and woman are increasingly requesting cesarean section for non-medical reasons (143). The debate is ongoing as the evidence supporting this is conflicting and much is derived from small studies, of heterogenous cohorts with differing and inconsistent definitions of incontinence. Epidemiological studies implicate parity associated with incontinence however it is less clear what the effect is of mode of delivery. Less pelvic floor damage seems occur after elective but not necessarily emergency cesarean section (18,19,144,145). With regard to urinary incontinence, some data suggest that cesarean is protective (27,146–148); however, others suggest that it is pregnancy itself that is the major risk factor (149,150). Elective cesarean section appears to prevent against mechanical trauma to the anal sphincter but not necessarily the urethral sphincter (151). However, elective cesarean section in not wholly protective even for anal incontinence (152). In addition, is has been estimated that 167 cesarean deliveries are needed to prevent one case of fecal incontinence (153). Therefore, before considering the potential benefits of cesarean delivery, they must be weighed against the potential risks for mother and child, including increased risk of postpartum hysterectomy, adhesions, ileus, placental implantation, problems in future pregnancies, and increased respiratory distress syndrome in the newborn (154,155). An answer to this question would really only come with women randomized to either vaginal birth or elective cesarean section, though this is of course impossible for clear ethical and practical reasons. The only study that gives a partial answer to this, it that of the term breech trial (149) where women with breech babies at term where randomized to an elective cesarean section or vaginal delivery. Women in the cesarean section arm of this study had a relative risk of 0.62 for stress incontinence. However, this data is short term and even if cesarean section were in the short-term protective, this protective effect diminishes with time and subsequent deliveries and factors such as ageing and the menopause may then be more relevant (156–158). A reanalysis of the EPINCONT study (158) has shown that women who have children at an older age are more likely to suffer from stress incontinence and this is supported by ultrasound studies which show an increase in odds of levator trauma of 10% for each year of delayed child bearing (159). These findings suggest that as women in Westernized societies delay childbearing, there will be a rise in the incidence of pelvic floor morbidity.

Given the lack of clarity with the present data, the focus should be on modifying potential risk factors that may impact on pelvic floor trauma. Pelvic floor exercises have been shown to reduce urinary incontinence and increase pelvic floor strength (160,161). Adequate training is required in recognition of perineal trauma and repair, intra- and postpartum bladder care (161). Training of birth attendants is important as inexperienced birth attendants will increase perineal damage (162,163). This should include skills such as choice and technique of instrumental delivery and use of episiotomy as it is known that even the angle and technique of the episiotomy can vary widely and may often be more midline than mediolateral in position (164). Easing the perineum with controlled delivery of the fetal head has also been shown to reduce the perineal trauma rate though this is often not used with the vogue for the "hands-off" approach employed by many birth attendants (165,166).

There are other modifiable factors that should also be addressed such as constipation and high body mass index (BMI), both of which were associated with an increased prevalence of urinary and anal incontinence (167,168). It may be prudent to consider active programs to promote a healthy prepregnancy BMI, not only for reducing pelvic floor morbidity but as this is known to be related to a higher risk of pregnancy complications including cesarean section.

For those women in whom postpartum incontinence and prolapse develops, treatment strategies and follow-up should be readily available and standardized protocols developed. There are now clear guidelines indicating the relevant therapies and investigations that could be used in these situations. Long term studies are required in assessing the outcome of interventions and treatments in women prior to and after delivery.

REFERENCES

1. MacArthur C, Lewis D, Bick D. Stress incontinence after childbirth. Br J Midwifery 1991; 1: 207–14.
2. Glazener CMA, Abdalla M, Stroud P, et al. Postnatal maternal morbidity: extent, causes, prevention and treatment. Br J Obstet Gynaecol 1995; 102: 282–7.
3. Sleep J, Grant A. West Berkshire perineal management trial: three year follow-up. BMJ 1987; 295: 749–51.
4. Sleep J, Grant A, Garcia J, et al. West Berkshire perineal management trial. BMJ 1984; 289: 587–90.
5. Andrews V, Thakar R, Sultan AH, Jones PW. Evaluation of postpartum perineal pain and dyspareunia- A prospective study. Eur J Obstet Gynecol Reprod Biol 2008; 137: 152–6.
6. Handa VL, Zyczynski HM, Burgio KL, et al. Pelvic floor disorders network. The impact of fecal and urinary incontinence on quality of life 6 months after childbirth. Am J Obstet Gynecol 2007; 197: 636,e1-6.
7. Brubaker L, Handa VL, Bradley CS, et al. Sexual function 6 months after first delivery. Obstet Gynecol 2008; 111: 1040–44.
8. Handa VL, Harris TA, Ostergard MD. Protecting the pelvic floor: obstetric management to prevent incontinence and pelvic organ prolapse. Obstet Gynecol 1996; 88: 470–8.
9. Nicholls C, Randall C. Vaginal Surgery. Baltimore: Williams and Wilkins, 1976.
10. Foldspang A, Lam GW, Elving L. Parity as a correlate of adult female urinary incontinence prevalence. J Epidemiol Comm Health 1992; 46: 595–600.
11. Milsom I, Ekelund P, Molander U, Arvidsson L, Areskoug B. The influence of age, parity, oral contraception, hysterectomy and menopause on the prevalence of urinary incontinence in women. J Urol 1993; 149: 1459–62.
12. Wilson PD, Herbison RM, Herbison GP. Obstetric practice and the prevalence of urinary incontinence three months after delivery. Br J Obstet Gynaecol 1996; 103: 154–61.
13. Viktrup L, Lose G. The risk of stress incontinence 5 years after first delivery. Am J Obstet Gynecol 2001; 185: 52–87.
14. Rortveit G, Daltveit AK, Hannestad YS, Hunskaar S. Urinary incontinence after vaginal delivery or caesarean section. N Engl J Med 2003; 348: 900–7.
15. Chaliha C, Digesu A, Hutchings A, Soligo M, Khullar V. Caesarean section is protective against stress urinary incontinence: an analysis of women with multiple deliveries. Br J Obstet Gynaecol 2004; 111: 754–5.
16. Sultan AH, Kamm MA, Hudson CN, Thomas JM, Bartram CI. Anal sphincter disruption during vaginal delivery. N Engl J Med 1993; 329: 1905–11.
17. Snooks SJ, Swash M, Setchell M, Henry MM. Injury to the innervation of pelvic floor sphincter musculature in childbirth. Lancet 1984; ii: 546–50.
18. Allen RE, Hosker GL, Smith ARB, Warrell DW. Pelvic floor damage and childbirth: a neurophysiological study. Br J Obstet Gynaecol 1990; 97: 770–9.
19. MacArthur C, Bick D, Keighley MRB. Faecal incontinence after childbirth. Br J Obstet Gynaecol 1997; 104: 46–50.
20. Ulmsten U, Ekman G, Giertz G, Malmstrom A. Different biochemical composition of connective tissue in continent and stress incontinent women. Acta Obstet Gynecol Scand 1987; 66: 455–7.
21. King J, Freeman R. Can we predict antenatally those patients at risk of postpartum stress incontinence. Neurourol Urodyn 1996; 15: 330–1.
22. Skoner M, Thompson WD, Caron VA. Factors associated with risk of stress urinary incontinence in women. Nurs Res 1994; 43: 301–6.

23. Thacker SB, Banta DH. Benefits and risks of episiotomy: an interpretative review of the English language literature, 1860–1890. Obstet Gynecol Surv 1983; 38: 322–38.

24. Madoff RD, Williams JG, Caushaj PF. Current concepts: fecal incontinence. N Engl J Med 1992; 362: 1002–7.

25. Klein MC, Gauthier RJ, Robbins JG, et al. Relationship of episiotomy to perineal trauma and morbidity, sexual dysfunction, and pelvic floor relaxation. Am J Obstet Gynecol 1994; 171: 591–8.

26. Thacker SB, Banta DH. Benefits and risks of episiotomy: an interpretative review of the English language literature, 1860–1890. Obstet Gynecol Surv 1983; 38: 322–38.

27. Eason E, Labreque M, Marcoux S, Mondor M. Effects of carrying a pregnancy and of method of delivery on urinary incontinence: a prosepctive cohort study. BMC Pregnancy and Childbirth 2004; 4: 4.

28. Signorello LB, Harlow BL, Chekos A, Repke JT. Postpartum sexual functioning and its relationship to perineal trauma: a retrospective cohort study of primiparous women. Am J Obstet Gynecol 2001; 184: 881–90.

29. Peschers UM, Schaer GN, DeLancey JOL, Schuessler B. Levator ani function before and after childbirth. Br J Obstet Gynaecol 1997; 104: 1004–8.

30. Gordon H, Logue M. Perineal function after childbirth. Lancet 1985; 2: 123–5.

31. Sartore A, Deseta F, Gianpaolo M, et al. The effects of mediolateral episiotomy on pelvic floor function after vaginal delivery. Obstet Gynecol 2004; 103: 669–73.

32. Kiff ES, Barnes RPH, Swash M. Evidence of pudendal neuropathy in patients with perineal descent and chronic constipation. Gut 1984; 5: 1279–82.

33. Dafnis E, Sabatini S. The effect of pregnancy on renal function: physiology and pathophysiology. Am J Med Sci 1992; 303: 184–205.

34. Lobel RW, Sand PK, Bowen LW. The urinary tract in pregnancy. In: Ostergard DR, Bent AE, eds. Urogynaecology and Urodynamics, 4th edn. Baltimore: Williams and Wilkins, 1996: 323.

35. Bennetts FA, Judd GE. Studies of the postpartum bladder. Am J Obstet Gynaecol 1941; 42: 419–27.

36. Seski AG, Duprey WM. Postpartum intravesical photography. Obstet Gynecol 1961; 18: 548–56.

37. Muellner SR. Physiological bladder changes during pregnancy and the puerperium. J Urol 1939; 41: 691–2.

38. Francis WJA. Disturbances of bladder function in relation to pregnancy. J Obstet Gynaecol Br Emp 1960; 67: 353–66.

39. Kerr-Wilson RHJ, Thompson SW, Orr JW, Davis RO, Cloud GA. Effect of labor on the postpartum bladder. Obstet Gynecol 1984; 64: 115–8.

40. Chaliha C, Kalia V, Monga A, Sultan AH, Stanton SL. Pregnancy, childbirth and delivery: a urodynamic viewpoint. Br J Obstet Gynaecol 2000; 107: 1354–9.

41. Parboosingh J, Doig A. Studies of nocturia in normal pregnancy. Obstet Gynecol Br Emp 1973; 80: 888–95.

42. Cutner A, Carey A, Cardozo LD. Lower urinary tract symptoms in early pregnancy. Br J Obstet Gynaecol 1992; 12: 75–8.

43. Cutner A. The lower urinary tract in pregnancy. MD Thesis, University of London, 1993.

44. Parboosingh A, Doig A. Renal nyctohemeral excretory patterns of water and solutes in normal human pregnancy. Am J Obstet Gynecol 1973; 116: 609–15.

45. Fischer W, Kittel K. Urine flow measurement in pregnancy and the puerperium. Zentralbl Gynakol 1990; 112: 593–9.

46. Myers DL, Scott RJ. Acute urinary retention and incarcerated retroverted gravid uterus. J Reprod Med 1995; 40: 487–90.

47. Saultz JW, Toffler WL, Shackles JY. Postpartum urinary retention. J Am Board Fam Pract 1991; 4: 341–4.

48. Andolf E, Iosif CS, Jorgensen C, Rydstrom H. Insidious urinary retention after vaginal delivery: prevalence and symptoms at follow-up in a population based study. Gynecol Obstet Invest 1994; 38: 51–3.

49. Yip S-K, Hin L-K, Chung TKH. Effect of duration of labor on postpartum postvoid residual bladder volume. Gynecol Obstet Invest 1998; 45: 177–80.

50. Carley ME, Carley JM, Vasdev G, et al. Factors that are associated with clinically overt postpartum urinary retention after vaginal delivery. Am J Obstet Gynecol 2002; 187: 430–3.

51. Khullar V, Cardozo LD. Bladder sensation after epidural analgesia. Neurourol Urodyn 1993; 12: 424–5.

52. Francis WJA. The onset of stress incontinence. J Obstet Gynaecol Br Emp 1960; 67: 899–903.

53. Viktrup L, Lose G, Rolff M, Barfoed K. The symptom of stress incontinence caused by pregnancy or delivery in primiparas. Obstet Gynecol 1992; 79: 945–9.

54. Chaliha C, Khullar V, Stanton SL, Monga AK, Sultan AHS. Urinary symptoms in pregnancy: are they useful for diagnosis? Br J Obstet Gynaecol 2002; 109: 1181–3.

55. Stanton SL, Kerr-Wilson R, Harris GV. The incidence of urological symptoms in normal pregnancy. Br J Obstet Gynaecol 1980; 87: 897–900.

56. Viktrup L, Lose G. Lower urinary tract symptoms 5 years after first delivery. Int Urogynecol J Pelvic Floor Dysfunct 2000; 11: 336–40.

57. Foldspang A, Hvidman L, Momssen S, Nielsen JB. Risk of postpartum urinary incontinence associated with pregnancy and mode of delivery. Acta Obstet Gynecol Scand 2004; 83: 923–7.

58. Dolan LM, Hosker G, Mallett VT, Allen RE, Smith ARB. Stress incontinence and pelvic floor neurophysiology 15 years after first delivery. Br J Obstet Gynaecol 2003; 110: 1107–14.

59. Ekstrom A, Altamn D, Wiklund I, Larrson C, Andolf E. Planned cesarean section versus planned vaginal delivery: comparison of lower urinary tract symptoms. Int Urogynecol J, 2008; 19: 459–65.

60. Chaliha C, Kalia V, Stanton SL, et al. Antenatal prediction of postpartum urinary and fecal incontinence. Obstet Gynecol 1992; 79: 945–9.

61. Wilson PD, Herbison RM, Herbison GP. Obstetric practice and the prevalence of urinary incontinence three months after delivery. Br J Obstet Gynaecol 1996; 103: 154–61.

62. Jackson S, Barry C, Davies G, et al. Duration of the second stage of labour and epidural analgesia: effect on subsequent urinary symptoms in primiparous women. Neurourol Urodyn 1995; 14: 498–9.

63. Dimpfl T, Hesse U, Schussler B. Incidence and cause of postpartum urinary stress incontinence. Eur J Obstet Gynecol Reprod Biol 1992; 43: 29–33.

64. Tezschner T, Sorensen M, Lose G, et al. Anal and urinary incontinence in women with obstetric anal sphincter rupture. Br J Obstet Gynaecol 1996; 103: 1034–40.

65. Viktrup L, Lose G. Epidural analgesia during labour and stress incontinence after delivery. Obstet Gynecol 1993; 82: 984–6.

66. Röckner G. Urinary incontinence after perineal trauma at childbirth. Scand J Caring Sci 1990; 4: 169–72.

67. Iosif S, Ulmsten U. Comparative urodynamic studies of continent and stress incontinent women in pregnancy and the puerperium. Am J Obstet Gynecol 1981; 140: 645–50.

68. Toews H. Intraurethral pressure in normal and stress incontinent women. Obstet Gynecol 1967; 29: 613–24.

69. Bunne G, Obrink A. Urethral closure pressure in stress: a comparison between stress incontinent and continent women. Urol Res 1977; 6: 127–34.

70. Schultze H, Wolansky D. Urethral wall pulsation in pregnant patients, continent and stress incontinent females. Zentralbl Gynakol 1990; 112: 19–22.

71. Perucchini D, DeLancey JOL, Ashton-Miller JA. Regional striated muscle loss in the female urethra: where is striated muscle vulnerable? Neurourol Urodyn 1997; 16: 407–8.

72. Toozs-Hobson P, Balmforth J, Cardozo L, Khullar V, Athanasiou S. Effect of mode of delivery on pelvic floor functional anatomy. Int Urogynecol J Pelvic Floor Dysfunct 2008; 19: 407–16.

73. Benness CJ, Barnick CG, Cardozo L. Normal urodynic findings in symptomatic women: who to believe, the patient or the test? Int Urogynecol J 1990; 1: 173–4.

74. Smith ARB, Hosker G, Warrell DW. The role of partial denervation of the pelvic floor in the aetiology of genitourinary prolapse and stress incontinence of urine: a neurophysiological study. Br J Obstet Gynaecol 1989; 96: 24–8.

75. Smith ARB, Hosker GL, Warrell DW. The role of pudendal nerve damage in the etiology of genuine stress incontinence in women. Br J Obstet Gynaecol 1989; 96: 29–32.

76. Deindl FM, Vodusek DB, Hesse U, Schussler B. Pelvic floor activity patterns: comparison of nulliparous continent and parous urinary stress incontinent women. Br J Urol 1994; 73: 413–7.

77. Peschers U, Schaer G, Anthuber C, DeLancey JOL, Schuessler B. Changes in vesical neck mobility following vaginal delivery. Obstet Gynecol 1996; 88: 1001–6.

78. Meyer S, Schreyer A, De Grandi P, Hohlfeld P. The effects of birth on urinary continence mechanisms and other pelvic floor characteristics. Obstet Gynecol 1998; 92: 613–8.

79. Athanasiou S, Boos K, Khullar V, Anders K, Cardozo L. Pathogenesis of genuine stress incontinence and urogenital prolapse. Neurourol Urodyn 1996; 15: 339–40.

80. Toozs-Hobson P, Balmforth J, Cardozo L, Khullar V, Athanasiou S. The effect of mode of delivery on pelvic floor functional anatomy. Int Urogynecol J 2008; 19: 407–16.

81. Meyer S, Bachelard O, De Gandi P. Do bladder neck mobility and urethral sphincter function differ during pregnancy compared with the non-pregnant state? Int Urogynecol J 1998; 9: 397–404.

82. Keane DP, Sims TJ, Bailey AJ, Abrams P. Analysis of the pelvic floor electromyography and collagen status in premenopausal nulliparous females with genuine stress incontinence. Neurourol Urodyn 1992; 11: 308–9.

83. Lavin JM, Smith ARB, Anderson J, et al. The effect of pregnancy on the connective tissue rectus sheath. Neurourol Urodyn 1997; 16: 381–2.

84. King J, Freeman R. Is antenatal bladder neck mobility a risk factor for postpartum stress incontinence? Br J Obstet Gynaecol 1998; 105: 1300–7.

85. Sultan AH, Kamm MA, Hudson CN, Bartram CI. Effect of pregnancy on anal sphincter morphology and function. Int J Colorect Dis 1993; 8: 206–9.

86. Kamm MA. Obstetric damage and faecal incontinence. Lancet 1994; 344: 730–3.

87. Law PJ, Kamm MA, Bartram CI. Anal endosonography in the investigation of faecal incontinence. Br J Surg 1991; 78: 312–4.

88. Zetterstrom JP, Lopez A, Anzen B, et al. Anal incontinence after vaginal delivery: a prospective study in primiparous women. Br J Obstet Gynaecol 1999; 106: 324–30.

89. Combs CA, Robertson PA, Laros RK. Risk factors for third-degree and fourth-degree perineal lacerations in forceps and vacuum deliveries. Am J Obstet Gynecol 1990; 163: 100–4.

90. Walker M, Farine D, Robin S, Ritchie J. Epidural analgesia, episiotomy and obstetric laceration. Obstet Gynecol 1991; 77: 668–71.

91. Henriksen TB, Bek KM, Hedegaard M, Secher NJ. Episiotomy and perineal lesions in spontaneous vaginal deliveries. Br J Obstet Gynaecol 1992; 99: 950–4.

92. Crawford LA, Quint EH, Pearl ML, DeLancey JO. Incontinence following rupture of the anal sphincter during delivery. Obstet Gynecol 1993; 82: 527–31.

93. Snooks SJ, Barnes PRH, Swash M, Henry MM. Damage to the innervation of the pelvic floor musculature in chronic constipation. Gastroenterology 1985; 89: 977–81.

94. Parks AG, Swash M, Urich H. Sphincter denervation in anorectal incontinence and rectal prolapse. Gut 1977; 18: 656–65.

95. Parks AG, Swash M. Denervation of the anal sphincter causing idiopathic ano-rectal incontinence. J R Coll Surg Edinb 1979; 24: 94–6.

96. Beersiek F, Parks AG, Swash AM. Pathogenesis of anorectal incontinence: a histometric study of anal sphincter musculature. J Neurol Sci 1979; 42: 111–27.

97. Lubowski DZ, Swash M, Nicholls RJ, Henry MM. Increase in pudendal nerve terminal motor latency with defaecation straining. Br J Surg 1988; 75: 786–8.

98. Snooks SJ, Swash M, Mathers SE, Henry MM. Effect of vaginal delivery on the pelvic floor: 5 year follow-up. Br J Surg 1990; 77: 1358–60.

99. Sultan AH, Kamm MA, Bartram CI, Hudson CN. Pudendal nerve damage during labour: prospective study before and after childbirth. Br J Obstet Gynaecol 1994; 101: 22–8.

100. Miller R, Bartolo DCC, Roe A, Cervero F, Mortensen NJ. Anal sensation and the continence mechanism. Dis Colon Rectum 1988; 31: 433–8.

101. Rogers J. Testing for and the role of anal rectal sensation. Baillières Clin Gastroenterol 1992; 6: 179–91.

102. Aitchinson M, Fisher BM, Carter K, et al. Impaired anal sensation and early diabetic faecal incontinence. Diabet Med 1991; 8: 960–3.

103. Ferguson GH, Redford J, Barrett JA, Kiff ES. The appreciation of rectal distension in fecal incontinence. Dis Colon Rectum 1989; 32: 964–7.

104. Miller R, Bartolo DCC, Mortensen NJ. Anorectal temperature sensation: a comparison of normal and continent patients. Br J Surg 1987; 74: 511–5.

105. Barrett JA, Brocklehurst JC, Kiff ES, Ferguson G, Faragher EB. Anal function in geriatric patients with faecal incontinence. Gut 1989; 30: 1224–51.

106. Small KA, Wynne JM. Evaluating the pelvic floor in obstetric patients. Aust N Z J Obstet Gynaecol 1990; 30: 41–5.

107. Cornes H, Bartolo DCC, Stirrat GM. Changes in anal canal sensation after childbirth. Br J Surg 1991; 78: 74–7.

108. Chaliha C, Bland JM, Monga A, Sultan AHS, Stanton SL. Anal function: effect of pregnancy and delivery. Am J Obstet Gynecol 2001; 185: 427–32.

109. Sultan AH, Kamm MA, Hudson CN, Bartram CL. Third degree obstetric anal sphincter tears: risk factors and outcome of primary repair. Br Med J 1994; 308: 887–91.

110. Klein MC, Gauthier RJ, Robbins JM, et al. Relationship of episiotomy to perineal trauma and morbidity, sexual dysfunction and pelvic floor relaxation. Am J Obstet Gynecol 1994; 171: 591–8.

111. Sultan AH, Kamm MA, Talbot IC, Nicholls RJ, Bartram CI. Anal endosonography for identifying external sphincter defects confirmed histologically. Br J Surg 1994; 81: 463–5.

112. Sultan AH, Kamm MA, Bartram CI, Hudson CN. Anal sphincter trauma during instrumental delivery. A comparison between forceps and vacuum extraction. Int J Gynecol Obstet 1993; 43: 263–70.

113. Oberwalder M, Connor J, Wexner SD. Meta-analysis to determine the incidence of obstetric anal sphincter damage. Br J Surg 2003; 90: 1333–7.

114. Abramowitz L, Sobhani I, Ganansia R, et al. Are sphincter defects the cause of anal incontinence after vaginal delivery? Results of a prospective study. Dis Colon Rectum 2000; 43: 590–6.

115. Varma A, Gunn J, Gardiner A, Lindow SW, Duthie GS. Obstetric anal sphincter injury: prospective evaluation of incidence. Dis Colon Rectum 1999; 42: 1537–43.

116. Fynes M, Donnelly V, Behan M, O'Connell PR, O'Herlihy C. Effect of second vaginal delivery on anorectal physiology and faecal continence: a prospective study. Lancet 1999; 354: 983–6.

117. Faltin DL, Boulvain M, Irion O, et al. Diagnosis of anal sphincter tears by postpartum endosonography to predict fecal incontinence. Obstet Gynecol 2000; 95: 643–7.

118. Poen AC, Felt-Bersma RJF, Dekker GA, et al. Third degree obstetric perineal tears: risk factors and the preventative role of mediolateral episiotomy. Br J Obstet Gynaecol 1997; 104: 563–6.

119. Shiono P, Klebanoff MA, Carey JC. Midline episiotomies: more harm then good? Obstet Gynecol 1990; 75: 765–70.

120. Signorello L, Harlo LB, Chekos AK, Repke JT. Midline episiotomy and anal incontinence: a retrospective cohort study. BMJ 2000; 320: 86–90.

121. Sangalli MR, Floris L, Faltin D, Weil A. Anal incontinence in women with third or fourth degree perineal tears and subsequent vaginal deliveries. Aust NZJ Obstet Gynecol 2000; 40: 244–8.

122. Fenner DE, Genberg B, Brahma P, Marek L, DeLancey JOL. Fecal and urinary incontinence after vaginal delivery with anal sphincter disruption in an obstetrics unit in the United States. Am J Obstet Gynecol 2003; 189: 1543–50.

123. Howard D, Davies P, Delancey J, Small Y. Differences in perineal laceration in Black and White primiparas. Obstet Gynecol 2000; 96: 622–4.

124. Goldberg J, Hyslop T, Tolosa J, Sultana C. Racial differences in severe perineal lacerations after vaginal delivery. Am J Obstet Gynecol 2003; 188: 1063–7.

125. Chiarelli P, Murphy B, Cockburn J. Fecal incontinence after high-risk delivery. Obstet Gynecol 2003; 102: 1299–305.

126. Bek KM, Laurberg S. Risks of anal incontinence from subsequent vaginal delivery after a complete obstetric anal sphincter tear. Br J Obstet Gynaecol 1992; 99: 724–6.

127. WHO Population Report. Healthier mothers and children through family planning programmes. Geneva: WHO, 1984; 27: J677.
128. Hayflick L. Theories of biological aging. Exp Gerontol 1985; 20: 145–59.
129. Yamauchi M, Woodley DT, Mechanic GL. Aging and crosslinking of skin collagen. Biochem Biophys Res Commun 1988; 152: 898–903.
130. Norton PA. Pelvic floor disorders: the role of fascia and ligaments. Clin Obstet Gynecol 1993; 36: 926–38.
131. Morley R, Cumming J, Weller R. Morphology and neuropathology of the pelvic floor in patients with stress incontinence. Int Urogynecol J 1966; 7: 3–12.
132. De Gregorio G, Hillemans HG, Quaas L, Mentzel J. Late morbidity following caesarean section: a neglected factor. Geburtshilfe Frauenheilkd 1988; 48: 16–9.
133. Chiaffarino F, Chatenoud L, Dindelli M, et al. Reproductive factors, family history, occupation and risk of urogenital prolapse. Eur J Obstet Gynecol Reprod Biol 1999; 82: 63–7.
134. O'Boyle AL, Woodman PJ, O'Boyle JD, Davis GD, Swift SE. Pelvic organ support in nulliparous pregnant and non-pregnant women: a case control study. Am J Obstet Gynecol 2002; 187: 99–102.
135. Dannecker C, Lienemann A, Fischer T, Anthuber C. Influence of spontaneous instrumental vaginal delivery on objective measures of pelvic organ support: assessment with pelvic organ prolapse quantification (POPQ) technique and functional cine magnetic resonance imaging. Eur J Obstet Gynecol 2004; 115: 32–8.
136. Delancey JO, Hurd WW. Size of urogenital hiatus in the levator hiatus muscles in normal women and women with pelvic organ prolapse. Obstet Gynecol 1998; 91: 364–8.
137. Athanasiou S, Chaliha C, Toozs-Hobson P, et al. Direct imaging of the pelvic floor muscles using two-dimensional ultrasound: a comparison of women with prolapse versus controls. BJOG 2007; 114: 882–9.
138. Tunn R, Paris S, Fischer W, Hamm B, Kuchinke J. Static magnetic resonance imaging of the pelvic floor muscle morphology in women with stress urinary incontinence and pelvic prolapse. Neurourol Urodyn 1998; 17: 579–89.
139. Kearney R, Miller J, Ashton-Miller J, Delancey J. Obstetric factors associated with levator ani muscle injury after vaginal birth. Obstet Gynecol 2006; 107: 144–9.
140. Dietz HP, Steensma AB. The role of childbirth in the aetiology of rectocele. Br J Obstet Gynecol 2006; 113: 264–7.
141. Dietz HP, Korda A. Which bowel symptoms are more strongly associated with a true rectocele? Aust NZJ Obstet Gynecol 2005; 45: 505–8.
142. Dietz HP, Lanzarone V. Levator trauma after vaginal delivery. Obstet Gynecol 2005; 106: 707–12.
143. Florica M, Stephansson O, Nordstrom L. Indications associated with increased cesarean section rates in the Swedish population. Int J Gynaecol Obstet 2006; 92: 182–5.
144. Fynes M, Donnelly V, O'Connell PR, O'Herlihy C. Caesarean delivery and anal sphincter injury. Obstet Gynecol 1998; 92; 496–500.
145. MacArthur C, Bick DE, Keighley MRB. Faecal incontinence after childbirth. Br J Obstet Gynaecol 1997; 104: 46–50.
146. Glazener CM, Herbison GP, Macarthur C, et al. New postnatal urinary incontinence: obstetric and other risk factors in primiparae. JOG 2006; 113: 208–17.
147. van Brummen HJ, Bruinse HW, van de Pol G, Heintz AP, van der Vaart CH. The effect of vaginal and cesarean delievry on lower urinary tract symptoms: what makes the difference? Int Urogynecol J Pelvic Floor Dysfunct 2007; 18: 133–9.
148. Farrell SA, Allen VM, Basket TF. Parturition and urinary incontinence in primiparas. Obstet Gynecol 2001; 97: 350–6.
149. Hannah ME, Whyte H, Hannah WJ, et al. Maternal outcomes at 2 years after planned cesarean section versus planned vaginal birth for breech presentation at term: the International randomised Term Breech Trial. Am J Obstet Gynecol 2004; 191: 917–27.
150. McKinnie V, Swift SE, Wang W, et al. The effect of pregnancy and mode of delivery on the prevalence of urinary and fecal incontinence. Am J Obstet Gynecol 2005; 193: 512–7.
151. Fitzpatrick M, O'Herlihy C. The effects of labour and delivery on the pelvic floor. Clin Obstet Gynecol 2001;15:63–79.
152. Lal M, Mann C, Callender R, Radley S. Does cesarean delivery prevent anal incontinence? Obstet Gynecol 2003; 101: 305–12.
153. Nelson R, Westercamp M, Furner S. A systematic review of the efficacy of cesarean section in the preservation of anal incontinence. Dis Colon Rectum 2006; 49: 1587–95.
154. Jackson N, Paterson-Brown S. Physical sequelae of caesarean section. Clin Obstet Gynecol 2001; 14: 49–61.
155. Bowers SK, Macdonald HM, Shapiro ED. Prevention of iatrogenic neonatal respiratory distress syndrome: elective repeat cesarean section and spontaneous labor. Am J Obstet Gynecol 1982; 143: 186–9.
156. Bollard RC, Gardiner A, Duthie GS. Anal sphincter injury, fecal and urinary incontinence. A 34 year follow-up after forceps delivery. Dis Colon Rectum 2003; 46: 1083–8.
157. Connolly TJ, Litman HJ, Tennstedt SL, Link CL, McKinlay JB. The effect of mode of delivery, parity and birth weight on risk of urinary incontinence. Int Urogynecol J Pelvic Fllor Dysfunct 2007; 18: 1033–42.
158. Rortveit G, Hannestad YS, Daltveit AK, Hunskaar S. Age and type-dependant effects of parity on urinary incontinence: the Norwegian EPINCONT study. Obstet Gynecol 2001; 98: 1004–10.
159. Dietz HP, Simpson JM. Does delayed childbearing increase the risk of levaotr injury in labour? Aus NZJ Obstet Gynecol 2007; 47: 491–5.
160. Reilly ETC, Freeman RM, Waterfield MR, et al. Prevention of postpartum stress incontinence in primigravidae with increased bladder neck mobility: a randomised controlled trial of antenatal pelvic floor exercises. Br J Obstet Gynaecol 2002; 1109: 68–76.
161. Harvey MA. Pelvic floor exercises during and after pregnancy: a systematic review of their role in preventing pelvic floor dysfunction. J Obstet Gynaecol Can 2003; 25: 487–98.
162. Andrews V, Sultan AH, Thakar R, Jones PW. Occult anal sphincter injuries—myth or reality? BJOG 2006; 113: 195–200.
163. Jander C, Lyrenas S. Third and fourth degree perineal tears. Predictor factors in a referral hospital. Acta Obstet Gynecol Scand 2001; 80: 256–61.
164. Andrews V, Sultan AH, Thakar R, Jones PW. Risk factors for obstetric anal sphincter injury: a prospective study. Birth 2006; 33: 117–22.
165. Parnell C, Langhoff-Roos J, Moller H. Conduct of labor and rupture of the sphincter ani. Acat Obstet Gynhecol Scand 2001; 80: 256–61.
166. Laine K, Pirhonen T, Rolland R, Pirhonen J. Decreasing the incidence of anal sphincter tears during vaginal delivery. Obstet Gynecol 2008; 111: 1053–7.
167. Boyles SH, Li H, Mori T, Osterweil P, Guise J-M. Effect of mode of delivery on the incidence of urinary incontinence in primiparous women. Obstet Gynecol 2009; 113: 134–41.
168. Burgio KL, Borello-France D, Richter HE, et al. Risk factors for fecal and urianry incontinence after childbirth: The childbirth and pelvic symptoms study. Am J Gastroenterol 2007; 102: 1998–2004.

55 Problems Associated with Sexual Activity
Swati Jha

INTRODUCTION

Female sexual dysfunction (FSD) is defined as a sexual desire, sexual arousal, orgasm, and/or sexual pain disorder which causes personal distress (Table 55.1). FSD is a relatively common health issue for women with a community prevalence of 30% to 50% (1). The wide range of the reported percentages depends on the impact of different concomitant factors on sexual function, such as interpersonal, emotional relationship and well-being, and psychological factors. Studies have shown that FSD and other sexual problems have been linked to a "diminished quality of life (QoL), low physical satisfaction, low emotional satisfaction, and low general happiness" (2). Women's sexuality and sexual function are very complex issues, strongly modulated by psychosocial situations and this necessitates a biopsychosocial approach for understanding the basis of dysfunction which has been dealt with elsewhere in this textbook. Physiological events such as pregnancy, childbirth, menopause, aging as well as gynecological conditions like infertility, prolapse, urinary incontinence (UI), and gynecological cancers, have an impact on sexual well-being. The interaction of these conditions with sexual health needs to be better understood to deal effectively with the problems as a whole.

Sexual dysfunction is highly prevalent in women attending urogynecological services with a prevalence of 50% to 64% (3,4). Furthermore, urogynecological surgery represents an important but underestimated cause of FSD. Different problems of the pelvic floor can impact on sexual activity in different ways. Interest in and publications about FSD are very recent (3).

In this chapter we review the correlation of common urogynecological conditions on sexual activity and the impact of their treatment.

URINARY INCONTINENCE

UI is a common condition and epidemiological studies suggest that it affects up to 41% of the adult female population (5). It is a health burden, and impacts on social, psychological, occupational, domestic, physical, and sexual well being (6–9). Women reporting lower urinary tract symptoms (LUTS) or UI complain of a deteriorating QoL in terms of social and psychological problems, and also of sexual dysfunctions in significantly greater numbers than the general healthy population, as reported in a recent cross-sectional study (10). Table 55.2 shows the prevalence of UI during sexual activity as shown in different population groups.

Complaints of stress urinary incontinence (SUI), overactive bladder (OAB), and LUTS have negative impact on all domains of sexual function (6,10). In this population of women, the symptoms per se, along with fear of odor, embarrassment, shame, loss of self-esteem and fear of, or actual occurrence of, incontinence are contributory factors. The most common sexual complaints in women with UI are low desire, vaginal dryness, and dyspareunia (11).

In women with SUI prevalence of coital incontinence ranges from 11% to 70% (12–15). Traditional teaching has been that urodynamic stress incontinence (USI) is associated with penetration incontinence and detrusor overactivity with orgasm incontinence (14); however, subsequent studies by Moran et al. (15) have failed to confirm this association. In their observational study USI was associated with high rates of penetration incontinence (80%), orgasm incontinence (93%), and a combination of the two (92%). Among the different types of UI, OAB has a particularly higher association with sexual dysfunction in various studies (16), which could be indicative of an underlying psychosomatic disorder (17). However studies assessing overall prevalence of sexual dysfunction in women with OAB and the impact on QoL remains controversial (18) whereas menopausal and partner status have been shown to be the better predictors (19).

In women with SUI, the impact of treating incontinence on sexual function is controversial. Surgical treatment in these patients may be curative of their coital incontinence but have the potential to cause undesired effects on sensation, blood flow, and the anatomy. These effects can affect sexual arousal and orgasm or cause dyspareunia.

Before the introduction of minimally invasive suburethral sling procedures, Burch colposuspension was regarded as the "gold standard" for the surgical correction of SUI. There is some data regarding the impact of colposuspension on sexual health. Moran et al. (20) evaluated 55 women with SUI who reported coital incontinence before undergoing colposuspension. Preoperative coital leakage occured in 65% with penetration, in 16% with orgasm, and 18% with both. After surgery, 81% of the women reported no coital incontinence. Baessler et al. (12) showed similar improvements in coital incontinence following a colposuspension.

The impact of midurethral slings, specifically tension-free vaginal tape (TVT) on female sexual function is unclear. Different studies have shown different outcomes, with some suggesting deterioration (21–24) of sexual function, some an improvement (25–27) whereas others were equivocal (28–31). Deterioration in function may be associated with dyspareunia (24), loss of libido, or partner associated discomfort. There have also been anecdotal reports of anorgasmia after TVT probably related to passage of the trochar and subsequent injury to the dorsal nerve of the clitoris (32). However, there seems to be a consensus that TVT reduces coital incontinence rates by three- to sixfold (24,28,33).

The transobturator tape appears to have an overall beneficial effect (32,34) on sexual function comparable to the retropubic approach (TVT) (35). In a comparison of the outside in and the inside out technique, reports are conflicting with one study suggesting the inside out (TVT-O) to be better (34) and another study showing the outside in technique to be superior (32).

In sexually active women with OAB and concurrent sexual dysfunction, sexual QoL, pelvic organ prolapse/urinary incontinence sexual questionnaire scores (PISQ), and anxiety states were all improved with corresponding improvement in OAB scores by treatment with anticholinergics (36).

PELVIC ORGAN PROLAPSE

Pelvic organ prolapse is a common medical problem in parous women and particularly with advancing age. As life expectancy increases, this is acquiring greater significance, and 20% of women on gynecology waiting lists in the United Kingdom are awaiting prolapse surgery demonstrating the enormity of this virtual pandemic. The incidence of prolapse requiring surgical correction in women who have had a hysterectomy is 3.6 per 1000 person years of risk; the cumulative risk is 1% at three years and 5% at 17 years after a hysterectomy (37).

A review of literature shows conflicting results on the impact of prolapse on sexual function, with some studies showing a deterioration of function and others showing no impact (11). In an observational study by Handa et al. looking at 1299 participants, 495 (38.1%) had evidence of pelvic floor disorders. Sexual complaints were significantly more common among women with pelvic floor disorders (53.2% vs. 40.4%, P < 0.01) and in a multiple regression model, UI was significantly associated with low libido [odds ratio (OR) 1.96], vaginal dryness (OR 2.11), and dyspareunia (OR 2.04), independent of age, educational attainment, and race. In contrast, pelvic organ prolapse was not associated with any sexual complaint. A study by Weber et al. (38) comparing 80 women with prolapse with or without incontinence and 30 controls (women with no prolapse) showed no diff in global sexual function score, vaginal dryness, dyspareunia, interest in sexual activity, or satisfaction with their sexual relationship. They concluded that women with prolapse and UI do not differ from continent women without prolapse in measures of sexual function and age is the most important predictor of sexual function. Burrows et al. (39) came to similar conclusions in their retrospective study of 352 women with prolapse. They also found that prolapse severity did not impact on sexual function. The study by Barber et al. (40) comparing the impact of prolapse and incontinence on sexual function found completely the opposite results. In their review of 343 community dwelling women with either symptomatic prolapse or incontinence, they found

Table 55.1 Classification of Female Sexual Dysfunction [DSM IV TR (Text Revision)] (119)

1. Sexual desire/interest disorders
2. Sexual arousal disorders
   Genital arousal disorder
   Subjective arousal disorder
   Combined arousal disorder
3. Orgasmic disorder
4. Dyspareunia and vaginismus
5. Persistent sexual arousal disorder

Table 55.2 Studies Showing Prevalence of Urinary Incontinence (UI) During Sexual Intercourse

Authors	Design and setting	Symptoms analyzed	% with UI during intercourse
Bo et al. (120)	RCT of women with SUI; Norway	UI during intercourse using BFLUTS	33%
Clark et al. (121)	48 women undergoing UDS;U.S.A.	Incontinence and other urinary symptoms during intercourse	56%
Gordon et al. (122)	100 consecutive women attending a clinic; Israel	Psychiatric assessment of sexual function	16%
Hilton (14)	324 sexually active women; U.K.	Standardized questionnaire	24%
Jackson et al. (123)	RCT of HRT in women with SUI; U.K.	UI during intercourse using BFLUTS	10%
Jha et al. (13)	Women with USI undergoing TVT; U.K.	ePAQ questionnaire	68%
Lam et al. (124)	2631 (random) women selected: 511 had SUI; Denmark	When they have SUI	2% of general group; 12% of women with SUI
Lemack et al. (21)	56 women; U.S.A.	UI with intercourse	11%
Moller et al. (125)	4000 randomly selected women from the community; Denmark	UI with intercourse	8% = sometimes 1.7% = weekly 0.4% = daily
Nygaard et al. (126)	224 random women: gynecology outpatient; U.S.A.	UI with penetration/orgasm	12.9%
Weber et al. (30)	81 sexually active women undergoing surgery; U.S.A.	UI with intercourse	22%
Vierhout et al. (127)	196 sexually active women attending clinic	UI with intercourse	34%

Abbreviations: RCT, randomized controlled trail; SUI, stress urinary incontinence; UDS, urodynamic studies; BFLUTS, Bristol female lower urinary tract symptoms; HRT, hormone replacement therapy; USI, Urodynamic stress incontinence, TVT, tension-free vaginal tape; ePAQ, electronic personal assessment questionnaire.

that prolapse was more likely to influence sexual function than UI. This study also demonstrated that treatment of prolapse was less likely to impact on change in sexual function whereas treatment of incontinence resulted in a mild improvement in sexual function.

Other studies have shown prolapse causes several problems with sexual function including discomfort, UI (40%) (both orgasm and penetration), obstruction, and dryness during intercourse. Women with prolapse were more likely to have urinary and or fecal incontinence during sexual activity, more dyspareunia, and fewer orgasms. They were also more likely to report negative emotional reactions associated with sex and higher rates of embarrassment leading to avoidance of sex (41). Presence of both prolapse and incontinence has a cumulative negative effect on sexual function, with libido, sexual excitement, and orgasm being significantly affected. Increasing severity of prolapse is associated with symptoms related to UI, voiding, defecatory, and sexual dysfunction, which do not necessarily correlate with the location of prolapse and therefore are not compartment-specific (42).

The problem with assessment of sexual function in the different studies reported in literature is that

1. different tools have been used in different studies;
2. studies cluster prolapse and incontinence under the same umbrella;
3. study groups are small; and
4. different types of prolapse clumped together (different compartments, diff grades).

There are a multitude of studies reporting on the impact of prolapse surgery on sexual function but the results are very conflicting with some being equivocal reporting no impact of prolapse correction on sexual function and others demonstrating a deterioration of sexual function following prolapse treatment. The cause of sexual dysfunction following vaginal surgery may be classified as organic and/or psychosocial (43). Organic causes are anatomical, physiological, vascular, neural, and hormonal. Psychosocial factors on the other hand such as life stressors, anxiety, and depression must be borne in mind. Altered perception of genital health after surgery, both by the woman and her partner, with associated apprehension and fear of damage to the internal organs, can also be contributory factors for a negative impact on sexual function.

Current treatment options for vaginal wall prolapse include pelvic floor muscle training (PFMT) (physiotherapy), use of topical hormone replacement therapy (HRT), use of mechanical devices (ring or shelf pessaries) and surgery, with or without mesh reinforcement. The impact of these different forms of treatment for prolapse on sexual function are discussed here.

Physiotherapy
In their systematic review looking at the benefits of PFMT, Hagen et al. (44) identified some benefit on sexual function in women with mild prolapse. But even more reassuringly women who were currently performing PFMT scored significantly better on several aspects of sexual function (45,46), and is therefore to be encouraged in women.

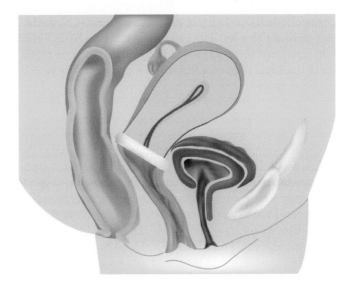

Figure 55.1 Ring pessary in situ: no interference with sexual activity.

Estrogen Therapy
There are no studies looking at the impact of estrogen therapy in women with prolapse or its impact on sexual function. However several studies have shown an individual improvement in symptoms of atrophic vaginitis which may negatively impact on sexual function even in the absence of prolapse, hence may be considered for that indication.

Pessaries
There are a variety of pessaries available, made of rubber, plastic, or silicone-based material. The commonest pessaries are the rings and shelf, but other types being increasingly used are the inflatable, the doughnut and the Gellhorn all of which have slightly different uses and specifications. A recent study by Kuhn et al. (47), demonstrated desire, lubrication, and sexual satisfaction significantly improved with pessary use, though orgasm remained unchanged (Fig. 55.1).

Surgery
Surgical correction of prolapse depends largely on the compartment which is affected. So for vaginal wall prolapse it may involve an anterior colporrhaphy/anterior vaginal wall repair, posterior colporrhaphy/posterior vaginal wall repair, or a vaginal hysterectomy. For a vaginal vault prolpase surgical correction may require a sacro-spinous fixation, an abdominal sacro-colpopexy, or an infracoccygeal procedures which may involve the use of trocar systems (e.g., apogee, post I-stop).

Richard TeLinde said, "Every surgeon of extensive and long experience will have to admit that he is not entirely and absolutely satisfied with the long term results of all his operations for prolapse and allied conditions." This is further substantiated by the repeat surgery rates for recurrent prolapse being in the region of 30%. In 1908, White said that "plastic gynecology remains the last unsolved problem of surgical gynecology," and this remains true even in the 21st century.

Though Weber et al. (30) identified a decrease in the vaginal dimensions after surgery for prolapse, this was associated with either no alteration in sexual function or a mild improvement. Anterior vaginal repair does not appear to impact adversely on postoperative sexual function or cause dyspareunia. Nevertheless, there are very few data confirming this paradigm. Weber (48) compared three surgical techniques for cystocele repair, the dyspareunia rate reduced from 30% preoperatively to 22% postoperatively.

Both Colombo (49) and van Geelen (50) found that anterior repair when compared to a Burch colposuspension for a cystocele did not predispose to dyspareunia. Though it was associated with significant vaginal shortening when compared to the Burch, this did not appear to impact on function unless combined with a posterior repair. Combining a posterior vaginal wall repair with anterior colporrhaphy significantly increased dyspareunia rates and there may be a place for doing the two procedures separately where feasible. This would also indicate that a prophylactic posterior repair should be avoided at the time of an anterior repair in sexually active women.

Studies looking at posterior vaginal wall defect are more confusing and, whereas earlier studies suggest dyspareunia and problems with intercourse (51) with a posterior repair, this is not substantiated in more recent studies and this could be due to a recognition of the problem and a change in technique (52). Levator ani plication is frequently implicated as the cause for dyspareunia due to post operative mid-vaginal narrowing (51,53,54). In contrast, improvement in dyspareunia have been reported with site-specific defect or midline plication procedures (55–57). In sexually active women, therefore, levator plication should be avoided where possible and surgical techniques aimed at avoiding narrowing of vaginal introitus adopted.

Vault prolapse surgery may be associated with postoperative dyspareunia and FSD. However, as this procedure often involves a concomitant repair, it is methodologically difficult to ascertain which specific procedure is causing sexual dysfunction. Maher et al. (58) in their comparison of the two most common procedures for vault prolapse found that whereas both abdominal sacrocolpopexy and vaginal sacrospinous fixation are highly effective in the treatment of vaginal vault prolapse, abdominal sacrocolpopexy has a lower rate of recurrent vault prolapse and dyspareunia compared to sacrospinous fixation. Baessler and Schuessler found that sacrocolpopexy was actually curative in women with dyspareunia and ceased in all but one of the nine patients among 33 consecutive women presenting with prolapse-related dyspareunia preoperatively (59). Postoperative dyspareunia is reported to be between 8% and 16% after sacrospinous fixation (60–62). When combined with a repair vaginal narrowing, excessive colpectomy occurring due to a concomitant repair procedures was identified as the most common cause of postoperative dyspareunia (63), but vaginal narrowing and pudendal nerve injury have also been implicated. Therefore in sexually active women a sacrocolpopexy is the preferred procedure.

Iliococcygeal fixation is also performed for vault prolapse. In a matched case-control study comparing sacrospinous to ileococcygeal fixation, Maher et al. (64) found no significant difference in the percentage of women who were sexually active (58% vs. 55%), who had dyspareunia (14% vs. 10%), or buttock pain (19% vs. 14%). It is well recognized that bilateral ileococcygeal fixation may result in shortening of the vagina by 2 to 3 cm. In sexually active women with vault prolapse and a short vagina, bilateral ileococcygeal fixation is contraindicated, as it may cause severe postoperative dyspareunia.

Mesh
The aims of using mesh in the repair of vaginal wall prolapse are to add additional support and to reduce the risk of recurrence, particularly for women with recurrent prolapse or with congenital connective tissue disorders (such as Ehlers–Danlos or Marfan's syndromes).

A recent study by Abdel Fatah et al. (65) looking at the complications of mesh reinforcement identified some very severe complications and therefore the need for caution when using synthetic materials in the absence of clear cut indications.

Milani R et al. (66) also demonstrated that though the use of mesh was associated with high success rates there was a very high rate of dyspareunia of 20% when used for anterior repair and 63% when used for posterior repair. This warrants extensive counseling and caution when using meshes in women who are sexually active. These results are further borne out by other studies though some studies are equivocal and some even demonstrate an improvement following the use of mesh in vaginal repair.

The verdict is still open on the impact that prolapse has on sexual function, and larger epidemiological studies are required to substantiate or refute the currently available conflicting evidence. This will also be partly achieved by the long term follow up of randomized controlled trials. When counseling women with a prolapse and particularly before treatment, these factors should feature in the discussion and aid decision making. This allows more realistic expectations from the treatments available, and avoids disappointment when those goals are not met. There remain many unanswered questions, but it is important to remember that the presence of anatomical defect does not imply dysfunction. The goal of pelvic surgery should be restoration of anatomic support without deleterious effects on visceral and sexual function. Data is currently limited on QoL and sexual function following both traditional and graft-reinforced anterior vaginal prolapse surgery; further research is required to determine whether surgical technique and type of graft used impact surgical outcome and complications before introduction into routine clinical practice. Women should be counseled and managed depending on current best available evidence.

URINARY TRACT INFECTIONS (UTIS)
The association of LUTS and sexual dysfunction is widely accepted. The incidence of UTIs in women who have become sexually active is about 3% per annum and about 4% of all LUT infections in this group are thought to be related to sexual activity and 60% in recurrent cases (67). Honeymoon cystitis refers to LUTS occuring after sexual intercourse. Bacteria are often pushed mechanically up the urethra and into the bladder during coitus. If they are not voided soon after, they multiply and may cause infection. The relative risk of UTI increased from 1.0 for unmarried women who had not been sexually active in the previous week to 9.0 for women who had had intercourse seven times during that period (68). The term

"honeymoon" was applied because, in the past, this was expected to be the time of first intercourse. The male urethra, being substantially longer, is not susceptible to the same problem. Some women are particularly sensitive to postcoital urinary tract dysfunction due to the development of a relatively high urethral pressure following intercourse. Of course, the condition of post-coital female lower UTI occurs at many times beyond the traditional "honeymoon"–from the onset of sexual activity into old age. This is further illustrated by the fact that nuns have a lower prevalence of bacteriuria than other populations of women in early adult life (69). Following intercourse urinary bacterial count is significantly raised in 30% of women (70) and Nicolle et al. (71) reported that both symptomatic and asymptomatic bacteriuria was more frequent the day after intercourse. Several behavioral factors have been shown to enhance the risk of UTI following sexual intercourse. These include deferred voiding after intercourse (72), frequent intercourse (67), low fluid intake (73), and deferred voiding after the initial urge to micturate (74). In addition, reduced lubrication and the use of spermicide coated condoms, and spermicides either alone or in conjunction with diaphragm have also been incriminated (75). Contraceptive diaphragms (by reducing urinary flow), spermicidal cream and the use of spermicidal-lubricated condoms can sometimes result in vaginal and urethral irritation hence the association. These risk factors were shown to have a detrimental effect in a large prospective study by Hooton and co-workers who examined a variety of risk factors for UTI in young women (76).

The initial management of postcoital UTIs includes several simple measures which may be effective. Close attention to perineal hygiene, change of coital technique, use of a vaginal lubricant, and avoidance of the contraceptive diaphragm may all be successful first-line measures. Women should be encouraged to drink fluid before anticipated sex to facilitate postcoital voiding. Ingestion of products containing cranberry (as juice or a supplement) has long been thought to afford protection against UTIs (77). Cranberries contain two substances (proanthocyanidines and fructose) which are thought to inhibit adhesion of infecting bacteria, particularly type 1 and type P fimbriated *Escherichia coli*, to the uroepithelium (78). A systematic review of the literature considered the role of cranberry in the setting of recurrent UTIs and found the relative risk of developing a UTI over six months while taking cranberry to be reduced to 0.61 (CI 0.4–0.91) compared to 1.0 for placebo or no treatment (79). The role of cranberry in prophylaxis against infection following intercourse, however, has yet to be established.

For women who do not respond to simple measures, regular or intermittent antibiotic prophylaxis is usually effective (80,81). A recent systematic review of the literature found evidence that in women with recurrent UTIs associated with sexual activity, postcoital ciprofloxacin is equally as effective as a continuous daily prescription and should be considered in this setting (82). There is evidence that local application of estrogen could be protective against infection in the context of recurrent UTIs in young women who are on oral contraceptives (83). When simple measures fail to alleviate postcoital cystitis, further investigation including investigation for

atypical organisms such as *Mycoplasma hominis* and *Ureaplasma urealyticum*, is often worthwhile. Chlamydia causing acute urethritis should also be ruled out. Underlying abnormalities such as voiding difficulties and vesicoureteric reflux should always be considered, and imaging of the renal tract with ultrasonography, intravenous urography or videocysto-urethrography may be necessary. It is also sometimes appropriate to perform a cysto-urethroscopy and or magnetic resonance imaging to exclude a urethral diverticulum or an intravesical foreign body such as a calculus.

PAINFUL BLADDER SYNDROME (PBS)
Interstitial cystitis (IC)/PBS is a chronic, debilitating disease of unknown etiology characterized by urinary frequency, urgency, nocturia, suprapubic pressure, and pain. The true prevalence of the condition ranges from 10 to 500 cases per 100,000 women depending on the strictness of the criteria used for the diagnosis (84,85). Studies suggest that most women with IC experience not only pelvic pain, but also dyspareunia, sexually related distress, and significant declines in desire and orgasm frequency (86,87). The prevalence of sexual dysfunction in these women is higher than previously estimated and substantially affects QoL and sexuality (88). Because multiple factors contributing to sexual dysfunction (including biopsychosocial comorbidities such as stress, abuse, or chronic illness) can be present in women with IC, a variety of treatments might be required. It is also important to consider that some typical IC treatments, such as antidepressants and opioids used to manage pelvic pain, can exacerbate sexual dysfunction. Hypertonic pelvic floor dysfunction is prevalent in patients with IC (89) and contracted muscles can result in dyspareunia, vulvodynia, and vaginismus. The association between IC and syndromes such as vestibulodynia and spontaneous or provoked vulvodynia is commonly reported. The magnitude of the association between vulvar and bladder symptoms is variable. This has obvious negative implications on sexual function and sexual functioning is in fact one of the strongest predictors of poorer QoL in patients diagnosed with refractory IC/PBS (90).

Several Studies have demonstrated an improvement in the dyspareunia and other levels of sexual function when PBS symptoms are alleviated either by intravesical injections of lidocaine, heparin, and sodium bicarbonate (91) or other pharmacological treatments (92) such as pentosan polysuphate. The pelvic floor muscles play an important role in female responsiveness and sexual function; thus, therapies aimed at treating the pelvic floor might be even more efficacious in improving sexual function, the woman's self-esteem, and her relationship with her partner. Some therapies that have been reported to be helpful include pelvic floor therapy, biofeedback, neuromodulation, and botulinum toxin type A (89).

FECAL INCONTINENCE
Anal incontinence is reported to affect 8% of women in the general population (93). Fecal incontinence is known to cause sexual dysfunction and this may be associated with anal sphincter injury related to birth trauma (94,95) or due to other causes such as neurological disorders. Fecal incontinence of

solid stool and depression related to fecal incontinence were correlated with poorer sexual function

Corrections of fecal incontinence irrespective of the mode of repair were associated with an improvement in sexual function in most studies (95,96). However, some studies actually suggest an equivocal impact on sexual function following a repair (97). Trowbridge (98) in his study showed that sexual function scores were not correlated with continence scores. But patients who had undergone an overlapping sphincteroplasty versus an end-to-end sphincteroplasty reported pain during intercourse 24% versus 4% of subjects (P = 0.04).

PREGNANCY, CHILDBIRTH, AND PERINEAL TRAUMA

Data on the impact of childbirth on sexual function is conflicting. There is a dearth of scientifically reliable data about the impact of childbirth on sexual function and the association with the different modes of delivery.

It is generally accepted that pregnancy itself is associated with reduced interest in sex, ranging from 57% to 75% (99,100). Sexual interest usually improves postpartum, but 23% to 57% of women still report reduced sexual interest at three months, and 21% to 37% at six months (101,102). Generally speaking women are less likely to be sexually active during pregnancy, particularly in advanced pregnancy (101) with only 26% having intercourse in the third trimester. This could be due to a reduction in the ability to reach orgasm with 60% of women experiencing orgasm through the second trimester (99) declining to 50% in the third trimester (101). Sexual function, which declined through pregnancy was not recovered postpartum (P = 0.017). The main predictor for poor sexual function in early pregnancy, was impaired body image, while in the postpartum period, worse urinary symptoms correlated with poor sexual function scores (103). Interestingly though sexual practices changed during pregnancy they returned to early pregnancy levels in the postpartum period.

It is widely reported that postpartum dyspareunia is associated with the mode of delivery with assisted vaginal delivery being predominantly incriminated (94,104–106) with at least a twofold increase in dyspareunia when compared to spontaneous vaginal delivery. Barret et al. reported that women delivered by caesarean section (C/S) were significantly less likely to report dyspareunia at three months postpartum than those with vaginal delivery (102). However, the same authors in a subsequent study, by employing a larger cohort with longer follow-up found dyspareunia was equivalent in both groups (107). Though a study by Buhling et al. (108) found the highest dyspareunia after operative vaginal delivery, and least with elective C/S, this decreased uniformly in each group by six months. Operative vaginal deliveries had a persistent rate of dyspareunia of 14%, but there was no difference between the spontaneous vaginal delivery group with an intact perineum and C/S (3.4% dyspareunia at 6 months). Interestingly, at three months postpartum, all of the patients reported "enjoyment at sexual intercourse" regardless of the mode of delivery (108). Perineal trauma with or without operative instrumental delivery was an important precursor of dyspareunia and the greater the tear even, with spontaneous vaginal delivery, the lower the

sexual desire (109). Women with an intact perineum or first-degree perineal tear six months postpartum were more likely to experience orgasm (94) than those with either second-, third-, or fourth-degree perineal tear.

Postpartum, sexual desire, and the ability to reach orgasm do improve but the main problems encountered and impacting on sexual function are sexual arousal, excitement, and lubrication (102). The risk of vaginal dryness and lubrication problems is increased with prolonged breast-feeding, which results in vaginal atrophy secondary to hypo-estrogenism. The latter is easily corrected with topical estrogens or nonhormonal lubricants.

Owing to the inconsistencies in the definition of FSD and use of heterogeneous and invalid tools for evaluation in most of the studies, it is difficult to draw a scientifically sound conclusion about the impact of mode of delivery on sexual health. Reports on the negative effect of vaginal childbirth on sexual health led to the concept of elective C/S to preserve sexual function. Many health care professionals also advocate this approach with 7% to 24% of obstetricians and 4.4% of midwives preferring elective C/S for themselves or their partner (110–112). Interestingly, urogynecologists scored even higher, with 45.5% opting for primary elective C/S (112).

HYSTERECTOMY

Hysterectomy is the commonest major gynecological operation in the United Kingdom. Theoretically it poses a risk not only to the intricate pelvic nerve plexus and damage to the autonomic nerve endings of the cervico-vaginal fascia hence impacting on orgasm or sensation during intercourse, but may also cause distortion of pelvic anatomy by shortening the vagina thereby resulting in dyspareunia. Historically, the uterus, "hystero," was believed to be the center of female sexuality and its removal may also have culture-dependent psychological effects leading to loss of self-esteem, female identity, and consequent FSD.

Following hysterectomy an overall improvement (113) in the different aspects of sexual function i.e., frequency of sexual relations, dyspareunia, orgasm, vaginal dryness, and sexual desire were noted. The route of hysterectomy appears to play no role. A prospective study by El-Thouky et al. (114) compared hysterectomies performed abdominally, vaginally, or laparoscopically found that patients reported significantly lower rates of deep dyspareunia (18.8%, 19.7%, and 26.3% reduction respectively) after surgery than before the operation, regardless of the routes and technique used.

The belief that the cervix is necessary to achieve orgasm or that total abdominal hysterectomy (TAH) leads to local innervation damage with subsequent impairment of sexual function is not supported by current evidence. This belief was held for several years following a study by Kilkku et al. which found women had a lower libido and orgasm following a TAH (115) when compared to a subtotal abdominal hysterectomy (STAH). However the same group subsequently reported an improvement in dyspareunia rates irrespective of the type of hysterectomy. Subsequent larger studies specifically comparing STAH and TAH (116) have also failed to identify a difference in sexual function.

CONCLUSION

In spite of the common presentation of sexual dysfunction in association with pelvic floor disorders, overall assessment by clinicians remains low and a recent survey of the members of the British Society of Urogynaecology demonstrated that only half of all clinicians routinely asked about FSD in the clinic and similar numbers at the postoperative follow up visit (117). Similar trends have been seen amongst the U.S. clinicians and a recent survey of members of the American Urogynecologic Society (AUGS) has shown that 77% and 76% of AUGS members enquired of FSD, respectively in similar situations (118). Lack of time, uncertainty about therapeutic options and older age of the patient were cited as potential reasons for failing to address sexual complaints as part of routine history. Clinicians dealing with women with these conditions need greater training to manage FSD in association with the underlying pathology.

Currently available evidence of pelvic floor problems and their impact on sexual function is conflicting. Greater and more robust research into different urogynecology conditions impacting on sexual function and their treatment is required. Assessment of patients with urogynecology problems firstly requires a history and direct enquiry into sexual function, but also requires the development of standardized tools with well defined end point to assess the severity of the problem.

REFERENCES

1. Mercer CH, Fenton KA, Johnson AM, et al. Sexual function problems and help seeking behaviour in Britain: national probability sample survey. BMJ 2003; 327: 426–7.
2. Sadovsky R, Nusbaum M. Sexual health inquiry and support is a primary care priority. J Sex Med 2006; 3: 3–11.
3. Pauls RN, Segal JL, Silva WA, Kleeman SD, Karram MM. Sexual function in patients presenting to a urogynecology practice. Int Urogynecol J Pelvic Floor Dysfunct 2006; 17: 576–80.
4. Geiss IM, Umek WH, Dungl A, et al. Prevalence of female sexual dysfunction in gynecologic and urogynecologic patients according to the international consensus classification. Urology 2003; 62: 514–18.
5. Jolleys JV. Reported prevalence of urinary incontinence in women in a general practice. Br Med J (Clin Res Ed) 1988; 296: 1300–2.
6. Aslan G, Koseoglu H, Sadik O, et al. Sexual function in women with urinary incontinence. Int J Impot Res 2005; 17: 248–51.
7. Fultz NH, Burgio K, Diokno AC, et al. Burden of stress urinary incontinence for community-dwelling women. Am J Obstet Gynecol 2003; 189: 1275–82.
8. Kelleher CJ, Cardozo LD, Khullar V, Salvatore S. A new questionnaire to assess the quality of life of urinary incontinent women. Br J Obstet Gynaecol 1997; 104: 1374–9.
9. Kizilkaya BN, Yalcin O, Ayyildiz EH, Kayir A. Effect of urinary leakage on sexual function during sexual intercourse. Urol Int 2005; 74: 250–5.
10. Salonia A, Zanni G, Nappi RE, et al. Sexual dysfunction is common in women with lower urinary tract symptoms and urinary incontinence: results of a cross-sectional study. Eur Urol 2004; 45: 642–8.
11. Handa VL, Harvey L, Cundiff GW, Siddique SA, Kjerulff KH. Sexual function among women with urinary incontinence and pelvic organ prolapse. Am J Obstet Gynecol 2004; 191: 751–6.
12. Baessler K, Stanton SL. Does Burch colposuspension cure coital incontinence? Am J Obstet Gynecol 2004; 190: 1030–3.
13. Jha S, Radley S, Farkas A, Jones G. The impact of TVT on sexual function. Int Urogynecol J Pelvic Floor Dysfunct 2009; 20: 165–9.
14. Hilton P. Urinary incontinence during sexual intercourse: a common, but rarely volunteered, symptom. Br J Obstet Gynaecol 1988; 95: 377–81.
15. Moran PA, Dwyer PL, Ziccone SP. Urinary leakage during coitus in women. J Obstet Gynaecol 1999; 19: 286–8.
16. Field SM, Hilton P. The prevalence of sexual problems in women attending for urodynamic investigation. Int Urogynecol J Pelvic Floor Dysfunct 1993; 4: 212–15.
17. Frewen WK. An objective assessment of the unstable bladder of psychosomatic origin. Br J Urol 1978; 50: 246–9.
18. Shaw C. A systematic review of the literature on the prevalence of sexual impairment in women with urinary incontinence and the prevalence of urinary leakage during sexual activity. Eur Urol 2002; 42: 432–40.
19. Patel AS, O'Leary ML, Stein RJ, et al. The relationship between overactive bladder and sexual activity in women. Int Braz J Urol 2006; 32: 77–87.
20. Moran P, Dwyer PL, Ziccone SP. Burch colposuspension for the treatment of coital urinary leakage secondary to genuine stress incontinence. J Obstet Gynaecol 1999; 19: 289–91.
21. Lemack GE, Zimmern PE. Sexual function after vaginal surgery for stress incontinence: results of a mailed questionnaire. Urology 2000; 56: 223–7.
22. Rogers RG, Kammerer-Doak D, Darrow A, et al. Sexual function after surgery for stress urinary incontinence and/or pelvic organ prolapse: a multicenter prospective study. Am J Obstet Gynecol 2004; 191: 206–10.
23. Yeni E, Unal D, Verit A, et al. The effect of tension-free vaginal tape (TVT) procedure on sexual function in women with stress urinary incontinence. Int Urogynecol J Pelvic Floor Dysfunct 2003; 14: 390–4.
24. Mazouni C, Karsenty G, Bretelle F, et al. Urinary complications and sexual function after the tension-free vaginal tape procedure. Acta Obstet Gynecol Scand 2004; 83: 955–61.
25. Elzevier HW, Venema PL, Nijeholt AA. Sexual function after tension-free vaginal tape (TVT) for stress incontinence: results of a mailed questionnaire. Int Urogynecol J Pelvic Floor Dysfunct 2004; 15: 313–18.
26. Ghezzi F, Serati M, Cromi A, et al. Impact of tension-free vaginal tape on sexual function: results of a prospective study. Int Urogynecol J Pelvic Floor Dysfunct 2006; 17: 54–9.
27. Jha S, Moran P, Greenham H, Ford C. Sexual function following surgery for urodynamic stress incontinence. Int Urogynecol J Pelvic Floor Dysfunct 2007; 18: 845–50.
28. Glavind K, Tetsche MS. Sexual function in women before and after suburethral sling operation for stress urinary incontinence: a retrospective questionnaire study. Acta Obstet Gynecol Scand 2004; 83: 965–8.
29. Maaita M, Bhaumik J, Davies AE. Sexual function after using tension-free vaginal tape for the surgical treatment of genuine stress incontinence. BJU Int 2002; 90: 540–3.
30. Weber AM, Walters MD, Piedmonte MR. Sexual function and vaginal anatomy in women before and after surgery for pelvic organ prolapse and urinary incontinence. Am J Obstet Gynecol 2000; 182: 1610–15.
31. Shah SM, Bukkapatnam R, Rodriguez LV. Impact of vaginal surgery for stress urinary incontinence on female sexual function: is the use of polypropylene mesh detrimental? Urology 2005; 65: 270–4.
32. Spinosa JP, Dubuis PY, Riederer BM. Transobturator surgery for female stress incontinence: a comparative anatomical study of outside-in vs inside-out techniques. BJU Int 2007; 100: 1097–102.
33. Ward K, Hilton P. Prospective multicentre randomised trial of tension-free vaginal tape and colposuspension as primary treatment for stress incontinence. BMJ 2002; 325: 67.
34. Elzevier HW, Putter H, Delaere KP, et al. Female sexual function after surgery for stress urinary incontinence: transobturator suburethral tape vs. tension-free vaginal tape obturator. J Sex Med 2008; 5: 400–6.
35. Murphy M, van Raalte H, Mercurio E, et al. Incontinence-related quality of life and sexual function following the tension-free vaginal tape versus the "inside-out" tension-free vaginal tape obturator. Int Urogynecol J Pelvic Floor Dysfunct 2008; 19: 481–7.
36. Rogers R, Bachmann G, Jumadilova Z, et al. Efficacy of tolterodine on overactive bladder symptoms and sexual and emotional quality of life in sexually active women. Int Urogynecol J Pelvic Floor Dysfunct 2008; 19: 1551–7.
37. Mant J, Painter R, Vessey M. Epidemiology of genital prolapse: observations from the Oxford Family Planning Association Study. Br J Obstet Gynaecol 1997; 104: 579–85.

38. Weber AM, Walters MD, Schover LR, Mitchinson A. Sexual function in women with uterovaginal prolapse and urinary incontinence. Obstet Gynecol 1995; 85: 483–7.

39. Burrows LJ, Meyn LA, Walters MD, Weber AM. Pelvic symptoms in women with pelvic organ prolapse. Obstet Gynecol 2004; 104(5 Pt 1): 982–8.

40. Barber MD, Visco AG, Wyman JF, Fantl JA, Bump RC. Sexual function in women with urinary incontinence and pelvic organ prolapse. Obstet Gynecol 2002; 99: 281–9.

41. Novi JM, Jeronis S, Morgan MA, Arya LA. Sexual function in women with pelvic organ prolapse compared to women without pelvic organ prolapse. J Urol 2005; 173: 1669–72.

42. Ellerkmann RM, Cundiff GW, Melick CF, et al. Correlation of symptoms with location and severity of pelvic organ prolapse. Am J Obstet Gynecol 2001; 185: 1332–7.

43. Srivastava R, Thakar R, Sultan A. Female sexual dysfunction in obstetrics and gynecology. Obstet Gynecol Surv 2008; 63: 527–37.

44. Hagen S, Stark D, Maher C, Adams E. Conservative management of pelvic organ prolapse in women. Cochrane Database Syst Rev 2004; 2: CD003882.

45. Beji NK, Yalcin O, Erkan HA. The effect of pelvic floor training on sexual function of treated patients. Int Urogynecol J Pelvic Floor Dysfunct 2003; 14: 234–8.

46. Dean N, Wilson D, Herbison P, et al. Sexual function, delivery mode history, pelvic floor muscle exercises and incontinence: a cross-sectional study six years post-partum. Aust N Z J Obstet Gynaecol 2008; 48: 302–11.

47. Kuhn A, Bapst D, Stadlmayr W, et al. Sexual and organ function in patients with symptomatic prolapse: are pessaries helpful? Fertil Steril 2009; 91: 1914–18.

48. Weber AM, Walters MD, Piedmonte MR, Ballard LA. Anterior colporrhaphy: a randomized trial of three surgical techniques. Am J Obstet Gynecol 2001; 185: 1299–304.

49. Colombo M, Vitobello D, Proietti F, Milani R. Randomised comparison of Burch colposuspension versus anterior colporrhaphy in women with stress urinary incontinence and anterior vaginal wall prolapse. BJOG 2000; 107: 544–51.

50. van Geelen JM, Theeuwes AG, Eskes TK, Martin CB Jr. The clinical and urodynamic effects of anterior vaginal repair and Burch colposuspension. Am J Obstet Gynecol 1988; 159: 137–44.

51. Kahn MA, Stanton SL. Posterior colporrhaphy: its effects on bowel and sexual function. Br J Obstet Gynaecol 1997; 104: 82–6.

52. Paraiso MF, Barber MD, Muir TW, Walters MD. Rectocele repair: a randomized trial of three surgical techniques including graft augmentation. Am J Obstet Gynecol 2006; 195: 1762–71.

53. Amias AG. Sexual life after gynaecological operations—II. Br Med J 1975; 2: 680–1.

54. Jeffcoate TN. Posterior colpoperineorrhaphy. Am J Obstet Gynecol 1959; 77: 490–502.

55. Maher CF, Qatawneh AM, Baessler K, Schluter PJ. Midline rectovaginal fascial plication for repair of rectocele and obstructed defecation. Obstet Gynecol 2004; 104: 685–9.

56. Glavind K, Madsen H. A prospective study of the discrete fascial defect rectocele repair. Acta Obstet Gynecol Scand 2000; 79: 145–7.

57. Kenton K, Shott S, Brubaker L. Outcome after rectovaginal fascia reattachment for rectocele repair. Am J Obstet Gynecol 1999; 181: 1360–3.

58. Maher CF, Qatawneh AM, Dwyer PL, et al. Abdominal sacral colpopexy or vaginal sacrospinous colpopexy for vaginal vault prolapse: a prospective randomized study. Am J Obstet Gynecol 2004; 190: 20–6.

59. Baessler K, Schuessler B. Abdominal sacrocolpopexy and anatomy and function of the posterior compartment. Obstet Gynecol 2001; 97(5 Pt 1): 678–84.

60. Colombo M, Milani R. Sacrospinous ligament fixation and modified McCall culdoplasty during vaginal hysterectomy for advanced uterovaginal prolapse. Am J Obstet Gynecol 1998; 179: 13–20.

61. Goldberg RP, Tomezsko JE, Winkler HA, et al. Anterior or posterior sacrospinous vaginal vault suspension: long-term anatomic and functional evaluation. Obstet Gynecol 2001; 98: 199–204.

62. Paraiso MF, Ballard LA, Walters MD, Lee JC, Mitchinson AR. Pelvic support defects and visceral and sexual function in women treated with sacrospinous ligament suspension and pelvic reconstruction. Am J Obstet Gynecol 1996; 175: 1423–30.

63. Holley RL, Varner RE, Gleason BP, Apffel LA, Scott S. Sexual function after sacrospinous ligament fixation for vaginal vault prolapse. J Reprod Med 1996; 41: 355–8.

64. Maher CF, Murray CJ, Carey MP, Dwyer PL, Ugoni AM. Iliococcygeus or sacrospinous fixation for vaginal vault prolapse. Obstet Gynecol 2001; 98: 40–4.

65. Abdel-Fattah M, Ramsay I. Retrospective multicentre study of the new minimally invasive mesh repair devices for pelvic organ prolapse. BJOG 2008; 115: 22–30.

66. Milani R, Salvatore S, Soligo M, et al. Functional and anatomical outcome of anterior and posterior vaginal prolapse repair with prolene mesh. BJOG 2005; 112: 107–11.

67. Stamatiou C, Bovis C, Panagopoulos P, et al. Sex-induced cystitis—patient burden and other epidemiological features. Clin Exp Obstet Gynecol 2005; 32: 180–2.

68. Hooton TM, Stapleton AE, Roberts PL, et al. Perineal anatomy and urine-voiding characteristics of young women with and without recurrent urinary tract infections. Clin Infect Dis 1999; 29: 1600–1.

69. Kunin CM, McCormack RC. An epidemiologic study of bacteriuria and blood pressure among nuns and working women. N Engl J Med 1968; 278: 635–42.

70. Buckley RM Jr, McGuckin M, MacGregor RR. Urine bacterial counts after sexual intercourse. N Engl J Med 1978; 298: 321–4.

71. Nicolle LE, Harding GK, Preiksaitis J, Ronald AR. The association of urinary tract infection with sexual intercourse. J Infect Dis 1982; 146: 579–83.

72. Strom BL, Collins M, West SL, Kreisberg J, Weller S. Sexual activity, contraceptive use, and other risk factors for symptomatic and asymptomatic bacteriuria. A case-control study. Ann Intern Med 1987; 107: 816–23.

73. Ervine C, Komaroff AL, Pass TM. Behavioural factors and urinary incontinence. J Am Med Assoc 1980; 243: 330–1.

74. Adatto K, Doebele KG, Galland L, Granowetter L. Behavioral factors and urinary tract infection. JAMA 1979; 241: 2525–6.

75. Handley MA, Reingold AL, Shiboski S, Padian NS. Incidence of acute urinary tract infection in young women and use of male condoms with and without nonoxynol-9 spermicides. Epidemiology 2002; 13: 431–6.

76. Hooton TM, Scholes D, Hughes JP, et al. A prospective study of risk factors for symptomatic urinary tract infection in young women. N Engl J Med 1996; 335: 468–74.

77. Ronald AR. Sex and urinary tract infections. N Engl J Med 1996; 335(Editorial): 511–12.

78. Zafriri D, Ofek I, Adar R, Pocino M, Sharon N. Inhibitory activity of cranberry juice on adherence of type 1 and type P fimbriated Escherichia coli to eucaryotic cells. Antimicrob Agents Chemother 1989; 33: 92–8.

79. Jepson RG, Craig JC. A systematic review of the evidence for cranberries and blueberries in UTI prevention. Mol Nutr Food Res 2007; 51: 738–45.

80. Stapleton A. Prevention of recurrent urinary-tract infections in women. Lancet 1999; 353: 7–8.

81. Pfau A, Sacks T, Engelstein D. Recurrent urinary tract infections in premenopausal women: prophylaxis based on an understanding of the pathogenesis. J Urol 1983; 129: 1153–7.

82. Albert X, Huertas I, Pereiro II, et al. Antibiotics for preventing recurrent urinary tract infection in non-pregnant women. Cochrane Database Syst Rev 2004; 3: CD001209.

83. Pinggera GM, Feuchtner G, Frauscher F, et al. Effects of local estrogen therapy on recurrent urinary tract infections in young females under oral contraceptives. Eur Urol 2005; 47: 243–9.

84. Diokno AC, Homma Y, Sekiguchi Y, Suzuki Y. Interstitial cystitis, gynecologic pelvic pain, prostatitis, and their epidemiology. Int J Urol 2003; 10(Suppl): S3–6.

85. Parsons M, Toozs-Hobson P. The investigation and management of interstitial cystitis. J Br Menopause Soc 2005; 11: 132–9.

86. Peters KM, Killinger KA, Carrico DJ, et al. Sexual function and sexual distress in women with interstitial cystitis: a case-control study. Urology 2007; 70: 543–7.

87. Ottem DP, Carr LK, Perks AE, Lee P, Teichman JM. Interstitial cystitis and female sexual dysfunction. Urology 2007; 69: 608–10.

88. Temml C, Wehrberger C, Riedl C, et al. Prevalence and correlates for interstitial cystitis symptoms in women participating in a health screening project. Eur Urol 2007; 51: 803–8.

89. Peters KM, Carrico DJ. Frequency, urgency, and pelvic pain: treating the pelvic floor versus the epithelium. Curr Urol Rep 2006; 7: 450–5.

90. Nickel JC, Tripp D, Teal V, et al. Sexual function is a determinant of poor quality of life for women with treatment refractory interstitial cystitis. J Urol 2007; 177: 1832–6.

91. Welk BK, Teichman JM. Dyspareunia response in patients with interstitial cystitis treated with intravesical lidocaine, bicarbonate, and heparin. Urology 2008; 71: 67–70.

92. Nickel JC, Parsons CL, Forrest J, et al. Improvement in sexual functioning in patients with interstitial cystitis/painful bladder syndrome. J Sex Med 2008; 5: 394–9.

93. Melville JL, Fan MY, Newton K, Fenner D. Fecal incontinence in US women: a population-based study. Am J Obstet Gynecol 2005; 193: 2071–6.

94. Signorello LB, Harlow BL, Chekos AK, Repke JT. Postpartum sexual functioning and its relationship to perineal trauma: a retrospective cohort study of primiparous women. Am J Obstet Gynecol 2001; 184: 881–8.

95. Lewicky CE, Valentin C, Saclarides TJ. Sexual function following sphincteroplasty for women with third- and fourth-degree perineal tears. Dis Colon Rectum 2004; 47: 1650–4.

96. Thornton MJ, Kennedy ML, Lubowski DZ, King DW. Long-term follow-up of dynamic graciloplasty for faecal incontinence. Colorectal Dis 2004; 6: 470–6.

97. Pauls RN, Silva WA, Rooney CM, et al. Sexual function following anal sphincteroplasty for fecal incontinence. Am J Obstet Gynecol 2007; 197: 618.e1–6.

98. Trowbridge ER, Morgan D, Trowbridge MJ, DeLancey JO, Fenner DE. Sexual function, quality of life, and severity of anal incontinence after anal sphincteroplasty. Am J Obstet Gynecol 2006; 195: 1753–7.

99. Sayle AE, Savitz DA, Thorp JM Jr, Hertz-Picciotto I, Wilcox AJ. Sexual activity during late pregnancy and risk of preterm delivery. Obstet Gynecol 2001; 97: 283–9.

100. Bogren LY. Changes in sexuality in women and men during pregnancy. Arch Sex Behav 1991; 20: 35–45.

101. Robson KM, Brant HA, Kumar R. Maternal sexuality during first pregnancy and after childbirth. Br J Obstet Gynaecol 1981; 88: 882–9.

102. Barrett G, Pendry E, Peacock J, et al. Women's sexual health after childbirth. BJOG 2000; 107: 186–95.

103. Pauls RN, Occhino JA, Dryfhout VL. Effects of pregnancy on female sexual function and body image: a prospective study. J Sex Med 2008; 5: 1915–22.

104. Lydon-Rochelle M, Holt VL, Martin DP, Easterling TR. Association between method of delivery and maternal rehospitalization. JAMA 2000; 283: 2411–16.

105. Glazener CM. Sexual function after childbirth: women's experiences, persistent morbidity and lack of professional recognition. Br J Obstet Gynaecol 1997; 104: 330–5.

106. Brown S, Lumley J. Maternal health after childbirth: results of an Australian population based survey. Br J Obstet Gynaecol 1998; 105: 156–61.

107. Barrett G, Peacock J, Victor CR, Manyonda I. Cesarean section and postnatal sexual health. Birth 2005; 32: 306–11.

108. Buhling KJ, Schmidt S, Robinson JN, et al. Rate of dyspareunia after delivery in primiparae according to mode of delivery. Eur J Obstet Gynecol Reprod Biol 2006; 124: 42–6.

109. Rogers RG, Borders N, Leeman LM, Albers LL. Does spontaneous genital tract trauma impact postpartum sexual function? J Midwifery Womens Health 2009; 54: 98–103.

110. MacDonald C, Pinion SB, MacLeod UM. Scottish female obstetricians' views on elective caesarean section and personal choice for delivery. J Obstet Gynaecol 2002; 22: 586–9.

111. Wright JB, Wright AL, Simpson NA, Bryce FC. A survey of trainee obstetricians preferences for childbirth. Eur J Obstet Gynecol Reprod Biol 2001; 97: 23–5.

112. Wu JM, Hundley AF, Visco AG. Elective primary cesarean delivery: attitudes of urogynecology and maternal-fetal medicine specialists. Obstet Gynecol 2005; 105: 301–6.

113. Rhodes JC, Kjerulff KH, Langenberg PW, Guzinski GM. Hysterectomy and sexual functioning. JAMA 1999; 282: 1934–41.

114. El Toukhy TA, Hefni M, Davies A, Mahadevan S. The effect of different types of hysterectomy on urinary and sexual functions: a prospective study. J Obstet Gynaecol 2004; 24: 420–5.

115. Kilkku P. Supravaginal uterine amputation vs. hysterectomy. Effects on coital frequency and dyspareunia. Acta Obstet Gynecol Scand 1983; 62: 141–5.

116. Thakar R, Ayers S, Clarkson P, Stanton S, Manyonda I. Outcomes after total versus subtotal abdominal hysterectomy. N Engl J Med 2002; 347: 1318–25.

117. Roos AM, Thakar R, Sultan AH, Scheer I. Female sexual dysfunction: are urogynecologists ready for it? Int Urogynecol J Pelvic Floor Dysfunct 2009; 20: 89–101.

118. Pauls RN, Kleeman SD, Segal JL, et al. Practice patterns of physician members of the American urogynecologic society regarding female sexual dysfunction: results of a national survey. Int Urogynecol J Pelvic Floor Dysfunct 2005; 16: 460–7.

119. Basson R, Althof S, Davis S, et al. Summary of the recommendations on sexual dysfunctions in women. J Sex Med 2004; 1: 24–34.

120. Bo K, Talseth T, Vinsnes A. Randomized controlled trial on the effect of pelvic floor muscle training on quality of life and sexual problems in genuine stress incontinent women. Acta Obstet Gynecol Scand 2000; 79: 598–603.

121. Clark A, Romm J. Effect of urinary incontinence on sexual activity in women. J Reprod Med 1993; 38: 679–83.

122. Gordon D, Groutz A, Sinai T, et al. Sexual function in women attending a urogynecology clinic. Int Urogynecol J Pelvic Floor Dysfunct 1999; 10: 325–8.

123. Jackson S, Shepherd A, Brookes S, Abrams P. The effect of oestrogen supplementation on post-menopausal urinary stress incontinence: a double-blind placebo-controlled trial. Br J Obstet Gynaecol 1999; 106: 711–18.

124. Lam GW, Foldspang A, Elving LB, Mommsen S. Social context, social abstention, and problem recognition correlated with adult female urinary incontinence. Dan Med Bull 1992; 39: 565–570.

125. Moller LA, Lose G, Jorgensen T. The prevalence and bothersomeness of lower urinary tract symptoms in women 40–60 years of age. Acta Obstet Gynecol Scand 2000; 79: 298–305.

126. Nygaard I, Milburn A. Urinary incontinence during sexual activity: prevalence in a gynecological practice. J Women's Health 1995; 4: 83–6.

127. Vierhout ME, Gianotten WL. Mechanisms of urine loss during sexual activity. Eur J Obstet Gynecol Reprod Biol 1993; 52: 45–7.

56 The Menopause
Timothy C Hillard

INTRODUCTION

The menopause is a biological event unique to humans. The average age of the menopause in Western women is approximately 52 years, a figure which has remained remarkably consistent over the last few hundred years. The term menopause was first coined in early nineteenth-century France at a time of radical social reform. In Victorian Britain there was little interest until around 1860. However at this stage the average woman would not expect to live many years past her menopause. Now with women living well into their 80s and beyond women can expect to live over a third of their life in the post-menopause. Consequently, over the last 50 years there has been an increasing interest in the effects of the menopause on long-term health, its effects on quality of life, and the potential treatments. In evolutionary terms the menopause was considered advantageous as it allowed women who were no longer fertile to look after their children's offspring and allow their children to continue breeding—the so called grandmother effect. The use of grandparents as child-minders to allow the mother to return to work could be considered a modern adaptation!

DEFINITIONS

The term "menopause" means the final menstrual period (from the Greek, *menos*—month, *pausos*—ending). It occurs as a result of loss of ovarian follicular activity leading to a fall in estradiol levels below the level needed for endometrial stimulation. Strictly speaking it can only be said to have occurred after 12 consecutive months of amenorrhea. Whilst the menopause can sometimes be a sudden event, for most women there is a gradual change in menstrual pattern in the years preceding the menopause as ovarian activity fluctuates which may be accompanied by troublesome symptoms; this is often called the "peri-menopause." The menopause, or final menstrual period, represents a watershed in the reproductive life of a woman as represented in the staging system described by the American Society for Reproductive Medicine in their Stages of Reproductive Ageing Workshop (STRAW) (Fig. 56.1) (1).

The term "climacteric" is often used synonymously with peri-menopause but means the phase of transition from the reproductive to the non-reproductive state, the menopause being a specific event within that phase.

A surgical menopause occurs when functioning ovaries are removed such as at hysterectomy for malignancy or severe endometriosis. A menopause may also be iatrogenically induced by other treatments such as radio or chemotherapy for malignancy or temporarily during treatment with gonadotropin releasing hormone (GnRH) analogues for a variety of conditions.

A "premature" menopause occurs if the menopause happens before the age of 45. This may either occur naturally, be induced following surgery or other treatments, or be for other reasons (see below). Women who have had a premature menopause are at an increased risk of a number of complications later in life and need special support.

ETIOLOGY

The ovaries produce three principal steroid hormones, estradiol, progesterone, and testosterone, although the latter plays no part in menstrual cycle control. Ovarian function and the normal menstrual cycle are controlled by the gonadotrophins, follicle stimulating hormone (FSH), and lutenizing hormone (LH), which are released from the anterior pituitary gland. Their release is controlled by the release of GnRH from the hypothalamus which in turn is governed by the negative feedback from circulating levels of estradiol, progesterone, and inhibin (a peptide hormone produced by the ovary).

A detailed description of reproductive physiology can be found in Speroff (2). In summary each ovary contains several million germ cell units (oocytes) which achieve maximal levels in-utero. There is a steady decline in these units over the pre-pubertal and reproductive years but the maturation of these follicular units during this time is one of the key components of ovulation, corpus luteum formation, and ovarian steroidogenesis. It is estimated that up to 1000 follicles fail for every one which matures to ovulation (Fig. 56.2). As the ovary ages the remaining follicles, which are probably the least sensitive to gonadotrophins and are increasingly less likely to mature, and so ovulation declines and ovarian function gradually fails. Eventually the level of estradiol production is no longer sufficient to stimulate endometrial proliferation and menopause ensues. Further decline in estradiol levels over subsequent years has effects on all estrogen responsive tissues (which are widespread throughout the body—see below). As a result the effects of ovarian failure are often noted before the last period and the effects can go on for many years. Menopause may only be a single event but it represents a significant change in a woman's hormonal milieu which has implications for her future health and quality of life—hence the importance of post-reproductive health for women.

The mean age of menopause in the western world is around 51 to 52 years and has been so since Greek times (3). There are significant variations around the world with some African and Asian communities reportedly having younger menopause (4). Certain genetic and environmental factors may influence age of menopause such as growth restriction in-utero, low weight gain in infancy, and poor nutrition in childhood and family history (5). Smoking may reduce the age of menopause by up to three years and women with Down's syndrome are also more likely to have an early menopause.

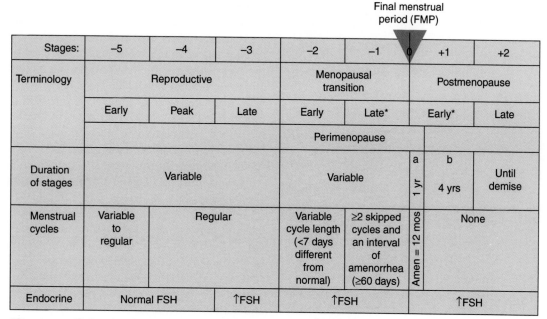

Stages:	–5	–4	–3	–2	–1	0	+1	+2
Terminology	Reproductive			Menopausal transition			Postmenopause	
	Early	Peak	Late	Early	Late*		Early*	Late
				Perimenopause				
Duration of stages	Variable			Variable		a 1 yr	b 4 yrs	Until demise
Menstrual cycles	Variable to regular	Regular		Variable cycle length (<7 days different from normal)	≥2 skipped cycles and an interval of amenorrhea (≥60 days)	Amen = 12 mos	None	
Endocrine	Normal FSH		↑FSH	↑FSH			↑FSH	

*Stages most likely to be characterized by vasomotor symptoms   ↑ = Elevated

Figure 56.1 STRAW staging system for reproductive ageing. *Abbreviations*: STRAW, Stages of Reproductive Ageing Workshop; FSH, follicle stimulating hormone. *Source*: From Ref. 1.

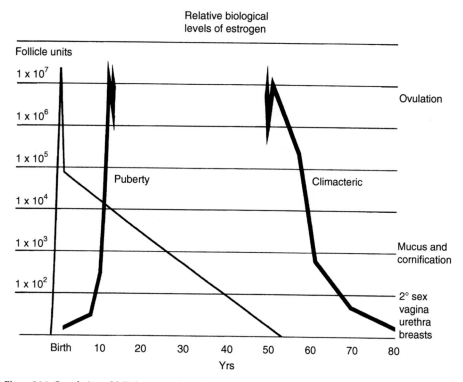

Figure 56.2 Correlation of follicle maturation, follicle availability, and estrogen production. *Source*: From Ref. 2.

A menopause that occurs before the age of 45 is known as a premature menopause. It probably accounts for 1% of women under 40 and 0.1% under 30. It one of the commoner causes of primary and secondary amenorrhea and should always be considered in the diagnosis. The implications of this endocrine failure can be very significant particularly at a young age. The cause of spontaneous premature ovarian failure is usually unknown, but there are a number of well established causes that should be excluded (Table 56.1). Either there may be something wrong with the ovaries themselves (primary ovarian failure), for example, certain chromosomal abnormalities or auto-immune disorders or something happens to the ovary, e.g., oophorectomy, radiotherapy or chemotherapy damage, or infection.

Table 56.1 Causes of Premature Ovarian Failure

Primary
Chromosome anomalies (e.g., Turner's, Fragile X)
Auto-immune disease (e.g., hypothyroidism, Addison's, myasthenia gravis)
Enzyme deficiencies (e.g., galactosemia, 17 α hydroxylase)
Follicle stimulating hormone receptor gene polymorphism

Secondary
Surgical menopause after bilateral oophorectomy
Chemotherapy or radiotherapy
Infections (e.g., tuberculosis, mumps, malaria, varicella)

Table 56.2 Effects of the Menopause in Different Time Frames

Short term
Vasomotor symptoms (e.g., hot flushes, night sweats)
Psychological symptoms (e.g., labile mood, anxiety, tearfulness)
Loss of concentration, poor memory
Joint aches and pains
Dry and itchy skin
Hair changes
Decreased sexual desire

Intermediate
Vaginal dryness, soreness
Dyspareunia
Sensory urgency
Recurrent urinary tract infections
Uro-genital prolapse

Long-term
Osteoporosis
Cardiovascular disease
Dementia

INVESTIGATIONS

When to Investigate

Usually the diagnosis of menopause is straightforward and does not require specific investigation. For example, a woman in her late 40s with oligomenorrhea and classical menopausal symptoms is almost certainly peri-menopausal and no blood tests are needed. Equally a woman in her mid 50s with at least 12 months amenorrhea has gone through the menopause and no specific tests are required to confirm that. However, in other clinical situations it can be helpful to confirm the diagnosis or perhaps more commonly to refute the diagnosis, e.g., in a woman in her mid 40s with vague symptoms who thinks she is going through the menopause. Here a normal FSH/LH levels will help to reassure that this is not the cause. It is mandatory, however, to investigate women suspected of undergoing a premature menopause. The implications of the diagnosis have major long-term consequences both in terms of long-term treatment and also potential fertility. The younger women (under 40) require detailed assessment and specialist assessment.

What Investigations

FSH measurements are the most useful for confirming the diagnosis. A level of >30 IU/L is considered diagnostic of menopause. However there is significant daily variation of FSH levels throughout the cycle and the results should be interpreted with caution and repeated if necessary. The tests are best done on day three to five of the cycle when FSH levels are usually at their lowest. To confirm that a woman with amenorrhea or who has been hysterectomized is menopausal two measurements at least two weeks and up to three months apart are recommended. FSH levels are no use in predicting when menopause will occur or assessing fertility status. Equally monitoring FSH levels on treatment is of little value. There is no value in using estradiol, progesterone, testosterone or LH levels in the diagnosis of menopause. Estradiol levels may be useful in monitoring treatment in certain situations.

Thyroid function (T4 and thyroid stimulating hormone) should be checked if there are any clinical suspicions as the symptoms of hypothyroidism can be confused with menopause or may explain poor response to estrogens. In resistant cases of intractable hot flushes 24-hour urinary collections of catecholamines (vanillylmandelic acid), 5 hydroxyindolacetic acid, and methylhistamine may be done to exclude rare causes such as phaeo-chromocytoma, carcinoid syndrome, and mastocytosis, respectively.

Further Assessment

The menopause presents an opportunity to screen for significant disease in later years and introduce appropriate preventative measures. There a wide range of investigations that can be performed:

- Breast screening and mammography
- Endometrial assessment of unscheduled bleeding
- Cardiovascular disease risk assessment
- Skeletal assessment including bone density estimation and fracture risk assessment

Whilst the majority of these are unlikely to be instituted by a uro-gynecologist some understanding is helpful. A more detailed description can be found in the British Menopause Society Handbook (6).

EFFECTS OF THE MENOPAUSE

The menopause can have significant effects throughout the body. The effects vary chronologically and are summarized in Table 56.2.

Menopausal Symptoms

Vasomotor symptoms, which usually manifest as hot flushes or night sweats, are the commonest symptoms of the menopause. Their exact cause is unknown but amongst the many theories it is hypothesized that a fall in circulating estrogen levels disrupts the control of the body's thermostat, located in the hypothalamus, leading to cutaneous vasodilatation and heat loss (7). Classically the hot flush only affects the upper trunk and head and neck. Recent renewed interest in the cause of the hot flush has implicated a possible role for serotonin and its receptors in the central nervous system (8). Certain triggers can be identified such as stress, spicy foods, alcohol, caffeine, and hot drinks although these are often very individual. Typically hot flushes start to occur a year or two before the menopause, peaking in frequency and intensity in the first year after menopause, and on average lasting for up to five years. However, they can continue for 20 or more years and some unfortunate individuals continue to flush all their lives (9).

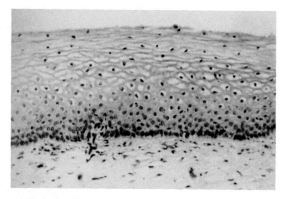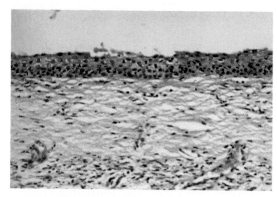

Figure 56.3 Vaginal epithelium in premenopausal woman (*left*) and postmenopausal (*right*) woman showing atrophic changes. *Source*: From Ref. 110.

About 70% of women in the west experience some form of vasomotor symptoms but their intensity varies enormously. For some women they are a minor nuisance but for others they can be very disabling and can have a major impact on their quality of life. Flushes occurring at night can lead to night sweats, which in turn disrupts sleep, which in turn leads to tiredness and can affect mood, concentration, and libido.

Psychological Symptoms

Symptoms such as irritability, depressed mood, anxiety, loss of memory and concentration, overwhelming tiredness, and mood swings are common around the menopause and there is peak prevalence of women seeking help from their general practitioner for this type of problem at this time (10). However, whether these problems are actually caused by ovarian failure or secondary to other menopausal symptoms or due to other co-exsistant factors is questionable. Several longitudinal studies have not demonstrated any association between depressed mood and the menopause transition (11,12). Women who report psychological symptoms at the menopause are more likely to have had previous psychological problems, poor health, premenstrual problems, and have current life stresses such as dependent relatives, relationship problems, and negative attitudes to ageing and the menopause (13). The menopause occurs at a time of life when there can be many other stressful events going on and in western society the woman is often the lynchpin that keeps many families together. The additional physical and emotional changes that occur at the menopause can put this balance under pressure and some women will struggle to cope. Whatever the underlying cause, many women do need additional support during this time and some may benefit from specific treatment for their symptoms such as hormone replacement therapy (HRT).

Genito-Urinary Problems

During the fourth to seventh weeks of fetal development the uro-genital sinus separates from the cloaca and develops into the bladder and proximal urethra in the upper part and the distal urethra and the vestibule of vagina in the lower part. This shared embryological origin explains why both the genital tract and the lower two-thirds of the urinary tract are rich in estrogen and progesterone receptors and why the loss of estrogen at the menopause can lead to the symptoms and signs of urogenital atrophy. Uro-genital atrophy is a common observation in post-

menopausal women which increases with age, but the prevalence of symptomatic atrophy is unclear. In a population-based study of Australian women observed over seven years, vaginal dryness was a complaint in 3% of premenopausal women, 4% of women in early menopause, but up to 47% of women three years or more into their menopause (14).

Vaginal atrophy results in loss of the normal architecture within the vaginal epithelium (Fig. 56.3), reducing its secretions, and elasticity and making it more prone to trauma, dryness, spontaneous bleeding, and infection. Clinically this manifests as vaginal dryness, itching, dyspareunia, vaginal pain, discharge, and bleeding. An increased incidence of sexually transmitted diseases is now being reported in postmenopausal women (15). In part this may be related to the increasing numbers of postmenopausal women restarting sexual activity but could also in part be due to the sharp reduction in the number of women who are now using estrogens (16).

A midlife peak of urinary symptoms around the menopause has also been reported by numerous epidemiological studies (17,18). Although loss of estrogen is not the principle cause in many of these, there is no doubt that atrophy of the distal urinary tract and in particular the urethra and trigone can lead to troublesome symptoms. Typically these women describe urinary frequency and dysuria in the absence of proven infection. Sometimes referred to as the "urethral syndrome," this is due to urethral atrophy and responds well to vaginal estrogens. Thinning of the urethral mucosa and trigone results in a more sensitive and trauma-prone bladder which in turn leads to sensory urgency and recurrent urinary tract infections, symptoms that respond well to local estrogen administration (19). Loss of estrogen also plays a role in more widespread pelvic floor dysfunction leading to weakening of the supporting tissues and ligaments, which may already be damaged by childbirth or other trauma, and thus contributing to the increased incidence of prolapse and stress urinary incontinence seen after menopause (20). Thinning of the urethral mucosa due to atrophy probably contributes to incomplete closure of the urethra, leading to a reduction in urethral closure pressure, and subsequent stress incontinence.

Sexual Dysfunction

Many women complain of loss of sexual desire or libido around the menopause. Whether this is directly due to a fall in estrogen or other simultaneous factors is the subject of considerable research. The term "female sexual dysfunction" is now in widespread use based on a classification system introduced by the International Consensus Development Conference on Female Sexual Dysfunction (21).

The U.S. National Health and Social Life Survey (22) reported that amongst 18 to 59 year olds sexual dysfunction was more prevalent in women (43%) than men (31%) and that the prevalence of sexual dysfunction rose from 42% to 88% during the menopausal transition. Dennerstein (11) found in an increased prevalence of sexual dysfunction but concluded that this was primarily secondary to vaginal atrophy and relationship difficulties. The underlying reasons behind sexual dysfunction are often multi-factorial. For many women sexual desire naturally decreases with age and the menopause may coincide with other stressful major life events. In addition, menopausal symptoms and vaginal atrophy may lead to tiredness and discomfort, there may be reduced response to sexual stimuli, more difficulty reaching orgasm and their male partners may also have reduced interest and have difficulty getting or maintaining an erection. This is undoubtedly a complex area but one that does require some understanding particularly in women presenting with other genital tract problems for whom maintaining sexual function is important.

Correction of physical symptoms, often with systemic or vaginal estrogens, may be sufficient in many cases to overcome the problem but in other women the causes are more complex and may benefit from psycho-sexual input. In western society the menopause is often viewed as a negative event and some women suffer with low self-esteem which undoubtedly does not help, but in some cultures the menopause can be associated with an increase in libido as the shackles of monthly bleeding and risk of pregnancy are finally cast off. The role of testosterone and other treatments are discussed later.

LONG TERM EFFECTS

Estrogen receptors are widespread throughout the body and the fall in circulating estradiol levels leads to a number of changes in a variety of organs and systems that can have notable effects on quality of life and a potentially major impact on long-term morbidity and mortality. These conditions often develop without obvious clinical manifestation in the early post-menopause but pose a significant economic burden for the future particularly with an increasingly ageing population. For women who undergo a premature menopause, the prolonged time they spend without estrogen increases the risk of these conditions developing at a younger age.

Osteoporosis

Osteoporosis is defined as "a skeletal disorder characterized by compromised bone strength predisposing to an increased risk of fracture" (23). Bone strength is principally a reflection of bone quality and bone density (Fig. 56.4). The latter is clinically most relevant as it can be readily measured and a woman's osteoporotic risk assessed using standard WHO criteria (Table 56.3). Osteoporosis is a major health problem for the western world that will only worsen as the population ages. The commonest sites of osteoporotic fracture are the neck of femur, wrist, and vertebrae but any long bone is susceptible. Osteoporosis is far more prevalent in women than men and it is estimated that as many as 50% of women will suffer an osteoporotic fracture at in their lifetime (24).

Bone density peaks in the mid-20s as a result of genetic and environmental influences, the levels start to decline in the mid 40s with an accelerated phase of around 6 to 10 years after menopause subsequent rate of bone loss. Thereafter there is a steady decline with advancing age. The accelerated post-menopausal loss is largely due to the loss of estrogen which

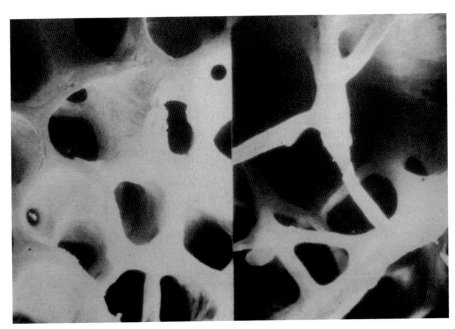

Figure 56.4 Electron micrograph of trabecular bone showing normal structure (*left*) and osteoporotic bone (*right*). *Source*: From Ref. 110.

Table 56.3 Definitions of Osteoporosis (WHO)

Description	Definition
Normal	BMD value between −1 and +1 SD of young adult mean (T score −1 to +1)
Osteopenia	BMD value between −1 and −2.5 SD of young adult mean (T score −1 to −2.5)
Osteoporosis	BMD value equal or below −2.5 SD of young adult mean (T score −2.5 or below)

Abbreviations: BMD, bone mineral density; T, .

has anti-resorptive actions. This results in an accelerated phase of bone resorption and loss of trabecular bone. The rapid fall in bone density immediately after the menopause has triggered a wide range of strategies to prevent osteoporosis over the last 30 years (25). Estrogen replacement has been proven to both reduce bone loss (26) and reduce the subsequent rate of hip fracture in low risk populations (27), and is thus an effective preventative treatment in appropriate individuals (see below).

Current strategies target preventative treatment at individuals identified as high risk of subsequent fracture rather than treating large sections of the population. Current models, such as the FRAX model from Sheffield (28), screen postmenopausal women for risk factors including age at menopause (premature menopause being particularly high risk). Those deemed as increased risk undergo dual energy X-ray absorptiometry bone scanning and those with low bone density are offered preventative treatment. There is much debate about when to start preventative treatment as long-term treatments have potential adverse effects and are costly. Recent NICE guidance favors a very limited role for preventative treatment in women under 75 except those with previous fracture (29). This is contrary to previous guidance based on a more clinical approach (30). Prevention of osteoporosis remains a lifelong strategy even if for some or most of that time no specific treatment is used. A detailed description of all the treatments and their potential role can be found elsewhere (25,26,31).

Coronary Heart Disease (CHD)

Whilst CHD is the single most common cause of death in women in the United Kingdom, it is relatively uncommon before the menopause. Menopausal status can be considered an independent risk factor (32) and after the menopause the risk increases considerably. There is a large body of evidence suggesting that estrogen has a protective influence against CHD (33). Early oophorectomy without additional estrogen is associated with a two to fourfold increased risk CHD compared to premenopausal women of a similar age (34) and large scale population studies over 20 years suggested that taking estrogens around the time of the menopause leads to a reduction in risk (35). Estrogens reverse many of the adverse changes in

cholesterol and other postmenopausal CHD risk factors (36) and also appear to reduce atherogenesis in animal studies (37). However, the large Women's Health Initiative (WHI) randomized trial did not show any convincing evidence that taking estrogen after the menopause has any CHD benefits (38). The mean age of women in this study was 63 years, but when the data were reanalyzed for those women under the age of 60 no harmful effect was found; indeed there was a suggestion of a beneficial effect (39). This is more consistent with the previous epidemiological data that estrogens are started around time of menopause they may have a beneficial effect on future CHD risk (40).

Dementia

Decline in cognitive function inevitably occurs with age but once this interferes substantially with social or occupational functioning it becomes dementia. The incidence of dementia, of which Alzheimer's is the commonest form, is increasing and doubles every five years after the age of 65 (41). Alzheimer's is much more common in women but the evidence for a role of estrogen and menopause in the patho-physiology of cognitive decline and dementia is conflicting; 36% to 62% of women reported memory changes during the menopause in two midlife studies (42,43) but natural menopause does not seem to be associated with objective loss of memory (44). However, early surgical menopause is associated with increased dementia risk in later life (45) and a meta analysis of postmenopausal estrogen use around the time of the menopause suggested that it may improve cognitive function and reduce the risk of Alzheimer's (46). Conversely, the WHI memory study reported an increased incidence of dementia with HRT usage; however, this was in a relatively old population (over 65 years), who would not normally expect to be starting estrogens (47). If estrogens do have any beneficial effect on cognitive function and dementia they probably need to be started around menopause but there is insufficient evidence at the moment to suggest this is a benefit of HRT.

MANAGEMENT

The menopause is a natural event and for many women there is no need to "manage" it at all, although awareness of the long term implications such as osteoporosis and cardiovascular disease should be part of good preventative medicine. However, for other women the menopause can be a difficult time and there are a variety of treatment options available. Whilst HRT is an extremely effective option it is only one of a number of possible approaches. For most women menopausal symptoms are relatively short lived and will settle within a few years but for some they will go on much longer and longer term treatment may be needed. The menopause is a hormonal milestone and provides an opportunity to establish firm strategies for the prevention of the long term disorders outlined above.

Lifestyle

Dealing with the effects of the menopause should be a holistic approach and those that do best will be those women who can grasp the opportunity to see it in a positive light. For many women the menopause can be a time of uncertainty and may be the first time they have sought professional help for themselves for many years. It is an ideal time to look at changes in diet and exercise and build for a healthy future to maximize their health potential. Smoking is associated with an earlier menopause, an increased risk of cardiovascular disease, lung cancer, and osteoporosis. Smoking cessation leads to a steady reduction in all the increased risks and should be encouraged as part of a health promotion strategy.

Diet

With the current epidemic of obesity in the western world, diet is something that all women will be familiar with. Body weight increases on average 1 kg/yr around menopause although this does not seem to be a direct effect of the menopause itself (48). In addition there are metabolic changes and changes in body fat distribution that shifts body fat from the hips and thighs (gynecoid) to the more android distribution (abdomen) (49). Thus it is particularly important women going through menopause eat sensibly and try and avoid excessive weight gain. A recommended diet should be rich in fruit and vegetables, whole grain, and high fiber foods, oily fish twice a week, saturated fat intake <10%, cholesterol <300 mg/day, alcohol intake no more than 1 unit/day, and sodium no more than 1 tsp a day (50). For women with obesity problems entering the menopause specialist dietary advice may be helpful. HRT is not associated with an increase in weight gain (51) although in some women it can increase fluid retention and over time may lead to a reversal of the body fat changes seen at menopause.

Exercise

Regular physical activity has positive effects on a variety of conditions and regular exercise, even of relatively low intensity, can be beneficial to cardiovascular risk (52). Exercise has a key role to play in the maintenance of bone health, not only does regular weight bearing exercise help to conserve bone density in the hip and spine it also helps to maintain muscle strength, joint flexibility, and overall balance, all factors that will reduce the risk of falls and subsequent fracture (53). Physical activity can be effectively used to reduce vasomotor symptoms (54) possibly by an effect on endorphins.

ALTERNATIVE AND COMPLEMENTARY THERAPIES

A wide variety of complementary and alternative medicines are used to improve menopausal symptoms, although robust evidence for the efficacy and safety of most of these products or methods is notably lacking (55). Despite this, the use of such treatments is widespread and increasing (56). In our own specialist clinic we identified that up to 40% of women were taking additional over the counter supplements for their menopausal symptoms and 10% were taking more than four different products concurrently (57). These products are currently unregulated in the United Kingdom and whilst the majority are likely to be harmless, a number of serious and potentially fatal interactions have been reported between herbal supplements and standard medications (58). By contrast, the use of phyto-estrogens, plant substances with similar activity to estrogen, appear to have some beneficial effects on both menopausal symptoms and bone prevention, although the effects are modest and inconsistent in the published literature (59). Further randomized controlled trials are needed.

HORMONE REPLACEMENT THERAPY

HRT is the mainstay of medical treatment available for troublesome menopausal symptoms and simply acts by replacing the hormones that are normally produced by the human ovary at physiological levels. Estrogen is the principal hormone and can either be given alone or in combination with progestogen, which should be given to all non-hysterectomized women. A third hormone, testosterone, can also be given in conjunction with estrogen.

Estrogen

There are a variety of different types of estrogen available, which can be given at varying doses and by different routes (60). For the vast majority of women, the type and route of administration are not important and, provided an adequate dose of estrogen is given, it is likely to be effective. However, there are some women who do not show an appropriate response and adjustment to a different type of estrogen may be helpful.

As with any treatment the lowest possible dose should be used. Previously 1 mg estradiol or 0.625 mg conjugated equine estrogen (CEE) were considered the lowest dose but there is now plenty of evidence from randomized controlled trials to indicate that very low or ultra low doses of HRT (0.3 mg CEE or 0.5 mg of estradiol) are effective in relieving menopausal symptoms (61,62). Their role in osteoporosis prevention is less clear but even the lowest doses appear to slow down the rate of bone loss (63).

Different routes of estrogen administration have different pharmacokinetic profiles. Non-oral routes, such as percutaneous and transdermal administration, do offer potential advantages in avoidance of the first-pass effect. Accordingly, in some situations, such as a personal or relevant family history of venous thrombosis or known liver abnormalities, the transdermal preparations, which have less effects on coagulation and hemostatic mechanisms, would appear to have a lower risk (64). However, oral estrogens, because of their first-pass effect, have potentially greater effects on lipids and lipoproteins, and glucose and insulin metabolism (60,65), so women with hypercholesterolemia or hyper-triglyceridemia may benefit more from oral estrogens. For the vast majority of patients, the route of administration is not important provided adequate estrogen levels are achieved. Non-oral routes tend to be more expensive and, for those women who need a progestogen, there can be logistical problems administering the progestogen component simultaneously. Whilst the majority of long-term studies on the benefits and risks of HRT have been conducted with oral estrogens (predominantly CEE), the absence of such studies on non-oral HRT does not mean that it can be assumed that the risks, or indeed the benefits, that apply to oral treatment do not equally apply to non-oral treatment.

Table 56.4 Different Progestogens Used in HRT

Norethisterone (transdermal)
Levonorgestrel (transdermal, intrauterine)
Dydrogesterone
Medroxyprogesterone acetate
Drospirenone
Micronized progesterone (rectally)
Cyproterone acetate (not available in United Kingdom)

Note: All are available orally. Additional routes are listed.

Table 56.5 Main Indications for Taking HRT

Menopausal symptoms
　Hot flushes night sweats
　Mood changes, irritability
　Loss of memory, concentration
　Joint aches and pains
Urogenital atrophy
Osteoporosis prevention

Progestogens

Giving unopposed estrogens to non-hysterectomized women substantially increases their risk of developing endometrial cancer (66). Progestogens added for at least 10 days per calendar month negate this risk (67). They can either be given cyclically, mimicking the natural 28 day cycle and resulting in a regular withdrawal bleed, or continuously to prevent any bleeding, so-called "no bleed" treatment. The latter is usually recommended for women who are clearly post-menopausal, whilst the former is usually prescribed for women who are peri-menopausal. Long cycle HRT can also be used where progestogen is added for two weeks every three months. Whilst this has potential advantages in limiting withdrawal bleeds to four per year, it carries an increased risk of breakthrough bleeding and potential endometrial abnormalities if continued longterm (68).

There are several different types of progestogen used in HRT (Table 56.4). Side effects are common, particularly in the first few months, and these may vary depending on the type and dose of progestogen used. Switching from one type of progestogen to another, or changing the route of administration can alleviate side effects in many cases. The advent of the levonorgestrel intra-uterine system has allowed many women who could not tolerate any of the available progestogen combinations to continue HRT safely. The use of progestogens in HRT has been reviewed (60,69).

Testosterone

Fifty percent of testosterone production in women is from the ovaries (the other 50% is from peripheral fat stores and the adrenals). Testosterone production is not generally affected by natural menopause although a decline in sex hormone-binding globulin may lead to a small rise in circulating free testosterone. However women who undergo a surgical or chemo-radiation induced menopause may become relatively testosterone deficient. Symptoms can be hard to determine specifically but classically are loss of libido, decreased sexual activity, fatigue, and reduced feelings of physical wellbeing (70). There are a number of potential treatment options which are discussed later.

Indications and Benefits of HRT

The majority of women start HRT for the relief of menopausal symptoms (Table 56.5). There is abundant evidence from randomized placebo-controlled studies that estrogen is effective in treating hot flushes (71), with improvement usually noted within four to six weeks. Comparative studies indicate that HRT is far more effective than non-hormonal preparations, such as clonidine and selective serotonin-reuptake inhibitors (72).

The symptoms of vaginal and uro-genital atrophy discussed above, respond well to systemic or vaginal estrogens (19,71,73). Treatment should be continued at a low maintenance dose, otherwise the symptoms tend to recur.

There is grade A evidence that HRT is effective in the prevention of postmenopausal bone loss and osteoporotic fractures at the spine and hip (26,74). Thus, women taking HRT for symptom relief will derive benefit as far as their bones are concerned. What has been more debatable is whether or not HRT should be prescribed for osteoporosis prevention alone. Despite strong evidence of its efficacy, the regulatory authorities have advised that HRT should not be used as a first-line treatment for osteoporosis prevention as the potential risks outweigh the benefits (75). Whilst this is clear cut in women over 60, the position for younger women is less clear (76). The long term efficacy and safety of alternatives for osteoporosis prevention, such as the bisphosphonates, have not been established in younger (<60 years) postmenopausal women (77) and there are increasing concerns about the long-term safety of these preparations (78). However, the regulatory authorities do emphasize that HRT or estrogen alone are the most appropriate treatments for osteoporosis prevention in women with premature ovarian failure under the age of 50 (75).

Over recent years there have been a number of high profile "scares" about HRT. A critical analysis of all grade A evidence regarding the benefits and risks of HRT is summarized in Table 56.6 (79).

Risks of HRT

Ever since the introduction of HRT there have been concerns that the prolongation of exposure to natural hormones may have an adverse effect on the breast and other estrogen-sensitive tissues. Yet, despite widespread use for several decades and numerous studies, there remains uncertainty and controversy about exactly what the risks are and how relevant they are to the majority of healthy post-menopausal women.

Breast Cancer

A large body of epidemiological studies have suggested that less than five years of HRT use in the early post-menopause does not increase breast cancer risk (80). Thereafter, there does appear to be a small increase in risk, dependent on years

Table 56.6 Risks, Benefits, and Uncertainties of HRT based on Grade A Evidence

Benefits	Risks
Vasomotor symptoms	Breast cancer
Urogenital symptoms	VTE
Sexual function	Stroke
Osteoporosis	Endometrial cancer
Colon cancer	
	Uncertainties
	Cardiovascular disease and stroke
	Alzheimer's
	Ovarian cancer
	Quality of life

Abbreviations: HRT, hormone replacement therapy; VTE, venous thromboembolism.
Source: British Menopause Society consensus statement. [Available from: www.thebms.org.uk].

of exposure. The magnitude of risk appears to be similar to that associated with late natural menopause (2.3% compared with 2.8% per year, respectively). A meta-analysis of all observational data prior to 1997 estimated that current use of any HRT for more than five years, when started over the age of 50, increased breast cancer risk by 1.35 (95% confidence interval 1.20–1.49) (80). In absolute numbers this equates to two to four extra breast cancer cases per 1000 women who use HRT from the age of 50 for five years. Women who start HRT early for premature menopause do not show this effect, suggesting that it may be the lifetime sex hormone exposure that is relevant. The WHI study (81), which is the largest randomized trial on HRT, reported a broadly similar risk to that seen in the epidemiological studies for combined estrogen and progestogen treatment, but also found no increase in risk over seven years with estrogen only treatment (82). There are conflicting reports about what happens to breast cancer risk after stopping HRT. A recent three-year follow-up of women who were in the WHI trial, claimed that the risk of breast cancer remains elevated for three years after treatment was stopped (83). However, these findings are at odds with other recent publications which imply the risk of breast cancer falls quickly after cessation of HRT (84,85).

The Million Women Study (MWS) which was a large observational study (85) reported an increased risk of breast cancer with all HRT regimens (i.e., unopposed estrogen and combined HRT). This was in marked contrast to the randomized WHI and another recent large observational study, both of which found no increased risk with unopposed estrogen (82,86). The design, results and interpretation of the MWS have been questioned (87).

In summary, otherwise healthy postmenopausal women in their late 40s and 50s wishing to take HRT should be reassured that the overall risk of developing breast cancer in the first few years as a result of their HRT is small. If they take estrogen alone, that risk is probably even lower. Overall other personal risk factors such as family history are likely to be more important predictive factors.

Endometrial Cancer

Unopposed estrogen replacement therapy increases endometrial cancer risk which is reduced by the addition of progestogens (66,67). When continued for more than five years cyclical progestogen addition does not completely eradicate this excess risk whilst continuous progestogen addition does (67). Thus, once a woman is clearly post-menopausal, she should be switched to a continuous combined (no bleed) regimen. Any abnormal bleeding on HRT should be investigated, although the likelihood of underlying malignancy is low.

Ovarian Cancer

Most of the limited data relate to estrogen alone and suggest a small increase in risk with very long term (>10 years) treatment (88,89). This increase does not seem apparent with combined therapy (90,91). There is currently insufficient evidence to recommend any alterations in HRT prescribing practice (79).

Venous Thromboembolism (VTE)

HRT increases the risk of VTE twofold, with the highest risk occurring in the first year of use (92). The background risk of VTE in women over 50 years not taking HRT is small (1.7/1000) (93), so the overall impact of this increase is low. However, the background risk is significantly increased in women who smoke, are obese, have an underlying thrombophilia such as Factor V Leiden, or who have previously suffered a VTE (92). Transdermal HRT has less impact on hemostatic mechanisms and appears to be associated with a lower risk of VTE (64,92,94), even in women with a thrombophilia, and thus may be the treatment of choice in this group.

Coronary Heart Disease

From the data discussed earlier it is clear there is a conflict between large scale epidemiological studies which have consistently shown that estrogens appears to have a protective effect on CHD and the more recent randomized trials which suggested a possible adverse effect (35,38). Subsequent detailed analysis of these and other data suggest that timing of the introduction of estrogen may be critical (95,96). For women starting HRT shortly after menopause, there may well be a protective effect on CHD, and this particularly appears to be the case for women undergoing premature menopause. However, in women many years past the menopause, starting HRT may have a detrimental effect, i.e., early benefit, late harm. There is no indication to use HRT specifically for cardiovascular disease protection (97).

Stroke

Small increases in the risk of stroke with both estrogen only and combined estrogen and progestogen were reported in the WHI study (38), although there was a significant age effect, with a relatively high risk in older women and no reported increase in the 50 to 59 age group. In general, the data suggest a trend towards a small increase incidence of stroke with HRT (97,98) and HRT should not be initiated for women over the age of 60, or those who have strong risk

Table 56.7 Additional Events Anticipated per 1000 Women on HRT for Five Years Aged 50–59 (MHRA 2004)

Condition	Placebo	Extra events (±SD)	
		E only	E + P
Breast cancer	16	0	+4 (±4)
Stroke	8	+2 (±2)	+1 (±1)
VTE	6	+1 (±1)	+4 (±3)

Abbreviations: HRT, hormone replacement therapy; VTE, venous thromboembolism; MHRA, Medicines and Healthcare Products Regulatory Agency; E, estrogen; P, progesterone.

factors for stroke or cardiovascular disease risk without carefully weighing up the potential risks against any potential benefits (Table 56.7).

Practical Considerations for Prescribing HRT

HRT is only one option for dealing with menopausal symptoms and other options can be considered (99). Yet, despite the recent controversies, HRT remains a clinically effective and cost-effective strategy for women with menopausal symptoms (100). For the majority of healthy symptomatic menopausal women the potential benefits will outweigh any small risks (75). However, like all treatments the risks and benefits should be weighed up individually with the patient before starting treatment.

Selecting which HRT regimen is a matter for the individual prescriber. If there are specific special circumstances, then a particular type or route of administration may be most appropriate. Follow-up should be arranged after a few months to check the treatment's effectiveness and side effects. It is common for women to have some problems in the first few months, and if these do not settle down, a change of treatment may be advisable. There are over 80 preparations available, but the majority of women respond well to whatever treatment they are given. A significant minority experience poor symptom control or side effects and a change of preparation may be needed, perhaps utilizing an alternative prgestogen (Table 56.4). Treatment should be started at the lowest appropriate dose and can be increased if there is no symptomatic improvement after a few months.

The duration of HRT use depends on the individual circumstances and indication for taking it. The "average" menopausal woman in her early 50s will probably only take it for one to two years, but there is no reason why she should not take it for longer if indicated. The Medicines and Healthcare Products Regulatory Agency recommend taking "the minimum effective dose" of HRT for the "shortest duration" without defining any specific length of time (75). Based on other recommendations, this has generally been interpreted as about five years, although in reality most women do not take it that long. However treatment can be continued for longer in women with persistent troublesome symptoms that adversely affect their quality of life. The exception to these recommendations is women who have undergone a premature menopause. In this group the risk/benefit balance is strongly in favor of them taking HRT at least up until the age of 50 as a true physiological replacement (75).

For all women their individual risk of VTE, stroke, and breast cancer should be appraised regularly and balanced against the benefits she is gaining from the treatment. For the majority of women, the overall increase in any risk will be very small and there are many women who opt to continue taking HRT for its benefits well into their 60s.

Stopping HRT should be done gradually reducing the dose to avoid rebound symptoms. At the same time positive lifestyle factors should be emphasized, such as diet and regular exercise. Vaginal estrogens can be added in if troublesome genitourinary symptoms persist. These are not absorbed systemically to any great extent and can be continued after HRT has been stopped without significant risk (101).

Reduced sexual desire is a common complaint around the menopause which can lead to distress and have a negative impact on psychological wellbeing and relationships (102). This is a complex area and there are often multiple factors that play a part (103). Menopausal symptoms and uro-genital atrophy should be treated with systemic or local estrogens and psycho-sexual counseling should be considered if appropriate. Testosterone supplementation appears to be effective in some women when combined with estrogen. Sub-dermal testosterone implants have been available for many years and seem to have beneficial effect on libido, particularly in oophorectomized women (104). However these need to be inserted under the skin under local anesthetic every six months. Transdermal testosterone (300 mcg) has proven efficacy in randomized trials (105,106) but is currently only indicated in the United Kingdom in women who have been oophorectomized and who are already taking estrogen replacement. However, it also appears to be effective in naturally menopausal women (107). Tibolone is a synthetic steroid with estrogenic, progestogenic, and androgenic activity with a licensed indication for women with loss of libido (108).

Contraception

Contraception should be continued until two years after the last period in women under 50 and one year in women over 50. Identifying the last menstrual period can be difficult, particularly if the woman is on hormonal contraception or HRT. HRT itself is not a contraceptive and serum FSH levels are not particularly reliable on HRT. The continuing use of condoms will reduce the incidence of sexually transmitted infections, particularly for those in new relationships. A full review of contraceptive choices for peri-menopausal women can be found elsewhere (109).

SUMMARY

The menopause is a time of significant physiological change which signifies the end of the reproductive phase of life. Whilst this can be a positive development for many women, for some women the menopause can be a difficult time with distressing symptoms that impact on their quality of life and relationships. The potential impact on long term health should also be considered and the menopause provides a good opportunity to improve lifestyle risk factors and put long term prevention strategies in place. Women with premature ovarian failure have particular needs and will often benefit from specialist support. A wide range of potential treatments are available for helping women through the menopause and beyond. HRT is only one option but is effective and has a large body of evidence supporting its use and its limitations. For the vast majority of healthy symptomatic menopausal women the benefit/risk balance is in favor of using it for a limited period. No two women's experience of the menopause is exactly the same and any advice or treatment should therefore be tailored to the needs of the individual woman.

REFERENCES

1. Soules MR, Sherman S, Parrott E, et al. Executive summary: Stages of Reproductive Ageing Workshop (STRAW). Fertil Steril 2001; 76: 874–8.
2. Speroff L, Glass RH, Kase NG. Clinical Gynecologic Endocrinology and Infertility. Baltimore, USA: Williams and Wilkins, 1990: 121–64.
3. Amunsdn DW, Diers CJ. The age of menopause in medieval Europe. Hum Biol 1973; 45: 605.
4. OlaOlorun F, Lawoyin T. Age menopause and factors associated with attainment of menopause in an urban community in Ibadan, Nigeria. Climacteric 2009; 12: 352–63.
5. Mishra GD, Cooper R, Tom SE, Kuh D. Early life circumstances and their impact on menarche and menopause. Womens Health 2009; 5: 175–90.
6. Rees M, Stevenson J, Hope S, et al. Management of the Menopause. London: British Menopause Society and RSM Press, 2009.
7. Freedman RR. Physiology of hot flashes. Am J Hum Biol 2001; 13: 453–64.
8. Berendsen HH. The role of serotonin in hot flushes. Maturitas 2000; 36: 155–64.
9. Stearns V, Ullmer L, Lopez JF, et al. Hot flushes. Lancet 2002; 360: 1851–61.
10. Bungay GT, Vessey MP, McPherson CK. Study of symptoms in middle life with special reference to the menopause. BMJ 1980; ii: 181–3.
11. Dennerstein L, Guthrie JR, Clark M, et al. A population based study of depressed mood in middle aged Australian born women. Menopause 2004; 11: 563–8.
12. Fugate Woods N, Mariella A, Sullivan Mitchell E. Depressed mood symptoms during the menopause transition: observations from the Seattle Midlife Women's Health Study. Climacteric 2006; 9: 195–203.
13. Hunter MS. Predictors of menopausal symptoms: psychological aspects. Ballieres Clin Endocrinol Metab 1993; 7: 34–45.
14. Dennerstein L, Dudley EC, Hopper JL, et al. A prospective population based study of menopausal symptoms. Obstet Gynecol 2000; 96: 351–8.
15. Drew O, Sherrard J. Sexually transmitted infections in the older woman. Menopause Int 2008; 14: 134–5.
16. Greenouse P. Increase in HIV in older women in relation to falling use of HRT– personal communication.
17. Hannestad YS, Rortveit G, Sandvik H, Hunskaar S. Epidemiology of incontinence in the county of Nord-Trondelag. A community based epidemiological survey of female urinary incontinence. The Norwegian EPICONT study. J Clin Epidemiol 2000; 53: 1150–7.
18. Hunskaar S, Lose G, Sykes D, Voss S. The prevalence of urinary incontinence in four European countries. BJU Int 2004; 93: 324–30.
19. Cardozo L, Lose G, McClish D, Versi E, de Koning Gans H. A systematic review of estrogens for recurrent urinary tract infections: third report of the hormones and urogenital therapy (HUT) committee. Int Urogynecol J 2001; 12: 15–20.
20. Versi E, Harvey MA, Cardozo LD, et al. Urogenital prolapse and atrophy at menopause: a prevalence study. Int Urogynecol J 2001; 12: 107–10.
21. Basson R, Berman J, Burnett A, et al. Report of the international consensus development conference on female sexual dysfunction: definitions and classifications. J Urol 2000; 163: 888–93.
22. Laumann EO, Paik A, Rosen RC. Sexual dysfunction in the United States: prevalence and predictors. JAMA 1998; 281: 537–44.
23. NIH. Consensus development panel on osteoporosis prevention, diagnosis and therapy. JAMA 2001; 285: 785–95.
24. Johnell O, Kanis J. Epidemiology of osteoporotic fractures. Osteoporos Int 2005; 16(Suppl 2): S3–7.
25. Poole KES, Compston JE. Osteoporosis and it management. BMJ 2006; 333: 1251–6.
26. Al-Azzawi F, Barlow D, Hillard T, et al. Prevention and treatment of osteoporosis in women. British Menopause Society Consensus Statement. Menopause Int 2007; 13: 178–81.
27. Cauley JA, Robbins J, Chen Z, et al. Women's Health Initiative Investigators. Effects of estrogen plus progestin on risk of fracture and bone mineral density: the Women's Health Initiative Randomised Trial. JAMA 2003; 290: 1729–38.
28. Kanis JA, Johnell O, Oden A, Johansson H, McCloskey E. FRAX and the assessment of fracture probability in men and women from the UK. Osteoporos Int 2008; 19: 385–97.
29. NICE. Alendronate, etidronate, risedronate, raloxifene and strontium ranelate for the primary prevention of osteoporotic fragility fractures in postmenopausal women. TA161 Oct 2008. [Available from: www.nice.org].
30. Guideline Development Group of the Royal College of Physicians. Royal College of Physicians Clinical Guidelines for the Prevention and Treatment of Osteoporosis. London: Royal College of Physicians, 1999.
31. Stevenson JC. Justification for the use of HRT in the long-term prevention of osteoporosis. Maturitas 2005; 51: 113–16.
32. Atsma F, Bartelink ML, Grobbee DE, van der Schouw YT. Postmenopausal status and early menopause as independent risk factors for cardiovascular disease: a meta analysis. Menopause 2006; 13: 265–79.
33. Mendelsohn ME, Karas RH. The protective effects of estrogen on the cardiovascular system. NEJM 1999; 340: 1801–11.
34. Lobo RA. Surgical menopause and cardiovascular risks. Menopause 2007; 14(Suppl 3): 562–6.
35. Stampfer MJ, Colditz GA. Estrogen replacement therapy and coronary heart disease: a quantitative assessment of the epidemiologic evidence. Prev Med 1991; 20: 47–63.
36. Stevenson JC. Metabolic effects of hormone replacement therapy. J Br Menopause Soc 2004; 10: 157–61.
37. Clarkson TB. Estrogens, progestins and coronary heart disease in cynomolgus monkeys. Fertil Steril 1994; 62(Suppl 6): 147S–51S.
38. Writing Group for the Women's Health Initiative Investigators. Risks and benefits of estrogen plus progestin in healthy postmenopausal women. Principal results from the Women's Health Initiative Randomized Controlled Trial. JAMA 2002; 288: 321–33.
39. Hsia J, Langer RD, Manson JE, et al. Conjugated equine estrogens and coronary heart disease. Arch Intern Med 2006; 166: 357–65.
40. Hodis HN. Assessing benefits and risks of hormone therapy in 2008: new evidence, especially with regard to the heart. Cleve Clin J Med 2008; 75(Suppl 4): S3–12.
41. Alzheimer's society. [Available from: www.alzheimers.org.uk].
42. Mitchell ES, Woods NF. Midlife women's attributions about perceived memory changes: observations from the Seattle Midlife Women's Health Study. J Wom Health Gend Base Med 2001; 10: 351–62.
43. Henderson VW, Dudley EC, Guthrie JR, et al. Estrogen exposures and memory at midlife: a population based study of women. Neurology 2003; 60: 1369–71.
44. Kok HS, Kuh D, Cooper R, et al. Cognitive function across the life course and the menopause transition in the British birth cohort. Menopause 2006; 13: 4–5.
45. Rocca WA, Bower JH, Maraganore DM, et al. Increased risk of cognitive impairment or dementia in women who underwent oophorectomy before menopause. Neurology 2007; 69: 1074–83.
46. Le Blanc ES, Janowsky J, Chan BK, Nelson HD. Hormone replacement therapy and cognition: systematic review and meta-analysis. JAMA 2001; 285: 1489–99.
47. Shumaker SA, Legault C, Rapp SR. Estrogen plus progestin and the incidence of dementia and mild cognitive impairment in postmenopausal women: the Women's Health Initiative Memory Study: a randomised trial. JAMA 2003; 289: 2651–62.
48. Guthrie JR, Dennerstein L, Dudley EC. Weight gain and the menopause: a 5 year prospective study. Climacteric 1999; 2: 205–11.

49. Ley CJ, Lees B, Stevenson JC. Sex and menopause associated changes in body fat distribution. Am J Clin Nutr 1992; 55: 950–4.

50. American Heart Association. [Available from: www.americanheart.org].

51. Davies KM, Heaney RP, Recker RR, et al. Hormones, weight change and menopause. Int J Obes Relat Metab Disord 2001; 25: 874–9.

52. Blair SN, Kampert JB, Kohl 3rd HW, et al. Influences of cardio-respiratory fitness and other precursors on cardiovascular disease and all-cause mortality in men and women. JAMA 1996; 276: 205–10.

53. Bonaiuti D, Shea B, Iovine R, et al. Exercise for preventing and treating osteoporosis in postmenopausal women. Cochrane Database Syst Rev 2002; 3: CD000333.

54. Daley AJ, Stokes-Lampard HJ, MacArthur C. Exercise to reduce vasomotor and other menopausal symptoms. Maturitas 2009; 63: 176–80.

55. Panay N, Rees M. Alternatives to HRT for the management of symptoms of the menopause (SAC Opinion Paper 6). [Available from: www.rcog.org.uk/womens-health/clinical-guidance/alternatives-hrt-management-symptoms-menopause].

56. Van der Sluijs CP, Bensoussan A, Liyanage L, Shah S. Women's health during mid-life survey: the use of complementary and alternative medicine by symptomatic women transitioning through menopause in Sydney. Menopause 2007; 14: 397–403.

57. Bell B, Hillard A, Hillard TC. An alternative approach: a survey of alternative methods used by women in a consultant led specialist menopause clinic. Menopause Int 2007; 13: 200–1

58. MHRA. Public health risks with herbal medicines: an overview. July 2008. [Available from: http://www.mhra.gov.uk/Howweregulate/Medicines/Herbalandhomoeopathicmedicines/Herbalmedicines/HerbalSafetyNews/CON009286].

59. Thompson Coon J, Pittler MH, Ernst E. The role of red clover (Trifolium pratense) isoflavones in women's reproductive health: a systematic review and meta-analysis of randomised clinical trials. Focus Altern Complement Ther 2003; 8: 544.

60. Kuhl H. Pharmacology of estrogens and progestogens: influence of different routes of administration. Climacteric 2005; 8(Suppl 1): 3–63.

61. Peeyananjarassri K, Baber R. Effects of low-dose hormone therapy on menopausal symptoms, bone mineral density, endometrium, and the cardiovascular system: a review of randomized clinical trials. Climacteric 2005; 8: 13–23.

62. Panay N, Ylikorkala O, Archer DF, et al. Ultra low dose estradiol and norethisterone acetate: effective menopause symptom relief. Climacteric 2007; 10: 120–31.

63. Ettinger B, Ensrud K, Wallace R, et al. Effects of ultra-low dose transdermal oestradiol on bone mineral density: a randomised clinical trial. Obstet Gynecol 2004; 104: 443–51.

64. Canonico M, Oger E, Plu-Bureau G, et al. Estrogen and Thromboembolism Risk (ESTHER) Study Group. Hormone therapy and venous thrombo-embolism among postmenopausal women: impact of the route of estrogen administration and progestogens: the ESTHER study. Circulation 2007; 115: 840–5.

65. Godsland IF. Effects of postmenopausal hormone replacement therapy on lipid, lipoproteins and apolipoprotein (a) concentrations: analysis of studies published from 1974–2000. Fertil Steril 2001; 75: 898–915.

66. Weiderpass E, Adami HO, Baron JA, et al. Risk of endometrial cancer following estrogen replacement with and without progestins. J Natl Cancer Inst 1999; 91: 1131–7.

67. The writing group for the PEPI trial. Effects of hormone replacement therapy on endometrial histology in postmenopausal women. The postmenopausal estrogen/progestin interventions (PEPI) trial. JAMA 1996; 275: 370–5.

68. Pukkala E, Tulenheimo-Silfvast A, Leminen A. Incidence of cancer among women using long versus monthly cycle hormonal replacement therapy, Finland 1994–1997. Cancer Causes Control 2001; 12: 111–15.

69. Whitehead MI, Hillard TC, Crook D. The role and use of progestogens. Obstet Gynecol 1990; 75: 59s–76s.

70. Mazer NA. Testosterone deficiency in women: etiologies, diagnosis and emerging treatments. Int J Fertil 2002; 47: 77–8.

71. Rymer J, Morris EP. Extracts from "clinical evidence": menopausal symptoms. BMJ 2000; 321: 1516–19.

72. Albertazzi P. Non-estrogenic approaches for the treatment of climacteric symptoms. Climacteric 2007; 10(Suppl 2): 115–20.

73. Suckling J, Lethaby A, Kennedy R. Local oestrogen for vaginal atrophy in postmenopausal women. Cochrane Database Syst Rev (Online) 2006; 4: CD001500.

74. Cauley JA, Robbins J, Chen Z, et al. for the women's health initiative investigators. Effects of estrogen plus progestin on risk of fracture and bone mineral density: the women's health initiative randomized trial. JAMA 2003; 290: 1729–38.

75. Medicines and Healthcare Products Regulatory Agency and Commission on Human Medicines. Hormone replacement therapy: updated advice. Drug Safety Update 2007; 1: 2–5.

76. Birkhauser MH, Panay N, Archer DF, et al. Updated recommendations for hormone replacement therapy in the peri- and postmenopause. Climacteric 2008; 11: 108–23.

77. Ott SM. Long-term safety of bisphosphonates. J Clin Endocrinol Metab 2005; 90: 1897–9.

78. Ruggiero SL, Mehrotra B, Rosenberg TJ, Engroff SL. Osteonecrosis of the jaws associated with the use of bisphosphonates: a review of 63 cases. J Oral Maxillofac Surg 2004; 62: 527–34.

79. Pitkin J, Rees MC, Gray S, et al. Managing the menopause: British menopause society council consensus statement on hormone replacement therapy. J Br Menopause Soc 2005; 11: 152–6.

80. Collaborative group on hormonal factors in breast cancer. Breast cancer and hormone replacement therapy: collaborative reanalysis of data from 51 epidemiological studies of 52,705 women with breast cancer and 108,411 women without breast cancer. Lancet 1997; 350: 1047–59.

81. Writing group for the Women's Health Initiative Investigators. Risks and benefits of estrogen plus progestin in healthy postmenopausal women. Principal results from the Women's Health Initiative Randomized Controlled Trial. JAMA 2002; 288: 321–33.

82. Stefanick ML, Anderson GL, Margolis KL, et al. Effects of conjugated equine estrogens on breast cancer and mammography screening in postmenopausal women with hysterectomy. JAMA 2006; 295: 1647–57.

83. Heiss G, Wallace R, Anderson GL, et al. Health risks and benefits 3 years after stopping randomized treatment with estrogen and progestin. JAMA 2008; 299: 1036–45.

84. Li CI, Daling JR. Changes in breast cancer incidence rates in the United States by histologic subtype and race/ethnicity, 1995 to 2004. Cancer Epidemiol Biomarkers Prev 2007; 16: 2773–80.

85. Million Women Study Collaborators. Breast cancer and hormone-replacement therapy in the Million Women Study. Lancet 2003; 362: 419–27.

86. Chen WY, Manson JE, Hankinson SE, et al. Unopposed estrogen therapy and the risk of invasive breast cancer. Arch Intern Med 2006; 166: 1027–32.

87. Whitehead M, Farmer R. The million women study: a critique. Endocrine 2004; 24: 187–93.

88. Beral V, Million Women Study Collaborators, Bull D, Green J, Reeves G. Ovarian cancer and hormone replacement therapy in the million women study. Lancet 2007; 369: 1703–10.

89. Greiser CM, Greiser EM, Doren M. Menopausal hormone therapy and risk of ovarian cancer: systematic review and meta-analysis. Hum Reprod Update 2007; 13: 453–63.

90. Anderson GL, Judd HL, Kaunitz AM, et al. Women's Health Initiative Investigators. Effects of estrogen plus progestin on gynecologic cancers and associated diagnostic procedures: the women's health initiative randomized trial. JAMA 2003; 290: 1739–48.

91. Danforth KN, Tworoger SS, Hecht JL, et al. A prospective study of postmenopausal hormone use and ovarian cancer risk. Br J Cancer 2007; 96: 151–6.

92. Gomes MPV, Deitcher SR. Risk of venous thromboembolic disease associated with hormonal contraceptives and hormone replacement therapy. Arch Intern Med 2004; 164: 1965–76.

93. Cushman M, Kuller LH, Prentice R, et al. for the Women's Health Initiative Investigators. Estrogen plus progestin and risk of venous thrombosis. JAMA 2004; 292: 1573–80.

94. Canonico M, Plu-Bureau G, Lowe GD, et al. Hormone replacement therapy and risk of venous thromboembolism in postmenopausal women: systematic review and meta-analysis. BMJ 2008; 336: 1227–31.

95. Salpeter SR, Walsh JM, Greyber E, et al. Mortality associated with hormone replacement therapy in younger and older women: a meta-analysis. J Gen Intern Med 2004; 19: 791–804.

96. Lobo RA. Postmenopausal hormones and coronary artery disease: potential benefits and risks. Climacteric 2007; 10(Suppl 2): 21–6.

97. International Menopause Society consensus statement: ageing, menopause, cardiovascular disease and HRT. Climacteric 2009; 12: 368–77.

98. Grodstein F, Manson JE, Stampfer MJ, et al. Postmenopausal hormone therapy and stroke. Arch Intern Med 2008; 168: 861–6.

99. Albertazzi P. Non-estrogenic approaches for the treatment of climacteric symptoms. Climacteric 2007; 10(Suppl 2): 115–20.

100. Zethraeus N, Borgstrom F, Jonsson B, Kanis J. Reassessment of the cost-effectiveness of hormone replacement therapy in Sweden: results based on the Women's Health Initiative Randomised Controlled Trial. Int J Technol Assess Health Care 2005; 21: 433–41.

101. Pitkin J, Rees M. Urogenital atrophy. Menopause Int 2008; 14: 136–7.

102. Graziotin A. Sexuality and the menopause. In: Studd J, ed. The Management of the Menopause. Annual Review. London: Parthenon, 1998.

103. Dennerstein L, Lehert P, Burger H. The relative effects of hormones and relationship factors on sexual function of women through the natural menopause transition. Fertil Steril 2005; 84: 174–80.

104. Montgomerie JC, Appelby L, Brincat M, et al. Effect of oestrogen and testosterone implants on psychological disorder in the climacteric. Lancet 1987; i: 297–9.

105. Simon J, Braunstein G, Nachtigall L, et al. Testosterone patch increases sexual activity and desire in surgically menopausal women with hypoactive sexual desire disorder. J Clin Endocrinol Metab 2005; 90: 5226–33.

106. Davis SR, van der Mooren MJ, van Lunsen RH, et al. Efficacy and safety of a testosterone patch for the treatment of hypoactive sexual desire disorder in surgically menopausal women: a randomized, placebo-controlled trial. Menopause 2006; 13: 387–96.

107. Shifren JL, Davis SR, Moreau M, et al. Testosterone patch for the treatment of hypoactive sexual desire disorder in naturally menopausal women: results from the INTIMATE NM1 Study. Menopause 2006; 13: 770–9.

108. Egarter C, Topcuoglu A, Vogl S, Sator M. Hormone replacement therapy with tibolone: effects on sexual functioning in postmenopausal women. Acta Obstet Gynecol Scand 2002; 81: 649–53.

109. Gebbie A. Contraception in the perimenopause. In: Tomlinson JM, Rees M, Mander A, eds. Sexual Health and the Menopause. London: RSM Press, 2005: 47–54.

110. Whitehead MI, Whitcroft SIJ, Hillard TC. Atlas of the Menopause. Lancashire, UK: Parthenon, 1993.

57 Sports and Fitness Activities

Jeanette Haslam, Kari Bø, and Philip Toozs-Hobson

INTRODUCTION

Although urinary incontinence (UI) has been regarded as a problem of the postmenopausal, multiparous woman, it has also been shown in various groups of nulliparous young females (1–4). Athletes who are usually thought of being fit have also been found to have a high prevalence rate of UI (5–7). Prevalence data vary between 12% and 52%, and may be explained by differences in definitions, study design, and populations. The most common type of UI in women is stress urinary incontinence (SUI) (8), defined as involuntary leakage on effort, exertion, sneezing, or coughing (9).

ASSESSMENT OF INCONTINENCE DURING PHYSICAL ACTIVITY

Usually the diagnosis of urodynamic SUI is made during assessment in a static position and interestingly the original International Continence Society (ICS) pad test did not involve physical activity at all. However, subsequent standards have evolved to include activities such as stair climbing and jumping (9,10). Often women who are active may have a significant problem with vigorous exercise yet the test fails to reproduce symptoms. Methodologic problems in study design have meant that there is a lack of studies describing bladder and urethral function during physical activity. James (11) used ambulatory bladder pressure measurements to demonstrate peaks of bladder pressure rise during running and jumping which occurred when the feet touched the ground. Although pressure rise was higher during coughing, some women were leaking only during exercise. Two studies (12,13) designed tests based on physical activities. These involved running, jumping jacks, standing up and lying down, and abdominal curls, which were found to be nine times as provocative as the ICS test involving physical activity. The authors concluded that assessment of the degree of SUI has to be physically provocative to detect SUI.

Two studies have looked at the incidence of symptoms in college students In the United states; Nygaard et al. reported that 7% of women admitted to urine loss only during sports, and that 40% and 17% first noted UI during sport while in high school or junior high school, respectively (5). The second study had a low response rate which highlighted the difficulty of carrying out epidemiology studies on this subject. Of the 18 schools and colleges approached only two colleges and one high school completed and returned surveys. One principal refused to distribute the surveys after angry phone calls from parents. Although 550 surveys were provided to agreeing participants, only 171 were distributed to athletes of which 86 were returned completed. Of the completing surveys 28% reported SUI symptoms, with more than 91% of the respondents having never heard of pelvic floor muscle exercises (PFME). The author concluded that student athletes require more education on the matter (14).

Kulseng-Hanssen and Klevmark (15) attempted to assess pressure changes by placing bladder and urethral transducer catheters in a silicon cuff and sutured it to the external urethral opening to keep it stable during activity. Figure 57.1 demonstrates measurements of a patient with SUI during jumping and coughing. In 16 of the patients, 115 leakage episodes were seen in 45 minutes. In 92 of these episodes, the maximum urethral pressure decrease was larger than the detrusor pressure increase. However, some patients complained of urinary leakage during strenuous exercise (running and jumping for longer periods), although leakage was undetected even in this test. Similar results were seen in the study of Bø et al. (16) where the test did not detect leakage in four subjects with convincing history of urinary leakage.

These findings are consistent with striated muscle fatigue of the urethral wall and pelvic floor muscles, which will vary and require vigorous and continuous activities in certain women to provoke the leakage they experience outside the laboratory. This theory is supported by a study of 12 young nulliparous women with symptoms of mild SUI, that after 90 minutes of strenuous physical activity that they had lower maximal voluntary PFM contractions. The authors concluded that this indication of PFM fatigue needs further investigation regarding its long term impact (17). These results were confirmed a study of 157 athletes, it was reported that urine loss was more frequent during the second part of training or competition (18).

Conversely there was no difference found in the time to fatigue of the PFM (defined as rate of force loss) in 26 parous continent volunteers compared with 20 parous patients with SUI. Muscular fatigue did not appear to be associated with SUI, but the normalized force taking account of body weight was significantly reduced in the SUI group (19); however, this study did not have an absolute to compare baselines so it was possible that the symptomatic women started from a compromised postion.

Comparing change in foot arch flexibility in 47 continent and incontinent varsity athletes, Nygaard et al. (20) demonstrated a significant decreased foot flexibility in incontinent women (p < 0.03). They suggested that how impact forces are absorbed may be one etiologic factor for stress incontinence, and that more research is required to understand how impact forces are transmitted to the pelvic floor. The high prevalence of urine loss in gymnasts may be explained by the extremely high impact during landing and take-off and the transmission of this pressure to the pelvic floor.

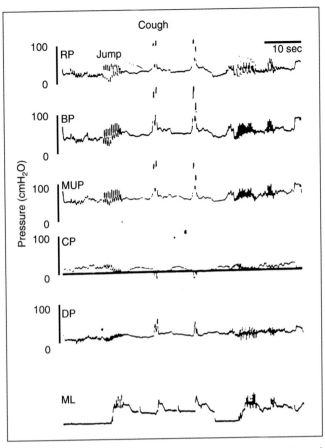

Figure 57.1 Trace from a stress incontinent patient during jumping and coughing. *Abbreviations*: BP, bladder pressure; CP, closure pressure; DP, detrusor pressure; ML, leakage; MUP, maximum urethral pressure; RP, rectal pressure. *Source*: Reproduced from Ref. 15.

PREVALENCE OF UI AMONG PARTICIPANTS IN SPORT AND FITNESS ACTIVITIES

SUI implies that urine loss occurs during an increase in abdominal pressure. Therefore, one may expect that women with this condition are likely to experience urine loss during participation in most forms of physical activity. Sedentary women are less exposed to physical exertions and therefore may prevent leakage from occurring, despite the underlying condition potentially being present. The literature on urine loss associated with sport and fitness activities is mostly based on epidemiologic studies.

Studies have demonstrated that SUI is common both among physical education/sport students, women who exercise for fitness, and female elite athletes with 26% of young physical education students reporting having urinary leakage during different forms of physical activity (21). A difference which was significant when compared to a group of sedentary nutrition students. It has also been shown that many physical activities—lifting, floor exercises, jogging, and the use of hydraulic exercise machines—although producing variable pressures were generally lower than those generated on cough. However individuals varied in the pressure exerted (22).

A further study of first year female students (n = 37) with a mean age 20.2 years demonstrated a prevalence of 38% of SUI symptoms. Eight of 13 women (61.5%) considered the leakage a social or hygienic problem (23), giving a prevalence using the former ICS definition of 21.6% for this population of physically fit, young, exercising nulliparous women. In this latter study, ambulatory urodynamic testing was used to verify urodynamic SUI. Seven women with symptoms were evaluated by urodynamics, and in six of seven urethral sphincter incompetence was confirmed. Mean leakage measured by pad test with standardized bladder volume was 12 g (range 0–46).

Nygaard et al. (4) studied incontinence and exercise in a group of 326 women presenting to private gynecology offices (response rate 50%). Eighty-nine percent were exercising at least once per week, with an average of three times per week for 30 to 60 minutes per session. Forty-seven percent reported some degree of UI.

Alenee's study (7) investigated the type of exercise and reported on 173 women participating in the high perineal impact sport of horse riding took place to determine if the subjects had increased sexual dysfunction and lower urinary tract symptoms (LUTS). Hundred and two female swimmers were used as a control as a low perineal impact sport. Bicycling habits were investigated in both groups as a possible confounding factor. It was found that the horseback riding did not increase the risk of female urinary tract nor show a connection to sexual dysfunction. However, there was a trend towards a protective association between horseback riding and stress incontinence (p = 0.0567). It was hypothesized that as equestrians carry their body weight in their stirrups part of the time, it may lead to strengthened pelvic floor musculature. It must also be noted that good posture in riding depends on good trunk stability perhaps implicating the role of the core stability musculature. The hardness of bicycle seat (p = 0.02) and years of cycling (p = 0.04) were associated with an increased prevalence for LUTS in women—this was thought to be related to neurological and vascular stress.

Further studies on type of sport were summarized in a systematic review (21) examining prevalence studies up to 2004, and found a variation in prevalence between sports, from zero in golfers up to 80% in high impact sports. The most quoted paper (4) asked women whether they had ever experienced urinary leakage during participation in sports and during coughing, sneezing, heavy lifting, walking to the bathroom, sleeping, and upon hearing the sound of running water. They rated frequency of leakage in a five-point scale. Twenty-eight percent reported urine loss while participating in their sports. There was a tendency in two-thirds of these women to be incontinent frequently rather than rarely. Sixteen percent were incontinent during practice sessions and 14% during competition. Forty-two percent reported urine loss during at least one of the activities of daily life, 18% more often than rarely. Twenty-one percent reported urine loss only during daily life and not during sports, and 7% noted incontinence only during sports. A similar study (23) compared prevalence of symptoms of UI in Norwegian elite athletes and age-matched controls and found a prevalence of 41% and 39% of SUI, and 16% and 19% of urge incontinence in athletes and controls, respectively.

A further study (24) looked at whether high impact activity contributes to later UI and compared former female Olympians who had competed in swimming (low impact) and gymnastics or track and field (high impact). One hundred and four women participated (response rate 51%). When doing their sport as Olympians, high impact athletes had higher prevalence (36%) compared to low impact athletes (4.5%). However, when studied more than 20 years after cessation of the sport, there was no significant difference in prevalence of incontinence between the groups. It was concluded that participation in regular, strenuous, high impact activity when younger did not predispose to significant urinary leakage later in life.

CONSEQUENCES OF SUI DURING PHYSICAL ACTIVITY

UI may lead to withdrawal from social activities and reduction of well-being (25). Norton et al. (26) reported that urinary leakage frequently interfered with daily life in more than 50% of their study group. Additionally, Fall et al. (27) reported that, in their study of women with incontinence, 42% had problems during sport and physical activities.

Bø et al. (28) showed that two-thirds of sedentary women with urodynamic SUI reported urinary leakage to be the cause of inactivity. Of 52 women participating in specific sport and fitness activities, 27 had withdrawn from one or more activities because of leakage. Of these 27 women, 19 had withdrawn from aerobic and dance activities, despite these being among the most popular fitness activities for women. They all reported that the major leakage occurred during high impact activities during the aerobics session, especially when performing "jumping jacks" (jumping with legs in subsequent abduction and adduction), which is one of the most commonly used high impact exercises in aerobic dance and general fitness programs.

This corresponds with the results of Nygaard et al. (4) where women reported leakage with running and high impact aerobics. Thirty percent of the exercisers noted incontinence during at least one type of exercise. Twenty percent of these women stopped doing the activity solely because of incontinence, 18% changed the way they performed an exercise, and 55% wore a pad during exercise. Frequency, time spent per session, and duration of a particular exercise had no significant impact on the prevalence.

Brown and Miller (29) concluded that UI was an important barrier to women's participation in physical activities. Regular physical activity is an important factor for women's health at all ages. Moderate physical activity can be one important factor in prevention of coronary heart disease, high blood pressure, osteoporosis, musculoskeletal diseases, obesity, breast and colon cancer, anxiety, and depression (30).

A broad population of women aged 18 to 60 years in U.S. households with mixed educational levels, income, and race were mailed questionnaires regarding UI and exercise. Three thousand five hundred and sixty two questionnaires were completed (68% response rate), of which 3,364 were analyzed. One in seven of the women experienced urine loss during exercise and one in eight perceived leakage to be a moderate barrier to exercise. This percentage increased to 85% in those

groups of women with more severe incontinence. Urine loss in the last 30 days was a predictor of barrier to participation in sport. Those with both symptoms of both stress and urge incontinence were more likely to perceive leakage as a barrier than those with either type alone. Overall, incontinence was a moderate or substantial barrier to exercise for 9.8% women, 25% of women perceiving at least monthly UI being a barrier to them participating in exercise (31).

In an Italian study of 679 women involved in non-competitive sporting activity, 101 (14.9%) women complained of UI of which 32 complained of UI only during sporting activities (31.7% of those with UI), 48 during daily life, and 21 in both circumstances. The highest rates of UI were in basketball, athletics, tennis, or squash. 10.4% abandoned favorite sport and 20% limited the way they practiced their sport (32).

CAN PHYSICAL ACTIVITY CAUSE UI?

Several risk factors have been suggested for development of female UI; hereditary weak connective tissue, weak or non-functional pelvic floor muscles, hormonal factors, dyssynergia between detrusor, and urethral smooth and striated muscle activity, pregnancy, vaginal delivery, heavy physical exertion, inactivity, obesity, cigarette smoking, menopause, and old age are frequently cited as being etiologic factors. To date there is little evidence supporting a strong causal effect for many of these factors. The reality is that UI has a multifactorial etiology in women, including failure of one or more factors to compensate for another weak factor. The speed and strength of the pelvic floor muscle contraction may be one such important factor (33).

Optimal pelvic floor muscle function implies a localization of the pelvic floor in an adequate anatomic position, with sufficient cross-sectional area to give structural support for the vagina, bladder, and the urethra in order to prevent descent during an increase in the abdominal pressure (34). The muscles have to be in a neurologic state of "readiness for action," allowing an appropriate quick and strong response, or be a part of a feed forward loop, contracting automatically simultaneously with, or before, the intra-abdominal pressure increase.

In a study of 331women, former elite athletes found them no more likely to have SUI or urge urinary incontinence later in life than a control group (n = 640) from the same geographical area in Norway. High impact sports seemed to make no difference to outcomes either at that time or later. However, urinary leakage during competitive sport was strongly associated with UI 15 years later. No such control group association could be determined as they were not questioned about their original continence status (35).

Pelvic Floor Muscles and Female Athletes

Typically, there are two theories about female athletes and pelvic floor muscles strength, which go in opposing directions (21). The first hypothesis is that general physical activity may lead to strengthening of the pelvic floor, thus making the pelvic floor muscles in female athletes stronger. To date, no research has verified this hypothesis. The fact that so many female athletes report SUI (21) actually contradicts this view.

This second theory is supported by the observations from translabial ultrasonography imaging in a group of 24 high-impact, frequent intense training (HIFIT) female athletes compared with 22 controls (36) demonstrating a higher mean diameter of the pubovisceral muscle (pubococcygeus + puborectalis), greater bladder neck descent and larger hiatal area on Valsalva maneuver in the athletes. The authors hypothesize the changes in connective tissue or muscle biomechanics occur prior to, or as a result of training.

The second hypothesis is that heavy exercise (e.g., marathon running with repetitive bouncing towards the pelvic floor or weight lifting) may overload the pelvic floor and weaken the muscles over time. Nichols and Randall (37) proposed that women exposed to chronic straining may have increased prevalence of genital prolapse because of connective tissue damage as a result of persistent intra-abdominal pressure increase. Nichols and Milley (38) suggested that the cardinal and uterosacral ligaments, pelvic floor muscles, and the connective tissue of the perineum may be damaged chronically because of repeatedly increased abdominal pressure due to, for example, manual work and chronic cough. According to this theory, strenuous exercise raising the abdominal pressure may contribute to development of SUI in women with a predisposition to incontinence.

This is supported by two linked studies (39,40) utilizing recruits to the U.S. military academy were examined prior to and after training. It was have found on first assessment that 50% of the women studied had stage 1 or 11 pelvic support and 19% reported UI (n = 147).

At the second examination after six weeks of various types of training, stage 1 support had increased from 46% to 54% and stage 2 from 2% to 22%. Of those undergoing paratrooper training, 14 of the 37 women had newly observed stage two prolapse. This therefore shows paratrooper training to be a significant risk factor for the development of stage 11 prolapse or decrease in pelvic support. The rate of incontinence post training had increased from 15% to 21%. But the researchers were unable to show a relationship between urine loss and paratrooper training. Davis and Goodman (41) also studied 512 female airborne infantry and found that nine developed UI during the training period. Urodynamic investigation demonstrated SUI in six of the women. All six demonstrated a definite cystourethrocele, a hypermobile vesical neck with loss of the posterior ureterovesical angle, and visible urine loss with Valsalva after the training period. Four reported feeling a tearing pain in their lower quadrant on impact during a parachute jump, and one subject related a similar event during heavy lifting and doing sit-ups. Parachute jumping is an extreme high impact activity, and from the data available today, it is not possible to conclude whether moderate to high impact activities can cause connective tissue or pelvic floor muscle damage. It is likely that there is a self-selection of continent women who undertake high impact sports and fitness activities.

Another contributing factor for SUI in female elite athletes may be hypothalamic amenorrhea due to either intensive exercise or eating disorders (or a combination of both), with resultant low estrogen levels (4). However, the association between low estrogen levels and prevalence of SUI is not clear (42). Most women in the studies of Nygaard et al. and Bø et al. who reported and demonstrated SUI had regular menstrual cycles (4,21). However, in the study by Bø and Sundgot-Borgen (23), a higher prevalence of SUI was found in those with eating disorders. Eating disorders may be associated with low estrogen levels.

Young mostly nulliparous women with a history of regular organized high impact trampoline training were found to have a higher prevalence of UI than normals. Those who only trained recreationally prior to the menarche had the same prevalence rate as the normal population. Relevant factors were: years of training after the menarche, training frequency, more advanced jumps and number of years trampolining (43). There is therefore an inference of dose response and hormonal considerations affecting the subjects. The most influential risk variable for urinary leakage in the group was an inability to stop midstream with constipation strongly associated (44).

Protection During Exercise to Prevent Leakage

Because of the health benefits of regular moderate exercise, it is important to emphasize that women should be encouraged to continue exercising despite their urinary leakage. However, they can be advised about changing to low impact activities; for example, walking, Nordic walking, dancing, low impact aerobics, step training, cycling, swimming, cross-country skiing, etc., which may carry a lower risk of precipitating symptoms.

Although the present evidence for the benefit of transversus abdominus (TrA) training with or without PFM training for the treatment of female UI is insufficient (45), TrA training is still advocated as an unproven possible contribution to the prevention of UI (Fig. 57.2). In which case a TrA contraction is facilitated by the patient adopting a comfortable position in a four point kneeling, supine crook, side, or prone lying ideally with the lumbar spine in a neutral position. The instruction is to slowly draw in the lower abdomen and hold the contraction for up to 10 seconds, repeated 10 times whilst breathing normally (46). A simultaneous contraction of the pelvic floor muscles should take place at the same time as the TrA contraction and any substitution strategies corrected. During exercise the woman should be encouraged to use specially designed

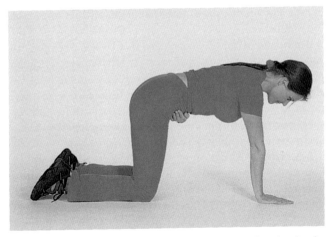

Figure 57.2 Training the transversus abdominis muscle. Hold one hand under the lower abdomen and lift the navel towards the spine without curving the back.

protection. Fortunately, some of the best protecting pads are now manufactured in small sizes, making active women more comfortable when wearing them while exercising. In addition, women may use urethral or vaginal devices to prevent leakage during physical activity (47,48). In the study of Glavind (49), six women with stress incontinence demonstrated total dryness when using a vaginal device during 30 minutes of aerobic exercise. However training of the TrA should not be seen as a substitution for PFME training. It has been shown that instructing contraction of the PFM is more effective than TrA contraction in reducing the levator hiatus in women with grade 1to 2 pelvic organ prolapse score. It is further recommended that a co-contraction of the PFM be confirmed prior to suggesting indirect training via the TrA (50).

TREATMENT

No studies have been found that evaluate any treatment methods for UI in a defined subgroup of athletes. Generally, the least invasive treatment should be tried first (51,52), with pelvic floor muscle training being the method recommended as first line treatment. In addition, as female elite athletes are mostly young and nulliparous, surgery is not recommended.

On reviewing the literature the Cochrane reviewers conclude that pelvic floor muscle training helps women with all types of incontinence although the women that benefit most are those with stress incontinence who exercise for three months or more. They further hypothesize that the treatment effect might be greater in younger women (in their 40s and 50s) who participate in a supervised PFMT program but this requires further investigation (53).

Bø et al. (28) demonstrated that after specific strength training of the pelvic floor muscles, 17 of 23 women had reduced leakage during jumping and running, and 15 during lifting. In addition, significant improvement was obtained while dancing, hiking, during general group exercise, and in an overall score on ability to participate in different activities (28). Measured with a pad test with a standardized bladder volume, tests comprising running, jumping jacks, and sit-ups showed a significant reduction in urine loss from a mean of 27 to 7.1 g $p < 0.01$ (54).

There appear to be no published data on the effect of pelvic floor muscle training in treatment of female elite athletes. However, as these women are accustomed to conducting regular training and are highly motivated for exercise, one would expect that the effect would be equally effective or even more effective in this specific group of women. Pelvic floor muscle training should be the first choice of treatment for several reasons: When conducted appropriately it has proved to be effective. It is physiological with no known side effects that can be very cost effective compared to other treatment modalities. The woman herself is able to control her health: she learns body awareness and, if successful, the training may enhance self-esteem and coping strategies.

CONCLUSIONS

SUI is prevalent in exercising women at all levels. This may well be because the activity "unmasks" a predisposition to leak as it is yet not possible to conclude whether strenuous physical activity may cause SUI or pelvic organ prolapse. Current understanding certainly suggests that more vigorous exercise is associated with higher rates of leakage and that women with such problems restrict their physical activities. More research is needed to understand how impact from different exercises may affect pelvic organs, connective tissue, and pelvic floor muscles. The effect of pelvic floor muscle training on elite athletes has not yet been evaluated. However, from current knowledge on the effect of pelvic floor muscle training, this is suggested as the first choice of treatment. Surgery, whilst outside the scope of this chapter is also in certain circumstances an appropriate option in these women.

REFERENCES

1. Jolleys J. Reported prevalence of urinary incontinence in women in a general practice. BMJ 1988; 296: 1300–2.
2. Bø K, Mæhlum S, Oseid S, Larsen S. Prevalence of stress urinary incontinence among physically active and sedentary female students. Scand J Sports Sci 1989; 11: 113–16.
3. Simeonova Z, Bengtsson C. Prevalence of urinary incontinence among women at a Swedish primary health care centre. Scand J Prim Health Care 1990; 8: 203–6.
4. Nygaard I, DeLancey JOL, Arnsdorf L, Murphy E. Exercise and incontinence. Obstet Gynecol 1990; 75: 848–51.
5. Nygaard I, Thompson FL, Svengalis SL, Albright JP. Urinary incontinence in elite nulliparous athletes. Obstet Gynecol 1994; 84: 183–7.
6. Eliasson K, Edner A, Mattsson E. Urinary incontinence in very young and mostly nulliparous women with a history of regular organised high-impact trampoline training: occurrence and risk factors. Int Urogynecol J 2008; 19: 687–96.
7. Alanee S, Heiner J, Liu N, Monga M. Horseback riding: impact on sexual dysfunction and lower urinary tract symptoms in men and women. Urology 2009; 73: 109–14.
8. Hunskaar S, Burgio K, Diokno A, et al. Epidemiology and natural history of urinary incontinence in women. Urology 2003; 62(Suppl 4A): 16–23.
9. Abrams P, Cardozo L, Fall M, et al. The standardization of terminology of lower urinary tract function: report from the Standardisation Subcommittee of the International Continence Society. Neurourol Urodyn 2002; 21: 167–78.
10. Abrams P, Blaivas JG, Stanton SL, Andersen JT. The standardisation of terminology of lower urinary tract function. Scand J Urol Nephrol Suppl 1988; 114: 5–19.
11. James ED. The behaviour of the bladder during physical activity. Br J Urol 1978; 50: 387–94.
12. Henalla SM, Kirwan P, Castleden DM, Hutchins CJ, Breeson AJ. The effect of pelvic floor muscle exercises in the treatment of genuine stress incontinence in women at two hospitals. Br J Obstet Gynaecol 1988; 95: 81–92.
13. Hagen RH, Kvarstein B, Bø K, Larsen S. A simple pad test with fixed bladder volume to measure urine loss during physical activity. International Continence Society Annual Meeting, Oslo. 1988; 88–9.
14. Carls C. The prevalence of stress urinary incontinence in high school and college-age female athletes in the midwest: implications for education and prevention. Urol Nurs 2007; 27: 21–4.
15. Kulseng-Hanssen S, Klevmark B. Ambulatory urethro-cystorectometry: a new technique. Neurourol Urodyn 1988; 7: 119–30.
16. Bø K, Stien R, Kulseng-Hanssen S, Kristoffersen M. Clinical and urodynamic assessment of nulliparous young women with and without stress incontinence symptoms: a case control study. Obstet Gynecol 1994; 84: 1028–32.
17. Ree ML, Nygaard I, Bø K. Muscular fatigue in the pelvic floor muscles after strenuous physical activity. Acta Obstet Gynecol Scand 2007; 86: 870–6.
18. Caylet N, Fabbro-Peray P, Marès P, et al. Prevalence and occurrence of stress urinary incontinence in elite women athletes. Can J Urol 2006; 13: 3174–9.

19. Verelst M, Leivseth G. Are fatigue and disturbances in pre-programmed activity of pelvic floor muscles associated with female stress urinary incontinence? Neurourol Urodyn 2004; 23: 143–7.

20. Nygaard IE, Glowacki C, Saltzman L. Relationship between foot flexibility and urinary incontinence in nulliparous varsity athletes. Obstet Gynecol 1996; 87: 1049–51.

21. Bø K. Urinary incontinence, pelvic floor dysfunction, exercise and sport. Sports Med 2004; 34: 451–64.

22. O'Dell KK, Morse AN, Crawford SL, Howard A. Vaginal pressure during lifting, floor exercises, jogging and use of hydraulic exercise machines. Int Urogynecol J 2007; 18: 1481–9.

23. Bø K, Sundgot-Borgen J. Prevalence of stress and urge urinary incontinence in elite athletes and controls. Med Sci Sports Exer 2001; 33: 1797–802.

24. Nygaard IE. Does prolonged high-impact activity contribute to later urinary incontinence? A retrospective cohort study of female Olympians. Obstet Gynecol 1997; 90: 718–22.

25. Papanicolaou S, Hunskaar S, Lose G, Sykes D. Assessment of bothersomeness and impact on quality of life of urinary incontinence in women in France, Germany, Spain and the UK. BJU Int 2005; 96: 831–8.

26. Norton P, MacDonald LD, Sedgwick PM, Stanton SL. Distress and delay associated with urinary incontinence, frequency, and urgency in women. BMJ 1988; 297: 1187–9.

27. Fall M, Frankenberg S, Frisen M, Larsson B, Petren M. 456 000 svenskar kan ha urininkontinens. Endast var fjærde søker hjelp før besværen. Laekartidningen 1985; 82: 2054–6.

28. Bø K, Hagen R, Kvarstein B, Larsen S. Female stress urinary incontinence and participation in different sport and social activities. Scand J Sports Sci 1989; 11: 117–21.

29. Brown W, Miller Y. Too wet to exercise? Leaking urine as a barrier to physical activity in women. J Sci Med Sport 2001; 4: 373–8.

30. Bouchard C, Shephard RJ, Stephens T. Physical activity, fitness, and health. Consensus Statement. Champaign, IL: Human Kinetics, 1993.

31. Nygaard I, Girts T, Fultz NH, et al. Is urinary incontinence a barrier to exercise in women? Obstet Gynecol 2005; 106: 307–14.

32. Salvatore S, Serati M, Laterza RM, et al. The impact of urinary stress incontinence in young and middle-age women practicing recreational sport activity: an epidemiological study. Br J Sports Med 2009; 43: 1115–8.

33. Lose G. Simultaneous recording of pressure and cross-sectional area in the female urethra: a study of urethral closure function in healthy and stress incontinent women. Neurourol Urodyn 1992; 11: 54–89.

34. Bø K. Pelvic floor muscle training is effective in treatment of stress urinary incontinence, but how does it work? Int Urogynecol J 2004; 15: 76–84.

35. Bø K, Sundgot-Borgen J. Are former female elite athletes more likely to experience urinary incontinence later in life than non-athletes? Scand J Med Sc Sports 2010; 20: 100–4.

36. Kruger JA, Dietz HP, Murphy BA. Pelvic floor function in elite nulliparous athletes. Ultrasound Obstet Gynecol 2007; 30: 81–5.

37. Nichols DH, Randall CL 3rd, eds. Vaginal Surgery. Baltimore: Williams and Wilkins, 1989.

38. Nichols DH, Milley PS. Functional pelvic anatomy: the soft tissue supports and spaces of the female pelvic organs. The Human Vagina. Amsterdam: Elsevier/North-Holland Biomedical Press, 1978; 21–37.

39. Larsen WI, Yavorek TA. Pelvic organ prolapse and urinary incontinence in nulliparous women at the United States military academy. Int Urogynecol J 2006; 17: 208–10.

40. Larsen WI, Yavorek T. Pelvic prolapse and urinary incontinence in nulliparous college women in relation to paratrooper training. Int Urogynecol J 2007; 18: 769–71.

41. Davis GD, Goodman M. Stress urinary incontinence in nulliparous female soldiers in airborne infantry training. J Pelvic Surg 1996; 2: 68–71.

42. Fantl JA, Cardozo L, McClish DK. Estrogen therapy in the management of urinary incontinence in postmenopausal women: a meta analysis. First report of the hormones and urogenital therapy committee. Obstet Gynecol 1994; 83: 12–18.

43. Eliasson K, Larsson T, Mattson E. Prevalence of stress incontinence in nulliparous elite trampolinists. Scand J Med Sci Sports 2002; 12: 106–10.

44. Eliasson K, Nordlander I, Larson B, Hammarström M, Mattsson E. Influence of physical activity on urinary leakage in primiparous women. Scand J Med Sci Sports 2005; 15: 87–94.

45. Bo K, Morkved S, Frawley H, Sherburn M. Evidence for the benefit of transversus abdominis training alone or in combination with pelvic floor muscle training to treat female urinary incontinence: a systematic review. Neurourol Urodyn 2009; 28: 368–73.

46. Jones RC. Pelvic floor stability and trunk muscle coactivation. In: Haslam J, Laycock J, eds. Therapeutic Management of Incontinence and Pelvic Pain, 2nd edn. London: Springer Verlag 2008; 99–104.

47. Thyssen HH, Lose G. Long-term efficacy and safety of a disposable vaginal device (continence guard) in the treatment of female stress incontinence. Int Urogynecol J 1997; 8: 130–3.

48. Staskin D, Bavendam T, Miller J. Effectiveness of a urinary control insert in the management of stress urinary incontinence; results of a multicenter study. Urology 1996; 47: 629–36.

49. Glavind K. Use of a vaginal sponge during aerobic exercises in patients with stress urinary incontinence. Int Urogynecol J 1997;8:351–3.

50. Bø K, Braaekken IH, Majida M, Engh ME. Constriction of the levator hiatus during instruction of pelvic floor or transversus abdominis contraction: a 4D study. Int Urogynecol J 2009; 20: 27–32.

51. Fantl JA, Newman DK, Colling J, et al. Urinary incontinence in adults: acute and chronic management. 2, update [96-0682]. Rockville, MD: U.S. Department of Health and Human Services, Public Health Service, Agency for Health Care Policy and Research, 1996; 1–154.

52. Wilson PD, Bø KH-SJ, Nygaard I, et al. Conservative treatment in women. In: Abrams P, Cardozo L, Khoury S, Wein A, eds. Incontinence. Plymouth, UK: Health Publication, 2002; 571–624.

53. Hay-Smith J, Dumoulin C. Pelvic floor muscle training versus no treatment, or inactive control treatments, for urinary incontinence in women. Cochrane collaboration. Cochrane database syst Rev 2006; (1): CD005654.

54. Bø K, Hagen RH, Kvarstein B, Jørgensen J, Larsen S. Pelvic floor muscle exercise for the treatment of female stress urinary incontinence: III. Effects of two different degrees of pelvic floor muscle exercise. Neurourol Urodyn 1990; 9: 489–502.

58 Anal Incontinence
Tony Mak and Simon Radley

INTRODUCTION

Anal incontinence is the involuntary loss of solid or liquid stool per rectum. It is personally and socially incapacitating and only a half of sufferers will volunteer their symptoms spontaneously if not asked directly (1). Although it affects men and women of all ages, incontinence is eight times more common in women than in men at the age of 45, implicating obstetric factors in the etiology. A study from Birmingham found that 4% of women develop fecal incontinence following childbirth (2). The focus of this chapter is on obstetric injuries, which are the underlying cause of anal incontinence in most women, but other causes must be considered (Table 58.1). The principles of management are broadly similar whatever the etiology. Vaginal delivery is the most important etiologic factor in postobstetric anal incontinence.

Two principal mechanisms are responsible for the development of fecal incontinence following vaginal delivery:

- direct injury to the sphincter muscle itself; and
- damage to the nerves supplying the pelvic floor or anal sphincter.

Less frequently, new symptomatic anal incontinence may occur in women following cesarean delivery.

PATHOGENESIS
Sphincter Injury

Direct damage to the sphincter muscles is responsible for anal incontinence in most of the women who present early after childbirth. Sphincter injuries are more common in primiparous women; new sphincter injuries are less common with subsequent deliveries (3). Up to 35% of primiparas have been reported to have sphincter injury, however some remain asymptomatic (4). Other risk factors or associations for sphincter injury include large babies, forceps delivery, a prolonged second stage of labor, and occipitoposterior presentation (5). Some authors have raised doubts on posterolateral episiotomy and claims that it does not protect against sphincter injury (6).

It has become clear that following vaginal delivery anal sphincter injuries may be unrecognized or misclassified as a less severe injury. When perineal examination is undertaken by a trained clinician immediately following delivery, the incidence of detected sphincter injury may be significantly increased (7). Some sphincter defects may be truly occult, occurring with minimal or no perineal injury, where the mechanism is likely to be tissue shearing during delivery. However, there is a notable variation in incidence of recognized third-degree tears between centers publishing their data (8). The observation that women with second-degree tears are the group most likely to develop anal incontinence postpartum (9)

further suggests that a proportion of anal sphincter injury remains undetected following delivery. Even when sphincter damage is recognized and repaired at the time of delivery, up to 85% of women still have identifiable sphincter defects and around 50% of women have some symptoms of anal incontinence (5).

The development of incontinence later in life is more likely to be multifactorial in origin, resulting from a combination of one or more factors including sphincter damage, progressive neuropathy, muscle atrophy, hormonal changes (10), and alteration in bowel function (11).

Neurologic Damage

Prolonged pudendal nerve motor terminal latencies (PNMTL) have been demonstrated in a third of primigravidae following vaginal delivery (12). These usually revert back to normal, but up to a third remain prolonged at six months. Prolonged PNMTL is not necessarily associated with incontinence. After emergency cesarean section late in labor, pudendal nerve latencies may be increased, implicating damage to the nerves supplying the pelvic floor or sphincter (13). In some women, electromyographic studies revealed increased fiber density in the external sphincter consistent with damage to sphincter innervation. Pudendal nerve damage and increased fiber density were seen more frequently in multiparae, suggesting that nerve damage may be cumulative with subsequent deliveries. The development of neurogenic incontinence is likely to be a progressive process, rather than an acute event at the time of delivery, and therefore may be exacerbated by subsequent deliveries or prolonged straining.

PATIENT ASSESSMENT

The maintenance of continence is a complex process involving an interrelationship between intestinal function, rectal sensitivity and compliance, and anal sphincter function. This in turn depends upon the integrity of sensory and motor neural pathways and the sphincter musculature itself. The anal sphincter complex comprises two muscles—an inner circular smooth muscle maintaining constant tone and largely responsible for resting anal canal tone (14), and an outer striated muscle under voluntary control which can be contracted to defer defecation when appropriate (15).

History

Careful questioning can give a clue to the etiology of incontinence. A change in bowel habit to increased frequency and looseness may precipitate anal incontinence and could be suggestive of underlying colorectal disease. Urgency of defecation with reduced warning time (sometimes to only a few minutes) indicates loss of voluntary muscle control and suggests damage

Table 58.1 Etiology of Fecal Incontinence

Traumatic
• Obstetric
• Accident/injury
• Surgical

Colorectal disease
• Rectal prolapse
• Inflammatory bowel disease
• Hemorrhoids
• Neoplasia
• Fistulae

Congenital
• Anal atresia

Neurological
• Cerebral
• Spinal
• Peripheral

Miscellaneous
• Impaction
• Behavioral
• Immobility

Table 58.3 Investigations for Anal Incontinence

Investigation	Information
Imaging/structural	
Colonoscopy/barium enema/sigmoidoscopy	Underlying colorectal pathology precipitating or contributing to incontinence
Endoanal ultrasound (EAUS)	Integrity of internal and external anal sphincter
	Thickness of internal anal sphincter
	Fistulae
Magnetic resonance imaging (MRI)	Integrity of internal and external anal sphincter
Functional	
Manometry	Resting anal canal pressure
	Voluntary squeeze pressure
	Involuntary squeeze pressure
	Functional anal canal length
Rectal sensation and compliance	Rectal hypo/hypersensitivity
	Normal or reduced compliance
Pudendal nerve motor terminal latency (PNMTL)	Damage to pudendal nerves

Table 58.2 St Mark's Incontinence Scoring System (16)

	Never	Rarely (<1/mo)	Sometimes (<1/wk)	Usually (<1/day)	Always (daily)
Solid	0	1	2	3	4
Liquid	0	1	2	3	4
Gas	0	1	2	3	4
Lifestyle	0	1	2	3	4
Need to wear plug/pad/change underwear for soiling				No 0	Yes 2
Taking constipating medicine				0	2
Lack of ability to defer defecation for 15 min				0	2
Total score = /24					

to the striated external anal sphincter or its nerve supply. Similarly, incontinence associated with vigorous activity or coughing suggests a deficiency of external sphincter function. Incontinence occurring between episodes of defecation with no call to stool, or the involuntary passage of flatus, indicates a poor anal canal resting tone and suggests damage or degeneration of the internal sphincter muscle. Inability to discriminate solid stool from flatus suggests damage to anorectal sensory pathways. Seepage or perineal soiling may be seen in situations where there is distortion of the anal canal by scarring or in the presence of a fistula. A careful medical history should be taken with specific attention to colonic function, previous anorectal surgery, and any potential causes of anal incontinence. An obstetric history should include details of birth weight, mode of delivery, length of labor, instrumental delivery, and details of any perineal trauma. Scoring systems, such as the St Marks score (16) (Table 58.2), Wexner score (also known as Cleveland Clinic Florida Incontinence scoring system) (17), and Birmingham bowel and urinary symptoms questionnaire (BBUSQ-22) (18) may be used to quantify anal incontinence and for audit or research (16). Their role may also include

assessing treatment outcome in terms of cure or improvement in symptoms.

Examination

Physical examination should include inspection of the perineum, noting scarring from previous surgery or obstetric trauma. Voluntary contraction of the external sphincter can be seen and defects in the sphincter may be observed. Gaping of the anus at rest or on gentle perineal traction suggests a low resting tone and impaired internal anal sphincter function. Descent of the perineum at rest with accentuation on straining suggests pelvic floor weakness, pudendal neuropathy, or both. Straining may also reveal an unsuspected rectal prolapse. Perineal sensation can be tested by light touch and pinprick. Digital examination will allow crude assessment of resting anal tone and voluntary squeeze pressure, and any sphincter defects may be palpable.

Investigation

Special investigations can provide useful information in the management of women with incontinence (Table 58.3). Presentation with new anal incontinence, particularly in middle age, may be precipitated by a change in frequency or consistency of stool. Routine examination of the colon by barium enema or colonoscopy should be carried out to detect the presence of colonic pathology such as neoplasia or colitis. Clinical assessment of the pelvic floor and anal sphincters should be combined with anorectal physiologic studies. Manometry allows measurement of functional anal canal length and of the resting and squeeze pressures. These provide objective evidence of internal and external anal sphincter function, respectively (19). Anal canal sensation can be tested using a stimulating electrode and may be transiently impaired by vaginal delivery. Rectal sensation and compliance are usually measured by balloon distension. It is important that the rectum is compliant for preservation of continence. Inflammatory bowel disease, radiation proctitis, rectal prolapse, and diabetes can affect the rectal capacity and compliance. Measurement of PNMTL assesses pudendal nerve function by stimulating the pudendal nerve on each side and measuring the evoked response in the external anal sphincter (20). Normal latencies do not necessarily exclude pudendal nerve damage.

Endoanal ultrasonography (EAUS) has revolutionized the understanding of anal canal anatomy (Figs. 58.1, 58.2). Both the internal and external anal sphincters can be visualized and EAUS is the investigation of choice for detection of defects in these sphincters (21). The detection of sphincter defects enables clinicians to select women to undergo surgical sphincter repair, and the accuracy of EAUS for detecting sphincter disruption has been validated by correlation with operative findings (22). Abnormal thinning of the internal sphincter can be measured accurately using EAUS; this may be indicative of idiopathic degeneration, whereas thickening of the muscle may be associated with prolapse syndromes.

Magnetic resonance imaging (MRI) using an endoanal coil provides excellent multiplanar views of the sphincter complex and can demonstrate defects in both the internal and external

anal sphincters. It is probably most useful in identifying abnormalities in the external anal sphincter, the outer border of which may be difficult to visualize using EAUS. Expertise in MRI of the sphincters is not widely available and most clinicians continue to rely on EAUS. Where both imaging facilities are available, one or both may be used for diagnosis since they are complementary.

MANAGEMENT

Early Recognition of Obstetric Injuries

Evidence of sphincter injury should be sought by careful bimanual examination in all women who have a perineal tear or who have had an instrumental delivery. This should be carried out by someone trained in the recognition of sphincter injury. In the United Kingdom, there are a number of courses specifically for training obstetricians in the identification and management of obstetric sphincter injuries. An adjunct to bimanual examination is the use of EAUS in the delivery suite immediately postpartum. This is acceptable to women and can be used to diagnose sphincter injury and to assess the integrity of any repair (23). Once recognized, repair of a sphincter injury should be carried out by someone adequately trained to do so, in an operating theatre under regional or general anesthetic. Training in repair of sphincter injury should be part of the obstetric training program as the adequacy of sphincter repair is related to the experience of the operator (24). At postnatal follow-up visits, women should be asked directly about anal incontinence as they are about other postpartum symptoms. Increased general awareness of the risk of postobstetric sphincter injury among midwifery and obstetric staff will also aid in the early diagnosis and treatment of anal incontinence. Early follow-up in a multidisciplinary clinic of women who have sustained obstetric trauma further increases the recognition of residual sphincter injury and enables effective early intervention where necessary (25).

Conservative Therapy

For most women, symptoms are relatively minor and should be managed conservatively, interventional procedures being reserved for those women with severe symptoms or in whom conservative measures fail.

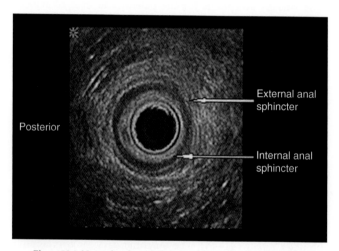

Figure 58.1 Normal endoanal ultrasound immediately postpartum.

Lifestyle

Attention to diet or the addition of a bulking agent such as ispaghula husk can improve symptoms in some individuals. Encouraging a daily routine for defecation may also help. The use of barrier creams to prevent excoriation of perianal skin as a result of stool leakage is encouraged.

Drugs

Antidiarrheal agents such as codeine phosphate or loperamide reduce colonic motility and increase fluid absorption, producing more manageable formed stools. However their side effects may include nausea, constipation, and abdominal cramping. The use of enemas or rectal washouts may help some women. The enema induces a bowel action and keeps the rectum empty between bowel movements.

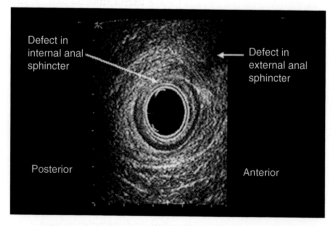

Figure 58.2 Defects in internal and external anal sphincters.

Amitriptyline at low dose may be of benefit for some women with anal incontinence. Study has demonstrated its value, particularly for those with faecal urgency and increased rectal sensitivity by increasing transit time and decreasing the amplitude and frequency of rectal motor complexes respectively (26).

There have been some reports of duloxetine hydrochloride helping women with fecal incontinence. Whether in the future this represents a viable treatment option remains to be seen.

Biofeedback

Biofeedback therapy can be helpful for some women with anal incontinence. It is a behavioral technique using equipment which provides auditory or visual feedback to alter physiologic events (27). The technique uses electromyography (EMG), where a sensing device monitoring external sphincter contraction is connected to a transducer producing an audio or visual response for the woman. The audiovisual record of sphincter activity assists the woman in recognizing strength and length of contraction. Using a balloon to distend the rectum, women are encouraged to improve sphincter contraction in response to decreasing rectal distension, so that over a period of time their response becomes automatic. These techniques are most useful for women who are well motivated, have some rectal sensation, and are able to contract the external sphincter voluntarily.

In a series of 100 patients treated with biofeedback, 43 regarded themselves as cured and 24 symptomatically improved (28). Interestingly, 27 of the 46 patients in this series with structural sphincter damage also reported cure or improvement.

Biofeedback is initially labor intensive requiring a dedicated therapist but can be carried out at home after training. It has the advantage of being painless, safe, and complementary to other interventions. Biofeedback training has been shown to improve functional outcome for women with persistent symptoms following sphincter repair (29). However, a more recent study has suggested that it is the therapist rather than the technique that is important to the outcome (30).

Anal Plug

Containment may be improved by the use of a disposable anal plug or tampon to enhance continence. The device expands after insertion and is removed to allow evacuation. Use of the anal tampon has been shown to improve continence scores and quality of life but only about half of patients found it comfortable to use on a regular basis (31). It has a role for those with severe symptoms who are awaiting (or are unsuitable for) surgery.

SURGERY

For some women conservative therapies will fail and surgical options need to be considered. Two categories of patient may be identified:

- women with evidence of a sphincter defect; and
- women where the sphincters are intact but weak, secondary to denervation or muscle atrophy.

In the first group, direct repair of the sphincter defect should be considered; in the second group, decision-making is more difficult, the surgical options more varied, and outcome less predictable.

Sphincter Repair

Sphincter repair is the operation of choice where there is a single defect of the external anal sphincter, either alone or in combination with a defect of the internal anal sphincter. Two different surgical techniques have been used: direct apposition and overlapping repair.

Sphincter repair by mobilization of the sphincter muscle, scar excision, and direct apposition resulted in a failure rate of around 40% (32), these poor results being attributed to the cutting out of sutures or retraction of the muscle ends. Parks and McPartlin subsequently modified this technique by identifying and repairing the torn internal anal sphincter separately and employing an overlapping repair of the muscle (33). Authors using the former technique along with an end-to-end repair have reported a significant reduction in incontinence (upto 8%) (34). Indeed, the results of two randomized controlled trials have shown both techniques to be similar (35,36).

Most studies seemed to be in-favor of immediate rather than delayed repair for third- or fourth-degree tears following delivery. Although both immediate (37) and delayed repairs (38) have demonstrated good results. Immediate repair would be more socially acceptable for the patient and delayed repairs should probably only be considered where there expertise is lacking at the time of injury.

The need for a defunctioning stoma following sphincter repair has been studied and is only necessary where there is significant perineal sepsis. A temporary stoma confers no benefit in terms of functional outcome and is associated with higher morbidity and longer hospital stay related to the stoma closure (39). Medical bowel confinement confers no benefit in terms of septic complications or functional outcome (40). Prophylactic broad spectrum antibiotics are used to prevent infection which may be linked to breakdown of the repair.

Review of published series shows that excellent or good results, with continence to solid and liquid stool, can be achieved in between 47% and 79% of patients undergoing sphincter repair (41–43). The outcome data for overlapping sphincter repair should, however, be interpreted with caution for a number of reasons. Many of the reported series are small, with patients recruited over several years, often involving several different operating surgeons and follow-up tends to be short. The groups of patients reported are often heterogeneous in terms of age, sex, and indication for repair. The frequent absence of standardized scoring systems or physiologic measurements to evaluate continence pre- and postoperatively does not allow series to be readily compared.

Outcome where there has also been damage to the internal sphincter is less certain. The importance of repairing the internal anal sphincter (when damaged) as well as the external sphincter has been highlighted during immediate repair of third degree tears (44). Such attention should probably also be applied to repairing a deficient internal anal sphincter during secondary repair. It is accepted, however, that internal sphincter defects may be more difficult to identify surgically and repair adequately, and soiling—together with incontinence to flatus—will remain a problem for some women.

Factors Predicting Outcome from Anal Sphincter Repair

A number of factors have been identified as predictive of outcome following anal sphincter repair.

Age and Body Habitus

Some authors have reported an adverse influence of increasing age on outcome (45). Although older age is not a contraindication to surgery (42,43), it should certainly be considered in preoperative counseling when discussing outcome. Obesity has also been recognized to worsen outcome following repair of anterior anal defects (45).

Pudendal Neuropathy

Prolonged PNMTL (unilateral or bilateral) have been shown by some to be predictive of a poorer outcome after sphincter repair (46). Although this finding may be useful in counseling women preoperatively, it should not necessarily be used to deny a woman operative correction of an obvious sphincter defect.

External Sphincter Atrophy

The detection by MRI scanning of atrophy of the external anal sphincter, which is characterized by thinning and fatty replacement, has been shown to adversely affect outcome following sphincter repair (47).

Failure of Sphincter Repair

Up to 10% of repairs may break down, resulting in persistent defects and poor functional results. Where such defects are identified, repeated sphincter repair may be successful (48). Since the operation may be technically more difficult and tissue quality poor, the outcome following repeated sphincter repair is less certain. Where failure has resulted from significant perineal sepsis, a temporary defunctioning colostomy may be required.

Long-Term Outcomes After Sphincter Repair

Most series report only short-term follow-up and interest has recently focused upon the long-term outcomes of sphincter repair. In a five-year follow-up study of incontinent women who had a overlapping repair for obstetric trauma, only four out of 38 were totally continent of solid and liquid stool and none was fully continent of stool and flatus (49). The overall success of the overlap method deteriorated with time. Whether the deterioration was due to progressive denervation of mobilized muscle or failure to repair internal sphincter defects adequately is uncertain. We however believe that sphincter repair remains the standard first approach for isolated defects, particularly in women presenting soon after obstetric injury (44). These women should be made aware that initial good results may not be permanent and that deterioration in continence may occur in the future.

Alternative Surgical Techniques

For women with symptomatic anal incontinence but an intact sphincter confirmed by imaging, other surgical options can be considered.

Sacral Nerve Modulation (SNM)

A novel approach to women with incontinence and weak but intact internal and external sphincters is to modulate the neurologic control of the anorectum. SNM was initially used in patients with detrusor instability and urinary retention in the 1980s (50). The observation of a simultaneous improvement in bowel symptoms in some of these patients led to its use by Matzel et al. in patients with anal incontinence in 1995 (51).

SNM involves chronic low-frequency electrostimulation of one of the sacral spinal nerves (S2, S3, or S4). The mechanism of action of SNM is uncertain: studies have demonstrated that SNM not only modifies somatic and autonomic nervous functions (52), but also central nervous system activity (53). However, the effect of SNM on the anal sphincter is inconsistent as some authors reported an increased anal resting tone and maximum anal squeeze pressure whilst others reported the contrary (54–56). Indeed, clinical studies on SNM have demonstrated improvement in continence in patients with external sphincter defects, suggesting the sphincter mechanism is not solely responsible for maintaining continence (57). The results of rectal sensitivity and compliance are also unclear and conflicting (54,58,59). Possible reasons include small sample size and the hetergeneous etiology of anal incontinence within sample groups. Anorectal physiological studies do not appear to be a useful predictor of outcome for SNM.

A major advantage of SNM is that it involves placement of a temporary electrode (Fig. 58.3), which can be used over a one to four week test period to measure response prior to embarking on surgical implantation of the permanent device. Sixty percent to eighty-eight percent of patients proceed to permanent implantation (Fig. 58.4) following the initial trial (60–62). A further advantage of SNM is that it does not involve any risk of direct surgical trauma to the sphincter mechanism itself. Morbidities associated with the procedure are less compared with other surgical techniques with a reported incidence ranging from 5% to 26% (52). Such morbidities are usually minor and include pain at implant site, seroma, excessive tingling in the vaginal région, and superficial wound infection (52).

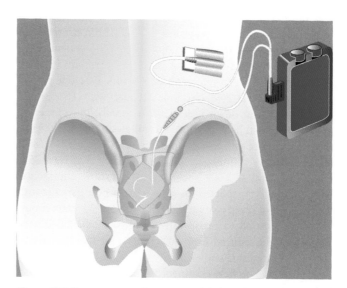

Figure 58.3 Temporary sacral nerve modulation *Source*: Courtesy of Medtronic, Watford, U.K.

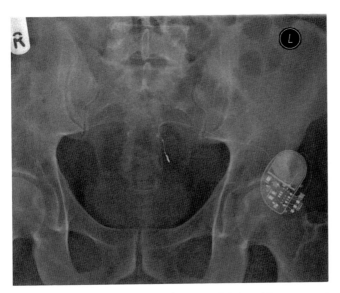

Figure 58.4 Radiograph showing sacral nerve modulation with a permanent implanted device.

A systematic review published in 2004 of the early results of SNM showed an improvement in anal incontinence in patients resistant to conservative treatment (63). A more recent randomized controlled study by Tjandra et al. has demonstrated SNM to be more effective than optimal medical therapy, with the SNM group reporting significantly less mean incontinent episodes per week (from 9.5 to 3.1) and mean incontinent days per week (3.3 to 1) compared to controls (from 9.2 to 9.4 and from 3.3 to 3.1 respectively) (62). Within the same institute and population sample, Chan et al. also demonstrated that SNM improved continence in patients with external anal sphincter defects of up to 120° of circumference (57).

Few studies have reported long-term results (minimum of at least 5–7 years) in SNM. In the national registry of the Italian group of sacral nerve stimulation, Altomare et al. (61) reported follow-up of 52 patients over a mean period of 74 months (range, 60–122). The group originally had 60 patients but two patients died of non-related disease to anal incontinence, six had the device removed due to persistent complications or progressive failure of therapeutic efficacy within the first two years of follow-up. Hence 52 out of 60 (86.7%) patients were available for review. Fifteen out of fifty-two patients (28.8%) continued to suffer from complications which include pain at site of implant (11.5%), electrode displacement (15.4%) and early battery run down (1.9%). Functionally, by comparing Wexner scores at both baseline and follow-up for 50 patients, the mean score decreased from 15 to 5.9 patients (18%) achieved 100% continence, 25 (50%) achieved at least 75% continence and 37 (74%) achieved at least 50% continence. Matzel et al. (64) reported the follow-up of nine patients with a minimum of seven years and mean period of 9.8 years (range 7–14). Compared to preoperative results, accidental loss of bowel content reduced from 40% to 0%, median number of incontinence episodes/week from 9 to 0.4 out of the 9 (44.4%) patients remained fully continent.

The application of sacral nerve stimulation to patients with anal incontinence continues to evolve. Encouragingly, SNM appears to be effective long term for patients with urinary incontinence but only continued evaluation will determine whether the same is true for women with anal incontinence.

Postanal Repair (PAR) and Total Pelvic Floor Repair (TPFR)
The operation of PAR aims to restore an adequate anorectal angle, which is of theoretical importance in maintaining continence. The long-term results from PAR are poor, with only a third of women maintaining continence at five-year follow-up. TPFR combines PAR with anterior sphincter plication and anterior levatoroplasty. Long-term follow-up indicates that TPFR rarely renders women fully continent, but around half have substantially improved continence and lifestyle (65).

The poor long-term success rates reflect progressive neuropathy or atrophy of the muscles and have led to a move away from PAR and TPFR as surgical options. These operations are, however, associated with low morbidity and thus may still have a role for women with significant symptoms who are unsuitable for more complex reconstructive procedures or who refuse a stoma.

Neosphincters
Muscle Transposition
It is possible to augment the anal sphincter with another striated muscle. The muscles most commonly used are gracilis or gluteus but others such as obturator internus have also been employed (66). Gracioplasty involves mobilization of the muscle from the inner thigh, which is wrapped around the anal canal and fixed to the contralateral ischial tuberosity. Continence is reliant upon the muscle wrap being tight enough to keep the anal canal closed, as coordinated voluntary contraction of the muscle itself is difficult. Gluteus transposition is a technically more demanding procedure but has the advantage that the muscles are easier to contract since the glutei are natural synergists of the anal sphincter. Results of unstimulated muscle transposition vary widely and it is now a rarely used technique. Bilateral gracioplasty may be useful where lack of local technical expertise or financial resources do not allow stimulated transposition.

Stimulated Muscle Transposition
The observation that by chronic stimulation muscle fibers could be converted from type II fast twitch to fatigue-resistant slow twitch fibers led to the development of the stimulated gracioplasty (67). The mobilization of the gracilis muscle and wrap are similar to that for unstimulated gracioplasty but involve identification of the nerve to gracilis and implantation of a stimulating electrode around the nerve trunk or its branches. The stimulator is placed in a subcutaneous pocket in the abdominal wall and the electrode wires tunneled to it. After satisfactory healing, a period of muscle stimulation is commenced until continuous stimulation results in sustained muscle contraction. The patient switches off the stimulator to allow the muscle to relax and enable defecation (68). Contraindications to stimulated gracioplasty include a history of perianal sepsis or crohn's disease. In addition, as the stimulator may interfere with pacemakers and implanted defibrillators, the technique may not be appropriate in these patients.

In a study of 52 patients undergoing stimulated graciloplasty, 73% were continent after a median follow-up of two years and success was associated with improved quality of life (68). Others have reported far less favorable results. Septic complications, hardware problems, and physiologic imbalance have led to the high failure rates reported in some series (66). Case selection is important; patients need to be well motivated and require careful preoperative assessment and counseling. The procedure has a recognized failure rate and may be associated with significant morbidity and scarring. In addition, patients may require significant input in terms of support for fine-tuning the stimulator.

Artificial Bowel Sphincter

When the sphincter muscles are irretrievably damaged or previous attempts at reconstruction have failed, the use of an artificial bowel sphincter may provide a simpler and less invasive approach than stimulated muscle transposition. The artificial sphincter prosthesis was developed from use in the treatment of urinary incontinence. It comprises a cuff which is implanted around the anus and a pressure-regulating balloon which is placed behind the rectus muscles and connected to a pump placed in the subcutaneous tissues of the labia. A temporary colostomy is not normally required. Cuff opening is controlled by squeezing the labial pump which empties the cuff to enable evacuation; the cuff then slowly refills from the pressure-regulating balloon over a number of minutes to close the anal canal.

Early reports of the purpose-designed artificial bowel sphincter indicated that excellent functional results can be achieved both in terms of improving continence scores and improving anal canal resting pressures without adversely affecting rectal function (69). An audit of the United Kingdom experience, however, showed that two-thirds of the sphincters implanted had required removal (70). Infection was the predominant cause and meticillin-resistant *Staphylococcus aureus* (MRSA) a common pathogen. Despite good functional outcomes in a proportion of patients, the future for the artificial sphincter remains uncertain. Early septic complications necessitate removal of the device in some patients and improvements in care directed at preventing infection are required. Long-term results reported by the minnesota group demonstrated that only 49% of 45 patients achieved a functional artificial sphincter, with infection being the main reason for failure. Where implantation was successful those patients did experience improved continence and quality of life (71).

Injectable Bulking Agents

The method of mechanical bulking of the anal sphincter has been used for fecal incontinence since 1993 (72). Injectable agents may have a role in those patients with internal anal sphincter defects or a gutter deformity of the anal canal which allows passive leakage of stool. A variety of different injectable bulking agents have been used; coaptite (calcium hydroxylapatite ceramic microspheres), contigen (collagen implant), durasphere (pyrolytic carbon-coated beads), ethylene vinyl alcohol, and textured silicone particles. Injections are usually made into the submucosal region or at the site of the sphincter defect. Morbidities described are low and range from pruritis ani, persistent anal discomfort to perianal sepsis (73). Recent systematic review on the efficacy and safety of injectable bulking agents for passive fecal incontinence indicated 13 case series studies and one randomized controlled trial. Although most studies reported statistical significant improvement in incontinence scores and quality of life, in the only randomized controlled trial, no statistical difference was found between the treatment and placebo arms (73). Whilst the injection of a bulking agent is a simple low morbidity procedure, their exact role remains to be defined.

Stomas

For some women who fail to respond to conservative or surgical treatments, a colostomy may be the only alternative to managing intolerable symptoms. In these individuals, a stoma should not be seen as a treatment failure and may allow many women to return to a near normal lifestyle. Colostomy irrigation is possible and may further improve their quality of life. Unfortunately, for a few women with a colostomy, persistent incontinence of mucus from the defunctioned rectum remains a problem and a proctectomy may be required.

SUMMARY

Careful assessment and investigation of anal incontinence can usually determine the underlying cause. Most women can be managed conservatively by a combination of dietary modification, medication, and biofeedback. Where conservative treatment fails, surgery may be considered. Women with sphincter defects may benefit from overlapping sphincter repair which offers good short-term functional results. They should be counseled that longer-term results are less certain. When sphincter repair fails or where the sphincter itself is intact but weak, a trial of SNM should be considered. PAR, TPFR, and unstimulated muscle transposition offer short-term improvement for many women. Stimulated muscle transposition and artificial sphincters can provide a more satisfactory solution, but may be associated with significant morbidity. For a few women who have failed all treatment modalities, diversion stomas may be recommended.

REFERENCES

1. Leigh RJ, Turnberg LA. Faecal incontinence: the unvoiced symptom. Lancet 1982; 1: 1349–51.
2. MacArthur C, Bick DE, Keighley MR. Faecal incontinence after childbirth. Br J Obstet Gynaecol 1997; 104: 46–50.
3. Fynes M, Donnelly V, Behan M, O'Connell PR, O'Herlihy C. Effect of second vaginal delivery on anorectal physiology and faecal continence: a prospective study. Lancet 1999; 354: 983–6.
4. Tan JJ, Chan M, Tjandra JJ. Evolving therapy for fecal incontinence. Dis Colon Rectum 2007; 50: 1950–67.
5. Sultan AH, Kamm MA, Hudson CN, Bartram CI. Third degree obstetric anal sphincter tears: risk factors and outcome of primary repair. BMJ 1994; 308: 887–91.
6. Kamm MA. Obstetric damage and faecal incontinence. Lancet 1994; 344: 730–3.
7. Groom KM, Paterson-Brown S. Can we improve on the diagnosis of third degree tears? Eur J Obstet Gynecol Reprod Biol 2002; 101: 19–21.
8. Johanson RB, Fernando RJ, Kettle C, et al. The "Repair" survey of the incidence of 3rd degree perineal tears in UK hospitals. unpublished data 2001.

9. Lal M, C HM, Callender R, Radley S. Does cesarean delivery prevent anal incontinence? Obstet Gynecol 2003; 101: 305–12.

10. Donnelly V, O'Connell PR, O'Herlihy C. The influence of oestrogen replacement on faecal incontinence in postmenopausal women. Br J Obstet Gynaecol 1997; 104: 311–5.

11. Donnelly VS, O'Herlihy C, Campbell DM, O'Connell PR. Postpartum fecal incontinence is more common in women with irritable bowel syndrome. Dis Colon Rectum 1998; 41: 586–9.

12. Snooks SJ, Setchell M, Swash M, Henry MM. Injury to innervation of pelvic floor sphincter musculature in childbirth. Lancet 1984; 2: 546–50.

13. Fynes M, Donnelly VS, O'Connell PR, O'Herlihy C. Cesarean delivery and anal sphincter injury. Obstet Gynecol 1998; 92: 496–500.

14. Bennett RC, Duthie HL. The functional importance of the internal anal sphincter. Br J Surg 1964; 51: 355–7.

15. Henry MM, Thomson JP. The anal sphincter. Scand J Gastroenterol Suppl 1984; 93: 53–7.

16. Vaizey CJ, Carapeti E, Cahill JA, Kamm MA. Prospective comparison of faecal incontinence grading systems. Gut 1999; 44: 77–80.

17. Jorge JM, Wexner SD. Etiology and management of fecal incontinence. Dis Colon Rectum 1993; 36: 77–97.

18. Hiller L, Bradshaw HD, Radley SC, Radley S. Criterion validity of the BBUSQ-22: a questionnaire assessing bowel and urinary tract symptoms in women. Int Urogynecol J Pelvic Floor Dysfunct 2007; 18: 1133–7.

19. Coller JA. Clinical application of anorectal manometry. Gastroenterol Clin North Am 1987; 16: 17–33.

20. Snooks SJ, Swash M, eds. Nerve Stimulation Techniques. London: Butterworths, 1985.

21. Tjandra JJ, Milsom JW, Schroeder T, Fazio VW. Endoluminal ultrasound is preferable to electromyography in mapping anal sphincteric defects. Dis Colon Rectum 1993; 36: 689–92.

22. Deen KI, Kumar D, Williams JG, Olliff J, Keighley MR. Anal sphincter defects. correlation between endoanal ultrasound and surgery. Ann Surg 1993; 218: 201–5.

23. Pretlove SJ, Thompson PJ, Guest P, Toozs-Hobson P, Radley S. Detecting anal sphincter injury: acceptability and feasibility of endoanal ultrasound immediately postpartum. Ultrasound Obstet Gynecol 2003; 22: 215–7.

24. The management of third- and fourth-degree perineal tears. London (UK): Royal College of Obstetricians and Gynaecologists (RCOG); 2007 Mar. 11 p. (Green-top guideline; no. 29).

25. Pretlove S, Thompson PJ, Toozs-Hobson PM, Radley S. The first 18 months of a new perineal trauma clinic. J Obstet Gynaecol 2004; 24: 399–402.

26. Santoro GA, Eitan BZ, Pryde A, Bartolo DC. Open study of low-dose amitriptyline in the treatment of patients with idiopathic fecal incontinence. Dis Colon Rectum 2000; 43: 1676–81; discussion 81-2.

27. MacLeod JH. Management of anal incontinence by biofeedback. Gastroenterology 1987; 93: 291–4.

28. Norton C, Kamm MA. Outcome of biofeedback for faecal incontinence. Br J Surg 1999; 86: 1159–63.

29. Jensen LL, Lowry AC. Biofeedback improves functional outcome after sphincteroplasty. Dis Colon Rectum 1997; 40: 197–200.

30. Norton C, Chelvanayagam S, Wilson-Barnett J, Redfern S, Kamm MA. Randomized controlled trial of biofeedback for fecal incontinence. Gastroenterology 2003; 125: 1320–9.

31. Mylonakis E, Radley S, Payton N, et al. The role of an intra-anal tampon for faecal incontinence: preliminary results of a prospective study. Colorectal Dis 2001; 3(Suppl 1): 82.

32. Blaisdell PC. Repair of the incontinent sphincter ani. Surg Gynecol Obstet 1940; 70: 692–7.

33. Parks AC, McPartlin JF. Late repair of injuries of the anal sphincter. Proc R Soc Med 1971; 64: 1187–9.

34. Fernando RJ, Sultan AH, Radley S, Jones PW, Johanson RB. Management of obstetric anal sphincter injury: a systematic review & national practice survey. BMC Health Serv Res 2002; 2: 9.

35. Fitzpatrick M, Behan M, O'Connell PR, O'Herlihy C. A randomized clinical trial comparing primary overlap with approximation repair of third-degree obstetric tears. Am J Obstet Gynecol 2000; 183: 1220–4.

36. Tjandra JJ, Han WR, Goh J, Carey M, Dwyer P. Direct repair vs. overlapping sphincter repair: a randomized, controlled trial. Dis Colon Rectum 2003; 46: 937–42; discussion 42–3.

37. Fernando R, Sultan AH, Kettle C, Thakar R, Radley S. Methods of repair for obstetric anal sphincter injury. Cochrane Database Syst Rev 2006; 3: CD002866.

38. Soerensen MM, Bek KM, Buntzen S, Hojberg KE, Laurberg S. Long-term outcome of delayed primary or early secondary reconstruction of the anal sphincter after obstetrical injury. Dis Colon Rectum 2008; 51: 312–7.

39. Hasegawa H, Yoshioka K, Keighley M. Randomised trial of faecal diversion of sphincter repair. Dis Colon Rectum 2000; 43: 961–5.

40. Nessim A, Wexner SD, Agachan F, et al. Is bowel confinement necessary after anorectal reconstructive surgery? A prospective, randomized, surgeon-blinded trial. Dis Colon Rectum 1999; 42: 16–23.

41. Laurberg S, Swash M, Henry MM. Delayed external sphincter repair for obstetric tear. Br J Surg 1988; 75: 786–8.

42. Engel AF, Kamm MA, Sultan AH, Bartram CI, Nicholls RJ. Anterior anal sphincter repair in patients with obstetric trauma. Br J Surg 1994; 81: 1231–4.

43. Oliveira L, Pfeifer J, Wexner SD. Physiological and clinical outcome of anterior sphincteroplasty. Br J Surg 1996; 83: 502–5.

44. Hayes J, Shatari T, Toozs-Hobson P, et al. Early results of immediate repair of obstetric third-degree tears: 65% are completely asymptomatic despite persistent sphincter defects in 61%. Colorectal Dis 2007; 9: 332–6.

45. Nikiteas N, Korsgen S, Kumar D, Keighley MR. Audit of sphincter repair. Factors associated with poor outcome. Dis Colon Rectum 1996; 39: 1164–70.

46. Baig MK, Wexner SD. Factors predictive of outcome after surgery for faecal incontinence. Br J Surg 2000; 87: 1316–30.

47. Briel JW, Stoker J, Rociu E, et al. External anal sphincter atrophy on endoanal magnetic resonance imaging adversely affects continence after sphincteroplasty. Br J Surg 1999; 86: 1322–7.

48. Pinedo G, Vaizey CJ, Nicholls RJ, et al. Results of repeat anal sphincter repair. Br J Surg 1999; 86: 66–9.

49. Malouf AJ, Norton CS, Engel AF, Nicholls RJ, Kamm MA. Long-term results of overlapping anterior anal-sphincter repair for obstetric trauma. Lancet 2000; 355: 260–5.

50. Oerlemans DJ, van Kerrebroeck PE. Sacral nerve stimulation for neuromodulation of the lower urinary tract. Neurourol Urodyn 2008; 27: 28–33.

51. Matzel KE, Stadelmaier U, Hohenfellner M, Gall FP. Electrical stimulation of sacral spinal nerves for treatment of faecal incontinence. Lancet 1995; 346: 1124–7.

52. Tjandra JJ, Lim JF, Matzel K. Sacral nerve stimulation: an emerging treatment for faecal incontinence. ANZ J Surg 2004; 74: 1098–106.

53. Braun PM, Baezner H, Seif C, et al. Alterations of cortical electrical activity in patients with sacral neuromodulator. Eur Urol 2002; 41: 562–6; discussion 6-7.

54. Roman S, Tatagiba T, Damon H, Barth X, Mion F. Sacral nerve stimulation and rectal function: results of a prospective study in faecal incontinence. Neurogastroenterol Motil 2008; 20: 1127–31.

55. Ganio E, Masin A, Ratto C, et al. Short-term sacral nerve stimulation for functional anorectal and urinary disturbances: results in 40 patients: evaluation of a new option for anorectal functional disorders. Dis Colon Rectum 2001; 44: 1261–7.

56. Koch SM, van Gemert WG, Baeten CG. Determination of therapeutic threshold in sacral nerve modulation for faecal incontinence. Br J Surg 2005; 92: 83–7.

57. Chan MK, Tjandra JJ. Sacral nerve stimulation for fecal incontinence: external anal sphincter defect vs. intact anal sphincter. Dis Colon Rectum 2008; 51: 1015–24; discussion 24-5.

58. Vaizey CJ, Kamm MA, Turner IC, Nicholls RJ, Woloszko J. Effects of short term sacral nerve stimulation on anal and rectal function in patients with anal incontinence. Gut 1999; 44: 407–12.

59. Ganio E, Ratto C, Masin A, et al. Neuromodulation for fecal incontinence: outcome in 16 patients with definitive implant. The initial Italian Sacral Neurostimulation Group (GINS) experience. Dis Colon Rectum 2001; 44: 965–70.

60. Koch SM, Melenhorst J, Uludag O, et al. Sacral nerve modulation and other treatments in patients with faecal incontinence after unsuccessful pelvic floor rehabilitation: a prospective study. Colorectal Dis 2009; 12: 334–41.

61. Altomare DF, Ratto C, Ganio E, et al. Long-term outcome of sacral nerve stimulation for fecal incontinence. Dis Colon Rectum 2009; 52: 11–7.

62. Tjandra JJ, Chan MK, Yeh CH, Murray-Green C. Sacral nerve stimulation is more effective than optimal medical therapy for severe fecal incontinence: a randomized, controlled study. Dis Colon Rectum 2008; 51: 494–502.

63. Jarrett ME, Mowatt G, Glazener CM, et al. Systematic review of sacral nerve stimulation for faecal incontinence and constipation. Br J Surg 2004; 91: 1559–69.

64. Matzel KE, Lux P, Heuer S, Besendorfer M, Zhang W. Sacral nerve stimulation for faecal incontinence: long-term outcome. Colorectal Dis 2008; 11: 636–41.

65. Korsgen S, Deen KI, Keighley MR. Long-term results of total pelvic floor repair for postobstetric fecal incontinence. Dis Colon Rectum 1997; 40: 835–9.

66. Niriella DA, Deen KI. Neosphincters in the management of faecal incontinence. Br J Surg 2000; 87: 1617–28.

67. Williams NS, Patel J, George BD, Hallan RI, Watkins ES. Development of an electrically stimulated neoanal sphincter. Lancet 1991; 338: 1166–9.

68. Baeten CG, Geerdes BP, Adang EM, et al. Anal dynamic graciloplasty in the treatment of intractable fecal incontinence. N Engl J Med 1995; 332: 1600–5.

69. Vaizey CJ, Kamm MA, Gold DM, et al. Clinical, physiological, and radiological study of a new purpose-designed artificial bowel sphincter. Lancet 1998; 352: 105–9.

70. Malouf AJ, Vaizey CJ, Kamm MA, Nicholls RJ. Reassessing artificial bowel sphincters. Lancet 2000; 355: 2219–20.

71. Parker SC, Spencer MP, Madoff RD, et al. Artificial bowel sphincter: long-term experience at a single institution. Dis Colon Rectum 2003; 46: 722–9.

72. Shafik A. Polytetrafluoroethylene injection for the treatment of partial fecal incontinence. Int Surg 1993; 78: 159–61.

73. Luo C, Samaranayake CB, Plank LD, Bissett IP. Systematic review on the efficacy and safety of injectable bulking agents for passive fecal incontinence. Colorectal Dis 2009; 12: 296–303.

59 Constipation

Nadia Ali-Ross and Anthony RB Smith

INTRODUCTION

Chronic constipation is not the consequence of a single disease entity but rather a symptom of many conditions. It may be associated with dietary deficiency of fiber or fluid, immobility, learned dysfunction, irritable bowel syndrome (IBS), drug induced slow transit (Table 59.1), medical conditions (Table 59.2), and pseudo-obstruction. The majority of these are managed in the primary care setting. A smaller proportion of people suffers with functional constipation and is classified as idiopathic slow transit constipation (STC), obstructed defecation, or a combination of these. Although infrequent bowel motions are often considered indicative of constipation, a U.K. population study involving 1455 people revealed that 99% of healthy subjects moved their bowels between three times per day to three times per week (1). The Rome consensus group has defined functional gastrointestinal disorders and recognized that there may be several features of constipation. They have defined constipation as the presence of at two out of a possible six criteria listed in Table 59.3. Recently the Rome 2 consensus has been updated to the Rome 3 consensus in an attempt to tighten the definition of constipation (2). The criteria themselves remain the same but the onset of symptoms should have begun at least six months prior to diagnosis (rather than 12 months in Rome 2) and must have been active for the preceding three months.

The prevalence of constipation in the female general population is reported between 2.8% and 35.4% (3–9). Higgins and Johanson estimated that 12% of the North American population fulfilled the Rome 2 criteria for constipation (4). There is great variation in the individual perception of constipation. Sandler and Drossman surveyed healthy young adults on their understanding of constipation (10). Half defined constipation as straining to pass feces, 44% considered it to be the passage of hard stool, 32% associated infrequent bowel movements with constipation, and 34% described it as the inability to defecate at will. Nyam et al. performed physiological studies on 1009 patients with severe chronic constipation and found 13% had STC, 25% had obstructed constipation, and 3% had a combination of the two (11). Obstructed constipation and combined STC with obstructed constipation are more common in women and often present with intractable symptoms. These women may require combined input from gynecologists, gastroenterologists, colorectal surgeons, urologists, physiotherapists, and nurse specialists.

This chapter reviews the normal physiology of defecation, the pathophysiology of STC and obstructed constipation, the epidemiology of constipation, clinical assessment, investigations, and treatment of constipation.

PHYSIOLOGY OF NORMAL COLONIC TRANSIT AND DEFECATION

Whole-gut transit time ranges between 12 and 120 hours (12). It is clearly influenced by age, genetic, racial, hormonal, and dietary factors. Ingested matter only spends a small proportion of time in the small intestine. A mean oro-cecal transit of 4.4 hours and colonic transit of 34 to 36 hours (upper range 72–88 hours) has been reported in healthy controls (11,13,14). Although transit times differ between men and women, these are not of clinical significance (15). The menstrual cycle has not been shown to influence colonic transit in women (12,16).

The colon has three purposes: (*i*) to conserve water and minerals; (*ii*) to enable bacteria to split dietary fiber into absorbable products; and (*iii*) to store and expel the residual feces at appropriate times. The colon receives 1000 to 2000 ml of isotonic chyme from the ileum each day and this is converted into approximately 250 ml of semi-solid feces. The bacterial fermentation of undigested carbohydrate in the colon contributes to nearly one-third of stool bulk. Unfermented fiber retains water and also contributes to stool mass. Higher stool bulk stimulates colonic peristalsis and facilitates transit through the colon. Feces are then stored in the rectum until defecation can take place.

Defecation involves the co-ordination of intact spinal and enteric neuronal systems with anal sphincter, pelvic floor, and abdominal musculature. The sensory and motor innervation of the anal sphincter complex and pelvic floor musculature is provided by the pudendal nerve, lumbar colonic nerves, and the L2–S4 nerve roots. The desire to defecate occurs when the critical stool volume exceeds rectal compliance. This triggers the recto-anal inhibitory reflex (RAIR) which causes the internal anal sphincter to relax. Defecation can only take place once the striated external anal sphincter and the puborectalis muscles relax. These are innervated by the pudendal nerve and are under voluntary control. Relaxation of puborectalis allows the anorectal angle to straighten facilitating the passage of stool into the anal canal. Relaxation of the external anal sphincter allows the evacuation of stool. During defecation, contraction of iliococcygeus and pubococcygeus cause the anococcygeal raphe to shorten and widen by virtue of the crisscross nature of its fibers. This has been proposed as a mechanism to allow dilatation of the organs traversing the urogenital hiatus promoting the passage of feces (17). Straining of the abdominal wall muscles (which increases intra-peritoneal pressure) and the peristaltic contractions of the colon have minor contributions to normal defecation. Squatting facilitates defecation better than sitting as the greater degree of hip flexion aids the straightening of anorectal angle. Elevation of the feet using a

Table 59.1 Drug-induced Constipation

Drug group/effect	Condition	Example
Opiates	Severe pain	Pethidine, diamorhine
	Terminal care	Oromorph, codeine, fentanyl
Anticholinergic	Overactive bladder	Oxybutynin
	Psychosis	Chlorpromazine
	Parkinson disease	Benzhexol
	Depression	Amytriptyline
	Allergy	Diphenhydramine (less with newer antihistamines)
Calcium channel blockers	Hypertension Ischemic heart disease	Verapamil
Sympathomimetics	Asthma	Terbutaline
Diuretics	Hypertension	Frusemide
Antidiarrheal therapy	Noninfective diarrhea	Loperamide, codeine
Antacids	Indigestion	Calcium containing agents
Supplements	Osteoporosis	Calchichew
	Anemia	Iron

Table 59.2 Medical Conditions Associated with Constipation

Mechanical obstruction	Colon cancer
	Stricture (diverticular disease, iatrogenic, idiopathic)
	Hirshsprung's disease
	Megarectum
	Fecal impaction (cognitive impairment, secondary to painful anal conditions)
Metabolic condition	Diabetes mellitus
	Hypothyroidism
	Hypocalcemia
	Hypokalemia
Neuropathy	Cerebro-vascular accident
	Spinal cord compression (tumor)
	Spinal injury (trauma)
	Nerve injury (obstetric trauma)
	Parkinson's disease
	Multiple sclerosis
Myopathies	Systemic sclerosis
	Amyloidosis
Miscellaneous	Immobility
	Depression
	Acquired cognitive impairment
	Learning difficulty
	Cardiac disease
	Pan-gut dysmotility

Table 59.3 The Rome 3 Consensus; Diagnostic Criteria for Functional Constipation

Must include two or more of the following:
- Straining during at least 25% of defecations
- Lumpy or hard stools in at least 25% of defecations
- Sensation of incomplete evacuation for at least 25% of defecations
- Sensation of anorectal obstruction/blockage for at least 25% of defecations
- Manual maneuvers to facilitate at least 25% of defecations (e.g., digital evacuation, support of the pelvic floor)
- Fewer than three defecations per week

Loose stools are rarely present without the use of laxatives

There are insufficient criteria for irritable bowel syndrome

Note: Criteria fulfilled for the last three months with symptom onset at least six months prior to diagnosis.

to do so, then the puborectalis and the external anal sphincters remain contracted and a reflex relaxation of iliococcygeus and pubococcygeus occurs which allows the urge to defecate to ease (17).

The neural control of the colon involves extrinsic innervation (sympathetic, parasympathetic, and somatic) and intrinsic innervation known as the enteric nervous system (myenteric and submucosal plexuses). The sympathetic nervous system (via the hypogastric nerve) promotes storage by reducing colonic contractions and enhancing anal tone. Conversely the parasympathetics (via vagus and pelvic splanchnic nerves) increase colonic motility. The enteric nervous system controls baseline tone and rhythmic ring contractions throughout the colon (18). The interstitial cells of Cajal (ICC) are abundant within the myenteric plexus and circular muscle of the colon. These are non-neuronal cells of mesenchymal origin and exhibit a pacemaker function.

Chronic constipation may be secondary to metabolic disorders (e.g., hypothyroidism, hypercalcemia, diabetes mellitus), neurological disease (e.g., Parkinson's, stroke, spinal injury, multiple sclerosis), drug interactions (e.g., opiates), or structural abnormalities (e.g., carcinoma of colon, megacolon). However, an organic cause cannot be demonstrated in many and these are termed functional constipation. The two main functional pathophysiologies are STC and obstructed defecation (with slow or normal colonic transit).

PATHOPHYSIOLOGY
Slow Transit Constipation
STC is usually associated with a lack of urge to defecate and often women with this condition are able to evacuate the rectum without straining. The term colonic inertia is inappropriately applied to all patients with STC as it does not distinguish between colonic stasis associated with reduced propagated colonic contractions and increased uncoordinated motor activity in the distal colon that slows the transit of feces. STC can be associated with unfavorable stool consistency, diet, hormonal fluctuations (e.g., pregnancy), and drugs. Neuromuscular pathology of the smooth muscle and abnormal

foot stool when sitting on the toilet can produce a similar effect.

Fecal continence is maintained by rectal compliance, tonic contraction of the anal sphincter complex, and the acute anorectal angle which is maintained by the sling of puborectalis muscle. If it is socially inappropriate to defecate despite a desire functioning of the enteric nervous system of the human intestine have also been implicated.

Idiopathic STC is not well understood. A recent study involving colectomy specimens in patients with STC showed decreased ICC on immunohistochemical staining (19). As these cells have a pacemaker action on the colon, this may explain the reduced colonic motility in STC. Decreased ICC density and reduction in the number and size of enteric nerve cells (moderate hypoganglionosis) have been demonstrated in other small histopathological studies of patients with severe STC requiring colectomy (20–23). It is not clear whether these studies demonstrate a causative association or are simply the result of chronic constipation or laxative treatment.

Gastrointestinal hormones, such as somatostatin and pancreatic glucagon, have been shown to be reduced in women with severe idiopathic constipation (24). This may influence gut motility but it is unknown whether this causes constipation or is secondary to another condition. Systemic hormones have also been implicated with STC. Constipation is a feature of hypothyroidism but is unlikely to be the only symptom of this condition. Altered serotonin signaling in the intestine has also been suggested as a cause of STC. Serotonin is produced by the enterochromaffin cells in the gut mucosa and when released it activates neural reflexes involved in intestinal secretions and motility. It is unknown whether reduced intestinal motility is mediated by decreased serotonin availability or reduced functional receptors (25).

Reduced follicular phase progestogen (adrenal in origin), luteal estradiol (ovarian in origin), and both follicular and luteal cortisol and testosterone have been shown in women with STC. It is not clear whether these findings are the cause of reduced motility, secondary to the slow gut transit, or simply co-incidental (26). However, around one-quarter of women reported constipation during pregnancy and in the three months postpartum (27). During pregnancy this is likely to be associated with slower gut transit secondary to the high levels of progestogen. In a small study of 15 women, slower oro-cecal transit times have been demonstrated in the third trimester compared to the postpartum period (28). Therefore, although normally sex hormones do not have a well defined effect on bowel, the much higher levels in pregnancy are likely to contribute to altered motility.

In a small proportion of patients both STC and obstructed defecation contribute to constipation. This is known as a combination syndrome and the STC component is thought to be secondary to the chronic obstruction.

Constipation-predominant IBS can be symptomatically similar to STC. However, the main difference is abdominal pain which is often associated with a change in bowel habit and stool consistency (Rome 3 definition IBS). Visceral hypersensitivity is a feature of IBS not STC although laxatives or severe fecal loading may cause pain in the latter group. Slow colonic transit is not consistently shown in patients with constipation-predominant IBS. Although colectomy is a valid treatment in severe STC, it is not therapeutic in IBS sufferers as abdominal bloating and pain persists. Therefore, distinguishing between these two subsets is important.

Obstructed Defecation

Obstructed defecation is also known as outlet delay, evacuatory disorders, dyschezia, animus, or pelvic floor dysfunction. It represents a group of structural and functional disorders of the anorectum which obstruct the process of defecation. In pure obstructed defecation the proximal colonic motility is normal. Uncommonly slow colonic transit occurs secondarily to obstruction and these women are categorized as having a combination syndrome.

Structural Disorders of the Anorectum

Mechanical causes of anal stenosis, such as carcinoma, stricture, previous surgery, rectal mucosal prolapse, rectal intussusception, and large enterocoeles can lead to obstructed defecation. Fecal impaction may occur secondary to reduced rectal sensation and high compliance. Learning difficulty, immobility in the elderly, and ignored desire to defecate (due to social or cultural reasons) may result in the accumulation of feces which becomes painful to pass due to the large volume. In the extreme this can result in fecal impaction and megarectum.

Obstructed defecation is a classical feature of Hirschsprung's disease (aganglionosis) which usually presents in infancy or childhood. Occasionally only a small portion of colon is affected which may not manifest until late teenage or early adulthood. The congenital aganglionic colonic segments can lead to the failure of relaxation of the internal anal sphincter due to the absent RAIR. This can result in a megacolon and megarectum.

Rectal prolapse and intussusception may cause mechanical obstruction to defecation and produce the sensation of incomplete evacuation. However, these are often difficult to identify by history or examination alone. Both can be associated with a solitary rectal ulcer. It is unclear whether rectal prolapse is the primary pathology that results in obstructed defecation or the result of chronic straining due to constipation.

Rectocoeles are common in women and often asymptomatic which explains why several studies have failed to demonstrate correlation between bowel symptoms and posterior vaginal prolapse. Soligo et al. found that women with posterior vaginal prolapse were twice as likely to suffer constipation compared to those without a posterior prolapse [odds ratio (OR) 2.3] (29). Mouristen and Larsen reported more severe posterior prolapse in women with bowel symptoms (30). Others have shown correlation between digital assistance of fecal evacuation and posterior vaginal prolapse (31,32). Disruption of the rectovaginal septum may cause specific evacuatory difficulty due to the forward bulging of the rectum into the vagina and the loss of continuity between the perineal body and levator ani (33). In such cases surgical repair of prolapse may resolve the obstructed defecation.

Enterocoeles may cause obstructed defecation due to extrinsic compression of the rectum and anorectal junction. Enterocoeles are associated with post-hysterectomy vault prolapse. Enterocoeles and sigmoidocoeles are five times more common in women who have undergone hysterectomy (34). Enterocoeles are recognized complications of retropubic colposuspension and the Manchester repair. Fecal incontinence may be more commonly associated with enterocoeles (30). Not all enterocoeles are symptomatic and some are a result of repeated straining due to constipation.

Weakness of the pelvic floor musculature and perineal body associated with obstetric trauma and chronic straining can give rise to the "descending perineum syndrome." The lack of support of the rectum and perirectal structures results in the anterior rectum protruding in to the anal canal causing obstructed defecation. This leads to straining and a sense of incomplete evacuation. Excessive descent of the perineum is noted during straining. In a large study of 1004 women, longer perineal bodies were associated with straining, digitations, and incomplete evacuation (35). Neuropathy, possibly due to stretch injury of the pudendal nerve, has been reported with chronic constipation and parturition (36–39). Pudendal nerve neuropathy has also been implicated in denervation of the external anal and urethral sphincters (39). Repeated straining may lead to denervation of external anal sphincter and puborectalis which may lead to fecal incontinence over time.

Proctalgia fugax and levator ani syndrome are rare conditions in which the predominant symptom is rectal pain in the absence of organic anorectal disease. The pathophysiology of these conditions remains poorly understood.

Functional Obstructed Defecation
Defecation normally involves co-ordinated relaxation of the puborectalis and external anal sphincter muscles in conjunction with raised intra-abdominal pressure and colonic peristalsis. Failure of relaxation or the paradoxical contraction of puborectalis leads to functional obstructed defecation (sometimes referred to as anismus, dyssynergic defecation, or pelvic floor dysfunction). Inadequate propulsive forces during attempted defecation may also cause dyssynergic defecation. The diagnostic criteria of functional obstructed defecation require the presence of functional constipation (Rome 3 criteria) and two signs of dyssynergic defecation [evidence of impaired evacuation based on balloon expulsion test or imaging; (i) inappropriate contraction of the pelvic floor or <20% relaxation of basal resting sphincter pressure measured by manometry, imaging, or electromyography (EMG); and (i) inadequate propulsive forces assessed by manometry or imaging] (40). Relaxation of puborectalis and the external anal sphincter are under voluntary control and failure or paradoxical contraction may represent an acquired or learned dysfunction. A high prevalence of sexual and physical abuse was reported in women with functional gastrointestinal disorders (41). This may represent subconscious somatization resulting in functional obstructed defecation in some women. However, contraction of the anal sphincter during defecation has been observed in normal subjects, which has led some clinicians to doubt dyssynergic defecation as an entity (42,43).

EPIDEMIOLOGY
Most studies have shown that constipation is more common amongst women than men (particularly obstructed defecation) and that the prevalence increases with age. The most marked increase occurs after 65 years of age (4). However, the age-related increase has been shown to occur earlier in women (9). Women with constipation are also more likely to seek medical care and use laxatives than men (6,9). Several studies have reported racial differences with more prevalent constipation in non-white populations (OR 1.1–2.9) (4–6). Constipation is also associated with low calorie intake, number of medications, opioid use, low income, and low education (4,6,44,45). Low fiber intake has not consistently been associated with constipation. However, most studies did not identify those who had increased dietary fiber as a treatment for constipation (45). The Department of Health recommends at least 18 g of fiber per day for adults although higher daily intakes have been suggested to reduce the risk of bowel cancer. Everhart et al. found that those with <5.2 g of fiber per day had a twofold increase risk of constipation (5).

Inactivity is often considered to be linked with constipation. This belief is based on the physiological reduction of bowel motility during sleep, increased bowel motility in athletes, and the high prevalence of constipation amongst the elderly and immobile. Everhart et al. reported that less physically active subjects reported more constipation in a longitudinal study involving 10,024 people (5). Others have failed to demonstrate any association with reduced activity and constipation or reduction in constipation with increased activity (46,47). It may be that physical activity does not influence all forms of constipation.

Hysterectomy has not consistently been shown to correlate with constipation and this is in part influenced by the variation in definition of constipation. Some women give a clear history of constipation from the post-operative period. It is unknown how many women have transient constipation during recovery. Prior et al. assessed bowel symptoms in 205 women before and after hysterectomy (mostly due to dysfunctional bleeding, fibroids, or prolapse) (48). They found that half the women with pre-operative bowel symptoms were cured or improved at six months but de novo symptoms of constipation-predominant IBS were reported in 10% and painless constipation in 2%. De novo symptoms were not more common in those who had undergone a vaginal hysterectomy compared to an abdominal procedure. This suggests that hysterectomy per se may be related to de novo constipation rather than pre-existing pelvic organ prolapse. However, another study involving questionnaires before and one year after abdominal hysterectomy did not show any significant changes in bowel symptoms (49). Self-reported constipation was found to be more common amongst women with symptomatic pelvic organ prolapse who had undergone a hysterectomy compared to those without a previous hysterectomy (54% vs. 31%) (50). Others have reported more frequent constipation in women with a previous vaginal or laparoscopic hysterectomy (34). Such women are likely to have a greater degree of pelvic organ support defect than women in whom the abdominal route was required. Therefore, it is unclear whether constipation is a feature of pelvic organ support defects or a post-operative complication of hysterectomy.

Constipation and Pelvic Organ Prolapse
There is recognized overlap between prolapse, bowel, and urinary symptoms. It is unclear whether these complaints simply share risk factors or are part of one disease spectrum. In a cross-sectional U.K. study involving healthy controls

(n = 266), women with urodynamic stress incontinence requiring surgery (n = 75), and women referred to secondary care for pelvic organ prolapse (n = 135), the rates of self reported constipation were 16%, 20%, and 40%, respectively (50). Soligo et al. found that women with posterior vaginal wall prolapse were twice as likely to report constipation (29). Others have demonstrated correlation between anterior but not posterior vaginal prolapse and constipation which suggests the association is not purely due to obstructed defecation but part of a spectrum of pelvic floor dysfunction (35).

Pudendal nerve neuropathy has been implicated in the etiology of pelvic organ prolapse and constipation (36,37,51,52). Spence-Jones et al. found that women with prolapse reported straining as a young adult more commonly than controls (61% vs. 4%) (39). This may indicate the effect of repeated stretching on the pudendal nerve resulting in denervation of the pelvic floor muscles which leads to prolapse and evacuatory difficulty. Childbirth is a recognized and unavoidable risk factor for pelvic organ prolapse (53–58). Therefore, constipation in pregnancy may be a potentially avoidable risk factor for prolapse (50).

CLINICAL HISTORY

Taking a thorough and careful history is essential to determine the features of constipation, what treatments have been tried, what bothers the patient, and what their expectations are. Although some patients find disclosing bowel habit embarrassing, the symptoms must be explored sensitively to determine bowel frequency, straining, slow defecation rather than straining, reduced rectal sensation (unaware of need to defecate), incomplete defecation, the need for digitation or perineal splinting, incontinence (solid, loose, or watery stool), soiling of underwear, and pain. Occasionally soft or watery fecal incontinence may represent overflow in cases of fecal impaction or excessive use of laxatives. A symptom diary may be more reliable than recollection. The Bristol stool chart can be useful in some cases. In order to individualize treatment, use of bowel specific quality of life tools is helpful to target the most bothersome symptoms (59). Identification of medical conditions (Table 59.2) or drug therapies (Table 59.1) associated with constipation may help explain the symptoms and direct treatment. Many patients with STC have a long history of opioid analgesics use due to chronic conditions or malignancy. Obviously analgesics are necessary and treatment must take this into account.

The clinician needs to distinguish between chronic constipation and a change in bowel habit or "red flag" symptoms such as rectal bleeding as the latter warrant investigation to exclude malignancy. Rectal prolapse, intussusception, and the solitary rectal ulcer syndrome may cause pain and bleeding in addition to constipation. When pain and bloating are main features, normal gut motility is likely. These symptoms are often associated with constipation predominant IBS. In patients with a megarectum, disturbed bladder function may occur secondary to compression. Concurrent symptoms of vomiting or a history of pseudo obstruction and malnutrition may indicate pan-intestinal dysmotility secondary to neuropathic or myopathic conditions.

STC is classically associated with:

- a lack of urge to defecate
- infrequent bowel movements
- good response to laxatives.

Obstructed defecation is associated with:

- prolonged defecation (up to one hour)
- rectal fullness
- sensation of anorectal obstruction
- tenesmus
- perineal splinting or digitations of vagina or rectum to assist evacuation
- symptoms of vaginal prolapse (vaginal bulge or dragging sensation)

In some women, STC and obstructed defecation co-exist and symptomatology may reflect this. However, symptom clusters are not diagnostic of the pathophysiology of constipation and overlap exists. A detailed obstetric history may reveal high vaginal parity, prolonged labors, obstetric trauma, and difficult deliveries which may cause obstructed defecation due to advanced uterine prolapse or enterocoele (extrinsic obstruction), rectocoele, and the descending perineum syndrome.

Clinical Examination

In most patients a general examination is not helpful. Rarely thyroid goiter may be obvious and should prompt screening for hypothyroidism. Neurological signs, such as lower limb weakness, may suggest a spinal lesion causing neuropathic constipation. Abnormal perineal and lower limb sensation may indicate a spinal cord lesion. Perineal innervation can also be assessed by the reflex contraction of the external anal sphincter to perianal stimulation (touch) or cough. A loss of this reflex suggests impaired innervation.

Abdominal examination may reveal distension and fecal loading. In women, the presence of abdominal hernias and stretch marks has been associated with pelvic organ prolapse and a gynecological examination should be performed (60,61). A history of obstructed defecation or vaginal prolapse should also prompt a vaginal and pelvic examination.

Inspection of the perineum in the left lateral position both at rest and during straining may reveal disruption of the integrity of the perineal body. Excessive descent during can be assessed subjectively during the Valsalva maneuver or straining. Normally the perineum should not descend below the bony outlet of the pelvis during straining. Perineometers have been used in the research setting to more objectively measure this but are not used in routine clinical practice. Gaping of anal opening at rest may suggest an underlying neurological problem. Hemorrhoids and rectal prolapse may be evident with straining and can cause constipation. Digital rectal examination is essential in women presenting with severe constipation. Rectal tumors, fissures, intussusception, and rectal mucosal prolapse may be found on examination. Proctoscopy or sigmoidoscopy can be useful when assessing rectal masses and can be performed in the clinic setting.

The tone and squeeze pressure of the anal sphincter should also be assessed as they may be abnormal in women with neurological or traumatic injury, often with a relevant obstetric history. The finger expulsion test involves the patient straining to expel the examining finger in the rectum. Rectal prolapse may become more obvious, as will excessive perineal descent, during straining. Paradoxical contraction of puborectalis and the external anal sphincter during strain is suggestive but not diagnostic of pelvic floor dyssynergy. A combined digital examination of the vagina and rectum allows assessment of contraction and tenderness of the levator ani and puborectalis.

Care must be used when interpreting examination findings as they can be misleading. Anxiety may cause the patient to strain inadequately or contract their pelvic floor muscles. Similarly women may not demonstrate the full extent of rectal or vaginal prolapse due to avoidance of straining for fear of incontinence. Positioning of the patient may also influence this. More severe pelvic organ prolapse has been demonstrated in the standing and sitting positions compared to dorsal lithotomy (62,63). More marked prolapse has been reported on the second vaginal examination by two blinded examiners (50). This suggests that repeated straining may produce greater pelvic organ descent due to the training effect of repeated straining (i.e., getting better at straining) or tissue plasticity. Physical activity before examination has also been found to reveal more severe prolapse (64). It is therefore important to recognize that vaginal and rectal prolapse may be underestimated at examination and maximal prolapse should be confirmed by the patient by sight or palpation if possible.

INVESTIGATION

Women with normal transit times and constipation usually respond well to dietary fiber and laxatives. Hence they do not require further investigation. Those with severe constipation due to STC or obstructed defecation, non-responsive to laxatives, or secondary to medical conditions may require investigation. The American Gastroenterology Association (AGA) published a diagnostic algorithm for the investigation of such patients. This is shown in Figure 59.1. The AGA Technical Review listed colon transit studies, anorectal manometry (ARM) and surface EMG as procedures of value in the investigation of constipation (15). Defecatory proctography, balloon expulsion tests, and rectal sensory testing were listed to be of possible value. These are all discussed below.

Blood Tests

Traditionally routine hematological, biochemical, and thyroid function tests have been recommended when investigating severe chronic constipation. A full blood count, urea and electrolytes, and inflammatory markers (C-reactive protein and erythrocyte sedimentation rate) may be abnormal in women with underlying metabolic disorders or malignancy associated with constipation. Hypercalcemia and hypothyroidism may also be associated with constipation. Diabetic neuropathy affects whole gut transit times and can result in constipation. In this group, glycosylated hemoglobin levels may identify those with poor diabetic control. Better control may alleviate some symptoms but is unlikely to cure constipation.

There is no clear evidence to support routine blood tests in patients presenting with severe constipation (65). Conversely there is no evidence to refute the need of these tests. Certainly, routine screening for hypothyroidism in the absence of specific symptoms (poor appetite, weight gain, cold intolerance, thinning of hair) or suspicion of goiter is considered unnecessary by some clinicians. The remaining blood tests may be

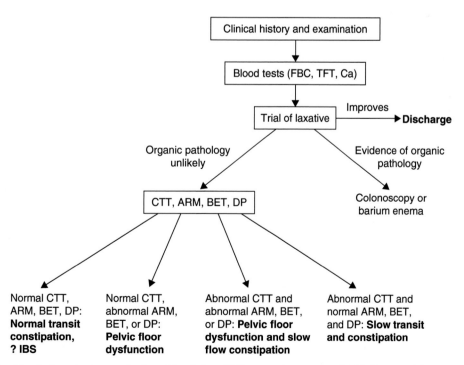

Figure 59.1 Diagnostic algorithm for investigating constipation. *Abbreviations:* ARM, anorectal manometry; BET, balloon expulsion test; Ca, calcium; CTT, colonic transit test; DP, defecation proctogram; FBC, full blood count; IBS, irritable bowel syndrome; TFT, thyroid function test. *Source:* Based on American Gastroenterological Association Guidelines, Ref. 15; adaptation by courtesy of Dr. Jason Goh.

helpful in directing investigation and treatment. In addition, they are cheap and simple to perform.

Endoscopy

Sigmoidoscopy and colonoscopy is necessary if underlying bowel tumors or organic pathology is suspected. A retrospective study of 563 patients with constipation undergoing endoscopy revealed 1.6% had colonic cancer and 14.4% had colonic adenomas (66). Megacolon and megarectum may be diagnosed on endoscopy although radiological tests are superior.

Barium Enema

Most patients with constipation will not require a barium enema. However, it can be used in conjunction with a sigmoidoscopy as an alternative to colonoscopy in the investigation of organic pathology or bowel tumors. It is a particularly useful imaging test for bowel dilatation such as megarectum (transverse diameter of rectum >6.5 cm at the pelvic brim) and megacolon. It will also show denervated bowel segments with proximal dilatation characteristic of Hirschsprung's disease.

Defecating Proctograms

Defecography is not used routinely to investigate constipation. It may be indicated if obstructed defecation is suspected and provides an assessment of the rate, process, and effectiveness of evacuation (Fig. 59.2). Barium paste is used in a variety of carrier mediums, such as oatmeal, to make a paste that approx-

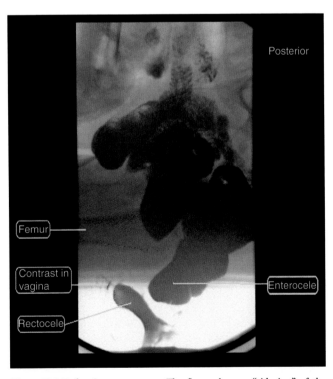

Figure 59.2 Defecating proctogram. The figure shows a "sideview" of the female pelvis with the rectum and sigmoid colon outlined by barium paste. Both a rectocele and an enterocele are clearly demonstrated. The investigations can be enhanced by estimating percentage contrast retention by the rectocele and by performing a simultaneous vaginogram. *Source*: Courtesy of Dr. Peter Guest.

imates feces. This is instilled into the rectum and the patient then defecates on a commode with static and dynamic radiological imaging. Functional obstruction due to failure of relaxation or paradoxical contraction of puborectalis can be identified by measurement of the anorectal angle during attempted defecation. Structural obstructed defecation due to anterior rectocoele, rectal prolapse, intussusception, enterocoeles, vault prolapse, and excess perineal descent can also be identified. The rate and completeness of defecation can be quantified by asking the patient to evacuate 100 ml of barium paste (or alternative low radiation isotope labeled stool) such as quickly as possible.

The accuracy of defecography has been questioned by several investigators (43). Poor inter-observer correlation has been shown in the measurement of the anorectal angle which is critical in the diagnosis of dyssynergic defecation. Although, the rates of evacuation and completeness are lower in subjects with severe constipation compared to normal controls, there is considerable overlap. In addition, rectal mucosal prolapse, intussusception, and perineal descent have been reported in asymptomatic subjects. Defecating proctograms may be helpful in diagnosing anterior rectocoeles in women who describe incomplete evacuation aided by digitation of the vagina or rectum. However, rectocoeles < 2 cm are considered normal in women (67). In addition, larger rectocoeles are not always associated with evacuatory difficulty. Furthermore, surgical correction may not improve defecation.

Dynamic MRI proctography avoids radiation and is non-invasive. However, it is costly and involves defecation in the supine position which is less physiological than using a commode. The development of erect MRI may give more insight into functional evaluation of the anorectum. Translabial (or introital) ultrasound scans are used by some gynecologists and colorectal surgeons as an alternative to defecography a sit is less invasive. Good correlation between translabial ultrasound and anterior and apical prolapse has been reported but only moderate correlation with posterior vaginal prolapse (68). Rectal prolapse and intussusception are also less reliably detected on translabial scanning compared to defecography (69).

Colonic Transit Studies

Colonic transit studies allow patients with slow and normal transit constipation to be objectively distinguished. This is essential before proceeding to colectomy as a treatment for STC. In addition, colonic transit studies may help identify regional delays such as the rectosigmoid in women with functional obstruction due to pelvic floor dysfunction (dyssynergy).

Historically whole gut transit time was measured by the time between ingestion and defecation of glass beads. Currently radiopaque markers are swallowed and abdominal X rays are usually taken at 12 and 120 hours (Fig. 59.3). Normal transit is most commonly defined as the retention of >20% of markers at 12 hours and <80% at 120 hours. The patient should ingest a high fiber diet (20–30 g/day) and avoid laxatives, enemas, or medication that affects the bowel during the study (15). Radiopaque markers of different shapes can be ingested on

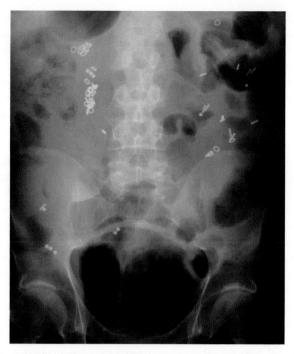

Figure 59.3 The shapes test to evaluate colonic transit. Six gelatin capsules, each containing 10 radiopaque polyurethane markers, are taken two at a time on three consecutive days. The marker shapes are as follows: day 1, spheres; day 2, small rods; day 3, rings. The patient then returns to hospital on day 6 to have an abdominal X ray, which is used to calculate the global and segmental transit times, based on the number and types of markers retained. *Source:* Reproduced by permission from Chaussade S, Roche H, Khyari A, et al. Measurement of colonic transit time: description and validation of a new methoed. Gastroenterol Clin Biol 1986; 10: 38509.

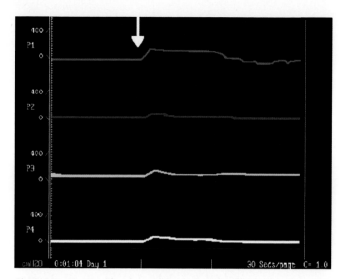

Figure 59.4 An example of a negative rectoanal inhibitory response in a patient with Hirshsprung's disease. Inflation of a balloon in the rectum (the start of inflation is marked by the arrow) fails to cause a corresponding relaxation of the anal canal. The manometric ports are positioned as follows: P1, rectum; P2, upper anal canal; P3, mid-anal canal; P4, low anal canal. *Source:* Courtesy of Ms. Joanne Hayes.

consecutive days to provide intermediate transit information on a single abdominal radiograph at 120 hours. These provide different transit studies in the same individual and are referred to as the "shapes test" (Fig. 59.3). A prolonged transit suggests increased colonic transit is it the main component of whole gut transit. However, small bowel transit and gastric emptying should be measured by radionucleotide or manometric tests before surgical treatment of STC.

Scintigraphy is less commonly used to assess transit times as it involves radiation exposure and is more costly in terms of equipment and personnel. This involves radioisotopes such as indium 111-diethylenetriamine pentaacetic acid or iodine 131. Technetium 99m can be added to measure gastric emptying and small bowel transit. The radioisotopes are swallowed after dissolving in water or incorporated in pH sensitive capsules that dissolve in the terminal ileum thus delivering the isotope to the colon. The progress of the isotope through the colon can be measured with a gamma camera and specific regional transit can be measured. This may be helpful in identifying pelvic floor dyssynergy and in turn guide treatment.

Anorectal Manometry

ARM is usually used to investigate fecal incontinence but may be helpful in some cases of severe constipation to diagnose pelvic floor dyssynergy or exclude Hirschsprung's disease. Anal canal pressures are measured at rest, during squeeze, whilst straining, and during simulated defecation. Water perfused catheters, solid tip microtransducers, or fluid filled balloons can be used to measure anal pressures. Resting pressure indicates the tonic activity of the internal and external anal sphincters and approximately 75% to 85% is due to the internal sphincter (15). Squeeze pressures are measured whilst the patient is asked to contract the external sphincter and therefore the pressure generated mainly reflects the external sphincter action. Resting and squeeze pressures are helpful in the investigation of incontinence rather than constipation. Rectal sensitivity to balloon distension may show hyposensitivity (sensory threshold and urgency threshold) and indicate an impaired innervation. It is unclear whether this may be the cause or a result of chronic constipation. Rectal sensory testing with electronic stimulation of the mucosa may allow neurological causes of constipation to be distinguished from functional constipation. However, this technique has not been validated for this use.

Anal canal relaxation during straining and coughing suggests that the RAIR is intact. The RAIR can be demonstrated during simulated defecation by rectal distension with a balloon. The presence of the RAIR excludes Hirschsprung's disease. Although the absence suggests Hirschsprung's disease, this may also occur in megarectum due to other causes (Fig. 59.4). It is noteworthy that in the presence of megarectum considerable rectal distension is needed before confirming that the RAIR is absent. Histological confirmation with full thickness rectal biopsies is necessary to diagnose Hirschsprung's disease. Manometry during attempted defecation of the rectal balloon may show high anal canal pressures suggesting paradoxical external anal sphincter contraction as is found in pelvic floor dyssynergy. However, it is well recognized that this can also been shown in healthy patients and may reflect anxiety and an inability to relax during the invasive test. Concomitant EMG of the external anal sphincter would confirm that the pressure rises are due to the external sphincter and further supports the diagnosis.

Pudendal Nerve Latency

EMG of the pelvic floor is predominantly used to investigate fecal incontinence. However, adhesive surface electrodes can be used to assess external anal sphincter activity during defecation (real or simulated) in severely constipated patients. A failure to relax suggests pelvic floor dyssynergy. Anal sponge electrodes may produce more reliable results than solid anal plugs as the latter is rigid and does not mould to the shape of the anal canal. Jones et al. found good agreement between surface EMG and balloon expulsion test in the assessment of dyssynergic defecatory patterns. EMG may have the additional advantage of providing visual or audible cues during biofeedback pelvic floor training.

Balloon Expulsion Test

The balloon expulsion test involves a latex balloon inserted into the rectum and filled with 50, 100, or 150 ml of water and subjects are then asked to pass this. Healthy individuals are able to do this indicating normal motor function. Inability to pass a 50 ml balloon in less than two minutes suggests a defecatory disorder which may be due to dyssynergy or structural obstruction. Although this test is not sensitive enough to guide treatment, it is simple to perform in a clinic setting and may identify those who need further investigation.

TREATMENT

Constipation due to systemic, neoplastic, or IBS conditions requires specific management and is not discussed here. The treatment of severe functional constipation varies with the pathophysiology and often involves a multidisciplinary team. STC is managed initially with patient education, lifestyle modification, dietary measures, and medical therapy. Severe intractable cases may require surgery. Constipation due to obstructed defecation is treated with biofeedback, relaxation exercises, and suppositories (rather than laxatives). Rarely in severe cases of pelvic floor dyssynergy is a diversionary colostomy performed when biofeedback and medical measures have failed. Surgery is indicated when there is a structural cause of obstruction such as rectocoele. Patients with a combination of STC and obstructed defecation should be reviewed after treatment of the obstructed defecation. However, there is a lack of high quality evidence for the treatment of severe constipation. This is in part due to the variation in the diagnostic criteria used, small study sizes, and few placebo-controlled randomized controlled trials (RCT).

The variety of treatment modalities used requires the involvement of various health care professionals such as general practitioners, physiotherapists, specialist nurses, dieticians, gastroenterologists, colorectal surgeons, and gynecologists. It is essential that individualized care is planned for each patient with recognition of what troubles the patient. Many therapies require a highly motivated patient and an understanding of the pathophysiology and the aims of the treatment will aid this. In addition, realistic treatment outcomes must be discussed from the beginning as some expectations such as daily bowel opening are unrealistic and will result in a poorly compliant disillusioned patient.

Dietary and Lifestyle Modification

Poor dietary intake of fluid and fiber may contribute to constipation and need to be addressed prior to embarking medical treatment. Correction of this may help with both STC and obstructed defecation. Hard, dry "pebbles" of stool suggests inadequate fluid intake. Reduction in fluid intake in healthy controls has been shown to reduce the stool frequency and mass. Increasing fluid intake has been shown to increase stool frequency in both controls and adults with self reported constipation (<3 bowel movements per week) (70). The increase was greater in those with constipation. In the elderly, a weak correlation between decreased fluid intake and constipation has been reported (47). Cautious increase in the fluid intake is needed in elderly patients with renal or cardiac failure. A fluid intake of 1.5 to 2 L a day is reasonable.

Inadequate dietary fiber is associated with lower stool mass, in part due to its physical mass and partly as it helps bind water. Therefore, stool can be more difficult to pass. The recommended daily fiber intake in the United Kingdom is 18 g/day although 20 to 35 g/day is suggested by some authorities for the treatment of constipation. Dietary fiber can be sourced from cereal, fruit, and vegetables (particularly green vegetables such as peas, spinach, and broccoli). Fresh fruit provide more fiber than fruit juices. Wheat bran is one of the most effective sources and each ounce provides approximately 12 g fiber. Two to six tablespoons can be added to each meal and taken with a glass of water. Ispaghula husk is another commonly used fiber supplement. A gradual increase in intake is recommended over several weeks to minimize abdominal bloating and flatulence due to the fermentation of the degradable fiber by colonic bacteria.

Other lifestyle modifications such as amending irregular eating habits and timing defecation may also be useful. Eating breakfast followed by defecation utilizes the gastro-colic reflex which is strongest in the mornings. This may be helpful in both STC and obstructed defecation. Although, maintaining physical activity is often recommended as a treatment for constipation, there is little evidence to support this (47). The use of bedpans in the elderly is discouraged wherever possible as this position requires more straining effort (71).

Medical Treatment

Many patients have already tried fiber supplements and laxatives before a diagnosis of functional constipation is made. Normal transit constipation will usually respond to fiber and laxatives. STC often responds well to laxatives but obstructed defecation can be exacerbated. Suppositories and enemas may be used to time defecation in women with structural or functional obstruction.

Laxatives

Bulking, osmotic, emollient, and stimulant laxatives are available and will be discussed in turn. Bulking laxatives such as psyllium, methylcellulose, bran, and calcium polycarbophil work by increasing fecal mass and absorbing water. This assists peristalsis and results in increased stool mass and reduced bowel frequency. Natural polysaccharides (e.g., psyllium) may be associated with more abdominal bloating due to fermentation by colonic bacteria than the synthetic preparations (e.g., methylcellulose). A review by the American College of Gastroenterology Chronic Constipation Taskforce reported that psyllium is effective in increasing stool frequency in patients with chronic constipation (grade B recommendation), but that there was insufficient evidence for other bulking agents (72).

Osmotic laxatives, such as polyethylene glycol (PEG) and lactulose, create an osmotic gradient with the gut drawing water into the lumen. Both PEG and lactulose effectively increase stool frequency and consistency in patients with chronic constipation (grade A recommendation) (72). Electrolyte imbalance and diarrhea can occur with these agents. However, low dose PEG was associated with less diarrhea than lactulose in a small well designed RCT (73). Currently a Cochrane review of lactulose versus PEG is being performed.

Emollient laxatives, such as sodium docusate, are surface-acting agents that reduce the surface tension allowing water to be absorbed more easily by the stool. Hence they are often called stool softeners. Although useful to treat occasional constipation, there is insufficient evidence for their use in chronic constipation. In addition, a comparative study showed that psyllium produced significantly better stool frequency than docusate (74). However, no difference in adverse effects between softeners and placebo has been reported (72).

Stimulant laxatives, such as senna and bisacodyl are thought to work by stimulation of the sensory nerves in the colon increasing motility and inhibiting water absorption by the intestinal mucosa. These drugs are useful in cases of occasional constipation but here is inadequate data to recommend their use in patients with chronic constipation (72). In addition, abdominal pain, electrolyte imbalance, and protein losing enteropathy have been reported with these agents. However, some patients find that intermittent use (e.g., three times per week) can be helpful. There is no evidence that long-term use of stimulant laxatives are associated with impaired colonic function, enteric damage, or increased risk of cancer (47).

Enemas/Suppositories
Glycerine or phosphate enemas can used to time defecation in patients with in patients with structural obstruction who do not wish surgery or in whom surgery has been unsuccessful. Although this may cause loose stool and incontinence, it may provide the patient with control over when they defecate in relation to their daily activities. Some patients with hard dry stool which has not improve with increased fluid and fiber or bulking agents find suppositories and enemas assist evacuation.

Prokinetics
Drugs such as metoclopramide and domperidone increase gut motility but appear to predominantly affect increased gastric emptying and upper intestinal motility. They have not been shown to be useful in the treatment of chronic constipation. Cisapride is a benzodiazepine with prokinetic action. However, concerns about safety led to its withdrawal in 2000. Misoprostol (a prostaglandin analogue) has also been used to improve bowel motility (75). However, it should be avoided in women who may become pregnant as it can lead to miscarriage. Erythromycin is macrolide antibiotic that acts on the motilin receptors in the intestinal tract (76). It is associated with increased upper gastrointestinal motility and reduced colonic transit time (77). Its role in the treatment of idiopathic chronic constipation and constipation predominant IBS is currently the subject of an ongoing Cochrane review.

Tegaserod is a partial 5-hydroxytryptamine (5HT) agonist which has been used in constipation predominant IBS and chronic idiopathic constipation. It was shown to improve the stool frequency, frequency of spontaneous complete evacuation, stool consistency, and reduce straining (grade A recommendation) (72,78). In March 2007, it was withdrawn from the market in the United States due to concerns about cardiovascular effects. It has since been re-introduced under a new investigational drug protocol. Prucalopride is also a 5HT agonist and has recently been shown to increase gut motility in placebo-controlled trials over a three month study period (79). However, long term efficacy and safety data is lacking at present.

Lubiprostone
This locally acting calcium channel activator stimulates a chloride rich secretion from the intestines. In comparison to placebo, it has been shown to increase the frequency of spontaneous bowel movements and reduce straining (80). However, long term safety and efficacy compared to other treatments for chronic constipation have yet to be established.

Botulinum Toxin A
Recently Botulinum A has been explored as a treatment for chronic constipation due to paradoxical contraction or failure of puborectalis to relax. In a small study involving 24 patients 60 to 100 units of botulinum A was injected into puborectalis (bilaterally) under ultrasound control. ARM and defecography revealed sustained improvement at two months (81). No fecal incontinence was reported in this series. Botulinum A may prove to be a useful treatment in patients with functional obstruction in whom biofeedback has failed. Repeated injections may be necessary.

Medical Treatment of Opioid-related Constipation
Chronic pain and terminal cancer care often involve opiate therapy which may produce constipation as a side effect. Opioids bind to receptors in the gut and central nervous system and can cause reduced gut motility. Fentanyl is reported to be less constipating than morphine (82). Ensuring adequate hydration and use of stool softeners such as sodium docusate will relieve this side effect in some patients. Others require osmotic laxatives such as PEG. Suppositories can be used if nausea prevents oral therapies. Opioid antagonists, such as naloxone, can be used in conjunction with the opiate analgesia to reduce constipation with reported minimal reduction in analgesia (83). Methylnaltrexone and alvimopan are new opioid antagonists that only work peripherally and hence do not interfere with pain control. Data on their full effectiveness is awaited but the evidence so far is promising (84).

Pregnancy Induced Constipation

STC occurs in some women in pregnancy. There is some evidence that constipation and pregnancy are risk factors for pelvic organ prolapse. As pregnancy and childbirth are non-modifiable risk factors, management of constipation may be particularly important in this group. It is unknown if treatment of pregnancy related constipation reduces the risk of prolapse. A Cochrane review reported that although stimulant laxatives were more effective than bulking agents, these were associated with more unacceptable side effects (abdominal pain and diarrhea) (85). Therefore bulking agents are recommended as first line treatment.

Bowel Retraining and Biofeedback

Biofeedback physiotherapy improves constipation due to pelvic floor dyssynergia in 60% and 80% patients (86–88). Women with symptoms of tenesmus, straining, and sensation of an anorectal blockage are reported to be more likely to respond to biofeedback. Women who needed to digitate to assist evacuation were more likely to fail (88). Biofeedback has not been shown to be helpful in the treatment of STC although some surgeons choose to explore this in patients with STC before undertaking radical surgery (89). The purpose of biofeedback is to retrain the patient to relax the pelvic floor during defecation which is confirmed by EMG and successful expulsion of a rectal balloon. The paradoxical contraction of the pelvic floor can be demonstrated to the patient during simulated defecation using manometry probes (such as anal plugs) or surface perianal/intrarectal EMG probes. Using this form of biofeedback they can then be taught how to relax appropriately and will be "rewarded" by expelling the rectal balloon. Chiarioni et al. showed that successful balloon expulsion occurred in 82% of patients with pelvic floor dyssynergia following a five-week biofeedback program compared to none prior to biofeedback (88). Biofeedback was superior to PEG in symptom improvement and anal EMG findings. Resolution of pelvic floor dyssynergia was confirmed on EMG in 83% of patients at six months and the effects of biofeedback were sustained at two years (88). A well designed RCT in patients with proven pelvic floor dyssynergia showed that instrumented biofeedback (with audible or visual reinforcement) was more effective than verbal instruction alone (87). In addition, biofeedback has been shown to be twice as effective as diazepam, a skeletal muscle relaxant, and placebo (87,88).

Pelvic floor physiotherapy may also be helpful in patients with excessive perineal descent that causes a structural obstruction to defecation. Strengthening of the pelvic floor muscles may ameliorate the degree of perineal descent and reduce the need to strain. Instrumented biofeedback may be helpful in some women although the physiotherapist provides verbal biofeedback by confirming levator ani contraction during the pelvic assessment. If the patient is unable to generate a contraction, electrical stimulation can be used to illustrate a levator ani contraction to the patient.

Complementary Medicine

Some patients with chronic idiopathic constipation try herbal remedies or alternative medicine such as acupuncture or colonic irrigation. There are no robust studies exploring these, with the exception of a small number involving acupuncture. A Cochrane review of the role of acupuncture is currently being performed (90).

Surgical Treatment

Slow Transit Constipation

Five percent of patients with severe STC seen in tertiary centers are estimated to go on to surgery as medical therapies fail (91). A thorough assessment of patients requiring surgery should be performed in all cases to confirm slow colonic transit (radioopaque markers), exclude abnormal upper gastrointestinal motility (scintillography or barium studies), exclude obstructed defecation (defecatory proctogram), and confirm an intact anal sphincter (ultrasound scan and manometry). Pre-operative psychological assessment is routine in some centers as psychological co-morbidity has been associated with poorer outcomes. Clear counseling with should outline that surgery is intended to cure constipation but may have no effect on other physical symptoms ,such as abdominal pain or bloating, or psychological complaints that may be perceived to be due to constipation.

When surgery is required for intractable STC, a total colectomy and ileorectal anastomosis is usually performed. The colectomy is performed at the level of the sacral promontory and care must be taken to preserve the presacral sympathetic nerves. In a series of 74 patients with STC who underwent a total colectomy and ileorectal anastomosis, excellent functional outcome was reported in all cases at five years (11). Ninety seven percent reported that they were satisfied with the surgical results and 90% reported good or improved quality of life. Poorer and more variable outcomes reported in earlier studies have been attributed to less rigorous pre-operative patient selection.

Subtotal colectomy, partial resection of the colon, and preservation of the sigmoid colon (whole or part) are associated with poorer outcomes as constipation can recur in the residual colon (92). Preservation of the caecum has also been associated with poorer outcome. Some surgeons treat severe STC with the antegrade continent enema (ACE) procedure in an attempt to avoid the more invasive colectomy. A conduit is created from the appendix, ileum, caecum, or colon and brought out onto the anterior abdominal wall. Patients are taught to irrigate the conduit thus reducing the time taken to evacuate the bowel and increasing bowel frequency. However, fecal incontinence can occur at the conduit. Other complications include stricture formation and failure. Lees et al. followed up 32 patients (at a median of 36 months) who underwent an ACE procedure due to STC, obstructed defecation, or both (93). The findings revealed that nearly 60% had the procedure reversed and half of these went on to have alternative surgery.

Obstructed Defecation

Structural obstruction due to Hirshsprung's disease is usually diagnosed in childhood and surgery depends on the length of the aganglionic segment. Anal myotomy may be suitable in cases of short segment disease whereas resection may be indicated if larger segments are involved.

Rectocoele Repair

The presence of a rectocoele does not indicate that it is the cause of obstructed defecation. However, a history of digitation of the posterior vagina to assist defecation is supportive. Surgical repair is often performed transvaginally by gynecologists although the technique is not standardized. The colporrhaphy may involve non-specific or defect-specific repair of the rectovaginal fascia. Some gynecologists routinely perform a levatorplasty as part of the posterior vaginal repair. Dysparuenia has been reported in up to 25% of women following a posterior vaginal repair (94). Many urogynecologists attribute this to levatorplasty and have largely abandoned this as a routine part of a transvaginal repair. However, dysparuenia has also been reported following transanal repair. Niemmen et al.) compared the transvaginal and transanal approaches in a small randomized trial and found no cases de novo dysparuenia in either group and similar improvement in sexual function with both techniques (95). The vaginal approach has been reported as superior to the transanal approach in the correction of the symptom of a bulge (95,96). However, others have reported similar improvement in vaginal bulge and obstructed defecation in the vaginal and transanal approaches (97,98) The transanal procedure involves an incision in the anterior rectal wall just above the dentate line to create a mucosal flap through which the rectovaginal septum is plicated. Excess rectal mucosa can be excised before suturing the flap back. Some surgeons believe that this results in better resolution of symptoms of tenesmus and straining. However, currently there is no strong evidence to recommend the transvaginal approach over the transanal or vice versa.

Transperineal repair of rectocoele may be useful if co-existent fecal incontinence requiring sphincter repair is present. Laparoscopic repair of rectocoele with mesh is a relatively new technique and not widely used. It involves more complex surgery with mobilization of the rectum but may afford better access to the rectovaginal septum (due to gaseous dissection) and correction of enterocoele and rectocoele. However, mesh infection or erosions are recognized complications.

Surgery for Rectal Prolapse and Intussusception

Surgical correction of rectal prolapse and intussusseption can be via the abdominal (open or laparoscopic), transperineal, or transrectal approach. Abdominal rectopexy using either suture or mesh fixation may be more effective in relieving obstructive symptoms if it is performed in conjunction with sigmoid resection. A Cochrane review of rectal prolapse surgery found that lower rates of post operative constipation occur with bowel resection and rectopexy (99). Higher post-operative constipation but less recurrent rectal prolapse occurred with division rather than preservation of the lateral ligaments (99). Predictably, laparoscopic surgery was associated with lower morbidity and shorter hospital stay than open abdominal surgery (99). In the presence of demonstrable vault prolapse or enterocoele, a sacrocolpopexy may be needed to prevent persistent post-operative obstructive symptoms.

Perineal procedures can be performed under regional anesthesia and are associated with less morbidity than abdominal procedures. Despite higher recurrence rates of rectal prolapse with perineal procedures, they are useful techniques in very elderly or medically unfit patients. Tou et al. review of complete rectal prolapse reported that there was insufficient data to determine superiority of abdominal or perineal techniques (99). Perineal rectosigmoidectomy (Altemeier procedure) involves the resection of prolapsed rectum and sigmoid and coloanal reanastomosis via the perineal approach. The subsequent fibrosis is thought to attach the lower rectum to the sacrum and may prevent recurrent prolapse. Comparison of perineal rectosigmoidectomy with harmonic scalpel resection and stapled reanastomosis with diathermy resection and hand-sewn reanastomosis showed recurrent prolapse in approximately 10% for both techniques (100). However, this was a small RCT involving 20 patients in each arm and improvement of obstructed defecation was not confirmed by proctography. Delormes procedure is also carried out via the perineal approach and involves stripping of the rectal mucosa and plication of the underlying muscle. Low morbidity has been reported with this technique but recurrent rectal prolapse has been described in 27% following a primary Delorme's procedure (101).

More recently, transrectal procedures to correct rectal prolapse have been developed. The stapled transanal rectal resection removes internally prolapsed rectum and rectocoele with a purpose designed stapler. Short term data suggests improvement in obstructed constipation with no recurrence of rectal prolapse (102). Complications of the procedure included fecal urgency, flatal incontinence, bleeding, and stenosis.

Sacral Nerve Stimulation (SNS)

SNS is an effective treatment in some people with fecal incontinence (103). Early results suggest that it has a place in the treatment of severe idiopathic STC and obstructed constipation in which conventional medical, biofeedback, and surgical treatment have failed. Successful neuromodulation of the sacral nerve plexus can be tested initially with temporary peripheral nerve stimulation to select patients who demonstrate improvement to go on to a permanent implant. The implants are inserted under general anesthesia and in comparison to colectomy are less invasive and reversible. Jarrett et al. performed a systematic review of two studies involving temporary peripheral nerve evaluation, two series involving permanent SNS implants, and a double-blind cross over study involving two patients (with STC) with permanent SNS (104). A total of 20 patients in the review had permanent SNS as a treatment of severe functional chronic constipation (STC, obstructed defecation, and IBS). An increased frequency of defecation, reduction in abdominal bloating, and improvement in constipation and quality of life scores was found in those with permanent SNS. Return of symptoms and reduction in the frequency of bowel movements occurred in one case series (n = 16) and the double-blind crossover study (n = 2) when the implant was switched "off" (105,106). A Cochrane review by Mowatt et al. agreed that the limited evidence available suggested that SNS was an effective treatment for constipation in some patients (103). More recently, a study of 19 women with STC, rectal outlet obstruction (excluding rectal prolapse) or both showed that 42% (n = 4 STC and n = 4 with

615

outlet obstruction) responded to the stimulation in the evaluation period (107). These women were fitted with a permanent pulse SNS and demonstrated sustained improvement in the Wexner constipation scores at a median of 11 months (108). One subject lost the response following traumatic dislodgement of the implant in a car crash.

In the future SNS implants may become first-line treatment in severe constipation when conservative measures have failed and before consideration of invasive and irreversible surgery. However, there is insufficient evidence to recommend this at present. Larger studies are required to fully evaluate this technique and safety. Adverse events such as dislodgement, pain, and infection have been reported.

CONCLUSION

Functional constipation is common in the general population and can produce severe intractable symptoms affecting quality of life. The etiology is varied and not fully understood. There is increasing evidence of abnormalities in the enteric nervous system in patients with STC. However, it is unknown whether this is a cause or effect of constipation. Treatment of STC involves dietary and medical therapy with surgery reserved for intractable cases. Obstructed defecation and combined STC and obstructed defecation are more prevalent in women. Laxatives are often unhelpful in structural obstruction although suppositories or enemas are useful in some patients. Surgery to correct prolapse (rectocoele, rectal prolapse, enterocoeles, or uterine prolapse) may be required. Functional obstruction due to paradoxical puborectalis contraction (or failure to relax) requires biofeedback and bowel retraining with diversionary surgery for severe intractable cases. SNS and botulinum A injections are exciting new developments in the treatment of dyssynergic defecation but need further evaluation. Greater refinement of our understanding of the etiology should lead to a refinement in the selection of treatment options. More robust evaluation of outcomes of treatment including quality of life measures will lead to progress in management.

There is recognized overlap in bowel, prolapse, and urinary symptoms in women with pelvic floor dysfunction. Straining due to constipation may be a risk factor for prolapse. This may be particularly important in pregnant women as parity itself is the strongest risk factor for prolapse. Therefore constipation in women, and especially during pregnancy, should be treated.

REFERENCES

1. Connell AM, Hilton C, Irvine G, et al. Variation in bowel habit in two sample populations. BMJ 1965; 2: 1095–9.
2. Drossman DA. The functional gastrointestinal disorders and the Rome 3 process. Gastroenterology 2006; 130: 1377–90.
3. Pare P, Ferrazzi M, Thompson WG, et al. An epidemiological survey of constipation in Canada: definitions, rates, demographics, and predictors of health care seeking. Am J Gastroenterol 2001; 96: 3130–37.
4. Higgins PD, Johanson JF. Epidemiology of constipation in North America: a systematic review. Am J Gastroenterol 2004; 99: 750–9.
5. Everhart JE, Go VLW, Johannes RS, et al. A longitudinal survey of self-reported bowel habits in the United States. Dig Dis Sci 1989; 34: 1153–62.
6. Stewart WF, Liberman JN, Sandler RS, et al. Epidemiology of constipation (EPOC) study in the United States: relation of clinical subtypes to sociodemographic features. Am J Gastroenterol 1999; 94: 3530–40.
7. Drossman DA, Li Z, Andruzzi E, et al. U.S. householder survey of functional gastrointestinal disorders. Dig Dis Sci 1993; 38: 1569–80.
8. Talley NJ, Weaver AL, Zinsmeister AR, et al. Functional constipation and outlet delay: a population-based study. Gastroenterology 1993; 105: 781–90.
9. Johanson JF, Sonnenberg A, Koch TR. Clinical epidemiology of chronic constipation. J Clin Gastroenterol 1989; 11: 525–36.
10. Sandler RS, Drossman DA. Bowel habits in young adults not seeking health care. Dig Dis Sci 1987; 32: 841–5.
11. Nyam DC, Pemberton JH, Ilstrup DM, Rath DM. Long-term results of surgery for chronic constipation. Dis Colon Rectum 1997; 40: 273–9.
12. Evans RC, Kamm MA, Hinton JM, Lennard-Jones JE. The normal range and a simple diagram for recording whole gut transit time. Int J Colorectal Dis 1992; 7: 15–17.
13. Notghi A, Hutchinson R, Kumar D, et al. Simplified method for the measurement of segmental colonic transit time. Gut 1994; 35: 976–81.
14. Bouchoucha M, Devroede G, Arhan P, et al. What is the meaning of colorectal transit time measurement? Dis Colon Rectum 1992; 35: 773–82.
15. Locke III GR, Pemberton JH, Phillips SF. AGA technical review of constipation. Gastroenterology 2000; 119: 1766–78.
16. Kamm Ma, Farthing MJ, Lenard-Jones JE. Bowel function and transit rate during the menstrual cycle. Gut 1989; 30: 605–8.
17. Shafik A. The role of the levator ani muscle in evacuation, sexual performance and pelvic floor disorders. Int Urogynecol J Pelvic Floor Dysfunct 2000; 11: 361–6.
18. Schermann M, Neunlist M. The human enteric nervous system. Neurogastroenterol Motil 2004; 16: 55–9.
19. Tong WD, Liu BH, Zhang LY, et al. Decreased interstitial cells of Cajal in the sigmoid colon of patients with slow transit constipation. Int J Colorectal Dis 2004; 19: 467–73.
20. Lee JI, park H, Kamm MA, Talbot IC. Decreased density of interstitial cells of Cajal and neuronal cells in patients with slow-transit constipation and acquired megacolon. J Gastroenterol Hepatol 2005; 20: 1292–8.
21. Wedel T, Spiegler J, Soellner S, et al. Enteric nerves and interstitial cells of Cajal are altered in patients with slow-transit constipation and megacolon. Gastroenterology 2002; 123: 1459–67.
22. Wang LM, McNally M, Hyland J, Sheahan K. Assessing interstitial cells of Cajal in slow-transit constipation using CD117 is a useful diagnostic test. Am J Surg Pathol 2008; 32: 980–5.
23. He CL, Burgart L, Wang L, et al. Decreased interstitial cells of Cajal volume in patients with slow-transit constipation. Gastroenterology 2000; 118: 14–21.
24. van der Sijp JRM, Kamm MA, Nightingale JMD, et al. Circulating gastrointestinal hormone abnormalities in patients with severe idiopathic constipation. Am J Gastroenterol 1998; 93: 1351–6.
25. Costedio MM, Hyman N, Mawe G. Serotonin and its role in colonic function and in gastrointestinal disorders. Dis Colon Rectum 2007; 50: 376–88.
26. Kamm MA, Farthing MJ, Lennard-Jones JE, et al. Steroid hormone abnormalities in women with severe idiopathic constipation. Gut 1991; 32: 80–4.
27. Bradley CS, Kennedy CM, Turcea AM, et al. Constipation in pregnancy: prevalence, symptoms and risk factors. Obstet Gynecol 2007; 110: 1351–7.
28. Wald A, Thiel DH, Hoechstetter L, et al. Effect of pregnancy on gastrointestinal transit. Dig Dis Sci 1982; 27: 1015–18.
29. Soligo M, Salvatore S, Emmanuel AV, et al. Patterns of constipation in urogynaecology: Clinical importance and pathophysiologic insights. Am J Obstet Gynecol 2006;195: 50–5.
30. Mouristen L, Larsen JP. Symptoms, bother, and POPQ in women referred with pelvic organ prolapse. Int Urogynecol J Pelvic Floor Dysfunct 2003; 14: 122–7.
31. Weber Am, Walters MD, Ballard LA, et al. Posterior vaginal wal prolapse and bowel function. Am J Obstet Gynecol 1998; 179: 1446–9.
32. Fialkow MF, Gardella C, Melville J, et al. Posterior vaginal defects and their relation to measures of pelvic floor neuromuscular function and posterior compartment symptoms. Am J Obstet Gynecol 2002; 187: 1443–8.

33. Glavind K, Marsden H. A prospective study of discrete fascial defect in rectocoele repair. Acta Obstet Gynecol Scand 2000; 79: 145–7.

34. Wiersma TG, Werre AJ, Den Hartog G, et al. Hysterectomy; the anorectal pitfall. A guideline for evaluation. Scand J Gastroenterol 1997; 223(Suppl): 3–7.

35. Kahn MA, Breitkopf CR, Valley MT, et al. Pelvic organ support study (POSST) and bowel symptoms; straining at stool is associated with perineal and anterior descent in a general gynecologic population. Am J Obstet Gynecol 2005; 192: 1516–22.

36. Snooks SJ, Barnes PR, Swash M, Henry MM. Damage to the innervations to the pelvic floor musculature in chronic constipation. Gastroenterology 1985; 89: 977–81.

37. Lubowski DZ, Swash M, Nichols RJ, Henry MM. Increased pudendal nerve terminal motor latency with defecation straining. Br J Surg 1988; 75: 1095–7.

38. Kiff ES, Barnes PR, Swash M. Evidence of pudendal neuropathy in patients with perineal descent and chronic straining at stool. Gut 1984; 25: 1279–82.

39. Spence-Jones C, Kamm MA, Henry MM, Hudson CM. Bowel dysfunction: a pathogenic factor in uterovaginal prolapse and urinary stress incontinence. BJOG 1994; 101: 147–52.

40. Bharaucha AE, Wald A, Enck P, Rao S. Functional anorectal disorders. Gastroenterology 2006; 130: 1510–18.

41. Drossman DA, Leserman J, Nachman G, et al. Sexual and physical abuse in women with functional or organic gastrointestinal disorders. Ann Intern Med 1990; 113: 828–33.

42. Crowell MD. Pathogenesis of slow transit and pelvic floor dysfunction; from bench to bedside. Rev Gastroenterol Disord 2004; 4: S17–27.

43. Diamant NE, Kamm MA, Wald A, Whitehead WE. AGA technical review on anorectal testing techniques. Gastroenterology 1999; 116: 735–60.

44. Sandler RS, Jordan MC, Shelton BJ. Demographic and dietary determinants of constipation in the US population. Am J Pub Health 1990; 80: 185–9.

45. Locke III GR, Pemberton JH, Phillips SF. AGA medical position statement; guidelines on constipation. Gastroenterology 2000; 119: 1761–6.

46. Tuteja AK, Taley NJ, Joos SK, et al. Is constipation associated with decreased physical activity in normally active subjects? Am J Gastroenterol 2005; 100: 124–9.

47. Muller-Lissner SA, Kamm MA, Scarpignato C, Wald A. Myths and misconceptions about chronic constipation. Am J Gastroenterol 2005; 100: 232–42.

48. Prior A, Stanley KM, Smith ARB, Read NW. Relation between hysterectomy and the irritable bowel: a prospective study. Gut 1992; 33: 814–17.

49. Weber AM, Walters MD, Schover LR, et al. Functional outcomes and satisfaction after abdominal hysterectomy. Am J Obstet Gynecol 1999; 181: 530–5.

50. Ali-Ross NS. Pelvic floor signs and symptoms in women with and without pelvic floor dysfunction. M.D. Thesis. University of Manchester, 2008.

51. Smith AR, Hosker GL, Warrell DW. The role of partial denervation of the pelvic floor in the aetiology of genitourinary prolapse and stress incontinence. A neurophysiological study. BJOG 1989; 96: 24–8.

52. Gilpin SA, Gosling JA, Warrell DW. The pathogenesis of genitourinary prolapse and stress incontinence of urine. A histological and histochemical study. BJOG 1989; 96: 15–23.

53. Lawrence JM, Lucacz ES, Nager CW, et al. Prevalence and co-occurrence of pelvic floor disorders in community-dwelling women. Am J Obstet Gynecol 2008; 111: 678–85.

54. Samuelsson EC, Arne Victor FT, Tibblin G, Svardsudd KE. Signs of genital prolapse in a Swedish population of women 20 to 59 years of age and possible related factors. Am J Obstet Gynecol 1999; 180(2 Pt 1): 299–305.

55. Progetto Group. Risk factors for genital prolapse in non-hysterectomized women around the menopause. Results from a cross-sectional study in menopausal clinics in Italy. Progetto Menopausa Italia Study Group. Eur J Obstet Gynecol Reprod Biol 2000; 93: 135–40.

56. Chiaffarino F, Chatenoud L, Dindelli M, et al. Reproductive factors, family history, occupation and risk of genital prolapse. Eur J Obstet Gynecol Reprod Biol 1999; 82: 63–7.

57. Mant J, Painter R, Vessey M. Epidemiology of genital prolapse: observations from the Oxford family planning association study. BJOG 1997; 104: 579–85.

58. Hendrix SL, Clark A, Nygaard I, et al. Pelvic organ prolapse in the Women's Health Initiative: gravity and gravidity. Am J Obstet Gynecol 2002; 186: 1160–6.

59. Lewis SJ, Heaton KW. Stool form scale a useful guide to intestinal transit time. Scand J Gastroenterol 1997; 32: 920–4.

60. Sayer TR, Dixon GL, Hosker GL, Warrell DW. A study of paraurethral connective tissue in women with stress incontinence of urine. Neurourol Urodyn 1990; 9:319–20.

61. Rinne KM, Kirkinen PP. What predisposes young women to genital prolapse? Eur J Obstet Gynecol Reprod Biol 1999; 84: 23–5.

62. Barber MD, Lambers A, Visco AG, Bump RC. Effect of patient position on clinical evaluation of pelvic organ prolapse. Obstet Gynecol 2000; 96: 18–22.

63. Visco AG, Wei JT, McClure LA, Handa VL, Nygaard IE. Effects of examination technique modifications on pelvic organ prolapse quantification (POP-q) results. Int Urogynecol J Pelvic Dysfunct 2003; 14: 136–40.

64. Ali-Ross NS, Smith ARB, Hosker G. The effect of physical activity on pelvic organ prolapse. BJOG 2009; 116: 824–8.

65. Rao SSC, Ozturk R, Laine L. Clinical utility of diagnostic tests for constipation in adults: a systematic review. Am J Gastroenterol 2005; 100: 1605–15.

66. Pepin C, Ladabaum U. The yield of lower endoscopy in patients with constipation: survey of a university hospital, a public county hospital and a veterans administration medical center. Gastrointest Endosc 2002; 56: 325–32.

67. Shorvon P, McHugh JS, Diamant NE, et al. Defecography in normal volunteers: results and implications. Gut 1989; 30: 1737–49.

68. Dietz HP, Haylen BT, Broome J. Ultrasound in the quantification of female pelvic organ prolapse. Ultrasound Obstet Gynecol 2001; 18: 511–14.

69. Perniola G, Shek C, Chong CC, et al. Defecation proctography and translabial ultrasound scan in the investigation of defecatory disorders. Ultrasound Obstet Gynecol 2008; 31: 567–71.

70. Jones PN, Lubowski DZ, Swash M, Henry MM. Is paradoxical contraction of puborectalis muscle of functional importance? Dis Colon Rectum 1987; 30: 667–70.

71. Anti M, Pignataro G, Armuzzi A, et al. Water supplementation enhances the effect of high-fibre diet on stool frequency and laxative consumption in adult patients with functional constipation. Hepatogastroenterology 1998; 45: 727–32.

72. Castledine G, Grainger M, Wood N, Dilley C. Researching the management of constipation in long-term care: Part 1. Br J Nurs 2007; 16: 1128–31.

73. Brandt L, Prather C, Schiller L, et al. An evidence-based approach to the management of chronic constipation in North America. Am J Gastroenterol 2005; 100(Suppl 1): S1–22.

74. Attar A, Lemann M, Ferguson A, et al. Comparison of a low dose polyethylene glycol electrolyte solution with lactulose for treatment of chronic constipation. Gut 1999; 44: 226–30.

75. McRorie JW, Daggy BP, Morel Jg, et al. Psyllium is superior to docusate sodium for treatment of chronic constipation. Aliment Pharmacol Ther 1998; 12: 491–7.

76. Roarty TP, Weber F, Soykan I, McCallum RW. Misoprostol in the treatment of chronic refactory constipation: results of a long-term open label trial. Aliment Pharmacol Ther 1997; 11: 1059–66.

77. Coulie B, Tack J, Peeters T, Janssens J. Involvement of two different pathways in the motor effects of erythromycin on the gastric antrum in humans. Gut 1998; 43: 395–400.

78. Landry C, Vidon N, Sogni P, et al. Effects of erythromycin on gastric emptying, duodeno-caecal transit time, gastric and biliopancreatic secretion during continuous gastric infusion of a liquid diet in healthy volunteers. Eur J Gastroenterol Hepatol 1995; 7: 797–802.

79. Evans BW, Clark WK, Moore DJ, Whorwell PJ. Tegaserod for the treatment of irritable bowel syndrome and chronic constipation. Cochrane Database Syst Rev 2007: CD003960. DOI: 10.1002/14651858. CD003960.pub3.

80. Camilleri M, Kerstens R, Rykx A, Vandeplassche L. A placebo-controlled trial of Prucalopride for severe chronic constipation. NEJM 2008; 358: 2344–54.

81. Johasson JF, Ueno R. Lubiprostone, a locally acting chloride channel activator, in adult patients with chronic constipation: a double blind placebo-controlled, dose ranging study to evaluate efficacy and safety. Aliment Pharmacol Ther 2007; 25: 1351–61.

82. Maria G, Cadeddu F, Brandara F, et al. Experience with type A botulinum toxin for treatment of outlet-type constipation. Am J Gastroenterol 2006; 101: 2570–5.

83. Tassinari D, Sartori S, Tamburini E, et al. Adverse effects of transdermal opiates treating moderate-severe cancer pain in comparison to long-acting morphine: a meta-analysis and systematic review of the literature. J Palliat Med 2008; 11: 492–501.

84. Sykes NP. An investigation of the ability of oral naloxone to correct opioid-related constipation in patients with advanced cancer. Palliat Med 1996; 10: 135–44.

85. McNichol ED, Boyce D, Schumann R, Carr DB. Mu-opioid antagonists for opioid-induced bowel dysfunction. Cochrane Database of Syst Rev 2008: CD006332. DOI: 10. 1002/14651858. CD 006332.

86. Jewell D, Young G. Interventions for treating constipation in pregnancy. Cochrane Database Syst Rev 2001: CD001142. DOI 10.1002/14651858. CD001142

87. Palssoon OS, Heyman S, Whitehead WE. Biofeedback treatment for functional anorectal disorders: a comprehensive efficacy review. Appl Psychophysiol Biofeedback 2004; 29: 153–74.

88. Heyman S, Scarlett Y, Jones K et al. Randomized, controlled trial shows biofeedback to be superior to alternative treatments for patients with pelvic floor dyssynergia-type constipation. Dis Colon Rectum 2007; 50: 428–41.

89. Chiarioni G, Whitehead WE, Pezza V, et al. Biofeedback is superior to laxatives for normal transit constipation due to pelvic floor dyssynergia. Gastroenterology 2006; 130: 657–64.

90. Chiarioni G, Salandini L, Whitehead WE. Biofeedback benefits only patients with outlet dysfunction, not patients with isolated slow transit constipation. Gastroenterology 2005; 129: 86–97.

91. Zhao H, Liu JP, Liu Z, Peng W. Acupuncture for chronic constipation. Cochrane Database of Systematic Reviews 2003, Issue 2 Art. CD 004117: DOI: 10.1002/14651858. CD004117.

92. Kamm MA, Hawley PR, Lennard-Jones JE. Outcome for colectomy for severe idiopathic constipation. Gut 1988; 29: 969–73.

93. Vasilevsky Ca, Nemer FD, Balcos EG, et al. Is subtotal colectomy a viable option in the management of chronic constipation? Dis Colon Rectum 1988; 31: 679–81.

94. Lees NP, Hodson P, Hill J, et al. Long-trem results of the antegrade continent enema procedure for constipation in adults. Colorectal Dis 2004; 6: 362–8.

95. Kahn MA, Stanton SI. Posterior colporrhaphy; its effects on bowel and sexual function. Br J Obstet Gynaecol 1997; 104: 882–6.

96. Niemmen K, Hiltunen K, Laitinen J, et al. Transanal or vaginal approach to rectocoele repair: a prospective randomized pilot study. Dis Colon Rectum 2004; 47: 636–42.

97. Kahn MA, Stanton SL, Kumar D, Fox SD. Posterior colporrhaphy is superior to the transanal repair for the treatment of posterior vaginal wall prolapse. Neurourol Urodyn 1999; 18: 329–30.

98. Zbar AP, Lienemann A, Fritsch H, et al. Rectocoele: pathogenesis and surgical management. Int J Colorectal Dis 2003; 18: 369–84.

99. Murphy VK, Orkin BA, Smith LE, Glassman LM. Excellent outcome using selective criteria for rectocoele repair. Dis Colon Rectum 1996; 39: 374–8.

100. Boccasanta P, Venturi M, Barbieri S, Roviaro G. Impact of new technologies on the clinical and functional outcome of Altemeier's procedure: a randomized controlled trial. Dis Colon Rectum 2006; 49: 652–60.

101. Watts AM, Thompson MR. Evaluation of Delorme's procedure as a treatment for full-thickness rectal prolapse. Br J Surg 2000; 87: 218–22.

102. Boccasanta P, Venturi M, Salamina G, et al. New trends in the surgical treatment of outlet obstruction; clinical and functional results of two novel transanal stapled techniques from a randomised controlled trial. Int J Colorectal Dis 2004; 19: 359–69.

103. Mowatt G, Glazener CM, Jarrett M. Sacral nerve stimulation for facela incontinence and constipation in adults. Cochrane Database of Systematic Reviews 2007: CD0044464. DOI: 10.1002/14651858.CD004464. pub2.

104. Jarrett MED, Mowatt G, Glazener CMA, et al. Systematic review of scaral nerve stimulation for faecal incontinence and constipation. Br J Surg 2004; 91: 1559–69.

105. Ganio E, Masin A, Ratto C et al. Sacral nerve modulation for chronic outlet constipation. [Available from: http://www.colorep.it]. [May 2003].

106. Kenefick NJ, Vaizey CJ, Cohen CRG, et al. Double-blind placebo-controlled crossover study of sacral nerve stimulation for idiopathic constipation. Br J Surg 2002; 89: 1570–1.

107. Holzer B, Rosen HR, Novi G, et al. Sacral nerve stimulation in patients with severe constipation. Dis Colon Rectum 2008; 51: 524–30.

108. Agachan F, Chen T, Pfeifer J, et al. A constipation scoring system to simplify evaluation and management of constipated patients. Dis Colon Rectum 1996; 39: 681–5.

60 Female Sexual Dysfunction
Irwin Goldstein

INTRODUCTION

On an average day in a female urology and urogynecology practitioner's office, patients will be examined who also have sexual health concerns (1–41). In fact, the sexual health problem may be highly associated, or indeed the primary health care problem (5,6,12,14,20,26,27,30,36,41–43).

To provide the best overall care, it is important that clinicians be familiar with the basic aspects of appropriate women's sexual health care delivery. Women's sexual problems may be associated with significant personal distress including a diminution of self-worth and self-esteem, a reduction in life satisfaction, and a decline in the quality of the relationship with her partner (13,22,42,43). In some women, a satisfying sex life may be important throughout most of their lives (13).

To appreciate women's sexual health care problems, it is relevant to understand the term "sexual health" (44). "Sexual health" refers to a state of physical, emotional, mental, and social well-being related to sexuality. Women have the right to a positive and respectful approach to sexuality and to sexual relationships, and to have pleasurable and safe sexual experiences, free of coercion, discrimination, and violence. For sexual health to be attained and maintained, the sexual rights of all women must be respected, protected, and fulfilled. Women have the right to sexual equity–the freedom from all forms of discrimination regardless of sexual orientation, age, race, social class, religion, or physical and emotional disability. Women also have the right to sexual pleasure, which is a source of physical, psychological, intellectual, and spiritual well-being (44).

Despite female urology and urogynecology practitioners having a unique position to understand the anatomy and physiology of the peripheral genitalia and pelvic floor constituents, they may still face multiple challenges while engaging their patients who present with primary urinary dysfunction but who also have sexual health concerns. Time is not the only constraint on developing effective strategies to manage their sexual health concerns; female urology and urogynecology clinicians have often received limited or no training in the diagnosis and treatment of women with sexual health concerns during medical school, residency, and/or sub-specialty training.

Furthermore, sexual medicine issues are usually complex and are, in general, secondary to individual interrelated psychological, physiological, and relationship issues molded with distinct couple dynamics. Psychological factors (7) include: previous sexual trauma and abuse (45–49), depression (50–53), psychoses, anxiety, distraction, sexual neuroses, sexual inhibitions or idiosyncrasies, and/or interpersonal relationship issues. Pertinent biological factors may involve aging (54,55), exposure to metabolic syndromes (8), hyperlipidemia (9),

obesity (8), diabetes (2,8,11,35), and hypothyroidism (8), urological conditions such as interstitial cystitis (34), post-radical cystectomy, recurrent urinary tract infections, overactive bladder (18,27,33,42,43), urinary incontinence (5,20,26,30,36), gynecological conditions such as endometriosis, uterine fibroids (15), aspects associated with prior hysterectomy, tissue weakness with organ prolapse (6,41), retroperitoneal masses (56), genital tissue sexually transmitted infections (12), inflammation, abnormal immunologic conditions, blunt or penetrating traumatic injury, sexual pain disorders (57–63), pregnancy and childbirth (64,65), vulvar dermatologic disorders (66), infertility issues (67), hormone replacement therapy and menopause (10,14,68–73), breast cancer (74–76), other medical problems such as rectal cancer (77), renal failure (78–81), headache (82), coronary artery disease and cardiovascular rehabilitation (83–85), sleep apnea (86), other sexual problems such as pelvic floor dysfunction (5,32,46,61), persistent genital arousal disorder (87–89), and female genital mutilation (90). Women's sexual health problems may also stem from the male partner (91–96); that is, should the male partner experience premature ejaculation, erectile dysfunction, inability to have an orgasm, Peyronie's disease, or prostate cancer, his sexual dysfunction can adversely effect his female partner's sexual health (91–96).

The objective of this chapter is to provide relevant evidence-based clinical information to help practitioners to diagnose and treat specific biologic-based sexual health pathophysiologies. Even though health care clinicians need to be holistic in managing women with sexual dysfunction and be aware that both psychological and biological issues cause sexual health problems, the this chapter concentrates on the biological aspects of how to identify pathologies associated with the sexual health concerns, and how to provide evidence-based safe and effective management strategies. A clinical biological-based paradigm (Fig. 60.1A and B) is presented founded on results derived from emerging basic science and evidence-based data derived from clinical research. In most cases women with sexual health concerns should consider undergoing concomitant psychological assessment and management by an appropriately trained specialist (97–100).

Clinicians who are particularly interested in women's sexual health or want to improve their clinical management skills may wish to become members of the International Society for the Study of Women's Sexual Health (ISSWSH), an international, multidisciplinary, academic, clinical, and scientific organization. The purposes of ISSWSH are to provide opportunities for communication among scholars, researchers, and practitioners about women's sexual health; to support the highest standards of ethics and professionalism in research, education, and clinical practice relative to women's sexual health; and to provide

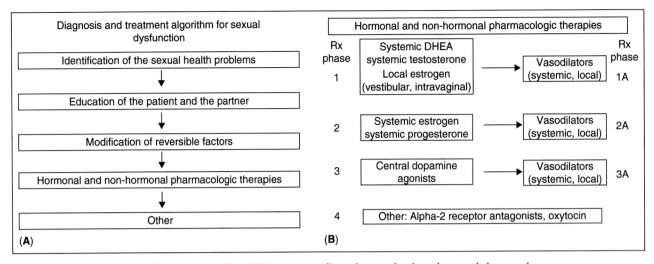

Figure 60.1 (**A**) Step care paradigm. (**B**) Step care paradigm—hormonal and non-hormonal pharmacotherapy.

the public with accurate information about women's sexual health. Interested healthcare professionals should visit the organization's website: http://www.isswsh.org.

DIAGNOSIS OF WOMAN WITH SEXUAL HEALTH CONCERN
History
There are limited consensed management paradigms for the diagnosis of women with sexual health complaints. As it concerns the biological-based sexual dysfunction, the most relevant aspect of the diagnosis is the history and physical examination.

Clinical history taking centers on three components: sexual, medical, and psychosocial aspects. The sexual history should begin with the patient describing the sexual problem. The following questions may be utilized to help obtain maximal descriptive information.

- Sexual problems are common in women who have urinary complaints, do you have any sexual problems?
- Do you ever experience problems with sexual interest, sexual arousal, and sexual orgasm?
- What is your current sexual functioning in terms of interest, arousal, and orgasm compared to when you were at peak sexual function?
- How long have you had the sexual problem?
- Does the sexual problem happen all the time?
- Does the sexual problem occur during partner-related sexual activity?
- Does the sexual problem occur during self-stimulation?
- In which situations is the sexual problem minimized? In which situations is the sexual problem maximized?
- Is the sexual problem associated with any degree of discomfort, tenderness, soreness or pain? If so, can you localize the site of the pain on a schematic diagram of a woman's genitalia?
- What tests have you already had in the evaluation of your sexual health concern?

- What treatments have you already received and what are the outcomes of the various treatments?
- How does the sexual problem effect you? How is your partner effected by the sexual problem?
- Does the sexual problem cause you to withdraw from partner-related sexual activity, from self-stimulated sexual activity or from the relationship? How would you feel if the sexual problem were cured?

It is relevant to inquire after the sexual health of the partner. For women with men, there may exist male sexual dysfunctions such as erectile dysfunction, early ejaculation, or an anatomical concern, such as Peyronie's disease.

Validated, reliable, standardized self-rated questionnaires (101–104) are useful to assist in identification of the presence or absence of the various domains of women's sexual dysfunction, such as sexual desire, sexual arousal, orgasm, and/or sexual pain. The most common such questionnaire is the female sexual function index (2,3,8,9,17,23,24,26,35,39). This self-reported patient screening tool is used to score symptoms against normative values for populations of women with and without sexual dysfunction. As in all areas of clinical medicine, the use of screening tools for clinical diagnosis has recognized limitations. The determination of particular psychological contributors or confounds, contextual conditions, and other features and characteristics that cause individual women their unique sexual concerns requires more traditional assessment through structured history and physical examination.

The medical history should include focused questions on any accompanying medical/surgical illnesses and/or the use of medications (18). Urogynecologic history-taking such as incontinence (5,20,26,30,36), frequent urinary tract infections, interstitial cystitis (34), pelvic surgeries, childbirth (64,65), abortions, episiotomy, abnormal prostatic acid phosphatase smears, sexually transmitted diseases (12), pelvic inflammatory disorder, endometriosis, fibroids (15), hysterectomy with or without oophorectomy, and menopausal status (10,14, 68–73) will have already been obtained.

Topics of importance in the medical history may include: (*i*) neurological illnesses such as spinal cord injury, headache (82), multiple sclerosis, or lumbosacral disc disease; (*ii*) chronic/medical illnesses such as diabetes (2,8,11,35), anemia, hyperlipidemia (9), coronary artery disease (83–85), or renal failure (78–81), (*iii*) endocrinologic conditions such as low estradiol (10,14), low progesterone, low testosterone (68,69,71), elevated prolactin, or low or elevated thyroid hormone (8); (*iv*) atherosclerotic vascular risk factor exposure such as hypertension, smoking or family history; (*v*) non-hormonal medication/recreational drug use such as antihypertensives, selective seratonin reuptake inhibitors antidepressants, over the counter drugs, street drugs, alcohol, or cocaine; (*vi*) hormonal medication use such as combined oral contraceptives, infertility drugs (67), or leuprolide acetate; (*vii*) pelvic/perineal/genital trauma such as pelvic fracture or bicycling injury; (*viii*) surgical history such as laminectomy, colon/rectalsurgery (77), or vascular bypass surgery and (*ix*) psychiatric history such as depression (50–53), panic, or anxiety.

Since sex steroid hormones are critical for genital structure and function, the medical history should routinely probe and evaluate for symptoms of estrogen deficiency (10,14) such as vaginal dryness, vaginal bleeding with minimal sexual contact, pain and soreness after sexual activity, hot flashes, and night sweats. Symptoms of androgen deficiency include fatigue, lack of energy, diminished skeletal muscle strength, depressed mood, falling asleep after meals, decreased athletic performance or lack of interest in sexual activity (68,69,71).

The psychosocial history should assess such issues as social factors, past sexual beliefs, past sexual abuse and trauma (45–49), depression (50–53), emotional concerns, and interpersonal relationship matters. Any past history of mood or psychiatric disorders should be identified.

One important caveat to history taking in women with sexual health concerns is that history-taking may be viewed in some women as actually the beginning of their treatment. Women are often empowered following the detailed discussion about their sexual health concerns. Women who have undergone detailed history-taking have initiated the first step in overcoming past failures to take action in this area. It is not uncommon for the discussion with the health care clinician to become a model of what is possible about sexual health conversation. Many patients will thereafter initiate a sexual health conversation with their partner, close friend, or family member.

Physical Examination
The physical examination for a woman with sexual health concerns should be tailored to the sexual medicine complaint obtained on history taking. For example, if during history-taking genital itching is a major sexual health problem, a careful assessment would follow for the presence of a genital dermatitis condition (66). If a woman with sexual health problems is under the age of 50 and has sexual pain, a careful physical examination should evaluate for the presence or absence of provoked vestibulodynia or vulvar vestibulitis syndrome (57–63). Similar complaints of sexual pain in a woman over 50 years of age should assess for the presence of vaginal atrophy with dryness, loss of rugae, mucosal thinning, pale hue, and lack of shiny vaginal secretions (10,14). The physical

examination should be performed ideally without menses and without intercourse or douching for twenty-four hours before the exam. If dysfunction occurs at a specific time, such as mid-cycle dyspareunia, the physical examination should be scheduled at the time of the sexual problem.

The genital-focused examination should be considered routine in the diagnosis of women's sexual health problems, but its personal character demands that a rational explanation exist for its inclusion in the diagnostic process. A focused peripheral genital examination is recommended in women with sexual dysfunction for complaints of dyspareunia, vaginismus, genital arousal disorder and combined arousal disorder, orgasmic disorder, pelvic trauma history, and any disease affecting genital health such as herpes or lichen sclerosis. The examiner may also assess for anal and vaginal tone, voluntary tightening of anus, and bulbocavernosal reflexes in women with suspected neurological disorders (105).

Patient consent to examination is particularly important. It is vital that the patient is aware of the purpose of the exam and understands that she has the final authority to terminate the physical examination, to ask questions, to have control over who is in attendance, and to understand the extent of the assessment. Inclusion of the sexual partner, with permission of the patient, is advantageous and provides needed patient support. Allowing the patient to observe any pathology via digital photography is often therapeutic, allowing, for the first time in many cases, an illustration and connection of a detected physical abnormality with the sexual health problem. If there exists a genital sexual pain history, the patient should point with her finger to the locations of the discomfort during the physical examination (68).

Independent of the gender of the examining health care clinician, it is strongly recommended that a female chaperone health care clinician be present in the examination room. The patient should wear a sheet to cover her lower torso. The patient should be placed in the lithotomy position and the examining health care clinician should use vulvoscopy (Fig. 60.2) with magnified vision and a focused light source (68).

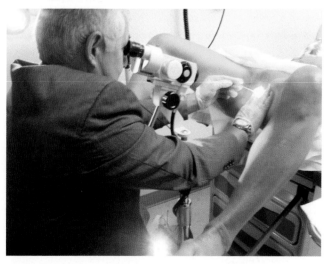

Figure 60.2 Vulvoscopy. The examining health care clinician should use vulvoscopy with magnified vision and a focused light source.

The first part of the examination involves inspection of the vulva and labia majora. Inspection of the vestibule requires retraction of the labia minora. Two gloved fingers are placed on either side of the clitoral shaft and using an upward force in the cephalic direction, the prepuce is retracted to gain full exposure of the glans clitoris, corona, and right and left frenulum emanating at 5:00 and 7:00 from the posterior portion of the glans clitoris (Figs. 60.3A and B). The labia minora are inspected for labial resorption and for their ability to meet in the midline posterior fourchette (Fig. 60.4A). The maximal labial width is recorded. Inspection of the urethral meatus is performed (Fig. 60.5A) and any erythema, stenosis or meatal prolapse (Fig. 60.5B) is noted. Using gauze to maximally retract the labia minora, the labial-hymenal junction is identified. A Q-tip cotton swab test is performed, gently applying pressure on the minor vestibular glands (Fig. 60.6A), documenting the quality of the discomfort or pain or erythema (Fig. 60.6B). The Q-tip cotton swab is placed at multiple locations in the vulva and vestibule (68).

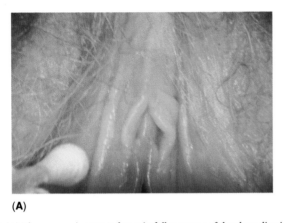 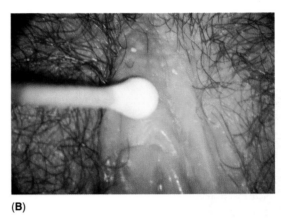

(A) (B)

Figure 60.3 (**A**) The prepuce is retracted to gain full exposure of the glans clitoris, corona, and right and left frenulum emanating at 5:00 and 7:00 from the posterior portion of the glans clitoris. (**B**) Vulvoscopic view of moderate clitoral phimosis.

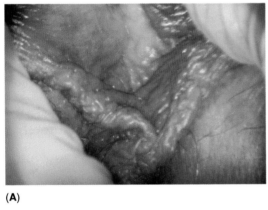 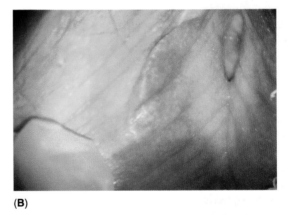

(A) (B)

Figure 60.4 (**A**) The labia minora are inspected for labial resorption and for their ability to meet in the midline posterior fourchette. (**B**) Labial resorption.

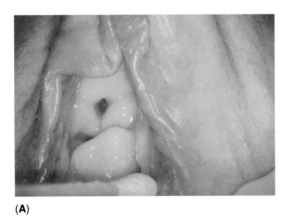 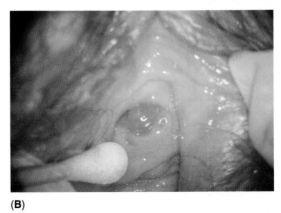

(A) (B)

Figure 60.5 (**A**) Inspection of the urethral meatus is performed. (**B**) Mild urethral prolapse.

622

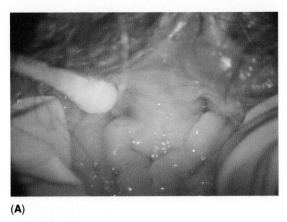 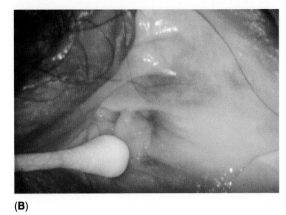

(A)   (B)

Figure 60.6 (**A**) A Q-tip cotton swab test is performed, gently applying pressure on the minor vestibular glands. This woman had no pain, no erythema overlying minor vestibular glands. (**B**) This woman had pain, discomfort, and erythema overlying minor vestibular glands.

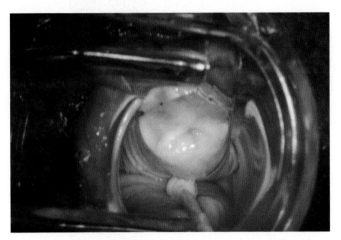

Figure 60.7 The peri-urethral tissue or G-spot region is inspected.

For the speculum examination, a warm, lubricated speculum is used. The peri-urethral tissue or G-spot region is inspected (Fig. 60.7). The vaginal wall is examined for the presence of vaginal rugae (Figs. 60.8A and 60.8B), inflammation, color and thickness of the vaginal walls, vaginal discharge, and any vaginal lesions. Vaginal smear and wet mount is obtained. Vaginal pH is recorded. Single digit palpation is achieved by gently placing a finger into the vaginal opening and depressing the bulbocavernosus muscle. A bimanual examination and evaluation of pelvic floor may be subsequently performed if indicated. Two fingers are placed against the lateral walls and the levators and underlying obturator are assessed for tenderness or taut bands. In addition, a bimanual examination can evaluate the integrity of the fornices, bladder, and urethral bases and pelvic organs. A rectovaginal examination can be performed if indicated (68,105).

A useful device to document objective data regarding the tone of a women's pelvic floor muscle is a perineometer (68). This tampon shaped electronic device is inserted into a woman's vagina and digitally records the relative resting tone and voluntary contraction tone of the pelvic floor muscles, with the pressures expressed in centimeters of water. Perineometry

testing, in concert with the patient's response to palpation, can serve as a basis for intervention by physical therapy and aides in evaluation of the success of programs such as biofeedback and graduated dilator use. Additional pelvic floor muscle testing may include: internal or external electromyography, urodynamic testing, pudendal nerve motor latency, or anal manometry (5,32,46,61).

Neurourological examination consists of sensory and reflex testing (105). The sensory neurologic exam evaluates the integrity of the three branches of the pudendal nerve including the dorsal nerve of the clitoris (sensation from the glans clitoris and clitoral shaft), the perineal nerve (sensation from the perineum and labia), and the inferior rectal nerve (sensation from the perianal skin). Testing is performed by assessing light touch (cotton ball or Q-tip) (Fig. 60.9A) and pin prick (sterile needle) (Fig. 60.9B). Testing sites include the right and left sides of the clitoral area, labia majora, labia minora, and perianal areas. The motor portion of the pudendal nerve is derived from the pelvic floor muscles. Sacral reflexes include the bulbocavernosus reflex and the anal wink reflex, and both sensory and motor arms of these reflexes are branches of the pudendal nerve. The afferent arm of the bulbocavernosus reflex is the dorsal nerve of the clitoris, and the efferent arm is the perineal nerve. The index and middle fingers are placed along the posterolateral aspect of either the right or left vaginal wall overlying the bulb of the clitoris, surrounded by the bulbocavernosus muscle. A gentle pinch of the glans clitoris with the opposite hand will elicit contraction of the bulbocavernosus muscle (Fig. 60.10). The examination is repeated with the examining fingers facing the opposite vaginal wall. The afferent and efferent arms of the anal wink reflex both arise from the inferior rectal nerve. The anal wink reflex is performed using the wooden shaft end of the Q-tip, and is assessed by touching the perianal skin, about 1 cm from the anus at the 3 o'clock and the 9 o'clock positions. Visible contraction of the anal sphincter will be noted after touching the skin (105).

Neurophysiological tests are not yet consensed so the history and physical examination remain the best methodology to screen for neurologic causes for female sexual dysfunction.

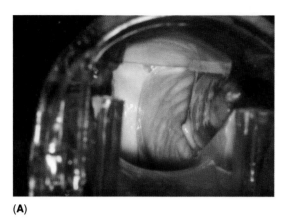
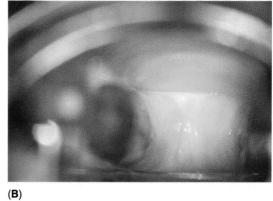

(A)   **(B)**

Figure 60.8 (**A**) The vaginal wall is examined for the presence of vaginal rugae. (**B**) Absent vaginal rugae.

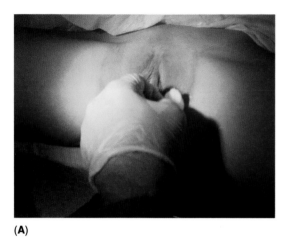
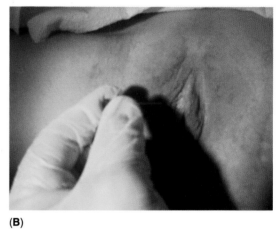

(A)   **(B)**

Figure 60.9 (**A**) Neurologic testing is performed by assessing light touch (cottonball or Q-tip) (**B**) and pinprick (sterile needle).

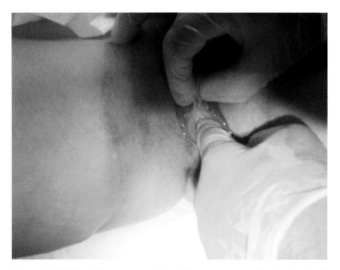

Figure 60.10 The afferent arm of the bulbocavernosus reflex is the dorsal nerve of the clitoris, and the efferent arm is the perineal nerve. The index and middle fingers are placed along the posterolateral aspect of either the right or left vaginal wall overlying the bulb of the clitoris, surrounded by the bulbocavernosus muscle. A gentle pinch of the glans clitoris with the opposite hand will elicit contraction of the bulbocavernosus muscle.

Objective sensory nerve testing may be performed with a biothesiometer (Fig. 60.11A). This quantitative sensory test measures vibratory perception thresholds (expressed in volts) and values are obtained in a non-genital reference site (pulp index finger) as well as in multiple genital sites such as the glans clitoris (dorsal nerve of the clitoris), and the right and left labia minora (the perineal nerve). Other quantitative sensory testing involves determination of hot and cold perception threshold values in these test sites (Fig. 60.11B) (68).

The health care clinician may also perform a complete physical, such as examining for a thyroid goiter, to rule out other co-morbid conditions that might be causing sexual dysfunction. A general physical exam is highly recommended in women with chronic illnesses, and as part of good medical care, including evaluation of blood pressure, heart rate, and a detailed breast exam.

Laboratory Testing

There is no consensus on recommended routine laboratory tests for the evaluation of women with desire, arousal, and orgasm sexual health concerns. Blood testing should be

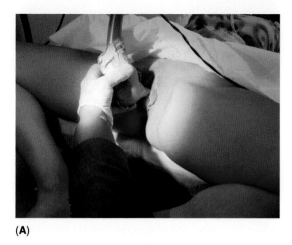
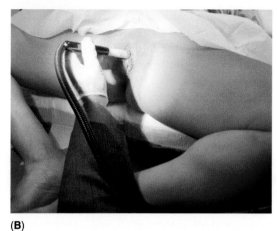

(A)   **(B)**

Figure 60.11 (**A**) A biothesiometer measures vibratory perception thresholds (expressed in volts) and quantitative sensory test values are obtained in a non-genital reference site (pulp index finger) as well as in multiple genital sites such as the glans clitoris (dorsal nerve of the clitoris), and the right and left labia minora (the perineal nerve). (**B**) Other quantitative sensory testing involves determination of hot and cold perception threshold values in these test sites.

dictated by clinical suspicion, especially the results of the history and physical examination. If appropriate, the health care clinician may assess multiple androgen and estrogen values (68) such as: dehydroepiandrosterone (DHEA) sulphate, androstenedione, total testosterone, free testosterone, sex hormone binding globulin (SHBG), dihydrotestosterone, estradiol, estrone, and progesterone. Pituitary function may be measured by obtaining luteinizing hormone (LH), follicle stimulating hormone (FSH), and prolactin. Thyroid stimulating hormone (TSH) should be measured to exclude subclinical thyroid disease (68).

There are multiple problems with the determination of serum hormone levels, especially testosterone (68,69,71). The normal ranges of testosterone concentration values for women of different age groups without sexual dysfunction are also not well defined. Testosterone levels reach a nadir during the early follicular phase, with small but less significant variation across the rest of the cycle. Testosterone assays are not uniformly sensitive or reliable enough to accurately measure testosterone at the low serum concentrations typically found in women. Free testosterone is clinically more important than total testosterone in sexual function because the vast majority of testosterone is bound to SHBG, and only a small amount of total testosterone is biologically available. The measurement of SHBG is relatively simple to perform with good reproducibility. Equilibrium dialysis is a highly sensitive assay for free testosterone; however, this method is not feasible for clinical practice. Measurement of free testosterone by analogue assays is unreliable. Free androgen may also be calculated using the free androgen index, defined as total testosterone (nmol/l) divided by SHBG (nmol/l). Calculated free testosterone may be determined and takes into account total testosterone, SHBG, and albumin. A calculator for this free testosterone is available online at http://www.issam.ch/freetesto.htm.

Sex steroid hormone actions are quite complex and involve critical enzymes and critical hormone receptors that also determine tissue exposure, tissue sensitivity, and tissue responsiveness. For example, in individuals there are variations in the amount and activity of critical enzymes such as 5 alpha-reductase and aromatase. In addition, individuals have variations in individual sex steroid hormone receptor sequencing. Thus, independent of the values of sex steroid hormones, the unique individual variations in critical enzymes and sex steroid hormone receptors result in individual differences in tissue exposure, tissue sensitivity, and tissue responsiveness. More research is needed in the blood testing of sex steroid hormones in women with sexual health concerns.

Although there is a lack of clinical consensus as to the value, specificity, and sensitivity of individual hormone blood tests, there are evidence-based, placebo-controlled, double-blind data supporting the efficacy of exogenous sex steroid hormone treatment in women with sexual health concerns (68–73). As such the prudent physician may wish to discuss with the patient the strategy of serial blood test surveillance testing to address safety concerns during such treatment.

Treatment
This goal of this section is to discuss the biologic-focused management of women who have sexual health issues (68). The ideal management of all women with sexual health concerns is holistic engaging psychologic and biologic strategies.

HORMONAL
Sex steroid hormones are critical for sexual structure and function. A number of studies have demonstrated that hormone therapy using systemic or local preparations improves sexual desire, arousal, orgasm, and frequency of sexual activity. Estrogen and androgen hormones act on estrogen and androgen receptors, respectively, which exist in high numbers in genital tissues, including the epithelial/endothelial cells and smooth muscle cells of the vagina, vulva, vestibule, labia, and urethra. Diminished estrogen production for natural or iatrogenic reasons renders women's genital tissues highly susceptible to atrophy. Physical examination of the postmenopausal woman's genitalia shows clitoral atrophy, phimosis, and nearly absent labia minora. The appearance of a woman's labia minora mirrors her level of estradiol, because these labia are exquisitely sensitive to estradiol. The urogenital area termed

the vestibule is very important in female sexual function because it contains organs that are sensitive to both estrogen and androgen. For example, the clitoral tissues and prepuce are androgen sensitive. The minor vestibular glands which are located in the labial-hymenal junction, are embryologically derived from the glands of littre, which are also androgen dependent. The glands of littre are located on the anterior surface of the urethra (68).

Studies have consistently reported that androgen sex steroid hormone values decline gradually and estradiol values decline abruptly in natural menopause or in menopause induced by chemotherapy or surgery. Hormone insufficiency states may also be caused by a number of clinical conditions and medications, including the use of oral contraceptive therapy or associated with infertility or endometriosis treatments (68).

Of importance, not all women have absent estradiol synthesis in the menopause. During menopause, ovarian estradiol production ceases in all women. However, estrogen continues to be synthesized in the periphery (e.g., skin, adipose tissue, bone, muscle) in postmenopausal women through conversion of androstenedione to estrone and testosterone to estradiol, but the amount of estradiol synthesized depends, in part, on the enzymatic activity of aromatase (68).

A host of structural changes and cellular dysfunctions occur in women's genital tissues as a result of estrogen deficiency. For example, estrogen deficiency specifically in the vagina leads to vaginal atrophy. One consequence is an alteration in the normally acidic vaginal pH that discourages the growth of pathogenic bacteria. The change to an alkaline pH value in the atrophic vagina leads to a shift in the vaginal flora, increasing the likelihood of discharge and odor. In an estrogen-rich environment, glycogen from sloughed epithelial cells is hydrolyzed into glucose and then metabolized to lactic acid by normal vaginal flora. In postmenopausal women, however, epithelial thinning reduces the available glycogen (10,14).

In addition to vaginal atrophy and a reduction in organ size, other signs of a decline in sex hormones in women include: vaginal dryness; no secretions or lubrication; pale or inflamed tissue; petechiae; epithelial/mucosal thinning; organ prolapse; changes in external genitalia; decreased tissue elasticity and loss of smooth muscle. Symptoms of women's sexual health concerns that the clinician may elicit when taking a history in a menopausal woman are: dyspareunia (57,60–63), vaginismus (58,59), coital anorgasmia, vaginal and/or urinary tract infections (pH imbalance), and overactive bladder/incontinence (5,20,26,30,36).

The use of systemic testosterone, systemic and/or local estrogen with or without systemic progesterone must be individualized to each patient's desires, wishes, requirements, and expectations (68,69,71). Systemic hormone therapy can successfully improve hot flushes, night sweats, and sleep disturbances that can otherwise markedly diminish afflicted women's body image and mood. Local hormone therapy can successfully improve vaginal lubrication dryness and dyspareunia. Alleviation of hormone deficiency-induced symptoms by systemic and/or localized sex steroid hormones can increase quality of life, desire, arousal, and orgasmic function (68).

The following represents a clinical paradigm for the evidence-based biologic-focused treatment of women with desire, arousal, and orgasm sexual health concerns. As discussed above, treatment is holistic and is based on the history, physical examination and laboratory tests. There is no one hormonal intervention that will be effective in all women with desire, arousal and orgasm sexual health concerns secondary, in part, to sex steroid hormone deficiency states (68).

Phase 1

It is important to emphasize that no single type of hormonal intervention or regimen will be effective in all women with desire, arousal, and orgasm sexual health concerns (68).

The hormonal abnormalities that are identified will determine which of the following four biologic treatment options women are offered in Phase 1. Based on blood test results, systemic androgen treatment may be achieved with systemic DHEA alone or systemic testosterone alone or a combination of both systemic androgens. Based on the history and physical examination, local estrogen treatment may be achieved with vestibular estradiol alone or intravaginal estradiol alone or a combination of both.

Systemic androgens (systemic DHEA and/or systemic testosterone) have been shown to improve mood, energy, stimulation, sensation, arousal, and orgasm in women with sexual health concerns. Limited clinical trials have examined the effects of systemic DHEA therapy on sexual function in women (106–108). Baulieu and colleagues (107) administered systemic DHEA (50 mg) or placebo to 140 women between the ages of 60 and 79 years for 12 months. Systemic DHEA treatment produced approximately a doubling of serum total testosterone concentration and also significantly increased skin hydration and bone density. Libido was increased after six months of treatment, sexual activity, and sexual satisfaction were both increased after 12 months (107).

Systemic testosterone has been used to treat women with sexual dysfunction since the 1940's (109). Transdermal patches or gels or subcutaneous pellets are being studied for their safety and efficacy in reducing sexual symptoms associated with testosterone insufficiency (68,69,71,109–112). Transdermal testosterone patches have been compared with placebo in estrogenized women who had undergone oophorectomy and hysterectomy. One study (110) showed that the 300-microgram testosterone patch was significantly more effective than the 150-microgram patch or placebo in improving frequency of sexual activity, pleasure, and fantasy during a 12-week period. Typically, the initial testosterone dose utilized to treat women with testosterone deficiency syndrome is one tenth of the dose used in men. After an interval of time, usually three months, the results of blood testing and clinical symptoms determine subsequent dosing.

One benefit of administering systemic DHEA and systemic testosterone is that these hormones will endogenously aromatize to estradiol, thus relieving hot flashes and night sweats without the administration of systemic estrogen (68).

Local estrogen, in the form of vaginal estradiol improves vaginal perfusion, lubrication, tissue tone, and elasticity, and restores the normal vaginal pH and vaginal health

(10,14,70,73,113–115). Vaginal estradiol also relieves dyspareunia, atrophic vaginitis, and vaginismus. Some systemic estradiol absorption occurs with all local vaginal estrogens and regular estradiol blood testing may be necessary in some women. Daily application of a film of vestibular estrogen is recommended as well, because it promotes the health of the frenulum (the most sensitive part of the external genitalia), labia minora, urethral meatus, hymenal tissue, and vestibular glands (10,14,113–115).

The human vagina consists of three layers of tissue: the epithelium (composed of squamous cells), the lamina propria, and the muscularis (inner circular and outer longitudinal smooth muscle) (10,14). The epithelium undergoes mild changes during the menstrual cycle. The lamina propria is replete with tiny blood vessels that become engorged with blood during sexual arousal, leading to lubrication. The smooth muscle of the muscularis enables the vagina to dilate and lengthen during penile penetration. Relaxation of that muscle leads to arousal. These three layers of tissue may function in an interrelated way. It is hypothesized that the blood vessels in the lamina propria that allow for lubrication are dependent on growth factors, and that the growth factors are derived from the muscularis. Postmenopausal atrophy of vaginal tissues may be due to decreased synthesis these growth factors resulting in diminished number of critical blood vessels in the lamina propria (10,14).

Increased vaginal blood flow is an indicator of sexual arousal (116). Genital swelling and lubrication are responses to increased clitoral and vaginal perfusion; increased length and diameter of the vaginal canal and clitoral corpora cavernosa; engorgement of the vagina wall, clitoris, and labia major and minora; and transudation of lubricating fluid from the vaginal epithelium. In animal studies (116), blood flow to the vagina was greatly reduced in the oophorectomized rats compared with the intact rats. Contrary to what one might expect, subphysiologic doses of estradiol increased vaginal blood flow in oophorectomized rats more than either physiologic or supraphysiologic doses. Ovariectomy deprived estradiol values caused the vaginal epithelium to thin down to a single layer. Subphysiologic doses of estradiol increased the thickness of the vaginal epithelium the most because the oophorectomized rats had more estrogen-alpha receptors in the epithelium than the intact animals. A small amount of estradiol delivered to tissue with many estrogen-alpha receptors produced a huge response. Thus, estradiol regulates estrogen receptors through a negative feedback system. The more estradiol that is available, the fewer estrogen receptors there are. The muscularis, the muscle that enables the vagina to lengthen and widen during sexual arousal, also atrophies without estrogen. In postmenopausal women who do not take hormone therapy, the vaginal epithelium, lamina propria blood vessels, and muscularis all decrease. Like the epithelium, the muscularis responds to estradiol by increasing in thickness (116).

Women with sexual dysfunction who are placed on Phase 1 treatment need to undergo surveillance blood tests after three months of therapy to monitor the patient's levels of estradiol, progesterone, DHEA, testosterone, androstenedione, dihydrotestosterone, FSH, LH, prolactin, and TSH as indicated.

Women with desire, arousal, and orgasm sexual health concerns whose symptoms of distress are not resolved satisfactorily with Phase 1 treatments may consider progressing to Phase 2 treatments.

Phase 2

In Phase 2, women receive systemic estrogen and/or systemic testosterone. Several clinical trials have shown that the distressing symptoms of vaginal atrophy associated with low estrogen states are ameliorated after estrogen therapy. Low doses of systemic bioidentical non-synthetic 17-beta estradiol reduced vaginal atrophy compared with placebo in healthy menopausal women (68,70,73). Systemic estrogen therapy can also successfully improve hot flushes, night sweats, and sleep disturbances that negatively affect body image, mood, and sexual desire. All efforts are made to keep serum estradiol levels between 30 and 50 ng/dl. Risks of systemic estrogen use include breast cancer, heart attack, and stroke. The concept of maintaining estradiol values at low levels is to reduce side effect risk while achieving a minimum efficacious dose (68).

In women with an intact uterus, systemic estrogen should always be opposed by a progestogen. All efforts are made to use a bioidentical non-synthetic progesterone and keep values in the range of 1 ng/dl (68).

Phase 3

In Phase 3, attention is given to the possible role of dopamine agonists in facilitating desire and orgasm sexual responses (117–119). Sexual motivation is encouraged, sustained, and ended by a number of central nervous system neurotransmitter and receptor changes induced, in part, by the action of sex steroids, androgens, estrogens, progestins, and the central neurotransmitter dopamine (117). The activation of dopamine receptors may be a key intermediary in the stimulation of incentive sexual motivation, and sexual reward. These neurotransmitter and receptor changes, in turn, activate central sexual arousal and desire. Contemporary animal research reveals that dopamine neurotransmitter systems may play a critical intermediary role in the central regulation of sexual arousal and excitation, mood, and incentive-related sexual behavior, in particular, in the motivational responses to conditioned external stimuli. In summary, the complex central neurochemical actions of steroid hormones stimulate sensory awareness, central sexual arousal, mood, and reward, and relate them to relevant individual's sexual experiences involving a partner, a place, and an action (117). In the future, the drug flibanserin is expected to be the first Food and Drug Administration-approved agent for the treatment of a women's sexual health problem, specifically hypoactive sexual desire disorder in premenopausal women. Flibanserin diminishes serotonin release by serotonin 1A agonism and also inhibits binding to the serotonin 2A receptor involved in inhibitory cortical outflow. Flibanserin further acts to increase the facilitator neurochemicals, dopamine, and noradrenalin. In balance, flibanserin use is associated with facilitated sexual behavior (117).

Bupropion, which is a noradrenaline and dopamine reuptake inhibitor with nicotinic antagonist properties originally marketed as an antidepressant, may have a beneficial effect on women with hypoactive sexual desire disorder (68,118,119). In a placebo-controlled trial, bupropion produced an increase in desire and frequency of sexual activity compared with placebo. However, frequency was correlated to total testosterone level at baseline and during treatment. A traditional starting dose is 100 mg bupropion per day generally taken in the AM. A new medication flibanserin is been studied for pre-menopausal women with hypoactive sexual desire disorder (118).

VASODILATORS

Basic science studies (120,121) investigating the physiology of sexual function utilizing female animal models support the role of nitric oxide-cyclic guanosine monophosphate –phosphodiesterase type five pathways in the peripheral arousal physiology of the clitoral corpus cavernosum, corpus spongiosum, vaginal epithelium, and vaginal lamina propria.

There have been several clinical studies (122–124) on selective phosphodiesterase type five inhibitors over the last few years, conducted with either pre-menopausal or post-menopausal women with arousal sexual health concerns as well as healthy women without sexual dysfunction. Many studies did not take into account the hormonal milieu of the subjects in the inclusion and exclusion criteria. An important point in treating women with arousal sexual health concerns is that an adequate sex steroid (androgen and estrogen) hormonal milieu is critical for benefits from selective phosphodiesterase type five inhibitor treatment. Several studies did assess safety and efficacy of selective phosphodiesterase type five inhibitors in subjects with a normal hormonal milieu.

A double-blind, crossover, placebo-controlled safety and efficacy study (122) with a selective phosphodiesterase type five inhibitor was performed in pre-menopausal women with normal ovulatory cycles and normal levels of steroid hormones who were affected by female sexual arousal disorder without hypoactive sexual desire disorder. Subjects were observed to benefit from treatment with the active selective phosphodiesterase type five inhibitor, showing improvement in sexual arousal, orgasm, frequency, and enjoyment of sexual intercourse versus placebo. Nurnberg found that sildenafil significantly improved sexual function—especially orgasm in women whose free testosterone values were in the normal range—in women who developed sexual health problems following use of selective serotonin reuptake inhibitors (124).

SEXUAL PAIN MANAGEMENT
Medical Therapy for Genital Sexual Pain Disorders

Biologic pathophysiologies resulting in woman's sexual health problems associated with sexual pain may occur in the clitoris, urethra, bladder, vulva, vestibule, vagina, and pelvic floor muscles.

Clitoris, Prepuce, and Frenulae

In women with focused clitoral pain, clitoral itching, or clitoral burning, careful inspection of the glans clitoris should be performed (125). Failure to visualize the whole glans clitoris with the corona is consistent with some degree (mild, moderate, or severe) of prepucial phimosis, based on the elasticity of the prepuce and its ability to retract on examination. Since phimosis may create a closed compartment, phimosis is often the underlying pathology in clitoral glans balanitis associated with recurrent fungal infections. Initial treatment may be conservative with topical estrogen and/or testosterone creams to see if the prepuce can be made more elastic and retractile. Topical antifungal agents such as nystatin or oral antifungal agents such as fluconazole may be considered. Infections can also be related to herpes virus, with appropriate treatment administered such as acyclovir. If conservative treatment fails due to the phimotic prepuce, surgical management by dorsal slit procedure should be considered (125).

Urethral Meatus

Gentle retraction of the labia minora should provide full view of the urethral meatus. Prolapse of the urethral mucosa out the urethral lumen is highly associated with estrogen deficiency states such as following bilateral oophorectomy, natural menopause, or following chemotherapy for malignancy. Clinical symptoms include urgency, frequency, and discomfort on urination and also spotting of blood which may be observed on the toilet paper after wiping following voiding. The abnormal voiding history is often accompanied by a unique sexual history. Women with urethral prolapse often have the ability to have full sexual pleasure and satisfaction during self-stimulation of the clitoris; however, during sexual activity with the partner or with a mechanical device, she experiences pain and/or urgency to urinate and/or inability to have orgasm secondary to distracting pain. Conservative treatment options include topical or systemic estrogens, although the risks and benefits of estrogen treatment need to be fully discussed.

Vulva/Vestibule

Genital sexual pain in the vulva/vestibule may be related to varied specific disorders (63,126,127). The treatment of any genital sexual pain disorder involves the multi-disciplinary team approach, and this is especially true for the disabling condition of vestibulodynia. Patient management includes education and support, especially regarding avoidance of contacts and practice of healthy vulval hygiene, pelvic floor physical therapy treatment, management of concomitant depression, and management of any associated neurologic, dermatologic, gynecologic, orthopedic, or urologic conditions. Medical management includes amitriptyline and/or gabapentin.

Provoked vestibulodynia is one of the most common causes of dyspareunia (63), especially in pre-menopausal women. The treatment includes conservative measures including education, support, counseling, physical therapy, and/or biofeedback. Elimination of the pain trigger should be performed. Topical estrogen and androgen creams and topical xylocaine creams and/or ointments should be considered. Systemic medications include tricyclic antidepressant or gabapentin. Correction of the sex steroid hormonal milieu should be considered.

The symptoms of atrophic vaginitis include vaginal dryness, dyspareunia, stinging, bleeding, and dysuria. On physical examination, women with atrophic vaginitis reveal vaginal mucosal changes. The classic healthy appearing vagina has a pink hue with vaginal folds and rugae that, when touched with

a Q-tip, reveals a shiny lubricating substance and, when rubbed with a Q-tip, does not bleed. In atrophic vaginitis, the vagina transforms to an unhealthy pale complexion, with a lack of vaginal folds and rugae, a lack of lubricating substance on the surface and the tissue bleeds with minimal contact. On wet mount, the microscopic examination reveals parabasal cells, increased white blood cells and absent background flora of lactobacilli. The vaginal pH is elevated to 6.0 to 7.0. The conservative treatment involves the use of local topical vestibular and/or intravaginal estradiol. There are multiple products on the market including intravaginal estradiol rings, intravaginal estradiol tablets, and estradiol creams (68).

Disorders of the female pelvic floor that result in bladder/ urethra dysfunction and/or sexual dysfunction, are common. Conservative therapies for hypersensitivity disorders of the pelvic floor are aimed at muscle re-education. An individualiszd pelvic floor rehabilitation program aimed at facilitating sexual comfort and pleasure for patients can be designed. Massage of the pelvic floor can be performed to elongate shortened muscles and decrease high tone spasm in such patients. Conservative therapies for low tone pelvic floor dysfunction are also aimed at muscle re-education. Pelvic floor muscle strengthening exercises, augmented with biofeedback and/ or electrical stimulation to the pelvic floor can be initiated. If this and other conservative treatment options fail, surgical procedures, including sling and tension-free vaginal tape placement provide cure rates as high as 95% when performed in appropriate candidates (5,32,46,61).

Role of the Pelvic Floor in Women's Sexual Function

Female urologists and urogynecologists are familiar with the diagnosis and treatment of women with disorders of the female pelvic floor (5,32,46,61). Normal function of the pelvic floor musculature is essential in maintaining appropriate sexual function. Both "low tone pelvic floor dysfunction or high-tone pelvic floor muscle dysfunction," can be closely associated with women's sexual health concerns. Hypotonus of the pelvic floor muscles, secondary to childbirth, trauma, and/or aging, is related to urinary incontinence during orgasm, vaginal laxity, and/or thrusting dyspareunia secondary to pelvic organ prolapse. Hypertonus of the pelvic floor secondary to childbirth, postural stressors, microtrauma, infection, adhesions, and surgical trauma and can contribute to symptoms of urinary retention, reduced force of stream, dysuria, urgency, penetrative dyspareunia ,and/or vaginismus.

The assessment of tone in the pelvic floor is determined by the woman's ability to isolate, contract, and relax the pelvic floor muscles. During a pelvic examination, a digital exam, by exerting light pressure on the lateral walls of the vagina, should assess whether the woman is asked to squeeze on the examining finger and to elevate the pelvic floor, without simultaneously contracting the abdominal, gluteal, or adductor muscle groups. If the patient is not able to produce sufficient muscle strength to compress the finger or is not able to sustain that pressure for several seconds, she may be exhibiting a low tone pelvic floor dysfunction pattern. If, conversely, the woman experiences muscle tenderness or pain when pressure is applied to the lateral vaginal wall or during an attempted squeeze

against resistance, she may be exhibiting a high tone pelvic floor dysfunction pattern. A perineometer or an electromyography probe, designed to measure muscle activity can verify these physical examination findings (5,32,46,61).

Hypersensitivity disorders involving the genitourinary tract represent a spectrum of symptoms and conditions that include chronic bacterial cystitis, urgency and frequency syndrome, sensory urgency, urethral syndrome, interstitial cystitis, vulval pain, vaginal pain, perineal, and pelvic pain. Hypersensitivity disorders, associated with hypertonus of the pelvic floor musculature, account for some of the concerns of female patients who present for evaluation of sexual health concerns. Sexuality is adversely affected for the majority of women with hypersensitivity disorders of the bladder, bowel, and vulva and high tone pelvic floor dysfunction. Those that are able to tolerate coitus often suffer a flare of their symptoms for days as a result of sexual activity, which then becomes a negative reinforcement for future sexual activity (5,32,46,61).

Weakness and laxity of the pelvic floor muscles represent a spectrum of symptoms and conditions that include women with pelvic organ prolapse with or without urinary or fecal incontinence. Risk factors include age, heredity, vaginal birth trauma, previous pelvic/vaginal surgery, history of radiation therapy, menopausal status, lifestyle factors such as strenuous lifting and chronic medical conditions including obstructive pulmonary disease, obesity, and constipation. Stress incontinence that occurs with increased intra-abdominal pressure and maneuvers such as sneezing, coughing, and straining, is related to abnormalities in urethral closure and poor pelvic muscle support. Sexuality is often adversely affected for women with severe low tone pelvic floor dysfunction, especially those with severe incontinence and prolapse where symptoms are a source of anxiety and interfere with the overall sense of sexual satisfaction. Women who experience incontinence during intercourse express concern about feeling undesirable, fearing embarrassment, and possibly infecting themselves or their partner (5,32,46,61).

Dermatologic Conditions such as Lichen Sclerosis/Lichen Planus

Lichen sclerosis (66) is a chronic genital dermatitis condition that is associated with varying intensity of symptoms including vulval itch and/or burning and various degrees of vulval scarring leading to narrowing of the introitus and dyspareunia. There is a wide variation in presentation symptoms. In some women, especially those not sexually active, there can be minimal symptoms and the patient may be unaware of the condition of lichen sclerosis for years. Alternatively, the burning and itching symptoms can be so intense as to severely interfere with sexual activity, day-to-day activities, and even sleep. If the scarring of lichen sclerosis involves the perianal area, the patient may also complain of perianal fissuring and painful defecation. The diagnosis of lichen sclerosis is suspected by physical examination showing white color genital, vulval and vestibular tissue with paleness, loss of pigmentation, and a characteristic "cigarette paper" wrinkling. Classically, the genital tissue changes do not involve the inside of the vagina and if they involve the perianal area, there is a traditional

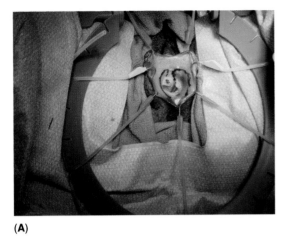

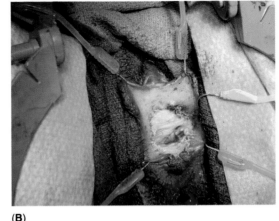

(A)   **(B)**

Figure 60.12 (**A**) Complete vestibulectomy with vaginal advancement flap includes excision of the vestibular mucosa adjacent to the urethral meatus/skene's glands region anteriorly, (**B**) excision of vestibular mucosa laterally and posteriorly with reconstruction including the posterior vaginal flap advancement.

"figure of eight" extension. The lichen sclerosis condition commonly involves the vestibule with associated labia minora atrophy and the vaginal introitus with loss of elasticity and narrowing (66).

Lichen planus is another chronic genital dermatitis condition, which is likely to have a pathophysiology related to varied altered immunologic disorders and as a result the presenting symptoms may vary widely.

Lichen planus may occur secondary to drugs, such as antihypertensives, diuretics, oral hypoglycemics, and non-steroidal anti-inflammatory agents, that may rarely induce a lichen planus-like eruption. One presentation is primarily associated with itching and does not result in scarring. Another is erosive and destructive. Overall patient complaints may include severe vulval itching, pain, burning, and irritation. Dyspareunia occurs secondary to vaginal introital scarring. Some types of lichen planus, unlike lichen sclerosis, may involve the vaginal mucosa. If there is vaginal involvement, a purulent malodorous discharge may be noted. Findings on physical examination of women with lichen planus vary widely. The pruritic type of lichen planus is associated with a purple color, and multiple papules and plaques on the vulva and vestibule. The erosive type is associated with vestibular ulcers, scarring, clitoris and labia minora atrophy, and occasionally destruction of the vagina has been reported (66).

Surgical Treatment for Neuroproliferative Vestibulodynia
Surgical intervention (126,127) for management of women with neuroproliferative vestibulodynia is offered to those who have failed initial conservative medical, psychological, and/or physical therapy focused treatment. Surgery is based on the hypothesis that the pathophysiology of neuroproliferative vestibulodynia, is associated with inflamed, irritated, and hypersensitive vestibular glandular tissue and related increased nerve density in the vestibular mucosa. Surgical success is therefore based on excision of this abnormal glandular and nerve tissue in the vestibule. In women with provoked vestibulodynia secondary to neuroproliferative vestibulodynia, the procedure entitled complete vestibulectomy with vaginal advancement flap includes excision of the vestibular mucosa

adjacent to the urethral meatus/skene's glands region anteriorly, excision of vestibular mucosa laterally, and posteriorly with reconstruction including the posterior vaginal flap advancement (Figs. 60.12A and B). This procedure is usually performed under general or regional anesthesia.

Complications include bleeding, infection, increased pain, hematoma, wound dehiscence, vaginal stenosis, scar tissue formation, and Bartholin duct cyst formation. During vestibulectomy, the vaginal advancement may cover the ostia of the Bartholin glands; however, the risk of post-operative Bartholin gland cysts is only 1%. As always with surgery, the risk of these complications can be reduced with appropriate surgical techniques. Various closure techniques have been described to minimize the risks of post-operative complications. Specifically, the vaginal advancement flap should be anchored by multiple subcutaneous mattress sutures of 3-0 Vicryl placed in an anterior-posterior direction and should be approximated to the perineum with interrupted stitches of 4-0 Vicryl (126,127).

Other Surgical Procedures
Distressing and disabling clitoral pain may occur secondary to phimosis of the clitoral prepuce and recurrent fungal balanitis of the clitoral glans or frenulae. If conservative treatment fails, a dorsal slit procedure (125) of the prepuce may be indicated to relieve the woman of the closed compartment perpetuating the recurrent fungal clitoral glans infection.

Distressing and disabling vestibular pain, urinary urgency and frequency and genital sexual pain may occur secondary to urethral prolapse. If conservative treatments fail, surgical excision of the prolapsed urethral mucosa may be indicated.

Distressing vulval/vestibular discomfort may occur secondary to a Bartholin's cyst. If conservative treatments fail, marsupialization of the cyst (128) may be indicated to enable drainage of the highly viscous and mucinous cyst fluid.

CONCLUSIONS
In a comprehensive textbook on Female Urology and Urogynecology, it is important and appropriate to have a detailed chapter on the biologic focused management of women's

sexual health concerns. Increasing numbers of health care clinicians will manage women with sexual health concerns since more and more women will expect and demand such management. In addition, those health care clinicians who want to maximize overall women's health care delivery will increasingly engage in management of women's sexual health concerns, in addition to the traditional focus on continence and urourological conditions. In the future, it will become increasingly more difficult for female urologists and urogynecologists to not provide at least first line sexual health care to women.

The basic premise of biologically focused management of women's sexual health concerns is that normal physiologic processes regulating sexual activity can be altered by biologic pathology. How each specific medical condition modulates woman's sexual health requires increased intensive basic science investigation. From the perspective of biology-focused clinicians, the essential principle guiding medical decision-making is identification of the underlying pathophysiology of the sexual dysfunction. If the biologic basis of the sexual health concern can be diagnosed by history and physical examination and laboratory testing, management outcome may be successfully directed to the source pathophysiology. Of the many challenges facing healthcare professionals today, the first is to improve the ability to accurately diagnose women with sexual health concerns and the second is to ensure that women receive the best evidence-based available management options. The biologically-focused clinician needs to have access to new developments in evidence-based, state-of-the-art data concerning biologically focused management strategies for women's sexual health concerns. As stated above, membership in specialized societies such as the ISSWSH will help the interested clinician achieve this goal.

REFERENCES

1. Bekker M, Beck J, Putter H, et al. The place of female sexual dysfunction in the urological practice: results of a Dutch survey. J Sex Med 2009. [Epub ahead of print].
2. Ogbera AO, Chinenye S, Akinlade A, Eregie A, Awobusuyi J. Frequency and correlates of sexual dysfunction in women with diabetes mellitus. J Sex Med 2009. [Epub ahead of print].
3. Goshtasebi A, Vahdaninia M, Rahimi Foroshani A. Prevalence and potential risk factors of female sexual difficulties: an Urban Iranian population-based study. J Sex Med 2009. [Epub ahead of print].
4. Serati M, Salvatore S, Uccella S, et al. Sexual function after radical hysterectomy for early-stage cervical cancer: is there a difference between laparoscopy and laparotomy? J Sex Med 2009; 6: 2516–22. Epub 2009.
5. Rivalta M, Sighinolfi MC, De Stefani S, et al. Biofeedback, electrical stimulation, pelvic floor muscle exercises, and vaginal cones: a combined rehabilitative approach for sexual dysfunction associated with urinary incontinence. J Sex Med 2009; 6: 1674–7. Epub 2009.
6. Kuhn A, Brunnmayr G, Stadlmayr W, Kuhn P, Mueller MD. Male and female sexual function after surgical repair of female organ prolapse. J Sex Med 2009; 6: 1324–34.
7. Clayton AH, Balon R. The impact of mental illness and psychotropic medications on sexual functioning: the evidence and management. J Sex Med 2009; 6: 1200–11. quiz 1212–3.
8. Veronelli A, Mauri C, Zecchini B, et al. Sexual dysfunction is frequent in premenopausal women with diabetes, obesity, and hypothyroidism, and correlates with markers of increased cardiovascular risk. A preliminary report. J Sex Med 2009; 6: 1561–8. Epub 2009.
9. Esposito K, Ciotola M, Maiorino MI, et al. Hyperlipidemia and sexual function in premenopausal women. J Sex Med 2009; 6: 1696–703. Epub 2009.
10. Nappi RE, Polatti F. The use of estrogen therapy in women's sexual functioning (CME). J Sex Med 2009; 6: 603–16. quiz 618–9.
11. Kim NN. Sex steroid hormones in diabetes-induced sexual dysfunction: focus on the female gender. J Sex Med 2009; 6(Suppl 3): 239–46. Review.
12. Graziottin A, Serafini A. HPV infection in women: psychosexual impact of genital warts and intraepithelial lesions. J Sex Med 2009; 6: 633–45. Epub 2009. Review.
13. DeRogatis LR, Graziottin A, Bitzer J, et al. Clinically relevant changes in sexual desire, satisfying sexual activity and personal distress as measured by the profile of female sexual function, sexual activity log, and personal distress scale in postmenopausal women with hypoactive sexual desire disorder. J Sex Med 2009; 6: 175–83.
14. Lara LA, Useche B, Ferriani RA, et al. The effects of hypoestrogenism on the vaginal wall: interference with the normal sexual response. J Sex Med 2009; 6: 30–9. Review.
15. Ertunc D, Uzun R, Tok EC, Doruk A, Dilek S. The effect of myoma uteri and myomectomy on sexual function. J Sex Med 2009; 6: 1032–8. Epub 2008.
16. Stuckey BG. Female sexual function and dysfunction in the reproductive years: the influence of endogenous and exogenous sex hormones. J Sex Med 2008; 5: 2282–90. Review.
17. Ferguson GG, Nelson CJ, Brandes SB, Shindel AW. The sexual lives of residents and fellows in graduate medical education programs: a single institution survey. J Sex Med 2008; 5: 2756–65. Epub 2008.
18. Hajebrahimi S, Azaripour A, Sadeghi-Bazargani H. Tolterodine immediate release improves sexual function in women with overactive bladder. J Sex Med 2008; 5: 2880–5. Epub 2008.
19. Lowenstein L, Pierce K, Pauls R. Urogynecology and sexual function research. How are we doing? J Sex Med 2009; 6: 199–204. Epub 2008.
20. Yang SH, Yang JM, Wang KH, Huang WC. Biologic correlates of sexual function in women with stress urinary incontinence. J Sex Med 2008; 5: 2871–9. Epub 2008.
21. Laumann EO, Waite LJ. Sexual dysfunction among older adults: prevalence and risk factors from a nationally representative U.S. probability sample of men and women 57–85 years of age. J Sex Med 2008; 5: 2300–11. Epub 2008.
22. Dennerstein L, Guthrie JR, Hayes RD, DeRogatis LR, Lehert P. Sexual function, dysfunction, and sexual distress in a prospective, population-based sample of mid-aged, Australian-born women. J Sex Med 2008; 5: 2291–9. Epub 2008.
23. Aslan E, Beji NK, Gungor I, Kadioglu A, Dikencik BK. Prevalence and risk factors for low sexual function in women: a study of 1,009 women in an outpatient clinic of a university hospital in Istanbul. J Sex Med 2008; 5: 2044–52. Epub 2008.
24. Song SH, Jeon H, Kim SW, Paick JS, Son H. The prevalence and risk factors of female sexual dysfunction in young korean women: an internet-based survey. J Sex Med 2008; 5: 1694–701.
25. Hayes RD, Dennerstein L, Bennett CM, et al. Risk factors for female sexual dysfunction in the general population: exploring factors associated with low sexual function and sexual distress. J Sex Med 2008; 5: 1681–93.
26. Cohen BL, Barboglio P, Gousse A. The impact of lower urinary tract symptoms and urinary incontinence on female sexual dysfunction using a validated instrument. J Sex Med 2008; 5: 1418–23. Epub 2008.
27. Myung SC, Lee MY, Lee SY, et al. Contractile changes of the clitoral cavernous smooth muscle in female rabbits with experimentally induced overactive bladder. J Sex Med 2008; 5: 1088–96. Epub 2008.
28. Mulhall J, King R, Glina S, Hvidsten K. Importance of and satisfaction with sex among men and women worldwide: results of the global better sex survey. J Sex Med 2008; 5: 788–95. Epub 2008.
29. Hayes RD, Dennerstein L, Bennett CM, Fairley CK. What is the "true" prevalence of female sexual dysfunctions and does the way we assess these conditions have an impact? J Sex Med 2008; 5: 777–87. Epub 2008.
30. Pace G, Vicentini C. Female sexual function evaluation of the tension-free vaginal tape (TVT) and transobturator suburethral tape (TOT) incontinence surgery: results of a prospective study. J Sex Med 2008; 5: 387–93.

31. Garcia S, Moreno S, Aponte H. Prevalence of sexual dysfunction in female outpatients and personnel at a Colombian hospital: correlation with hormonal profile. J Sex Med 2008; 5: 1208–13. Epub 2008.

32. Voorham-van der Zalm PJ, Lycklama A, Nijeholt GA, et al. Diagnostic investigation of the pelvic floor: a helpful tool in the approach in patients with complaints of micturition, defecation, and/or sexual dysfunction. J Sex Med 2008; 5: 864–71. Epub 2008.

33. Mehta A, Bachmann G. Premenopausal women with sexual dysfunction: the need for a bladder function history. J Sex Med 2008; 5: 407–12. Epub 2007.

34. Nickel JC, Parsons CL, Forrest J, et al. Improvement in sexual functioning in patients with interstitial cystitis/painful bladder syndrome. J Sex Med 2008; 5: 394–9. Epub 2007.

35. Olarinoye J, Olarinoye A. Determinants of sexual function among women with type 2 diabetes in a Nigerian population. J Sex Med 2008; 5: 878–86. Epub 2007.

36. Elzevier HW, Putter H, Delaere KP, et al. Female sexual function after surgery for stress urinary incontinence: transobturator suburethral tape vs. tension-free vaginal tape obturator. J Sex Med 2008; 5: 400–6. Epub 2007.

37. Clayton AH. Epidemiology and neurobiology of female sexual dysfunction. J Sex Med 2007; 4(Suppl 4): 260–8.

38. Derogatis LR, Burnett AL. The epidemiology of sexual dysfunctions. J Sex Med 2008; 5: 289–300. Epub 2007.

39. Oniz A, Keskinoglu P, Bezircioglu I. The prevalence and causes of sexual problems among premenopausal Turkish women. J Sex Med 2007; 4: 1575–81.

40. Parish WL, Laumann EO, Pan S, Hao Y. Sexual dysfunctions in urban china: a population-based national survey of men and women. J Sex Med 2007; 4: 1559–74. Epub 2007.

41. Zucchi A, Costantini E, Mearini L, et al. Female sexual dysfunction in urogenital prolapse surgery: colposacropexy vs. hysterocolposacropexy. J Sex Med 2008; 5: 139–45. Epub 2007.

42. Coyne KS, Margolis MK, Jumadilova Z, et al. Overactive bladder and women's sexual health: what is the impact? J Sex Med 2007; 4: 656–66.

43. Coyne KS, Margolis MK, Brewster-Jordan J, et al. Evaluating the impact of overactive bladder on sexual health in women: what is relevant? J Sex Med 2007; 4: 124–36.

44. Available from: http://www.who.int/reproductive-health/gender/sexual_health.html

45. Schulte-Herbrüggen O, Ahlers CJ, Kronsbein JM, et al. Impaired sexual function in patients with borderline personality disorder is determined by history of sexual abuse. J Sex Med 2009. [Epub ahead of print].

46. Beck JJ, Elzevier HW, Pelger RC, Putter H, Voorham-van der Zalm PJ. Multiple pelvic floor complaints are correlated with sexual abuse history. J Sex Med 2009; 6: 193–8.

47. Rellini A. Review of the empirical evidence for a theoretical model to understand the sexual problems of women with a history of CSA. J Sex Med 2008; 5: 31–46. Epub 2007.

48. Rellini A, Meston C. Sexual function and satisfaction in adults based on the definition of child sexual abuse. J Sex Med 2007; 4: 1312–21.

49. Elzevier HW, Voorham-van der Zalm PJ, Pelger RC. How reliable is a self-administered questionnaire in detecting sexual abuse: a retrospective study in patients with pelvic-floor complaints and a review of literature. J Sex Med 2007; 4(4 Pt 1): 956–63.

50. Yang JC, Park K, Eun SJ, et al. Assessment of cerebrocortical areas associated with sexual arousal in depressive women using functional MR imaging. J Sex Med 2008; 5: 602–9. Epub 2008.

51. Clayton A, Kornstein S, Prakash A, Mallinckrodt C, Wohlreich M. Changes in sexual functioning associated with duloxetine, escitalopram, and placebo in the treatment of patients with major depressive disorder. J Sex Med 2007; 4(4 Pt 1): 917–29.

52. Nelson CJ, Shindel AW, Naughton CK, Ohebshalom M, Mulhall JP. Prevalence and predictors of sexual problems, relationship stress, and depression in female partners of infertile couples. J Sex Med 2008; 5: 1907–14. Epub 2008.

53. Chen KC, Yeh TL, Lee IH, et al. Age, gender, depression, and sexual dysfunction in Taiwan. J Sex Med 2009. [Epub ahead of print].

54. Bitzer J, Platano G, Tschudin S, Alder J. Sexual counseling in elderly couples. J Sex Med 2008; 5: 2027–43. Epub 2008.

55. Smith LJ, Mulhall JP, Deveci S, Monaghan N, Reid MC. Sex after seventy: a pilot study of sexual function in older persons. J Sex Med 2007; 4: 1247–53.

56. Yildiz F, Camuzcuoglu H, Toy H, Terzi A, Guldur ME. A rare cause of difficulty with sexual intercourse: large retroperitoneal leiomyoma. J Sex Med 2009. [Epub ahead of print].

57. Landry T, Bergeron S. How young does vulvo-vaginal pain begin? Prevalence and characteristics of dyspareunia in adolescents. J Sex Med 2009; 6: 927–35. Epub 2009.

58. Yasan A, Akdeniz N. Treatment of lifelong vaginismus in traditional Islamic couples: a prospective study. J Sex Med 2009; 6: 1054–61. Epub 2009.

59. Dogan S. Vaginismus and accompanying sexual dysfunctions in a Turkish clinical sample. J Sex Med 2009; 6: 184–92.

60. Sutton KS, Pukall CF, Chamberlain S. Pain, psychosocial, sexual, and psychophysical characteristics of women with primary vs. secondary provoked vestibulodynia. J Sex Med 2009; 6: 205–14.

61. Rosenbaum TY, Owens A. The role of pelvic floor physical therapy in the treatment of pelvic and genital pain-related sexual dysfunction (CME). J Sex Med 2008; 5: 513–23.

62. Desrosiers M, Bergeron S, Meana M, et al. Psychosexual characteristics of vestibulodynia couples: partner solicitousness and hostility are associated with pain. J Sex Med 2008; 5: 418–27. Epub 2007.

63. Goldstein AT, Burrows L. Vulvodynia. J Sex Med 2008; 5: 5–14.

64. Pauls RN, Occhino JA, Dryfhout VL. Effects of pregnancy on female sexual function and body image: a prospective study. J Sex Med 2008; 5: 1915–22. Epub 2008.

65. Erol B, Sanli O, Korkmaz D, et al. A cross-sectional study of female sexual function and dysfunction during pregnancy. J Sex Med 2007; 4: 1381–7. Epub 2007.

66. Burrows LJ, Shaw HA, Goldstein AT. The vulvar dermatoses. J Sex Med 2008; 5: 276–83. Epub 2008.

67. Khademi A, Alleyassin A, Amini M, Ghaemi M. Evaluation of sexual dysfunction prevalence in infertile couples. J Sex Med 2008; 5: 1402–10. Epub 2007.

68. Goldstein I. Current management strategies of the postmenopausal patient with sexual health problems. J Sex Med 2007; 4(Suppl 3): 235–53.

69. Panzer C, Guay A. Testosterone replacement therapy in naturally and surgically menopausal women. J Sex Med 2009; 6: 8–18. quiz 19–20.

70. Cayan F, Dilek U, Pata O, Dilek S. Comparison of the effects of hormone therapy regimens, oral and vaginal estradiol, estradiol + drospirenone and tibolone, on sexual function in healthy postmenopausal women. J Sex Med 2008; 5: 132–8. Epub 2007.

71. Kingsberg SA, Simon JA, Goldstein I. The current outlook for testosterone in the management of hypoactive sexual desire disorder in postmenopausal women. J Sex Med 2008; 5(Suppl 4): 182–93.

72. Alatas E, Yagci B, Oztekin O, Sabir N. Effect of hormone replacement therapy on clitoral artery blood flow in healthy postmenopausal women. J Sex Med 2008; 5: 2367–73. Epub 2008.

73. Nijland EA, Weijmar Schultz WC, Nathorst-Boös J, et al. LISA study investigators. Tibolone and transdermal E2/NETA for the treatment of female sexual dysfunction in naturally menopausal women: results of a randomized active-controlled trial. J Sex Med 2008; 5: 646–56.

74. Alder J, Zanetti R, Wight E, et al. Sexual dysfunction after premenopausal stage I and II breast cancer: do androgens play a role? J Sex Med 2008; 5: 1898–906. Epub 2008.

75. Krychman ML, Stelling CJ, Carter J, Hudis CA. A case series of androgen use in breast cancer survivors with sexual dysfunction. J Sex Med 2007; 4: 1769–74. Epub 2007.

76. Huyghe E, Sui D, Odensky E, Schover LR. Needs assessment survey to justify establishing a reproductive health clinic at a comprehensive cancer center. J Sex Med 2009; 6: 149–63. Epub 2008.

77. Breukink SO, Wouda JC, van der Werf-Eldering MJ, et al. Psychophysiological assessment of sexual function in women after radiotherapy and total mesorectal excision for rectal cancer: a pilot study on four patients. J Sex Med 2009; 6: 1045–53. Epub 2008.

78. Filocamo MT, Zanazzi M, Li Marzi V, et al. Sexual dysfunction in women during dialysis and after renal transplantation. J Sex Med 2009. [Epub ahead of print].

79. Tavallaii SA, Fathi-Ashtiani A, Nasiri M, et al. Correlation between sexual function and postrenal transplant quality of life: does gender matter? J Sex Med 2007; 4: 1610–8. Epub 2007.

80. Ketta E, Cayan F, Akbay E, Kiykim A, Cayan S. Sexual dysfunction and associated risk factors in women with end-stage renal disease. J Sex Med 2008; 5: 872–7. Epub 2007.

81. Lew-Starowicz M, Gellert R. The sexuality and quality of life of hemo-dialyzed patients–ASED multicenter study. J Sex Med 2009; 6: 1062–71. Epub 2008.

82. Larner AJ. Transient acute neurologic sequelae of sexual activity: headache and amnesia. J Sex Med 2008; 5: 284–8. Epub 2007.

83. Kazemi-Saleh D, Pishgou B, Assari S, Tavallaii SA. Fear of sexual intercourse in patients with coronary artery disease: a pilot study of associated morbidity. J Sex Med 2007; 4: 1619–25.

84. Kazemi-Saleh D, Pishgou B, Farrokhi F, et al. Gender impact on the correlation between sexuality and marital relation quality in patients with coronary artery disease. J Sex Med 2008; 5: 2100–6. Epub 2008.

85. Günzler C, Kriston L, Harms A, Berner MM. Association of sexual functioning and quality of partnership in patients in cardiovascular rehabilitation–a gender perspective. J Sex Med 2009; 6: 164–74.

86. Onem K, Erol B, Sanli O, et al. Is sexual dysfunction in women with obstructive sleep apnea-hypopnea syndrome associated with the severity of the disease? A pilot study. J Sex Med 2008; 5: 2600–9. Epub 2008.

87. Waldinger MD, van Gils AP, Ottervanger HP, Vandenbroucke WV, Tavy DL. Persistent genital arousal disorder in 18 Dutch women: Part I. MRI, EEG, and transvaginal ultrasonography investigations. J Sex Med 2009; 6: 474–81. Epub 2008.

88. Korda JB, Pfaus JG, Goldstein I. Persistent genital arousal disorder: a case report in a woman with lifelong PGAD where serendipitous administration of varenicline tartrate resulted in symptomatic improvement. J Sex Med 2009; 6: 1479–86. Epub 2009.

89. Waldinger MD, Schweitzer DH. Persistent genital arousal disorder in 18 Dutch women: Part II. A syndrome clustered with restless legs and over-active bladder. J Sex Med 2009; 6: 482–97. Epub 2008.

90. Catania L, Abdulcadir O, Puppo V, et al. Pleasure and orgasm in women with female genital mutilation/cutting (FGM/C). J Sex Med 2007; 4: 1666–78.

91. Fisher WA, Eardley I, McCabe M, Sand M. Erectile dysfunction (ED) is a shared sexual concern of couples I: couple conceptions of ED. J Sex Med 2009. [Epub ahead of print].

92. Rubio-Aurioles E, Kim ED, Rosen RC, et al. Impact on erectile function and sexual quality of life of couples: a double-blind, randomized, place-bo-controlled trial of tadalafil taken once daily. J Sex Med 2009; 6: 1314–23.

93. Knoll N, Burkert S, Kramer J, Roigas J, Gralla O. Relationship satisfaction and erectile functions in men receiving laparoscopic radical prostatectomy: effects of provision and receipt of spousal social support. J Sex Med 2009; 6: 1438–50.

94. Conaglen JV, Conaglen HM. The effects of treating male hypogonadism on couples' sexual desire and function. J Sex Med 2009; 6: 456–63.

95. Garos S, Kluck A, Aronoff D. Prostate cancer patients and their partners: differences in satisfaction indices and psychological variables. J Sex Med 2007; 4: 1394–403. Epub 2007.

96. Rosen RC, Althof S. Impact of premature ejaculation: the psychological, quality of life, and sexual relationship consequences. J Sex Med 2008; 5: 1296–307. Epub 2008.

97. Levine SB. The first principle of clinical sexuality. J Sex Med 2007; 4(4 Pt 1): 853–4.

98. Woo JS, Brotto LA. Age of first sexual intercourse and acculturation: effects on adult sexual responding. J Sex Med 2008; 5: 571–82. Epub 2008.

99. Harris JM, Cherkas LF, Kato BS, Heiman JR, Spector TD. Normal variations in personality are associated with coital orgasmic infrequency in heterosexual women: a population-based study. J Sex Med 2008; 5: 1177–83. Epub 2008.

100. Brotto LA, Basson R, Luria M. A mindfulness-based group psychoeducational intervention targeting sexual arousal disorder in women. J Sex Med 2008; 5: 1646–59.

101. Clayton AH, Goldfischer ER, Goldstein I, et al. Validation of the decreased sexual desire screener (DSDS): a brief diagnostic instrument for general-ized acquired female hypoactive sexual desire disorder (HSDD). J Sex Med 2009; 6: 730–8. Epub 2009.

102. DeRogatis LR, Allgood A, Rosen RC, et al. Development and evaluation of the women's sexual interest diagnostic interview (WSID): a structured interview to diagnose hypoactive sexual desire disorder (HSDD) in standardized patients. J Sex Med 2008; 5: 2827–41. Epub 2008.

103. Davison SL, Bell RJ, La China M, Holden SL, Davis SR. Assessing sexual function in well women: validity and reliability of the Monash women's health program female sexual satisfaction questionnaire. J Sex Med 2008; 5: 2575–86. Epub 2008.

104. Derogatis L, Clayton A, Lewis-D'Agostino D, Wunderlich G, Fu Y. Validation of the female sexual distress scale-revised for assessing distress in women with hypoactive sexual desire disorder. J Sex Med 2008; 5: 357–64. Epub 2007.

105. Yang CC. The neurourological examination in women. J Sex Med 2008; 5: 2498–501.

106. Baulieu E-E. Dehydroepiandrosterone (DHEA): a fountain of youth? J Clin Endocrinol Metab 1996; 81: 3147–51.

107. Baulieu E-E, Thomas G, Legrain S, et al. Dehydroepiandrosterone (DHEA), DHEA sulfate, and aging: contribution of the DHEA Study to a sociobiomedical issue. Proc Natl Acad Sci USA 2000; 97: 4279–84.

108. Arlt W, Callies F, Van Vlijmen JC, et al. Dehydroepiandrosterone replacement in women with adrenal insufficiency. N Eng J Med 1999; 341: 1013–20.

109. Loeser A. Subcutaneous implantation of female and male hormone in tablet from in women. The British Medical Journal 1940; 1: 479–82.

110. Shifren JL, Braustein GD, Simon JA, et al. Transdermal testosterone treatment in women with impaired sexual function and oophorectomy. N Engl J Med 2000; 343: 682–8.

111. Lobo RA, Rosen RC, Yang HM, Block B, Van Der Hoop RG. Comparative effects of oral esterified estrogens with and without methyltestosterone on endocrine profiles and dimensions of sexual function in postmeno-pausal women with hypoactive sexual desire. Fertil Steril 2003; 79: 1341–52.

112. Lobo RA, Rosen RC, Yang HM, Block B, Van Der Hoop RG. Comparative effects of oral esterified estrogens with and without methyltestosterone on endocrine profiles and dimensions of sexual function in postmeno-pausal women with hypoactive sexual desire. Fertil Steril 2003; 79: 1341–52.

113. Buckler H, Al-Azzawi F. The UK VR multicentre trial group. The effect of a novel vaginal ring delivering oestradiol acetate on climacteric symptoms in postmenopausal women. BJOG 2003; 110: 753–9.

114. Barentsen R, van de Weijer PHM, Schram JHN. Continuous low dose estradiol released from a vaginal ring versus estriol vaginal cream for urogenital atrophy. Eur J Obstet Gynecol Reprod Biol 1997; 71: 73–80.

115. Rioux JE, Devlin C, Gelfand MM, Steinberg WM, Hepburn DS. 17beta-estradiol vaginal tablet versus conjugated equine estrogen vaginal cream to relieve menopausal atrophic vaginitis. Menopause 2000; 7: 156–61.

116. Giraldi A, Marson L, Nappi R, et al. Physiology of female sexual function: animal models. J Sex Med 2004; 1: 237–53.

117. Pfaus JG. Pathways of sexual desire. J Sex Med 2009; 6: 1506–33.

118. Clayton AH, Warnock JK, Kornstein SG, et al. A placebo-controlled trial of bupropion SR as an antidote for selective serotonin reuptake inhibitor-induced sexual dysfunction. J Clin Psychiatry 2004; 65: 62–7.

119. Segraves RT, Clayton A, Croft H, Wolf A, Warnock J. Bupropion sustained release for the treatment of hypoactive sexual desire disorder in premenopausal women. J Clin Psychopharmacol 2004; 24: 339–42.

120. Park K, Moreland RB, Goldstein I, Atala A, Traish A. Sildenafil inhibits phosphodiesterase type 5 in human clitoral corpus cavernousum smooth muscle. Biochem Biophys Res Commun 1998; 249: 612–7.

121. Burnett AL, Calvin DC, Silver RI, Peppas DS, Docimo SG. Immunohis-tochemical description of nitric oxide syntheses isoforms in human clitoris. J Urol 1997; 158: 75–8.

122. Caruso S, Intelisano G, Lupo L, Agnello C. Premenopausal women affected by sexual arousal disorder treated with sildenafil: a double-blind, crossover, placebo-controlled study. Br J Obstet Gynaecol 2001; 108: 623–8.

123. Caruso S, Intelisano G, Farina M, Di Mari L, Agnello C. The function of sildenafil on female sexual pathways: a double-blind, cross-over, placebo-controlled study. Eur J Obstet Gynecol 2003; 110: 201–6.

124. Nurnberg GH, Hensley PL, Heiman JR, et al. Sildenafil treatment of women with antidepressant-associated sexual dysfunction: a randomized controlled trial. JAMA 2008; 300: 395–404.

125. Goldstein I. Doral slit surgery for clitoral phimosis. J Sex Med 2008; 5: 2485–8.

126. Goldstein AT, Klingman D, Christopher K, Johnson C, Marinoff SC. Surgical treatment of vulvar vestibulitis syndrome: outcome assessment derived from a postoperative questionnaire. J Sex Med 2006; 3: 923–31.

127. Goldstein AT. Surgery for vulvar vestibulitis syndrome. J Sex Med 2006; 3: 559–62.

128. Lowenstein L, Solt I. Bartholin's cyst marsupialization. J Sex Med 2008; 5: 1053–6.